Orthopaedic Basic Science

Orthopaedic Basic Science

Edited by
Sheldon R. Simon, MD
Judson Wilson Professor and Chief of Orthopaedic Surgery
The Ohio State University
Columbus, Ohio

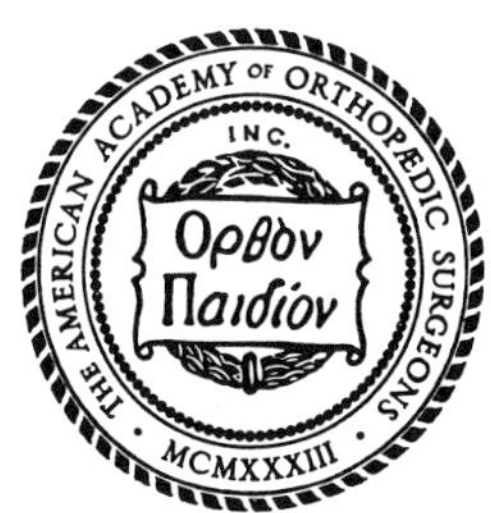

American Academy
of Orthopaedic Surgeons

Library of Congress Cataloging-in-Publication Card No.: 9374320

ISBN 0-89203-059-3 Soft Cover
0-89203-079-8 Hard Cover

This book is printed on recycled paper.

Acknowledgements

American Academy of Orthopaedic Surgeons

Executive Director:
Thomas C. Nelson

Director, Division of Education:
Mark W. Wieting

Director, Department of Publications:
Marilyn L. Fox, PhD

Senior Editor:
Bruce A. Davis

Associate Senior Editors:
Joan R. Abern
Jane Baque

Production Manager:
Loraine Edwalds

Assistant Production Manager:
Kathy M. Brouillette

Editorial Assistants:
Sharon Duffy
Sophie Tosta

Publications Secretaries:
Geraldine Dubberke
Em Lee Lambos

Technical Illustration:
Stephen J. Brady
David R. Schumick

Composition:
Carlisle Communications

Manufacturing:
Port City Press

Table of Contents

Contributors

Hannu Alaranta, MD, PhD
Associate Professor, Head of the Rehabilitation Unit
The Invalid Foundation
Helsinki, Finland

Kai-Nan An, PhD
Professor of Bioengineering
Chair, Division of Orthopedic Research
Mayo Clinic and Mayo Medical School
Rochester, Minnesota

Steven P. Arnoczky, DVM
Wade O. Brinker Professor of Surgery
Director, Laboratory for Comparative Orthopaedic Research
College of Veterinary Medicine
Michigan State University
East Lansing, Michigan

Hannu T. Aro, MD, PhD
Acting Associate Professor and Vice-Chairman, Department of Surgery
University of Turku
Turku, Finland

C. Andrew L. Bassett, MD
Professor Emeritus, Orthopaedic Surgery
Bioelectric Research Center
Columbia University
Riverdale, New York

Thomas M. Best, MD, PhD
Research Associate, Orthopaedic Surgery
Duke University Medical Center
Durham, North Carolina

Sue C. Bodine, PhD
Assistant Professor, Department of Orthopaedics
University of California, San Diego
La Jolla, California

Mark E. Bolander, MD
Senior Associate Consultant, Department of Orthopedics
Mayo Clinic
Rochester, Minnesota

Lawrence B. Bone, MD
Associate Professor, Department of Orthopaedics
SUNY Buffalo
Buffalo, New York

Adele L. Boskey, PhD
Professor of Biochemistry
The Hospital for Special Surgery
New York, New York

Carl T. Brighton, MD, PhD
Paul B. Magnuson Professor of Bone and Joint Surgery
University of Pennsylvania School of Medicine
Philadelphia, Pennsylvania

Joseph A. Buckwalter, MD
Professor of Orthopaedic Surgery
University of Iowa
Iowa City, Iowa

Jean C. Burge, PhD, RD
Assistant Professor, Division of Medical Dietetics
College of Medicine
The Ohio State University
Columbus, Ohio

James H. Campbell, MS
Director, Orthotics and Prosthetics
Department of Orthopaedic Surgery
Cleveland Clinic Foundation
Cleveland, Ohio

Edmund Y.S. Chao, PhD
Professor, Vice Chairman for Research
Johns Hopkins University
Department of Orthopaedic Surgery
Baltimore, Maryland

Gail S. Chorney, MD
Assistant Professor, Orthopaedic Surgery
Columbia University, College of Physicians and Surgeons
New York, New York

Charles C. Clark, PhD
Assistant Director of Research
Department of Orthopaedic Surgery
University of Pennsylvania School of Medicine
Philadelphia, Pennsylvania

Andrew J. Cosgarea, MD
Assistant Professor, Orthopaedic Surgery
Ohio State University
Columbus, Ohio

Thomas A. Einhorn, MD
Professor of Orthopaedics
Director of Orthopaedic Research
The Mount Sinai School of Medicine
New York, New York

John L. Esterhai, Jr., MD
Associate Professor of Orthopaedic Surgery
University of Pennsylvania School of Medicine
Philadelphia, Pennsylvania

Richard Fischer, MD
Assistant Professor of Orthopaedic Surgery
The Ohio State University
Columbus, Ohio

Donald C. Fithian, MD
Director, Knee and Sports Medicine Fellowship
San Diego Kaiser Permanente
Clinical Instructor
University of California, San Diego
San Diego, California

Louis Flancbaum, MD, FACS, FCCM
Associate Professor of Surgery and Anesthesiology
Chief, Section of Critical Care and Trauma
Director, Nutrition Support Service
The Ohio State University College of Medicine
Columbus, Ohio

Evan L. Flatow, MD
Herbert Irving Assistant Professor of Orthopaedic Surgery
Associate Chief, The Shoulder Service
New York Orthopaedic Hospital
Columbia-Presbyterian Medical Center
New York, New York

Robert J. Foster, ScD
Department of Orthopaedic Surgery
Columbia University
New York, New York

Joel Frazier, MD
Assistant Professor of Surgery
The Ohio State University
Columbus, Ohio

Gary E. Friedlaender, MD
Professor and Chairman
Department of Orthopaedics and Rehabilitation
Yale University School of Medicine
New Haven, Connecticut

Robert F. Gagel, MD
Chief, Endocrinology Section
MD Anderson Cancer Center
Houston, Texas

William E. Garrett, Jr., MD, PhD
Associate Professor of Orthopaedic Surgery and Cell Biology
Duke University Medical Center
Durham, North Carolina

Victor M. Goldberg, MD
Chairman and Charles H. Herndon Professor
Department of Orthopaedics
Case Western Reserve University
Cleveland, Ohio

Steven A. Goldstein, PhD
Professor of Surgery (Orthopaedics)
Director of Orthopaedic Research
University of Michigan Medical School
Ann Arbor, Michigan

Wilson C. Hayes, PhD
Maurice E. Mueller
Professor of Biomechanics
Harvard Medical School
Boston, Massachusetts

Mark C. Horowitz, PhD
Associate Professor in Orthopaedics and Rehabilitation
Yale University School of Medicine
New Haven, Connecticut

Joseph P. Iannotti, MD, PhD
Associate Professor, Orthopaedic Surgery
University of Pennsylvania School of Medicine
Philadelphia, Pennsylvania

Frederick S. Kaplan, MD
Associate Professor of Orthopaedic Surgery and Medicine
Chief of the Division of Metabolic Bone Diseases
University of Pennsylvania School of Medicine
Philadelphia, Pennsylvania

Christopher Keading, MD
Assistant Professor
The Ohio State University
Columbus, Ohio

Tony M. Keaveny, PhD
Senior Research Associate
Orthopaedic Biomechanics Laboratory
Beth Israel Hospital and Harvard Medical School
Boston, Massachusetts

Janet L. Kuhn, PhD
Assistant Professor of Surgery (Orthopaedics)
University of Michigan Medical School
Ann Arbor, Michigan

Nancy E. Lane, MD
Assistant Professor of Medicine
Division of Rheumatology
University of California at San Francisco
San Francisco, California

Richard L. Lieber, PhD
Associate Professor, Department of Orthopaedics
Biomechanical Sciences Graduate Group
San Diego, California

Louis Lipiello, PhD
Professor and Director, Orthopaedic Research
University of Nebraska Medical Center
Omaha, Nebraska

Alan S. Litsky, MD, ScD
Assistant Professor of Orthopaedics and Biomedical Engineering
Director, Orthopaedic Biomaterials Laboratory
Ohio State University
Columbus, Ohio

Tyler S. Lucas, MD
Resident, Department of Orthopaedics
Mount Sinai School of Medicine
New York, New York

Henry J. Mankin, MD
Edith M. Ashley Professor of Orthopaedic Surgery
Harvard Medical School
Boston, Massachusetts

Eugene R. Mindell, MD
Professor, Department of Orthopaedic Surgery
State University of New York at Buffalo
Buffalo, New York

Robert W. Molinari, MD
Chief Resident, Orthopaedics
Mount Sinai School of Medicine
New York, New York

Van C. Mow, PhD
Professor of Mechanical Engineering and Orthopaedic Bioengineering
Columbia University
New York, New York

Michael Muha, MD
Hand Surgery Fellow
Department of Orthopaedics
The Ohio State University
Columbus, Ohio

Barry S. Myers, MD, PhD
Assistant Professor, Department of Biomedical Engineering
Assistant Research Professor, Division of Orthopaedic Surgery
Duke University Medical Center
Durham, North Carolina

Robert F. Ostrum, MD
Assistant Professor, Orthopaedic Surgery
The Ohio State University
Columbus, Ohio

Jacquelin Perry, MD
Professor of Orthopaedics
University of Southern California
Los Angeles, California

Malcolm H. Pope, DMSc, PhD
McClure Professor of Orthopaedic Research
Department of Orthopaedics and Rehabilitation
University of Vermont
Burlington, Vermont

Peter M. Quesada, PhD
Assistant Professor
Orthopaedics and Biomedical Engineering
The Ohio State University
Columbus, Ohio

Eric L. Radin, MD
Director, Bone and Joint Center
Henry Ford Hospital
Detroit, Michigan

Anthony Ratcliffe, PhD
Associate Professor, Department of Orthopaedic Surgery
Columbia University
New York, New York

Sheldon R. Simon, MD
Judson Wilson Professor and Chief of Orthopaedic Surgery
The Ohio State University
Columbus, Ohio

Myron Spector, PhD
Professor of Orthopedic Surgery (Biomaterials)
Brigham and Women's Hospital
Harvard Medical School
Boston, Massachusetts

Dempsey S. Springfield, MD
Visiting Orthopaedic Surgeon
Massachusetts General Hospital
Boston, Massachusetts

Marc F. Swiontkowski, MD
Professor and Vice Chairman, Department of Orthopaedics
University of Washington
Seattle, Washington

Jennifer S. Wayne, PhD
Assistant Professor
Medical College of Virginia
Virginia Commonwealth University
Richmond, Virginia

James N. Weinstein, DO
Endowed Professor, Department of Orthopaedic Surgery
University of Iowa College of Medicine
Director, Spine Diagnostic and Treatment Center
Iowa City, Iowa

Savio L-Y. Woo, PhD
Albert Ferguson, Jr. Professor and Vice Chairman for Research
Musculoskeletal Research Center
Department of Orthopaedic Surgery
University of Pittsburgh
Pittsburgh, Pennsylvania

Reviewers

Kai-Nan An, PhD
Professor of Bioengineering
Chair, Division of Orthopedic Research
Mayo Clinic and Mayo Medical School
Rochester, Minnesota

James R. Andrews, MD
Medical Director
American Sports Medicine Institute
Birmingham, Alabama

Mark E. Bolander, MD
Senior Associate Consultant, Department of Orthopedics
Mayo Clinic
Rochester, Minnesota

Lawrence B. Bone, MD
Associate Professor, Department of Orthopaedics
SUNY Buffalo
Buffalo, New York

Adele L. Boskey, PhD
Professor of Biochemistry
The Hospital for Special Surgery
New York, New York

Joseph A. Buckwalter, MD
Professor of Orthopaedic Surgery
University of Iowa
Iowa City, Iowa

John Joseph Callaghan, MD
Professor of Orthopaedic Surgery
University of Iowa
Iowa City, Iowa

Charles C. Clark, PhD
Assistant Director of Research
Department of Orthopaedic Surgery
University of Pennsylvania School of Medicine
Philadelphia, Pennsylvania

Laurence E. Dahners, MD
Professor, University of North Carolina at Chapel Hill
Chapel Hill, North Carolina

Mark C. Gebhardt, MD
Associate Professor of Orthopaedic Surgery
Harvard Medical School
Boston, Massachusetts

M. Mark Hoffer, MD
Professor and Chief, Department of Orthopaedics
University of California at Irvine
Irvine, California

Joshua J. Jacobs, MD
Assistant Professor, Department of Orthopaedic Surgery
Rush-Presbyterian-St. Luke's Medical Center
Chicago, Illinois

Herbert Kaufer, MD
Professor and Chairman of the Division of Orthopedic Surgery
University of Kentucky
Lexington, Kentucky

Joseph M. Lane, MD
Professor and Chairman, Orthopaedic Surgery
University of California Los Angeles
Los Angeles, California

David Pienkowski, PhD, MBA
Assistant Professor
Director, Orthopaedic Research Laboratory
University of Kentucky School of Medicine
Lexington, Kentucky

Michael S. Pinzur, MD
Professor, Department of Orthopaedic Surgery
Loyola University Medical Center
Maywood, Illinois

George T. Rab, MD
Professor of Orthopaedic Surgery
Chief, Pediatric Orthopaedic Surgery
University of California, Davis
Sacramento, California

Clinton T. Rubin, PhD
Professor and Director, Musculo-Skeletal Research Laboratory
Department of Orthopaedics, Health Sciences Center
State University of New York
Stony Brook, New York

Thomas Santner, PhD
Professor and Chair, Department of Statistics
The Ohio State University
Columbus, Ohio

Harry B. Skinner, MD, PhD
Professor of Orthopaedic Surgery
University of California, San Francisco
San Francisco, California

E. Shannon Stauffer, MD
Professor and Chairman
Division of Orthopaedics and Rehabilitation
Southern Illinois University School of Medicine
Springfield, Illinois

Laura A. Timmerman, MD
Assistant Professor, Sports Medicine
Department of Orthopaedic Surgery
University of California Davis School of Medicine
Sacramento, California

Stephen B. Trippel, MD
Assistant Professor of Orthopaedic Surgery
Harvard Medical School
Boston, Massachusetts

Frank C. Wilson, MD
Kenan Professor of Surgery and Chief, Division of Orthopaedics
University of North Carolina at Chapel Hill School of Medicine
Chapel Hill, North Carolina

Preface

In the past several decades the clinical practice of orthopaedics has advanced markedly. These advances are based in large part on the concurrent explosion in knowledge of the basic sciences of the musculoskeletal system. Many studies, reviews, and books have been written that describe in detail the individual areas of neuromusculoskeletal knowledge. Yet, a single comprehensive text in this area has been lacking. Recognizing this need, the American Academy of Orthopaedic Surgeons has published this text. Its purpose is to assemble in one place many of the essentials of these fields.

The present text is an outgrowth of the Academy's previous publication, *Orthopaedic Science: A Resource and Self Study Guide for the Practitioner.* That text represented a compilation of the many previous Academy workshops for basic science educators in orthopaedics. This publication, *Orthopaedic Basic Science,* expands on that syllabus, broadening its scope of topics and detailing and updating the material in a more comprehensive fashion. Because the fields it covers are so dynamic and difficult to succinctly present in total at any given moment, this book has gone through many philosophic changes and reorganizations since its inception several years ago.

Orthopaedic Basic Science contains 13 chapters that mirror the changes that have occurred in neuromusculoskeletal science in the past 20 years. Knowledge of the basic science of bone has become so voluminous as to require three separate chapters. Information on organ tissues, such as nerve and muscle, and the field of kinesiology has expanded to the point where they warrant recognition in their own distinct chapters. The major discoveries currently being made in molecular biology have led to its inclusion in the chapter that also provides current understanding of the pathophysiologic processes of bone and soft tissue tumors. Another major change relates to the growth in knowledge of physics and engineering and appreciation of their importance in providing basic understanding of the way in which the musculoskeletal system works, an understanding that is the basis of much current orthopaedic clinical practice. This change has led to integrating engineering and biologic material within each chapter, as well as to the inclusion of separate biomechanics and biomaterials chapters. These chapters will be especially useful because the health science curriculums of most schools do not include the fundamental principles and knowledge of these disciplines. A separate chapter about other medical conditions affecting orthopaedic practice has been included to provide basic knowledge of problems the clinician faces on a daily basis. The use of statistics in acquiring true knowledge in the biologic sciences has become more significant. Statistics has become such a necessary part of orthopaedics as to warrant review of its principles and applications in a separate chapter.

In each area of basic science addressed, the editors of this volume have attempted to provide information considered to be established theory or fact, while minimizing those hypotheses and data considered to be conjectural or too new to be fully verified. *Orthopaedic Basic Science* has been written primarily to address the needs of educators and residents in orthopaedic surgery. With this in mind, illustrations have been carefully selected to augment the text and are available in a slide set for teaching purposes.

The content of *Orthopaedic Basic Science* should also be of value to all clinicians, scientists, and ancillary health personnel whose efforts relate to the neuromusculoskeletal system. Over 30% of the clinical problems seen in everyday practice by primary care physicians relate to this system. This system also forms a major part of the practice of radiologists, rheumatologists, neurologists, and physiatrists, as well as physical and occupational therapists and those practicing veterinary medicine. It is hoped that this book will help these professionals to gain a better understanding and knowledge of the basic science of the neuromusculoskeletal system, and that they will find it helpful in their respective practices. The editorial board of this book, its authors, the Academy, and I do not consider this book to be all-inclusive. Rather, it is our desire to provide a useful, comprehensive, and accessible synthesis of the basic knowledge in orthopaedics.

Much effort by a large number of individuals was expended to assure that this book meets this goal. An editorial board was formed to assist me in its production. Each member had the responsibility of specific chapter(s), as well as of defining the overall content and publication of the book.

Because the subject matter of each chapter is so broad, each chapter editor selected a group of authors to contribute and assist in developing that chapter's text. When this process was completed, each chapter underwent extensive review. The first review was performed by me and at least three other members of the editorial board (chapter main editors). When we felt the contents of a given chapter were appropriate in range and depth for our principal audience (residents), we sent the chapter for outside review to experts in the respective content area and to academic orthopaedists responsible for residency training, in whose program no expertise in the given chapter was locally available. We asked content experts to assess the accuracy, quality, and depth of information in the chapter, and in some cases to contribute to the chapter they had reviewed. We asked academic orthopaedists involved with resident training whether the chapter was appropriate for their teaching purposes and whether it was in a form that was readable and understandable to themselves and to residents. Expert reviewers, who made a significant contribution to a chapter's content, are listed among chapter authors. For their valuable contributions and generous efforts, the editorial board, all contributors, and all reviewers are acknowledged in the front of this book.

Considerable effort was expended to provide both medical and copy editing in an attempt to make *Orthopaedic Basic Science* as comprehensive and cohesive as possible. To encourage information synthesis and enhance readability, the content is not directly cross-referenced with bibliographic citations. However, books and articles that will amplify the subject matter and enhance the reader's understanding thereof are listed at the end of each chapter. A complete reference bibliography was strongly considered but rejected for fear of being too voluminous, requiring cross-referencing and omitting valuable citations. A glossary has been included for those who are not familiar with the terminology.

As noted above, this book would not have come into fruition without the able assistance of many people. I would also like to acknowledge the contributions of Elly Castrodale and Barbara Suver in my office. Much of the line art was provided by Stephen J. Brady and David R. Schumick in the Medical Illustration Department at Ohio State University.

The publication process was overseen by the Academy's Publications Department under the direction of Marilyn Fox, PhD. The entire project was managed with considerable skill and diligence by Joan Abern, associate senior editor, who was also responsible for the copy editing. Bruce Davis, senior editor, and Jane Baque, associate senior editor, assisted her in this process. Production was overseen by Loraine Edwalds, production manager, with the able assistance of Kathy Brouillette, assistant production manager, and Sharon Duffy and Sophie Tosta, editorial assistants. Word processing was done by Geraldine Dubberke, Em Lee Lambos, and Sharon O'Brien.

Sheldon R. Simon, MD
Medical Editor

Chapter 1
Form and Function of Articular Cartilage

Henry J. Mankin, MD
Van C. Mow, PhD
Joseph A. Buckwalter, MD
Joseph P. Iannotti, MD, PhD
Anthony Ratcliffe, PhD

Chapter Outline

Introduction

Articular cartilage, the resilient load-bearing material of diarthrodial joints, provides joints with excellent friction, lubrication, and wear characteristics required for continuous gliding motion. It also serves to absorb mechanical shock and spread the applied load onto the bony supporting structures below. Under normal physiologic conditions, articular cartilage can perform these essential biomechanical functions with little damage over seven or eight decades. However, this tissue may be damaged by trauma or by chronic and progressive degenerative joint diseases. Although articular cartilage is a metabolically active tissue, it has a limited capacity for repair. Eventually, these disorders can cause severe and progressive disabilities of the joint, culminating in the degradation of the cartilage and destruction of the articular surface. At this point, total or partial joint replacements are required to restore pain-free mobility to the affected joint. Although joint-replacement procedures have revolutionized orthopaedic surgery, they come as the treatment of end-stage degenerative joint disease after much prolonged suffering by the patient. New research on articular cartilage, based on recent advances in the understanding of articular cartilage biology, composition, metabolism, molecular and ultrastructural organizations, and biomechanical properties, offers hope for the development of biologically based repair procedures as alternatives to prosthetic joint replacements in the treatment of degenerative joint diseases and joint injuries. The goal of generating a viable substitute for articular cartilage through tissue engineering concepts now appears to be achievable in the near future. Thus, it is important to provide a firm understanding of the structure and function of normal and diseased articular cartilage. This chapter presents a review of current understanding of articular cartilage, and forms the basis for understanding how the degenerative and repair processes may occur.

Composition and Organization of Normal Articular Cartilage

The Structure of Articular Cartilage

Articular cartilage consists primarily of a large extracellular matrix (ECM) with a sparse population of highly specialized cells (chondrocytes) distributed throughout the tissue. The primary components of the ECM are proteoglycans, collagens, and water, with other proteins and glycoproteins present in lower amounts. These all combine to provide the tissue with its unique and complex structure and mechanical properties.

The structure and composition of the articular cartilage vary throughout its depth (Fig. 1), from the articular surface to the subchondral bone. These differences can include cell shape and volume, collagen fibril diameter and orientation, and proteoglycan concentration. The cartilage can be divided into four zones: the superficial zone, the middle or tran-

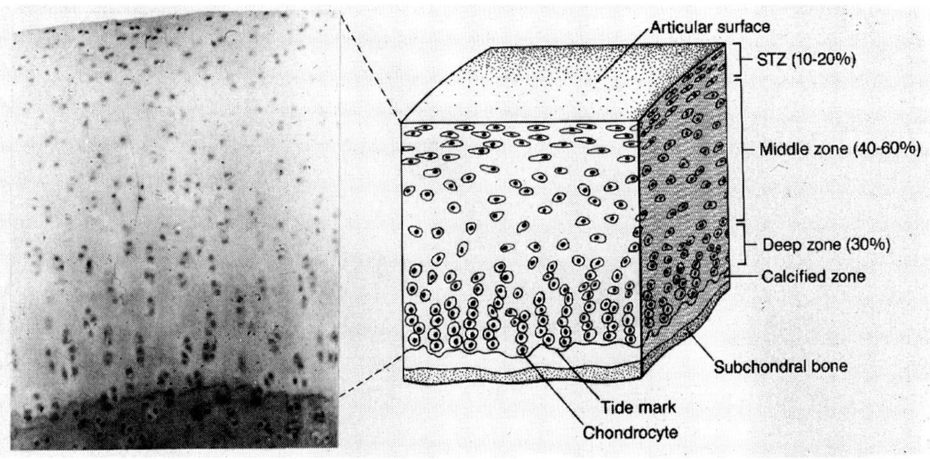

Figure 1
Left, Histologic section of normal adult articular cartilage showing even Safranin O staining and distribution of chondrocytes. **Right,** Schematic diagram of chondrocyte organization in the three major zones of the uncalcified cartilage, the tidemark, and the subchondral bone. (Reproduced with permission from Mow VC, Proctor CS, Kelly MA: Biomechanics of articular cartilage, in Nordin M, Frankel VH (eds): *Basic Biomechanics of the Musculoskeletal System,* ed 2. Philadelphia, Lea & Febiger, 1989, pp 31–57.)

sitional zone, the deep zone, and the zone of calcified cartilage.

The superficial zone is the uppermost zone of the cartilage and forms the gliding surface. The thin collagen fibrils are arranged parallel to the surface, the chondrocytes are elongated with the long axis parallel to the surface, and the proteoglycan content is at its lowest level. The middle, or transition, zone contains collagen fibers with a larger diameter and less apparent organization, and the chondrocytes have a more rounded appearance. The deep zone contains the highest concentration of proteoglycans and the lowest water content; the collagen fibers have a large diameter and are organized vertical to the joint surface. The chondrocytes are spherical and often are arranged in a columnar fashion. The deepest layer, the zone of calcified cartilage, separates the hyaline cartilage from the subchondral bone. It is characterized by small pyknotic cells distributed in a cartilaginous matrix heavily encrusted with apatitic salts. Histologic staining with hematoxylin and eosin shows a wavy bluish line, called the tidemark, which separates the deep zone from the calcified zone.

In addition to these articular surface-to-bone zonal distinctions, the ECM is divided into pericellular, territorial, or interterritorial regions, depending on its proximity to the chondrocyte (Fig. 2). These regions differ in their content (collagen, proteoglycan, and other matrix components), and the collagen fibril diameter and organization. The pericellular matrix is a thin layer adjacent to the cell membrane and completely surrounds the chondrocyte. The matrix contains primarily proteoglycans and other noncollagenous matrix components; almost no collagen fibrils appear to be present. The territorial matrix surrounds the pericellular matrix, and it is characterized by thin collagen fibrils that, at the boundary of the territorial matrix, appear to form a fibrillar network that is distinct from the outer interterritorial matrix. Recent studies have reintroduced the term chondron to encompass the chondrocyte and its pericellular and territorial matrices. The interterritorial matrix is the largest of the matrix regions, and contributes the majority of the material properties of the articular cartilage. It encompasses all of the matrix between the territorial matrices of the individual cells or clusters of cells and contains the large collagen fibers and the majority of the proteoglycans.

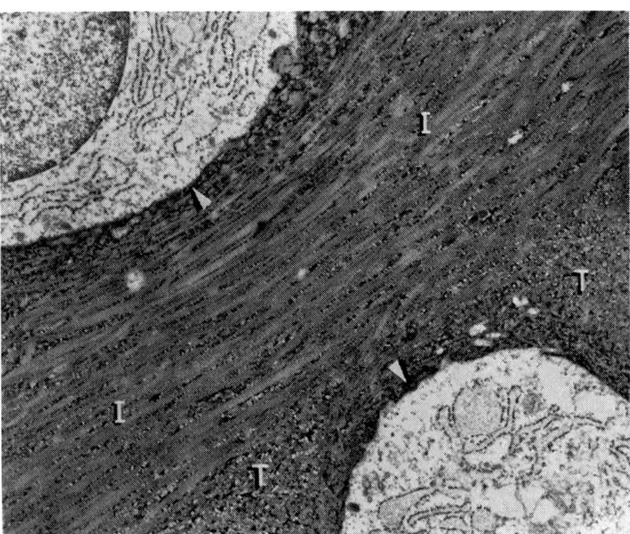

Figure 2
Electron microscopic view (8700 X) of mature rabbit articular cartilage from the radial zone of the medial femoral condyle. Micrograph shows cytoskeletal elements, and pericellular matrix (arrow), territorial matrix (T), and interterritorial matrix (I). The pericellular matrix lacks cross-striated collagen fibrils, whereas the territorial matrix has a fine fibrillar collagen network. The collagen of the interterritorial matrix has coarser fibers, and they tend to be parallel. (Reproduced with permission from Buckwalter JA, Hunziker EB: Articular cartilage biology and morphology, in Mow VC, Ratcliffe A (eds): *Structure and Function of Articular Cartilage.* Boca Raton, FL, CRC Press, 1993.)

Chondrocytes

The synthesis and maintenance of the articular cartilage depend on the chondrocytes. They are derived from mesenchymal cells, which differentiate in development to the chondrocyte phenotype. In growth, these cells generate the large amount of ECM, and in mature tissue, where they occupy less than 10% of the total tissue volume, these cells are responsible for the maintenance of this matrix. The chondrocytes are metabolically active, and are able to respond to a variety of environmental stimuli. These stimuli include soluble mediators, such as growth factors, interleukins, and pharmaceutical agents; matrix composition; mechanical loads; and hydrostatic pressure changes. Although the chondrocytes generally maintain a stable matrix, the response to some factors (for example, interleukin 1) may lead to degradation of the ECM. However, the transport of other messages commonly used to regulate many body processes is likely to be limited. The cartilage has no nerve supply; therefore, neural impulses cannot provide information, and the immune responses (cellular and humoral) are likely not to occur in cartilage because both monocytes and immunoglobulins tend to be excluded from the tissue by their size.

The Chemistry of Articular Cartilage

Because the chondrocytes of articular cartilage occupy only a small proportion of the total volume

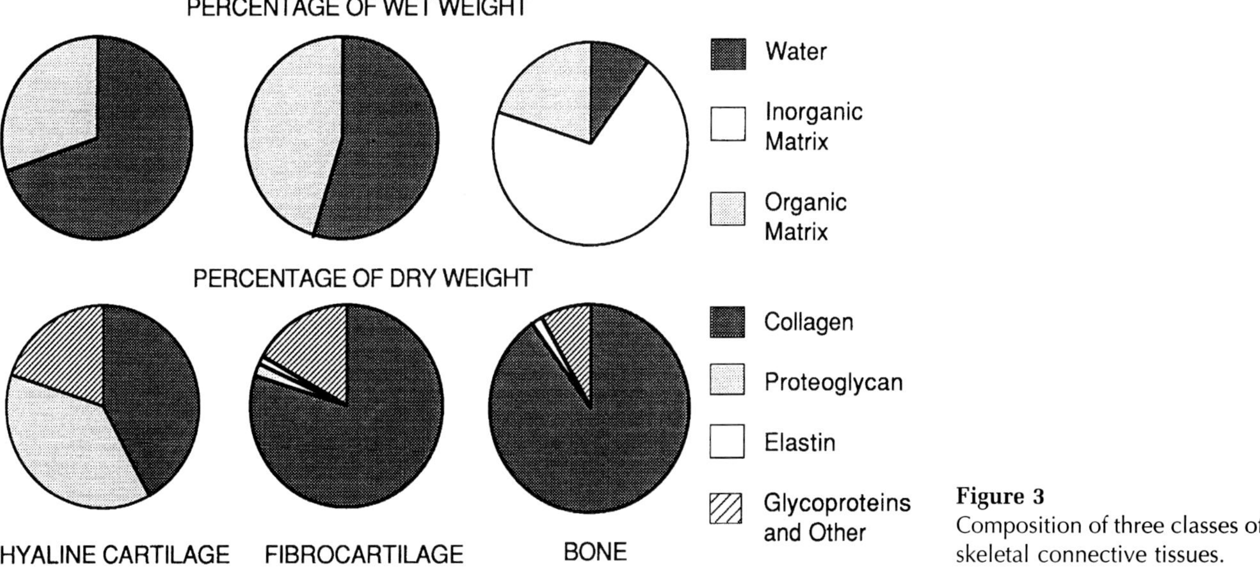

Figure 3
Composition of three classes of skeletal connective tissues.

of the tissue, its chemistry primarily reflects the composition of the matrix. Normal cartilage has water contents ranging from 65% to 80% of its total wet weight (Fig. 3, Table 1). The remaining wet weight of the tissue is accounted for principally by two major classes of macromolecular materials, collagens and proteoglycans. Several other classes of biochemical molecules, including lipids, phospholipids, proteins, and glycoproteins, make up the remaining portion of the extracellular matrix. Although their precise role in the extracellular matrix has not yet been determined, it is important to recognize that there are other constituents beside collagens and proteoglycans. Their function will certainly be elucidated as more information becomes available.

Table 1
Biochemical composition of articular cartilage

Component	% Wet Weight
Quantitatively Major Components	
Water	65 to 80
Collagen (type II)	10 to 20
Aggrecan	4 to 7
Quantitatively Minor Components (less than 5%)*	
Proteoglycans	
- biglycan	
- decorin	
- fibromodulin	
Collagens	
- type V	
- type VI	
- type IX	
- type X	
- type XI	
Link protein	
Hyaluronate	
Fibronectin	
Lipids	

*Although these components are present in lower overall amounts, they may be present in similar molar amounts compared to type II collagen and aggrecan (for example, link protein), and may have major roles to play in the functionality of the matrix.

Water in Articular Cartilage

Water is the most abundant component of normal articular cartilage, making up from 65% to 80% of the wet weight of the tissue. During the early phases of osteoarthritis, water content may increase to over 90% before total disintegration of the tissue occurs. A small percentage of this water is contained in the intracellular space, about 30% is associated with the intrafibrillar space within the collagen, and the remainder is contained in the molecular pore space of the ECM. Inorganic salts, such as sodium, calcium, chloride, and potassium, are dissolved in the tissue water. Water content is nonhomogeneously distributed throughout cartilage, decreasing in concentration from approximately 80% at the surface to 65% in the deep zone. Most of the water may be moved through the tissue or squeezed out from the tissue by applying a pressure gradient across the tissue or by compressing the solid matrix. Frictional resistance against this flow through the molecular size pores of the ECM is very high, and thus the permeability of the tissue is very low. This frictional resistance and the pressurization of the water within the ECM are the two basic mechanisms from which articular cartilage derives its ability to support very high joint loads (see the section on "Biomechanics of Articular Cartilage"). The flow of water through the tissue and across the articular surface also promotes the transport of nutrients, and provides a source of lubricant for the joint. The fluid mechanics of water flow through cartilage is governed by mechanical and physicochemical laws. From these laws, it is possible to show that very large pressures are required to move water through the ECM. For example, to move water at a rate of 17.5 μm/s (very slow) through normal cartilage, a pressure of 1 MPa (145 psi) is required. Conversely, if water is flowing through cartilage at this rate, a pressure differential of 1 MPa must be developed across the tissue. To appreciate the magnitude of this pressure, note that the pressure in an automobile tire usually is not greater than 30 psi (0.21 MPa).

The affinity of articular cartilage for water derives mostly from the hydrophilic nature of proteoglycans, and less from collagen. Water will wet materials made of pure collagen as a result of capillary or surface tension effects. This is a relatively weak physical mechanism. The ability of proteoglycans to attract water involves three physicochemical mechanisms, two of which are very strong and have been thoroughly characterized: (1) Donnan osmotic pressure, which is caused by the interstitial free-floating counter-ions (for example, Ca^{2+}, Na^{+}) required to neutralize the charges on the proteoglycans; (2) electrostatic repulsive forces that are developed between the fixed negative charges along the proteoglycan molecules; and (3) the entropic tendency of the proteoglycan to gain volume in solution. For articular cartilage, the degree of hydration is determined by a balance of the total swelling pressure (the sum of these three effects) exerted by the proteoglycans, and the constraining forces developed within the strong collagen network surrounding the trapped proteoglycans. Thus, when water is in contact with either of these macromolecules, a cohesive and strong solid gel is formed, which allows the tissue to hold its water with avidity.

Collagens in Articular Cartilage

Collagens are structural macromolecules found as major constituents of the ECM (Table 2). At this writing, there are 15 distinct collagen types composed of at least 29 genetically distinct chains. All members of the collagen family contain a characteristic triple helical structure that may constitute the majority of the length of the molecule, or may be interrupted by one or more nonhelical domains. Over 50% of the dry weight of articular cartilage consists of collagen. The major cartilage collagen, which represents 90% to 95% of the total, is known as type II. However, the articular cartilage matrix also contains types V, VI, IX, X, and XI. In general, the main function of collagen in articular cartilage is to provide the tissue's tensile properties and to immobilize the proteoglycans within the ECM. Collagen fibers in cartilage are generally thinner than those seen in tendon or bone, and this may, in part, be a function of their interaction with the relatively large amount of proteoglycan in this tissue. The fibers in articular cartilage vary in width from 10 to 100 nm, although their width may increase with age and disease. Originally, their macro-organization indicated tension-resisting arcades, but recent studies show that the fibers have a less ordered organization, especially in the middle zones of the tissue, where the fibers appear to be randomly distributed (Fig. 4).

Table 2
Types of collagen

Type	Tissue	Polymeric Form
Class 1 (300-nm triple-helix)		
Type I	Skin, bone, etc.	Banded fibril
Type II	Cartilage, disk	Banded fibril
Type III	Skin, blood vessels	Banded fibril
Type V	With type I	Banded fibril
Type XI (1α, 2α, 3α)	With type II	Banded fibril
Class 2 (basement membranes)		
Type IV	Basal lamina	Three-dimensional network
Type VII	Epithelial basement membrane	Anchoring fibril
Type VIII	Endothelial basement membrane	Unknown
Class 3 (short-chain)		
Type VI	Widespread	Microfilaments, 110-nm banded aggregates
Type IX	Cartilage (with type II)	Cross-linked to type II
Type X	Hypertrophic cartilage	Unknown
Type XII	Tendon, other?	Unknown
Type XIII	Endothelial cells	Unknown

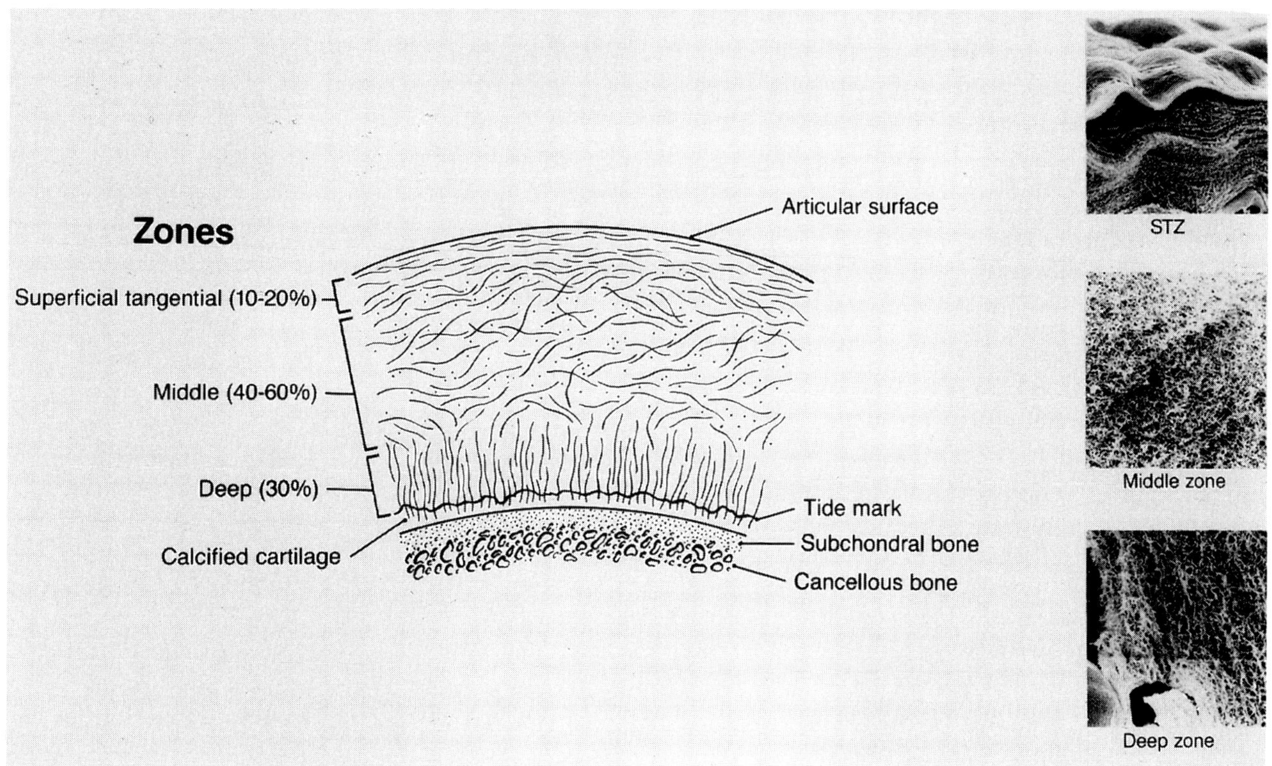

Figure 4
Left, Diagram of collagen fiber architecture in a sagittal cross section showing the three salient zones of articular cartilage. **Right,** Scanning electron micrographs that show actual arrangements of collagen in the three zones. (Reproduced with permission from Mow VC, Proctor CS, Kelly MA: Biomechanics of articular cartilage, in Nordin M, Frankel VH (eds): *Basic Biomechanics of the Musculoskeletal System,* ed 2. Philadelphia, Lea & Febiger, 1989, pp 31–57.)

Figure 5 shows the stages of collagen fibril formation and the typical dense banding pattern seen under the electron microscope. The triple helix, which is characteristic of all collagens, is composed of three polypeptide chains (α chains). The amino acid composition of the chains includes large quantities of glycine (~33% of total residues) and proline (~25% of total residues). Because of their proline content, each of these chains exhibits a characteristic left-handed helical configuration, and in the triple helix, each is wound around a common axis in a right-handed helical configuration to create a structure uniquely designed to resist tensile forces. Collagen also contains hydroxyproline, hydroxylysine, and glycosylated (either galactosyl- or galactosylglucosyl-) hydroxylysine. The amino acid sequence for the triple helical region of collagen can be represented by $(\text{Gly-Xaa-Yaa})_n$, where Xaa and Yaa can be any other amino acid, but frequently are proline and hydroxyproline, respectively. This location of glycine, the smallest amino acid, is an absolute steric requirement for the triple helical structure because a functional group of every third residue occupies the interior of the helix. The failure to maintain this prescribed sequence results in collagens, such as type IX, which contain interruptions in the triple helix. The presence of hydroxyproline is a requirement for the stability of the collagen helix at body temperature because it allows the formation of intramolecular hydrogen bonds along the length of the molecule. Hydroxylysine participates in the formation of covalent cross-links that principally stabilize collagen fibrillar assemblies; the role of glycosylated hydroxylysine is unknown, although it has been postulated to play a role in regulating collagen fibril assemblies and collagen fibril diameters.

Cartilage collagens exist as both homotrimers in which all three α chains are identical (for example, types II and X) and heterotrimers in which all three α chains are different (for example, types VI, IX, and XI). Because each α chain is the product of a distinct gene, cartilage collagens are encoded by at least ten different genes on at least four different chromosomes. One of the type XI chains appears to be a form of α1(II).

Some of the collagens (for example, type II) appear to be distributed uniformly throughout the

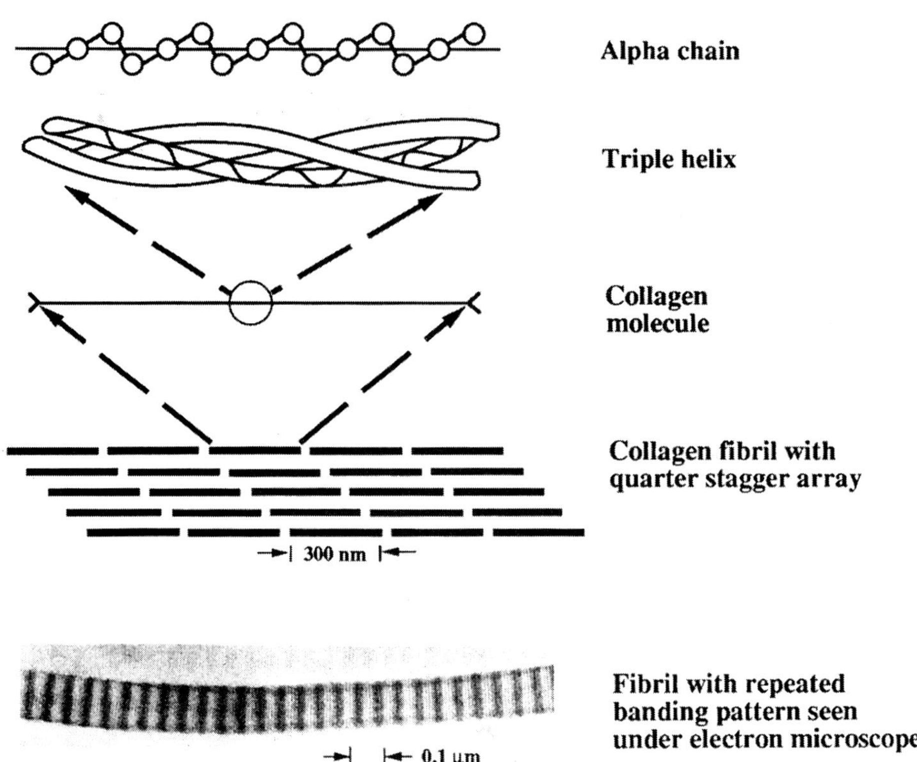

Figure 5
A scheme for the formation of collagen fibrils. The triple helix is made from three α chains, forming a procollagen molecule. Outside the cell the N- and C-terminal globular domains of the α chains are cleaved off to allow fibril formation, which occurs in a specific quarter-staggered array that ultimately results in the typical banded fibrils seen under electron microscopy. (Reproduced with permission from Mow VC, Zhu W, Ratcliffe A: Structure and function of articular cartilage and meniscus, in Mow VC, Hayes WC (eds): *Basic Orthopaedic Biomechanics.* New York, Raven Press, 1991, pp 143–198.)

cartilaginous matrix, whereas others (for example, types VI, IX, and XI) may be localized to specific areas. The prototypical organization of collagen monomers (tropocollagen in the older literature) is shown in Figure 5. In the extracellular matrix, monomers containing an uninterrupted triple helix align head-to-tail and side-by-side in a quarter-staggered array such that overlaps and holes are created in the three-dimensional (3-D) structure. This type of alignment results in the characteristic banding pattern of the fibrillar collagens. In cartilage, this organization is typical of type II collagen. Type XI collagen can also form fibrils, albeit thinner, and currently it is thought that these structures can act as nuclei for the deposition of type II collagen. Type IX collagen, because of interruptions in its triple helical domains, does not form fibrillar structures on its own, but it associates with the surface of the fibrils to form a novel heterotypical cartilage collagen fiber. Recent studies have shown that in addition to covalent cross-links between chains of type II collagen, there are links between types II and IX, and between chains of type XI collagen. Such an extensive network of cross-links undoubtedly contributes to the relative insolubility of these cartilage collagens.

The macromolecular organization of type VI collagen is quite different from those described above because its triple helical domain represents less than half of the molecular mass and is capped at both the amino and carboxyl termini by noncollagenous domains. These monomers readily aggregate into antiparallel tetramers that align end-to-end to form beaded microfibrils stabilized by disulfide bonds. Thus, type VI collagen can be readily extracted from cartilage using chaotropic (for example, guanidine HCl) and reducing agents. On the other hand, type X collagen appears to exist extracellularly in the form of fine fibrous mats. The roles of collagen types VI and X in articular cartilage are not yet known, but type VI appears to be localized to the pericellular capsule of the chondrons and type X to the deep calcified zone of mature joints. Type VI collagen may be important in tethering the chondrocyte to its pericellular matrix, whereas type X may play a role in the mineralization process that occurs just above the underlying subchondral bone.

Collagen Cross-links of Articular Cartilage

The collagens of cartilage appear to be present as a cross-linked network. This intra- and intermolecular cross-linking is thought to add 3-D stability to the network and is likely to contribute to the tensile properties of the tissue. The chemical cross-links prevalent in articular cartilage are the trifunctional hydroxypyridinium cross-links formed by hydroxylysine aldehydes being changed to 3-hydroxypyridinium residues. There are several chemical intermediates in the formation of the final mature cross-links, and their formation in cartilage may take several weeks. Data from recent studies have shown that every type IX collagen molecule in cartilage is cross-linked to type II collagen. Therefore, stabilizing the collagen network by linking the type II collagen fibrils has been proposed to be a function of type IX collagen.

Proteoglycans in Articular Cartilage

Proteoglycans are complex macromolecules that, by definition, consist of a protein core to which are linked extended polysaccharide (glycosaminoglycan) chains (Fig. 6). Proteoglycans were formerly called protein-polysaccharides or mucopolysaccharides and this term still is used to describe some inherited storage disorders.

Eighty to 90% of all proteoglycans in cartilage are of the large, aggregating type, called aggrecan (Fig. 6). They consist of a large, extended protein core to which are attached up to 100 chondroitin sulfate and 50 keratan sulfate glycosaminoglycan chains. The protein core of aggrecan is large (molecular weight 2.25 kd) and complex, and has several distinct globular and extended domains. One extended domain contains the majority of the keratan sulfate glycosaminoglycan chains, and is adjacent to the longest extended region, which has the chondroitin sulfate chains attached with some keratan sulfate chains interspersed. Finally, some small oligosaccharides are also attached along the protein core. At the N-terminal end of the protein core, one of the globular domains (G1) has the specific function of binding to hyaluronate (Fig. 7). The functions of the other globular domains of aggrecan are unknown. A separate, smaller molecule called link protein binds to both the G1 domain of aggrecan and the hyaluronate, stabilizing the bond and, thus, forming an aggrecan-hyaluronate-link protein complex. The noncovalent interactions of this complex are so strong that without proteolytic degradation this binding can be regarded as almost irreversible. Because each hyaluronate chain is long and unbranched (it, too, is a glycosaminoglycan), many aggrecan molecules can bind to a single chain of hyaluronate to form a large proteoglycan aggregate. Aggregate size can vary with age and disease state, but each aggregate can contain up to 200 aggrecan molecules. This is the way that the large proteoglycans are thought to become immobilized within the collagenous network of the cartilage.

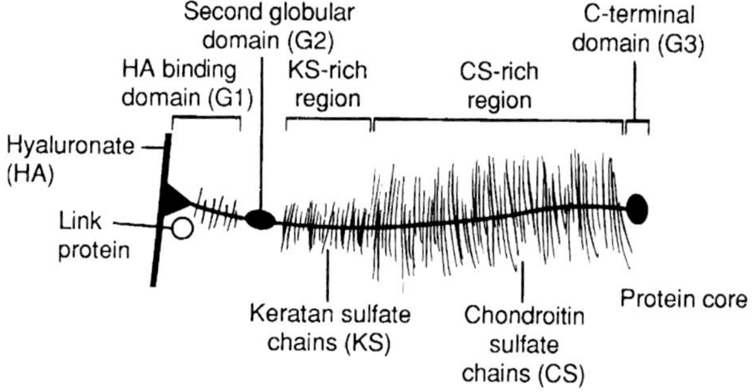

Figure 6
A schematic diagram of the aggrecan molecule and its binding to hyaluronate. The protein core has several globular domains (G1, G2, and G3), with other regions containing the keratan sulfate and chondroitin sulfate glycosaminoglycan chains. The N-terminal G1 domain is able to bind specifically to hyaluronate. This binding is stabilized by link protein.

The other proteoglycans in cartilage are genetically distinct, containing different core proteins. These include two small proteoglycans termed biglycan and decorin, both of which have a protein core of approximately 30 kd. Biglycan contains two dermatan sulfate chains, and decorin contains only one. Decorin is located on the surface of collagen fibrils and is thought to be involved with the control of fibrillogenesis. In addition, type IX collagen usually carries a chondroitin sulfate chain and, thus, is also a proteoglycan. Despite the relatively small contribution of small proteoglycan molecules to the mass of proteoglycans, there are nearly as many small proteoglycan molecules in cartilage as there are large ones. Thus, the small proteoglycans are not minor components of the tissue and almost certainly play major, though not yet defined, roles in the tissue. Fibromodulin (50 to 65 kd) is another small proteoglycan present in cartilage and contains keratan sulfate.

The proteoglycans of articular cartilage are not homogeneously distributed throughout the depth of the tissue. The surface superficial zone is rich in collagen and relatively poor in proteoglycans. In the transitional zone, the concentration of proteoglycans increases, and they are more homogeneously distributed. In the deep zone, the distribution is more variable. Around each chondrocyte in the pericellular matrix there is an approximately twofold increase in proteoglycan concentration, compared to that in the matrix distant from the cells. Whatever their distribution, concentrations and types of proteoglycans in cartilage will change with age and with disease.

Glycosaminoglycans consist of long-chain, unbranched, repeating disaccharide units. Three major types have been found in cartilage proteoglycans: (1) chondroitin sulfate 4- and 6-isomers; (2) keratan

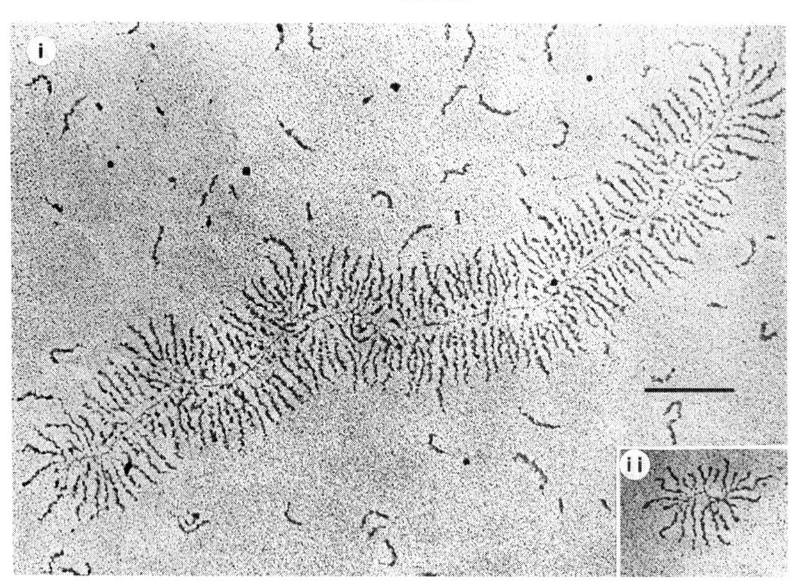

Figure 7
Top, A diagram of the aggrecan molecules arranged as a proteoglycan aggregate. Many aggrecan molecules can bind to a chain of hyaluronate, forming macromolecular complexes that effectively are immobilized within the collagen network. **Bottom,** Electron micrographs of bovine articular cartilage proteoglycan aggregates from (i) skeletally immature calf and (ii) skeletally mature steer. These show the aggregates to consist of a central hyaluronic acid filament and multiple attached monomers (bar = 500 μm). (Reproduced with permission from Buckwalter JA, Kuettner KE, Thonar EJ: Age-related changes in articular cartilage proteoglycans: Electron microscopic studies. *J Orthop Res* 1985;3:251–257.)

sulfate; and (3) dermatan sulfate (Fig. 8). The chondroitin sulfates are the most prevalent glycosaminoglycans in cartilage. They account for 55% to 90% of the total population, depending principally on the age of the subject or the presence of osteoarthritis. Each chain is composed of 25 to 30 repeating disaccharide units, giving an average chain weight of 15 to 20 kd. The keratan sulfate constituent of articular cartilage, which resides primarily in the large, aggregating proteoglycan, is not as well defined as the chondroitin sulfates. The keratan sulfate composition and degree of sulfation vary in human articular cartilage, and may be altered with age. Keratan sulfate chains from human articular cartilage are shorter than those of the chondroitin sulfates, with an average molecular weight of 5 to 10 kd. Hyaluronate is also a glycosaminoglycan, but, unlike those described above, it is not sulfated. A further distinguishing feature of this glycosaminoglycan is that it is not bound to a protein core, and, therefore, is not part of a proteoglycan. In cartilage it is present as an unbranched chain that can be very large (greater than 1 x 10^6 kd). Hyaluronate serves as an anchoring point for the aggrecan molecules, and as many as 200 can bind to one chain of hyaluronate to form a large proteoglycan aggregate.

On all glycosaminoglycans found in cartilage, carboxyl (COOH) and/or sulfate (SO_4) groups occur along the chain (Fig. 8). In solution, these groups become ionized (COO^- and SO_3^-), and in the physiologic environment, they require positive counterions such as Ca^{2+} and Na^+ to maintain overall electroneutrality. These free-floating ions within the interstitial water give rise to the Donnan osmotic pressure effect. Also, because the proteoglycans are packed to within one fifth of their free-solution volume in the tissue, the fixed-charge groups are spaced 10 to 15 Å apart, resulting in a strong charge-to-charge repulsive force. The magnitude of this repulsive force also depends on the concentration of the counterions present in the tissue. These two

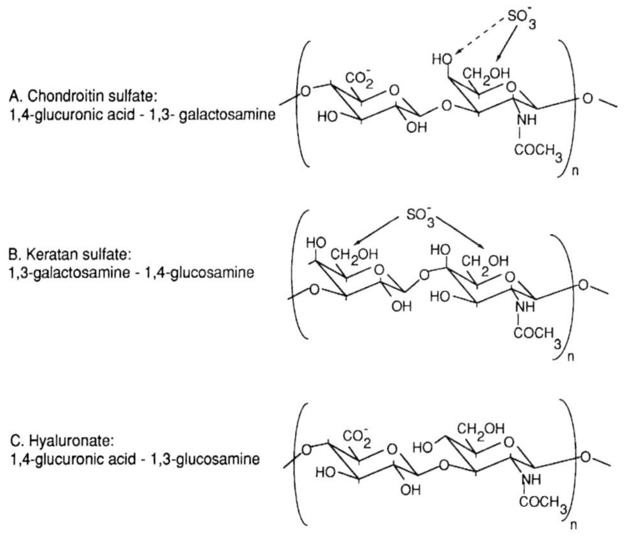

A. Chondroitin sulfate:
1,4-glucuronic acid - 1,3- galactosamine

B. Keratan sulfate:
1,3-galactosamine - 1,4-glucosamine

C. Hyaluronate:
1,4-glucuronic acid - 1,3-glucosamine

Figure 8
Chemical formula and structure of three primary glycosaminoglycans present in articular cartilage. (Adapted from Wight TN, Heinegård DK, Hascall VC: Proteoglycans: Structure and function, in Hay ED (ed): *Cell Biology of the Extracellular Matrix,* ed 2. New York, Plenum Press, 1991, pp 45–78.)

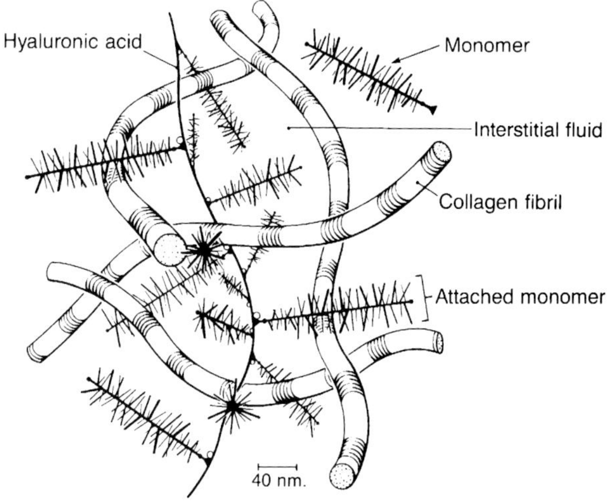

Figure 9
Molecular organization of the solid matrix of articular cartilage as a fiber-reinforced composite solid matrix. The swelling pressure exerted by the proteoglycan keeps the collagen network inflated. (Reproduced with permission from Mow VC, Proctor CS, Kelly MA: Biomechanics of articular cartilage, in Nordin M, Frankel VH (eds): *Basic Biomechanics of the Musculoskeletal System,* ed 2. Philadelphia, Lea & Febiger, 1989, pp 31–57.)

physical forces are predominantly responsible for the swelling pressure of cartilage.

Figure 9 depicts the composite nature of the porous-permeable, collagen-proteoglycan solid matrix. Undoubtedly, the size of the proteoglycans would arrest or minimize diffusion or hydrodynamic convective transport of these molecules through the ECM because of steric exclusion or intermolecular frictional effects. Thus, within the ECM, the size, structural rigidity, and molecular conformation of the charged proteoglycans trapped in the interfibrillar space will influence the mechanical behavior of articular cartilage. The size and complex organization of the proteoglycans also are known to promote proteoglycan-proteoglycan networking and proteoglycan-collagen interactions. This networking capacity enhances the ability of cartilage to maintain structural rigidity and adds to the stiffness and strength of the ECM. The lack of covalent bonds between the proteoglycan and collagen may be necessary to allow the collagen fibers to slide easily through the proteoglycan gel. In that way the collagen may resist the tensile stresses developed within the matrix during variable loading conditions. (See the chapter on biomechanics.)

Other Matrix Components

Three adhesive materials, chondronectin, anchorin CII, and fibronectin, are involved in the interactions between collagen fibrils and chondrocytes. Anchorin CII is part of a family of adhesive cell-surface macromolecules known as calpactins. Integrins are transmembrane molecules on the outer surface of the cell that form sites where the cell attaches to the surrounding matrix. On the inner surface of the cell, the integrins serve as sites of attachment to the cytoskeletal proteins. Integrins are important in transmembrane signaling of environmental and mechanical stimuli to the interior of the cell, and as such they play a fundamental role in the interaction of cells with their environment. Integrins also are thought to interact directly with the collagen fibril surrounding the chondrocyte. Fibronectin has been found to be associated with osteoarthrotic cartilage.

Lipids, which form 1% or less of the wet weight of human adult articular cartilage, are found in both the cells and the matrix. Their exact function is not yet known, but they vary with age and the presence of osteoarthrosis. Phospholipase A_2 is an enzyme that has sparked interest in the last few years. This enzyme may be important both in arachidonic acid metabolism and in the degradative pathway. Pericellular osmiophilic matrix vesicles measure 50 to 250 nm, contain apatitic calcific nodules, and are found in the radial zone. These vesicles appear to increase with age and may play a role in the pathogenesis of osteoarthrosis. Investigators have defined several other matrix proteins (for example, cartilage matrix protein) that may account for up to 15% of the dry weight; although none have been assigned a function.

Metabolism of Articular Cartilage

Metabolism in the strict sense deals with both synthesis (anabolism) and degradation (catabolism). A surprisingly active level of metabolism exists in articular cartilage. One of the factors that led to the general impression that articular cartilage was inert was the early demonstration that although articular cartilage had a well-defined glycolytic system, oxygen use was considerably lower in articular cartilage than in other tissues. This difference subsequently was established to be related to the sparse cell population rather than to a lack of metabolic activity. Nevertheless, there remains little doubt that articular cartilage uses principally the anaerobic pathway for energy production. Chondrocytes synthesize and assemble the cartilaginous matrix components and direct their distribution within the tissue. This synthetic apparatus is complex and involves synthesis of proteins by the standard genetic pathway, synthesis of glycosaminoglycan chains and their addition to the appropriate protein cores, and secretion of the completed molecules into the extracellular matrix. The final incorporation of its components into the matrix also appears to depend on the chondrocyte. All of these actions take place under avascular and, at times, anaerobic conditions, with considerable variation in local pressure and physicochemical states. In addition, the chondrocyte directs an active internal remodeling system for portions of the proteoglycan and probably the collagen by means of an elaborate series of degradative enzymes.

The maintenance of a normal extracellular matrix depends on the chondrocytes being able to balance the rates of synthesis of matrix components, the components' appropriate incorporation into the matrix, and their degradation and release from the cartilage. The cells do this by responding to their chemical and mechanical environments. Soluble mediators (for example, growth factors, interleukins), matrix composition, mechanical loads, hydrostatic pressure changes, and electric fields can all influence the metabolic activities of the chondrocytes. The response of the chondrocytes usually will maintain a stable matrix. However, in some cases the response of the cells can lead to a change of matrix composition and ultrastructural organization, and eventually to cartilage degeneration.

Proteoglycan Synthesis

Many investigators have clearly demonstrated that the chondrocyte is responsible for the synthesis, assembly, and sulfation of the proteoglycan molecule (Fig. 10). At the molecular level, this activity begins with proteoglycan gene expression and the transcription of the messenger RNA (mRNA) from the DNA within the nucleus. In the endoplasmic reticulum the mRNA is translated and the protein is synthesized at the ribosome. The protein core is then transported to the Golgi complex, where the glycosaminoglycan chains are added. Although the addition appears to be very specific and well coordinated, little is known about how the cell controls these events. Chondroitin/dermatan sulfate chains are attached to specific serine residues in the sequence Ser-Gly via a unique tetrasaccharide:

```
                                              |
-glucuronic acid-galactose-galactose-xylose-ser
                                              |
```

The repeating disaccharide glucuronic acid-galactosamine is then added to this linkage region; in dermatan sulfate, some of the glucuronic acid residues are subsequently isomerized to iduronic acid. On the other hand, keratan sulfate chains are attached to either serine or threonine by a different sequence:

```
-galactose-glucosamine
                     |              |
                     galactosamine-ser(thr)
                     |              |
   sialic acid-galactose
```

The repeating disaccharide galactose-glucosamine is then added to the linkage region galactose. All of the carbohydrate constituents of glycosaminoglycan chains are added one sugar at a time. While the chains are being elongated, hexosamine residues of both chondroitin/dermatan sulfate and keratan sulfate chains are being sulfated. All of the above steps are posttranslational enzymic reactions and, therefore, are not under direct genetic control. For this reason, the lengths of the glycosaminoglycan chains are quite polydispersed. Once glycosylation is complete, the proteoglycan molecules are secreted into the extracellular matrix. The protein core may represent as little as 10% of the completed molecule. Thus, the addition of the glycosaminoglycan chains and the other oligosaccharides as posttranslational modifications offers tremendous opportunity for variations in the final composition of the completed molecule. This is certainly reflected during aging and disease, and can offer significant variability of the structure of the molecules synthesized at any one time.

Synthesis of some of the proteoglycans by the chondrocyte appears to occur at a rapid rate and is affected by numerous endogenous and exogenous environmental alterations. Studies have shown that such diverse physical and pathologic states as lacerative injury; osteoarthritis; altered interstitial hydrostatic pressure; stresses, strains, and flows in the tissue; varied oxygen tension; pH alteration; calcium concentration; substrate or serum concentration; growth hormones; insulin-like growth factor-I;

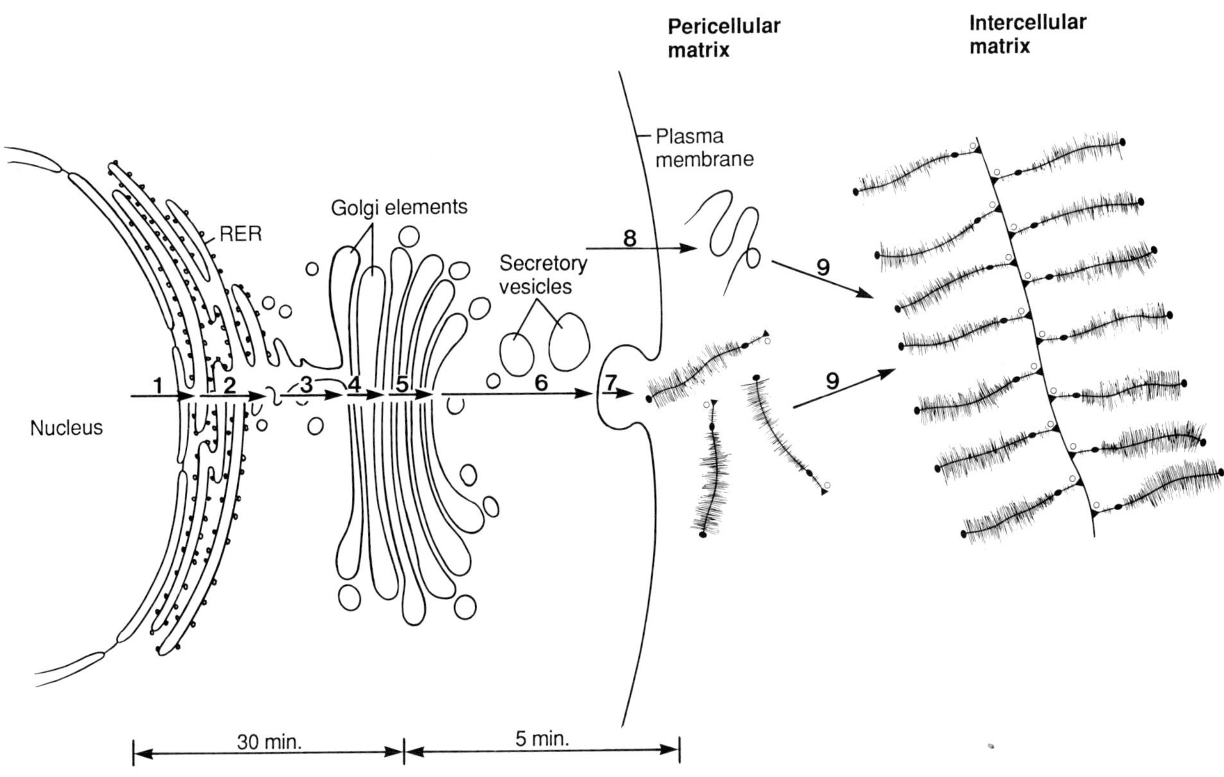

Figure 10
Diagram depicting the various stages involved in the synthesis and secretion of aggrecan and link protein by a chondrocyte. (1) The transcription of the aggrecan and link protein genes to mRNA. (2) The translation of the mRNA in the rough endoplasmic reticulum (RER) to form the protein core of the aggrecan. (3) The newly-formed protein is transported from the RER to (4) the cis and (5) medial-trans Golgi compartments where the glycosaminoglycan chains are added to the protein core. (6) On completion of the glycosylation and sulfation, the molecules are transported via secretory vesicles to the plasma membrane, where (7) they are released into the extracellular matrix. (8) Hyaluronate is synthesized separately at the plasma membrane. (9) Only in the extracellular matrix can aggrecan, link protein, and hyaluronate come together to form proteoglycan aggregates.

ascorbate; vitamin E; cortisol; prostaglandins; diphosphonates; salicylates and several other nonsteroidal anti-inflammatory drugs; hyaluronate; uridine diphosphate; xyloside; synovial tissue; and a variety of other factors have significant effects on the rate of synthesis of the proteoglycans. These data suggest that the control mechanisms for proteoglycan synthesis are extraordinarily sensitive to stimuli of a biochemical, mechanical, and physical nature. It is also evident that the turnover rate for a small fraction of the proteoglycans is quite rapid. This rapidity seems far in excess of that necessary merely to compensate for any attrition that may occur in cartilage in a joint that operates in an almost frictionless state. These data strongly suggest the presence of an elaborate internal remodeling system for proteoglycan synthesis, which is presumed to be dictated by circumstances other than attrition.

Proteoglycan Catabolism

In normal tissue, in repair processes, and in degradation, proteoglycans of articular cartilage are continually being broken down and released from the cartilage. This activity is regarded as a normal event in maintenance of normal tissue; it can occur as part of remodeling in repair processes, and in degenerative events it appears to occur at an accelerated rate. The rate of catabolism can be affected by soluble mediators and by loading of the cartilage. For example, interleukin 1 will accelerate proteoglycan degradation, and immobilization of a joint will cause rapid loss of proteoglycans from the cartilage matrix.

Current understanding of proteoglycan breakdown in articular cartilage comes from studies of aggrecan and proteoglycan aggregates. The heterogeneity of proteoglycans in articular cartilage is likely to be derived from some limited enzymatic cleavage of the protein core. A major cleavage site of the protein core is between the G1 and G2 domains (Fig. 11), separating the part of the proteoglycan involved in aggregation (binding to hyaluronate and link protein) from the part that contains the glycosaminoglycan chains. The free glycosaminoglycan-containing fragment, although it is large, is able to

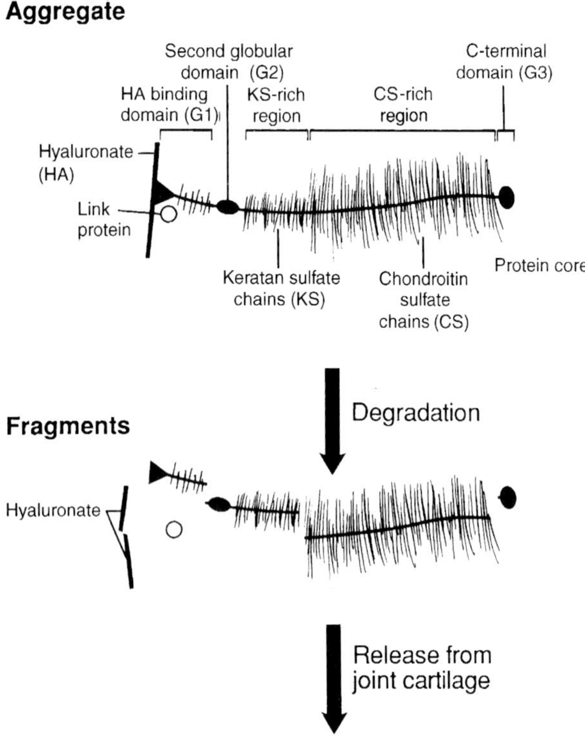

Figure 11
Representation of the mechanism of degradation of proteoglycan aggregates in articular cartilage. The major proteolytic cleavage site is between the G1 and G2 domains, making the glycosaminoglycan-containing portion of the aggrecan molecule nonaggregating. This fragment can now be released from the cartilage. Other proteolytic events can result in G1 domain and link protein also disaggregating and leaving the cartilage.

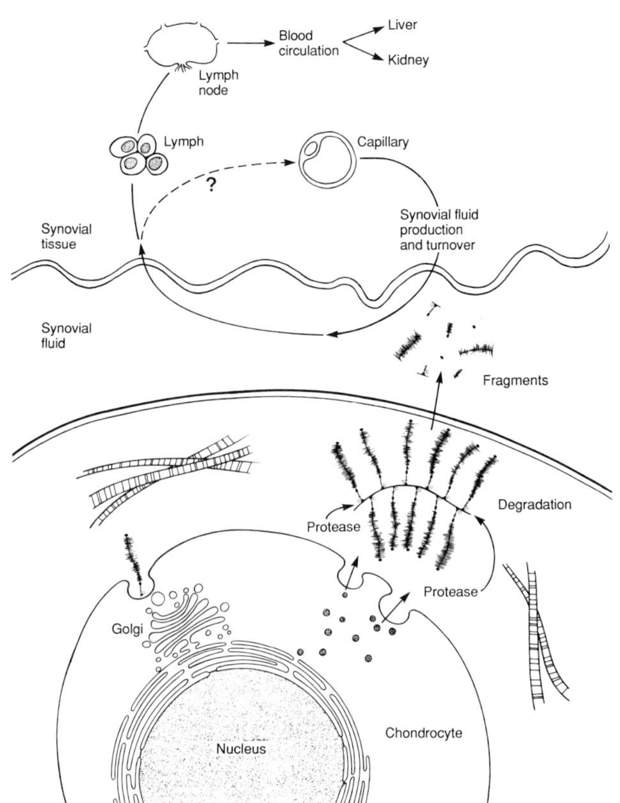

Figure 12
Schematic representation of the metabolic events controlling the proteoglycans in cartilage. The chondrocytes synthesize and secrete aggrecan, link protein, and hyaluronate, and they become incorporated into functional aggregates. Enzymes released by the cells break down the proteoglycan aggregates. The fragments are released from the matrix into the synovial fluid, and from there the fragments are taken up by the lymphatics and moved into the circulating blood.

pass through the matrix and leave the cartilage. This appears to be an efficient mechanism of turnover of the large proteoglycan. The G1 domain and link protein also are susceptible to proteolytic degradation and can thus be released from the cartilage. These fragments can be found in synovial fluid, from which they are taken up through the synovium to the lymphatic system (Fig. 12). The glycosaminoglycan chains can be found further along in this system, in the bloodstream, and even in the urine. The levels of proteoglycan fragments in the body fluids can be quantified, and, at least in synovial fluid, it is thought that these levels can indicate catabolic activities ongoing in the cartilage of that joint. It is hoped that this type of analysis may offer some diagnostic and prognostic help in the clinical evaluation of early degenerative joint disease.

Collagen Synthesis

Collagen of articular cartilage is much more stable than the proteoglycan. However the collagen network is subject to metabolism, and in osteoarthritic cartilage, or cartilage that has undergone lacerative injury, the collagen turnover can be increased. Most knowledge about collagen synthesis has come from studies of the major fibrillar types (for example, types I to III) (Fig. 13). In a manner identical to that for other secretory proteins, mRNA for the constituent α chains is translated to form a polypeptide containing a signal sequence and noncollagenous propeptide domains on both the amino and carboxy termini flanking the collagenous domain. The nascent chains are extruded into the cisterna of the rough endoplasmic reticulum where the signal peptide is immediately removed, and where the posttranslational events of propeptide glycosylation, proline and lysine hydroxylation, lysine glycosylation, and triple helix formation occur. The latter step, which is propagated in a carboxy to amino terminal direction, is obligatory for the procollagen molecule to enter the secretory apparatus. It is useful to note that the hydroxylation

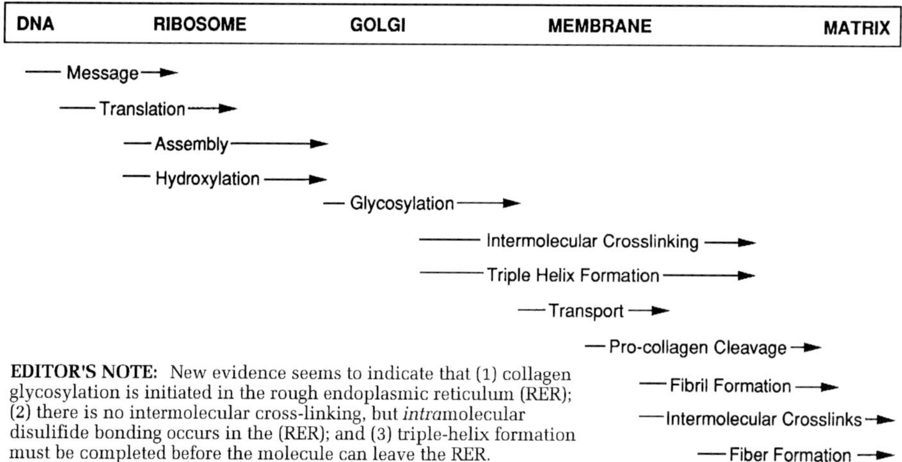
DNA
RIBOSOME
GOLGI
MEMBRANE
MATRIX
Message
Translation
Assembly
Hydroxylation
Glycosylation
Intermolecular Crosslinking
Triple Helix Formation
Transport
Pro-collagen Cleavage
Fibril Formation
Intermolecular Crosslinks
Fiber Formation
EDITOR'S NOTE: New evidence seems to indicate that (1) collagen glycosylation is initiated in the rough endoplasmic reticulum (RER); (2) there is no intermolecular cross-linking, but intramolecular disulifide bonding occurs in the (RER); and (3) triple-helix formation must be completed before the molecule can leave the RER.

Figure 13
The events involved in the synthesis of collagen, showing the intracellular sites that are used for each procedure. (Reproduced with permission from Mankin HJ, Brandt KD: Biochemistry and metabolism of articular cartilage in osteoarthritis, in Moskowitz RW, Howell DS, Goldberg VM, et al (eds): *Osteoarthritis: Diagnosis and Medical/Surgical Management,* ed 2. Philadelphia, WB Saunders, 1992, pp 109–154.)

reactions require vitamin C as one cofactor and that deficiencies (for example, scurvy) can result in alterations in collagen synthesis. After secretion, the propeptides are cleaved from both ends of the triple helical domain, and the resultant collagen molecules can self-assemble into the fibrillar arrays discussed previously. The final step in this process is covalent cross-link formation, which is catalyzed by the enzyme lysyl oxidase.

In cartilage, the above steps are generally followed by types II and XI collagen. For each of the other cartilage collagen types, there are variations on this process. Types VI, IX, and X collagen, for example, retain their noncollagenous terminal domains after secretion, and these unprocessed forms are used in subsequent matrix interaction. In addition, type IX collagen has a single site that usually contains a chondroitin sulfate chain, which probably is added intracellularly in the Golgi compartment. Finally, recent evidence has uncovered another level of complexity in cartilage collagen synthesis at the transcription level where collagen types II and IX can be alternatively spliced to yield slightly different products in different tissues.

Collagen Catabolism

As yet little is known about the mechanisms of collagen breakdown. In normal cartilage it occurs only at a very slow rate, although in degenerative cartilage and in cartilage undergoing repair and remodeling (for example in growth), there is now evidence for accelerated breakdown of the collagen network. The mechanism of breakdown may be enzymatic, with the metalloproteinase collagenase able to specifically cleave the triple helix of collagen, or mechanical.

Growth Factors and Articular Cartilage

Recently, cartilage biochemists have begun to define the response of articular cartilage to polypeptide growth factors, and it has become apparent, even at this early phase, that these agents play a major role in the regulation of the synthetic processes of normal cartilage. In addition, it has been speculated that these growth factors may even have a greater role in the osteoarthritic process. The methods by which these agents act on the chondrocyte have not been elucidated fully, but appear to be related principally to interaction with cell surface receptor sites on the responsive cells. In the case of at least two of these agents (insulin-like growth factor-I and insulin), competitive binding is present, which may alter the end result. For most of the factors, however, the cell receptor is highly specific and the response is dictated by the concentration of the growth factor and the number of receptors on the cell. The various growth factors are discussed below.

Platelet-derived Growth Factor (PDGF)

This factor is a major growth material for connective tissue cells. PDGF is a 30-kd glycoprotein that consists of a dimer of disulfide-bonded A and B polypeptide chains. Various isoforms have been identified and seem to have different activities. Although several studies have suggested that PDGF has a mitogenic effect on chondrocytes, the method of action is not clear nor does it seem likely that this material is active in the joint under normal conditions. In osteoarthritis and, especially, in lacerative injury a greater likelihood exists for the role of these peptides in healing.

Fibroblast Growth Factor (basic) (b-FGF)

This material, like many of the other factors, comes from multiple sources. In the past, the peptide coming from the pituitary was referred to as cartilage growth factor, and that generated by the cartilage was called cartilage-derived growth factor. It is now evident that these are identical to b-FGF, which acts in connective tissues principally as a very powerful mitogen. Studies have shown that b-FGF alone is a powerful stimulator of DNA synthesis in adult articular chondrocytes in culture. This material, although contributory to matrix production, seems less active unless it is introduced with other materials, such as insulin. Recent studies have shown that b-FGF markedly stimulates repair of cartilage slices in an in vivo rabbit model.

Insulin-like Growth Factor-I (IGF-I)

Perhaps the best studied of the growth factors, insulin, IGF-I, and IGF-II are three homologous peptides that bind with varying affinity to three distinct receptors on the cells. IGF-I and IGF-II are structurally homologous to proinsulin, almost the same size (70 and 67 amino acids), and share about 65% homology. IGF-I, formerly known as somatomedin-C, has been found to stimulate DNA and matrix synthesis in growth plate, in immature cartilage, and, more recently, in adult articular cartilage. There is little evidence to suggest that these growth factors are synthesized by articular cartilage, and it is unknown whether IGF is produced locally or in the liver. IGF-I is more effective when co-administered with other factors, including b-FGF, but not insulin. Recent evidence suggests that IGF-I maintains a steady state for proteoglycan synthesis in adult tissue.

Transforming Growth Factor-beta (TGF-β)

TGF-β is a 25-kd protein composed of two identical polypeptides linked by disulfide bonds. It shares its receptor with no other factors and is known to exist in at least five isoforms. Numerous cellular activities have been attributed to this material in relation to bone and more recently cartilage, and not all of these are stimulatory. The material seems to potentiate the stimulation of DNA synthesis by b-FGF, epidermal growth factor, and IGF-I rather than initiating it de novo. Recent studies have shown that TGF-β is synthesized locally by the chondrocytes and appears to stimulate proteoglycan synthesis and, at the same time, suppress type II collagen synthesis. There is now evidence to suggest that, in addition to its other functions, TGF-β is responsible for stimulating the formation of tissue inhibitor of metalloproteinase (TIMP) and plasminogen activator inhibitor-1, two materials believed to prevent the degradative action of stromelysin and plasmin.

The Degradative Enzymes of Articular Cartilage

The breakdown of the cartilage matrix in normal turnover, and in degradative events, appears to be by the action of proteolytic enzymes (proteinases) that are synthesized by the chondrocytes. This is part of the complex orchestration of events performed by the chondrocytes to maintain the normal cartilage matrix. It is likely that the overactivity of some of these enzymes is ultimately responsible for cartilage degradation in osteoarthritis and rheumatoid arthritis. The most important proteinases thought to be involved in cartilage turnover are shown in Figure 14. The major groups are metalloproteinases (collagenase, gelatinase, and stromelysin) and the cathepsins (cathepsins B and D).

The metalloproteinases derive their name from the fact that their activity depends on the presence of zinc in the active site. Collagenase is highly specific in its action on collagen, because it is the only enzyme that can cleave the triple helical part of the molecule, at a single site three quarters of the way along the molecule from the amino terminus. Gelatinase cleaves the denatured α-chains generated by prior collagenase activity. Stromelysin can act on type II collagen within the nonhelical domain, and can also act on type IX collagen. Breakdown of the protein core of aggrecan has been thought to be a major activity of stromelysin. Although it cleaves the protein core between the G1 and G2 domains (as occurs in normal aggrecan breakdown), the specific cleavage products identified in vivo and in vitro cannot be assigned to stromelysin. The possibility therefore remains that another, yet to be defined, enzyme is responsible for the cleavage of aggrecan, or that stromelysin acts together with another enzyme.

The activities of these metalloproteinases appear to be controlled by two mechanisms, their activation and their inhibition. Collagenase, stromelysin, and gelatinase are all synthesized as latent enyzmes (proenzymes), and they require activation outside of the cell by enzymatic modification. Plasmin, produced from plasminogen by the activity of a plasminogen activator, can activate collagenase. Stromelysin can super-activate collagenase to produce maximal activity. The mechanisms of activation for prostromelysin and progelatinase remain to be determined. The active enzymes can be inhibited irreversibly by TIMP, which also is secreted by the chondrocyte. The molar ratios of metalloproteinases and TIMP will determine whether there is net metalloproteinase activity.

A second group of enzymes present in articular cartilage are the cathepsins that have the capacity to degrade aggrecan. These have been identified as

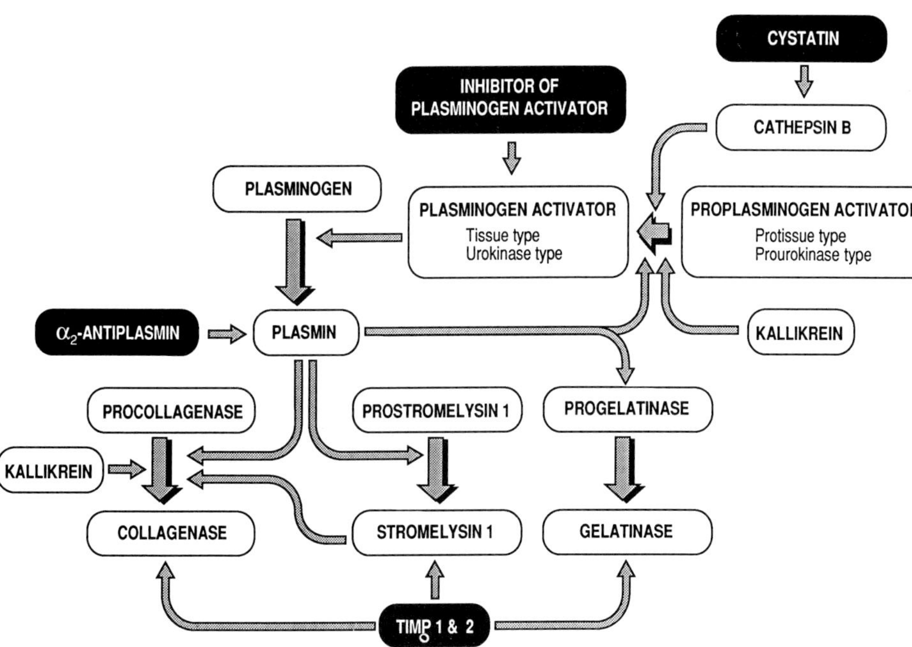

Figure 14
The proteolytic enzymes, their activators and inhibitors involved in the catabolism of articular cartilage matrix. (Reproduced with permission from Mow VC, Ratcliffe A, Poole AR: Cartilage and diarthrodial joints as paradigms for hierarchical structures. *Biomaterials* 1992; 13:67–97.)

cathepsins D and B, and both are known to occur in articular cartilage. Of some concern, however, has been the low pH optima at which these acid cathepsins act (pH 5.5), because it may exclude them from having a major role in the degradation of proteoglycan in the interterritorial matrix. However, there is some evidence that low pH can be achieved in the cartilage, possibly in the pericellular matrix; therefore, the ability of acid pH optimum enzymes to participate in cartilage metabolism cannot be excluded.

Immature Articular Cartilage and the Effects of Aging

Unlike many other body tissues, immature articular cartilage differs considerably from adult articular cartilage. On gross inspection, the cartilage from an immature animal appears blue-white in color, presumably because of the reflection of the vascular structures in the underlying immature bone, and is relatively thick. The thickness appears to be primarily a function of the dual nature of the cartilage mass, which serves not only as a cartilaginous articular surface for the joint but also as a microepiphyseal plate for endochondral ossification of the underlying bony nucleus of the epiphysis.

On histologic examination, it is apparent that immature articular cartilage is considerably more cellular than the adult tissue, and numerous studies have corroborated the increased number of cells per unit volume or mass (Fig. 15, *left*). The hypercellularity appears fairly uniform throughout the immature cartilage, and little variation is noted in cell density. The structural organization of the tissue also differs from that of adult cartilage in that the zonal characteristics show major variation, particularly in the lower zones. The gliding or tangential layer remains evident in immature cartilage, although the surface cells are somewhat larger and less discoid than those seen in adult cartilage. The midzone is wider and contains a larger number of randomly arranged cells. In the lower zones, however, the orientation differs markedly; at about the halfway mark in the distance from the surface to the underlying bone, the chondrocytes are arranged in irregular columns and, at further depth, the columniation becomes more evident. The cells in these columns show characteristics consistent with their participation in the process of diagonal division. With further distance from the surface, the cells are increased in size and show shrunken pyknotic nuclei and large intracytoplasmic vacuoles that have been demonstrated to contain glycogen. Vascular buds from the underlying bone invade the cartilage columns in a pattern resembling the zone of provisional calcification of the epiphyseal plate.

When immature articular cartilage is examined by light microscopy, mitotic figures are readily noted, and all stages of mitosis can be seen. Cell replication is not uniformly present throughout the tissue, however. In the very young animal, the mitotic activity occurs in two distinct zones. One lies subjacent to the surface and presumably ac-

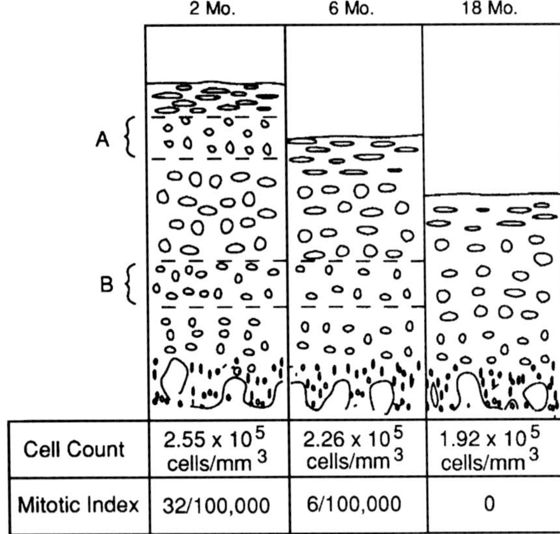

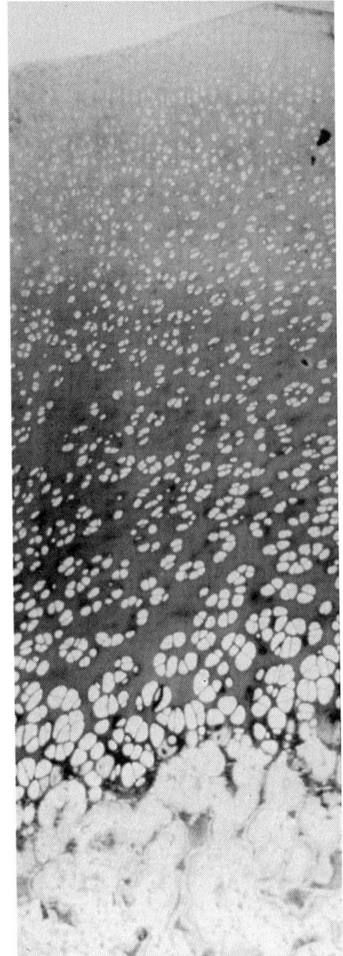

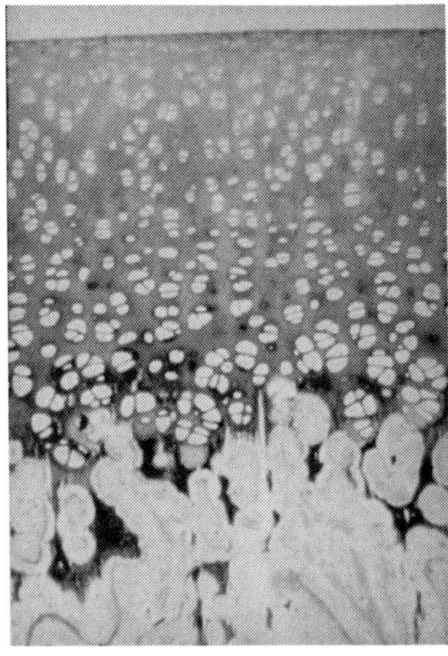

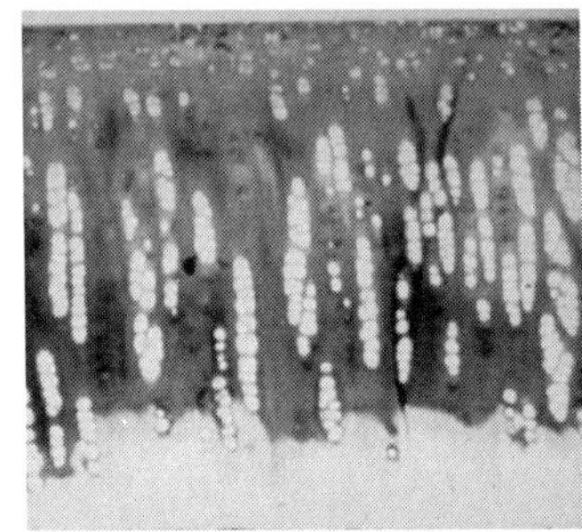

Figure 15
Left, Estimates of number density of chondrocytes in immature, maturing and adult articular cartilage. **Right,** Histologic sections of immature, maturing, and adult articular cartilage showing changes in thickness and cellular population. (Photomicrograph provided by EB Hunziker, 1990, Bern, Switzerland.)

counts for the growth of the cellular complement of the articular portion of the cartilage mass; the second lies below this region and consists of a narrow band of cells that morphologically resemble the proliferative zone of the microepiphyseal plate of the subjacent bony nucleus. Figure 15, *right,* shows the changes observed in rabbit articular cartilage. It should be noted that a two-month-old rabbit is immature; a six-month one, pubertal; and an 18-month one, a young adult. As the animal ages and approaches maturity, the pattern of cell replication changes. The mitotic activity is confined to the area just above the zone of vascular invasion in the lowermost portion of the cartilage, which now demonstrates a diffuse calcification. No evidence for cell replication can be found in the more superficial regions.

In the adult animal, mitotic activity ceases with the development of a well-defined calcified zone, the tidemark, and, in some species, with closure of the epiphyseal plate. Careful search of normal articular cartilage from adult animals of numerous species has failed to demonstrate mitotic figures, and ^{3}H-thymidine studies have not demonstrated grains over the nucleus indicating DNA replication. Although it has been suggested that the chondrocyte may divide by amitotic division, there is only limited evidence for such an activity, and cytophotometry and cytofluorometry have failed to demonstrate evidence of nuclear polyploidy in the adult tissue (Fig. 15, *right*).

In recent years, investigations have demonstrated significant variation in the chemistry of articular cartilage with advancing age. Water content appears to be relatively high in immature animals and slowly diminishes to a standard figure that remains constant throughout most of adulthood. The collagen content of fetal articular cartilage is considerably lower than that of mature animals. The collagen concentration climbs to adult levels shortly after birth, and it is maintained throughout the life of the animal. The principal chemical changes that occur in articular cartilage matrix with advancing age appear to be in the proteoglycans. Proteoglycan content in articular cartilage is highest at birth and diminishes slowly through the period of immaturity. The protein core and the glycosaminoglycan chains are longer in immature animals. As the animal approaches adolescence and maturity, the average length of the proteoglycan protein core becomes less, probably because of enzymatic cleavage of the resident proteoglycan population, near the C-terminal end of the protein core, and the lengths of the glycosaminoglycan chains, particularly those of chondroitin sulfate, diminish. Although an extraordinarily high concentration of chondroitin 4-sulfate has been noted in immature animals, a fairly rapid diminution in the value is noted with aging. Furthermore, with advancing age, the total chondroitin sulfate concentration falls and that of keratan sulfate increases until at approximately age 30 in humans, keratan sulfate represents 25% to 50% of the total glycosaminoglycans. This value then remains constant through old age. It should be noted that aggregation appears to diminish with advancing age, possibly on the basis of an alteration in the core protein or link protein, but this does not appear to be a result of any change in the concentration of hyaluronate. Synthesis of proteoglycans in vitro is diminished for rabbit and bovine articular chondrocytes from mature animals, which is consistent with a maintenance process of the extracellular matrix after its remodeling during growth, development, and maturation.

Biomechanics of Articular Cartilage

The chapter on biomechanics and the glossary will be helpful to the reader who is not familiar with the terminology and the constructs of biomechanics.

The Biphasic Nature of Articular Cartilage

The articular cartilage of diarthrodial joints is subject to high loads applied statically, cyclically and repetitively for many decades. Thus, the structural molecules, that is, collagen, proteoglycan, and other quantitatively minor molecules, must be organized into a strong, fatigue-resistant, and tough solid matrix capable of sustaining the high stresses and strains developed within the tissue from these loads. In terms of material behavior, this solid matrix is described as being porous and permeable, and very soft. Water, 65% to 80% of the total weight of the tissue, resides in the microscopic pores, and this water may be caused to flow through the porous-permeable solid matrix by a pressure gradient or by matrix compaction. Thus, the biomechanical properties of articular cartilage are understood best when the tissue is viewed as a biphasic material, composed of a solid phase and a fluid phase. Because of technical difficulties, early studies on cartilage biomechanics have generally ignored the water component of the tissue. Over the past decade, however, a theory has been developed, which is capable of describing the biphasic deformational behaviors of hydrated-soft tissues such as cartilage. This theory has been used to describe the experimentally measured behaviors of articular cartilage, as well as to calculate interstitial fluid flow and stresses and strains in the collagen-proteoglycan solid matrix. The material coefficients can be calculated from the experimental data by using the biphasic theory, and these define the intrinsic behavior of the collagen-proteoglycan solid matrix and its frictional resistance against interstitial fluid flow. Within this theoretical framework, the structure-function relationships of the collagen-proteoglycan solid matrix of normal cartilage, and changes of these intrinsic material properties in osteoarthritic cartilage, are determined.

Permeability of Articular Cartilage

For many years now, permeation studies have shown that water is capable of flowing through the cartilage when a pressure gradient is imposed. In this simple experiment, a tissue sample of thickness h is subjected to an applied pressure gradient ($\Delta P/h$) across the specimen. The rate of volume discharge Q across the permeation area A is related to the hydraulic permeability coefficient k by Darcy's law, which expresses a direct linear proportionality between Q and ($\Delta P/h$), $Q = kA(\Delta P/h)$. The permeation speed V is related to Q by the expression $V = Q/A\phi^f$ where ϕ^f, the porosity of the tissue (65% to 80%), is defined as the ratio of the interstitial fluid volume V^f to the total tissue volume V^T. Results from this permeation experiment showed that for normal cartilage and meniscus, the permeability coefficient k ranges from 10^{-15} to 10^{-16} m^4/Ns. The diffusive drag coefficient K is inversely related to the permeability coefficient k and is given by the following simple equation: $K = (\phi^f)^2/k$. Because the porosity ϕ^f for cartilage ranges from 0.65 to 0.80, K ranges from 10^{14} to 10^{15} Ns/m^4. This very large drag coefficient indicates that any interstitial fluid flow will cause large drag forces to be generated within the tissue. In turn, very high pressures are required to move the water through cartilage; a flow speed of 17.5 μm/s requires a pressure gradient of 1 MPa (or 145 psi).

Water also will flow through the porous-permeable solid matrix as the tissue is compressed. In this case, the compressive stress causes the solid matrix to be compacted, raising the pressure in the interstitium, and forcing the fluid out of the tissue. The rate of efflux is controlled by the drag force generated during flow. In general, the manner with which an applied load is shared between the fluid phase (hydrodynamic pressure) and the solid phase (stress in the solid matrix) is determined, among other things, by the volumetric ratios within the tissue, that is, the porosity ϕ^f and solidity ϕ^s ($= V^s/V^T$, where V^s is the volume of the solid matrix), the loading rates, and the type of loading (tension, compression, and shear). The load-carrying capacity of each phase is determined by balancing the frictional drag forces against the elastic forces at each point within the tissue. For example, flow of fluid through a highly permeable, stiff solid matrix would cause little frictional drag force or fluid pressurization. A compressive stress acting on such a material would be supported predominantly by the stress developed within the solid matrix, for example, a highly porous rigid steel filter. Conversely, flow of fluid through a soft solid matrix with very low permeability would cause high frictional drag forces and require high hydrodynamic pressures to maintain a significant flow. In this case, fluid pressure provides a significant component of total load support, thus minimizing the stress acting on the solid matrix. Such is the case for normal articular cartilage.

Articular cartilage permeability, as calculated using Darcy's law, is based on data obtained from permeation experiments. This permeability decreases nonlinearly with compression ϵ_c (Fig.16). This strain-dependent permeability effect serves to regulate the response of cartilage to compression by preventing rapid and excessive fluid exudation from the tissue with compressive loading, and by promoting interstitial fluid pressurization for load support. It also regulates the ability of cartilage to dissipate energy during cyclic loading. There are two reasons for this nonlinear effect: (1) as the tissue is compressed, the water content or porosity is reduced; and (2) as the tissue is compressed, the density of the negative charges on the proteoglycan (COO^- and SO_3^-) in the interstitium is increased (see below for a discussion on swelling pressure). Because proteoglycan is the main reason why water is held so tightly within the interstitium of cartilage, an increase in its concentration would act to decrease permeability. These observations have been verified experimentally by correlating the permeabilities of different osteoarthritic cartilages with tissue water and proteoglycan contents. Indeed, there is a strong direct relationship between permeability and water content, and an inverse relationship between permeability and proteoglycan content.

Flow-Dependent Viscoelasticity of Articular Cartilage in Compression

Articular cartilage is viscoelastic, that is, it will exhibit a time-dependent behavior when subjected to a constant load or constant deformation. When a constant compressive stress (load/area) is applied to the tissue, its deformation will increase with time, that is, it will creep until an equilibrium value is reached (Fig. 17, *top*). Similarly, when the tissue is deformed and held at a constant strain, the stress will rise to a peak, followed by a slow stress-relaxation process until an equilibrium value is

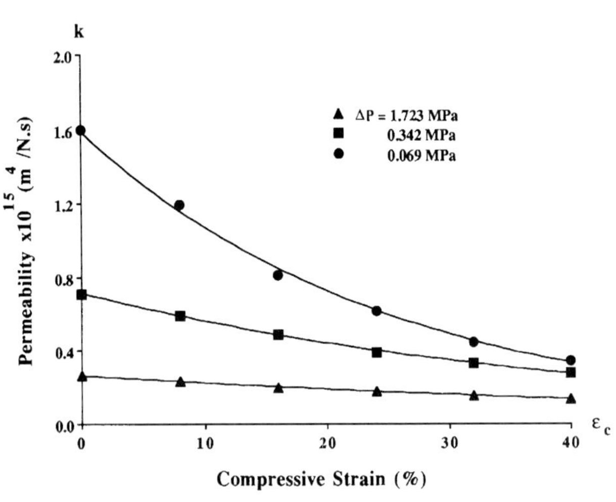

Figure 16
Permeability of normal bovine articular cartilage showing nonlinear strain dependence and pressure dependence. The decrease of permeability with compression acts to retard rapid loss of interstitial fluid during high joint loadings. (Reproduced with permission from Mow VC, Zhu W, Ratcliffe A: Structure and function of articular cartilage and meniscus, in Mow VC, Hayes WC (eds): *Basic Orthopaedic Biomechanics.* New York, Raven Press, 1991, pp 143–198.)

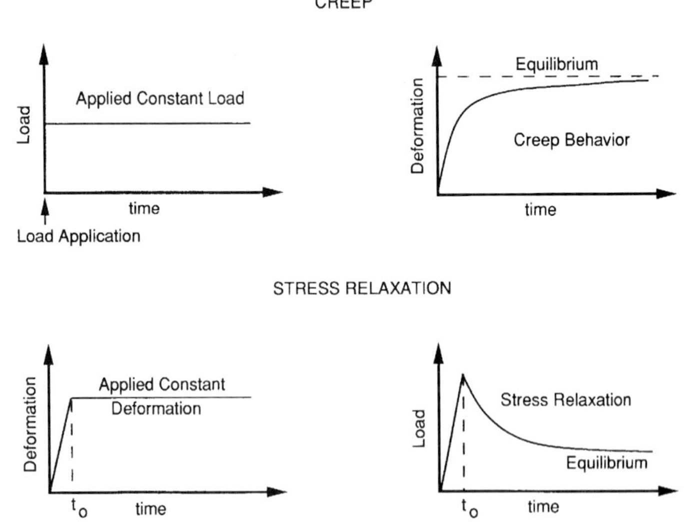

Figure 17
Top, Creep of a viscoelastic material under constant loading. **Bottom,** Stress rise during a ramp-displacement compression of a viscoelastic material and stress relaxation under constant compression. (Reproduced with permission from Mow VC, Ratcliffe A, Poole AR: Cartilage and diarthrodial joints as paradigms for hierarchical structures. *Biomaterials* 1992;13:67–97.)

reached (Fig. 17, *bottom*). In polymeric materials, these viscoelastic behaviors arise from the frictional force generated by the sliding motion of long-chain molecules within the material, resulting in internal energy dissipation. In articular cartilage, however, there are two mechanisms responsible for viscoelasticity: a flow-independent and a flow-dependent mechanism. The flow-independent viscoelastic behavior of the collagen-proteoglycan matrix of cartilage derives from intermolecular friction, and this is measured with a pure shear experiment in which no fluid flow occurs within the tissue. The flow-dependent mechanism depends on interstitial fluid flow and pressurization, as discussed above. It is now known that the drag resulting from interstitial fluid flow is the main contributor to the compressive viscoelastic behavior of cartilage (Fig. 18).

Interstitial fluid pressure is generated in cartilage during loading (compression), and it combines with matrix compression in supporting the applied load. However, under constant load, as creep continues, the load support is gradually transferred from the fluid phase (as the fluid pressure dissipates) to the solid phase. Typically, for normal cartilage, this equilibration process takes 2.78 to 5.56 hours to achieve. At equilibrium the fluid pressure vanishes, and load support is provided entirely by the compressed collagen-proteoglycan solid matrix. It has been experimentally determined that this equilibrium compressive strain is related linearly to the applied compressive stress. The proportionality constant of this linear relationship defines the equilibrium compressive modulus. Typically, this compressive modulus of the solid matrix of normal articular cartilage ranges from 0.4 to 1.5 MPa. Table 3 provides the Poisson's ratio, compressive aggregate modulus, and permeability coefficients for articular cartilage from the lateral condyle and patellar groove of young normal humans, steers, beagles, greyhounds, cynomolgus monkeys, and New Zealand white rabbits.

Because of the long equilibration time, articular cartilage is almost always dynamically loaded under physiologic conditions, that is, no equilibrium state occurs because the joints are always moving, even during sleep. Thus, fluid pressurization almost always will occur within the tissue. It is likely, then, that in normal articular cartilage, fluid pressurization is the dominant physiologic load-support mechanism in diarthrodial joints. This unique behavior of cartilage occurs only because the solid matrix is very soft and has a very low permeability.

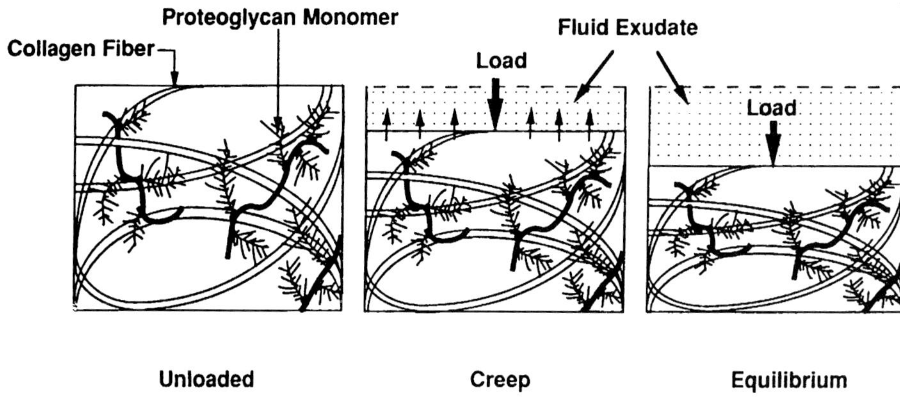

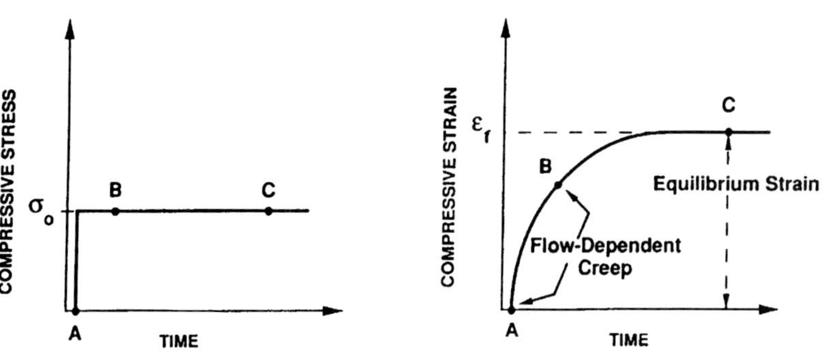

Figure 18
Biphasic creep behavior of a hydrated-soft tissue such as articular cartilage during compression. Rate of creep is governed by the rate at which fluid may be forced out from the tissue, which, in turn, is governed by the permeability and stiffness of the porous-permeable, collagen-proteoglycan solid matrix.

Table 3
Average Poisson's ratio, compressive aggregate modulus, and permeability coefficient of lateral condyle cartilage and patellar groove cartilage

	Human*	Bovine*	Canine*	Monkey*	Rabbit*
Poisson's Ratio (ϑ)					
Lateral Condyle	0.10	0.40	0.30	0.24	0.34
Patellar Groove	0.00	0.25	0.09	0.20	0.21
Compressive Aggregate Modulus (MPa)					
Lateral Condyle	0.70	0.89	0.60	0.78	0.54
Patellar Groove	0.53	0.47	0.55	0.52	0.51
Permeability Coefficient ($10^{-15}m^4/N \bullet s$)					
Lateral Condyle	1.18	0.43	0.77	4.19	1.81
Patellar Groove	2.17	1.42	0.93	4.74	3.84

* Animals are young normal humans; 18 months to 2-year-old steers; mature beagles and greyhounds; mature cynomolgus monkeys; and mature New Zealand white rabbits.

The known values of normal articular cartilage permeability and compressive modulus have been used in calculations to determine that fluid pressure supports, by far, the larger part of the applied load. In fact, the ratio of load supported by the fluid pressure to that supported by the solid matrix stress is greater than 20 to 1 in normal articular cartilage.

Physiologically, the most common finding of early human osteoarthritic cartilage is a gain of water content and a loss of proteoglycan content. It is known from the permeability experiments that these compositional changes would increase tissue permeability. The increase of tissue permeability would diminish the fluid pressurization mechanism of load support in cartilage and, thus, require the collagen-proteoglycan solid matrix to bear more of the load. It can now be appreciated why these changes could be so detrimental for the long-term survival of cartilage in the highly loaded environment of diarthrodial joints.

Flow-Independent Viscoelastic Shear Properties of Articular Cartilage

The random organization of the collagen architecture through the middle and deep zones of the tissue contributes significantly to the shear properties of articular cartilage. Stretching of these randomly dispersed collagen fibrils and shearing of the entrapped proteoglycan molecules provide cartilage with its shear stress-strain response (Figs. 4 and 19). No interstitial fluid flow occurs under pure shear because no pressure gradients or volume changes are developed within the tissue. Thus, the pure shear experiment provides a direct method to determine the flow-independent viscoelastic properties of artic-

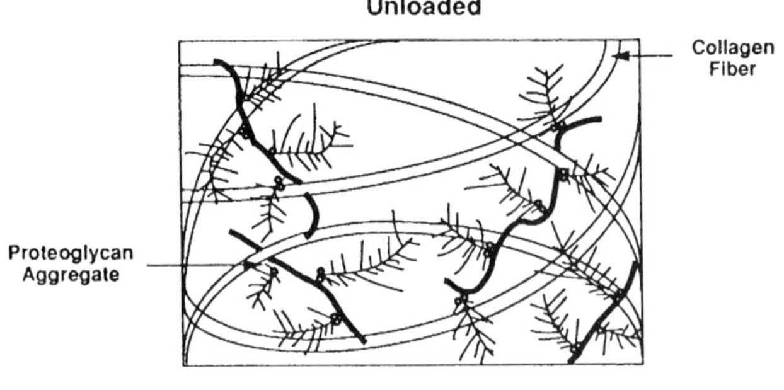

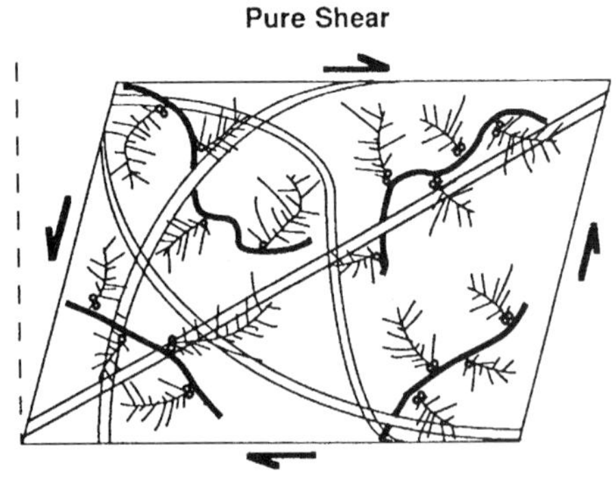

Figure 19
Schematic depiction of how the collagen-proteoglycan solid matrix may act under shear. The randomly dispersed fibers are stretched during shear **(bottom)** to provide the shear rigidity to the tissue. (Reproduced with permission from Buckwalter JA, Mow VC: Cartilage repair in osteoarthritis, in Moskowitz RW, Howell DS, Goldberg VM, et al (eds): *Osteoarthritis: Diagnosis and Medical/Surgical Management,* ed 2. Philadelphia, WB Saunders, 1992, pp 71–107.)

ular cartilage. For normal human and bovine articular cartilage, the equilibrium shear moduli have been determined to range from 0.05 to 0.30 MPa.

To assess the flow-independent viscoelastic properties, a dynamic (sinusoidal) pure shear experiment must be performed. In these experiments, the magnitude of the dynamic shear modulus $|G^*(\varphi)|$ and tan δ are measured. The dynamic shear modulus is a measure of the intrinsic shear stiffness of the solid matrix at any given frequency φ, and tan δ is a measure of the viscoelastic energy dissipation in the tissue during a cycle of shear. A value of $\delta = 0°$ represents a purely elastic material with no energy dissipation, while a value of $\delta = 90°$ represents a purely viscous material that is highly dissipative. The value of $|G^*|$ depends on the frequency of oscillation, and it has been measured to vary from 0.2 to 2.5 MPa with increasing frequency from 0.01 to 20 Hz; the corresponding values of δ range from 20° to 9° in an inverse manner with increasing frequency. The effects of compression on cartilage are to stiffen the tissue in shear and make it less dissipative. Again, this nonlinear effect is important in that the resistance of cartilage to shear stress increases with compression.

How does shear stress arise in cartilage when the articular surface is nearly frictionless? Consider the simple act of compressing a strip of cartilage. The tissue not only would be compressed in the direction of the applied load, but also would expand in the transverse direction; this is Poisson's ratio effect. If one surface of the strip is firmly attached to a rigid surface, such as the deep zone cartilage to the tidemark in situ, then the cartilage cannot expand freely at this interface. To prevent its expansion, a shear stress must be imparted onto the articular cartilage at the interface by the hard, bony substrate. Indeed, it has been shown that by compressing articular cartilage on bone, the shear stress attains a maximum value at the tidemark. Also, it is well known that high compressive loads, such as those that occur during blunt impact, will cause articular cartilage to be sheared off of the bone. The fact that any materials with a Poisson's ratio other than zero will spread in the transverse direction during compression means that tensile stresses and strains will also be developed within the material. For cartilage, these tensile stresses and strains may be sufficiently large to cause collagen fiber and network damage at the articular surface.

The low values of δ (9° to 20°) for articular cartilage as compared with ~70° for solutions of pure concentrated proteoglycan networks indicate that the collagen-proteoglycan solid matrix of articular cartilage is more elastic and less dissipative than the pure concentrated proteoglycan solutions. The collagen-proteoglycan matrix is, however, considerably more viscoelastic and dissipative than is collagen alone, with $\delta \sim 4.0°$ for a highly collagenous tissue such as canine medial collateral ligament. Figure 20 provides a comparison of energy dissipation for collateral ligament, articular cartilage, and proteoglycan solutions. In addition, the dynamic shear modulus $|G^*|$ of pure proteoglycan solutions indicates that the proteoglycan-collagen matrix is approximately 10^5 times stiffer than pure solutions of proteoglycan-proteoglycan networks alone. These differences lead to the conclusion that proteoglycan-proteoglycan networks in solution add little to the observed stiffness and elasticity of articular cartilage in shear. Furthermore, these results indicate that the stiffness and energy dissipation properties of cartilage in shear are provided by the proteoglycan-collagen structure present in the tissue, not by the proteoglycan-proteoglycan network. Thus, it is most likely that the networking capacity of proteoglycans functions to maintain the inflated spatial form of the collagen network in the extracellular matrix, and not to provide any appreciable stiffness in shear (Figs. 9 and 19).

Tensile Properties of Articular Cartilage

A change of volume always occurs when a piece of material is stretched (increase) or compressed (decrease). Thus, in any tensile experiment, both flow-dependent and flow-independent viscoelastic mechanisms contribute to the response of cartilage in tension. If specimens are stretched at extremely slow rates, or if the force response to stretch is obtained at equilibrium, both mechanisms of vis-

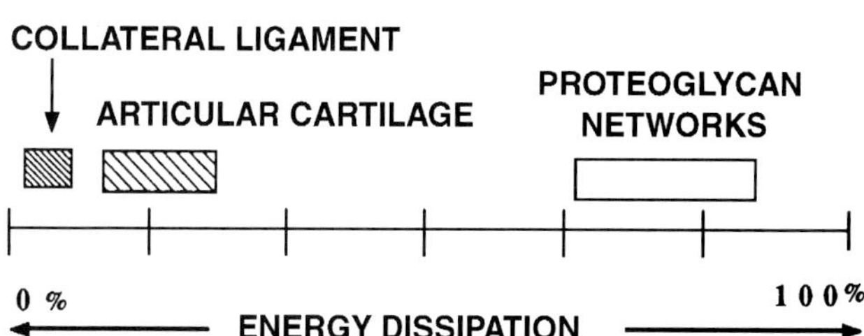

Figure 20
Diagram providing comparison of energy dissipation in a material composed predominantly of collagen (collateral ligament), a material composed of a collagen and proteoglycan mix (articular cartilage), and pure proteoglycans. (Reproduced with permission from Buckwalter JA, Mow VC: Cartilage repair in osteoarthritis, in Moskowitz RW, Howell DS, Goldberg VM, et al (eds): *Osteoarthritis: Diagnosis and Medical/Surgical Management,* ed 2. Philadelphia, WB Saunders, 1992, pp 71–107.)

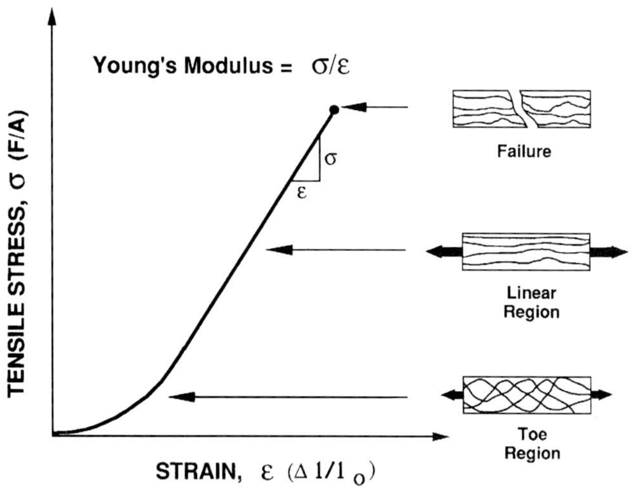

Figure 21
Representation of how the collagen network in a fibrous composite material such as articular cartilage might function during tension. (Reproduced with permission from Buckwalter JA, Mow VC: Cartilage repair in osteoarthritis, in Moskowitz RW, Howell DS, Goldberg VM, et al (eds): *Osteoarthritis: Diagnosis and Medical/Surgical Management,* ed 2. Philadelphia, WB Saunders, 1992, pp 71–107.)

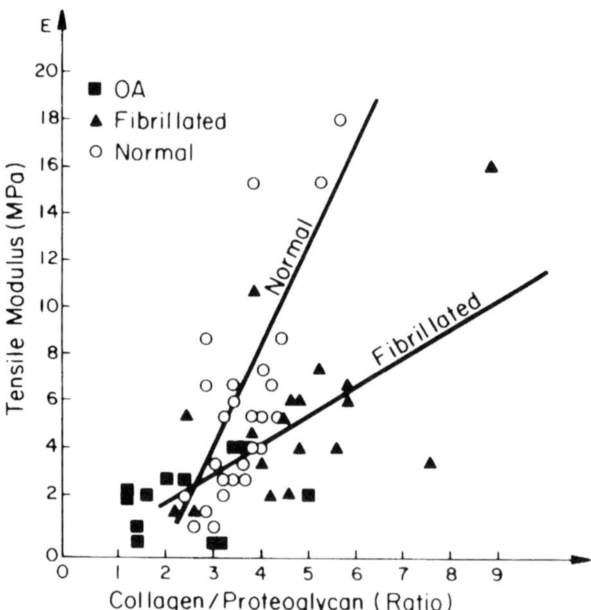

Figure 22
Variation of human knee joint cartilage tensile stiffness for normal, mildly fibrillated, and osteoarthritic (OA) tissue (from a site adjacent to frank OA lesions). (Reproduced with permission from Akizuki S, Mow VC, Muller F, et al: The tensile properties of human knee joint cartilage I: Influence of ionic conditions, weight bearing, and fibrillation on the tensile modulus. *J Orthop Res* 1986;4:379–392.)

coelasticity will be defeated. The intrinsic tensile response of the collagen-proteoglycan solid matrix has been measured in such slow strain-rate or equilibrium experiments. Figure 21 shows a typical tensile stress-strain curve for articular cartilage, with a toe region followed by a linear response. The proportionality constant in the linear portion of the stress-strain curve is called the tensile modulus, and it reflects the stiffness of the collagen network in tension. The tensile modulus of articular cartilage may vary from 5 to 50 MPa, depending on the location, depth, and orientation of the test specimen relative to the split line direction, surface fibrillation, or compositional changes. From numerous studies, it is known that samples from the superficial zone of articular cartilage are always stiffer than middle and deep zone samples because of the high concentration and high degree of orientation of collagen fibrils in this zone. Tensile stiffness decreases as mild fibrillation moves toward end-stage osteoarthritic degenerative changes (Fig. 22). The tensile moduli of normal and mildly fibrillated human articular cartilage correlate well with collagen content and ratio of collagen to proteoglycan present in the tissue. Figure 23 provides a comparison of the tensile, compressive, and shear properties of some important hydrated connective soft tissues.

Physicochemical Forces Responsible for Cartilage Swelling

Swelling is defined as the ability of a material to gain (or to lose) in size or weight when soaked in a solution. This swelling occurs as a result of the chemical or physical nature of the material. For articular cartilage the reason for the swelling often is referred to as physicochemical because it is derived mainly from the charged nature of the proteoglycan component of the tissue. In cartilage, the proteoglycans contain one or two negative charge group(s) on each dimeric hexosamine (for example, SO_3^- and COO^-; Fig. 8), and these groups are spaced 10 to 15 Å apart. For normal articular cartilage, the total fixed charge density ranges from 0.1 to 0.5 mEq/ml at physiologic pH; for osteoarthritic cartilage, it drops dramatically as a result of proteoglycan loss from the tissue. Because each of these negative charges requires an opposite (positive) charge to maintain electroneutrality, the total ion concentration inside the tissue must be greater than the ion concentration in the external bathing solution. The maximum difference occurs when the tissue is equilibrated in a very dilute external electrolyte solution. This imbalance of ion concentrations gives rise to an internal swelling pressure greater than the pressure in the external bath. The extent of swelling is limited by the stress generated in the solid matrix to resist its expansion.

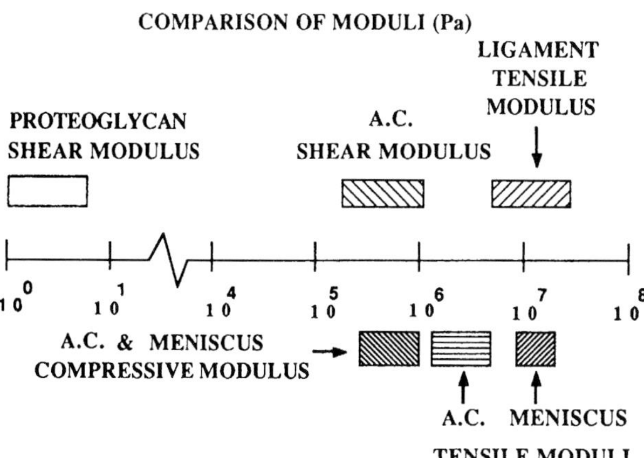

Figure 23
Comparison of tensile, compressive and shear properties for common connective tissues. (Reproduced with permission from Buckwalter JA, Mow VC: Cartilage repair in osteoarthritis, in Moskowitz RW, Howell DS, Goldberg VM, et al (eds): *Osteoarthritis: Diagnosis and Medical/Surgical Management*, ed 2. Philadelphia, WB Saunders, 1992, pp 71–107.)

The swelling pressure caused by the counterions in association with the fixed charge density is known as the Donnan osmotic pressure, and it usually is denoted by the symbol π. Because the charge groups fixed on the collagen-proteoglycan solid matrix are very close to each other, large charge-to-charge repulsive forces generate a chemical expansion stress T_c, which also causes swelling. Thus, at equilibrium, the total swelling pressure P_s in cartilage is given by $P_s = \pi + T_c$. This equation provides a convenient way to visualize the underlying chemical or physical forces contributing to the total swelling pressure P_s.

Both forces can be modulated by changing the external electrolyte (for example, NaCl) concentration. The ideal osmotic pressure law is given by $\pi = RT\Delta c$, where R is the universal gas constant, T is the absolute temperature, and Δc is the difference of ion concentrations between the interstitium and the external bathing solution. This difference of ion concentrations is determined by the fixed charge density c^F of proteoglycans within the interstitium, and the electrolyte concentration c* in the external bathing solution. First, according to the Donnan equilibrium ion distribution law, for a tissue equilibrated in a monovalent salt (NaCl) solution under ideal conditions, the concentration c of Na^+ in the interstitium is given by the simple quadratic equation $c(c + c^F) = (c^*)^2$. The difference Δc between the total ion concentration of NaCl in the interstitium and the external solution is $\Delta c = (2c + c^F) - 2c^*$, and it may be calculated from the Donnan equilibrium ion distribution law. The Donnan osmotic pressure p may be determined from the idealized law for osmotic pressure. From this analysis, a bit of reflection will show that as c* becomes large, Δc will vanish and π will become zero. In other words, when cartilage is bathed in a high concentration salt solution (hypertonic), the Donnan osmotic pressure becomes negligible, causing the tissue to shrink and lose water. Conversely, when cartilage is bathed in a low concentration salt solution (hypotonic), Δc will become large, causing the tissue to swell and gain water.

Recently, the chemical-expansion stress T_c (for a tissue in equilibrium with an external solution with NaCl concentration c*) has been described by an exponentially decaying function of c* given by $T_c = a_o c^F \exp(-\kappa c^*)$, where a_o and κ are specific tissue coefficients defining this property of the porous-permeable solid matrix. This law states that the chemical-expansion stress increases linearly with increasing proteoglycan concentration within the interstitium in the equilibrated state c^F and decreases exponentially with increasing counterion concentration c* in the external bathing solution.

For normal cartilage equilibrated in physiologic saline (0.15M NaCl), the total swelling pressure P_s has been calculated to range from 0.1 to 0.25 MPa, and the Donnan osmotic pressure component π is estimated to contribute up to 50% of the total swelling pressure P_s. The contribution of the swelling pressure toward load support, when normal cartilage is at a compressed equilibrium state, depends on the applied load. For a lightly loaded tissue, the swelling pressure may contribute significantly to the load support. But for highly loaded tissues, and certainly for dynamically loaded tissues in which interstitial fluid pressurization dominates, the contribution of this swelling pressure to load support is difficult to assess.

Equilibrium Swelling Behavior of Articular Cartilage

The physicochemical forces along a proteoglycan would cause the molecule to assume a stiff, fully-extended configuration in an infinitely dilute solution. Under these circumstances, the free-solution volume of the proteoglycan is limited only because the stiffness of the molecule itself resists the swelling forces. In cartilage, however, the proteoglycans are trapped and entangled within the interfibrillar space, and compacted to within a volume that is one fifth of the free-solution volume. As a result of interactions between collagen fibrils, such as cross-linking, and interactions between collagen, proteoglycans, and other molecules, the solid matrix of articular cartilage is strong and cohesive. Thus, in the tissue, the swelling pressure P_s is resisted by the stresses developed in the solid matrix where both collagen and proteoglycan share the load. It is likely that, in situ, collagen provides most of the resistance to the swelling pressure. This heuristic description is suggested in the schematic depiction of the collagen-proteoglycan composite matrix for cartilage (Fig. 9).

Recently, it has been shown that at free-swelling equilibrium, the stress tensor σ^s acting in the solid matrix has three equal normal stress components given by $\sigma^s = P_s$. For an elastic solid matrix, the dilatation $\Delta V/V_0$ (volumetric change per unit volume) produced by the swelling pressure is given by $P_s = B(\Delta V/V_0)$, where B is the elastic bulk modulus of the solid matrix, which may be measured by material testing methods described above and in the chapter on biomechanics. This simple equation may be used to calculate $\Delta V/V_0$ at every point within the tissue as well as for the tissue as a whole. Determination of $\Delta V/V_0$ results in some important conclusions: (1) A swelling pressure will exist within the articular cartilage, which is the sum of a Donnan osmotic pressure π and a chemical-expansion stress T_c; $P_s = \pi + T_c$. This swelling pressure will cause the porous-permeable, collagen-proteoglycan solid matrix to expand and imbibe water. (2) The elastic stiffness, more specifically the bulk modulus B of the solid matrix resists the swelling pressure. If the collagen network is damaged in any manner, swelling, that is, gain in volume or water, will occur. (3) Loss of proteoglycans resulting in a decrease of P_s will not necessarily mean a loss of water because more space is available within the interstitium for water, and the loss of proteoglycans will alter the elastic bulk modulus of the porous-permeable solid matrix to allow greater expansion. However, an increase of tissue hydration in early osteoarthritic cartilage is a universal experimental finding. Clearly, then, from the dilatation law $\Delta V/V_0 = P_s/B$, the bulk modulus B of the solid matrix must be decreasing faster than the swelling pressure P_s during the early stages of osteoarthritis. In other words, during early osteoarthritic cartilage changes, the loss of swelling pressure is less severe than the compromise in mechanical properties of the solid matrix. Each molecular, compositional, and ultrastructural change of collagen, proteoglycan, and other quantitatively minor glycoproteins, which compose and organize the solid matrix, has a specific influence on solid matrix properties. Thus, in recent decades, the biochemistry and molecular structure of major components of normal and diseased articular cartilages have been studied intensely. Concomitantly, changes of cartilage material properties during early osteoarthritis in animal models of the disease and in human cartilage specimens obtained at necropsy also have been the object of much investigation. Table 4 provides the mechanoelectrochemical swelling properties of articular cartilage.

Table 4
Summary of mechanoelectrochemical swelling properties of articular cartilage

c^F(mEq/ml)	P_s(MPa)	a_o(MPa/(mEq/ml))	$\kappa(M^{-1})$
0.01–0.50	0–0.25	2.5 (0–10)*	7.5 (0–10)*

*The range of values shown are estimates.

Physiology of Normal and Diseased Articular Cartilage

The Nutrition of Articular Cartilage

The source of nutritive materials for articular cartilage is somewhat of an enigma. Because the tissue is avascular in adult life, most investigators believe that nutrients diffuse through the matrix either from the surrounding synovial fluid or from the underlying bone. Experimental evidence suggests that in immature animals a portion of the nutrient that enters articular cartilage does so by diffusion from the permeable underlying bony substrate. In the adult, however, this type of diffusion disappears or becomes severely limited with the appearance of the tidemark and a heavy deposition of apatite in the calcified zone, leaving the synovial fluid as the most likely source of nutrition. The extremely small calculated pore size (estimated to be 50 Å) of the superficial zone should permit only low molecular weight components of the fluid (less than 20 kd) to diffuse into the tissue. Measured diffusion times range from ten seconds to one hour depending on the molecular weight, structure, size, and charge of the molecules diffusing through the tissue. However, molecules from the synovial fluid (for example, interleukin-1 and the prostaglandins) and some growth factors appear to move unrestricted through the tissue. Further, fragments of proteoglycans and other matrix components, generated by proteolytic activity in normal turnover and in degeneration, are able to leave the tissue rapidly. Normal joints contain very small amounts of synovial fluid. For example, even in a large joint such as the normal knee, there is less than 4 ml of synovial fluid, which forms a coating over the articular surfaces of the joint just 10 to 20 mm thick. Yet, sufficient nutrients and oxygen from the metabolically active synovium reach the chondrocytes, presumably by diffusion through the cartilage matrix via the synovial fluid.

Mechanosignal Transduction in Articular Cartilage

Articular cartilage is also an aneural tissue. Impulses that normally regulate many of the body processes cannot provide information to cartilage. Cellular and humoral immune responses also are not likely to occur in cartilage, because both monocytes and immunoglobulins tend to be excluded from the tissue by virtue of their size. Thus, if transport of such messages does occur, it may be considerably slower than in more vascular tissue. In theory at least, chondrocytes receive only limited information regarding the rest of the body state via the standard neural, lymphatic, or humoral pathways. On the other hand, if the cell is, as most believe, pressure or deformation sensitive, it may derive considerable information from alterations in the stresses and strains that act on the membrane as a result of alteration of the physical forces acting on the tissue. A large number of recent studies have resulted in reports on the effects of pressure, stresses, and strains on chondrocyte metabolism in vitro and the effects of joint instability and joint immobilization on cartilage degeneration and chondrocyte metabolism. These reports indicate that articular cartilage remodels quickly following alterations of mechanical stimuli to the tissue in vivo, and can change its metabolic activities in vitro. Thus, acts such as loading, unloading, or movement of the joint appear to serve as a principal stimuli to biochemical alterations in the cartilage and, ultimately, to its biomechanical properties. How the chondrocytes detect their mechanical environment and convert the information received to changes in specific gene expression in the nucleus is unknown, although it is thought that integrins, which are molecules that span the plasma membrane and are connected to the intracellular cytoplasm, are likely to be involved.

Effects of Joint Motion and Loading on Articular Cartilage

Joint loading and motion are required to maintain normal adult articular cartilage composition, structure, and mechanical properties. The type, intensity, and frequency of loadings necessary to maintain normal articular cartilage vary over a broad range. When the intensity or frequency of loading exceeds or falls below these necessary levels, the balance between synthesis and degradation processes will be altered, and changes in the composition and microstructure of cartilage could ensue.

Reduced joint loading, in the form of rigid immobilization or casting, leads to atrophy or degeneration of the cartilage. The effects can be separated into those occurring in contact areas and those occurring in noncontact areas. The use of external fixation to effect continuous and static compression of two opposing cartilage surfaces in the absence of normal joint motion may produce severe degenerative lesions and chondrocyte death in the area of contact. The severity of damage depends on the magnitude and duration of loading. Changes in the noncontact areas resulting from rigid immobilization include fibrillation, decreased proteoglycan content and synthesis, and altered proteoglycan conformation, such as a decrease in the size and amount of aggregate. These changes result, in part, because normal nutritive transport to cartilage from the synovial fluid by means of diffusion and convection has been diminished. With immobilization by casting or strapping, a limited range of joint motion is maintained in the absence of normal weightbearing forces. Animal studies have indicated that immobilizing the joint for as little as four weeks will produce many of the atrophic changes of rigid immobilization, such as increased water content, reduced proteoglycan content, and synthesis and macromolecular conformation of proteoglycan, although no collagen changes occur during these early periods. However, the severity of the changes caused by mild immobilization is significantly reduced. In addition, the mechanical properties of articular cartilage will be compromised with immobilization. Fluid flux and deformation in response to compression will increase, although these changes are minimal in areas where some level of joint contact is maintained. Normal tensile properties are maintained, reflecting the biochemical finding that proteoglycan rather than collagen is affected primarily by reduced joint motion and loading. All of these biochemical and biomechanical changes are, at least in part, reversible on remobilization of the joint after casting, although the extent of this recovery decreases with increasing periods of joint immobilization.

Increased joint loading, either through excessive use, increased magnitudes of loading, or impact, will also affect articular cartilage. Catabolic effects can be induced by a single-impact or repetitive trauma, and may serve as the initiating factor for progressive degenerative changes. Moderate running exercise increases the proteoglycan content and compressive stiffness, decreases the rate of fluid flux during loading, and may also increase the thickness of articular cartilage. In contrast, in canine studies, strenuous exercise produces fibrillation of the matrix and decreased proteoglycan content and aggregate size. However, no significant mechanical property changes are observed in dogs in response to periods of strenuous exercise up to 30 weeks.

Disruption of the intra-articular structures, such as menisci or ligaments, will alter the forces acting on the articular surface in both the magnitude and areas of loading. The resulting joint instability is associated with profound and progressive changes in the biochemical composition and mechanical properties of articular cartilage. In experimental animal models, responses to transection of the anterior cruciate ligament or meniscectomy have included fibrillation of the cartilage surface, increased hydration, changes in the proteoglycan content, reduced number and size of proteoglycan aggregates, joint capsule thickening, and osteophyte formation. It seems likely that some of these changes result from the activities of the chondrocytes, because their rates of synthesis of matrix components, breakdown of matrix components, and secretion of proteolytic enzymes are all increased. Changes in the mechanical properties also have been observed together with these histologic and biochemical composition changes. Significant and progressive decreases in the tensile and shear modulus have been observed in response to transection of the anterior cruciate ligament. Furthermore, decreases in the compressive modulus and increases in the hydraulic permeability occur in response to joint instability, which will produce increased matrix deformation, elevated fluid flux under physiologic loading, and diminution of the fluid pressurization effect of load carriage. There is evidence of increased chondrocyte mitotic and anabolic activity in joint instability, although these elevated chondrocyte responses are insufficient to repair early damage and to inhibit progression of cartilage degeneration. Rather, it appears that the increased anabolism is outpaced by an elevated catabolism, which is activated in models of altered joint loading.

The specific mechanisms by which joint loading influences chondrocyte function remain unknown, although various mechanical, physicochemical, and electrical transduction mechanisms have been proposed. Matrix deformation will produce fluid and ion flow, which may facilitate chondrocyte nutrition and chemical transduction signals, and chondrocyte deformation, which may directly control the metabolic activity. Deformation and fluid flow will lead to changes in the local charge density within the matrix, resulting in an electric potential that may serve as an electric transduction mechanism. In vitro studies have shown that loading of the cartilage matrix can cause all of these mechanical, electric, and physicochemical events, but thus far it has not been shown clearly which signals are most important in stimulating the anabolic and catabolic activity of the chondrocytes.

The Problems of Articular Cartilage Repair

Repair of cartilage refers to the replacement of damaged or lost cells and matrix with new cells and matrix. The repaired tissue often restores neither the original structure nor function of articular cartilage. For other tissues, the most common form of repair tissue, referred to as scar tissue, consists of densely packed collagen fibrils and scattered fibroblasts. Scar tissue can be remodeled over a prolonged period of time with cells and matrix macromolecules being replaced and reorganized, and with the composition of the extracellular matrix modified. In most tissues, type I collagen is the predominate matrix macromolecule of the mature scar. In many tissues, including skin, the dense fibrous scar tissue restores the structural integrity of the tissue and may restore normal function. Occasionally, repair fails, and the injured or lost tissue is not replaced and the function is not restored.

Under most circumstances, musculoskeletal tissues other than cartilage repair the lost or injured tissue, and the defect is filled with new cells and an extracellular matrix that closely resemble the original tissue. This repair tissue can restore normal or near normal function. Repair of significant defects in articular cartilage is rarely, if ever, this successful. Factors that limit the response of cartilage to injury include a lack of blood vessels and a lack of cells in the tissue that can repair defects of any significant size. Lack of blood vessels prevents new cells from entering the site of tissue injury, and lack of a population of undifferentiated mesenchymal cells prevents cartilage from initiating a healing response in the same way as the other tissues. When cartilage injury or disease penetrates the blood vessels in the subchondral region, cells that can repair tissue defects enter the injury site. These cells, however, do not consistently repair the injury with a tissue that has the unique composition, structure, and material properties of normal articular cartilage matrix. Cartilage alone among the primary musculoskeletal tissues (bone, dense fibrous tissue, and articular cartilage) has an extracellular matrix macromolecular framework consisting primarily of type II fibrillar collagen, large elaborate cartilage proteoglycans, and possible cartilage-specific noncollagenous proteins. Following most injuries, the cells responsible for repair do not produce these cartilage macromolecules in amounts sufficient to create a cohesive and strong extracellular matrix, and they fail to organize the molecules to create a matrix structure like that of articular cartilage.

Lack of Blood Supply

Normally, repair of significant musculoskeletal tissue defects begins with inflammation and requires a population of cells that migrate into the injury site, proliferate, and synthesize a new matrix. Because adult cartilage lacks blood vessels, disruption of the tissue does not cause the important processes derived from hemorrhage, fibrin clot formation, or movement of inflammatory cells to the site of tissue damage. Injured cells and platelets release mediators that can promote the vascular response to injury and stimulate cell migration and proliferation. The inflammatory cells may help remove necrotic tissue and, as they do so, release mediators that stimulate migration of mesenchymal cells capable of invading a fibrin clot, proliferating, differentiating into a wide range of connective tissue cells, and synthesizing a new matrix. The occurrence of these events during inflammation is critical for initiation of effective tissue repair.

Lack of Undifferentiated Cells

In addition to lacking blood vessels, cartilage lacks undifferentiated cells within the tissue that can migrate, proliferate, and participate in the repair response. The only cell type found in articular cartilage, the highly differentiated chondrocyte, has limited capacity for proliferation or migration because chondrocytes are encased within the tissue (Fig. 1). During cartilage growth, chondrocytes proliferate rapidly but the rate of cell division declines with increasing age until, in normal mature articular cartilage, few if any chondrocytes show signs of mitotic activity. Following cartilage injury or in osteoarthritis some chondrocytes proliferate, but this response is very limited, and there is no evidence that the cells migrate through the matrix to the site of tissue damage or deterioration.

Chondrocytes in the tissue also may have limited capacity for increasing matrix synthesis. In normal mature cartilage, chondrocytes synthesize sufficient matrix macromolecules to maintain the matrix, and they can increase their rate of matrix synthesis in response to injury or osteoarthritic changes. However, chondrocytes do not synthesize sufficient matrix to repair significant tissue defects, and the matrix macromolecules they do synthesize change with increasing age. The size of cartilage aggrecan and aggregates declines with increasing fetal age, and, with skeletal maturity, the size of the cartilage proteoglycans further decreases and the molecules become more variable in size. These age-related changes in matrix proteoglycans may adversely affect the cartilage, and it is not known if mature chondrocytes can be stimulated to produce the larger, more uniform proteoglycans. Another factor that may limit the ability of mature cartilage to repair tissue defects is that the number of chondrocytes declines during aging, thus reducing the capacity of the tissue to repair itself.

Response of Articular Cartilage to Superficial Lacerations

Experimental lacerations of articular cartilage perpendicular to the cartilage surface may resemble the earliest visible lesions of osteoarthritis (OA). The earliest visible articular cartilage degeneration begins with fraying of the superficial zone. With time, vertical clefts and fissures appear and become progressively deeper, giving the affected tissue an irregular fibrillated appearance. In the most superficial regions, proteoglycan is lost from the matrix. Perhaps in response to the loss of matrix proteoglycan, chondrocytes proliferate, forming clusters or clones, and begin to synthesize increased amounts of matrix macromolecules. However, the chondrocytes do not migrate into the areas of the defects nor does the matrix they synthesize fill the defects. As the deterioration of the matrix progresses, fragments of cartilage may tear loose and be released into the joint, leaving deeper regions exposed. Eventually, more tissue is lost, exposing subchondral bone and resulting in eburnation. The inability of the chondrocytes to repair the damaged tissue or to prevent further damage allows the disintegration of the articular surface to progress until only a hard, eburnated bone remains.

Superficial laceration injuries to articular cartilage that do not cross the tidemark generally do not heal. The earliest laceration injury experiments date back to Hunter in the mid 18th century. Despite recent suggestions to the contrary, performing intracartilaginous lacerative surgery through the arthroscope does not stimulate cartilage healing any more than surgery done in an open procedure; and using a shaver, laser, or cautery doesn't change the results for all the hundreds of studies described for similar injuries created with a knife. If the injury to mature cartilage is superficial, it will not heal. Conversely, lacerations of mature cartilage perpendicular to the surface only kill chondrocytes at the site of the injury, and the created matrix defects remain without progression. Thus, these lesions could remain at the joint surface unaltered, presumably for the life of the joint (Fig. 24).

Why do superficial lacerations behave this way? First, these lesions do not cause hemorrhage or initiate an inflammatory response. Also, fibrin clots rarely form on exposed surfaces of normal cartilage. Platelets do not bind to the damaged cartilage and a fibrin clot does not appear; nor do inflammatory cells, invading capillaries, or undifferentiated mesenchymal cells. Chondrocytes near the injury may proliferate and form clusters or clones and synthesize new matrix, but the chondrocytes do not migrate into the lesion, the new matrix they produce remains in the immediate region of the chondrocytes, and their proliferative and synthetic activity fails to provide new tissue to repair the damage. This repair phase is initially brisk. It is, however, limited in scope and duration, disappearing within a matter of weeks.

Superficial lacerations made tangential or parallel to the articular surface follow a similar course.

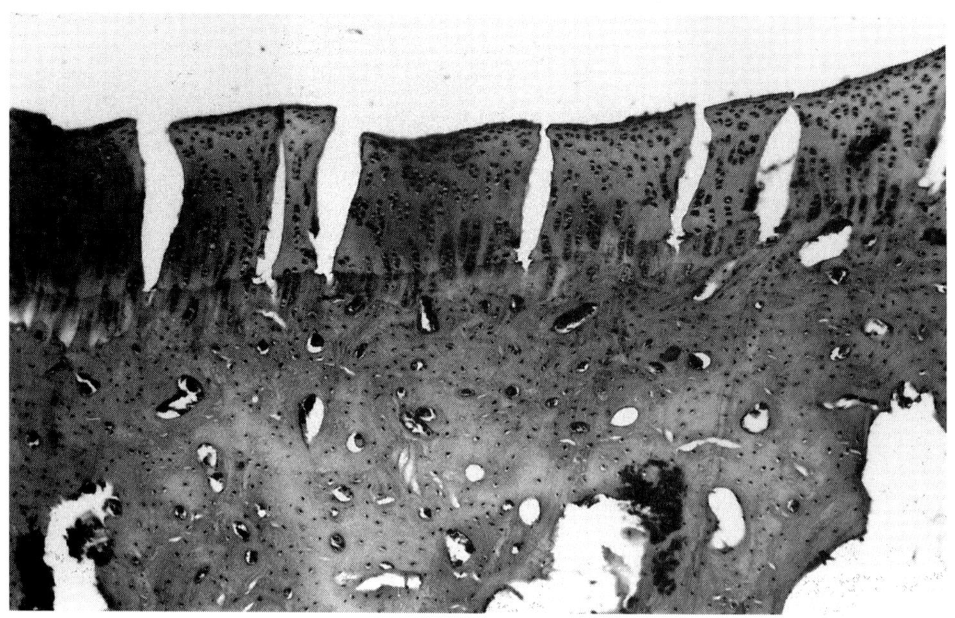

Figure 24
Light micrograph showing multiple laceration defects in rabbit articular cartilage six months after injury. These defects did not penetrate the subchondral bone. The chondrocytes have not migrated into the defects or formed a new matrix. (Reproduced with permission from Buckwalter JA, Mow VC: Cartilage repair in osteoarthritis, in Moskowitz RW, Howell DS, Goldberg VM, et al (eds): *Osteoarthritis: Diagnosis and Medical/Surgical Management,* ed 2. Philadelphia, WB Saunders, 1992, pp 71–107.)

Some cells directly adjacent to the lacerations die whereas others show evidence of proliferation and increased matrix synthesis. A thin layer of new matrix may form over the surface, but there is no evidence of significant repair, although the remaining tissue does not degenerate.

Results from experimental studies of repair of injuries limited to cartilage clearly demonstrate the inability of chondrocytes to repair cartilage defects. However, they also show that limited experimental injuries to normal articular surfaces in normal synovial joints generally do not progress to full-thickness loss of cartilage. Thus, it appears that the existence of the superficial cartilage lesions alone will not cause OA in otherwise normal joints and that the progression of superficial osteoarthritic lesions results either from an abnormality of the cartilage in the osteoarthritic joint or from other factors associated with the disease.

Mechanical Injury to Articular Cartilage and Subchondral Bone

The repair of cartilage defects that penetrate the subchondral bone (an osteochondral defect) may depend to some extent on the severity of injury as measured by the volume of tissue or surface area injured, and on the location of the injury in the joint. Experimental studies indicate that repair of larger osteochondral defects generally is less predictable and less complete than repair of smaller defects.

Another factor that may influence osteochondral repair is the age of the individual. Although possible age-related differences in healing of synovial joint injuries have not been investigated thoroughly, it is known that fractures heal more rapidly in children, and chondrocytes from skeletally immature animals proliferate and synthesize larger cartilage proteoglycans than those from mature animals. Thus, it is possible that osteochondral injuries and perhaps chondral injuries in very young people have the potential to heal more effectively than similar injuries in skeletally mature or elderly individuals. It is known, though not very well publicized, that immature cartilage does have a blood supply, albeit very limited.

Mechanical injury that disrupts bone as well as articular cartilage causes hemorrhage, fibrin clot formation, and inflammation. Soon after creation of the defect, a fibrin clot fills the injury site and inflammatory cells migrate into the clot. In addition to these visible differences between injuries limited to cartilage and injuries that penetrate subchondral bone, there is another important difference. Injury to bone and the subsequent clot formation release growth factors, proteins that influence multiple cell functions including migration, proliferation, differentiation, and matrix synthesis. Bone matrix contains a number of growth factors, and platelets release at least two important growth factors, PDGF and TGF-β. At present, the role of growth factors in cartilage repair has not been defined clearly. It is likely that the growth factors stimulate migration of undifferentiated mesenchymal cells or fibroblast-like cells into the clot and that the local concentrations and types of growth factors in the tissue defect influence the proliferative and synthetic activity of these cells. Within as little as two weeks after osteochondral injury, some of these mesenchymal cells have assumed the rounded form of chondrocytes and have begun to produce a matrix that contains type II collagen and a relatively high concentration of proteoglycans. Six to eight weeks after injury, the tissue within the chondral portion of the defect contains a relatively high proportion of chondrocyte-like cells and a matrix consisting of type II collagen, proteoglycans, and some type I collagen. Simultaneously, cells within the bone portion of the defect form immature bone, fibrous tissue, and cartilage with a hyaline matrix. The bone formation restores the original level of subchondral bone but rarely, if ever, progresses into the chondral portion of the defect. In general, by six months after injury the subchondral bone defect has been repaired with a tissue that consists primarily of bone, but also contains some regions of fibrous tissue and hyaline cartilage. In contrast, the chondral defect rarely is repaired completely, and although it contains a higher proportion of hyaline-appearing cartilage than the bony portion of the defect, it also contains substantial amounts of fibrous tissue. In many instances the composition and structure of the chondral repair tissue are intermediate between those of hyaline cartilage and fibrocartilage.

In most injuries the chondral repair tissue begins to show evidence of fibrillation, loss of cells with the appearance of chondrocytes, and loss of the hyaline-appearing matrix in less than one year. The remaining cells usually have the appearance of fibroblasts, and the surrounding matrix consists of densely packed collagen fibrils. However, the fate of cartilage repair tissue is not always progressive deterioration. Occasionally, the repair tissue persists and appears to function satisfactorily as an articular surface for a prolonged period of time. It may even remodel until it more closely resembles normal articular cartilage. The reasons why some repair tissue persists for a prolonged period of time while most repair tissue deteriorates remain unknown. Because of this, many orthopaedic surgeons continue to drill joint surfaces into the bleeding bone in their attempt to restore a hyaline articular surface.

The striking difference in the differentiation of the repair tissue in the chondral and bony parts of the same defect suggests that the different environments in the two regions of the defect cause the same type of repair cells to produce different types of tissue. It is not clear whether the differences in the environment in the two regions of the same defect are mechanical, biologic, electric, or related to unknown factors. However, the differentiation of the repair tissue in the chondral defect suggests that there is potential for directing the cartilage repair response toward restoration of an articular surface.

Figure 25, *top left,* shows a light micrograph of a well-formed repair tissue filling an osteochondral defect in a rabbit knee eight weeks after surgery. No graft material has been used in this defect to promote repair. The repair tissue stained well with Safranin O, indicating that a significant component of the extracellular matrix is proteoglycan, although the cellular organization is quite different from those of normal cartilage (Fig. 1). The subchondral bone seems to have been formed and closed. Figure 25, *top right,* is a higher magnification of the same healed defect, showing a rough articulating surface and a lack of Safranin O staining near the surface. Figure 25, *bottom left,* a photomicrograph of repair tissue six months after surgery. Note the well-formed tidemark in this repair tissue. However, in this section, Safranin O staining is streaked and the extracellular matrix now appears fibrillar. Typical surface defects have begun to appear. Figure 25, *bottom right,* is a photomicrograph at a higher magnification, showing fragmentation of rabbit cartilage repair one year after the injury. Clinically, it is known that, for the majority of cases, repair tissue in large osteochondral defects goes on to degeneration.

Material Properties of Cartilage Repair Tissue

The material properties of fibrocartilaginous repair tissue have not been extensively studied, but clinical experience suggests that in most patients the long-term performance of this tissue is inferior to that of normal articular cartilage. Studies have been performed on rabbits in which the compressive viscoelastic properties of metatarsal phalangeal joint cartilage were compared with those of repair tissues obtained from arthroplasties. The arthroplasty repair tissue always deformed more easily than normal cartilage, and this result correlated with the lower proteoglycan concentration of the repair tissues. In several studies on larger animals (pigs), the fibrocartilage repair tissue in osteochondral defects did not possess the same biomechanical properties as normal cartilage, and this repair tissue swelled excessively when bathed in physiologic Ringer's solution. A recent report of a detailed study indicates that osteochondral healing at a high weight-bearing area of a primate knee joint does not produce a repair tissue with material properties similar to those of normal articular cartilage. More specifically, repair tissues have a solid matrix with lower elastic modulus and higher permeability than those of normal tissues. Both of these qualities act to negate the fluid-pressure load-carrying capacity of the tissue, which was discussed earlier in this chapter. Another important finding from this study is that passive motion treatment of the injured joint did not enhance the quality of the healing tissue.

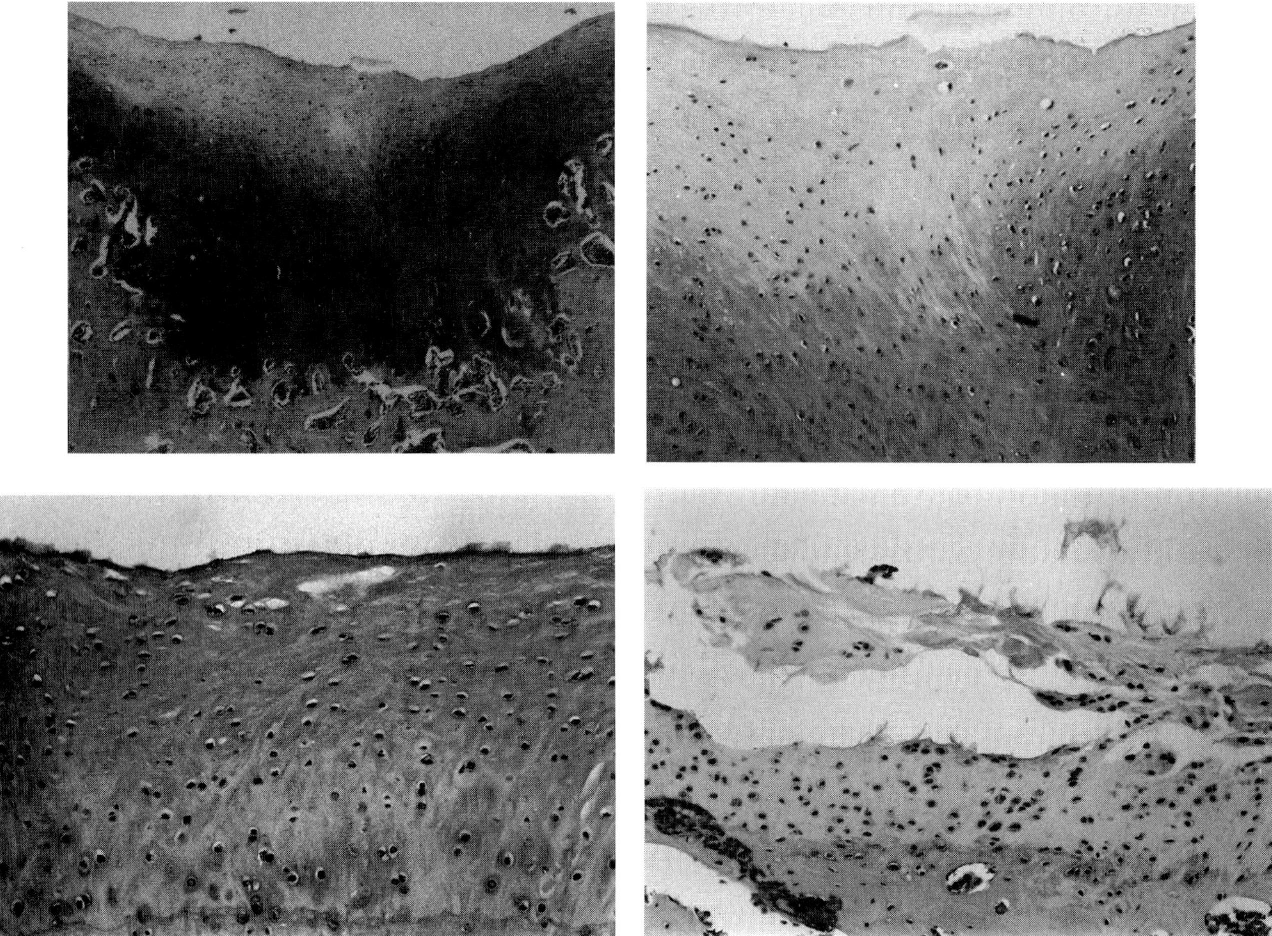

Figure 25
Top left, Light micrograph of a well-formed repair tissue filling an osteochondral defect in a mature rabbit, eight weeks after surgery. The dark staining by Safranin O indicates the presence of glycosaminoglycans. **Top right,** Mild fibrillation of the surface is seen at higher magnification. **Bottom left,** A well-formed defect after six months, with irregular Safranin O staining in the interterritorial matrix. **Bottom right,** Fragmentation of rabbit repair tissue one year after surgery. (Reproduced with permission from Buckwalter JA, Mow VC: Cartilage repair in osteoarthritis, in Moskowitz RW, Howell DS, Goldberg VM, et al (eds): *Osteoarthritis: Diagnosis and Medical/Surgical Management,* ed 2. Philadelphia, WB Saunders, 1992, pp 71–107.)

The differences in material properties between repair cartilage and normal cartilage may help explain the frequent deterioration of repair cartilage over time. Presumably, these differences can be explained by examination of the repair cartilage matrix, composition, and organization. In normal cartilage, the collagen meshwork gives the tissue its form and tensile strength and restrains the swelling of proteoglycans. The increased swelling of repair cartilage may reflect a lack of organization of the collagen fibrillar network. Inspection of repair cartilage shows that the orientation of the collagen fibrils does not follow the pattern seen in normal articular cartilage. Specifically, in most regions of repair cartilage the interterritorial matrix collagen fibrils appear to have a random orientation relative to the articular surface, rather than having different orientations in the superficial, middle, and deep zones. Another possible explanation of the increased swelling of repair cartilage is that the repair tissue may fail to establish the normal relationships between proteoglycans and the collagen network. This might occur because of formation of a different type of collagen, a lack of organization of the collagen network, insufficient concentrations of necessary adhesive molecules, or the presence of molecules that interfere with assembly of a normal articular cartilage matrix. Either a lack of organization of the collagen network or a failure to establish the normal relationships between the collagen and proteoglycans might make the repair tissue less durable. In addition, the inferior material properties of repair cartilage, including decreased stiffness, will subject the tissue to increased strain fields during joint use, thereby causing progressive structural damage.

Response of Articular Cartilage to Blunt Impact

Mammalian articular cartilages, by their very nature and in response to functional demands, can accommodate single or multiple moderate and, occasionally, high impact loads. A number of studies have addressed the effects of either a single excessive high-impact force causing injury to the cartilage without a break in the surface, or repetitive below-trauma-threshold loads causing an accumulation of damage to the cartilage by a repeated application of the load. From these studies, it is evident that cartilage can be damaged by either loading process, and that the damage caused may be significant. Chondrocyte death, matrix damage, fissuring of the surface, injury to the underlying bone, and thickening of the tidemark region can occur. At a certain threshold of impact loading, the cartilage may be sheared off of the subchondral bone before massive bony damage occurs. This phenomenon has been reported, and is widely regarded as the cause of basal layer degeneration of articular cartilage. These basal layer alterations have led to observed remodeling of the deep zone cartilage.

Perhaps the most provocative aspect of these studies is the suggestion that impact, especially in repetitive multiple injuries, leads to thickening or progressing of the tidemark, increasing the thickness of the calcified zone, and, ultimately, to an advance and even reduplication of the tidemark at the expense of articular cartilage thickness. These changes also may stiffen the cartilage-bone junction. Alterations in these parameters (thinning of cartilage and stiffening of the subchondral bone) have been hypothesized to lead to changes in the stresses and strains acting within the cartilage during normal function and, with time, to lead to osteoarthritic changes. According to this hypothesis, these changes in the calcified and subchondral tissues on which the articular cartilage rests are critical and necessary for the progression of articular cartilage damage observed in osteoarthritis.

Osteoarthritis

Definition and Pathology

Osteoarthritis is the most prevalent clinical entity within the domain of the orthopaedist. The clinical picture is well-documented, is easily recognized on the basis of physical examination and radiographic imaging, and, if necessary, can be confirmed by arthroscopy. Despite the familiarity of clinicians with this common disease, the name itself is a source of controversy. Although the term osteoarthrosis describes an involvement of bone and cartilage from initially mechanical causes with associated inflammation, most orthopaedists and rheumatologists use the term osteoarthritis to describe an inflammatory process involving bone and cartilage. Both terms are preferable to the less accurate older term "degenerative joint disease." Often, to avoid controversy, the disease is termed OA. Biochemically and metabolically there is no evidence for degeneration in the early phases of the disease. The process, although characterized by articular cartilage damage, is highly proliferative. The term hypertrophic arthritis, introduced to distinguish OA from atrophic arthritis, an old term for rheumatoid arthritis, is archaic. In this chapter, osteoarthritis or its abbreviation, OA, will be used.

Although articular cartilage is a hardy tissue, able to carry out its tasks of strenuous load bearing for a lifetime, it may become mechanically damaged and thus less functional. Most physicians are aware that joints can fail from either mechanical or biochemical causes. OA commonly is associated with aging, although for many older individuals, aging cartilage remains perfectly healthy with adequate composition and structural and material properties. Few studies on aging cartilage have been reported because of difficulties in obtaining the materials and in setting up a good statistical design for the study, and for studies that have been reported, it is difficult to tell if the reported changes are a result of aging or of disease. Nevertheless, in recent years, investigators studying cartilage from human and animal models with OA have defined the histologic, biochemical, metabolic, and biomechanical changes that are recognized as important in understanding the nature of these processes.

OA is a slowly progressive monoarticular or, less commonly, polyarticular disorder of unknown etiology and obscure pathogenesis. The condition generally occurs late in life, principally affecting both load-bearing and weightbearing joints, such as the hands, knees, hips, and shoulder. Clinically, OA is characterized by pain, swelling, deformity, osteophyte formation, enlargement of the joints, and limitation of motion. Pathologically, the disease is characterized by fissuring and focal erosive cartilage lesions (Fig. 26), cartilage loss and destruction (Fig. 27), subchondral bone sclerosis (Fig. 28), and cyst and large osteophyte formation at the margins of the joint (Fig. 29). OA appears to originate in the cartilage, and the virtually pathognomonic changes in that tissue are progressively more severe as the disease advances. It is always associated with structural aberrations in the underlying bone.

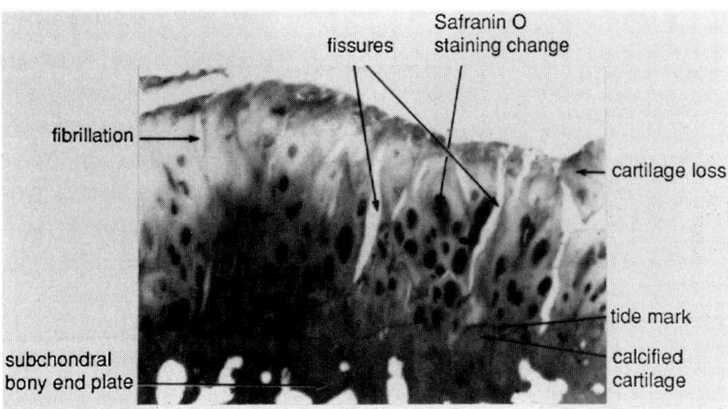

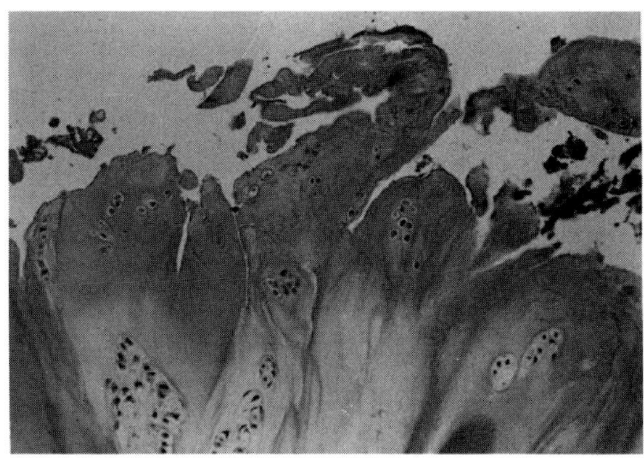

Figure 26
Left, Low power magnification of a section of a humeral glenohumeral head of osteoarthritic (OA) cartilage removed at surgery for total shoulder replacement. Note the significant fibrillation, vertical cleft formation, the tidemark, and the subchondral bony end plate. **Right,** A higher power magnification of surface fibrillation showing vertical cleft formation and widespread large necrotic regions of the tissue devoid of cells. Clusters of cells, common in OA tissues, are also seen.

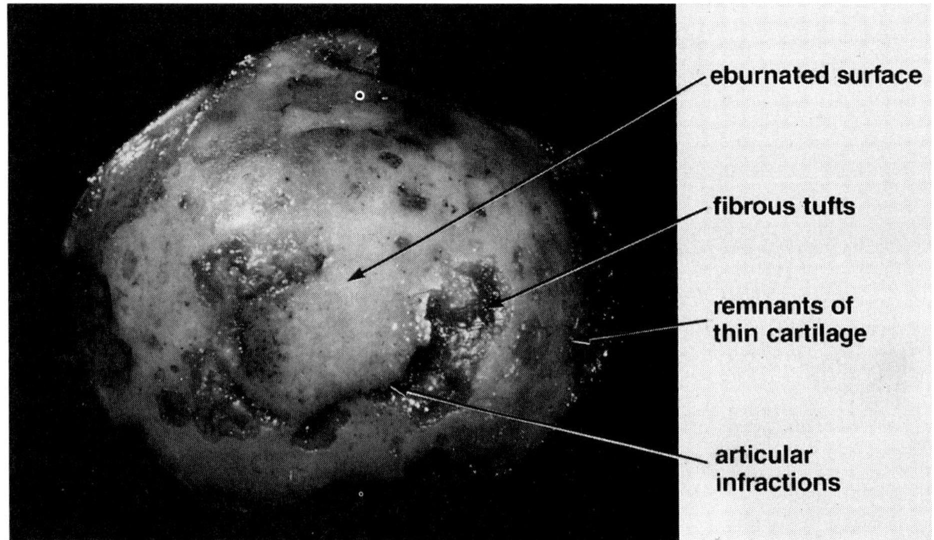

Figure 27
Macro-photograph showing total loss of articular cartilage on a human humeral head. The bone is eburnated and pitted. Regions showing remnants of cartilage are also present.

Joint Capsule

Gross examination of an OA joint demonstrates that other structures are also affected. The joint capsule is usually thickened and occasionally adheres to the deformed underlying bone. This condition probably accounts for the limitation of movement. Histologic examination of the capsule, particularly in advanced disease, also demonstrates focal areas of inflammatory infiltrate, neovascularity, and, in some areas, a hyalinization, amyloid deposition, and sparse cellularity. The synovial lining in an OA joint may show mild to moderate inflammatory changes, which when compared with those of rheumatoid arthritis, are thought to be secondary. The surface of the affected synovium is generally hypervascular and hemorrhagic. During OA, the synovium shows a pattern ranging from nearly normal tissues with only slight thickening of the subsynovial tissues and duplication of the synovial layer to tissues with marked thickening, villous formation, inflammatory change, and neovascularity. These, however, normally occur at a later stage of the disease.

Bone Changes

Consistent with the Greek root "osteo-" in the name of the disease, the bones in OA joints often show remarkable changes (Fig. 29). Although considerable remodeling of the underlying bone is evident from alterations in gross structure, thickening

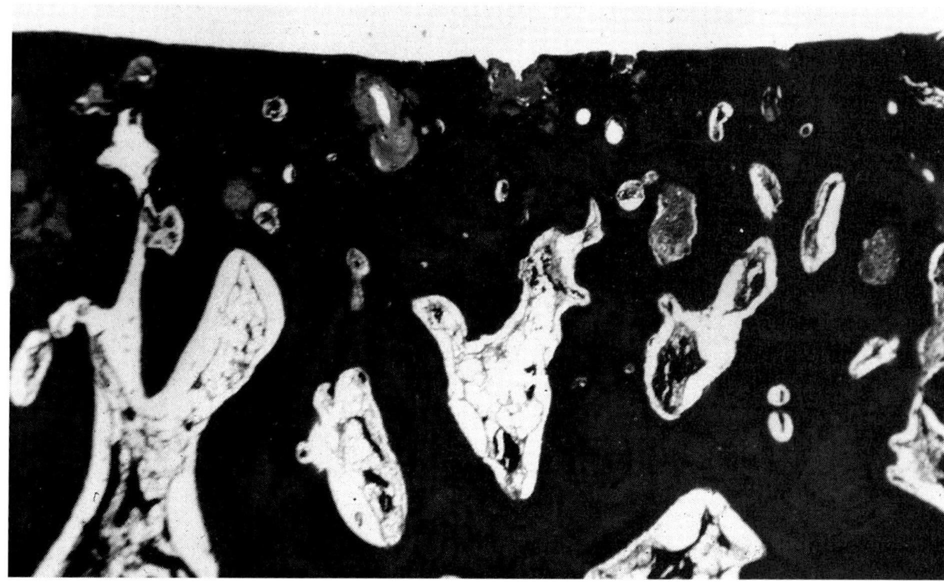

Figure 28
A histologic section of an eburnated section of bone with a dense sclerotic appearance.

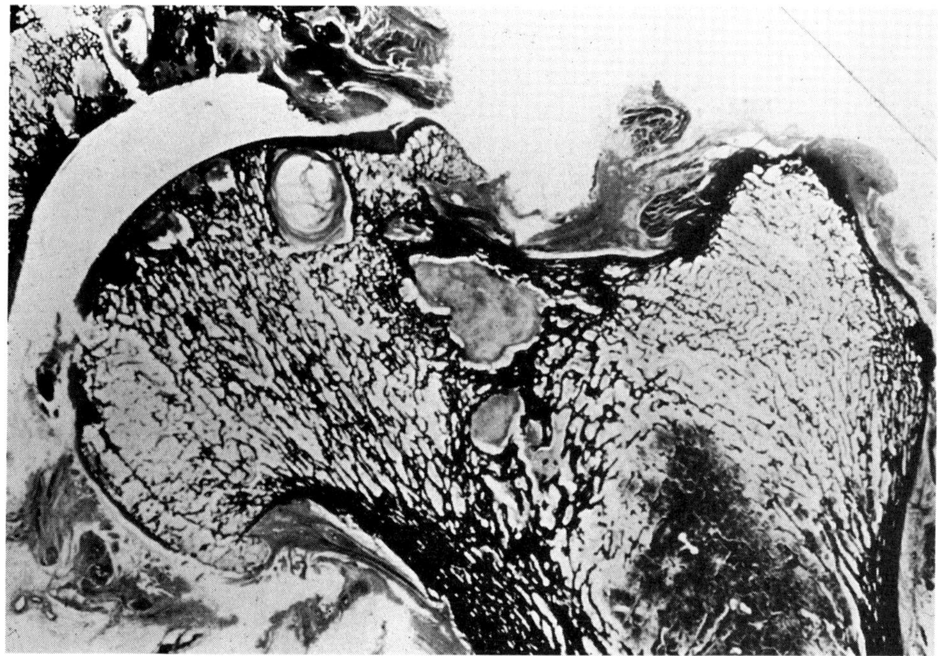

Figure 29
A macro section of an osteoarthritic human femoral head demonstrating a large cyst subjacent to the superior aspect of the head, sclerotic bone formation, and a large osteophyte at the inferior border. The acetabulum also shows similar bony reactions.

of the cortices, and changes in trabecular stress lines, the bone of the joint itself shows the most striking changes. The most severe changes are found at the point of maximum pressure against the opposing cartilage surface. After total denudation of the cartilage has occurred, a dense sclerosis with fibrous and fibrocartilage tufts at the surface and evidence for new bone formation may be seen (Figs. 27 to 29). Despite the OA subchondral hypervascularity, strongly supported by angiography and bone scans of this region, small islands and, sometimes, large segments of osteonecrotic bone are often encountered.

Osteophyte Formation

These bony structures, a cardinal feature of the disease, arise from the bony margins of the osseous components of the joint, surround it, and significantly alter its bony contours (Fig. 29). The majority of articular osteophytes are covered with apparently normal hyaline cartilage. This has been thought of as a biologic way to resurface the diseased joint. Careful examination of the bone often shows extensive thickening of the cortex, bony sclerosis frequently having prominent cement lines, and dilated vascular spaces that may penetrate the lower layers of the cartilage. Cysts of the bone appear as loose, sparsely cellular amorphous regions that stain poorly with hematoxylin and eosin.

Cysts

OA cysts (Fig. 29), another cardinal feature of the disease, frequently develop within the OA bone. The cysts usually are located quite close to the joint surface, although they occasionally appear at a considerable distance from the cartilage, even extending into the metaphyseal areas. The margins of the cysts are sclerotic, which helps to distinguish them from the cysts seen in patients with rheumatoid arthritis. The cysts on cut surfaces contain a glairy, homogeneous, clear or cloudy gelatinous material with a consistency resembling that found within ganglions adjacent to tendon sheaths.

Fibrillation

The gross appearance of hyaline articular cartilage in an OA joint shows a highly variable pattern and is markedly focal in the lesion areas (Fig. 26). In some areas, the cartilage shows softening and a yellowish or brownish discoloration, while in other areas the normally smooth glistening surface appears as a soft velvety felt work. Remnants of old irregularly scarred or ulcerated cartilage may lie adjacent to a pebble-grained newly formed material, which is dull white in color and lacks the smooth surface characteristic of ordinary hyaline cartilage. Ulcerations, fissures, and cracks appear on the surface and, at times, are so extensively focally denuded as to reveal the underlying sclerotic and eburnated subchondral bone (Fig. 27).

Histologic changes in OA articular cartilage are a striking feature of the disease. The earliest alterations include surface erosion and irregularities, deep fissures, and alterations in the staining of the matrix (Fig. 26, *left*). The tidemark, when identifiable, often shows irregularities, duplication, and discontinuities, and often is perforated with blood vessels. As the disorder progresses, the surface layer becomes more fragmented, and short vertical clefts often descend through the gliding zone of the cartilage into the transitional zone (Fig. 26). Deep horizontal clefts can sometimes be identified. A usual pattern is extension of the vertical clefts deep into the cartilage with horizontal components. The matrix shows greater irregularity in staining even with hematoxylin and eosin. With metachromatic stains, such as toluidine blue or Alcian blue, or an orthochromatic stain, such as Safranin O, a patchy, progressive depletion of color can be detected (Fig. 26, *left*). Initially confined to the surface areas, it extends to the deeper layers. Initially in the interterritorial areas and subsequently in the territorial regions, a staining alteration occurs, which closely parallels the progressive depletion of proteoglycan. As the disease advances, the focal fragmentation of the joint surface becomes greater, the clefts deeper (descending as far as the calcified zone), and the matrix staining even more irregular and depleted. Finally, at end stage, only wisps of cartilage are left clinging to the denuded eburnated sclerotic subchondral bone (Fig. 27).

Biochemical Alterations in the Cartilage in OA

DNA Content Cell counts and measurements of the quantity of DNA per unit tissue show considerable variation in OA, depending on the site tested and extent of the disease. Usually, however, DNA concentrations are near normal or slightly increased in OA. This supports the concept that, despite a reduction in tissue volume, the cell count is reasonably well maintained. Some of the chondrocyte clones show intense activity when studied autoradiographically using ^{3}H-cytidine, while others may show little or no evidence of RNA metabolism and are probably dead or dying. As the disease worsens, the tissues become hypocellular and, eventually, all cellular substance is lost over large areas of the diseased tissue.

Water The water content of articular cartilage has been the subject of numerous studies. These have demonstrated an increase in water content of OA cartilage that is statistically significant, although it is only a few percentage points over that of normal tissues. At first, this finding seemed inconsistent with the fact that the concentration of proteoglycans, which constitute approximately 4% to 7% of the wet weight of normal cartilage, is significantly reduced in later stages of OA. Several hypotheses put forth to explain this observation have been discussed. Several other possible explanations, along the ultrastructural line, also have been offered for the observed increase of hydration. One possibility is that removal of the proteoglycan opens up water-binding sites on the collagen that were otherwise obscured, and that these sites hold water better than the collagen-proteoglycan gel. A second possibility is that removal of some of the proteoglycan present in the interstitium allows the remainder to uncoil, thereby increasing both its negatively charged domain and its hydrophilic character. No matter how the phenomenon is explained, OA tissue always swells (gains water or size) relative to normal tissue.

Proteoglycan The proteoglycans of OA articular cartilage also have been studied intensely. It has been established that the proteoglycan content of OA cartilage is diminished and that this decrease appears to be directly proportional to the severity of the disease. Since these initial studies, additional investigations have been undertaken in an attempt to define the nature of the proteoglycan macromolecule present in OA articular cartilage, particularly in relation to aggregation, glycosaminoglycan chain length, and distribution of the glycosaminoglycans. Evidence exists for a marked increase in chondroitin sulfate concentration, especially chondroitin 4-sulfate, with a diminution in the concentration of keratan sulfate. One explanation for this alteration is that the articular chondrocytes in OA cartilage synthesize proteoglycans more usually found in immature cartilage. Another explanation is the possibility of an asymmetric degradation of the proteoglycan moiety that could selectively attack the hyaluronate-binding region of the macromolecule or possibly the keratan sulfate-containing region. A third possible explanation is supported by the finding of two populations of proteoglycans in cartilage: a larger one, rich in chondroitin sulfate, and a smaller one, with increased concentrations of keratan sulfate. Keratan sulfate has been shown to be reduced in OA, perhaps reinforcing the concept that during the early stages of the disease, cartilage more closely resembles immature than adult cartilage.

As described above, in normal cartilage, the aggrecans, which consist of a core protein and glycosaminoglycan side chains, usually exist in the form of very large aggregates in which they are linked at specific binding sites to a long-chain filament of hyaluronic acid in the presence of link proteins (Figs. 6 and 7). Results from many studies have shown that: (1) proteoglycan appears to be considerably more extractable from OA articular cartilage than from normal cartilage; (2) a higher percentage of the cartilage proteoglycan exists in the nonaggregating form; and (3) conversely, a smaller proportion of the proteoglycans are aggregated. These changes suggest that increased proteolytic activity attacks both the free terminal end of the aggrecan and the protein-rich portion (Fig. 11), thus reducing the chain length and damaging the hyaluronate-binding region of the core protein to the extent that, when additional hyaluronate is added, no aggregation occurs. Link proteins appear to be normal in character, but are quickly lost from OA cartilage, while hyaluronate is only moderately reduced.

Collagen The collagen of OA cartilage may show some marked variations in the size and arrangement of the fibers, usually demonstrating a much less orderly network. This variation allows for swelling of the surface with increased water. Nevertheless, no change in the concentration of collagen in early OA cartilage has been demonstrated. In severe OA, when the cartilage is almost totally destroyed, the collagen content must fall along with that of other constituents, but the relative concentration of collagen in relation to total mass (net weight, dry weight, or per microgram of DNA) is increased appreciably, reflecting a rapid loss of proteoglycan relative to collagen during the progression of the disease. This loss is reflected in the collagen network tensile stiffness and strength, which have been shown to be significantly reduced as cartilage moves from normal to mildly fibrillated to OA cartilage.

A question as to whether the collagen of OA cartilage remains as type II has arisen in recent years. Conflicting evidence exists, but the consensus suggests that the newly formed cartilage collagen, which attempts to repair the disease's defect, is mostly type II rather than type I. Type I collagen may be increased slightly, particularly in the osteophyte region. Scientists are just beginning to assess the variation in types IV, V, IX, and X collagen in OA. Such alterations may explain some of the characteristics of the disease and, perhaps, how these characteristics might influence the water content and proteoglycan distribution within the tissue.

Other Materials Severe OA-like changes occur in patients with alkaptonuric ochronosis or hemachromatosis. These disorders seem to occur in relation to a tanning of the collagen fiber present as a result of the deposition in the cartilage substance of molecules of homogentisic acid or hemosiderin. A more subtle form of chemical disorder has been suggested by recent studies that note the increased frequency of joint cartilage calcification (chondrocalcinosis articularis) in OA. A considerable body of data has evolved, which demonstrates increased calcium pyrophosphate in the joint; increased numbers of membrane-bound, calcium-containing vesicles; and increased alkaline phosphatase concentration in cartilage from some patients with OA. The relationship of these alterations to the pathogenesis of the disease is obscure, but one theory suggests that the midzones of the tissue are stiffened and more prone to mechanical injury.

Material Property Changes During OA

Alterations in cartilage composition, molecular structure, and ultrastructural organization are known to produce significant degradation of the material properties of cartilage. To start with, from the swelling theory result $\Delta V/V = P_s/B$ and the hydration data (that is, there is generally a gain in tissue water content during OA), it can be concluded that the compositional and structural changes of OA cartilage always affect the mechanical properties of the solid matrix to a greater extent than they do the swelling pressure. Why this is so is, at present, unknown. The tensile stiffness and strength of the solid matrix have been measured and correlated with the collagen/proteoglycan ratio (Fig. 22). There is a significant drop of cartilage tensile stiffness with increasing severity of lesion, although much more collagen than proteoglycan is present. This change probably reflects damage to the collagen network. In a recent study on a canine OA model based on transection of the anterior cruciate ligament, it was found that the tensile stiffness was reduced by 50% at four months after surgery, water content increased by 7.5%, collagen content decreased by 25%, and collagen cross-link density decreased by 11%. These results show that, as early as four months after surgery, there are dramatic changes of cartilage collagen composition and tensile properties. In a similar series of studies, it was found that the equilibrium shear modulus in the experimental knee joints was reduced by 65% at six weeks, with a slight bit of progression at 12 weeks. The dynamic modulus $|G^*|$ of cartilage in this canine OA model was reduced by 62%, with a slight recovery at 12 weeks. The energy dissipation δ was significantly increased at six and 12 weeks. These results indicate a general loosening of collagen-proteoglycan solid matrix in early OA cartilage.

Typically, the increase in water content in early OA cartilage is associated with the loss of proteoglycan and an increase in the collagen/proteoglycan ratio (Fig. 22). From the biphasic nature of cartilage, it can be anticipated that water content of the tissue is a major factor determining its compression properties. Figure 30 shows the effects of increased water content and decreased total glycosaminoglycan content in human knee joint cartilage. The loss of the equilibrium compressive modulus results from an increase in porosity and a decrease in fixed charge density (swelling pressure). Also associated with these changes is an increased permeability (Fig. 31). An interesting finding from these studies is that the permeability does not increase linearly with porosity ϕ^f, but increases quadratically. This functional dependence clearly shows how important it is for the tissue to maintain normal levels of hydration because of its accentuated effect on permeability. All these findings support the hypothesis that, compositionally and structurally, altered cartilage during OA will have inferior material properties, causing it to lose its ability to support the loads of joint articulation. More specifically, the altered cartilage will lose its fluid pressurization mechanism of load support, which is important for it to maintain normal function in the joint. Eventually, failure of this load-bearing material occurs as arthritis develops. Thus, it is seen that the hydration of cartilage plays a pivotal role in the biomechanical function of the tissue.

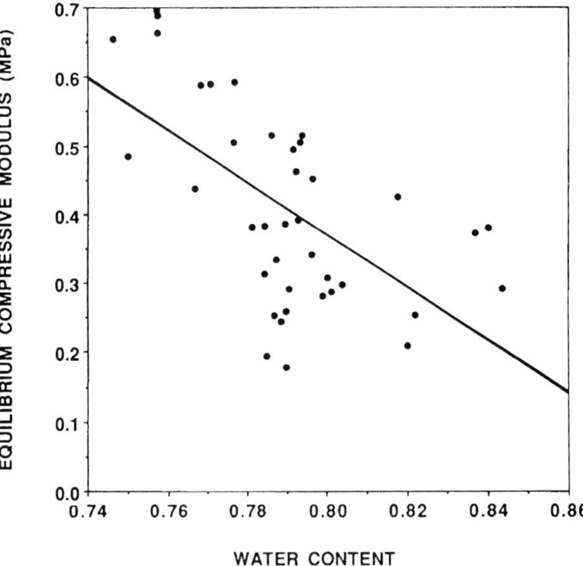

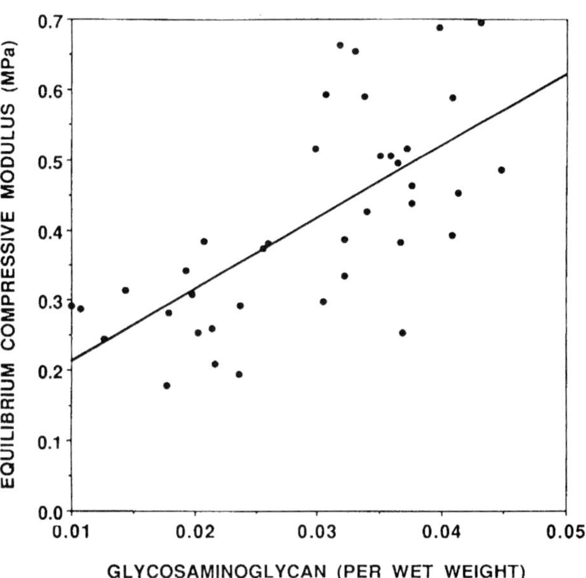

Figure 30
Top, Decrease of equilibrium compressive modulus with increasing water content for human knee joint cartilage. **Bottom,** Increase of equilibrium compressive modulus with increasing glycosaminoglycan content.

The Metabolism of OA Cartilage

Perhaps the most controversial issue in the biochemical study of OA cartilage has been the assessment of the metabolic rate of the tissue as compared with that of normal tissue. The early hypotheses suggested that the process consisted of a passive mechanical erosion by wear and tear of a relatively inert tissue. Therefore, it would seem logical that the cells would show no signs of degeneration and decreased synthetic activity as the dis-

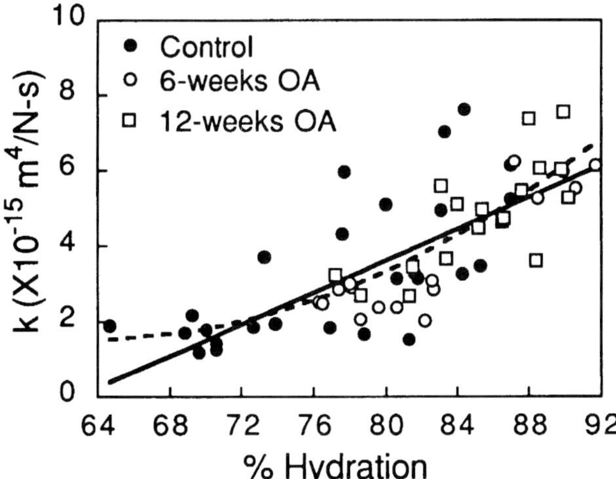

Figure 31
Change of canine knee joint cartilage water content and permeability six and 12 weeks after the anterior cruciate ligament has been transected. Note the statistical data follow the trend predicted by theory, indicating that permeability varies with the square of the hydration.

ease progressed. In fact, chondrocytes from OA human joints are considerably more active metabolically than those from normal articular cartilage. Furthermore, regardless of the material used to trace proteoglycan synthesis (radioactive sulfate or glucosamine), the rates of incorporation are not only higher in diseased than in normal tissue, but appear to parallel the severity of the disease process. In a recent study, hyaluronate synthesis was found to be markedly increased in OA, which seems unusual in view of the decreased aggregation and the diminished concentration of hyaluronate. Considering the data, it seems reasonable that: (1) the hyaluronate that is synthesized is abnormal and, hence, does not allow aggregation; or (2) the excess synthesis is a response to a rapid degradation of the synthesized product.

Collagen Synthesis and Breakdown The collagen of articular cartilage is considered to be much more stable than the proteoglycan, but several metabolic studies have shown that collagen synthesis varies with the severity of the disease. The rate of collagen synthesis is increased, but it is not established whether all of the collagen synthesized can be incorporated into the collagenous matrix in a manner that will maintain the integrity of the matrix. Information on the catabolism of the collagen network in OA is limited. The network is disrupted, but overall loss is limited. Further studies have shown, at least in several animal models, that the material synthesized is type II rather than type I collagen, supporting the concept that the repair tissue in OA is hyaline cartilage rather than fibrocartilage.

Another minor constituent protein of cartilage, fibronectin, has been discovered to show significant increments in both concentration and rate of synthesis in OA. The significance of this finding is currently unknown.

Proteoglycan Synthesis and Breakdown Proteoglycan synthesis has been found to be elevated in OA cartilage. This elevation generally is regarded as a mechanism used by the chondrocytes for matrix repair—a repair event that ultimately is doomed to failure. Animal studies have shown this synthesis to be one of the first biochemical events that occurs in the early development of OA. The proteoglycans synthesized are similar to those in normal cartilage, but they appear to have slightly longer chondroitin sulfate chains, which suggests that there are some fundamental changes in the synthesis mechanisms in OA chondrocytes. This observation is supported by recent data obtained using a monoclonal antibody to chondroitin sulfate, which shows that the chondroitin sulfate chains in OA cartilage have subtle but potentially important structural differences.

However, the decrease in the overall proteoglycan content in OA tissue leads to the conclusion that the proteoglycan breakdown rate has increased. This is indeed the case, and the increased rate of proteoglycan breakdown is a major metabolic change in OA cartilage, particularly at the early stages of development of the joint disease. However, no difference has been shown between the molecular mechanisms involved in proteoglycan breakdown in normal tissues, and those in accelerated degradation. It therefore seems that the increased rate of catabolism is caused by increased activities of enzymes already present and active in normal tissue. The proteolytic fragments are released from the cartilage into the synovial fluid, and then are cleared by the lymphatics. Recent studies indicate that the detection of significantly elevated levels of proteoglycan in synovial fluids, particularly at early stages of OA, may represent a means for detection and monitoring of the disease. The maintenance of the cartilage matrix is, therefore, a balance between the rates of synthesis and breakdown, and cartilage degradation appears to be an imbalance of these two events.

DNA Synthesis Studies of DNA synthesis in OA cartilage have shown both mitotic activity and increased ^{3}H-thymidine incorporation, particularly in the cells of the chondrocyte clones. This finding is supported by electron microscopic studies of the OA cartilage. All of these data indicate that the articular chondrocyte in OA "turns on the switch" for DNA synthesis and makes new cells that presumably become metabolically active. The rate of DNA synthesis appears to vary directly with the morphologic severity of the process up to a point of failure, after which the rate falls.

Degradative Enzymes in Osteoarthritic Articular Cartilage

Despite the findings that the rates for synthesis of proteoglycan, collagen, and DNA are all increased, OA is a disorder that produces inexorable and sometimes rapid cartilage degradation. The catabolic activity of the tissue, thus, can be extraordinarily high and can ultimately dominate the picture. The degradation of articular cartilage by enzymes has been the subject of many studies. Much of the work has been directed at determining which enzymes are present in the cartilage, and what are their in vitro activities. The determination of which specific enzyme is responsible for a specific degradative event has been elusive, partly because there has been a lack of enzyme inhibitors with the specificity to provide this information.

The enzymes found in articular cartilage include the metalloproteinases collagenase, gelatinase, and stromelysin, the serine proteases, including tissue plasminogen activator, elastase, and cathepsin G; and the cathepsins B and D. The activities of the metalloproteinases are controlled by the presence of their specific inhibitor, TIMP.

Levels of metalloproteinases and the cathepsins B and D are increased in OA cartilage. The increase in collagenase and gelatinase activities appears to correspond to the observed disruption of the collagenous network. The increased activity of stromelysin, which is likely to use the proteoglycans as a major substrate, corresponds to the increased release of proteoglycan from the articular cartilage. This enzyme also has recently been shown to degrade type IX collagen in cartilage and, thus, may play an important role in the disruption of the collagen network. The level of TIMP is not increased, and it even may be decreased in OA cartilage. This phenomenon provides support for the hypothesis that the balance of the levels of enzyme and inhibitor dictates the rate of matrix degradation, and that in OA degradation of the matrix is the result of an imbalance of these. Good evidence for the involvement of the cathepsins B and D in cartilage matrix degradation is lacking.

An important mediator of cartilage degradation, particularly in inflammatory events, is interleukin-1. Although this material may originate in the monocytes of inflamed joints, it also has been found to be synthesized by chondrocytes as a paracrine activity. Interleukin-1 enhances enzyme synthesis and activation of a number of enzyme systems in the cartilage including latent collagenase, stromelysin, and gelatinase and a tissue plasminogen activator (Figs. 14 and 32). Plasminogen is presumed to be synthesized by the chondrocyte or is contributed by the synovial cell transudation to enter the matrix. The stimulation of collagenase and stromelysin production by interleukin-1 is thought to be important in elevating the catabolic events in cartilage.

Etiology of OA

The exact cause of OA is not currently known. The disorder has no single cause and follows no common final pathway, but by a variety of means reaches a common end stage. Considerable specula-

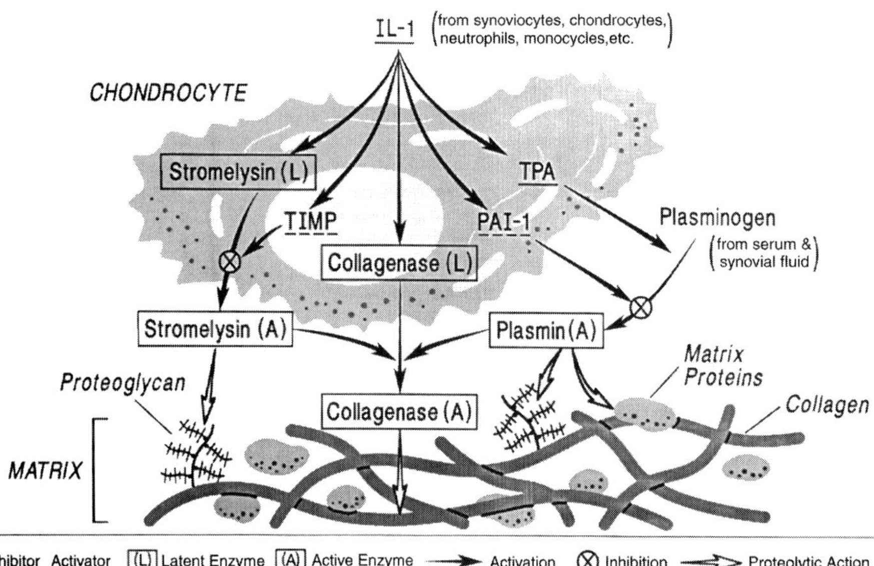

Figure 32
The cascade of enzymes, their activators and inhibitors involved in interleukin 1-stimulated degradation of articular cartilage.

tion exists concerning various factors that may contribute to the initiation, perpetuation, and pathogenesis of the disorder. The following factors have been considered significant.

Aging There is little doubt that OA is more common in the elderly and is, in fact, virtually unknown in children. But the aging changes in articular cartilage have not been clearly differentiated from those of OA, and the disease is not a natural consequence of aging. The occurrence of posttraumatic OA in young adults precludes the possibility that age-related changes in cartilage are prerequisite in the development of the disease.

Alterations in Matrix Structure Although secondary changes occur in matrix structure during the progress of OA, little support is offered for the concept that such changes are primary and lead to the eventual development of the disease. A recent observation of an alteration in the genetic structure of type II collagen in certain families provides some evidence for an inherited basis of OA.

Alterations in Cellular Activity There is no doubt that the metabolic activity of the OA chondrocyte is abnormal, and that its differences are phenotypic and dependent on the environment. The question arises, however, as to whether these changes are primary or merely alterations (presumably permanent) that occur when the cells are stimulated either acutely or chronically by some initiating factors for the disease. A large body of data indicates that altered stresses and strains in the solid matrix, osmotic pressure, streaming potential, and a whole host of other physical factors may play a role in modulating chondrocyte activities. The specific mechanism of signal transduction at the cellular level is unknown.

Alterations in Mediators Humoral, synovial, and cartilage-derived chemical mediators and mechanical stimuli play a major role in the regulation of synthetic processes. Ample evidence exists to demonstrate that such factors may have a significant effect on the cell. Factors such as interleukin-1 can produce profound, specific alterations in the metabolism of chondrocytes, severely diminishing anabolism while enhancing catabolism. The relative contribution of these factors in the progression of OA is not yet clear.

Altered Joint Mechanics It seems obvious that an ankle fracture, which is not reduced and leaves the joint incongruent, will in a short time lead to classic OA, and that chronic states, such as recurrent dislocation of the patella, congenital dislocation of the hip, and joint alterations as a result of osteonecrotic collapse, etc. will frequently lead to an OA lesion. OA may result from some mechanical insult, but the evolution of the process is so slow that it is manifested only in later years, or OA may result from a low level repetitive insult that is difficult to identify. Excessive joint laxity due to traumatic ligamentous injury or excessive joint tightness secondary to diseased or surgically shortened ligaments can lead to chronic asymmetric cartilage loading and result in OA.

Immune Responses Recent evidence suggests that some cartilaginous matrix proteins are unrecognized by the immune system as autogenous. When they escape from the cartilage into the synovial fluid, the local lymphocytic elements identify them as antigens. This may explain why a minor injury to the cartilage may initiate or perpetuate a local (synovial) autoimmune synovial inflammation. But such minor injuries are not associated with any chronic processes, nor do these joints develop OA.

Summary

Current understanding of articular cartilage has been derived from a massive worldwide effort, which includes detailed studies in the disciplines of biology, biochemistry, biomechanics, and pathology of the tissue. Equally important are the contributions made by interdisciplinary studies involving orthopaedic surgeons and basic scientists. Only a brief introduction has been presented here. The exciting aspect of cartilage research is that many of the topics discussed in this chapter were not even thought of a decade or so ago. Much progress still needs to be made before a clear conception of the most important aspects of articular cartilage function can be ascertained, and a definitive etiology of OA evolves. The material presented in this chapter should provide the reader with a basic knowledge of current and future articular cartilage research.

Selected Bibliography

General Reference Texts

Hay ED (ed): *Cell Biology of the Extracellular Matrix,* ed 2. New York, Plenum Press, 1991.

Kuettner KE, Schleyerbach R, Peyron JG, et al (eds): *Articular Cartilage and Osteoarthritis.* New York, Raven Press, 1992.

Mankin HJ, Brandt KD: Biochemistry and metabolism of articular cartilage in osteoarthritis, in Moskowitz RW, Howell VC, Goldberg VM, et al (eds): *Osteoarthritis: Diagnosis and Medical/Surgical Management,* ed 2. Philadelphia, WB Saunders, 1992, pp 109–154.

Mow VC, Hayes WC (eds): *Basic Orthopaedic Biomechanics.* New York, Raven Press, 1991.

Woo SL-Y, Buckwalter JA (eds): *Injury and Repair of the Musculoskeletal Soft Tissues.* Park Ridge, IL, American Academy of Orthopaedic Surgeons, 1988.

Structure of Articular Cartilage

Buckwalter JA, Hunziker EB: Articular cartilage biology and morphology, in Mow VC, Ratcliffe A (eds): *Structure and Function of Articular Cartilage.* Boca Raton, FL, CRC Press, 1993.

Clarke IC: Articular cartilage: A review and scanning electron microscope study: 1. The interterritorial fibrillar architecture. *J Bone Joint Surg* 1971;53B:732–750.

Clark JM: The organization of collagen in cryofractured rabbit articular cartilage: A scanning electron microscopic study. *J Orthop Res* 1985;3:17–29.

Schenk RK, Eggli PS, Hunziker EB: Articular cartilage morphology, in Kuettner KE, Schleyerbach R, Hascall VC (eds): *Articular Cartilage Biochemistry.* New York, Raven Press, 1986, pp 3–22.

Scott JE: Proteoglycan:collagen interactions in connective tissues. Ultrastructural, biochemical, functional and evolutionary aspects. *Int J Biol Macromol* 1991;13:157–161.

Physicochemistry of Articular Cartilage

Maroudas A: Tissue composition and organization, in Maroudas A, Kuettner K (eds): *Methods in Cartilage Research.* London, Academic Press, 1990, pp 209–239.

Mow VC, Ratcliffe A, Poole AR: Cartilage and diarthrodial joints as paradigms for hierarchical materials and structures. *Biomaterials* 1992;13:67–97.

Biomechanics of Articular Cartilage

Anderson DD, Brown TD, Radin EL: The influence of basal cartilage calcification on dynamic juxtaarticular stress transmission. *Clin Orthop* 1993;286:298–307.

Brown TD, Radin EL, Martin RB, et al: Finite element studies of some juxtaarticular stress changes due to localized subchondral stiffening. *J Biomech* 1984;17:11–24.

Grodzinsky AJ: Mechanical and electrical properties and their relevance to the physiological processes, in: Maroudas A, Kuettner K (eds): *Methods in Cartilage Research.* London, Academic Press, 1990, pp 275–311.

Mow VC, Holmes MH, Lai WM: Fluid transport and mechanical properties of articular cartilage: A review. *J Biomech* 1984;17:377–394.

Mow VC, Zhu W, Ratcliffe A: Structure and function of articular cartilage and meniscus, in Mow VC, Hayes WC (eds): *Basic Orthopaedic Biomechanics.* New York, Raven Press, 1991, pp 143–198.

Biology of Articular Cartilage

Helminen HJ, Kiviranta I, Tammi M, et al (eds): *Joint Loading: Biology and Health of Articular Structures.* Bristol, UK, Wright-Butterworth Scientific, 1987.

Palmoski MJ, Brandt KD: Running inhibits the reversal of atrophic changes in canine knee cartilage after removal of a leg cast. *Arthritis Rheum* 1981;24:1329–1337.

Palmoski MJ, Brandt KD: Effects of static and cyclic compressive loading on articular cartilage plugs in vitro. *Arthritis Rheum* 1984;27:675–681.

Stockwell RA: *Biology of Cartilage Cells.* Cambridge, UK, Cambridge University Press, 1979, pp 7–29.

Stockwell RA: Structure and function of the chondrocyte under mechanical loading, in Helminen HJ (ed): *Joint Loading: Biology and Health of Articular Structures.* Bristol, UK, Wright-Butterworth Scientific, 1992, pp 126–148.

Water Content

Armstrong CG, Mow VC: Variations in the intrinsic mechanical properties of human articular cartilage with age, degeneration, and water content. *J Bone Joint Surg* 1982;64A:88–94.

Mankin HJ, Thrasher AZ: Water content and binding in normal and osteoarthritic human cartilage. *J Bone Joint Surg* 1975;57A:76–80.

Maroudas A, Bayliss MT, Venn MF: Further studies on the composition of human femoral head cartilage. *Ann Rheum Dis* 1980;39:514–523.

Proteoglycans

Hardingham TE, Fosang AJ: Proteoglycans: Many forms and many functions. *FASEB J* 1992;6:861–870.

Lohmander S: Proteoglycans of joint cartilage: Structure, function, turnover and role as markers of joint disease. *Baillieres Clin Rheumatol* 1988;2:37–62.

Mow VC, Zhu W, Lai WM, et al: The influence of link protein stabilization on the viscometric properties of proteoglycan aggregate solutions. *Biochim Biophys Acta* 1989;992:201–208.

Muir H: Proteoglycans as organizers of the (inter)cellular matrix. *Biochem Soc Trans* 1983;11:613–622.

Rosenberg LC, Buckwalter JA: Cartilage proteoglycans, in Kuettner KE, Schleyerbach R, Hascall VC (eds): *Articular Cartilage Biochemistry.* New York, Raven Press, 1986, pp 39–58.

Roughley PJ: Structural changes in the proteoglycans of human articular cartilage during aging. *J Rheumatol* 1987;14:14–15.

Link Protein

Baker JR, Caterson B: The isolation of 'link proteins' from bovine nasal cartilage. *Biochim Biophys Acta* 1978;532:249–258.

Hardingham TE: The role of link-protein in the structure of cartilage proteoglycan aggregates. *Biochem J* 1979;177:237–247.

Collagen of Cartilage

Bruckner P, Vaughan L, Winterhalter KH: Type IX collagen from sternal cartilage of chicken embryo contains covalently bound glycosaminoglycans. *Proc Natl Acad Sci USA* 1985;82:2608–2612.

Eyre DR, Wu JJ, Apone S: A growing family of collagens in articular cartilage: Identification of 5 genetically distinct types. *J Rheumatol* 1987;14:25–27.

Mayne R, Irwin MH: Collagen types in cartilage, in Kuettner KE, Schleyerbach R, Hascall VC (eds): *Articular Cartilage Biochemistry.* New York, Raven Press, 1986, pp 23–38.

Nimni ME, Harkness RD: Molecular structures and functions of collagen, in Nimni ME (ed): *Collagen, Vol 1 Biochemistry.* Boca Raton, FL, CRC Press, 1988, pp 1–78.

van der Rest M, Garrone R: Collagen family of proteins. *FASEB J* 1991;5:2814–2823.

Fibronectin of Cartilage

Brown RA, Jones KL: The synthesis and accumulation of fibronectin by human articular cartilage. *J Rheumatol* 1990;17:65–72.

Burton-Wurster N, Horn VJ, Lust G: Immunohistochemical localization of fibronectin and chondronectin in canine articular cartilage. *J Histochem Cytochem* 1988;36:581–588.

Lipids of Cartilage

Bonner WM, Jonsson H, Malanos C, et al: Changes in the lipids of human articular cartilage with age. *Arthritis Rheum* 1975;18:461–473.

Ohira T, Ishikawa K, Masuda I, et al: Histologic localization of lipid in the articular tissues in calcium pyrophosphate dihydrate crystal deposition disease. *Arthritis Rheum* 1988;31:1057–1062.

Vignon E, Mathieu P, Louisot P, et al: Phospholipase A2 activity in human osteoarthritic cartilage. *J Rheumatol Suppl* 1989;18:35–38.

Other Proteins of Cartilage

Fife RS, Palmoski MJ, Brandt KD: Metabolism of a cartilage matrix glycoprotein in normal and osteoarthritic canine articular cartilage. *Arthritis Rheum* 1986;29:1256–1262.

Metabolism of Articular Cartilage

Mankin HJ, Brandt KD: Biochemistry and metabolism of articular cartilage in osteoarthritis, in Moskowitz RW, Howell DS, Goldberg VM, et al (eds): *Osteoarthritis: Diagnosis and Medical/Surgical Management,* ed 2. Philadelphia, WB Saunders, 1992, pp 109–154.

Mankin HJ, Johnson ME, Lippiello L: Biochemical and metabolic abnormalities in articular cartilage from osteoarthritic human hips: III. Distribution and metabolism of amino sugar-containing macromolecules. *J Bone Joint Surg* 1981;63A:131–139.

Oegema TR Jr, Thompson RC Jr: Metabolism of chondrocytes derived from normal and osteoarthritic human cartilage, in Kuettner KE, Schleyerbach R, Hascall VC (eds): *Articular Cartilage Biochemistry.* New York, Raven Press, 1986, pp 257–271.

Osborn KD, Trippel SB, Mankin HJ: Growth factor stimulation of adult articular cartilage. *J Orthop Res* 1989;7:35–42.

Ratcliffe A, Tyler JA, Hardingham TE: Articular cartilage cultured with interleukin 1: Increased release of link protein, hyaluronate-binding region and other proteoglycan fragments. *Biochem J* 1986;238:571–580.

Sandy JD, Brown HL, Lowther DA: Control of proteoglycan synthesis: Studies on the activation of synthesis observed during culture of articular cartilages. *Biochem J* 1980;188:119–130.

Treadwell BV, Mankin HJ: The synthetic processes of articular cartilage. *Clin Orthop* 1986;213:50–61.

Trippel SB, Ehrlich MG, Lippiello L, et al: Characterization of chondrocytes from bovine articular cartilage: I. Metabolic and morphological experimental studies. *J Bone Joint Surg* 1980;62A:816–820.

Enzymes of Cartilage

Campbell IK, Piccoli DS, Butler DM, et al: Recombinant human interleukin-1 stimulates human articular cartilage to undergo resorption and human chondrocytes to produce both tissue- and urokinase-type plasminogen activator. *Biochim Biophys Acta* 1988;967:183–194.

Gunja-Smith Z, Nagase H, Woessner JF Jr: Purification of the neutral proteoglycan-degrading metalloproteinase from human articular cartilage tissue and its identification as stromelysin matrix metalloproteinase-β. *Biochem J* 1989;258:115–119.

Nguyen Q, Murphy G, Roughley PJ, et al: Degradation of proteoglycan aggregate by a cartilage metalloproteinase: Evidence for the involvement of stromelysin in the generation of link protein heterogeneity in situ. *Biochem J* 1989;259:61–67.

Sandy JD, Brown HL, Lowther DA: Degradation of proteoglycan in articular cartilage. *Biochim Biophys Acta* 1978;543:536–544.

Yamada H, Stephens RW, Nakagawa T, et al: Human articular cartilage contains an inhibitor of plasminogen activator. *J Rheumatol* 1988;15:1138–1143.

Cartilage and Aging

Bayliss MT: Age-related changes in the stoichiometry of human articular cartilage proteoglycan aggregates, in Maroudas A, Kuettner K (eds): *Methods in Cartilage Research.* London, Academic Press, 1990, pp 220–222.

Buckwalter JA, Kuettner KE, Thonar EJ: Age-related changes in articular cartilage proteoglycans: Electron microscopic studies. *J Orthop Res* 1985;3:251–257.

Front P, Aprile F, Mitrovic DR, et al: Age-related changes in the synthesis of matrix macromolecules by bovine articular cartilage. *Connect Tissue Res* 1989;19:121–133.

Martel-Pelletier J, Pelletier JP: Neutral metalloproteases and age related changes in human articular cartilage. *Ann Rheum Dis* 1987;46:363–369.

Cartilage Injury and Repair

Buckwalter JA, Cruess RL: Healing of the musculoskeletal tissues, in Rockwood CA Jr, Green DP,

Bucholz RW (eds): *Fractures in Adults,* ed 3. Philadelphia, JB Lippincott, 1991, Vol 1, pp 181–222.

Buckwalter JA, Mow VC: Cartilage repair in osteoarthritis, in Moskowitz RW, Howell DS, Goldberg VM, et al (eds): *Osteoarthritis: Diagnosis and Medical/Surgical Management,* ed 2. Philadelphia, WB Saunders, 1992, pp 71–107.

Donohue JM, Buss D, Oegema TR Jr, et al: The effects of indirect blunt trauma on adult canine articular cartilage. *J Bone Joint Surg* 1983;65A:948–957.

Mankin HJ: Current concepts review: The response of articular cartilage to mechanical injury. *J Bone Joint Surg* 1982;64A:460–466.

Mitchell N, Shepard N: Effect of patellar shaving in the rabbit. *J Orthop Res* 1987;5:388–392.

Mow VC, Ratcliffe A, Rosenwasser MP, et al: Experimental studies on repair of large osteochondral defects at a high weight bearing area of the knee joint: A tissue engineering study. *J Biomech Eng* 1991;113:198–207.

Mow VC, Setton LA, Ratcliffe A, et al: Structure-function relationships for articular cartilage and effects of joint instability and trauma on cartilage function, in Brandt KD (ed): *Cartilage Changes in Osteoarthritis.* Indianapolis, IN, University of Indiana Press, 1990, pp 22–42.

O'Driscoll SW, Keeley FW, Salter RB: Durability of regenerated articular cartilage produced by free autogenous periosteal grafts in major full-thickness defects in joint surfaces under the influence of continuous passive motion: A follow-up report at one year. *J Bone Joint Surg* 1989;70A:595–606.

Salter RB, Simmonds DF, Malcolm BW, et al: The biological effect of continuous passive motion on the healing of full-thickness defects in articular cartilage: An experimental investigation in the rabbit. *J Bone Joint Surg* 1980;62A:1232–1251.

Wakitani S, Kimura T, Hirooka A, et al: Repair of rabbit articular surfaces with allograft chondrocytes embedded in collagen gel. *J Bone Joint Surg* 1989;71B:74–80.

Osteoarthritis

Dean DD, Martel-Pelletier J, Pelletier JP, et al: Evidence for metalloproteinase and metalloproteinase inhibitor imbalance in human osteoarthritic cartilage. *J Clin Invest* 1989;84:678–685.

Ehrlich MG, Armstrong AL, Treadwell BV, et al: The role of proteases in the pathogenesis of osteoarthritis. *J Rheumatol* 1987;14:30–32.

Kuettner KE, Schleyerbach R, Peyron JG, et al: *Articular Cartilage and Osteoarthritis.* New York, Raven Press, 1992.

Mankin HJ, Dorfman H, Lippiello L, et al: Biochemical and metabolic abnormalities in articular cartilage from osteo-arthritic human hips: II. Correlation of morphology with biochemical and metabolic data. *J Bone Joint Surg* 1971;53A:523–537.

Moskowitz RW, Howell DS, Goldberg VM, et al (eds): *Osteoarthritis: Diagnosis and Medical/Surgical Management,* ed 2. Philadelphia, WB Saunders, 1992.

Radin EL: Factors influencing the progression of osteoarthrosis, in Ewing JW (ed): *Articular Cartilage and Knee Joint Function.* New York, Raven Press, 1990, pp 301–309.

Ryu J, Treadwell BV, Mankin HJ: Biochemical and metabolic abnormalities in normal and osteoarthritic human articular cartilage. *Arthritis Rheum* 1984;27:49–57.

Setton LA, Mow VC, Pita JC, et al: Altered structure-function relationships for articular cartilage in human osteoarthritis and an experimental canine model, in van den Berg WB (ed): Proc 19th ESOA Symp, Noordijkerhout, Holland. Switzerland, Birkhauser Verlag, 1992.

Telhag H: Nucleic acids in human normal and osteoarthritic articular cartilage. *Acta Orthop Scand* 1976;47:585–587.

Chapter 2
Anatomy, Biology, and Biomechanics of Tendon, Ligament, and Meniscus

Savio L-Y Woo, PhD
Kai-Nan An, PhD
Steven P. Arnoczky, DVM
Jennifer S. Wayne, PhD
Donald C. Fithian, MD
Barry S. Myers, MD, PhD

Chapter Outline

Introduction

The injury and repair of soft tissue in and about diarthrodial joints remain significant problems in the practice of orthopaedics. With an increased interest in athletic activities and an increased use of high speed, energy-efficient transportation, soft-tissue injuries are playing an increasingly important role in clinical practice. Such injuries produce both acute and chronic disability and, although once thought to be of minor consequence, have been shown to lead to joint degeneration. The knee meniscus is, perhaps, the best example of this. Given the increasing span of human life, together with the increase in frequency of such soft-tissue injury, prevention of its sequelae and consequent chronic disability is likely to be more significant in the future.

This chapter is a review of the structure and function of three biologic soft tissues, tendon, ligament, and meniscus. Each structure is discussed in its own section. The anatomy, microanatomy, biology, and biomechanics of the structure are presented and attention is drawn to the role of these basic sciences in the clinical practice of orthopaedics. The text also depicts the hierarchical structural organization of joints and the ways that organization influences the behavior of the structure as a whole. That is, a joint is a structure composed of a group of components. These components, like the meniscus or a ligament, are themselves structures with components, like fascicles and fiber bundles, composed ultimately of collagen and other materials. To understand the behavior of the structure as a whole, it is necessary to look through this hierarchy to the smallest constituents and their biologic and biomechanical characteristics. It is also necessary to reassemble this information to understand the more relevant clinical questions.

In biologic systems, where the anatomic organization is hierarchical, the distinction between material and structural properties often depends on the reader's perspective. Both the mechanical and structural properties need to be studied and their interactions understood. For example, a ligament may be thought of as a uniform solid cylinder whose structural properties depend on the shape of the cylinder and the ligament's material properties.

A thicker ligament made of a material with a lower elastic modulus may have the same structural stiffness as a thinner ligament made from a material with a higher elastic modulus. Elastic modulus, being a mechanical property, changes as a result of the degree of organization of the ligament's fascicles and, ultimately, collagen molecules. Stiffness, being a structural property, changes as a result of changes in the material properties or changes in the geometry of the structure.

Another concept that is important to the understanding of joint mechanics is the degrees of freedom of a body. The degrees of freedom is the number of parameters needed to fully describe the position of a body. For example, the tibia requires six degrees of freedom to fully describe its location relative to the femur. Three describe the location of the tibial plateau (anteroposterior, superoinferior, and mediolateral positions). An additional three describe the orientation of the tibia relative to the femur (flexion-extension angle, valgus-varus angle, and internal-external rotation angle). Thus, full understanding of the motions of the knee, or any joint, requires an understanding of all six degrees of freedom of that joint.

Tendon

Anatomy

Morphologically, the tendon is a complex composite material consisting of collagen fibrils embedded in a matrix of proteoglycans associated with a relative paucity of cells. Fibroblasts, the predominant cell type within tendon, are arranged in long parallel rows in the spaces between the parallel collagen bundles. The cell bodies are rod or spindle-shaped and oriented in rows when seen microscopically in a longitudinally derived section (Fig. 1). When viewed in cross section, the cell's outlines appear as dark, star-shaped figures between the collagen bundles (Fig. 2). The cytoplasm of the fibroblasts stains darkly with basic dyes and contains a clear centrosome adjacent to the single round

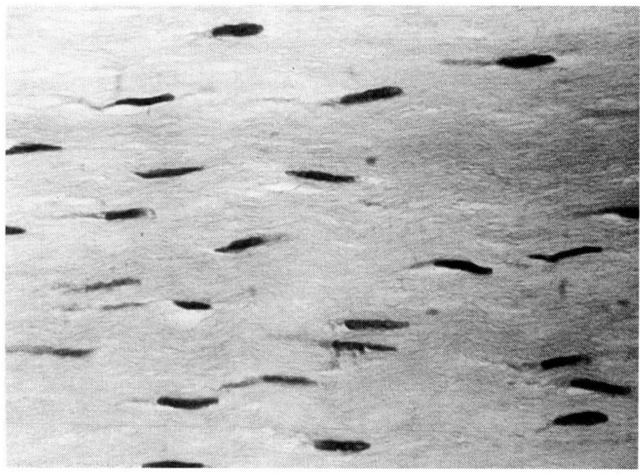

Figure 1
Photomicrograph of a longitudinal section of a human flexor tendon showing the spindle-shaped fibroblasts (H&E, X250).

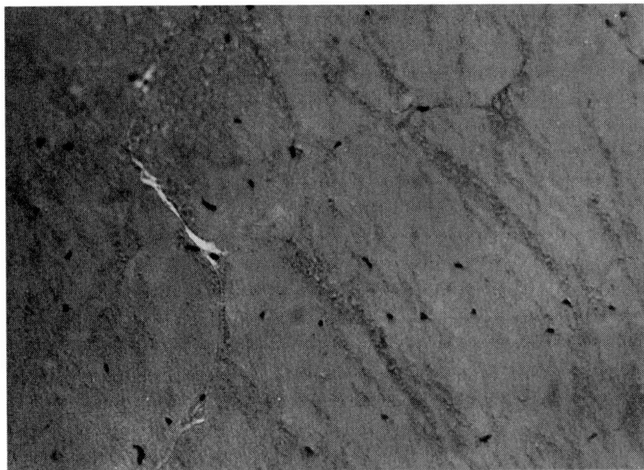

Figure 2
Photomicrograph of a cross section of a human flexor tendon showing the star-shaped fibroblasts with cytoplasmic processes extending between collagen bundles (H&E, X250).

nucleus. Although the borders between successive cells in a row are distinct, the lateral borders of the cells are indistinct as a result of thin cytoplasmic processes that extend between collagen bundles (Fig. 3).

The major constituent of tendon is type I collagen (86% dry weight). Collagen contains a high concentration of glycine (33%), proline (15%), and hydroxyproline (15%). Thus, almost two-thirds of the primary structure of the collagen chain consists of these three amino acids. Hydroxyproline, a derivative of the incorporated proline, is almost unique to collagen. Hydroxylysine makes up 1.3% of collagen dry weight and is also unique to the molecule.

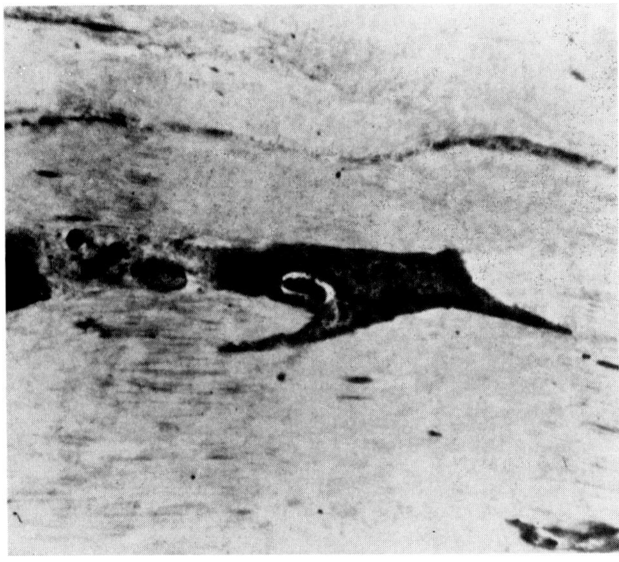

Figure 3
Electron micrograph of fibroblast (X4000).

The secondary structure of collagen relates to the arrangement of each chain in a left-handed configuration, and in its tertiary structure three collagen chains are combined into a collagen molecule. In type I collagen, there are two identical polypeptide chains called α1(I) and one slightly different chain called α2(I) or simply α2. The three chains are coiled together in a right-handed triple helix held together by hydrogen and covalent bonds (Fig. 4).

The quaternary structure of collagen relates to the organization of collagen molecules into a stable, low energy biologic unit based on a regular association of adjacent molecules' basic and acidic amino acids. By arranging adjacent collagen molecules in a quarter-stagger, oppositely charged amino acids are aligned. The fact that a great deal of energy and, therefore, force is required to separate these molecules accounts in part for the strength of the structure. In this way collagen molecules combine to form ordered units of microfibrils (five collagen molecules), subfibrils, and fibrils (Fig. 5). These units are arranged in closely-packed, highly-ordered parallel bundles that are oriented in a distinct longitudinal pattern. At this level, proteoglycans and glycoproteins in association with water are incorporated in a matrix, binding the fibrils together to form fascicles (Fig. 6).

The fascicles within the tendon are bound together by loose connective tissue, the endotenon,

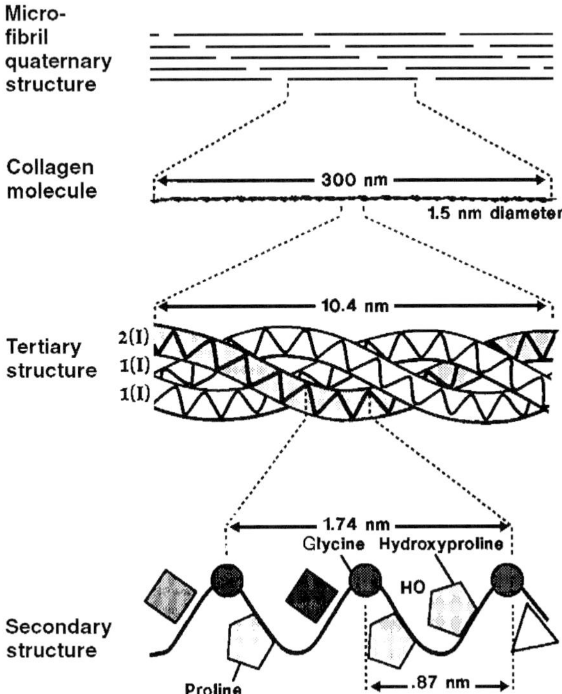

Figure 4
Schematic drawing of structural organization of collagen into the microfibril.

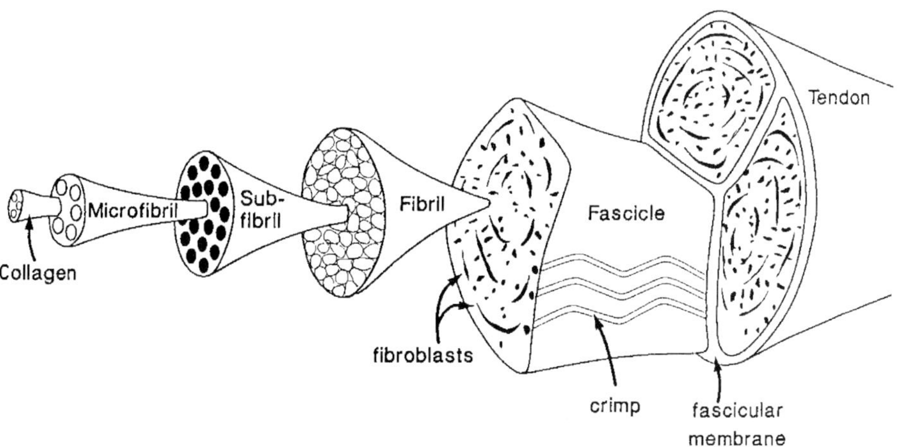

Figure 5
Schematic representation of the microarchitecture of a tendon. (Adapted with permission from Kastelic J, Baer E: Deformation in tendon collagen, in Vincent JFV, Currey JD (eds): *The Mechanical Properties of Biologic Materials.* Cambridge, Cambridge University Press, 1980, pp 397–435.)

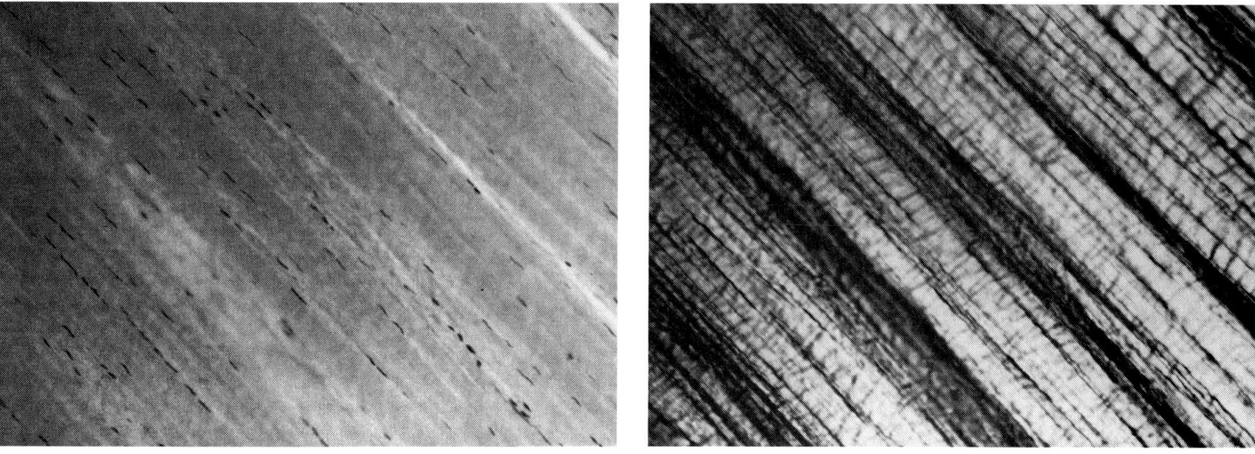

Figure 6
Left, Photomicrograph of a longitudinal section of a human flexor tendon. Note the parallel rows of fibroblasts lying between the collagen bundles. **Right,** Photomicrograph of same section under polarized light microscopy, illustrating the parallel, longitudinally arranged collagen bundles (H&E, X100).

which permits longitudinal movement of collagen fascicles and supports blood vessels, lymphatics, and nerves (Fig. 7). Tendons typically carry tensile forces (tractions). However, at regions where tendons wrap around an articular surface, large compressive stresses are produced. Interestingly, tendons in these regions assume a cartilage-like appearance. Tendons that bend sharply, such as the flexor tendons of the hand, are enclosed by a tendon sheath that acts as a pulley and directs the path of the tendon (Fig. 8). A bifoliate mesotenon originates on the side of the bend opposite from the pulley friction surface and joins the epitenon that covers the surface of the tendon. The sliding of this type of tendon is assisted by synovial fluid, which is extruded from the parietal synovial membrane and from the visceral synovial membrane or epitenon (Fig. 9). Tendons not enclosed within a sheath move in a straight line and are surrounded by a loose areolar connective tissue called the paratenon, which is continuous with the tendon.

Tendons receive their blood supply from vessels in the perimysium, the periosteal insertion, and the surrounding tissue via vessels in the paratenon or mesotenon. Tendons surrounded by paratenon have been referred to as vascular tendons, and those surrounded by a tendon sheath, as avascular tendons. In tendons surrounded by a paratenon, vessels enter from many points on the periphery and anastomose with a longitudinal system of capillaries (Fig. 10). The vascular pattern of a flexor tendon within a tendon sheath is quite different. Here the

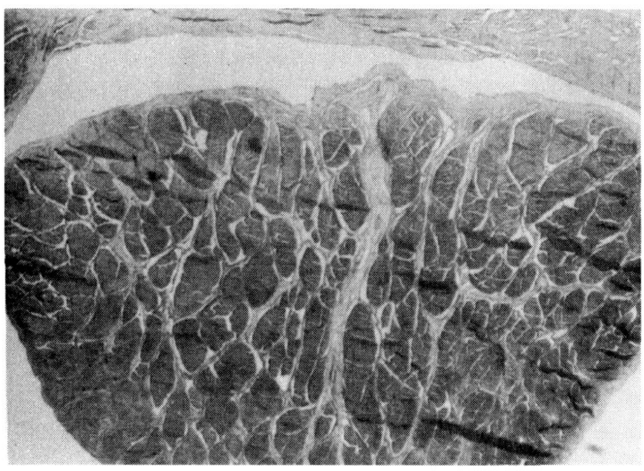

Figure 7
Photomicrograph of a cross section of a human flexor tendon showing the connective tissue (endotenon) that surrounds the fascicles of the tendon (H&E, X25).

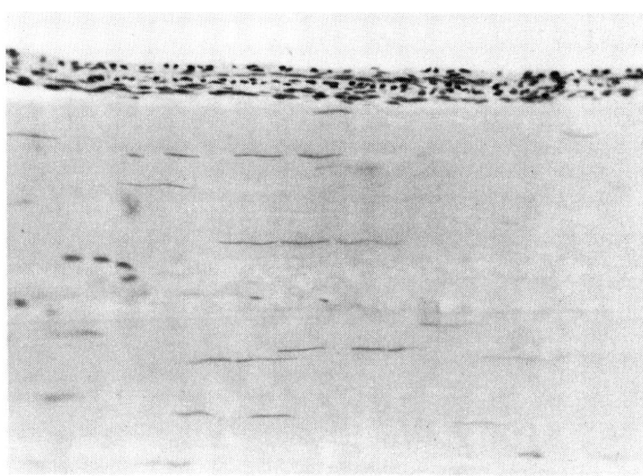

Figure 9
Longitudinal section of a human flexor tendon illustrating the epitenon on the surface of the tendon (H&E, X125).

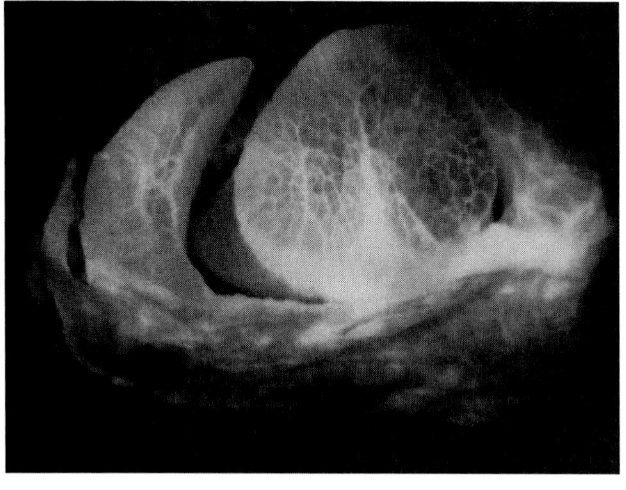

Figure 8
Cross section of a human flexor tendon (flexor digitorum superficialis, flexor digitorum profundus) at the midportion of the proximal phalanx of the third digit. The endotenon tissue of the profundus is clearly visible.

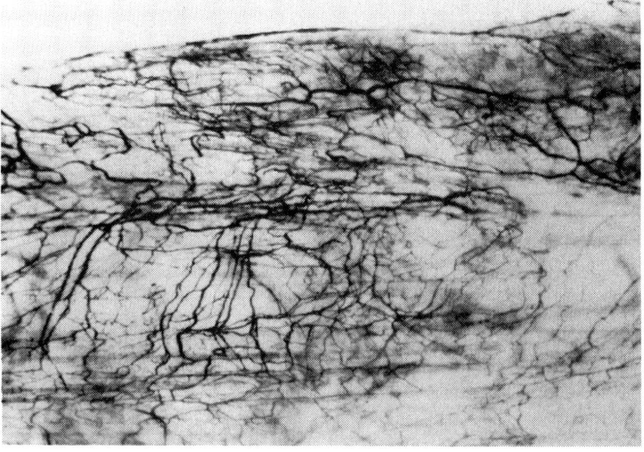

Figure 10
India ink injected (Spalteholz technique) calcaneal tendon of a rabbit, illustrating the vasculature of a paratenon-covered tendon. Vessels enter from many points on the periphery and anastomose with a longitudinal system of capillaries.

mesotenons are reduced to vincula (Fig. 11). This avascular region has led a variety of investigators to propose a dual pathway for tendon nutrition: a vascular pathway and, for the avascular regions, a synovial (diffusion) pathway. The concept of diffusional nutrition is of primary clinical significance in that it implies that tendon healing and repair can occur in the absence of adhesions (that is, a blood supply).

Biomechanics

The chapter on biomechanics and the glossary will be helpful to the reader who is not familiar with the terminology and the constructs of biomechanics.

Tensile Properties

Tendon possesses one of the highest tensile strengths of any soft tissue in the body, both because collagen is the strongest of fibrous proteins and because these fibers are arranged parallel to the direction of tensile force. The material properties of tendon depend mainly on the mechanical properties and architecture of the collagen fibers, elastin fibers, and proteoglycans.

The material properties of tendon, its stress-strain relationship, are similar to those of other collagenous soft tissues such as ligament and skin. The stress-strain curve begins with a toe region, in which the tendon stretches (strains) easily, without

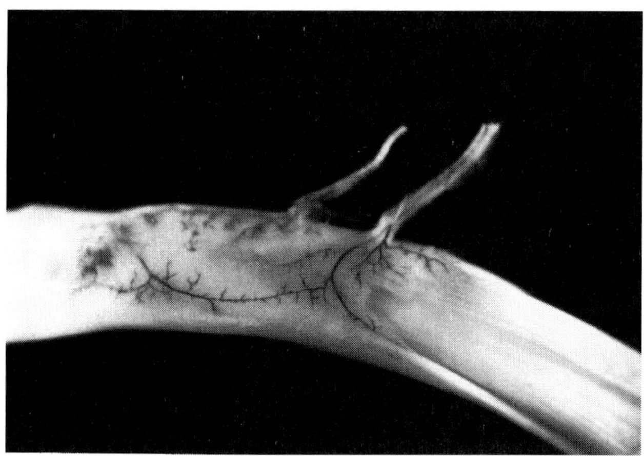
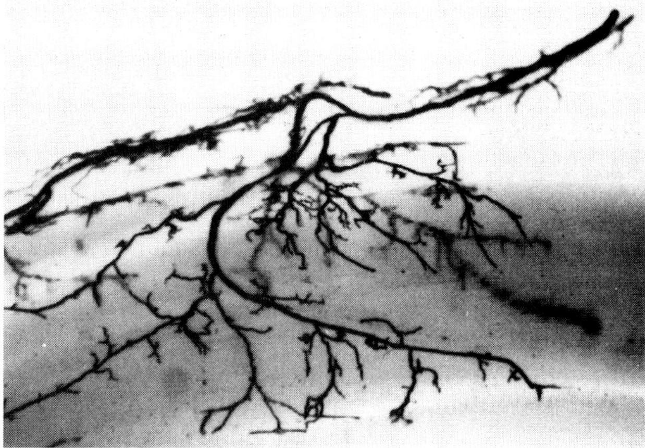

Figure 11
Left, India ink injected specimen illustrating the vascular supply of the flexor digitorum profundus in a human through the vinculum longus. **Right,** Close-up of specimen (Spalteholz technique) showing the extent of the blood supply from the vinculum longus. The vessels in the vinculum divide into the dorsal, proximal, and distal branches, giving off vertical vascular loops into the tendon substance.

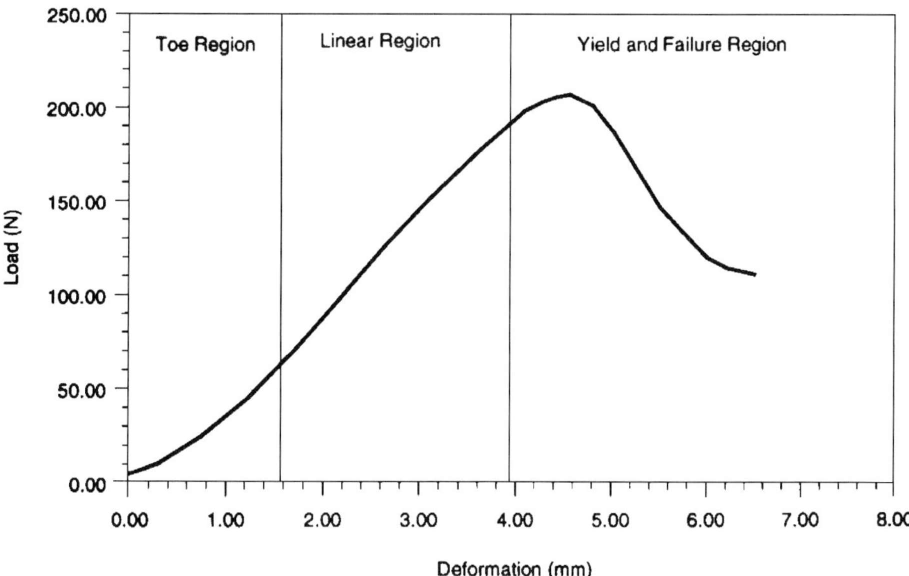

Figure 12
Basic stress-strain or load-deformation curve for tendon.

much force (Fig. 12). This behavior has been attributed to the straightening of the crimped fibrils and the orienting of the fibers in the direction of loading. The toe region is rather small in tendon because the collagen fibers are nearly parallel with the long axis of the tendon, and less realignment is required. In addition, the toe region decreases with age because the amount of crimp decreases with age.

As strains are increased, the toe region is followed by a fairly linear (straight) region, the slope of the line in this region has been used to represent the elastic modulus of the tendon. Following the linear region, at large strains, the stress-strain curve can end abruptly or curve downward as a result of irreversible changes (failure) or permanent stretching in the tendon. Thus, to fully describe the stress-strain curve, the slope of the linear region (the elastic modulus), the maximum stress (ultimate tensile strength) and strain (ultimate strain), and the area under the curve (the strain energy density to failure) are required.

Many factors affect these parameters. It has been found that, in animals, the ultimate tensile strength of tendons ranges from 45 to 125 MPa. In

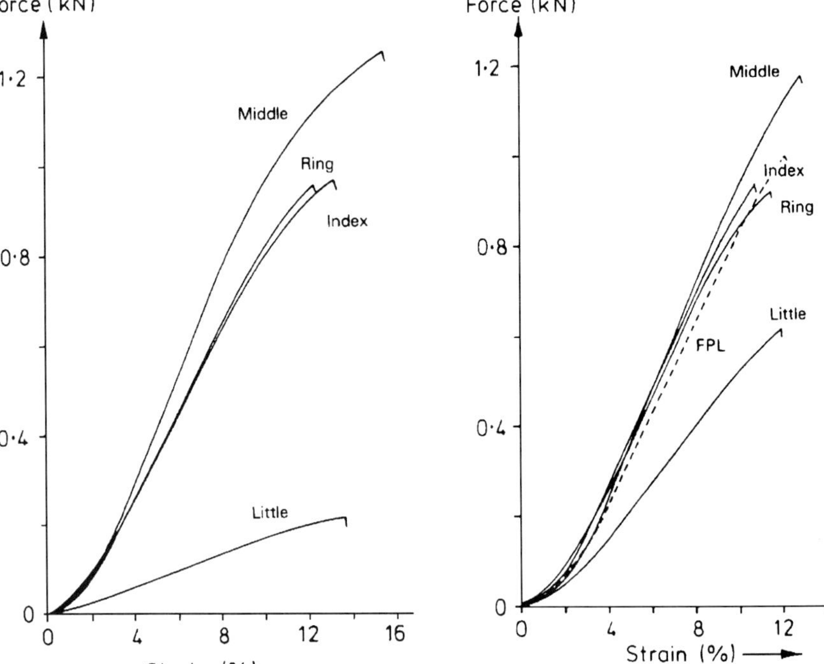

Figure 13
Left, Mean tensile behavior of tendons of flexor digitorum superficialis. **Right,** Mean tensile behavior of tendons of flexor digitorum profundus and flexor pollicis longus. (Reproduced with permission from Pring DJ, Amis AA, Coombs RRH: The mechanical properties of human flexor tendons in relation to artificial tendons. *J Hand Surg (Br)* 1985;10:331–336.)

humans, the elastic modulus ranges from 1.2 to 1.8 GPa, the ultimate tensile strength of tendons ranges from 50 to 105 MPa, and the ultimate strain ranges from 9% to 35%. The elastic strain energy recovered when a tendon is unloaded is 90% to 96% per cycle at physiologically relevant strain rates, indicating that tendons do not waste much energy during activity. In particular, the structural properties of human flexor tendons have been studied extensively (Fig. 13). Average breaking forces are 0.965, 1.252, 0.955, and 0.212 kN for the flexor superficialis of the index, middle, ring, and little fingers, respectively (1 kN = 223 pounds). Failure strains are in the range of 11% to 15%.

Tendons, like all other soft tissues, have viscoelastic material properties. In other words, their elongation depends not only on the amount of force, but also on the rate and history of force application. Tendons exhibit stress relaxation, creep, and hysteresis as a result of viscoelasticity. When performing a cyclic test by repeated loading and unloading of a tendon, the stress-strain curve shifts to the right (becomes less stiff, Fig. 14). This is important physiologically, because the loading of tendons encountered in activities of daily living usually is cyclic. The viscoelastic response will regulate not only the tension, but also the elongation and, thus, the characteristics of muscle contraction. For example, in an isometric contraction, the length of the muscle-tendon unit remains constant; however, because of creep, the tendon elongates, allowing the muscle to shorten. Physiologically, the change in length of the muscle decreases the rate of muscle fatigue. Thus, tendon creep increases muscle performance in an isometric contraction.

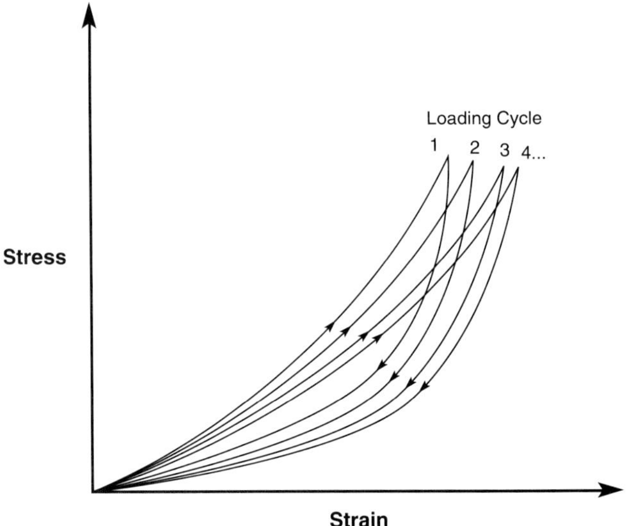

Figure 14
During cyclic loading of tendon, the stress-strain curve gradually shifts to the right. Usually, after 10 cycles, the curves become quite repeatable and steady.

Like those of other collagenous tissues, the properties of tendon are strain-rate dependent. An increased elongation speed (a higher strain rate) makes the tendon stiffer. However, for tendons, this strain-rate dependency is not as pronounced as it is for other soft tissues. The sensitivities of tensile strength, ultimate strain, and strain energy to strain rate have been studied for rat tail tendons at high (720%/s) and low (3.6%/s) strain rates. At a high strain rate of loading, the onset of permanent stretching was delayed, resulting in an increased ultimate strain and tensile strength (Fig. 15). These viscoelastic characteristics are thought to be a result of the viscous properties of the interfibrillar matrix of mucopolysaccharides (ground substance). Tendon, which contains more collagen and less ground substance than other soft tissues, demonstrates fewer viscoelastic effects and is more purely elastic than other soft tissues.

Factors Affecting Mechanical Properties

Many factors have been identified that influence the tensile properties of tendons. They include the viscoelastic effects discussed above, the anatomic location, the amount of activity, and the age of the tendon.

Anatomic location Tendons from different anatomic locations experience different biomechanical and biologic environments. Not surprisingly, tendon structural properties vary with location. The tensile strength and stiffness of the digital flexor tendons of adult miniature swine are about twice those of the digital extensor tendons. Further, the hysteresis of extensor tendons is twice as large as that of the digital flexor tendons. These differences increase with age and maturation (Fig. 16). At birth, the digital flexor and extensor tendons have identical material properties. The reason for the change in tendon properties with location is probably multifactorial. One hypothesis is that the cross-link stabilization that occurs in collagen during growth and aging, which results in increased stiffness and strength, takes place more rapidly in the flexor tendons than in the extensor tendons. This change may also be influenced by the level of stress experienced in vivo. Further, biochemical analysis shows that the digital flexors have a much higher collagen concentration than the digital extensors.

Exercise Exercise has a positive long-term effect on the structural and mechanical properties of swine tendons. The stiffness, ultimate tensile strength, and weight of the tendons increase as a result of long-term exercise training. The crimp angle and crimp length have been found to be influenced significantly by exercise. Exercise may also enhance collagen synthesis; this possibility is confirmed by results of biochemical studies of collagen metabolism after physi-

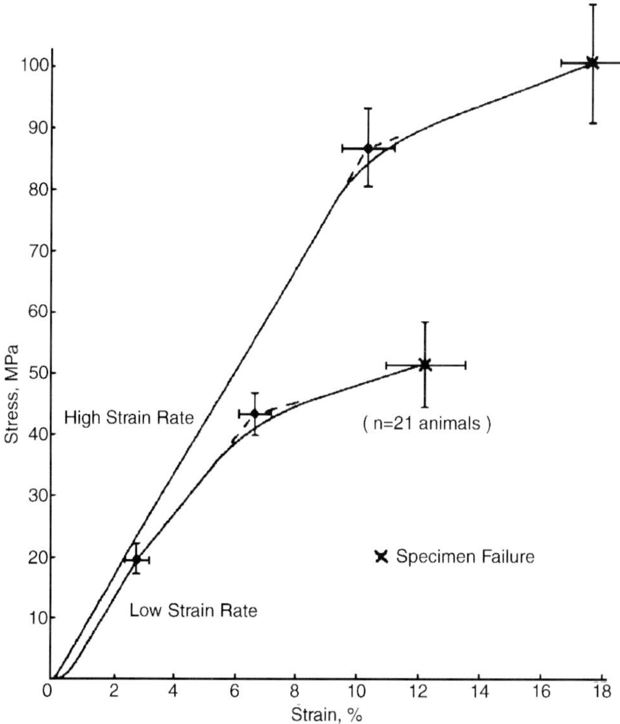

Figure 15
The tensile response of mature rat tail tendon at high (720%/s) and low (3.6%/s) strain rates. (Reproduced with permission from Haut RC: Age-dependent influence of strain rate on the tensile failure of rat-tail tendon. *J Biomech Eng* 1983;105:298.)

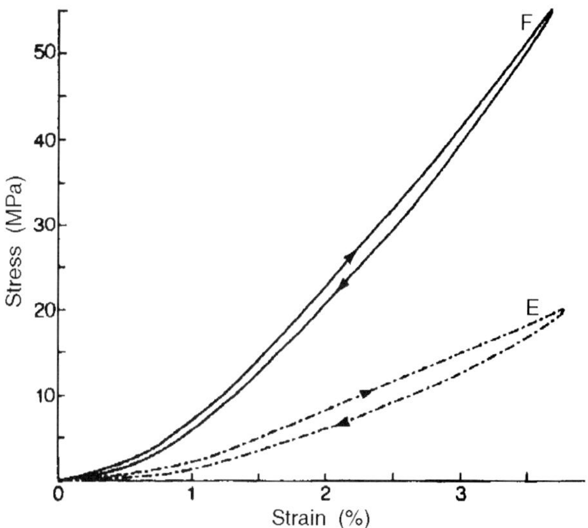

Figure 16
Examples of stress-strain curves obtained from digital flexor (F) and extensor (E) tendons of adult pigs. Arrows show loading and unloading directions. Elastic modulus values at peak stress are 1.8 and 0.7 GPa, and hysteresis values are 7% and 19%, respectively. (Reproduced with permission from Shadwick RE: Elastic energy storage in tendons: Mechanical differences related to function and age. *J Appl Physiol* 1990;68:1036.)

cal stress. Furthermore, tendons subjected to exercise have a high percentage of thick collagen fibrils. The thick fibrils can be expected to withstand greater tensile forces than thin fibrils because they contain a higher number of intrafibrillar covalent cross-links.

Age Age has a great influence on the mechanical properties of tendons. An age-related decrease in crimp angle decreases the toe region of the stress-strain curve. The stiffness and modulus within the linear region increase up to skeletal maturity and then remain constant. Before maturity, the linear region is followed by a single yield region in which irreversible elongation and structural damage take place (Fig. 17). A near-zero modulus is observed in this yield region. After maturity, this single yield plateau is not as obvious and is replaced by two distinct yield regions. The ultimate stress and strain also increase with maturation.

Experimental Considerations in Tensile Testing of Tendons

There are a number of technical difficulties associated with the experimental measurement of tensile properties of tendons, which readers should be aware of and appreciate when reviewing results reported in the literature.

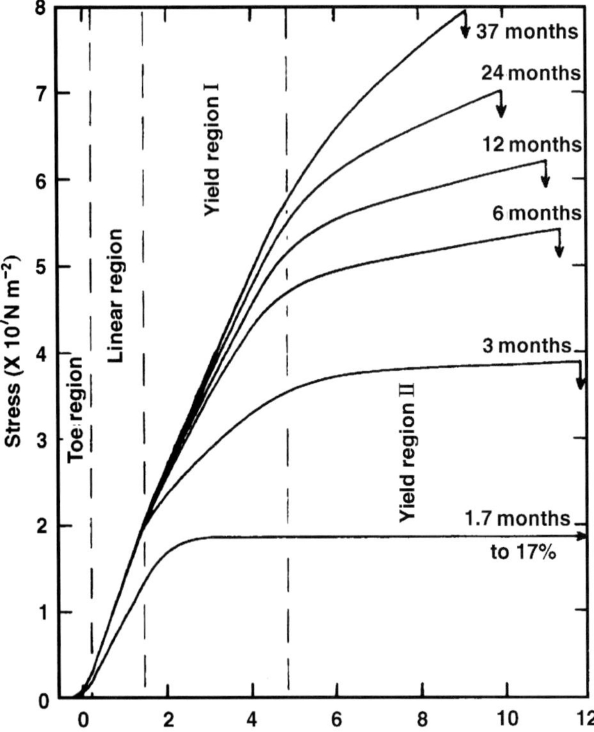

Figure 17
Stress-strain behavior of rat tail tendon as a function of age. (Adapted with permission from Kastelic J, Baer E: Deformation in tendon collagen, in Vincent JFV, Currey JD (eds): *The Mechanical Properties of Biologic Materials.* Cambridge, Cambridge University Press, 1980, pp 397–435.)

Testing environment The environment in which tendons are tested, including the specimen hydration and the temperature, affect the measured mechanical properties. Collagenous tissue swells in water and physiologic saline, and swells markedly in acid solution with an associated decrease in tendon stiffness. On the other hand, dehydration of the tendon causes it to stiffen and increases the failure stress. Temperature influences mechanical behavior, and elevated temperatures (39°C to 45°C) may cause irreversible structural damage. Results of a study on the effects of temperature on human digital tendons indicated the creep rate to be temperature dependent. The stiffness of canine Achilles and patellar tendons decreased significantly from 23°C to 49°C. A quantitative relationship also has been demonstrated between temperature and the viscoelastic properties of the canine medial collateral ligament.

Gripping the tendon Slipping of the tendon in the test grips has been a significant problem in experimental biomechanics for a long time. This slipping produces falsely large elongation measurements and may suggest failure at erroneously low forces. For small tendons such as rat tails, methods in which two looped ends are jammed into a hole or methods that involve wrapping the ends around a cylindric surface give satisfactory results with no slippage or tearing of the tendon in the grips. For larger tendons, special treatment of the ends is required. Methods in which the tendon ends are bound with wire, suture, or adhesive material have been used. Freezing the tendon ends into a fluid medium has been another successful method for securing test specimens with minimal structural damage.

Strain measurement In some studies, the movement between the clamps has been used to represent the elongation of a specimen. Unfortunately, slippage frequently results in erroneous measurements of tendon elongation. This method also assumes that the strain in the tendon is uniform along its length; however, it has been demonstrated that the distribution of strain is not uniform throughout the test specimens. Usually, the strain near the clamps is greater than twice the midsubstance strain. It is preferable to use an extensometer, which can provide strain measurements of the middle substrate of the tendon during testing. Optical methods that depend on either surface markers or markers inserted into the tendon can also be adopted for these measurements.

The initial length The definition of the initial length used in strain calculations (the gauge length) has a considerable effect on the reported mechanical properties because small forces produce large changes in length (strains) in the initial portion of the test as a result of the low stiffness of the toe region. Initial length affects not only the strain measurements but also the stiffness and modulus calculations. To help standardize testing, the gauge length usually is defined either based on observation of the morphologic appearance of the specimen in situ, or by the application of a small initial force (a preload).

Test specimen geometry The measured tensile strength of the whole tendon is usually lower than that of single fibers or fiber bundles. Two reasons for this phenomenon have been suggested. First, it is more difficult to grip thicker tendons; slippage must be prevented without causing structural damage and premature failure at the clamps. Second, the stress in thicker tendons is distributed more unevenly among the tendon fibers, leading to the sequential failure of fiber bundles.

Cross-sectional area for stress measurement Tensile stress is the tensile force divided by the cross-sectional area. An accurate measure of cross-sectional area is, therefore, of great importance. In early studies, gravimetric methods were used. In others, histologic sections have been used to measure area; however, this usage does not allow for the study of injury, because the specimen is destroyed to determine its area. Mechanical methods to measure width and thickness, with area obtained by assuming some cross-sectional shape such as a rectangle or ellipse, have also been used. These methods suffice for geometrically simple structures but produce large errors for structures with complex geometries.

Noncontact methods have the advantage of not deforming the material to measure its area, and these methods can be used for more complex geometries. They are, however, considerably more expensive. Noncontact methods generally involve an optical system and an image reconstruction technique. These include the shadow amplitude method, the profile method, and the laser micrometer method.

Biomechanical Modeling of Tendons

Characterization and prediction of the behavior of the body is the primary function of biomechanical models. The use of relatively simple mathematical expressions to describe the behavior of a component (a tendon) allows construction of a larger model (a joint). The relevance of modeling to orthopaedics stems from the prospective use of models to evaluate the effects of a therapeutic intervention, and to aid in the design of prosthetics and instrumentation. To characterize the force-elongation or stress-strain relationships, called a constitutive relationship, a variety of mathematical functions are considered to best represent the empirically obtained data. In general, stress σ has been related to strain ε in the power function,

$$\sigma = a\varepsilon^{b} \quad \textbf{(Eq. 1)}$$

or logarithm function,

$$\sigma = a + b \log \varepsilon \quad \textbf{(Eq. 2)}$$

in which a and b are constant.

This type of description treats the response of the tendon as nonlinear and elastic; that is, stress depends only on strain, and not on time. Cyclic loading, relaxation, and creep tests can be performed to characterize the viscoelastic responses. For example, a cyclic elastic modulus (the ratio of stress and strain at different frequencies) can be determined from cyclic testing and used to understand how rate of loading affects the stress-strain behavior. The relaxation function (measured stress versus time divided by the initial stress) can be derived from stress relaxation data and a similar creep function can be determined in the creep test. These functions describe the way in which stress and strain change with time.

The viscoelastic properties of tendon commonly have been described with the quasi-linear viscoelastic theory. This theory combines the elastic functions relating stress and strain with the relaxation function relating stress and time. With this theory, the stress at any time, from any strain, can be determined mathematically. This theory has proven to be very useful in characterizing not only tendon, ligament, and smooth and cardiac muscle, but also the structural responses of the intervertebral disk and the cervical spine as a whole.

Tendon Injury, Healing, and Repair

Tendon injury occurs as a result of direct trauma, laceration or contusion, and indirect trauma, tensile overload. Direct trauma frequently involves injury with sharp tools. Although direct injury can involve any tendon, it is of special importance to the hand and upper extremity, because of both its frequent incidence and its critical role in hand function. The healing process following direct injury has been studied extensively, and it has been shown to be intimately related to the inflammatory process and, therefore, to tendon vascularity.

Indirect injury mechanisms are multifactorial and depend heavily on anatomic location, vascularity, and skeletal maturity, as well as the magnitude of the applied forces. When the force (stress) in the muscle-tendon-bone complex exceeds the tolerance of this structure, injury (failure) occurs in the weakest link. Most tendons can withstand tensile forces larger than can be exerted by their muscles or sustained by the bones. As a result, avulsion fractures and tendon ruptures at the muscle tendon junction occur much more commonly than midsubstance tendon ruptures. In the flexor tendons of the hand, for example, avulsion of the bony insertion of the tendon occurs mainly in young adults during athletic events, and the ring finger is injured most often (75%). While the risk for injury depends on the forces applied and the strength of the tendon, it is interesting to note that the flexor digitorum profundus of the ring finger is significantly weaker than that of the long and index fingers.

Indirect injury to the tendon midsubstance requires the presence of preexisting pathology during the mechanical overload. This requirement is supported by the study of a number of different tendon injuries. Achilles tendon rupture typically occurs in middle-aged individuals engaged in a strenuous activity. The rupture is abrupt, frequently accompanied by a popping sensation, and many patients have no previous history of injury or discomfort. Histologic study of these injuries reveals a pathologic pattern described as angiofibrotic hyperplasia. This pattern suggests that a degenerative process or a failure of normal tendon remodeling has taken place prior to rupture. Relative avascularity, inflammatory disease, and other local factors also contribute to midsubstance ruptures. For example, extensor pollicis longus midsubstance rupture occurs as a result of attrition of the tendon against a bony prominence in rheumatoid arthritis patients. Tendon attrition in the absence of inflammation also is cited frequently as a factor in midsubstance rupture. For example, attrition of the rotator cuff and biceps brachii against the anteroinferior aspect of the acromion have long been thought to contribute to rupture of these tendons.

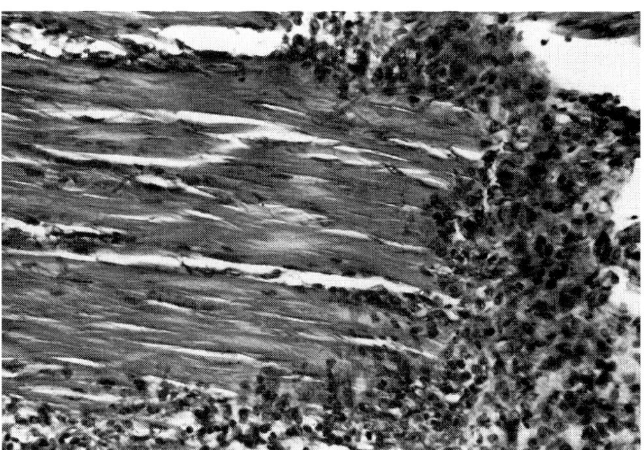

Figure 18
Longitudinal section of a rat calcaneal tendon three days after surgical transection and suture reapposition. Note the predominance of inflammatory cells in the wound. Some fibroblasts may be noted (H&E, X125; Courtesy of Dr. Scott Wolfe, New York).

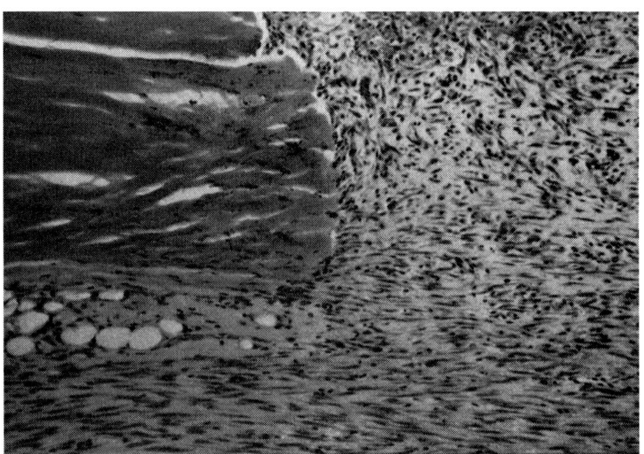

Figure 19
Longitudinal section of a rabbit tendon one week after surgical transection and suture reapposition. Note the increase of fibroblasts from the paratenon migrating into the wound (H&E, X100; Courtesy of Dr. Larry Stein, University of Illinois).

Healing Process In A Paratenon Covered (Vascular) Tendon

After the paratenon and tendon are incised, the wound fills with inflammatory products, blood cells, nuclear debris, and fibrin (Fig. 18). This tissue has no tensile strength. During the first week, proliferating tissue from the paratenon penetrates the gap between the tendon stumps and fills it with undifferentiated and disorganized fibroblasts. Capillary buds invade the area and together with the fibroblasts compose the granulation tissue between the tendon ends (Fig. 19).

Collagen synthesis can be detected as early as the third day. The process begins with an increased concentration in the protein mucopolysaccharides, which aids in the polymerization of the monomeric collagen. The endoplasmic reticulum of the fibroblasts synthesizes a precursor of collagen. This triple chain helix depends on heat-sensitive hydrogen bonds to connect the hydroxyl groups of hydroxyproline to the ketoimide groups of other amino acids. In this milieu, the collagen molecules begin to polymerize into fibrils. These fibrils progressively accumulate more collagen molecules until they have increased in size to become histologically visible thin wavy forms.

After two weeks, the tendon stumps appear to be fused by a fibrous bridge. Dramatic fibroblast proliferation and collagen production in the granu-

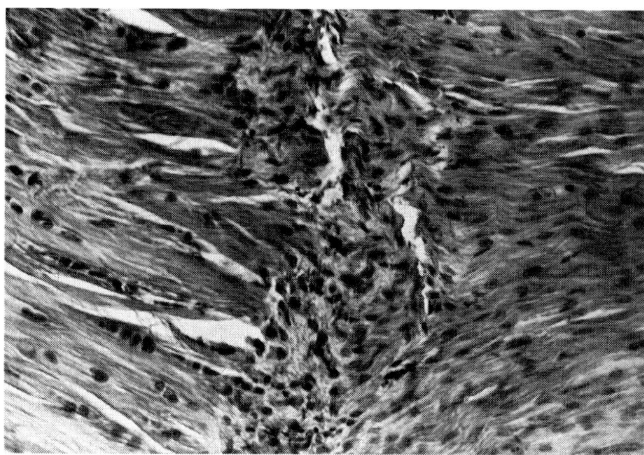

Figure 20
Longitudinal section of a rat calcaneal tendon two weeks after surgical transection and suture reapposition. Collagen fibers continue to migrate into the wound and are oriented perpendicular to the long axis of the tendon (H&E, X125; Courtesy of Dr. Scott Wolfe, New York).

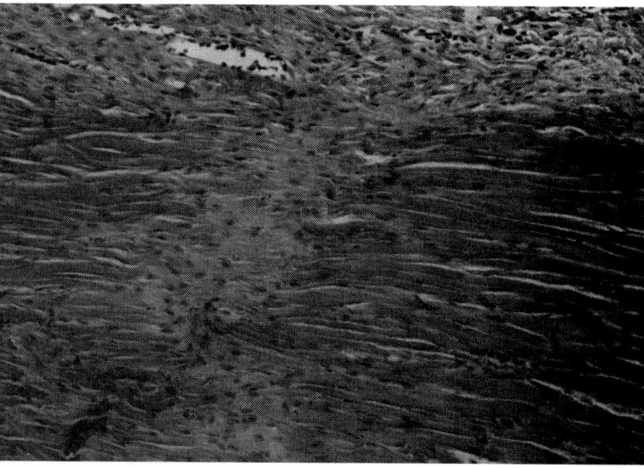

Figure 21
Longitudinal section of a rat calcaneal tendon 21 days after surgical transection and suture reapposition. The collagen within the wound neotendon begins to show evidence of longitudinal orientation.

lation tissue continue. The growth and migration of the collagen fibers between the tendon stumps are oriented perpendicular to the long axis of the tendon (Fig. 20). In an animal model, type I collagen production in the wound, documented by radiolabeled proline uptake, increases to 15 to 22 times normal. This rate of synthesis decreases slowly over a period of several months.

Histologically, the tendon stumps show a marked increase in fibroblast and vascular proliferation and a decrease in other cellular reactions. Fibroblasts and collagen fibers bridge the gap and physically unite the tendon ends. The fibrovascular tissue migrating from the paratendinous tissue blends with the epitenon to form the tendon callus (Fig. 21). During the third and fourth weeks, fibroblasts and collagen fibers near the tendon begin to orient themselves along the long axis of the tendon as a result of stress (Fig. 22). Only the collagen near the tendon reorganizes; the more distant scar tissue remains unorganized. The reorientation of collagen fibers is called secondary remodeling.

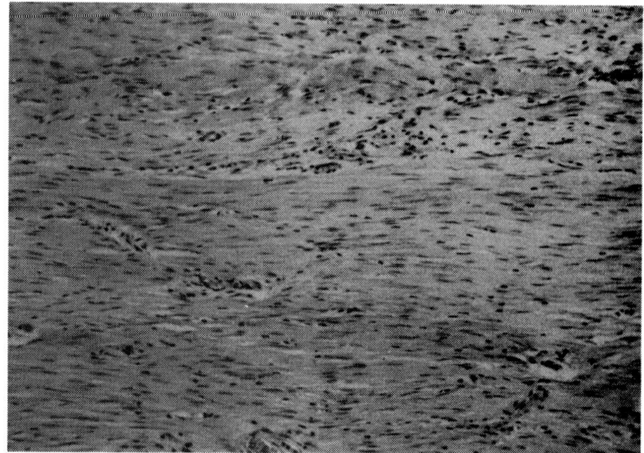

Figure 22
Longitudinal section of a rabbit tendon 28 days after transection and suture reapposition. Note the increased cellularity and vascularity within the repair neotendon and the longitudinal orientation of the collagen bundles (H&E, X100; Courtesy of Dr. Larry Stein, University of Illinois).

The two important factors of secondary remodeling, the increase in the biomechanical properties and the reduction in the mass of scar tissue, continue for many months. Tensile strength increases as a result of both the increasing degree of organization of the collagen fibers along the lines of stress and an increase in the number of intermolecular bonds between collagen fibers. Ultimate force increases despite the decrease in total mass of the scar (that is, a reduced cross-sectional area to resist force). Monomeric collagen production, fibril reorientation, and cross-linking all depend on the presence of applied stresses in the tendon. In the absence of stress, collagen production decreases, and remodeling does not occur. As the healing proceeds, remodeling continues until by the twentieth week there is minimal histologic difference in vascularity and cellularity between the scar and the normal tendon.

Healing Process In A Sheathed (Avascular) Tendon

The healing of a tendon that is enclosed by a tendon sheath has been a controversial topic for many years. Data from early investigations suggested that healing of these tendons was affected by granulation from the tendon sheath. Incised digital flexor tendons in the dog healed by means of a scar produced by fibroblasts derived from the tendon sheath and surrounding tissues. The tendon cells themselves played no active role in this repair. However, results of recent experimental investigations have demonstrated that tendon cells appear to have intrinsic capabilities of repair. Flexor tendons in cell culture are able to participate in the repair process; a tissue cap forms on the lacerated tendon ends by means of proliferation and migration of cells from the epitenon and endotenon (Fig. 23).

In this study, the flexor tendons of rabbits were transected through 90% of their thickness and placed in cell culture. At three weeks, cells from the epitenon migrated into the wound site and differentiated into phagocytes or macrophages. These chains of migrating epitenon cells were frequently joined together via desmosomes. Within the endotenon there was an increase in the number of cells. The cells looked like metabolically active fibroblasts that had well-formed granular endoplasmic reticulum with dilated cisternae containing electron-dense material, indicative of protein synthesis. By six weeks, the number of phagocytes within the repair site had increased. By nine weeks, cellular activity at the repair site continued, and cells migrating from the epitenon retained a phagocytic appearance. The fibroblasts within the endotenon also continued to show evidence of metabolic activity, and an extracellular matrix of collagen fibrils in various stages of polymerization was evident. Thus, two cellular processes are involved: phagocytosis by differentiated epitenon fibroblasts and collagen synthesis by cells of the endotenon.

It appears, therefore, that, in the proper environment, the tendon itself is capable of repair. In repaired tendons treated with controlled passive motion, this intrinsic response, originating from the epitenon, predominates. In the immobilized tendon, however, healing occurs through the ingrowth of connective tissue from the digital sheath and cellular proliferation of the endotenon (Fig. 24).

Tendon Repair

Issues surrounding tendon repair are numerous, and a detailed discussion is beyond the scope of this chapter. Suture material, the type of suture repair, knotting of sutures, continuous passive motion, weightbearing, and, of course, the nature and location of the injury, all impact on the quality of the tendon repair.

There are numerous suture techniques that take advantage of the mechanical strength of the tendon. For example, sutures passed between fascicles are easily pulled out. Sutures placed parallel to the tendon also pull out of the tendon at low forces. This observation has led to the development of current techniques in which a suture is passed perpendicular to the tendon before passing it across the injury; that is, parallel to the tendon (Fig. 25). In vitro evaluations have shown that perpendicularly passed sutures result in stronger tendon-suture-tendon constructs. These constructs typically fail by

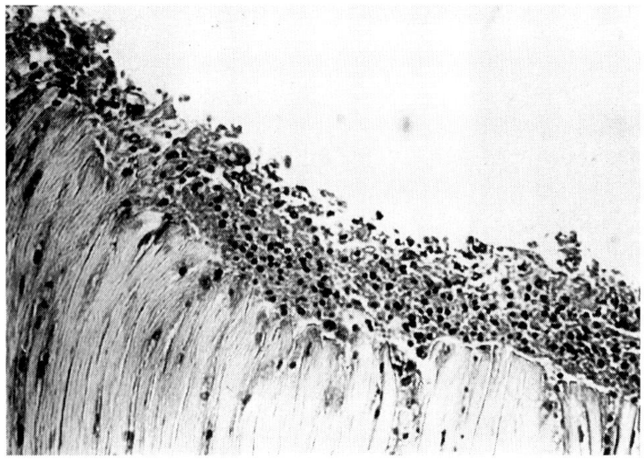

Figure 23
Photomicrograph of monkey flexor tendon after six weeks on culture, showing focal area of cellular proliferation. Note the apparent cellular migration from within the endotenon matrix at the tendon end (Courtesy of Dr. P. R. Manske, St. Louis).

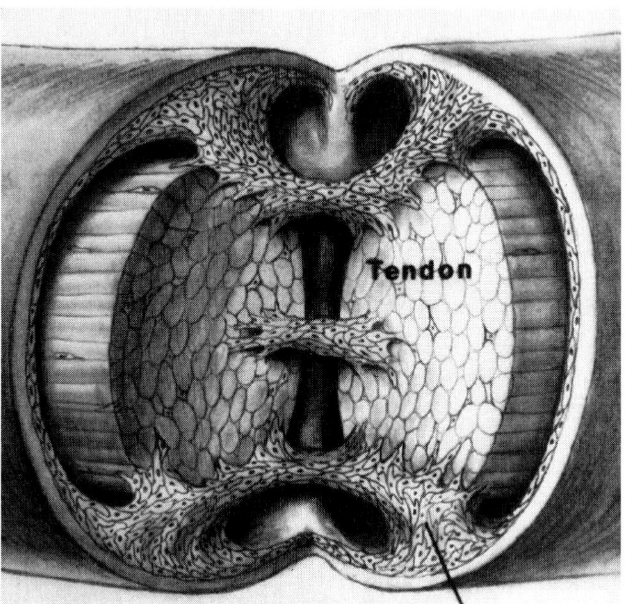

Figure 24
Schematic drawing of an immobilized tendon illustrating extrinsic and intrinsic repair (Courtesy of Dr. R. H. Gelberman, Boston).

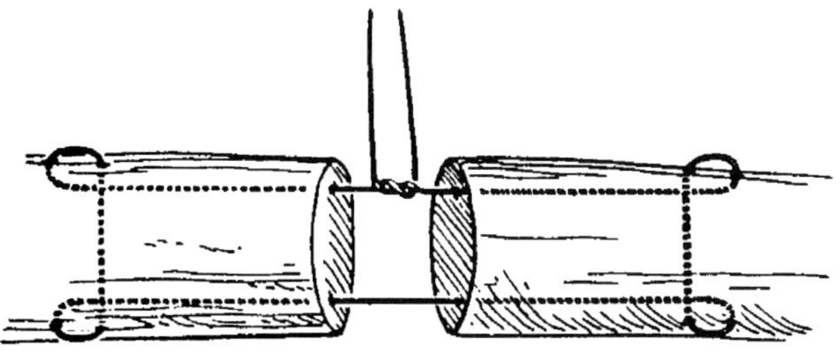

Figure 25
Schematic drawing of a tendon repair. The perpendicular portion of the suture increases the strength of the repair without compromising tendon vascularity. (Adapted with permission from Kleinert HE, Schepel S, Gill T: Flexor tendon injuries. *Surg Clin North Am* 1981;61:267–286.)

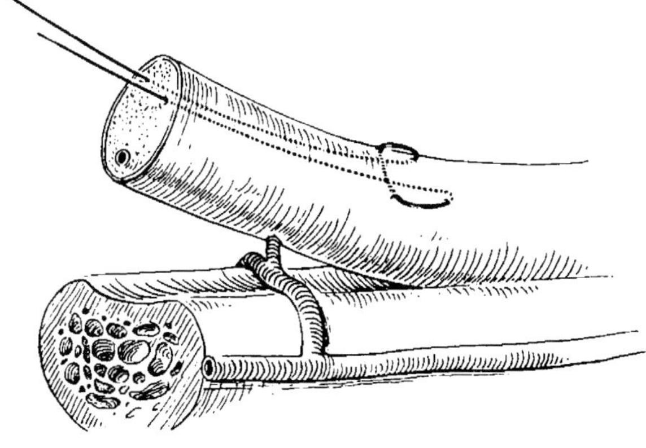

Figure 26
Schematic drawing of a suture placed in the volar surface of the tendon to avoid injury to the longitudinal vessels. (Reproduced with permission from Kleinert HE, Stilwell JH, Netscher DT: Complications of tendon surgery in the hand, in Sandzen SC Jr (ed): *Current Management of Complications in Orthopaedics: The Hand and Wrist.* Baltimore, MD, Williams & Wilkins, 1985, pp 206–227.)

suture rupture, indicating that the suture-tendon interface strength exceeds the strength of the suture.

Suture repair must also minimize gap formation between the tendon stumps, because even small gaps have been shown to adversely affect outcome. The ability of a construct to resist gap formation depends on the geometry of the construct, the amount of tension placed on the suture, and on viscoelastic creep that occurs not only in the tendon, but also in many suture materials. The resistance to gap formation as a mechanical parameter and modified repair techniques to minimize gap production have been evaluated in in vitro studies. The importance of the peripheral epitendinous suture to the repair strength and the resistance to gap formation have been noted.

Mechanical strength alone, however, is an insufficient measure of the likelihood of success, because mechanical strength at the expense of blood flow will compromise repair. For example, the placement of sutures in the volar aspect of the tendon has been advocated to avoid injury to the dorsally located intrinsic longitudinal vessels (Fig. 26).

Animal studies have provided valuable insight into many of these variables. These studies also allow for histologic and biochemical evaluation of the repair process. Limitations in animal studies include the large number of variables that merit evaluation, the variations in healing potential of the animal, the expense of long-term follow-up, and the difficulty in controlling the rehabilitation process. Determination of the optimal rehabilitation regimen remains a challenge in tendon repair. Early weight-bearing or aggressive early active mobilization of repaired tendon has been shown to result in rupture and gap formation because of the early weakness of the repair. However, carefully controlled early passive mobilization stimulates the repair and improves the strength of the tendon in the first few months following repair. Additionally, small motions applied early have been shown to reduce the number of adhesions associated with tendon healing. Thus, an optimum level of stress and motion exists that promotes healing without resulting in additional damage to the repairing tendon.

Tendon Transfer

Tendon transfers require considerable clinical experience and acumen. Indications for tendon transfers are numerous and include peripheral nerve injury and replacement of ruptured tendons in rheumatoid patients and patients with central nervous system disorders such as cerebral palsy. Considerations for transfer include the absence of inflammation and edema, the mobility of the joints, adequacy of the tissue bed, adequacy of skin coverage, and the potential for an effective line of action of the transferred tendon.

While these and many other factors contribute to the selection and staging of tendon transfers, the primary biomechanical considerations for the donor muscle include the expendability, excursion, and strength of the muscle being transferred. The expendability of a muscle depends on the particular clinical condition of the patient. Tendon excursion is proportional to the number of sarcomeres connected in series in the muscle; that is, it is proportional to the length of the muscle. Effective tendon excursion includes the sum of the contraction length from rest plus the traction length from rest plus the effect of intercalary joints (tenodesis effect). The tenodesis effect refers to the effective increase in excursion of a tendon that can occur when it crosses two joints.

The maximum contractile force of a muscle depends on the number of myosin-actin cross bridges acting in parallel. (In the clinical literature, this quantity is frequently misnamed the muscle power or muscle strength.) Therefore, the muscle force is proportional to the muscle's cross-sectional area. Muscle is capable of exerting a force of approximately 35 N/cm^2 of midmuscle belly cross section. Although the size of muscles varies considerably from patient to patient, the comparable size of muscles in a given patient remains relatively constant. For example, the flexor carpi radialis has the same contractile force as the pronator teres and half the contractile force potential of the flexor carpi radialis. Based on these concepts, the capacity of the muscle to do work, the product of the force and the distance through which it acts, is proportional to the product of the muscle's length and cross-sectional area. Therefore, the capacity of the muscle to do work is proportional to the mass of the muscle.

The relationship between the excursion and force of the muscle must be coupled with the needs of the recipient joint, including adequate joint torque generation and adequate range of motion. These relationships depend both on the properties of the muscle and on the insertion site of the tendon. Insertion of the muscle away from the axis of rotation of the joint increases the joint torque that the muscle can produce (torque = force × perpendicular distance). However, the range of motion decreases as the angular rotation is approximately equal to the total excursion/distance to the joint axis of rotation. Thus, for a given muscle, joint torque and range of motion have an inverse relationship governed by the insertion site of the tendon.

To select an appropriate tendon for transfer, two lists should be created: one of needed functions and one of working tendons. Nonexpendable tendons are removed from the list. The remaining tendons then can be connected to the needed functions based on the force and excursion needs of the transfer. Selection of an appropriate transfer for particular deficits has been studied extensively.

Ligament

Anatomy

Classified as a dense connective tissue, ligaments are grossly and microscopically similar to tendons. Ligaments are short bands of tough, flexible fibrous connective tissue, which connect bones or support viscera. Grossly, ligaments appear as band- or cable-like structures with few distinguishing landmarks. Closer examination reveals a high level of hierarchical organization. Ligaments contain rows of fibroblasts within parallel bundles of an extracellular matrix composed primarily of type I collagen fibers (70% dry weight). Elastin, a fibrillar protein that affects the mechanical properties, is also present in both tendon and ligament in very small amounts (less than 1% dry weight). In some ligaments, the flaval and nuchal ligaments of the spine in particular, elastin forms the primary structural component, resulting in considerably different mechanical properties from nonelastin dominated ligaments.

The collagen matrix is composed of fibrils that are 150 to 250 nm in diameter and are grouped into fibers that are 1 to 20 µm in diameter, which, in turn, make up a subfascicular unit that is 100 to 250 µm in diameter. These subfascicular units are surrounded by a loose band of connective tissue known as the endotenon. Three to 20 subfasciculi bind together to form fasciculi, which range in diameter from 250 µm to several millimeters and are surrounded by an epitenon. Fascicles can be spirally wound, as in the anterior cruciate ligament (ACL), or they can pass directly from bone to bone, as in collateral ligaments. Unlike the smaller subunits, no molecular bonds connect the fascicles and, thus, they are free to slide relative to each other. The entire group of fascicles that form the ligament are surrounded by the paratenon.

Ligament insertion into bone represents a transition from one material to the other. Insertions are classified as either direct or indirect, the latter being considerably more common. Direct insertions contain morphologically distinct superficial and deep fibers. The superficial fibers of the insertion join with the periosteum. The deep fibers of the insertion attach at a 90° angle to the bone (Fig. 27). The transition of deep fibers from ligament to bone occurs in four distinct phases: ligament, fibrocartilage, mineralized fibrocartilage, and bone. The size of each zone varies with particular ligaments; however, the total length of the transition zone is less than 1 mm. Indirect insertions consist largely of a superficial layer that inserts into the periosteum at acute angles (Fig. 28). Sharpey fibers, collagen fibers that originate in the bone and terminate in the periosteum, may play a role in securing the indirect ligament insertion. A few deep fibers are present in indirect insertions, which insert directly into bone with the four distinct zones of direct insertions.

As in the case of tendons, the mechanical properties of ligaments are based on the anatomic features of crimping and of biochemical bonding between structural subcomponents. Ligaments differ from tendons in a number of ways. Ligaments contain a lower percentage of collagen and a higher percentage of ground substance than tendons. The collagen in ligaments also is organized more randomly than that

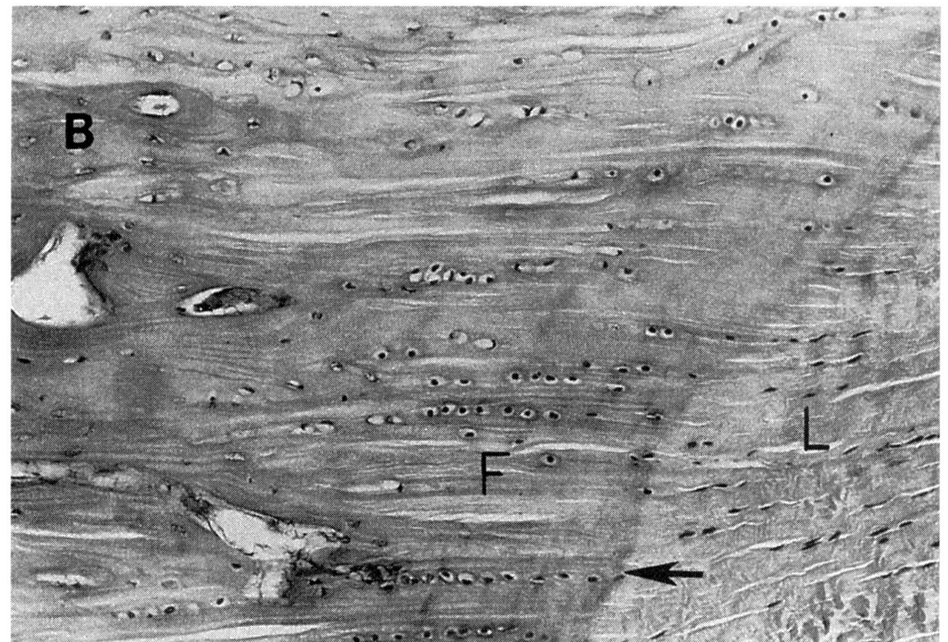

Figure 27
Femoral insertion of a rabbit MCL is typical direct insertion. The deep fibers of the ligament (L) pass into the bone (B) through a well-defined zone of uncalcified and calcified fibrocartilage (F). (Reproduced with permission from Woo SL-Y, Gomez MA, Sites TJ, et al: The biomechanical and morphological changes in the medial collateral ligament of the rabbit after immobilization and remobilization. *J Bone Joint Surg* 1987;69A:1200–1211.)

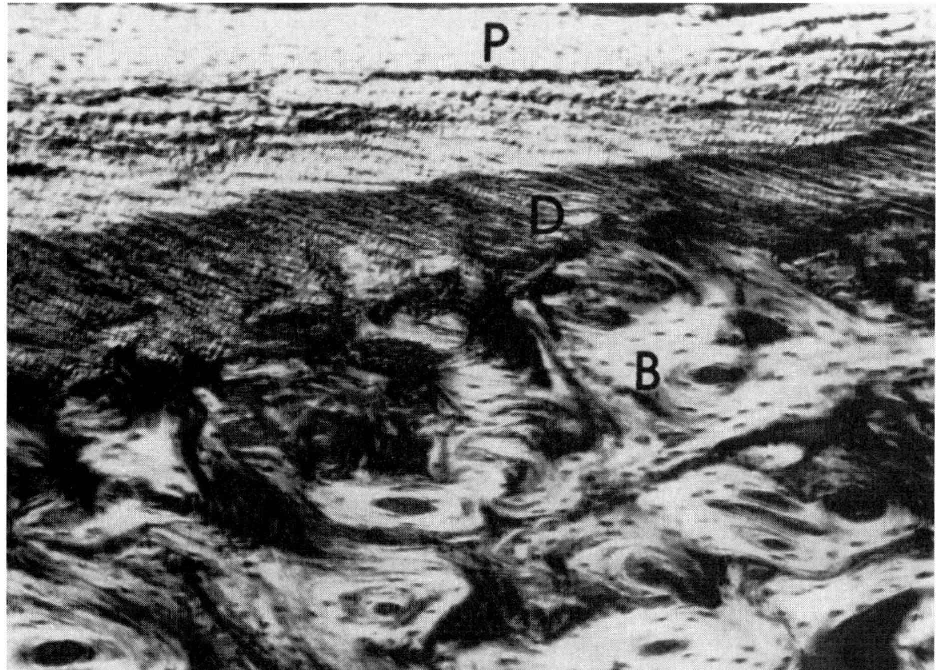

Figure 28
Indirect insertion of a rabbit MCL into the tibia showing superficial fibers (P) inserting into periosteum, and the deep fibers (D) inserting obliquely into bone (B). (H&E, X50; reproduced with permission from Woo SL-Y, Gomez MA, Sites TJ, et al: The biomechanical and morphological changes in the medial collateral ligament of the rabbit after immobilization and remobilization. *J Bone Joint Surg* 1987;69A:1200–1211.)

in tendons. Whereas tendon fibers are nearly all oriented along the long axis of the tendon, ligament fibers form a more weaving pattern.

Compared with surrounding tissues, ligaments appear to be hypovascular. Histologic study reveals, however, that throughout the ligament substance there is a uniform microvascularity, which originates from the insertion sites of the ligament. Despite the small size and limited blood flow of this vascular system, it is of primary importance in the maintenance of the ligament. Specifically, by providing nutrition for the cellular population, this vascular system maintains the continued process of matrix synthesis and repair. In its absence, damage from normal activities accumulates (fatigue), and the ligament is at risk for rupture.

Ligaments, which were once thought to be without innervation, have been shown in both human and animal studies to have a variety of specialized nerve endings. Evidence of pain fibers in spinal facet capsular ligaments has been demonstrated in histochemical studies. Innervation of a variety of ligaments including the medial collateral ligament (MCL) and ACL, which play a role in proprioception and nocioception, has been identified in other studies.

Biomechanics

General Tensile Properties

Tensile testing of ligaments involves measurements of force (or load) and elongation, generally from a bone-ligament-bone complex. For example, the femur-MCL-tibia complex (FMTC) is used to tensile test the MCL (Fig. 29). Like that of tendon, the load-elongation curve of the bone-ligament complex can be divided into an initial low stiffness region, the toe region, followed by a high stiffness region. Thus, ligament has a nonlinear, strain stiffening structural response. This behavior has been attributed to the undulating pattern (crimp) of the collagen fibrils and to the nonuniform recruitment of the individual fibers. During stretch, small initial forces produce large elongation because the crimp is easily straightened, after which much larger forces are needed for further stretch to cause the fibrils themselves to begin to elongate. Because of the varying degrees of crimping and the different orientations among the fibrils, each fibril uncrimps and begins to resist stretch at a different elongation of the ligament. As elongation is increased, more fiber bundles become uncrimped and oriented in the direction of loading. This recruitment of fibers produces a gradual increase in ligament stiffness.

Ligaments also display time and history dependent (viscoelastic) behavior that reflects the interactions of collagen and ground substance. That is, the stress in the ligament depends not only on the strain but also on time. The time dependence is illustrated by the phenomena of creep, stress relaxation, and hysteresis. History dependence means that the shape of the load-elongation curve will vary depending on the previous loading. For example, during cyclic loading and unloading of a ligament between two limits of elongation, the loading (top) and unloading (bottom) curves from one cycle follow different paths, and the area enclosed by the loop represents energy loss called hysteresis (Fig. 30). With increasing numbers of cycles, the peak force decreases. Eventually, after many cycles, the loading and unloading curves become similar to those in the previous cycle.

Creep and stress relaxation have a number of clinical implications. During ACL reconstruction, the initial force applied to tension the graft decreases over time as a result of stress relaxation. Stress relaxation in the human ACL and patellar tendon (PT) from young donors reduces graft forces to approximately 80% of their initial value after one hour. Thus, the amount of tension remaining in the graft postoperatively depends on the viscoelastic characteristics of the graft. These properties also are used to advantage during intraoperative spinal distraction. By applying the distraction in small steps separated by a few minutes, the peak forces applied to the instrumentation and its insertions on the vertebra can be reduced over 50% because of vertebral soft-tissue creep.

An additional viscoelastic effect in soft tissues, including ligament, tendon, and the intervertebral disk, is preconditioning. Following long periods of

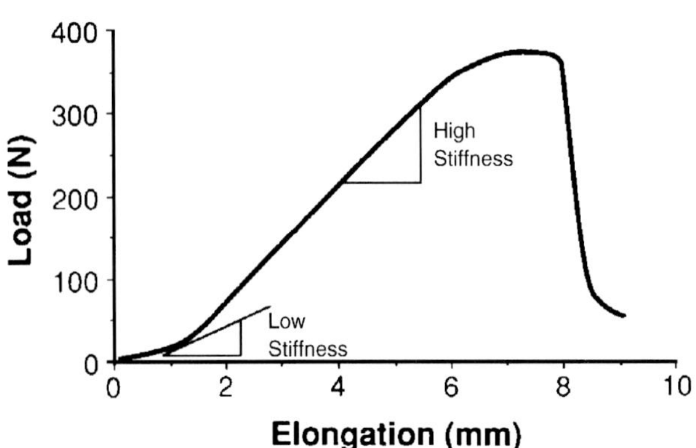

Figure 29
Typical load-elongation curve from tensile testing of a ligament, showing a region of low stiffness (toe region) and a region of high stiffness.

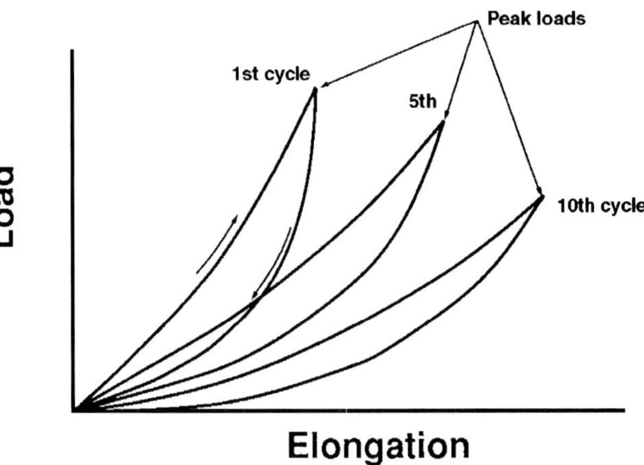

Figure 30
Typical loading (top) and unloading (bottom) curves from cyclic tensile testing of knee ligaments. The two nonlinear curves from any one cycle form a hysteresis loop. The area between the curves, called the area of hysteresis, represents the energy losses within the tissue.

inactivity (hours), the soft tissues imbibe additional fluid. The first few applications of force to the tissue extrude this extra fluid. Thus, the first few cycles following inactivity show greater stiffness and hysteresis energy loss than subsequent cycles. Following this warm-up, the behavior of the tissues becomes more repeatable. This cycling is called preconditioning and is an important part of biomechanical test protocols.

In addition to their being nonlinear and viscoelastic, a profound variation in the properties of ligaments has been found, which is based on species, anatomic location, biochemistry, previous exposure to stress, immobilization, age, and skeletal maturation. To further complicate understanding of the biomechanics of ligaments, significant differences in ligament mechanical properties can be observed based on the experimental technique used to study them. Difficulties are similar to those encountered in the study of tendon, and include gripping of ligaments, strain measurement, definition of the initial length, determination of the cross-sectional area, and others. Because of these complexities, it is impossible to use a single mechanical value to represent all ligaments. The following section presents current understanding of many of these factors, with particular attention to the ligaments of the knee.

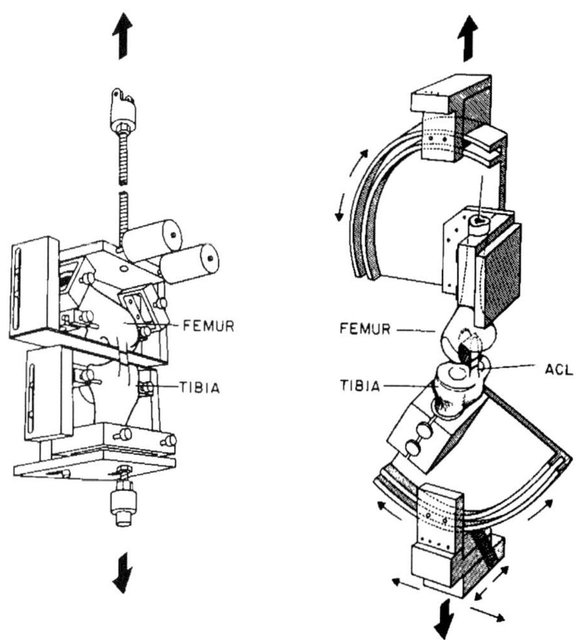

Figure 31
Anatomic preparations and testing system used to evaluate the MCL **(left)** and the ACL **(right).** The figure demonstrates the complexity of the test apparatus required to obtain meaningful in vitro data. (Reproduced with permission from Woo SL-Y, Newton PO, MacKenna DA, et al: A comparative evaluation of the mechanical properties of the rabbit medial collateral and anterior cruciate ligaments. *J Biomech* 1992;25:377–386.)

Mechanical Properties of Knee Ligaments

Because of their frequent involvement in knee injuries and different healing responses, extensive research has been devoted to contrasting the MCL and ACL. The two differ anatomically; the MCL is an extra-articular ligament that is relatively flat, whereas the intra-articular ACL has fibers that twist along the long axis of the ligament. Because of these anatomic differences, different experimental systems are required to evaluate these structures (Fig. 31). There are also histologic, ultrastructural, and biochemical differences. The structural properties for the human ACL and MCL are similar; the ultimate load, or load at failure, for both is between 340 and 390 N. The posterior cruciate ligament (PCL) is stronger, however, requiring 780 N to failure. The material properties of the human ACL, PCL, and lateral collateral ligament (LCL) are also similar, in contrast to those of the PT, which are quite different. The material properties of the rabbit medial and lateral portions of the ACL are similar to each other, but different from those of the MCL. The elastic modulus between 4% and 7% strain is approximately two times greater for the MCL than the ACL. The tensile strength of the MCL is over 70% greater than that of the medial ACL fascicles that fail midsubstance.

The higher modulus and tensile strength of the MCL compared to those of the ACL are attributed, in part, to morphologic differences. Rabbit MCL consists of more densely packed fiber bundles that have a lower frequency crimp pattern than the ACL. The sub-fascicular area fraction of collagen is significantly greater for the MCL than the ACL. Thus, the MCL has more force-bearing collagen fibers per unit area than the ACL. The mean fibril diameter is also greater for the MCL than the ACL, and larger diameter fibrils are believed to provide greater resistance to elongation.

Factors Influencing the Properties of Ligaments

A wide variety of factors influence the material properties of ligaments. Important factors in vivo include age, degree of maturation, rate of elongation, and the direction of the applied forces. Additional in vitro factors, which play an important role in the experimental evaluation of ligaments and the use of ligaments for surgical repair, include the above as well as temperature and freezing and sterilization techniques.

Strain rates The structural and material properties of ligament tend to increase with increasing rates of elongation (strain rates). This effect was studied in immature and mature rabbit MCL using elongation rates of 0.008 to 113 mm/s, which correspond to strain rates of 0.01 to over 200%/s. The structural properties differed between the lowest and highest strain rates, with larger differences occurring in the immature rabbits (Fig. 32). The ultimate load and energy absorbed were 2.3 and three times greater for the highest strain rate than for the lowest strain rate, respectively. The material properties followed similar trends, but the increases were less marked, especially for the mature group, in which the tensile strength of the MCL increased only 40% from the lowest to the highest strain rate (Fig. 33). Studies of the ACL at slow (0.003 mm/s), medium (0.3 mm/s), and fast (113 mm/s) elongation rates showed similar effects. Small differences were observed in the modulus between the slow and medium rates, but the modulus at the fast extension rate was 30% higher.

The influence of strain rate on injury has caused significant debate. Although clinical injuries to ligaments usually occur at high strain rates, many experimental studies use low to medium rates and do not produce midsubstance failure of the ligament. Several authors attribute this to the use of lower strain rates. Data from recent studies suggest that the status of the insertions, not the strain rate, may be the primary determinant of the type of injury produced in vitro.

Skeletal maturity Data from rabbit studies show a significant increase in the structural and mechanical properties of ligaments with skeletal maturation. Twofold, fourfold, and tenfold increases in linear stiffness, ultimate force, and energy absorbed at failure, respectively, are observed as the animals age from 3½ to 8½ months; physeal closure occurs at seven months. The modulus of the ligament substance also increases 5% to 15% during maturation (Fig. 34).

The modes of failure, that is, types of injury, also change with skeletal maturation. MCLs from rabbits with open epiphyses fail by tibial avulsion; MCLs from skeletally mature rabbits tear in the ligament substance. Thus, the insertion is the weakest link prior to physeal closure, and the ligament substance is the weakest link after closure. Histologic examination shows that active remodeling of the insertions and incomplete insertion of the deep ligamentous fibers into bone prior to maturation are possible causes of the avulsions. Stress relaxation is also more prominent in immature ligaments. Interestingly, immobilization interferes with the normal increase of ligament structural properties with skeletal maturity. Thus, the structural properties of immobilized, skeletally immature rabbit MCL decrease as the animal ages, unlike those of normal MCL, in which the strength increases with age until maturation.

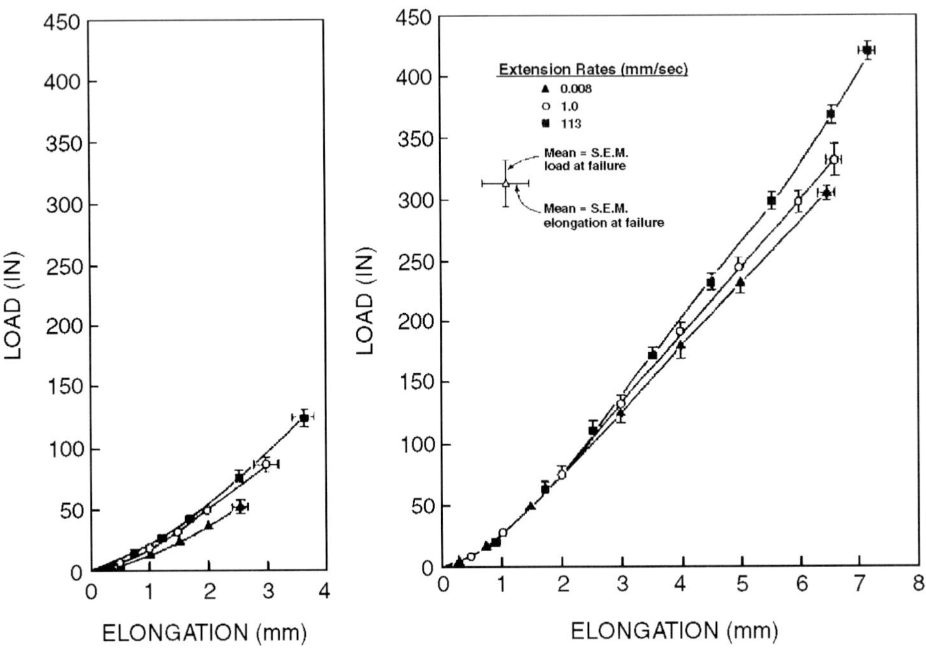

Figure 32
The structural properties (load-elongation curves) of the FMTC of skeletally immature **(left)** and mature **(right)** rabbits as a function of extension rate. (Reprinted with permission from Woo SL-Y, Peterson RH, Ohland KJ, et al: The effects of strain rate on the properties of the MCL in skeletally immature and mature rabbits: A biomechanical and histological study. *J Orthop Res* 1990;8:712–721.)

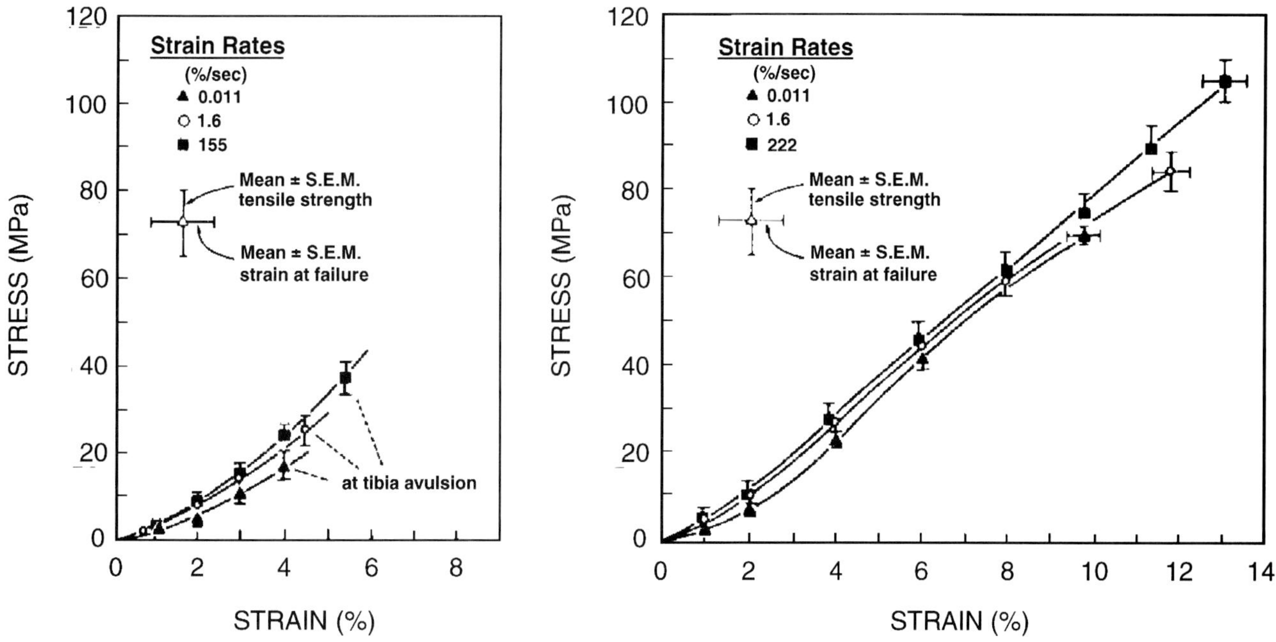

Figure 33
The material properties (stress-strain curves) of the MCL substance from skeletally immature **(left)** and mature **(right)** rabbits, and the influence of the rate of stretching of the ligament (strain rate) on the material properties. (Reproduced with permission from Woo SL-Y, Peterson RH, Ohland KJ, et al: The effects of strain rate on the properties of the MCL in skeletally immature and mature rabbits: A biomechanical and histological study. *J Orthop Res* 1990;8:712–721.)

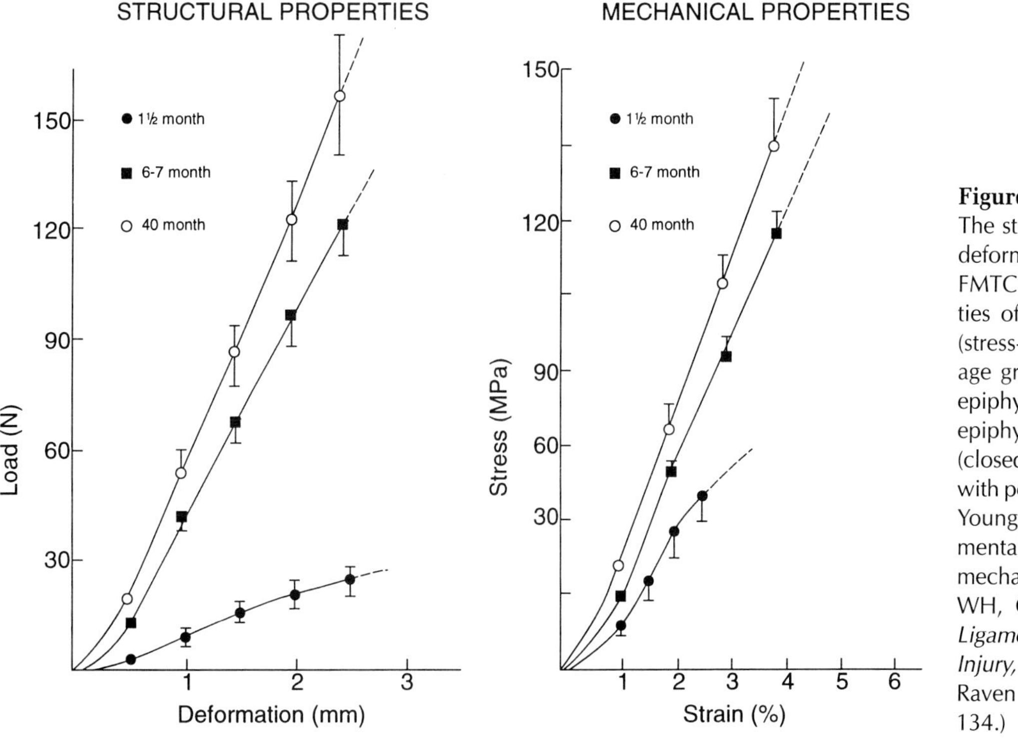

Figure 34
The structural properties (load-deformation curves) of the FMTC and the material properties of the ligament substance (stress-strain curves) for three age groups: 1½ months (open epiphysis), 6–7 months (closed epiphysis), and 40 months (closed epiphysis). (Reproduced with permission from Woo SL-Y, Young EP, Kwan MK: Fundamental studies in knee ligament mechanics, in Daniel D, Akeson WH, O'Connor JJ (eds): *Knee Ligaments: Structure, Function, Injury, and Repair.* New York, Raven Press, 1990, pp 115–134.)

Age In recent investigations of human femur-ACL-tibia complex (FATC), values of structural properties of FATCs from young human donors have been significantly higher than those from older donors. The stiffness and ultimate load for the young ACLs, ages 22 to 35 years, are reported as 242 ± 28 N/mm and 2160 ± 157 N, respectively, which are over threefold greater than for older specimens (Fig. 35).

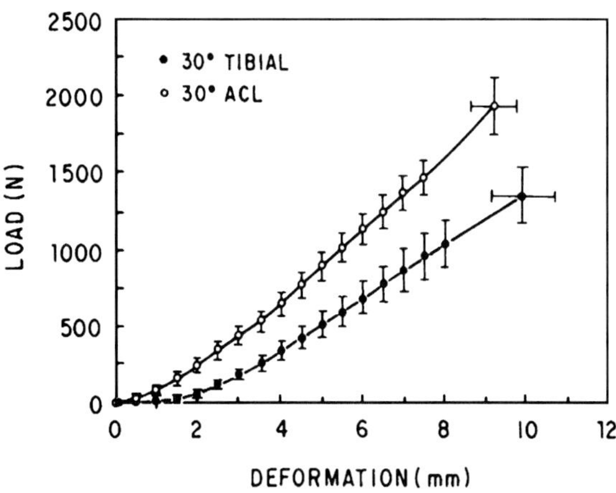

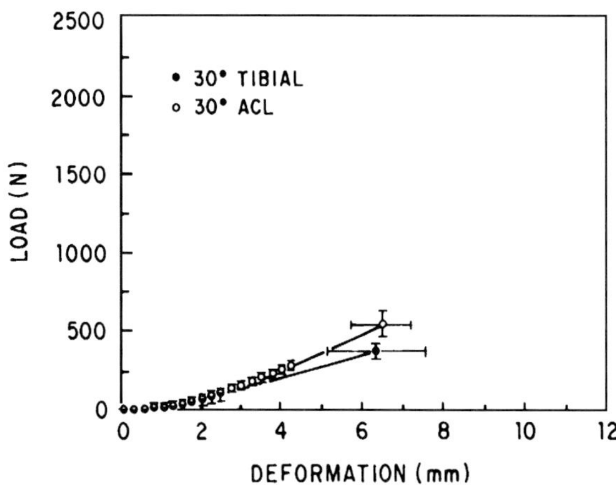

Figure 35
The structural properties (load-deformation curves) for the FATC tested at 30° of flexion along the tibial and ACL axes for younger **(left)** and older specimens **(right)**. (Reproduced with permission from Woo SL-Y, Adams DJ: The tensile properties of the human anterior cruciate ligament (ACL) and ACL graft tissues, in Daniel D, Akeson WH, O'Connor JJ (eds): *Knee Ligaments: Structure, Function, Injury, and Repair.* New York, Raven Press, 1990, pp 279–289.)

The values obtained for FATCs from younger donors should be used as a guideline for the strength requirements of ACL replacements.

Knee orientation and loading direction Because ligaments are structures and not simple materials, the direction of applied force and the initial position of the ligament have a large influence on the ligament's behavior; this is especially true of the ACL. The complex arrangement of the fiber bundles of the ACL makes uniform loading of the entire ligament cross section impossible. Applying the force in the direction of the ACL tenses a greater proportion of the fiber bundles than when the force is applied in any other direction. For example, the strength and stiffness of the FATC are greater when tested in the ligament direction than when tested in the tibial direction. In human cadaveric studies, the ultimate force was approximately 2,200 N for specimens tested in the ACL direction and 1,600 N when tested in the tibial direction (Fig. 36). The linear stiffness was approximately 240 and 220 N/mm for specimens tested in the ACL and tibial directions, respectively.

Data from rabbit studies show that ultimate force for the FATC decreases with increasing knee flexion when force is applied in the tibial direction. Other structural properties behave similarly. In contrast, flexion angle does not affect ACL strength when the force is applied in the ACL direction. Similar results are reported in canine studies.

Storage by freezing The effect of freezing on ligaments is of interest because freezing is a necessity during many biomechanical experiments and because freezing affects tissue allografts. One method used for freezing is to store knees with muscle and other tissues left intact to prevent dehydration. Each knee is double-wrapped in saline-soaked gauze, sealed in an airtight plastic bag, and frozen to -20°C. No significant differences in the structural proper-

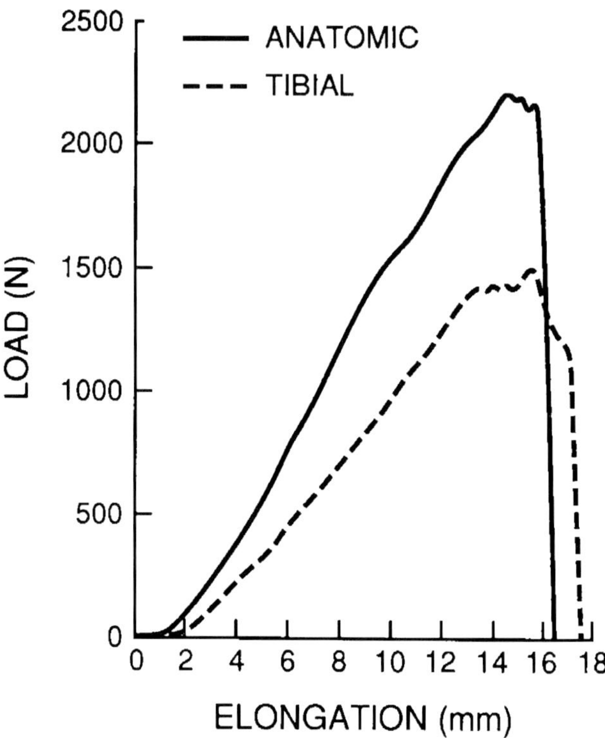

Figure 36
Typical load-displacement curves for the FATC tested along the ligament and tibial axes. (Reproduced with permission from Woo SL-Y, Hollis JM, Adams DJ, et al: Tensile properties of the human FATC: The effects of specimen age and orientation. *Am J Sports Med* 1991;19:217–225.)

ties of the FMTC or the material properties of the MCL have been noted between fresh rabbit knees and those frozen using this method. The one exception, which occurs during the first few cycles of loading and unloading, is a decrease in the area of hysteresis that becomes insignificant with further cycling. Similar results have been reported in other soft tissues.

Testing environment The in vitro environment has profound effects on ligament behavior. Maintenance of specimen hydration is of primary importance to the study of soft tissues. Temperature also has been shown to be of importance, although to a lesser degree than hydration. Increases in temperature from 2°C to 37°C resulted in a decrease in stiffness and a decrease in hysteresis energy. These factors have led many investigators to immerse their specimens in a physiologic saline bath where pH and temperature are closely controlled.

Contribution Of Ligaments To Joint Mechanics

Joint motion is a combination of translations and rotations that is determined by ligament forces, joint contact forces, externally applied forces, and muscle activity. This interaction allows joints to have a smooth motion as well as the ability to withstand large external forces. The nonlinear behavior of ligaments is uniquely suited to this task. In normal activities, ligaments are in the low stiffness region of the load-elongation curve and exert small forces on the joint. If the joint is subjected to excessively large forces, the ligament moves into the high stiffness region and produces large forces in an effort to limit excessive joint motion and provide protection to the joint.

Each ligament is not responsible for restraining only one particular motion, but rather contributes to joint stability in a number of motions referred to as primary and secondary stabilization. Typical primary stabilizers include the MCL resisting valgus angulation, the ACL resisting anterior tibial translation, and the PCL resisting posterior tibial translation. As secondary or passive stabilizers, ligaments play an important role in diagnosis of knee injury. Although many studies are performed using application of a single force, such as an anterior drawer force or a varus-valgus angulation, joint motions are generally three-dimensional, and the resistance encountered represents combinations of primary and secondary stabilization.

For example, the MCL has been reported to be a principal stabilizer of valgus knee angulation, although in some studies the ACL has been given a minor role. However, the contribution of the MCL and the ACL to valgus stability depends on the method used to evaluate it. Tests in which only varus-valgus angulation and proximodistal and mediolateral translation are permitted, called three degrees of freedom tests, which occur during a physical exam, demonstrate that an absent MCL produces valgus instability. This would suggest that the MCL is the primary stabilizer of valgus rotation. However, tests in which all motions except flexion-extension are permitted, five degrees of freedom tests, as might occur in normal gait, do not demonstrate valgus instability in the presence of an isolated MCL injury. Valgus instability in the five degrees of freedom test is present when the MCL is associated with an ACL injury. Thus, the injured MCL does not cause valgus instability, as long as the ACL remains intact.

An ACL-deficient knee is much more problematic in terms of total joint stability than the MCL-deficient knee. Midsubstance tears of the ACL, unlike ruptures of the MCL, generally will not heal, and produce knee instability in the majority of cases. Muscle strengthening can compensate for some of the instability, but most young, active patients do not return to the same level of activity because of the frequent occurrence of giving-way. Gait patterns appear to be affected, and muscle atrophy often is observed. Over time, the changes from normal joint kinematics frequently cause meniscal tears and joint degeneration. This scenario has led the orthopaedic community to advocate surgical intervention and has prompted investigators to perform in-depth studies of normal and ACL-deficient knee kinematics and reconstruction techniques.

The Effects of Immobilization, Remobilization, and Exercise

Rehabilitation regimens after musculoskeletal injuries often include immobilization to protect the afflicted tissues from further damage during the early healing phases. However, the side effects of immobilization are quite detrimental. Increases in joint stiffness caused by synovial adhesions and proliferation of fibro-fatty connective tissue have been observed clinically following immobilization. Joint contracture also has been hypothesized to be the result of new collagen fibrils forming interfibrillar contacts that restrict normal parallel sliding of fibers in ligaments. Quantitative assessment of joint stiffness in animals, following nine weeks of immobilization, demonstrated that large increases in torque and energy are required to extend the joints.

Ligament properties are also compromised by immobilization. Drastic decreases in the structural properties of rabbit MCL are observed after nine weeks of knee joint immobilization. The tensile load required for failure (ultimate load) of the FMTC is about 33%, and the energy absorbed at failure is only 16% of the contralateral nonimmobilized control (Fig. 37). Both tensile strength and elastic modulus of the MCL also are decreased with immobilization.

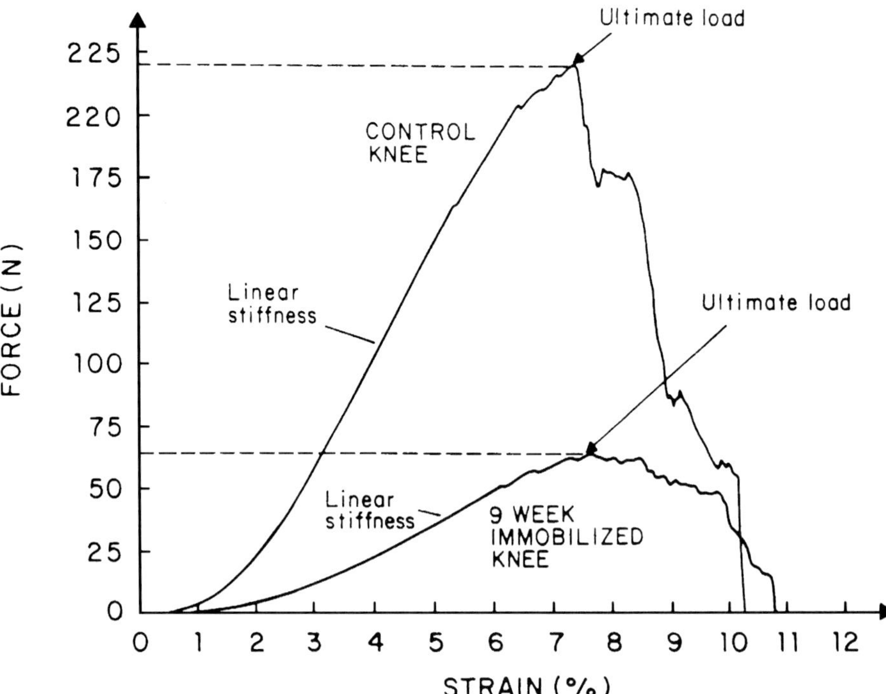

Figure 37
Force-strain curves of rabbit FMTC from control and immobilized limbs. (Reproduced with permission from Woo SL-Y, Gomez MA, Woo YK, et al: Mechanical properties of tendons and ligaments. II. The relationship of immobilization and exercise on tissue remodeling. *Biorheology* 1982;19:397–408.)

The decreases in structural properties of the bone-ligament-bone complex in rabbits are caused by a combination of changes to the insertions and to the ligament substance itself. Histologic evaluation of the MCL insertions following immobilization reveals marked disruption of the deep fibers inserting into bone. Osteoclastic activity results in subperiosteal bone resorption for the tibial insertion but little change to the femoral insertion. This resorption correlates with an increasing occurrence of failure by tibial avulsion in immobilized knees. Similar decreases in the properties of the ACL and FATC occur in primates. Investigators have observed subperiosteal resorption at both the femoral and tibial insertions.

The resumption of joint motion leads to a rather slow reversal in the effects of immobilization on the structural properties of the FMTC and FATC. The ultimate load and energy absorbed at failure of these two complexes reach 80% to 90% of control at one year. Histologic evidence of new bone formation at the ligament insertion reveals that the time required to return to normal is much longer than the immobilization period. In contrast, the material properties of the MCL substance return to normal after nine weeks of remobilization. These data illustrate a delayed recovery of the insertion compared to the ligament substance. Based on these data, the remobilization period should be on the order of months, following only a few weeks of immobilization.

The properties of the ligament substance and the insertion also are affected by exercise. Short-term exercise regimens, ranging from treadmill walking to running and swimming, have been studied by using various animal models and tend to show an increase in mechanical and structural properties. Following 12 months of exercise, the structural properties of the FMTC from swine increased when normalized to body weight. When exercised animals were compared to controls, a 38% increase in ultimate load and a 14% increase in stiffness were observed. The tensile strength and ultimate strain increased 20% and 10%, respectively.

Lifelong exercise consisting of treadmill running with an 11-kg backpack did not produce changes in the structural properties of the beagle MCL. Load-elongation curves of the FMTC between exercised and nonexercised, age-matched complexes were similar. The linear stiffness, ultimate load, ultimate elongation, and energy absorbed at failure were unaffected by the exercise, and only minimal changes in the material properties were observed. Although surprising, the lack of improvement in the structural/material properties might be attributed to the processes of aging, which could have masked the positive effects of exercise.

A relationship between different levels of stress and ligament properties undoubtedly exists. A representation of this relationship, derived from the results of the various studies, is depicted in Figure 38. Immobilization significantly compromises both the structural properties of the bone-ligament-bone complex and the material properties of the ligament, with weakening being more pronounced in the insertions. The material properties of ligament substance return to control levels after a short period of

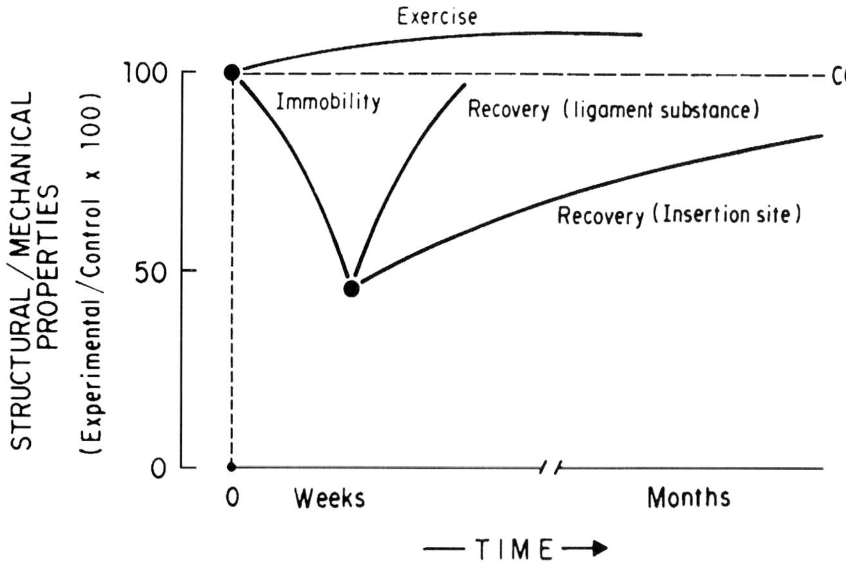

Figure 38
A schematic representation of the time course and magnitude of effects of various stress levels on the structural and mechanical properties of ligaments. (Reproduced with permission from Woo SL-Y, Gomez MA, Sites TJ, et al: The biomechanical and morphological changes in the medial collateral ligament of the rabbit after immobilization and remobilization. *J Bone Joint Surg* 1987;69A:1200–1211.)

remobilization, but the insertions require a much longer period of recovery to regain their previous properties. Thus, the complex remains weak, and avulsion injuries are more likely during this interval.

The changes in properties resulting from exercise or increased tension are not analogous to the marked decrease during immobilization or increase with remobilization. Although the properties are enhanced in response to exercise and increased tension, only moderate improvements are seen. Animal species, age, and sex, as well as the type, intensity, and length of the exercise activity contribute to minor variations in results.

Healing of Ligaments

Ligamentous injuries are classified into three grades or degrees. Grade I injuries, mild sprains, are an overstretching of the tissue without disruption. Although the tissue is grossly intact, microscopic examination reveals small hemorrhages and tearing, and electron microscopy reveals a pattern described as overstretched springs. Grade II injuries, moderate sprains, show gross tears and hemorrhages. Although continuity of the ligament is maintained, strength is greatly reduced. Grade III injury represents complete disruption of the ligament.

Inflammation and Healing of Ligaments

The healing of extra-articular ligaments is analogous to the repair process of other vascular tissues. Following injury there is exudation of blood and associated blood products from disrupted vessels, organization of a fibrin clot, vascularization of this fibrin scaffold, proliferation of cells, synthesis of an extracellular matrix, and, finally, remodeling of the repair tissue. Although this repair process occurs as a continuum, it has been divided into individual phases based on the morphologic and biochemical events that occur.

Phase I: Inflammation Following complete ligament disruption, the torn ends of the ligament retract and usually have an irregular mop-end appearance. In the extra-articular environment, damaged capillaries within the ligament and adjacent tissues produce a hematoma that fills the gap created by the retraction of the ligament ends. In response to the injury and their exposure to the fibrin clot, potent vasodilators, histamine, serotonin, bradykinins, and prostaglandins, are released. Bradykinins, in addition to vasodilation, increase capillary permeability, allowing transudation of fluid and movement of inflammatory cells into the extracellular space. The inflammatory mediators, in combination with the injured tissue and the forming coagulum initiate the healing process. These events usually occur during the first 72 hours following injury.

Histologically, inflammatory cells and erythrocytes fill the injured area. Leukocytes (polymorphonuclear cells and lymphocytes) migrate through capillary walls and disrupted blood vessels. This migration is followed by a gradual appearance of monocytic cells that, along with macrophages, begin phagocytosis of necrotic tissue. Capillary endothelial buds proliferate in the wound in response to an angiogenic factor secreted by the macrophage.

Toward the end of the inflammatory stage, fibroblast proliferation begins to occur. Thought to arise from undifferentiated mesenchymal cells, these fibroblasts produce a matrix of proteoglycan and collagen, forming a rudimentary scar. Considerable remodeling of the collagen takes place in this phase, with synthesis slightly exceeding degradation. Although most of the newly synthesized collagen scar is type III, a small amount of type I is produced. Type III collagen is thought to be responsible for early stabilization of the collagen meshwork, and type I collagen is more important to the long-term matrix properties.

Phase II: Matrix and cellular proliferation Matrix and cellular proliferation occurs over the next six weeks and is accompanied by increasing organization of the fibrin clot. The gap between the torn ligament ends is filled with a friable, vascular granulation tissue, and the fibroblast is the predominant cell type. At this stage, the scar is highly cellular and contains macrophage and mast cells in addition to fibroblasts. Vascular endothelial capillary buds communicate with adjacent capillaries in a diffuse network. Active collagen synthesis occurs during this phase in both the proliferating scar and the adjacent normal tissue. However, collagen concentration remains low because of the less dense, woven organization of the collagen framework. Spaces in this framework are thought to be filled with water and other extracellular components. Type I collagen is now the predominant matrix component, and the concentration of glycosaminogylcans also is increased. These biochemical changes correlate with an increase in the mechanical strength of the scar.

Phases III and IV: Remodeling and maturation After several weeks a gradual transition between the proliferative and remodeling phases takes place. There is a relative decrease in the cellularity and vascularity of the scar and an increase in its collagen density. In addition, polarized light microscopy of the ligament scar reveals a more organized collagen arrangement, with the collagen becoming aligned along the axis of the ligament.

Biochemically, there is a decrease in active matrix synthesis during this phase, and the biochemical profile of the matrix shifts toward that of normal ligament. While the collagen content of the healing ligament plateaus, the tensile strength of the ligament continues to increase. This increase is thought to reflect collagen reorganization, cross-linking, and other changes in the matrix. In an animal model, the scar formation is sufficient histologically at six weeks, and many have proclaimed complete healing on that basis. It should be noted, however, that while the ligament ends may appear to be united, several months are required for the scar tissue to remodel to achieve complete morphologic normalcy.

The ligament scar remains slightly disorganized and hypercellular. It is thought that as much as 12 months or more may be required to complete remodeling. Factors that influence healing and repair are numerous and include both host factors (biology) and biomechanics.

The above description of ligament healing relates predominantly to the collateral ligaments as an example of extra-articular ligament healing. Their anatomic location affords them direct access to the adjacent soft tissue vascular supply. In addition, the anatomy confines the scar to the gap between the torn ligament ends, effectively closing the gap and facilitating healing. In the intra-articular environment, the cruciate ligaments are not afforded this advantage. Results of experimental studies have shown that while the ACL has a profuse vascular response following injury, spontaneous repair does not occur. One of the many reasons could be the dilution of the hematoma by the synovial fluid, preventing the formation of a fibrin clot and, thus, the initiation of the healing mechanism.

Clinical and Biomechanical Aspects of Extra-Articular Ligament Healing and Repair

Clinical outcome following isolated tears of collateral ligaments generally is good. However, some investigators postulate that surgical repair is required, because the torn ends of the ligament form a gap that is filled by scar tissue rather than by true ligament. The possibility of reduced recovery time with the use of surgical repair and immobilization also has caused some to advocate primary surgical repair. However, clinical and experimental results reveal that nonoperative treatment achieves an equally good outcome.

Nonoperative treatment of grade III isolated MCL injury is preferable to surgical repair. In a prospective clinical trial, a total of 33 patients divided between surgical repair and nonrepair had equal clinical outcomes at 2.4 years; however, the 11.3-week rehabilitation period for the conservatively managed group was significantly reduced from the 14.9 weeks for the surgical group. Subsequent studies using the canine model support this finding and provide insight into the repair potential of the ligament. Specifically, at six weeks, the valgus rotations of the nonrepaired and repaired MCL were significantly higher than those of the control. However, at 12 and 48 weeks, the nonrepaired group had near normal valgus rotation, whereas that of the surgical group was larger than normal. The structural properties of the nonrepaired ligaments were also superior to those of the surgically repaired ligaments throughout the study and approached those of the controls at 48 weeks (Fig. 39). Despite the normal structural properties of the nonrepaired ligaments, the material properties of both the repaired and nonrepaired MCL were considerably weaker than those of the control. Tensile strength reached only 60% of control at one year. Histologically, this cor-

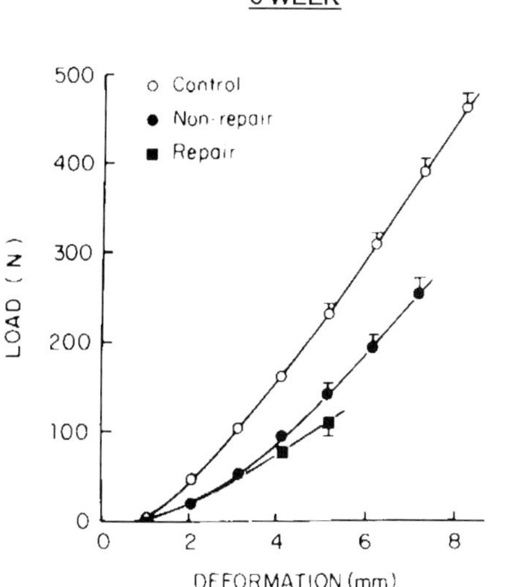

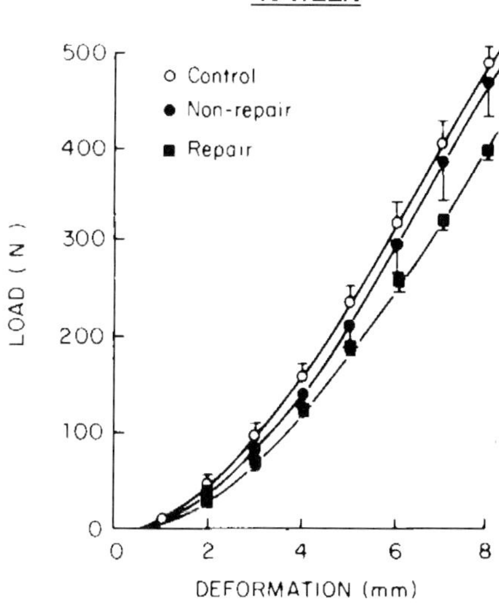

Figure 39
Structural properties of the repaired and nonrepaired canine FMTC at six and 48 weeks postoperatively. The controls are shown for comparison. (Reproduced with permission from Woo SL-Y, Horibe S, Ohland KJ, et al: The response of ligaments to injury: Healing of the collateral ligaments, in Daniel D, Akeson WH, O'Connor JJ (eds): *Knee Ligaments: Structure, Function, Injury, and Repair.* New York, Raven Press, 1990, pp 351–364.)

relates with a more irregular orientation of the collagen fibers.

Ligament reapposition following injury has short-term benefit in animal studies. When rabbit MCL is sutured and the healing response compared to that of MCL with a midsubstance gap, ultimate load and stiffness of the FMTC for the sutured group are greater than for the gap group up to 14 weeks postoperatively. Histologic analysis also reveals a less cellular and more organized collagen for the sutured group at three and six weeks postoperatively. The larger the gap, the greater the decrease in ultimate load and ultimate tensile strength. Both clinical experience and experimental studies demonstrate that nonoperative treatment of the isolated torn MCL is preferable to surgical repair. However, the healing does appear to depend on the size of the gap between the torn ends of the ligament. This fact suggests that the surrounding fascia likely maintain the torn MCL ends in close proximity, thereby yielding the satisfactory healing response of the isolated MCL injury without repair.

Allograft replacements for the MCL have been considered for severe injuries. In animal studies, they have been found to have long-term viability; however, the properties of the allograft are reduced from those of normal tissue. Fresh-frozen allograft FMTC were used to replace the MCL in the rabbit model. The highest ultimate load and energy absorbed at failure by the allograft occurred at three weeks and gradually decreased over time. Between 12 and 48 weeks posttransplantation, the ultimate load was only 50% to 60% of control and the energy absorbed at failure was 30% of that absorbed by the control FMTC. The tensile strength and modulus of the allograft were 30% and 30% to 40% of control, respectively, at 12 weeks. The allograft tissue was viable and vascular, but seemed to reach a new equilibrium that was different from normal. Its properties neither improved nor deteriorated once this equilibrium was reached. The central portion of fresh-frozen canine PT allografts have also been studied as MCL replacements. After a period of immobilization and remobilization, microangiographic and histologic evaluation revealed all reconstructed ligaments to be viable after one year of implantation. The ultimate load, that is, the load to failure, reached 71% of control at this time point, but the tensile strength was only 44% of control.

The management of MCL injury in the presence of ACL injury is a more complicated clinical problem. Of primary importance to this problem is the role of the ACL in stabilizing the MCL-deficient knee. As discussed earlier, the MCL is the primary stabilizer in constrained (three degrees of freedom) valgus rotation of the knee. In less constrained (five degrees of freedom) motion, as would occur during normal activities, valgus instability occurs only after ACL sectioning. Thus, valgus instability caused by a torn MCL can be compensated by the contributions of the remaining structures, the ACL in particular. However, loss of the ACL results in significant valgus instability. Therefore, the effects on MCL healing of transection of the ACL were investigated in a canine model. Although all MCL healed, the valgus rotation and mechanical properties of the healing MCL failed to recover to normal levels. Thus, MCL healing is dependent on ACL function.

Short-term joint immobilization in combined ACL-MCL injury reduces instability but has a negative effect on the FMTC strength in the rabbit model. Immobilized and nonimmobilized groups were compared at three, six, and 14 weeks postoperatively. The immobilized knees were similar to the normal knee, but the nonimmobilized knee had significant instability. However, the ultimate load in nonimmobilized MCL was significantly greater than in immobilized MCL. Joint immobilization was therefore believed to be of limited value for the combined MCL-ACL ruptures.

Clinical and Biomechanical Aspects of Intra-articular Ligament Replacement

Because midsubstance ACL tears usually do not heal, and the long-term sequelae of ACL-deficient knees include meniscal damage with secondary osteoarthritic changes, surgical intervention using autografts, allografts, or synthetic substitutes often is indicated. To develop and evaluate ACL replacements requires knowledge of the tensile properties of the ACL. In addition, the role of the ACL in controlling the normal rolling-sliding kinematics of the knee makes understanding its geometry, length, insertions, and intrinsic tension of primary importance to surgical reconstruction.

Although synthetic substitutes have been used as ACL replacements, by far the most popular replacements are biologic tissue grafts because of the potential for graft remodeling and integration into the joint. Experimental studies of the structural properties of the femur-graft-tibia complex have found the linear stiffness and ultimate load to be low in the initial postoperative period, and then to increase with time. Exposure of the graft material to excessive forces during the early remodeling phase, when it is weak, may be detrimental to the graft. Thus, understanding the biomechanical properties of grafts postoperatively is of primary importance to ACL reconstruction.

Autografts Various tissues, including the central and medial third of the bone-PT-bone complex, iliotibial tract (ITT), semitendinosus tendon, and gracilis tendon, have been employed as ACL replacements. The bone-PT-bone graft is presently the most popular graft because it has high ultimate load and bone blocks for direct bony fixation.

The time course of the remodeling process for PT grafts has been studied in various animal models such as the canine, sheep, goat, rabbit, and monkey. The general trend for the remodeling of PT autografts is for the ultimate load to reach 30% to 40% of the control FATC after one to two years, with some degree of increased anteroposterior joint translation and articular degeneration. For example, patellofemoral degenerative changes and increased anteroposterior joint translation were found in goats' knees reconstructed with a central one third PT. Structural properties were very low during the first few weeks after transplantation, but increased with time. Linear stiffness and ultimate load reached 35% and 45% of the control FATC, respectively, at 12 months. Similar findings were noted in a monkey model. In a canine model, the grafts were found to have an ultimate load less than 10% of the control FATC at the time of implantation because of fixation site weakness. At three months, the ultimate load increased to 20%, and at 20 months to 30% of control. In a rabbit model, the medial one third PT was used to replace the ACL. The structural properties of the autografts appeared to plateau at 30 weeks when the ultimate load and stiffness were 15% and 24% of the control FATC, respectively, and the anteroposterior knee laxity remained as high as twice that of control knees at one year.

When the ITT was used as a free graft in a canine model, however, the ultimate load of the femur-graft-tibia complex was only 157 N (23% of the control FATC value) after four years of implantation. The stiffness and ultimate load of the donor ITT were found to be 22% and 41%, respectively, of the control FATC. Eight weeks after implantation, the ultimate load had dropped to 15% of control. In a canine model, the stiffness and ultimate load of a pedicled ITT graft were reported to be 45% and 40% of the control FATC at one year. The semitendinosus tendon, after 26 weeks of implantation, was found to fail at loads less than 15% of the control FATC.

In all reconstruction studies, attention should be paid to the control values to which grafts are compared. In some studies, the initial properties of the graft are used as a control while in others the normal FATC is used. In addition, the structural properties of the FATC depend strongly on the orientation of the ligament during tensile testing. Thus, low values for the control FATC because of poor alignment of the ligament in the test apparatus can make a reconstruction procedure appear more successful. It is, therefore, of critical importance to evaluate both the absolute values and the normalized control values to determine the potential success of the procedure.

A report of a clinical study of central third PT autografts covered 80 reconstructions with a minimum two-year follow-up. Ninety-five percent of the knees no longer gave way, and 76% had 3 mm or less anterior drawer differences from the untreated knee. For those patients with more than 3-mm differences, an additional ligamentous instability subsequently was found. After arthroscopically obtaining biopsies of PT autografts in patients, the process can be categorized into four phases: synovial envelopment, zero to six months after surgery; fibrous tissue ingrowth, six to 12 months; transformation into ligament-like tissue, 12 to 18 months; and maturation of striated ligament-like structure.

For the fibrous ingrowth phase, the graft is surrounded by an abundantly vascular synovial tissue with increased cellularity, and the transformation phase is characterized by a decrease in vascularity and longitudinal arrangement of collagen bundles. It should be noted, however, that arthroscopic biopsies are generally obtained from the surface of the graft, which may not reflect the characteristics of the entire graft.

Allografts The morbidity associated with autograft procedures and the potentially limitless supply of allogeneic tissues has increased interest in allografts. Allograft ACL and other tissues, including Achilles tendon, have been evaluated as grafts with or without bony insertions. Allografts usually are preserved by deep-freezing or freeze-drying. Tissue typically is sterilized using cobalt irradiation or cold ethylene oxide gas. Because these processes can alter the properties of the allograft, a complete understanding of these effects is necessary.

Deep-freezing without drying has little or no effect on the mechanical properties of either ligament or tendon. To simulate the freezing effects caused by tissue-bank storage, in situ ACL of the goat was subjected to several freeze-thaw cycles. No significant differences in the ultimate load, stiffness, or modulus were noted between the treated and control ligaments 26 weeks following treatment. Freeze-drying of flexor tendons has been shown to decrease tendon strength; however, the effects of freeze-drying other biologic tissues are contradictory. For example, freeze-drying human PT, Achilles tendon, and fascia lata did not change their biomechanical properties when compared to those of fresh-frozen tissues.

Sterilization with cold ethylene oxide gas and low-dosage irradiation (2 Mrad) do not appear to change the mechanical properties of allografts, whereas sterilization with greater than 3 Mrad irradiation does. The dimensions of the bone-PT-bone complex did not change from control after 2 or 3 Mrad of cobalt irradiation. However, a decreasing trend in the structural and mechanical properties was observed, which became significant at the 3-Mrad dose. Significantly reduced ultimate tensile strength was noted with 3 Mrad of cobalt irradiation. Irradiation also alters tissue morphology. After 2 Mrad irradiation, human PTs were visibly crimped, and the collagen fascicles were separated. Despite these detrimental effects, the use of higher radiation dosages currently is being considered because of concerns that 3 Mrad is not sufficient to sterilize an allograft.

In vivo animal studies of allografts also have been performed. Nine months after implantation of fresh-frozen FATC allografts in the canine, ultimate loads were approximately 15% of normal canine FATC. The stiffness and ultimate load values were 35% and 25% of control, and anteroposterior translation was significantly greater in the reconstructed knee one year after implantation of a freeze-dried ACL allograft-bone complex. At one year, fresh-frozen PT allografts were reported to have an ultimate load that was 29% of control FATC.

In a clinical study of ACL reconstruction using freeze-dried, ethylene oxide-sterilized, bone-PT-bone allografts, there was a high failure rate and a significant rate of graft dissolution in 36 patients with up to two years follow-up. Radiographic examination showed joint space narrowing and the presence of osteophytes. Histologic evaluation of failed grafts demonstrated an inflammatory response with tissue necrosis and a lack of cellularity and collagen organization. To help understand the basis for graft dissolution, the production of interleukin-1 (IL-1) by synoviocytes exposed to deep frozen or freeze-dried, ethylene oxide-sterilized PT allografts in vitro was assessed. A significantly elevated production of IL-1 was found in the freeze-dried, ethylene oxide-treated tendon, whereas the deep frozen tendon was not different from the control. Because IL-1 is a potent mediator of inflammation, the elevated levels of IL-1 in vitro suggest an inflammatory basis for dissolution of freeze-dried, ethylene oxide-treated graft tendons in vivo.

Biomechanical Considerations in ACL Reconstruction Techniques

Once an ACL graft is chosen, numerous factors exist that affect its long-term function. In vitro studies have begun to address such issues as the effects of graft placement and initial graft tension on joint kinematics, length patterns of the graft, and the tension in the graft during a specified knee motion.

Graft placement Various methods of graft placement have been evaluated as a means of obtaining minimal changes in graft length and tension during passive flexion-extension of the knee. (This sometimes is mistakenly called isometry.) Obviously, the concept of isometry is oversimplified, because even the natural ACL is not isometric but has different fiber bundles that change their lengths with normal motion. (In flexion, the anterior bundles accept greater stress and strain, whereas in extension, the opposite occurs.) In a surgical context, this concept can refer only to preventing large changes in graft length and, thus, graft tension, which would render the reconstruction a failure.

Graft fixation to the tibia usually is obtained by drilling a tunnel through the tibia to the ACL insertion. Femoral fixation differs with the chosen procedure. The over-the-top method attaches the graft to the femur after routing it through the intercondylar notch and over the posterior surface of the lateral femoral condyle. This placement usually leads to significant increases in graft length as well as graft tension when the knee is near full extension. In the anatomic or double-tunnel method, the graft is passed through a tunnel in the femur. With this method, changes in length patterns during passive knee flexion-extension are reduced.

The length patterns of the cruciate ligaments in the sagittal plane can be modeled using a crossed four-bar linkage. The four bars represent the two cruciate ligaments and the femoral and tibial bones between the ligament attachment sites. Using this model, the length changes of the ACL replacement depend more on the femoral attachment site than the tibial site. Similar results were found in a study of human cadaver knees. Using the anatomic femoral insertion and moving the tibial attachment point in the mediolateral direction had minimal effects on ACL length. However, positioning the tibial insertion 7.5 mm anteriorly increased the ACL length by 5 to 8 mm. Using the anatomic tibial insertion and moving the femoral attachment resulted in much larger changes in length. A posterior shift of 5 mm made the ACL length longer in extension and shorter in flexion by 5 to 7 mm, and the opposite behavior was found when moving the femoral attachment 5 mm anteriorly. Thus, small changes in insertion site location, particularly that of the femoral insertion, can have a profound effect on graft length and, therefore, graft tension.

Initial graft tension Slight adjustments in the initial tension can significantly alter joint kinematics and graft tension during knee motion. A small initial tension will not provide joint stability, and a large tension can cause excessive graft forces that compromise the survivability of the replacement. Clinically, many advocate an initial tension near 20 N. The subject is still under debate, however, because the force in the normal ACL is unknown, and the initial graft tension significantly decreases shortly after tensioning as a result of viscoelastic effects.

The effect of an initial tension of 1 N or 39 N on PT autografts in the canine model was examined. After three months, no differences were found in anteroposterior joint instability or in ultimate load and stiffness of the bone-graft-bone complex. However, the autografts tensioned to 39 N demonstrated some histologic evidence of degeneration.

Graft augmentation The concern over initial graft weakness and the possibility of failure in the early postoperative period has prompted interest in the use of ligament augmentation devices (LADs) to provide temporary support. Data from some in vitro studies have suggested that the addition of an LAD to a reconstruction leads to improved initial anterior stability and reduced graft forces. However, in vivo studies have not demonstrated significant initial benefit, and graft vascularity has been shown to decrease in the presence of an LAD. Theoretically, the beneficial reduction in force provided by the LAD initially may also shield the graft from the forces and motion that are necessary for tissue remodeling and repair. Contradictory results currently are being presented in the literature, and the benefit of using devices such as the polypropylene LAD has yet to be demonstrated. Thus, while the use of the LAD may ultimately be advocated, the appropriate time remains unknown.

Augmentation may also take the form of a combined intra-articular and extra-articular reconstruction. The effectiveness of an extra-articular reconstruction alone, or in conjunction with an intra-articular reconstruction was studied in vitro. An isolated extra-articular reconstruction, using the anterolateral femorotibial ligament/iliotibial band tenodesis, was found to overconstrain internal tibial rotation with knee flexion, and normal anterior stability was not achieved. The combined procedure produced anterior tibial displacements and internal tibial rotations similar to those produced by an isolated intra-articular reconstruction, although the strains in the ACL graft were found to be decreased, suggesting that force sharing between the two constructs had taken place. Clinical studies in which patients who had an isolated intra-articular reconstruction were compared with those who had a combined procedure revealed no significant differences in anterior laxity and Cybex muscle strength analysis. No differences were found in anterior drawer using the KT-1000 arthrometer, the Lachman test, and the pivot-shift test. However, 42% of the knees that underwent the combined procedure were either painful or swollen laterally.

Meniscus

Once described as functionless remains of leg muscle, the menisci are now known to be integral components of the knee joint. Follow-up of patients with total meniscectomy reveals radiographic changes in 70% and significant arthritic lesions in 20% of cases within three years. Long-term follow-up (greater than 20 years) shows virtually all patients developing arthrosis. The early radiographic degenerative changes following meniscectomy, which include joint space narrowing, flattening of the marginal aspect of the condylar articular surface, and the formation of an osteophytic ridge on the involved femoral condyle were described in 1948. Increased subchondral bone density in the medial tibial plateau also is observed five to ten years following partial and total medial meniscectomy. The severity of the degenerative changes appears proportional to the amount of meniscus removed. Further, while not universally accepted, the long-term prognosis appears to be worse in the younger population. This realization has resulted in a renewed interest in the basic science of the meniscus.

Anatomy

Gross Anatomy

The menisci are actually extensions of the tibia, which serve to deepen the articular surfaces of the tibial plateau to better accommodate the femoral condyles. The peripheral border of each meniscus is thick, convex, and attached to the inside capsule of the joint; the innermost border tapers to a thin free edge. The proximal surfaces of the menisci are concave and in contact with the condyles of the femur; the distal surfaces are flat and rest on the tibial plateau (Fig. 40).

The semicircular medial meniscus is 3.5 cm in length and is wider posteriorly than it is anteriorly. The anterior horn is attached to the tibia plateau near the intercondylar fossa anterior to the ACL. The posterior fibers of the anterior horn merge with the transverse ligament, which connects the anterior horns of the medial and lateral menisci. The posterior horn is attached to the posterior intercondylar fossa of the tibia between the lateral meniscus and the PCL. The most superficial layers of the meniscus join to the capsule along the entire length of the meniscus. The tibial attachment is referred to as the coronary ligament. The femoral and tibial attachments are enlarged at the midpoint by the insertion of the deep fibers of the MCL.

The lateral meniscus is almost circular, covers a larger portion of the tibial surface than the medial meniscus, and is approximately the same width from front to back (Fig. 41). The anterior horn inserts on the tibia anterior to the intercondylar eminence and posterior to the ACL. The posterior horn attaches posterior to the intercondylar eminence of the tibia and anterior to the insertion of the medial meniscus. A loose connective tissue attaches the superficial portions of the lateral meniscus to the capsular ligament; however, these fibers do not attach to the lateral collateral ligament. The femoral medial condyle attachment to the posterior horn includes the anterior and posterior meniscofemoral ligaments of Humphrey and Wrisberg, respectively, which originate near the origin of the PCL.

Microanatomy and Biochemistry

The meniscus is fibrocartilaginous, composed of an interlacing network of collagen fibers, pro-

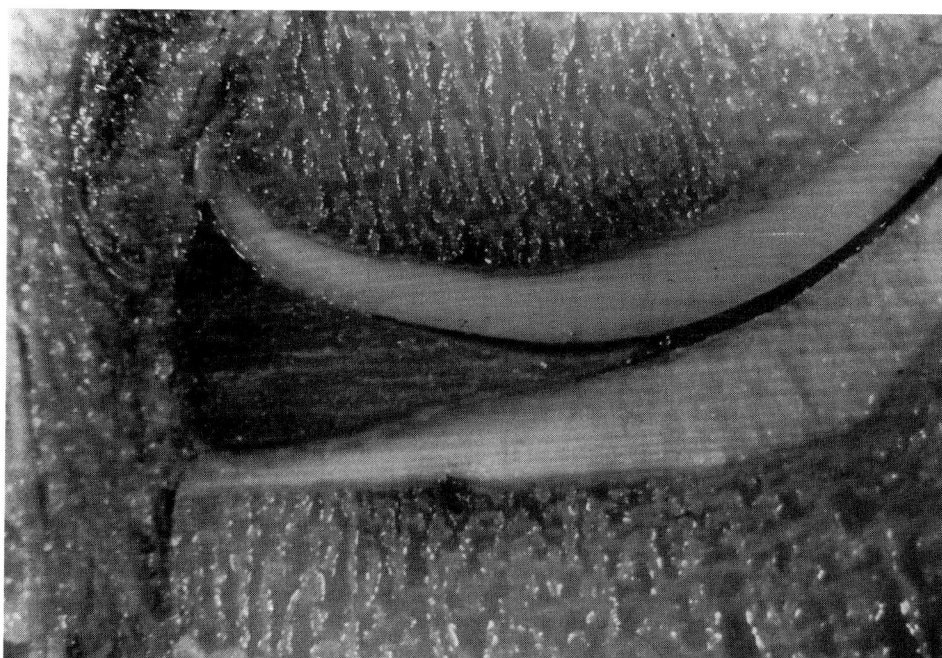

Figure 40
Frontal section of the medial compartment of a human knee illustrating the articulation of the menisci with the condyles of the femur and tibia. (Reproduced with permission from Warren RF, Arnoczky SP, Wickiewicz TL: Anatomy of the knee, in Nicholas JA, Hershman EB (eds): *The Lower Extremity and Spine in Sports Medicine.* St. Louis, CV Mosby, 1986, vol 1, pp 657–694.)

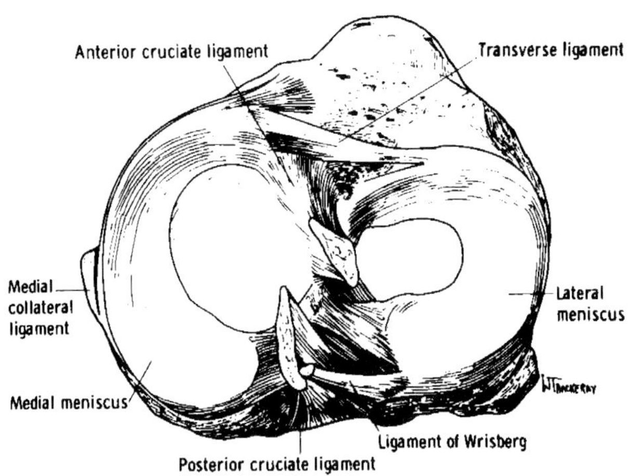

Figure 41
Drawing of a human tibial plateau showing the relative size and attachments of the medial and lateral menisci. (Reproduced with permission from Warren RF, Arnoczky SP, Wickiewicz TL: Anatomy of the knee, in Nicholas JA, Hershman EB (eds): *The Lower Extremity and Spine in Sports Medicine.* St. Louis, CV Mosby, 1986, vol 1, pp 657–694.)

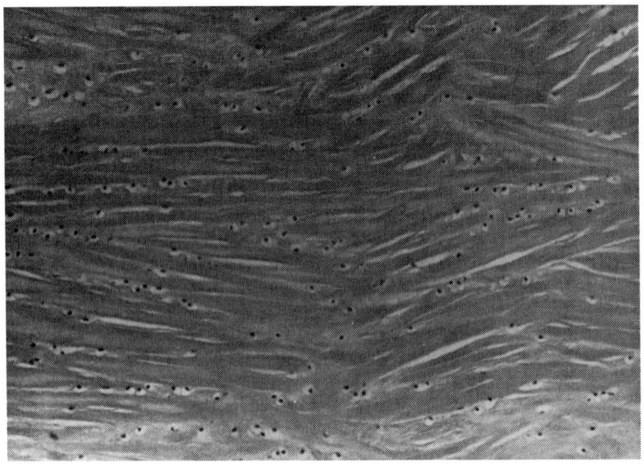

Figure 42
Photomicrograph of a longitudinal section of human meniscus showing the histologic appearance of meniscal fibrocartilage (H&E, X100).

teoglycans and glycoproteins, and interspersed cells (Fig. 42).

The cells of the meniscus are responsible for synthesis and maintenance of the extracellular matrix. These cells, which may be fibroblasts, chondrocytes, or a mixture of both, have been termed fibrochondrocytes. Two histologic types have been identified: a fusiform cell in the superficial zone and an ovoid cell in the remainder of the meniscus. Although the fusiform cells resemble fibroblasts, they are situated in lacunae and also resemble chondrocytes from the superficial zone of articular cartilage. Both cell types contain abundant endoplasmic reticulum and Golgi complexes. Mitochondria are infrequent, however, suggesting an anaerobic metabolism or very limited metabolic demands.

The extracellular matrix is primarily type I collagen (55% to 65% dry weight). Collagen types II, III, V, and VI also have been identified, and make up an additional 5% to 10% of the dry weight. These fibers are oriented primarily in a circumferential direction; however, a few small fibers are oriented in the radial direction. Although the functional significance of the radial fibers is unknown, some believe they 'tie' the circumferential fibers together, thus restraining motion between the circumferential bundles (Fig. 43). Subsequent study has revealed three layers of meniscal organization: a superficial layer of mesh-like fibers with a primarily radial orientation, a surface layer just beneath the superficial layer with irregularly aligned collagen bundles, and a middle layer or deep zone of larger fibers oriented in a parallel, circumferential direction (Fig. 44). The deep zone fibers, which constitute the bulk of meniscal substance, are grouped together into large fascicles that run parallel to the periphery of the meniscus. These fascicles are 50 to 150 mm in diameter and appear to be continuous with those of the anterior and posterior horns, which anchor the menisci firmly to bone.

The extracellular matrix also contains proteoglycans and glycoproteins, although only about

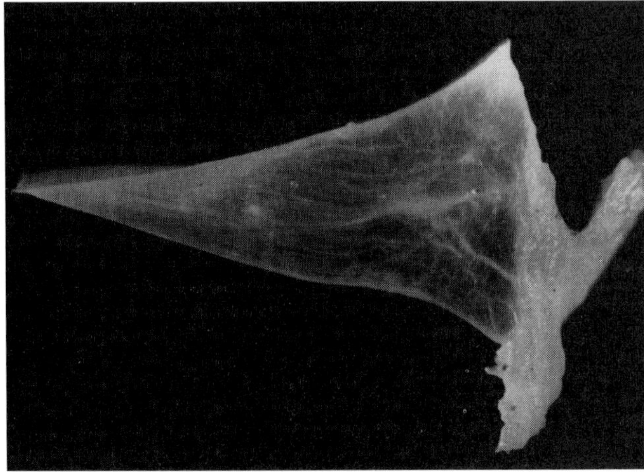

Figure 43
Cross section of a lateral meniscus showing the radial orientation of fibrous ties within the substance of the meniscus. (Reproduced with permission from Arnoczky SP, Torzelli PA: The biology of cartilage, in Hunter LY, Funk FJ Jr (eds): *Rehabilitation of the Injured Knee.* St. Louis, CV Mosby, 1984, pp 148–209.)

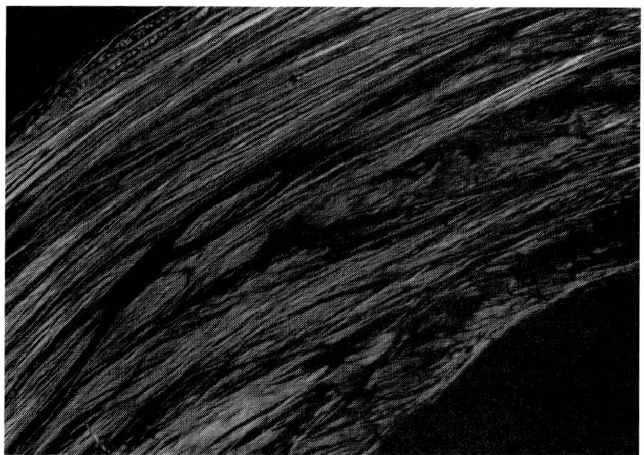

Figure 44
Photomicrograph of a longitudinal section of a meniscus under polarized light demonstrating the orientation of the coarse, deep, circumferentially oriented collagen fibers.

10% of that in hyaline cartilage. The quantity varies with age and location within the tissue, being present in greater quantity in the inner third of the meniscus and in the anterior horns of both the medial and lateral menisci. The glycosaminoglycans of the adult human consist of chondroitin 6-sulfate (40%), chondroitin 4-sulfate (10% to 20%), dermatan sulfate (20% to 30%), and keratin sulfate (15%). These form aggregates made up of 100 to 200 glycosaminoglycan monomers attached to a single backbone of hyaluronic acid. The binding of the monomers to the hyaluronate is stabilized by link protein, which has been identified in the meniscus. Elastin also has been identified in the extracellular matrix (0.6% dry weight). In addition, adhesive glycoproteins such as type IV collagen, fibronectin, and thrombospondin have been measured and may play a role in the organization of the extracellular matrix.

The substance of the meniscus is not always uniform, and the incidence of inhomogeneities increases with age. This is evident from magnetic resonance imaging studies in which there is nonuniform signal from the interior of the body of the meniscus. The altered signal does not communicate with the surface of the meniscus and is not associated with tears or clinically significant abnormal function. Autopsy studies of menisci with these changes reveal menisci that are grossly normal on the surface, but have degenerative changes within the body.

The menisci obtain their relatively sparse vascular supply from branches of the medial and lateral geniculate arteries, both inferior and superior. Branches from these vessels form a circumferentially arranged perimeniscal plexus that supplies the peripheral border of the meniscus. Radial branches directed toward the center of the joint arise from this plexus and penetrate approximately 10% to 30% of the width of the meniscus. The middle geniculate artery, along with branches of the medial and lateral geniculate arteries, supply the meniscus through the vascular synovial covering of the anterior and posterior horn attachments. These vessels penetrate the horns and give rise to short vessels that end in terminal capillary loops. A reflection of synovium is also present throughout the peripheral attachment of the menisci (an exception is the posterolateral portion of the lateral meniscus adjacent to the popliteal tendon). This synovial fringe extends approximately 2 mm over the articular surface and contains small, terminally looped vessels.

Innervation of the meniscus is restricted to the peripheral two thirds of the structure and includes type I and type II nerve endings. These fibers are concentrated primarily in the horns, with a considerably lower concentration in the meniscal body. It has been postulated that these fibers are sensory and may play a role in proprioception.

Biomechanics of Meniscus Function

The Contributions of the Meniscus to Joint Mechanics

It is now well established that intact menisci are necessary for normal knee joint function. The menisci play a role in load-distribution, shock absorption, and joint lubrication. The normal menisci are responsible for transmission of 50% of knee joint force when the knee is in extension, and 85% to 90% of the joint force when the knee is in flexion. Menisci also serve as secondary stabilizers against anteroposterior translation. Medial meniscectomy profoundly alters the forces and stresses across the knee joint. The changes include reduced contact area by at least 50% to 70%, increased peak stress and stress concentration, and decreased shock absorption. It is likely that loss of meniscus as a result of either partial or total meniscectomy allows overloading of the involved articular cartilage with subsequent joint degeneration.

During heel strike, impact generates a stress wave that propagates through the tibia and knee joint. Studies by a number of investigators have demonstrated that the meniscus attenuates these stress waves by as much as 20%. This is particularly important, considering that animal models of osteoarthritis have been based on repetitive impact loading. Menisci may also play a role in joint stability, although this role is uncertain. Some investigators have suggested that meniscectomy increases joint laxity; many others believe that it does not.

Certainly, in the presence of ligamentous insufficiency, the menisci have been shown to assist in joint stabilization.

The knee, like other synovial joints, is able to move at a wide range of rates in the presence of large forces with minimal friction between the contact surfaces. This is the result of a variety of lubrication mechanisms to which the meniscus contributes significantly. The entrapped water in the meniscus makes up 74% of the total weight. Under compression, much of this fluid is free and is thought to be extruded into the joint space, increasing the available fluid lubricant (weeping lubrication). Removal of the meniscus decreases the effectiveness of this process, which, while not proven, may contribute to the degenerative process.

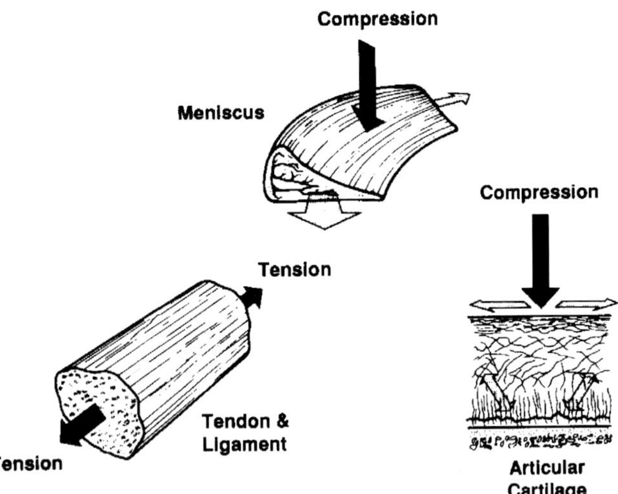

Figure 45
Tendons and ligaments function primarily under tension. Meniscus, while loaded in compression, sustains large radial and circumferential tensile stress because of its shape and its location in the joint. Loading of articular cartilage in compression causes tension in the surface and in the deeper zones as well. Collagen fiber orientation reflects the tensile loads experienced by each tissue. (Reproduced with permission from Mow VC, Fithian DC, Kelly MA: Fundamentals of articular cartilage and meniscus biomechanics, in Ewing JW (ed): *Articular Cartilage and Knee Joint Function: Basic Science and Arthroscopy.* New York, Raven Press, 1990, pp 1–18.)

Mechanical Properties of Meniscus and its Constituents

The most important mechanical properties of collagen fibers are their tensile stiffness and strength. They make their greatest contribution to tissue material properties when they are aligned along the direction of the largest (principal) tensile stress, as is the case in tendons and ligaments. Although the nature of loading and stress in articular cartilage and meniscus is more complex (Fig. 45), the basic assumption that collagen fibers tend to align with the principal tensile stresses seems to be valid. During loading, radial (extrusive) forces are resisted by firm attachments to the tibia at the anterior and posterior horns. This produces large circumferentially oriented hoop tensile stress. The collagen ultrastructure of meniscus with circumferential and radial fiber orientation, thus, tends to reflect the local tensile stresses within the tissue.

Proteoglycans also contribute to the mechanical behavior of meniscus. The high fixed-charge density and like-charge repulsion cause proteoglycans to be stiffly distended in the matrix, providing the tissue with a high capacity to resist compressive forces. In addition, these negatively charged molecules attract many positive counterions in the aqueous bath, creating a Donnan osmotic pressure that further resists compressive load. Proteoglycans are immobilized within the collagen fibrillar meshwork by the formation of large aggregates.

Mechanically, the matrix may be considered to be biphasic, composed of a solid phase (26% total weight) and a fluid phase (74% total weight). The solid matrix consists mostly of collagen, proteoglycans, and other noncollagenous proteins; its behavior is that of a fiber-reinforced porous-permeable composite material. The fluid phase consists of water and interstitial electrolytes, and most of this phase may be forced to flow through the porous-permeable solid matrix by a hydraulic pressure gradient and matrix compaction (Fig. 46). The flow of water through the porous-permeable matrix plays an important mechanical role in governing the behavior of the tissue. A biphasic theory has been used to determine the contribution each phase makes to the overall mechanical properties. In this theory, the intrinsic properties of the solid matrix along with interstitial fluid flow govern the deformability of the tissue. The creep and stress relaxation responses are determined by the frictional drag of fluid flow through the porous matrix. Viscoelastic shear responses result from molecular relaxation effects from motion of the long-chain polymers such as collagen and proteoglycans. The component of viscoelasticity caused by interstitial fluid flow is known as the biphasic viscoelastic behavior, and the component of viscoelasticity caused by molecular motion is known as the flow-independent or intrinsic viscoelastic behavior solid matrix. With this model, the elastic modulus of meniscus was found to be 0.411 MPa, less than half that of cartilage. The permeability was found to be $8.13 \times 10^{-16} m^4/N{\cdot}s$, one sixth that of cartilage. Thus, meniscus is softer and less permeable than cartilage.

Creep and stress relaxation are of the utmost importance in understanding the functional charac-

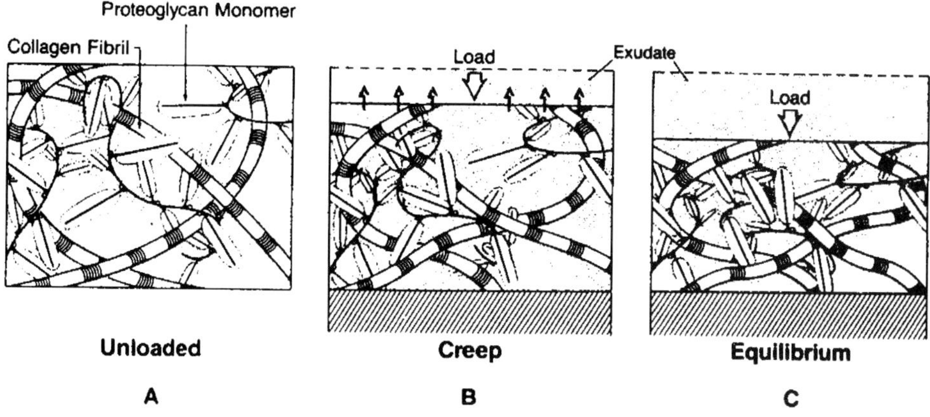

Figure 46
Compressive creep of cartilage is due to fluid exudation. Rate of creep is controlled by tissue permeability (B) and equilibrium is determined by the intrinsic stiffness of the collagen-proteoglycan solid matrix (C).

teristics of meniscus. When the joint is loaded over a long period of time, the contact area gradually increases as a result of creep, spreading the compressive force over a larger area and, thereby, reducing the stress. Stress relaxation makes it difficult to maintain high stresses in the collagen-proteoglycan solid matrix for extended periods of time. Stress may reach high levels momentarily, but interstitial fluid redistribution will always occur to decrease the tissue stress with time. The related meniscal properties of creep and stress-relaxation are thus important in the load distribution and shock absorption roles of the menisci.

The meniscus is believed to sustain significant shear stress under normal loading conditions. Its response to shear may be important in the development of vertical and horizontal tears. Bovine meniscus has been studied under oscillating pure shear conditions. On average, the meniscus is one sixth to one tenth as stiff in dynamic shear as articular cartilage. Bovine meniscus is anisotropic under dynamic shear. The anisotropy reflects the organization of the collagen fibers in the matrix. The tissue is 20% to 33% stiffer when the shear is perpendicular to the coarse fiber bundles than when it is parallel to them. Increasing the shear strain rate has a stiffening effect on the matrix, which has been observed for cartilage.

Compressive forces in the knee generate tensile stresses in the meniscus. The tensile stress-strain curve of meniscal tissue resembles those of other collagenous tissues. Studies of bovine meniscus have shown that the tissue has roughly ten times the elastic modulus in the direction of the collagen fiber bundles (7.55 MPa) that it has at right angles to them (0.78 MPa). That is, bovine meniscus is highly anisotropic. Investigators have also compared the tensile properties of circumferentially oriented specimens from the surface to those of the deep layers of bovine menisci. Specimens from the surface were neither as stiff nor as strong as those from the deep layers. Similarly, specimens from the inner one third of the medial meniscus of steers are significantly less stiff in tension than specimens from the peripheral two thirds. This difference is consistent with differences in composition and collagen fiber architecture.

Similarly, there are significant regional variations in the tensile stiffness and strength of normal human meniscus tested in the circumferential direction (Fig. 47). These variations are not explained by differences in biochemical composition of the matrix, which showed little variation among the regions studied. Rather, patterns of tensile stiffness appear to follow fiber-bundle architecture, which suggests that collagen ultrastructure and intermolecular interactions, such as collagen cross-linking, are

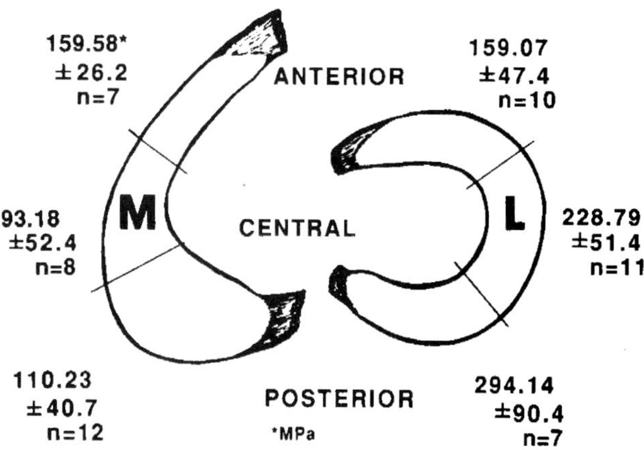

Figure 47
Circumferential tensile stiffness and strength are lower in the posterior medial meniscus than in the anterior horn or lateral meniscus (mean ± SD, MPa). (Reproduced with permission from Fithian DC, Kelly MA, Mow VC: Material properties and structure function relationships in the meniscus. *Clin Orthop* 1992;252:19–31.)

the predominant factors influencing the tensile response of the meniscus.

Recent work has shown that radial fibers strongly influence the behavior of meniscus under radially applied tension. In the posterior horn of bovine medial meniscus, radial fibers are present in greater numbers and have a more horizontal orientation than in the anterior horn (Fig. 48). This regional variation in radial fiber structure is reflected in the greater mean tensile stiffness and strength of samples from the posterior region. When bundles of radial fibers were included in radially oriented specimens undergoing tensile testing, tensile stiffness and strength increased tenfold to values close to those observed for circumferential specimens. Thus, it would appear that radial fibers, although far fewer in number and less regular in distribution and orientation, possess tensile properties similar to those of circumferential fibers. It has been observed that when the tissue fails in circumferential tension, the plane of failure is frequently the interface between two adjacent circumferential fiber bundles, and the failure proceeds in shear along this weak plane (Fig. 49). For radial samples, failure generally begins with breakage of individual fibers, then propagates along the interface between the radial fibers and the surrounding matrix. The disposition of fibers, both radial and circumferential, is, therefore, an important factor in the morphology of meniscal tears.

Modeling of Meniscal Function

The functions of the menisci are determined not only by their material properties and geometry but also by the shape of the femoral and tibial condyles, their position in the joint, anatomic attachments (constraints), and the magnitude and direction of the force applied to the knee. A completely accurate model of the meniscus must include all these factors. Early attempts at modeling have demonstrated the need for a more accurate representation of the mechanical properties of the meniscus than that of a linear elastic material. Material nonlinearity, anisotropy, and biphasic flow effects must all be taken into account for construction of a realistic structural model of the meniscus.

In addition, constraints on meniscal displacement along the periphery must be considered. Because the menisci are wedge-shaped and occupy the periphery of the joint, axial loading of the knee creates extrusive forces that tend to displace the meniscus from the joint. The strong insertions at the anterior and posterior horns prevent this displacement. Thus, although the primary function of the meniscus may be to bear compressive forces, it does so by supporting enormous tensile stresses directed in the circumferential direction. Evidence exists that the attachments between the medial meniscus and MCL are also important in constraining the motion of the medial meniscus.

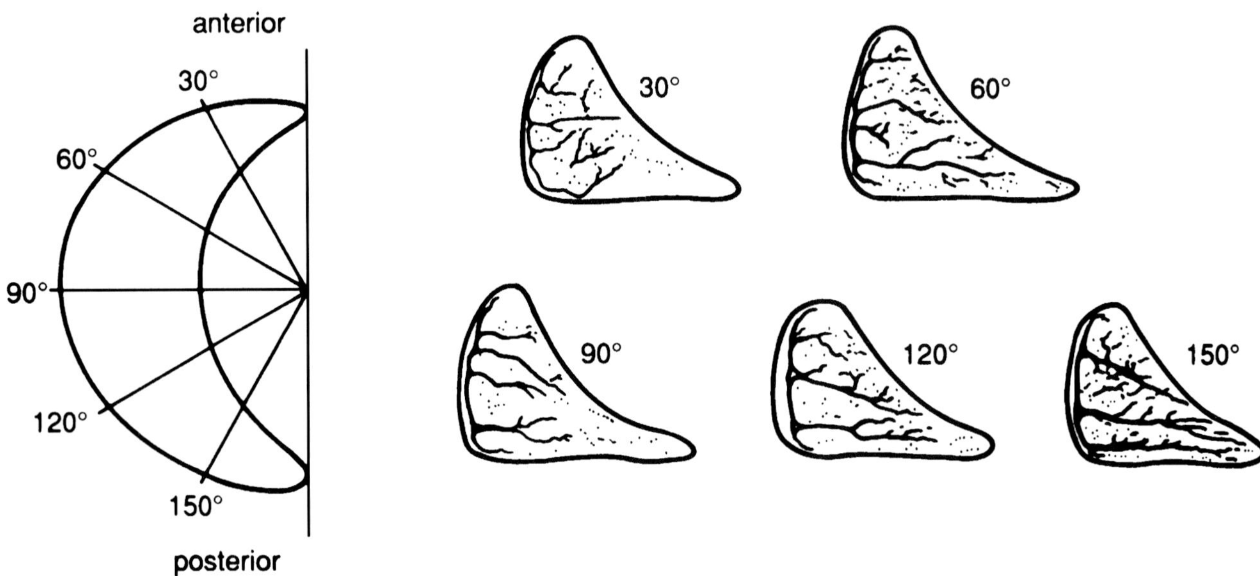

Figure 48
Radial fibers in the deep zone of bovine medial meniscus weave among the larger bundles of circumferentially-oriented fibers. The arrangement and density of radial fibers vary in different regions of the meniscus. (Reproduced with permission from Kelly MA, Fithian DC, Chern KY, et al: Structure and function of the meniscus, in Mow VC, Ratcliffe A, Woo SL-Y (eds): *Biomechanics of Diarthrodial Joints.* New York, Springer-Verlag, 1990; vol 1, p 194.)

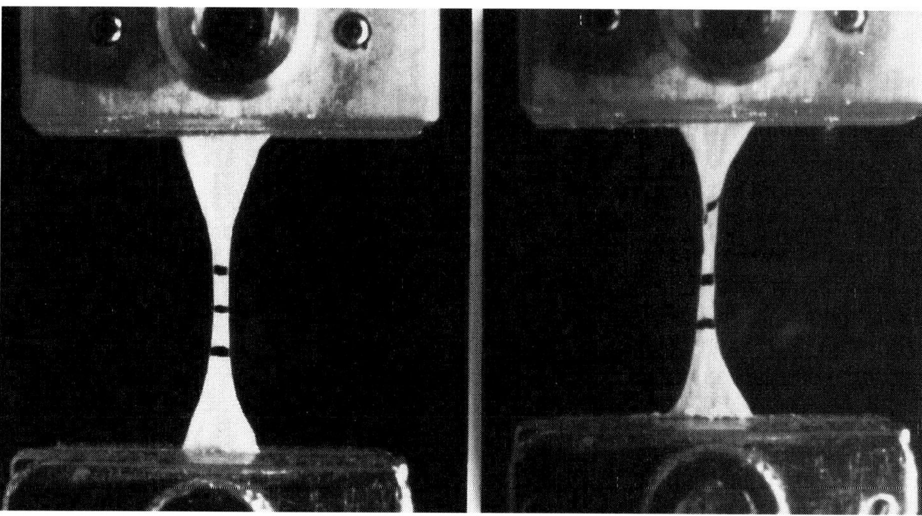

Figure 49
Failure of meniscus in circumferential tension. As individual fibers begin to fail, a plane of cleavage develops between adjacent fiber bundles. The orientation of the tear produced in this manner, thus, is parallel to the bundles.

An accurate model for the meniscus should allow predictions of its response under various loading conditions in the intact joint. An axisymmetric biphasic finite element model (a computational method for determining stress and strain) and experimentally derived material properties for normal human and bovine meniscus recently were used to predict strain distributions within the meniscus. It was found that predicted axial (vertical) strains were compressive, radial and circumferential strains were tensile, and radial strains in some instances reached as high as 25%. Predictions were generally within an order of magnitude (a factor of 10) of experimentally measured failure strains.

Meniscal Injury, Healing, Regeneration, Repair, and Replacement

Meniscal injury is common in young active individuals and occurs through direct contact and noncontact mechanisms. Greater than 60% of knees with an acute traumatic hemarthrosis have been found to have a meniscal lesion. Direct contact with the knee is less common and is usually associated with other injuries, particularly ACL injury and tibial plateau fracture from automotive-pedestrian impacts. Noncontact meniscal injuries occur as a result of joint loading during rapid changes in velocity or axial rotation or as a combination of a squatting and twisting movement. Soccer, track and field, and downhill skiing are the most common sources of meniscal injuries in athletes. Of these, injuries to the medial meniscus are three times more common than those to the lateral meniscus. Longitudinal tears, vertical tears that run anteroposteriorly, are the most common traumatic injury (30% to 50%). Extension of a longitudinal tear into the anterior and posterior horns produces a bucket-handle tear. Transverse vertical tears are much less frequent, typically occur in the middle third of the meniscus, and extend in a radial direction. These can extend anteriorly or posteriorly, becoming flap tears. Other injuries include oblique tears, mixed or complex tears, detachment (disinsertion), and degenerative injury. Degenerative injury is more common in the population over age 40, can occur spontaneously, and frequently produces horizontal cleavage tears.

The vascular portions of the meniscus are capable of a repair response similar to that of other connective tissues: exudation, organization, vascularization, cellular proliferation, and remodeling. Following injury within the vascular zone of the meniscus, a fibrin clot forms. Vessels from the capillary plexus proliferate into the fibrin scaffold together with undifferentiated mesenchymal cells. This fibrovascular scar tissue adheres to the torn surfaces and becomes continuous with normal fibrocartilage. Perimeniscal and synovial fringe vessels penetrate the scar and support the healing process. Experimental studies have shown that lesions of the vascular portion of the meniscus heal within ten weeks. However, remodeling of the scar to normal-appearing fibrocartilage requires several months. The strength of this repair tissue with time has yet to be determined. In contrast, the avascular region does not have reparative abilities. Data from a number of animal studies have indicated that injuries in the avascular zone do not stimulate a healing response from the meniscal cells, suggesting that the healing response depends on the vasculature.

The subject of meniscal regeneration following meniscectomy is controversial. Regrowth of a structure that is similar in shape and texture to meniscus following total meniscectomy has been seen in rabbits, sheep, and dogs. This initially fibrous material undergoes a metaplastic process, yielding fibrocartilage over a seven-month period. For this process to occur, the entire meniscus or a sufficiently large portion of tissue to expose the peripheral vasculature must be resected. Similar results have been observed in humans following total meniscectomy; however, the frequency and extent of the regeneration have not been established. Not surprisingly, lesions in the avascular regions do not produce this response. Synovectomy, which removes the synovial fringe, results in a complete failure to regenerate the meniscus, indicating the importance of this tissue to regeneration. Thus, both the synovial and peripheral meniscal vasculature contribute to the regenerative process.

Despite the inability of menisci to regenerate in the avascular zone, a remodeling process has been observed after partial meniscectomy. It has been suggested that this process is probably the result of accretion of tissue from adjacent extrameniscal sources. Initially the tear is filled with fibrin clot and cells that probably are of a synovial origin; the cells eventually elaborate a homogeneous matrix. This tissue then undergoes a remodeling process leaving a tissue that is grossly and microscopically similar to fibrocartilage. It should be noted that this remodeling occurs successfully in only 67% of cases studied and appears to be directly related to the presence of a hemarthrosis. This relationship is consistent with results of tissue culture studies, which demonstrate that meniscofibrochondrocytes proliferate and form matrix in response to factors present in hematoma (platelet-derived growth factor). In experimental and clinical studies in which an exogenous fibrin clot has been used to support the healing process, good results were reported. The use of collagen scaffolding has also been advocated based on histologic and biochemical studies. Additional experimental studies in the dog have also led to suggestions for the use of allograft meniscal replacement. Much remains to be done in this area of research.

Repair of meniscal injuries has been indicated for lesions greater than 1 cm within the vascular zone. Other indications for repair include all meniscal tears except in situations where the repair would replace less than 25% of the missing area. Contraindications for repair include short, stable tears (less than 1 cm), partial thickness tears (less than 50% of the vertical height), and shallow radial tears (less than 3 mm in depth). Unfortunately, most injuries occur outside the vascular zone, and meniscal repair and regeneration are limited. Efforts to evaluate the extent of the blood supply and methods to encourage vascular ingrowth into the avascular region to improve healing are currently being investigated. These include vascular synovial pedicle flaps, vascular access channels, synovial abrasion, and the use of exogenous fibrin clot to stimulate healing. Initial clinical results with synovial abrasion appear encouraging; however, the extent and quality of the repair are not yet fully understood. Thus, while the importance of meniscus to the knee joint function has been demonstrated, the choice and criteria for meniscal repair and replacement remain topics of future interest.

Selected Bibliography

Tendon Biomechanics

Abrahams M: Mechanical behaviour of tendon in vitro: A preliminary report. *Med Biol Eng* 1068;5:433–443.

Berchuck M, Andriacchi TP, Bach BR, et al: Gait adaptations by patients who have a deficient anterior cruciate ligament. *J Bone Joint Surg* 1990;72A:871–877.

Betsch DF, Baer E: Structure and mechanical properties of rat tail tendon. *Biorheology* 1980;17:83–94.

Carlstedt CA, Skagervall R: A model for computer-aided analysis of biomechanical properties of the plantaris longus tendon in the rabbit. *J Biomech* 1986;19:251–256.

Cohen RE, Hooley CJ, McCrum NG: Viscoelastic creep of collagenous tissue. *J Biomech* 1976;9:175–184.

Danielsen CC: Mechanical properties of native and reconstituted rat tail tendon collagen upon maturation in vitro. *Mech Ageing Dev* 1987;40:9–16.

Draganich LF, Vahey JW: An in vitro study of anterior cruciate ligament strain induced by quadriceps and hamstrings forces. *J Orthop Res* 1990;8:57–63.

Fung YC: Stress-strain-history relations of soft tissuc in simple elongation, in Fung YC, Perrone N, Anliker M (eds): *Biomechanics: Its Foundations and Objectives.* Englewood Cliffs, NJ, Prentice Hall, 1972, pp 181–208.

Gupta BN, Subramanian KN, Brinker WO, et al: Tensile strength of canine cranial cruciate ligaments. *Am J Vet Res* 1971;32:183–190.

Haut RC, Little RW: A constitutive equation for collagen fibers. *J Biomech* 1976;5:423–430.

Haut RC: The influence of specimen length on the tensile failure properties of tendon collagen. *J Biomech* 1986;19:951–955.

Haut RC: Age-dependent influence of strain rate on the tensile failure of rat-tail tendon. *J Biomech Eng* 1983;105:296–299.

Hubbard RP, Chun KJ: Mechanical responses of tendons to repeated extensions and wait periods. *J Biomech Eng* 1988;110:11–19.

Kastelic J, Baer E: Deformation in tendon collagen, in Vincent JFV, Curry JD (eds): *The Mechanical Properties of Biological Materials.* Cambridge, Cambridge University Press, 1980, pp 397–435.

Matthews LS, Ellis D: Viscoelastic properties of cat tendon: Effects of time after death and preservation by freezing. *J Biomech* 1968;1:65–71.

Michna H, Hartmann G: Adaption of tendon collagen to exercise. *Int Orthop* 1989;13:161–165.

Müller W: *The Knee: Form, Function, and Ligament Reconstruction.* Berlin, Springer-Verlag, 1983.

Noyes FR, Butler DL, Grood ES, et al: Biomechanical analysis of human ligament grafts used in knee ligament repairs and reconstructions. *J Bone Joint Surg* 1984;66A:344–352.

Pradas MM, Calleja RD: Nonlinear viscoelastic behaviour of the flexor tendon of the human hand. *J Biomech* 1990;23:773–781.

Pring DJ, Amis AA, Coombs RR: The mechanical properties of human flexor tendons in relation to artificial tendons. *J Hand Surg* 1985;10B:331–336.

Shadwick RE: Elastic energy storage in tendons: Mechanical differences related to function and age. *J Appl Physiol* 1990;68:1033–1040.

Torp S, Arridge RGC, Armeniades CD, et al: Structure-property relationships in tendon as a function of age, in Atkins EDT, Keller A (eds): *Structure of Fibrous Biopolymers.* London, Butterworth, 1975, pp 197–221.

VanBrocklin JD, Ellis DG: A study of the mechanical behavior of toe extensor tendons under applied stress. *Arch Phys Med* 1965;46:369–373.

Woo SLY, Gomez MA, Inoue M, et al: New experimental procedures to evaluate the biomechanical properties of healing canine medial collateral ligaments. *J Orthop Res* 1987;5:425–432.

Woo SLY: Mechanical properties of tendons and ligaments: I. Quasi-static and nonlinear viscoelastic properties. *Biorheology* 1982;19:385–396.

Woo SLY, Gomez MA, Woo YK, et al: Mechanical properties of tendons and ligaments: II. The relationships of immobilization and exercise on tissue remodeling. *Biorheology* 1982;19:397–408.

Wood TO, Cooke PH, Goodship AE: The effect of exercise and anabolic steroids on the mechanical properties and crimp morphology of the rat tendon. *Am J Sports Med* 1988;16:153–158.

Yasuda K, Sasaki T: Exercise after anterior cruciate ligament reconstruction: The force exerted on the tibia by the separate isometric contractions of the quadriceps or the hamstrings. *Clin Orthop* 1987;220:275–283.

Yasuda K, Sasaki T: Muscle exercise after anterior cruciate ligament reconstruction: Biomechanics of the simultaneous isometric contraction method of the quadriceps and the hamstrings. *Clin Orthop* 1987;220:266–274.

Tendon Injury, Healing, and Repair

Gelberman RH, Botte MJ, Spiegelman JJ, et al: The excursion and deformation of repaired flexor tendons treated with protected early motion. *J Hand Surg* 1986;11A:106–110.

Gelberman RH, Woo SLY, Lothringer K, et al: Effects of early intermittent passive mobilization on healing canine flexor tendons. *J Hand Surg* 1982;7A:170–175.

Manske PR, Lesker PA: Biochemical evidence of flexor tendon participation in the repair process: An in vitro study. *J Hand Surg* 1984;9B:117–120.

Nirschl RP: Rotator cuff tendinitis: Basic concepts of pathoetiology, in Barr JS Jr (ed): *Instructional Course Lectures, XXXVIII.* Park Ridge, IL, American Acadamy of Orthopaedic Surgeons, 1989, pp 439–445.

Potenza AD: Concepts of tendon healing and repair, in American Acadamy of Orthopaedic Surgeons, *Symposium on Tendon Surgery in the Hand.* St. Louis, CV Mosby Co, 1975, pp 18–47.

Seradge H: Elongation of the repair configuration following flexor tendon repair. *J Hand Surg* 1983;8A:182–185.

Shino K, Inoue M, Horibe S, et al: Reconstruction of the anterior cruciate ligament using allogeneic tendon: Long term followup. *Am J Sports Med* 1990;18:457–465.

Shino K, Kawasaki T, Hirose H, et al: Replacement of the anterior cruciate ligament by allogeneic tendon graft: An experimental study in the dog. *J Bone Joint Surg* 1984;66B:672–681.

Wade PJ, Muir IF, Hutcheon LL: Primary flexor tendon repair: The mechanical limitations of the modified Kessler technique. *J Hand Surg* 1986;11B:71–76.

Ligament Biomechanics

Amiel D, Frank C, Harwood F, et al: Tendons and ligaments: A morphological and biochemical comparison. *J Orthop Res* 1984;1:257–265.

Burks RT: Gross anatomy, in Daniel DM, Akeson WH, O'Connor JJ (eds): *Knee Ligaments: Structure, Function, Injury, and Repair.* New York, Raven Press, 1990, pp 59–76.

Butler DL, Kay MD, Stouffer DC: Comparison of material properties in fascicle-bone units from human patellar tendon and knee ligaments. *J Biomech* 1986;19:425–432.

Danto MI, Woo SLY: The mechanical properties of skeletally mature rabbit anterior cruciate ligament and patellar tendon over a range of strain rates. *J Orthop Res* 1993;11:58–67.

Figgie HE III, Bahniuk EH, Heiple KG, et al: The effects of tibial-femoral angle on the failure mechanics of the canine anterior cruciate ligament. *J Biomech* 1986:19:89–91.

Hart RA, Woo SL, Newton PO: Ultrastructural morphometry of anterior cruciate and medial collateral ligaments: An experimental study in rabbits. *J Orthop Res* 1992;10:96–103.

Kennedy JC, Hawkins RJ, Willis RB, et al: Tension studies of human knee ligaments: Yield point, ultimate failure, and disruption of the cruciate and tibial collateral ligaments. *J Bone Joint Surg* 1976:58A: 350–355.

Kennedy JC, Roth JH, Mendenhall HV: Presidential Address: Intraarticular replacement in the anterior cruciate ligament-deficient knee. *Am J Sports Med* 1980;8:1–8.

Laros GS, Tipton CM, Cooper RR: Influence of physical activity on ligament insertions in the knees of dogs. *J Bone Joint Surg* 1971;53A:275–286.

Lyon RM, Akeson WH, Amiel D, et al: Ultrastructural differences between the cells of the medial collateral and the anterior cruciate ligaments. *Clin Orthop* 1991;272:279–286.

Myers BS, McElhaney JH, Doherty BJ: The viscoelastic responses of the human cervical spine in torsion: Experimental limitations of quasi-linear theory, and a method for reducing these effects. *J Biomech* 1991;24:811–817.

Noyes FR: Functional properties of knee ligaments and alterations induced by immobilization: A correlative biomechanical and histological study in primates. *Clin Orthop* 1977;123:210–242.

Noyes FR, DeLucas JL, Torvik PJ: Biomechanics of anterior cruciate ligament failure: An analysis of strain rate sensitivity and mechanisms of failure in primates. *J Bone Joint Surg* 1974;56A:236–253.

Tipton CM, Matthes RD, Maynard JA, et al: The influence of physical activity on ligaments and tendons. *Med Sci Sports* 1975;7:165–175.

Trent PS, Walker PS, Wolf B: Ligament length patterns, strength and rotational axes of the knee joint. *Clin Orthop* 1976;117:263–270.

Viidik A: Elasticity and tensile strength of the anterior cruciate ligament in rabbits as influenced by training. *Acta Physiol Scand* 1968;74:372–380.

Viidik A, Sandqvist L, Mägi M: Influence of postmortal storage on tensile strength characteristics and histology of rabbit ligaments. *Acta Orthop Scand Suppl* 1965;79:1–38.

Woo SLY, Gomez MA, Sites TJ, et al: The biomechanical and morphological changes in the medial collateral ligament of the rabbit after immobilization and remobilization. *J Bone Joint Surg* 1987;69A:1200–1211.

Woo SLY, Hollis JM, Adams DJ, et al: Tensile properties of the human femur-anterior cruciate ligament-tibia complex: The effects of specimen age and orientation. *Am J Sports Med* 1991;19:217–225.

Woo SLY, Hollis JM, Roux RD, et al: Effects of knee flexion on the structural properties of the rabbit femur-anterior cruciate ligament-tibia complex. *J Biomech* 1987;20:557–563.

Woo SLY, Newton PO, MacKenna DO, et al: A comparative evaluation of the mechanical properties of the rabbit medial collateral and anterior cruciate ligaments. *J Biomech* 1992;25:377–386.

Woo SLY, Ohland KJ, Weiss JA: Aging and sex-related changes in the biomechanical properties of the rabbit medial collateral ligament. *Mech Ageing Dev* 1990;56:129–142.

Woo SLY, Orlando CA, Camp JF, et al: Effects of postmortem storage by freezing on ligament tensile behavior. *J Biomech* 1986;19:399–404.

Woo SLY, Peterson RH, Ohland KJ, et al: The effects of strain rate on the properties of the medial collateral ligament in skeletally immature and mature rabbits: A biomechanical and histological study. *J Orthop Res* 1990;8:712–721.

Healing and Reconstruction of Ligaments

Andrish JT, Woods LD: Dacron augmentation in anterior cruciate ligament reconstruction in dogs. *Clin Orthop* 1984;183:298–302.

Arnoczky SP, Warren RF, Ashlock MA: Replacement of the anterior cruciate ligament using a patellar tendon allograft: An experimental study. *J Bone Joint Surg* 1986;68A:376–385.

Ballock RT, Woo SLY, Lyon RM, et al: Use of patellar tendon autograft for anterior cruciate ligament reconstruction in the rabbit: A long term histologic and biomechanical study. *J Orthop Res* 1989;7:474–485.

Biden E, O'Connor JJ: Experimental methods used to evaluate knee ligament function, in Daniel DM, Akeson WH, O'Connor JJ (eds): *Knee Ligaments: Structure, Function, Injury, and Repair.* New York, Raven Press, 1990, pp 135–151.

Butler DL: Anterior cruciate ligament: Its normal response and replacement. *J Orthop Res* 1989;7:910–921.

Butler DL, Sheh MY, Stouffer DC, et al: Surface strain variation in human patellar tendon and knee cruciate ligaments. *J Biomech Eng* 1990;112:38–45.

Bylski-Austrow DI, Grood ES, Hefzy MS, et al: Anterior cruciate ligament replacements: A mechanical study of femoral attachment location, flexion angle at tensioning, and initial tension. *J Orthop Res* 1990;8:522–531.

Cho KO: Reconstruction of the anterior cruciate ligament by semitendinosus tenodesis. *J Bone Joint Surg* 1975;57A:608–612.

Clancy WG Jr, Narechania RG, Rosenberg TD, et al: Anterior and posterior cruciate ligament reconstruction in rhesus monkeys. *J Bone Joint Surg* 1981;63A:1270–1284.

Draganich LF, Reider B, Ling M, et al: An in vitro study of an intraarticular and extraarticular reconstruction in the anterior cruciate ligament deficient knee. *Am J Sports Med* 1990;18:262–266.

Engebretsen L, Lew WD, Lewis JL, et al: Mechanics of repair of the anterior cruciate ligament: A cadaveric study of ligament augmentation. *Acta Orthop Scand* 1989;60:703–709.

France EP, Paulos LE, Rosenberg TD, et al: The biomechanics of anterior cruciate allografts, in Friedman MJ, Ferkel RD (eds): *Prosthetic Ligament Reconstruction of the Knee.* Philadelphia, WB Saunders, 1988, pp 180–185.

Gibbons MJ, Butler DL, Grood ES, et al: Effects of gamma irradiation on the initial mechanical and material properties of goat bone-patellar tendon-bone allografts. *J Orthop Res* 1991;9:209–218.

Goodfellow J, O'Connor J: The mechanics of the knee and prosthesis design. *J Bone Joint Surg* 1978;60B:358–369.

Grood ES, Hefzy MS, Lindenfield TN: Factors affecting the region of most isometric femoral attachments: Part 1. The posterior cruciate ligament. Part II. The anterior cruciate ligament. *Am J Sports Med* 1989;17:197–216.

Haut RC, Powlison AC: The effects of test environment and cyclic stretching on the failure properties of human patellar tendons. *J Orthop Res* 1990;8:532–540.

Hefzy MS, Grood ES: Sensitivity of insertion locations on length patterns of anterior cruciate ligament fibers. *J Biomech Eng* 1986;108:73–82.

Holden JP, Grood ES, Butler DL, et al: Biomechanics of fascia lata ligament replacements: Early postoperative changes in the goat. *J Orthop Res* 1988;6:639–647.

Hoogland T, Hillen B: Intra-articular reconstruction of the anterior cruciate ligament: An experimental study of length changes in different ligament reconstructions. *Clin Orthop* 1984;185:197–202.

Horibe S, Shino K, Nagano J, et al: Replacing the medial collateral ligament with an allogenic tendon graft: An experimental canine study. *J Bone Joint Surg* 1990;72B:1044–1049.

Hurley PB, Andrish JT, Yoshiya S, et al: Tensile strength of the reconstructed canine anterior cruciate ligament: A long-term evaluation of the modified Jones technique. *Am J Sports Med* 1987;15:393.

Indelicato PA: Non-operative treatment of complete tears of the medial collateral ligament of the knee. *J Bone Joint Surg* 1983;65A:323–329.

Inoue M, McGurk-Burleson E, Hollis JM, et al: Treatment of the medial collateral ligament injury: I. The importance of anterior cruciate ligament on the varus-valgus knee laxity. *Am J Sports Med* 1987;15:15–21.

Jackson DW, Grood ES, Arnoczky SP, et al: Freeze dried anterior cruciate ligament allografts: Preliminary studies in a goat model. *Am J Sports Med* 1987;15:295–303.

Jackson DW, Grood ES, Cohn BT, et al: The effects of in situ freezing on the anterior cruciate ligament: An experimental study in goats. *J Bone Joint Surg* 1991;73A:201–213.

Jones KG: Reconstruction of the anterior cruciate ligament: A technique using the central one third of the patellar ligament. *J Bone Joint Surg* 1963;45A:925–932.

Larson RV, Sidles JA, Matsen FA, et al: Isometric ligament insertions in the knee. *Am J Sports Med* 1987;15:394.

Lew WD, Engebretsen L, Lewis JL, et al: Method for setting total graft force and load sharing in augmented ACL grafts. *J Orthop Res* 1990;8:702–711.

McPherson GK, Mendenhall HV, Gibbons DF, et al: Experimental, mechanical and histologic evaluation of the Kennedy ligament augmentation device. *Clin Orthop* 1985;196:186–195.

Mott HW: Semitendinosus anatomic reconstruction for cruciate ligament insufficiency. *Clin Orthop* 1983;172:90–92.

Noyes FR, Grood ES: The strength of the anterior cruciate ligament in humans and rhesus monkeys: Age-related and species-related changes. *J Bone Joint Surg* 1976;58A:1074–1082.

O'Brien SJ, Warren RF, Pavlov H, et al: Reconstruction of the chronically insufficient anterior cruciate ligament with the central third of the patellar ligament. *J Bone Joint Surg* 1991;73A:278–286.

O'Donoghue DH, Frank GR, Jeter GL, et al: Repair and reconstruction of the anterior cruciate ligament in dogs: Factors influencing long term results. *J Bone Joint Surg* 1971;53A:710–718.

Odensten M, Gillquist J: Functional anatomy of the anterior cruciate ligament and a rationale for reconstruction. *J Bone Joint Surg* 1985;67A:257–262.

Penner DA, Daniel DM, Wood P, et al: An in vivo study of anterior cruciate ligament graft placement and isometry. *Am J Sports Med* 1988;16:238–243.

Roberts TS, Drez D Jr, McCarthy W, et al: Anterior cruciate ligament reconstruction using freeze-dried, ethylene oxide-sterilized, bone-patellar tendon-bone allografts: Two year results in thirty-six patients. *Am J Sports Med* 1991;19:35–41.

Sabiston P, Frank C, Lam T, et al: Transplantation of the rabbit medial collateral ligament: II. Biomechanical evaluation of frozen/thawed allografts. *J Orthop Res* 1990;8:46–56.

Silvaggio VJ, Fu FH, Georgescu HI, et al: The induction of IL-1 by freeze dried ethylene oxide treated bone-patellar tendon-bone allograft wear particles: An in vitro study. *Arthroscopy*, in press.

Thomas ED, Gresham RB: Comparative tensile strength study of fresh, frozen, and freeze-dried human fascia lata. *Surg Forum* 1963;14:442–443.

van Rens TJ, van den Berg AF, Huiskes R, et al: Substitution of the anterior cruciate ligament: A long-term histologic and biomechanical study with autogenous pedicled grafts of the iliotibial band in dogs. *Arthroscopy* 1986;2:139–154.

Vasseur PB, Rodrigo JJ, Stevenson S, et al: Replacement of the anterior cruciate ligament with a bone-ligament-bone anterior cruciate ligament allograft in dogs. *Clin Orthop* 1987;219:268–277.

Webster DA, Werner FW: Mechanical and functional properties of implanted freeze-dried flexor tendons. *Clin Orthop* 1983;180:301–309.

Woo SLY, Buckwalter JA: Ligament and tendon autografts and allografts, in Friedlaender GE, Goldberg VM (eds): *Bone and Cartilage Allografts: Biology and Clinical Applications.* Park Ridge, IL, American Academy Orthopaedic Surgeons, 1991, pp 103–121.

Woo SLY, Inoue M, McGurk-Burleson E, et al: Treatment of the medial collateral ligament injury: II. Structure and function of canine knees in response to differing treatment regimens. *Am J Sports Med* 1987;15:22–29.

Woo SLY, Young EP, Ohland KJ, et al: The effects of transection of the anterior cruciate ligament on healing of the medial collateral ligament: A biomechanical study of the knee in dogs. *J Bone Joint Surg* 1990;72A:382–392.

Yasuda K, Tomiyama Y, Ohkoshi Y, et al: Arthroscopic observations of autogeneic quadriceps and patellar tendon grafts after anterior cruciate ligament reconstruction of the knee. *Clin Orthop* 1989;246:217–224.

Yoshiya S, Andrish JT, Manley MT, et al: Graft tension in anterior cruciate ligament reconstruction: An in vivo study in dogs. *Am J Sports Med* 1987;15:464–470.

Yoshiya S, Andrish JT, Manley MT, et al: Augmentation of anterior cruciate ligament reconstruction in dogs with prostheses of different stiffnesses. *J Orthop Res* 1986;4:475–485.

Meniscus

Cox JS, Nye CE, Schaefer WW, et al: The degenerative effects of partial and total resection of the medial meniscus in dogs' knees. *Clin Orthop* 1975;109:178–183.

Dandy DJ, Jackson RW: The diagnosis of problems after meniscectomy. *J Bone Joint Surg* 1975;57B:349–352.

DeHaven KE: Decision-making factors in the treatment of meniscus lesions. *Clin Orthop* 1990;252:49–54.

Fairbank TJ: Knee joint changes after meniscectomy. *J Bone Joint Surg* 1948;30B:664–670.

Jackson JP: Degenerative changes in the knee after meniscectomy. *J Bone Joint Surg* 1967;49B:584.

Mow VC, Arnoczky SP, Jackson DW (eds): *Knee Meniscus: Basic and Clinical Foundations.* New York, Raven Press, 1992.

Ricklin P, Ruttimann A, Del Buono MS (eds): *Meniscus Lesions, Diagnosis, Differential Diagnosis and Therapy,* ed 2. New York, Thieme-Stratton, 1983.

Tapper EM, Hoover NW: Late results after meniscectomy. *J Bone Joint Surg* 1969;51A:517.

Meniscal Anatomy

Adams ME, Ho YA: Localization of glycosaminoglycans in human and canine menisci and their attachments. *Connect Tissue Res* 1987;16:269–279.

Adams ME, Muir H: The glycosaminoglycans of canine menisci. *Biochem J* 1981;197:385–389.

Arnoczky SP, Warren RF: Microvasculature of the human meniscus. *Am J Sports Med* 1982;10:90–95.

Bullough PG, Munuera L, Murphy J, et al: The strength of the menisci of the knee as it relates to their fine structure. *J Bone Joint Surg* 1970;52B:564–567.

Fife RS: Identification of link proteins and a 116,000-Dalton matrix protein in canine meniscus. *Arch Biochem Biophys* 1985;240:682–688.

Hardingham TE, Muir H, Kwan MK, et al: Viscoelastic properties of proteoglycan solutions with varying proportions present as aggregates. *J Orthop Res* 1987;5:36–46.

Hascall VC, Hascall GK: Proteoglycans, in Hay ED (ed): *Cell Biology of Extracellular Matrix.* New York, Plenum Press, 1981, pp 39–63.

Biomechanics of Meniscus Function

Ahmed AM, Burke DL: In-vitro measurement of static pressure distribution in synovial joints: Part 1. Tibial surface of the knee. *J Biomech Eng* 1983;105:216–225.

Armstrong CG, Mow VC: Biomechanics of normal and osteoarthrotic articular cartilage, in Straub LR, Wilson PD Jr (eds): *Clinical Trends in Orthopaedics.* New York, Thieme-Stratton, 1982, pp 189–197.

Arnoczky SP, Adams ME, DeHaven KE, et al: Meniscus, in Woo SL-Y, Buckwalter JA (eds): *Injury and Repair of the Musculoskeletal Soft Tissues.* Park Ridge, IL, American Academy of Orthopaedic Surgeons, 1988, pp 487–537.

Aspden RM, Yarker YE, Hukins DW: Collagen orientations in the meniscus of the knee joint. *J Anat* 1985;140:371–380.

Buckwalter JA, Rosenberg LC: Electron microscopic studies of cartilage proteoglycans: Direct evidence for the variable length of the chondroitin sulfate-rich region of proteoglycan subunit core protein. *J Biol Chem* 1982;257:9830–9839.

Chern KY, Zhu W, Mow VC: Anisotropic viscoelastic shear properties of meniscus. *Adv Bioeng* 1989;15:105–106.

Eyre DR, Wu JJ: Collagen of fibrocartilage: A distinctive molecular phenotype in bovine meniscus. *FEBS Lett* 1983;158:265–270.

Fithian DC, Zhu WB, Ratcliffe A, et al: Exponential law representation of tensile properties of human meniscus. *Proc Inst Mech Eng* 1989;5:85.

Hardingham TE, Muir H: Hyaluronic acid in cartilage and proteoglycan aggregation. *Biochem J* 1974;139:565–581.

Hardingham TE: The role of link-protein in the structure of cartilage proteoglycan aggregates. *Biochem J* 1979;177:237–247.

Hayes WC, Bodine AJ: Flow-independent viscoelastic properties of articular cartilage matrix. *J Biomech* 1978;11:407–419.

Huiskes R, Chao EY: A survey of finite element analysis in orthopedic biomechanics: The first decade. *J Biomech* 1983;16:385–409.

Hukins DW, Aspden RM, Yarker YE: Fibre reinforcement and mechanical stability in articular cartilage. *Eng Med* 1984;13:153–156.

Kwan MK, Lai WM, Mow VC: Fundamentals of fluid transport through cartilage in compression. *Ann Biomed Eng* 1984;12:537–558.

Linn FC, Sokoloff L: Movement and composition of interstitial fluid of cartilage. *Arthritis Rheum* 1965;8:481–494.

Mow VC, Fithian DC, Kelly MA: Fundamentals of articular cartilage and meniscus biomechanics, in Ewing JW (ed): *Articular Cartilage and Knee Joint Function: Basic Science and Arthroscopy.* New York, Raven Press, 1990, pp 1–18.

Mow VC, Holmes MH, Lai WM: Fluid transport and mechanical properties of articular cartilage: A review. *J Biomech* 1984;17:377–384.

Mow VC, Kuei SC, Lai WM, et al: Biphasic creep and stress relaxation of articular cartilage in compression? Theory and experiments. *J Biomech Eng* 1980;102:73–84.

Mow VC, Rosenwasser MP: Articular cartilage: Biomechanics, in Woo SLY, Buckwalter JA (eds): *Injury and Repair of the Musculoskeletal Soft Tissues.* Park Ridge, IL, American Academy of Orthopaedic Surgeons, 1988, pp 427–463.

Muir H: Proteoglycans as organizers of the extracellular matrix. *Biochem Soc Trans* 1983;11:613–622.

Proctor CS, Schmidt MB, Whipple RR, et al: Material properties of the normal medial bovine meniscus. *J Orthop Res* 1989;7:771–782.

Radin EL, Ehrlich MG, Chernack R, et al: Effect of repetitive impulsive loading on the knee joint of rabbits. *Clin Orthop* 1978;131:288–293.

Rosenberg LC, Buckwalter JA, Coutts R, et al: Articular cartilage, in Woo SLY, Buckwalter JA, (eds): *Injury and Repair of the Musculoskeletal Soft Tissues.* Park Ridge, IL, American Academy of Orthopaedic Surgeons, 1988, pp 401–482.

Sauren AAHJ, Huson A, Schouten RY: An axisymmetric finite element analysis of the mechanical function of the meniscus. *Int J Sports Med* 1984;5:93S–95S.

Seedhom BB, Hargreaves DJ: Transmission of the load in the knee joint with special reference to the role of the menisci: Part II. Experimental results, discussion and conclusions. *Eng Med* 1979;8:220–228.

Shrive NG, Lam TC, Damson E, et al: A new method of measuring the cross-sectional area of connective tissue structures. *J Biomech Eng* 1988;110:104–109.

Shrive NG, O'Connor JJ, Goodfellow JW: Load-bearing in the knee joint. *Clin Orthop* 1978;131:279–287.

Voloshin AS, Wosk J: Shock absorption of meniscectomized and painful knees: A comparative in vivo study. *J Biomed Eng* 1983; 5:157–161.

Walker P, Amstutz HC, Rubinfield M: Canine tendon studies: II. Biomechanical evaluation of normal and regrown canine tendons. *J Biomed Mater Res* 1976;10:61–76.

Yasui K: Three dimensional architecture of normal human menisci. *J Jpn Orthop Assoc* 1978;52:391.

Meniscal Injury, Healing, Regeneration, Repair, and Replacement

Arnoczky SP, McDevitt CA, Schmidt MB, et al: The effect of cryopreservation on canine menisci: A biochemical, morphologic, and biomechanical evaluation. *J Orthop Res* 1988;6:1–12.

Arnoczky SP, Milachowski KA: Meniscal allografts: Where do we stand?, in Ewing JW (ed): *Articular Cartilage and Knee Joint Function: Basic Science and Arthroscopy.* New York, Raven Press, 1990, pp 129–136.

Arnoczky SP, Warren RF, McDevitt CA: Meniscal replacement using a cryopreserved allograft: An experimental study in the dog. *Clin Orthop* 1990;252:121–128.

Nikolaou PK, Seaber AV, Glisson RR, et al: Anterior cruciate ligament allograft transplantation: Long-term function, histology, revascularization, and operative technique. *Am J Sports Med* 1986;14:348–360.

Stone KR, Rodkey WG, Webber RJ, et al: Meniscal regeneration with copolymeric collagen scaffolds: In vitro and in vivo studies evaluated clinically, histologically, and biochemically. *Am J Sports Med* 1992:20:104–111.

Stone KR, Rodkey WG, Webber RJ, et al: Future directions: Collagen-based prostheses for meniscal regeneration. *Clin Orthop* 1990;252:129–135.

Chapter 3
Anatomy, Physiology, and Mechanics of Skeletal Muscle

William E. Garrett, Jr, MD, PhD
Thomas M. Best, MD, PhD

Chapter Outline

Chapter Outline

Skeletal muscle constitutes the single largest tissue mass in the body, making up 40% to 45% of the total body weight. It is a composite structure that consists of muscle cells, organized networks of nerves and blood vessels, and an extracellular connective tissue matrix (Fig. 1). This framework is necessary to support the structure against injury and to organize the individual units into tissues and organs that can contract efficiently to produce joint movement and locomotion. The structure and function of skeletal muscle have intrigued man throughout the ages. With its enormous adaptive potential, variability, and dependability, skeletal muscle has been the subject of many theories and complex philosophic schemes to explain the fascinating aspects of animal movement. In the last few centuries, and particularly in recent years, knowledge of skeletal muscle has expanded rapidly.

Muscle Structure and Function

Histologic Organization

The basic structural element of skeletal muscle is the muscle fiber. It is a syncytium of many cells fused together with multiple nuclei. The fiber runs from tendon or bone across one or more joints into a tendon of insertion, which connects to bone. The fiber is a single very long "cell," but usually is much shorter than the length of the muscle because of its oblique orientation to the muscle axis. Fiber arrangement can be parallel or oblique to the long axis of the muscle (Fig. 2). The latter arrangement includes pennate, bipennate, multipennate, or even more complex fiber arrangements.

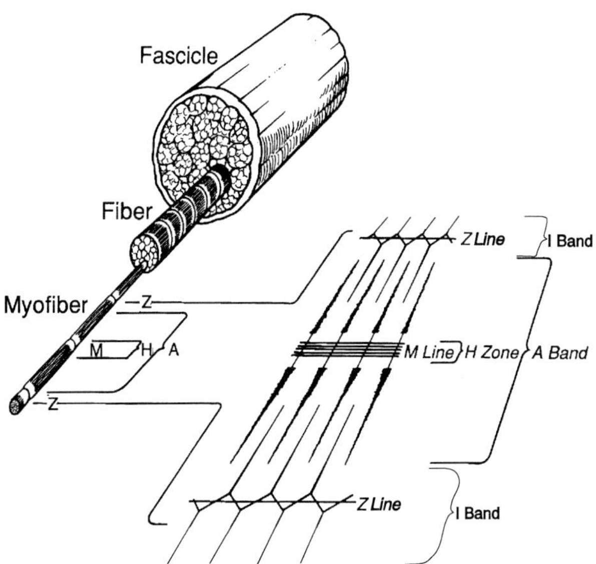

Figure 1
Schematic drawing of the structural design of human skeletal muscle.

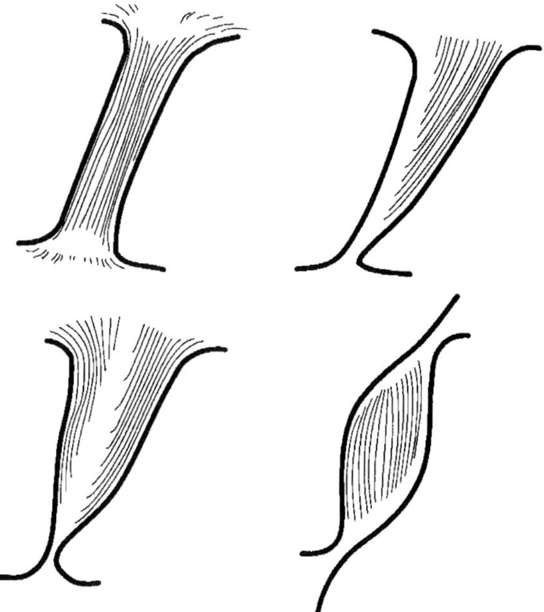

Figure 2
Muscle fiber architecture. **Top left,** Parallel. **Top right,** Unipennate. **Bottom left,** Bipennate. **Bottom right,** Fusiform.

Muscle fibers are organized histologically by the surrounding connective tissue. This framework serves to bind the contractile units together to provide for integrated motion among the fibers. The endomysium is the delicate connective tissue surrounding individual fibers. In turn, fibers are arranged together as fascicles, which are large enough to be visible to the naked eye. The connective tissue surrounding fascicles is called the perimysium and that surrounding the whole muscle is called the epimysium. This membrane covers the muscle loosely to allow for the length changes that occur in muscle. Blood vessels supplying the fibers also are arranged in the connective tissue with enough redundancy to allow for changes in length during the contraction-extension cycle of a muscle.

In addition to a highly organized pattern at the microscopic level, muscle fibers have a highly organized architectural arrangement. Fiber arrangement within the muscle is an important determinant of its functional and contractile properties (Fig. 3). As muscle fibers shorten, the muscle's volume usually is assumed to be constant. Consequently, the tendon moves only along the axis of pull, and fibers become more pennated (α increases, Fig. 3, *bottom right*). Therefore, the fiber and tendon shortening are not colinear, and the force along the axis of the tendon is reduced by cos α. Although this pennated arrangement results in a reduction of the muscle fiber force transmitted to the tendon, it permits a larger

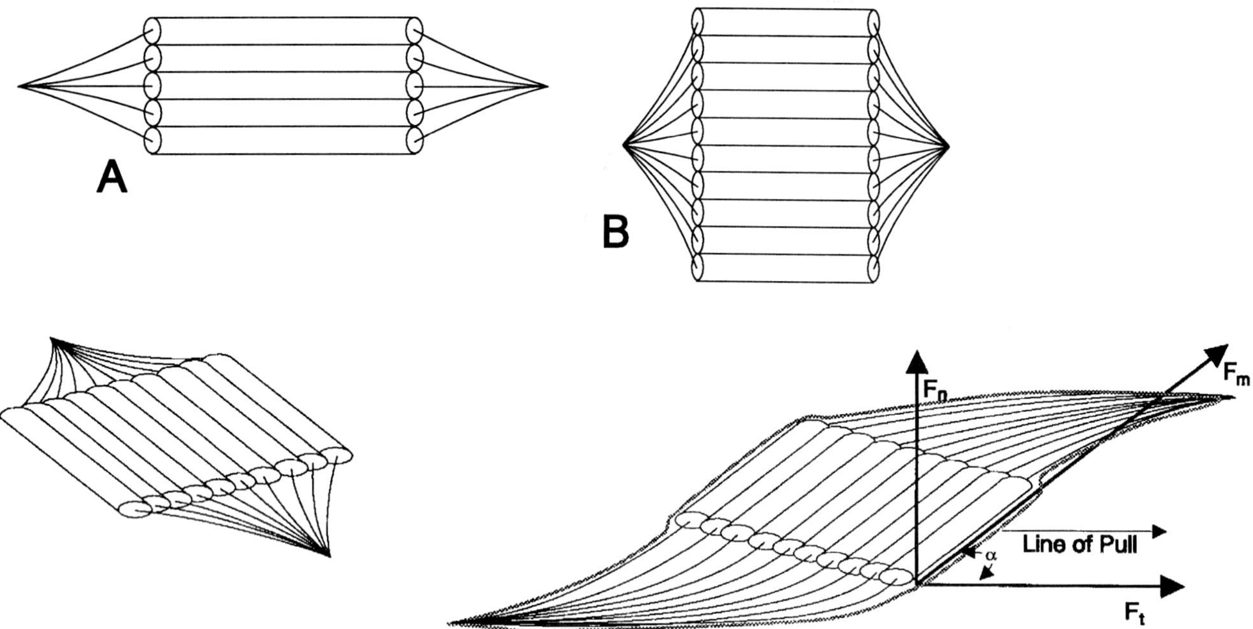

Figure 3
The effects of muscle architecture on force development and length change. **Top,** The length of A is twice that of B; the cross-sectional area of A equals that of B; the maximum force of A is one-half that of B and the maximum length change of A is twice that of B. **Bottom left,** The force is diminished only by a small factor when fibers are arranged in a pennate fashion. **Bottom right,** The effect of fiber angle pennation on whole-muscle force. α = angle of pennation; F_m = muscle force; F_n = normal component; F_t = tangential component.

number of fibers to be packed in a smaller cross-sectional area. In general, maximal force production of a muscle is proportional to its physiologic cross-sectional area (PCSA), but the total amount and speed of shortening are proportional to individual muscle fiber length. A muscle needed more for force production might have many short fibers arranged in a pennate fashion. However, the same amount of muscle tissue could be arranged in fewer but longer fibers when more shortening and less force are required of the muscle. In general, the architectural arrangement of its muscle fibers is quite specific to the task of a muscle in the body and is one of the primary mechanisms used for specificity of function.

In clinical practice a muscle made ineffective by direct trauma or denervation may be substituted by the transfer of another muscle-tendon unit. It is necessary to have a tendon with suitable size and length to allow transfer. Because the ability of the muscle to shorten and to generate force is largely determined by the number, size, and architectural arrangement of the muscle fibers within the muscle belly, it is important to match the characteristics desired of the deficient muscle with those of the transferred muscle.

Cytology of the Muscle Fiber

Individual muscle fibers are surrounded by a plasma membrane known as the sarcolemma. External to this membrane is a separate basement membrane that is a connective tissue structure 100 to 200 nm thick. Electron microscopy shows that this membrane consists of an inner layer, the lamina rara or lucida, and an outer, more dense layer, the lamina densa. The basement membrane then merges with a reticular layer and the extracellular matrix. This basement membrane contains a number of protein and carbohydrate components contributed by both the muscle fiber and fibroblasts. Among its components are collagen, laminin, fibronectin, and other specific glycoproteins. The basement membrane, the reticular layer, and the close layer of matrix and collagen fibers together constitute the endomysium, which is well supplied with capillaries.

Each striated muscle fiber contains numerous nuclei, which typically are located at the periphery of the fiber immediately beneath the sarcolemma. In addition, separate cells called satellite cells lie along the surface of the muscle at the periphery of each fiber. These cells are thought to be stem cells capable of proliferation and regeneration in the event of damage to the muscle fibers.

A muscle fiber contains a sarcoplasm that includes the contents of the sarcolemma exclusive of the nuclei. The sarcoplasm is similar to the cytoplasm of other cell types and, therefore, contains a cellular matrix and organelles. These organelles include the Golgi apparatus found near many of the nuclei and the mitochondria, which are abundant near the nuclei. The other important organelle is the sarcoplasmic reticulum, a continuous system of membrane that corresponds to the endoplasmic reticulum of other cell types. Other components of the sarcoplasm include lipid droplets, glycogen, and myoglobin.

Nerve-Muscle Interaction

Skeletal muscle is under the control of a nerve that enters the muscle at its motor point. Each nerve cell axon then branches many times, and every muscle fiber is contacted by one nerve terminal. This point of contact is called the motor end plate (Fig. 4) and is the site of cellular communication between the nervous system and skeletal muscles. Together a single nerve axon and all muscle fibers it contacts constitute a motor unit. Muscle fibers belonging to a single motor unit are not necessarily adjacent; adjacent muscle fibers can belong to different motor units. Both the number of muscle fibers within a motor unit and the number of motor units within a given muscle are quite variable. Where fine motor control and coordinated movements are necessary, for example, the extraocular muscles, there may be as few as 10 muscle fibers per motor unit. Yet in large muscles, such as the gastrocnemius, there may be more than 1,000 muscle fibers in a single motor unit. The size of the motor unit is also related to the size of the motor axon and to the size of the cell body in the anterior gray horn of the spinal cord. In addition, motor unit size is related to the fiber type and physiology of muscle, as will be discussed below.

A motor unit is stimulated to contract by an electrical impulse, or action potential, which originates from the cell body of the nerve. This potential is propagated down the entire length of the axon from the spinal cord to the peripheral skeletal muscle. The nerve forms a synapse with the muscle at a specialized region known as the motor end plate. An electrical impulse passing along the cell membrane of the axon is transformed to a similar electrical signal in the membrane of the muscle fiber. This transmission is not achieved by direct electrical transmission; the process involves chemical transmission across a gap of extracellular space separating the two membrane systems. As the axon approaches the muscle at the synapse, it loses its myelin sheath and the entire terminal axon is covered by a Schwann cell, a connective tissue cell surrounding nerve fibers (Fig. 4). The nerve terminal spreads out over an area of the muscle membrane called the sole plate. An axon terminal and muscle membrane interdigitate across a series of membrane foldings called primary synaptic folds, which greatly amplify the area of membrane juxtaposed between nerve and muscle. At all times the muscle membrane is separated from the nerve

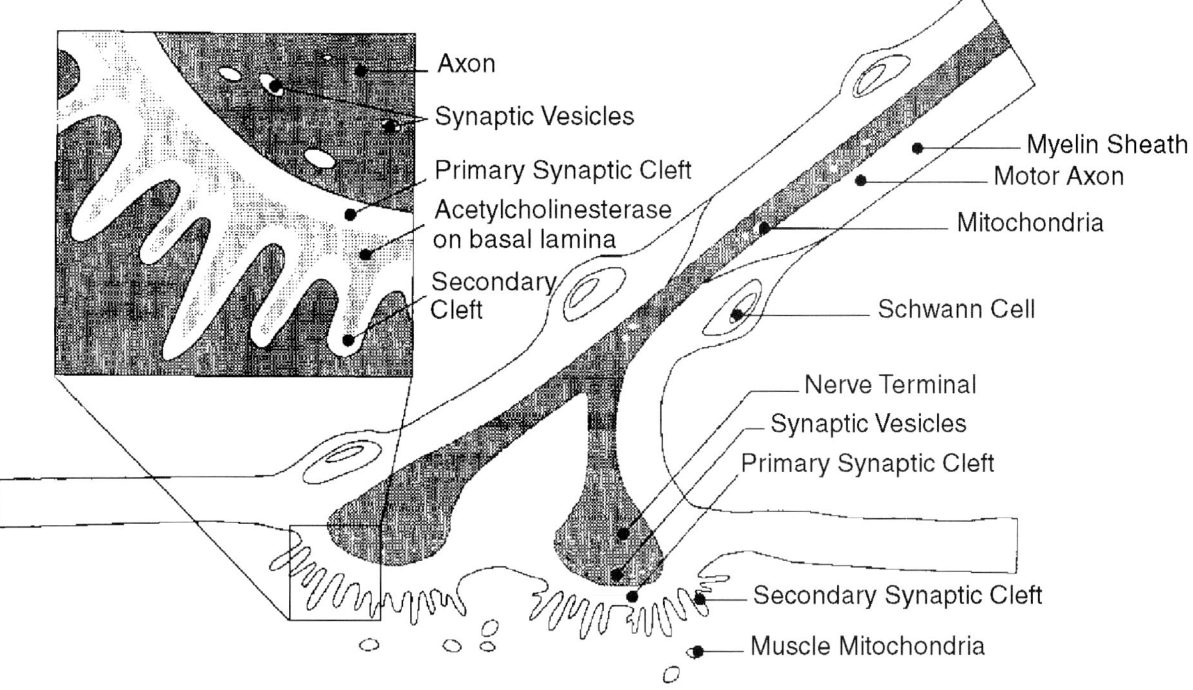

Figure 4
Schematic representations of the motor end plate.

membrane by a space of approximately 50 nm, called the synaptic cleft.

The nerve and muscle membranes are not in direct contact, and signals are passed from nerve to muscle by chemical transmitters. The chemical acetylcholine is stored in the presynaptic axon in small membrane-bound sacs called vesicles. When the electrical impulse arrives in the terminal axon, the membrane allows the flow of calcium ions into the cell. An increase in the intracellular calcium concentration causes the vesicles to fuse with the terminal axon membrane and to release acetylcholine into the synaptic cleft. The acetylcholine must then diffuse across the synaptic cleft and bind to a specific receptor on the surface of the muscle membrane. The binding of the acetylcholine to its receptor allows currents to flow into the muscle membrane and depolarize the cell. Depolarization triggers an action potential that passes the length of the muscle membrane. The action potential in the muscle membrane is similar to the action potential in a nerve. The acetylcholine is deactivated by the enzyme acetylcholinesterase or other less specific cholinesterases located in the extracellular space and associated with the basement membrane. The breakdown products may be reabsorbed by the terminal axon to be used in the resynthesis of additional transmitter.

Various pharmacologic and physiologic processes influence the neuromuscular junction. Alpha-tubocurarine binds to the acetylcholine receptors and makes impulse transmission impossible. This agent was discovered initially as a poison used on the arrows of South American Indian tribes to paralyze an animal, and today it is commonly used as a paralyzing anesthetic agent. Succinylcholine and many other compounds can exert a similar effect on muscle by various interactions with the receptor. Succinylcholine actually binds to the receptor and causes temporary depolarization of the muscle membrane, followed by failure of impulse transmission.

Other pharmacologic agents can inhibit acetylcholinesterase and lead to continued high concentrations of acetylcholine at the synapse. These agents can be used to help reverse the effects of paralyzing agents or to treat diseases characterized by deficient interactions between acetylcholine and its receptor. Myasthenia gravis is a disease characterized by severe muscle weakness that is particularly evident following muscle fatigue. The basic pathophysiology is a shortage of acetylcholine receptors, which probably is caused by an autoimmune reaction against the receptors. Cholinesterase inhibitors, such as neostigmine and edrophonium, allow a longer life for acetylcholine and, therefore, more chance for it to interact with receptors before hydrolysis of the molecule. The effects of these medically useful agents are, of course, reversible. There are also compounds that alter the cholinesterase irreversibly. These anticholinesterase compounds include the highly toxic nerve gases used in chemical warfare and in certain insecticides. The toxicity of these irreversible agents limits their clinical usefulness.

Muscle Membrane System

Muscle fibers are long cells, and electrical activity at the surface is far away from the central portions of these fibers. Following depolarization of the end plate, the electrical impulse passes down the muscle membrane to reach the interior of the muscle by an intricate membrane system (Fig. 5). This extensive system facilitates communication of the surface signals into the depths of the muscle fiber, permitting rapid signal impulse throughout the cell. Transverse tubules penetrate from the surface into the fibers near the level of the A-band and I-band junction in mammalian muscle. These tubules are generally directed perpendicularly to the axis of the cells and are therefore termed transverse. The transverse tubules interact with another large system of membrane-bound sacs called the sarcoplasmic reticulum, which stores calcium inside its membrane system and, therefore, out of the muscle cytoplasm. The membranes of the sarcoplasmic reticulum actively accumulate calcium from the muscle cytoplasm. An electrical impulse originating within the muscle membrane and tubular systems causes the momentary release of calcium from the

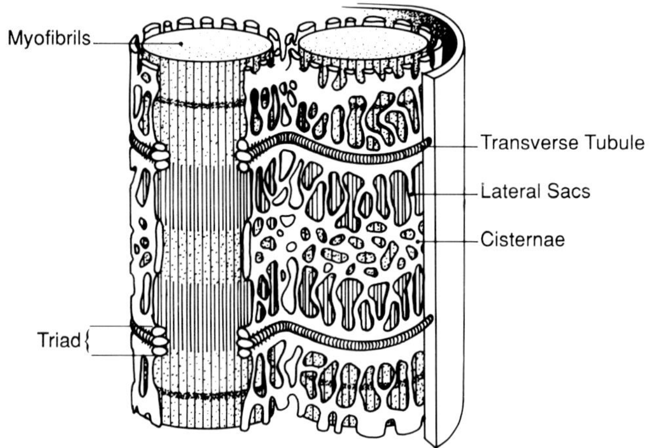

Figure 5
Details of the sarcoplasmic reticulum (SR), the system of membranes responsible for transmission of the electrical signal from one muscle cell to the next. An action potential moving over the surface of the fiber passes down the transverse tubules and causes Ca^{2+} release from the outer vesicles of the SR.

sarcoplasmic reticulum into the muscle cytoplasm. Calcium release is the trigger that causes the contractile proteins to interact and to generate force. The membrane system, including the surface membrane, transverse tubules, and sarcoplasmic reticulum, provides a mechanism for rapid conduction of an electric signal from the cell surface throughout the entire fiber. This system allows for more concurrent release of calcium, synchronized interactions of muscle proteins, and subsequent production of force.

The sarcoplasmic reticulum is specialized for somewhat different functions. The portion that abuts the transverse tubules is called the junctional sarcoplasmic reticulum. Usually the transverse tubule is linked to two sacs of the junctional reticulum in a structure called a triad. Bridging structures connect the three separate membrane systems. Electrical impulses in the tubules will cause calcium release from this sarcoplasmic reticulum. Other specializations of the sarcoplasmic reticulum include fenestrated and tubular membranous structures placed throughout the cell.

The sarcoplasmic reticulum contains specific enzymes for sequestration of calcium into the membrane system and out of the sarcoplasm. Control of the intracellular calcium concentration is the mechanism for regulating the on-off contractile function of the contractile proteins. The calcium adenosine triphosphatase (ATPase) protein is a distinct membrane protein. Calsequestrin and another glycoprotein with a high affinity for calcium are other protein components of the sarcoplasmic reticulum.

Structural Proteins of Muscle

The proteins responsible for force production in the presence of calcium form highly ordered structures in the muscle cytoplasm. On observation of histologic sections of muscle, it is clear that a high degree of order exists, and that there is a repeating structural array of longitudinal fibers with a discrete cross-striated appearance. If the plasma membrane and basement membranes of a muscle fiber are disrupted, the internal structures of the cell are seen to consist of many long, slender, parallel elements called myofibrils. The long myofibrils are about 1 μm in diameter and have a distinct banding pattern. The patterns in the individual myofibrils are usually in register in the muscle fiber. This gives the entire fiber a striated appearance by light microscopy, giving rise to striated muscle as the descriptive term for skeletal muscle. Within the fiber and within the individual myofibrils, there is a regular arrangement of alternating light and dark bands with a repeating period of 2 to 3 μm. The ordered structure is explained by the molecular structure of the contractile proteins.

The fibril is composed of repeating units called sarcomeres (Fig. 6). The fine structure of the sarcomere can be seen with the electron microscope. There are repeating light and dark bands; each of the bands is bisected by a more darkly staining line. The dark band or A-band is composed primarily of paral-

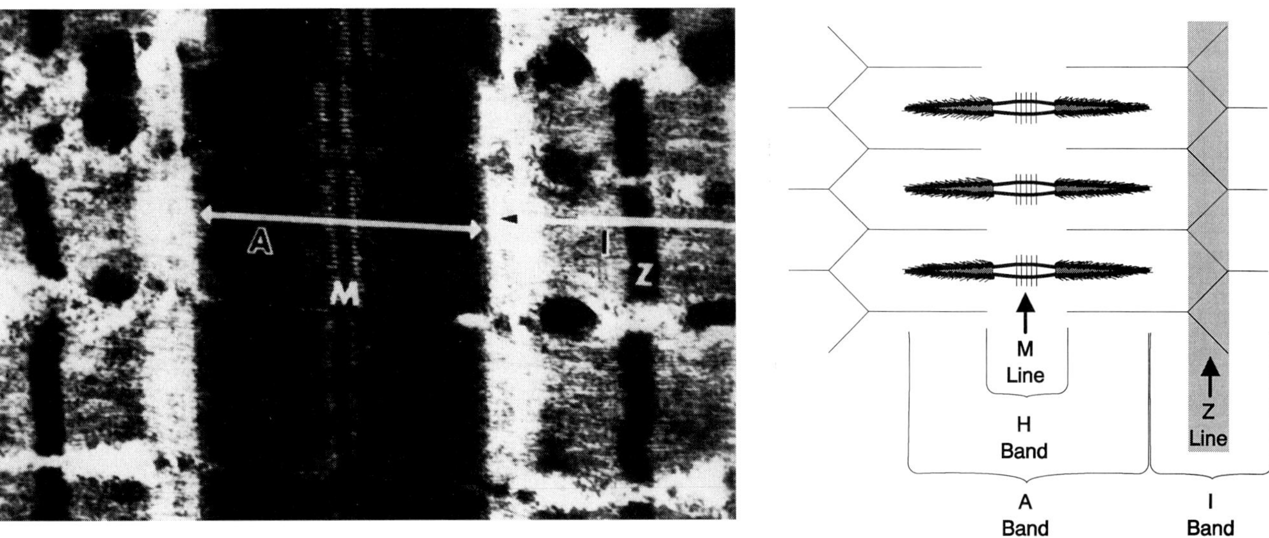

Figure 6
Left, Electron micrograph of skeletal muscle illustrating the striated, banded appearance. **Right,** the basic functional unit of skeletal muscle, the sarcomere.

lel thick filaments in register with a central set of interconnecting filaments called the M-line. The thick filaments are composed primarily of the protein myosin. Myosin is a hexameric molecule, molecular weight of about 500,000, composed of two large isomers known as heavy chains and four smaller polypeptides called light chains (Fig. 7). The molecule has a long relatively insoluble helical portion that polymerizes to form the backbone portion of the thick filament. There are also two associated globular portions of the molecule called cross-bridges, which project from the backbone of the thick filament. These globular proteins can be enzymatically cleaved from the helical portion of the myosin molecule and are soluble in physiologic solutions. The myosin projections are the enzymatic portion of the molecule; they are capable of binding to the thin filaments and are capable of hydrolyzing adenosine triphosphate (ATP). In addition to myosin, there are other proteins that make up the thick filaments. Among these are C-protein, M-protein, and titin. Titin is a large (10^6 dalton) protein that is involved in the tiny filamentous connections between the ends of the thick filaments to the Z-line. Additionally, M-protein, myosin, and creatine kinase are associated with thick filaments at the M-line. Creatine kinase catalyzes the phosphorylation of adenosine diphosphate (ADP) to form ATP and may be important in maintaining the supply of energy molecules to the cross-bridges. The functions of the minor proteins of the A-band are not well characterized.

The I-band is composed of thin filaments in register and joined at their axial center by the interconnecting Z-line (Fig. 8). The thin filaments are made up primarily of molecules of the protein actin. The thin filaments are approximately 1.0 μm long; the protein and the filament size are highly conserved. Actin monomers are arranged in a helical fashion on the thin filaments with an axial separation of 5.5 nm between subunits and a helical repeat of approximately 77 nm. Two other proteins associated with the thin filaments are troponin and tropomyosin, which will be discussed below. Other proteins associated with the Z-line include alpha-actinin, desmin, zeugmatin, and filamin. The Z-line is a highly organized structure that interconnects the thin filaments in a very precise array. The thick filaments of the A-band are arranged in a hexagonal lattice. A-bands and I-bands interdigitate so that the thin filaments are located at the trigonal points of the hexagonal lattice of thick filaments. The cross-bridges project from the thick filaments toward the thin filaments at regular intervals of approximately 14.3 nm.

The guiding hypothesis for muscle shortening calls for the cross-bridges from the thick filaments to reach out and attach to the thin filaments. Cross-bridges use the energy made available from the hydrolysis of ATP to undergo a conformational change and, by some mechanism, cause the thick filaments to slide past the thin filaments. The cross-bridges cycle many times as they release from the actin on the thin filament, spring back to their initial conformation, and are ready to repeat the process in rapid succession. Both actin and myosin molecules have a recognizable polarity, which is essential to muscular contraction. To allow shortening of the

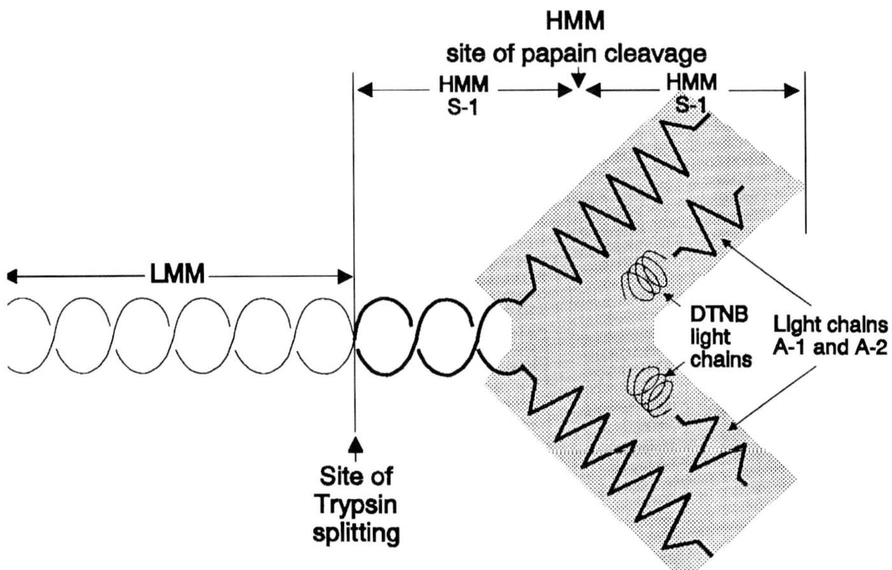

Figure 7
Schematic drawing of myosin molecule showing subunit structure. The heavy-chain component possesses the ATP-ase activity and the light chain confers solubility properties of the molecule. HMM = heavy meromyosin; LMM = light meromyosin.

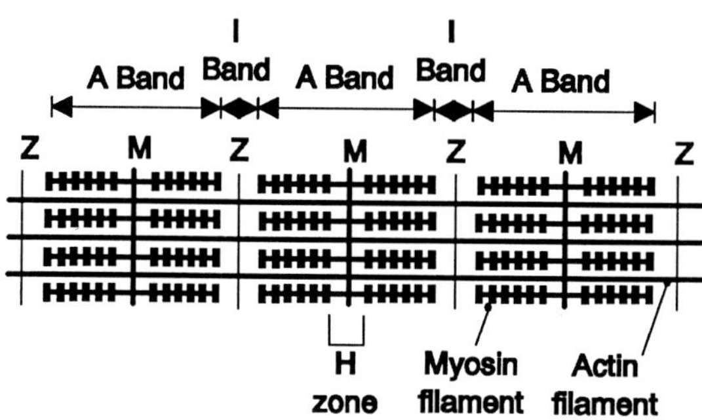

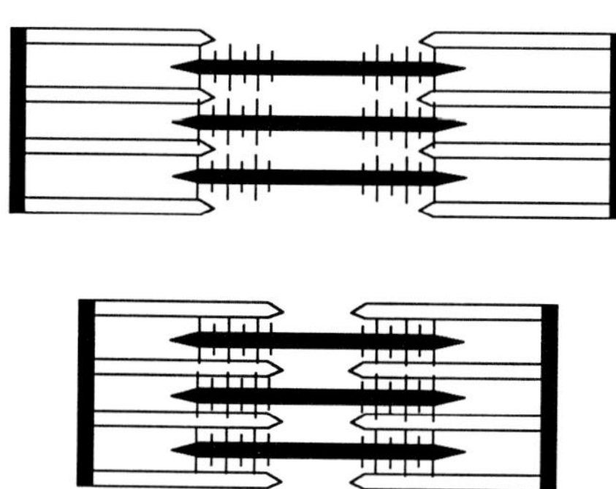

Figure 8
Schematic indicating the sliding of thick and thin filaments that occurs when a muscle is stretched. Note the constancy of the lengths of both thick and thin filaments. (Adapted with permission from Carlson FD, Wilkie DR: *Muscle Physiology.* New Jersey, Prentice Hall, 1974.)

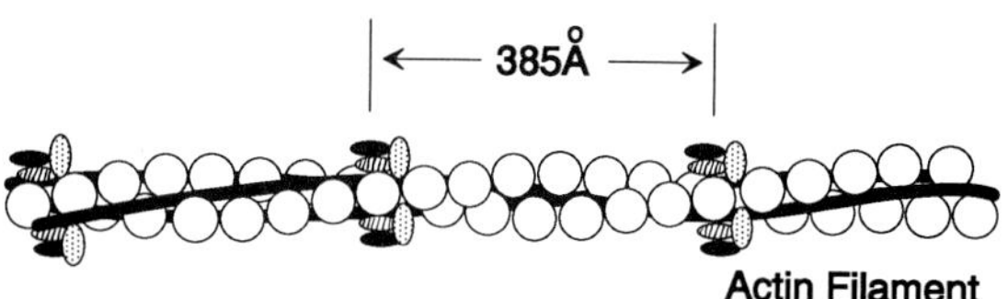

Figure 9
Features of regulation of muscle contraction. Structure of actin is represented by two chains of beads in a double helix. The troponin complex consists of calcium-binding protein (TN-C, black); inhibitory protein (TN-I, cross-hatched); and protein binding to tropomyosin (TN-T, stippled). The tropomyosin (dark line) lies in each groove of the actin filament.

sarcomere, the polarity must be different in the thick filaments on either side of the M-line so that the thick filament arrays of the I-bands on either side of the A-band are pulled toward each other and toward the center of the A-band. Similarly, the thin filaments must have opposite polarity on either side of the Z-line so that they are pulled in between the thick filaments by the cross-bridges to allow shortening and force production (Fig. 8). These features form the basis of the well-known sliding filament-swinging cross-bridge theory of muscle contraction.

How does calcium regulate this process? Troponin and tropomyosin are regulatory proteins linked to the actin molecules (Fig. 9). Tropomyosin is an approximately 41-nm-long helical molecule that is situated on the thin filament in such a manner that it prevents the cross-bridges from binding to the actin. The two main subunits of the molecule are the alpha and beta polypeptide chains, which differ mainly in their cysteine content and electrophoretic mobility. The ratio of these two subunits varies among fiber types. Troponin is the calcium-sensitive regulatory protein that can induce a conformational change in tropomyosin and, thereby, allow cross-bridge association with actin. Troponin has three subunits: troponin-I is inhibitory and can block actin-myosin interaction; troponin-T binds to tropomyosin; and troponin-C can bind calcium. A high enough concentration of calcium in the sarcoplasm will allow binding of calcium to troponin-C. A conformational change then removes the troponin-I from its inhibitory position and allows for actin and myosin interaction, with subsequent ATP hydrolysis and initiation of muscle contraction. When calcium is no longer available to the troponin, its conformation reverts and the tropomyosin shifts back to create a stearic block to the cross-bridges.

The physiology of the above activity is as follows. A single electrical impulse passes down an axon to its motor end plates, chemical transmission occurs at the synapses, and electrical potentials are generated in the muscle membranes. These electrical potentials pass along the muscle surface and into the fibers via the transverse tubules, resulting in calcium release from the sarcoplasmic reticulum. Calcium binds to the thin filaments and causes conformational changes that allow interactions between thick and thin filaments. Using the energy from the hydrolysis of ATP, the cross-bridges cycle and cause the sarcomeres to attempt to shorten or to resist stretch by pulling the thin filament arrays into the thick filament arrays. The contractile proteins interact, resulting in muscle contraction and force production. Following completion of the electrical event, muscle relaxation occurs by active transport of the calcium into the longitudinal tubules of the sarcoplasmic reticulum. This results in calcium dissociation from troponin and a conformational change in tropomyosin to prevent further cross-bridge attachment.

Muscle Contraction or Action

The cellular events in the process of muscle activation can now be considered at the level of the whole neuromuscular organ system along with the physiologic basis for muscle contraction. Traditionally, it has been important to define the conditions under which muscle is activated, because many parameters are felt to influence its contraction.

For the most part, muscle has been studied under conditions of controlled length or tension. In isometric (same length) testing, muscle length is held constant, and the resultant force is measured. Alternatively, in isotonic (same load) testing, a muscle is activated to shorten against a constant load, while length changes with time are assessed. More recently, muscle has been evaluated under isokinetic (same speed) activation, which the load accommodates to maintain a constant velocity of shortening or lengthening.

Muscle activation results in force generation within the muscle. If the resisting load is less than the force generated by the muscle, then the muscle will shorten; this condition is termed concentric action (or contraction). If the resisting force is greater than that generated by the muscle, the muscle will lengthen; this is termed eccentric action (or contraction). Some confusion has been generated by the traditional use of the term muscle contraction. Muscle can be activated and lengthened simultaneously. Rather than call this condition an eccentric (or lengthening) contraction, it is, perhaps, less confusing to call it eccentric action. However, contraction usually refers to the action of activated muscle whether its length is decreasing, constant, or increasing.

Conditions of nerve activation can be controlled to produce a single stimulus, repetitive stimuli at constant frequencies, or stimuli in other desired modes. For a single activation, the muscle tension can be seen to rise quickly and then fall back to baseline in a variable amount of time, usually less than 200 ms. This physiologic event is called a muscle twitch, the tension response by a muscle to a single nerve stimulus (Fig. 10). There is no increment in tension as a result of repetitive stimuli if a second nerve action potential arrives after the tension in response to the first action potential has returned to the baseline and the membrane has stabilized. All that happens is that another twitch occurs. However, if the nerve stimulation frequency increases such that successive action potentials arrive before the contractile tension resulting from the previous stimulus has returned to the baseline, the tension can rise above the tension of a single twitch. As the stimulation frequency increases, the tension in the muscle displays a summation effect that, with higher frequencies of stimulation, approaches a

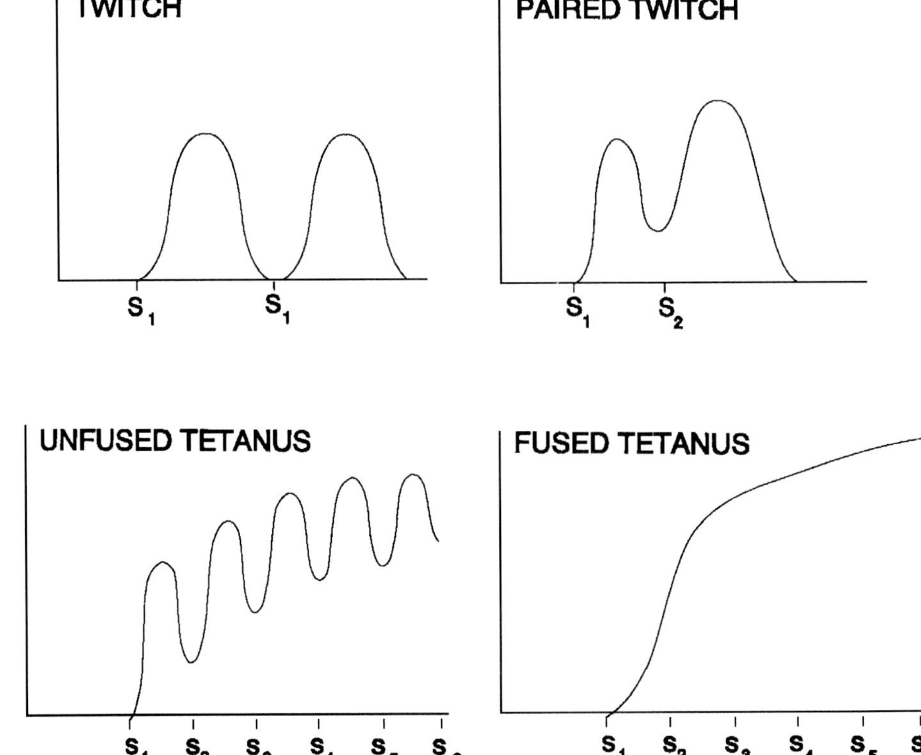

Figure 10
Twitch and tetanus. As the frequency of stimulation is increased, muscle force rises to an eventual plateau level known as fused tetanus.

maximum level called a tetanus. The tension generated during tetanus can be several times that of a twitch, making the alteration of stimulation frequency a powerful mechanism under control of the central nervous system (CNS) for altering tension. Stimulation frequencies needed to achieve tetanic stimulation vary from 40 to 300 Hz for different muscles and species.

The force of muscle contraction can be increased either by altering the frequency of stimulation to make the same motor units work harder or by involving more motor units (recruitment). It is now believed that these phenomena occur together, resulting in a very ordered and sequential recruitment of motor units and regulation of activation frequency to optimize muscle contraction and limb motion. The relative contribution of these two mechanisms to increasing force production varies among different muscles. For example, in muscles such as the abductor pollicis, motor unit recruitment is probably maximum when the force reaches about 30% of maximum; whereas, in muscles such as the biceps brachii, motor unit recruitment is felt to occur up to 85% of the maximum force.

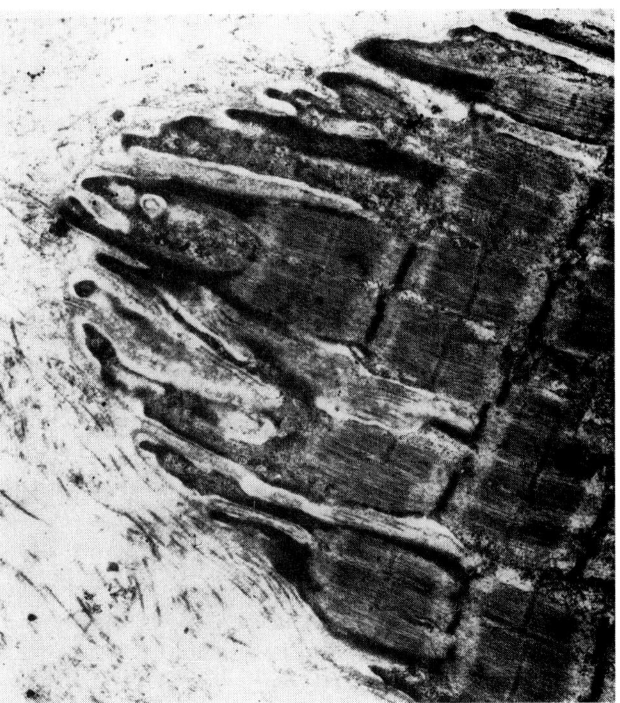

Figure 11
The myotendinous junction. Electron micrograph of a myotendinous junction section longitudinally. Myofilaments distal to the terminal Z disk end in a series of filaments bounded by a folded plasmalemma. (Reproduced with permission from Tidball JG: Myotendinous junction: Morphological changes and mechanical failure associated with muscle cell atrophy. *Exp Mol Pathol* 1984;40:1–12.)

Myotendinous Junction

The force generated within muscle fibers must be transmitted to the tendon to produce limb movement and human locomotion. The area responsible for this force transmission is the myotendinous junction, a region of highly folded membranes at the muscle-tendon interface (Fig. 11). This folding increases junctional surface area by ten to 20 times. Because stress is proportional to force and inversely related to contact area, the large increase in membrane area within this region results in a corresponding decrease in the stresses. In addition, the stresses are changed from tensile to shear because the membranes are aligned nearly parallel with the axis of the muscle and the tendon.

The structural and molecular organization of the myotendinous junction is being studied in more detail. The thin filaments appear to terminate beneath the muscle plasma membrane within subsarcolemmal densities that seem to be involved with the binding of the contractile proteins to the cell membranes. At least two cytoskeletal proteins, vinculin and talin, are thought to be involved in the molecular chain linking the thin filaments to the extracellular structural proteins. A separate structural link must actually traverse the cell membrane of the muscle. The likely molecular link is a large transmembrane glycoprotein called integrin, which has an affinity for both the intracellular and extracellular structural proteins and exists within the cell membrane at the myotendinous junction. On the extracellular side of the junction is a well-developed basement membrane seen easily by electron microscopy. At this region, the forces generated by the myofibrils and passed across the cell membrane are thought to be linked to the extracellular collagen fibers of the tendon. Among the proteins present in the basement membrane are fibronectin, laminin, type IV collagen, and M1 antigen. Some of these proteins have a molecular affinity for the collagen of the tendon.

Fiber Types and Adaptability of Muscle

The Motor Unit

A motor unit includes a single alpha motoneuron axon and the muscle fibers it innervates. All muscle fibers in a single motor unit have the same contractile and metabolic properties, implying that the muscle fiber type is related to its interaction with its motor nerve. Different fiber or motor unit types are widely recognized, and they have dis-

Table 1
Characteristics of human skeletal muscle fiber types

	Type I	Type IIA	Type IIB
Other Names	Red, slow twitch (ST) Slow oxidative (SO)	White, fast twitch (FT) Fast oxidative glycolytic (FOG)	Fast glycolytic (FG)
Speed of contraction	Slow	Fast	Fast
Strength of contraction	Low	High	High
Fatigability	Fatigue-resistant	Fatigable	Most fatigable
Aerobic capacity	High	Medium	Low
Anaerobic capacity	Low	Medium	High
Motor unit size	Small	Larger	Largest
Capillary density	High	High	Low

tinctly different physiologic, structural, and histochemical properties (Table 1). For example, chicken muscle exists in distinctly different fiber types as noted by color (dark or white) and taste. More recent observations of different muscle fiber types have been aided greatly by the use of histochemical stains. Histochemical staining allows differentiation of muscle fibers based on the reactivity of muscle structural proteins and metabolic pathways in response to incubation in appropriate chemical reactants. Serial sections can then be used to compare the properties of the same fiber after exposure to other histochemical stains and to routine histologic techniques.

The most useful histochemical techniques for distinguishing fiber types are those based on the ability of myosin to hydrolyze ATP and those based on the enzymes and substrates of the different metabolic pathways in muscle fibers. The enzyme which hydrolizes ATP is referred to as actomyosin ATPase, or more commonly the ATPase. Differences in the specific ATPase activities of myosin are a result of the existence of several forms of this protein. Myosin from muscles that develop tension slowly (slow twitch muscles) is acid stable and alkaline labile, whereas the opposite is true for muscles that develop tension quickly (fast twitch muscles). According to the sliding filament hypothesis, myosin is the most important contractile protein because it hydrolyzes the ATP to yield the energy for formation of the actomyosin complex. Furthermore, the activity of the myosin ATPase correlates closely with the intrinsic speed of muscle shortening. Much of the regulation and alteration of skeletal muscle phenotypes involves the myosin molecule, and the relative size of a muscle fiber appears to be related to the type of myosin expressed. Relatively large fibers express primarily fast myosin, whereas relatively small fibers express slow myosin.

Histochemical stains have allowed profiling of several sets of fibers according to the structural, biochemical, and physiologic characteristics of the fiber types. There are also subtle differences in the myofibrillar structure. At least three separate motor unit profiles are widely accepted, although available evidence and classification schemes make it clear that there is significant overlap and that other fiber types might also be considered.

The type I or slow-oxidative fiber is characterized histochemically by a light reaction to myosin ATPase stains at alkaline conditions and a heavy reaction to the enzymes and substrates of oxidative metabolic pathways. Physiologically this fiber type has slower contraction and relaxation times than other fiber types. The contraction time of a muscle relates to the rate at which force is developed after electrical stimulation (for example, fast or slow), and relaxation time relates to the rate of decline of force in the muscle following cessation of stimulation. Type I motor units, those with type I fibers, are extremely resistant to fatigue. Structurally, there are more mitochondria in these fibers as well as more capillaries per fiber.

Type II motor units can be subdivided into several subgroups; however, two main subgroups usually are considered, types IIA and IIB. The type IIB or fast glycolytic motor unit has the fastest contraction time and is the least resistant to fatigue. As expected from its physiologic characteristics, this type has a well-developed glycolytic metabolic capacity and a less well-developed oxidative system. The type IIB motor unit has the largest number of muscle fibers per motor unit, the largest axon, and the largest cell body.

Intermediate between type I and type II motor units are the type IIA or fast oxidative glycolytic motor units. Their contraction times are faster than type I but slower than type IIB. Similarly, their fatigue resistance lies between that of type I and IIB motor units. In IIA motor units, both the oxidative and glycolytic pathways are well developed. Axon size and the number of muscle fibers per motor unit in type IIA motor units also rank between type I and IIB motor units. Distinctions in physiologic, histochemical, and biochemical properties are less distinct between IIA and IIB fibers than between either of them and type I fibers. Biochemically, the structural proteins in the sarcomere are also distinct. Myosin, tropomyosin, and troposin have distinct structural isomers with different fiber types. Recent investigations have shown more heterogeneity in the structural proteins than had been expected.

Most mammalian carnivores, including humans, also have a type IIc fiber, which is most prominent in the jaw muscle. It has a unique myosin with physiologic and histochemical properties intermediate in the spectrum, between type IIA and type IIB fibers. At birth, up to 10% of muscle fibers may be type IIc; this declines to approximately 2% after the first year of life. As a result, it is often felt that the type IIc fiber is an undifferentiated fiber. During physical training there may be as many as 10% of these fibers present in some muscles of endurance athletes. Their presence has yet to be explained, although it is felt by some that this fiber type represents a transitional form between types I and II fibers.

Motor units and fiber types are recruited into activity by the CNS in an orderly fashion according to size. The smaller motor units, composed predominantly of type I fibers, are recruited first, whereas the largest motor units, composed of type IIB fibers, are recruited primarily with exercise of higher intensity, and the type IIA fibers or motor units are intermediate in size and order of recruitment. This seems quite reasonable considering the metabolic, physiologic, and anatomic characteristics of the different motor units. Motor units of small force, slow speed, and good endurance are involved first; with more intensity, type IIA motor units having more speed and force and relatively good endurance are added; and for the most intense exercise, the type IIB motor units with high speed, high force, but little endurance are added to the other motor units. Biochemistry studies of muscle glycogen depletion patterns in man have supported this concept. It has been shown that low intensity exercise results in significant glycogen depletion in the type I fibers with little change in type II fibers. Conversely, high intensity exercise produces glycogen depletion in both fiber types, but it is more severe in the type II fibers.

Correlation of Fiber Type With Performance

Most human muscles are composed of a mixture of the muscle fiber types discussed above, whereas some animal muscles are composed of a single muscle fiber type. The tonic or postural muscles, for example, soleus, are usually situated closer to the bony skeleton and have a greater proportion of type I fibers. In contrast, the phasic or faster contracting muscles lie in a more superficial position and have a higher proportion of type II fibers. However, individual variations in fiber type composition are often quite large, and biopsies of the vastus lateralis muscle may vary to the extent that more than 90% of the muscle fibers are either type I or type II fibers. In addition, significant variations in fiber type percentages occur at different locations within the same muscle for a given individual. Thus, significant skepticism should be displayed when interpreting the results of studies showing changes in fiber type proportions in response to different exercise regimens.

The physiologic properties of a muscle largely reflect the specific types and concentrations of proteins within the muscle. Inherent fiber type differences appear to be related to performance capacity, especially where speed of contraction and endurance or fatigability are concerned. Muscle biopsies from successful sprinters are much more likely to show a preponderance of type II fibers. Similarly, distance runners are highly inclined towards having predominantly type I fibers. Athletes in those sports requiring the extremes of speed and endurance often display a fiber type profile that is consistent with current knowledge of fiber type differences. However, it remains unknown at this time if these fiber distributions are genetically based or are a response to sustained extremes of training.

In addition, isokinetic dynamometers can be used to evaluate the ability of individuals to perform motor tasks requiring speed or endurance for which they have not trained, and muscle biopsy indicates a correlation between performance and fiber type. Those with a higher percentage of type I fibers will generally exhibit more endurance, whereas those with more type II fibers will demonstrate more torque at higher speeds. There is overlap, however, and fiber type is only one of many factors relevant to performance capacity. Most sports are neither purely speed nor endurance oriented, and fiber type percentage provides little correlation with performance. In addition, athletes without a fiber type composition that might be considered ideal are still able to excel at speed and endurance sports. Therefore, the utility of a biopsy in selecting athletes for sport is not generally accepted.

Mutability of Fiber Types

Various forms of overload can bring about adaptation of all components of the motor unit including the muscle fiber itself, the neuromuscular junction, and the corresponding alpha motoneuron. This biologic plasticity of muscle typically results in a logical alteration of both the morphology and the function of the muscle fiber, which is consistent with the hypothesis that muscle adapts to the function it performs. This polymorphism of the skeletal muscle fiber also exists in smooth muscle and cardiac muscle. A variety of stimuli including cross-reinnervation, electrical stimulation, hypergravity stress, thyrotoxicosis, compensatory hypertrophy, and exercise have been studied to elucidate mechanisms for this adaptive response.

Extreme conditions, beyond those usually encountered in rigorous training, can lead to fiber type interconversions. Studies have shown that a nerve to predominantly type I muscle can be cut and reconnected to the distal cut end of a predominantly type II muscle. Similarly, the proximal end of a nerve to a type II muscle can be connected to a type I muscle. Both result in a logical alteration in the expression of fiber types. With time, there is an extensive, but not complete, conversion of the fiber type characteristics of the muscle to reflect the fiber types usually supplied by the new motor nerve. Even without interchanging the nerves, the fiber type characteristics of a muscle can be altered to a new profile by changing the frequency at which the muscle is stimulated. Type II muscles driven by external stimulation of the nerve at the low frequencies characteristic of type I muscles can undergo fiber type interconversions. Clearly, there is a complex interaction between the nerve, the muscle, and their pattern of use by the CNS that can lead to interconversions between type I and II fibers.

Caution must be taken in drawing conclusions about the potential adaptive response of human muscle to exercise. The experimental protocols used in the above studies bear little resemblance to physical activity of humans. It is generally accepted that in humans the relative percentages of type I or type II fibers are established genetically without a great deal of capacity for change. However, within the type II fiber population there is ample evidence for interconversion of types IIA and IIB fibers. For example, endurance training appears to be able to increase the percentage of type IIA fibers at the expense of type IIB fibers. Strength training without an emphasis on endurance conditioning may correspondingly increase the percentage of type IIB fibers. Certainly, the differences and boundaries between types IIA and IIB fibers are less than those between types I and II fibers.

Energetics of Muscle

Phosphagens

The immediate chemical energy source for muscle contraction is the ATP molecule (Fig. 12). This molecule consists of an adenosine moiety attached to three serial inorganic phosphate moieties; the terminal two phosphate bonds are high-energy bonds that, on hydrolysis, make a significant amount of chemical energy available to support biologic reactions. When the terminal phosphate of ATP is hydrolyzed, ADP and inorganic phosphate are formed, and energy is released. The second high-energy phosphate bond may be hydrolyzed, resulting in the formation of adenosine monophosphate (AMP) and inorganic phosphate and, again, the release of the energy of the phosphate bond.

Although ATP is used as the energy source for muscle contraction, most studies show little change in the level of ATP in activated muscle even after enough time to hydrolyze all available ATP. The muscle cell has mechanisms for maintaining the concentration of ATP. Another source of high energy phosphate bonds, the molecule creatine phosphate (CP), has a bond energy even higher than that in ATP. However, CP cannot be used directly by the cells as a source of energy; instead, it is used to synthesize ATP from ADP. The enzyme creatine kinase found in muscle catalyzes transfer of the high-energy phosphate bond of CP to ADP by the reaction

$$\text{ADP} + \text{CP} \rightarrow \text{ATP} + \text{Creatine}$$

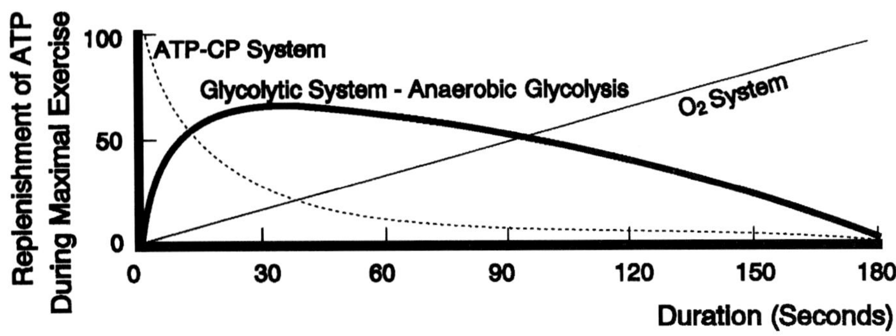

Figure 12
Energy sources for anaerobic activity.

In addition, a second enzyme, myokinase, maintains ATP concentration by the reaction

$$ADP + ADP \rightarrow ATP + AMP$$

The total energy available from ATP hydrolysis is approximately enough to allow a person to sprint for less than 50 yards. If the energy available from all the stored forms of high-energy phosphate compounds (phosphagens) is considered, there is enough energy to run approximately 200 yards.

Normal activity levels and, especially, the extremely high activity levels of athletic participation rely on metabolic processes that can replenish the supply of phosphagens to support muscle contraction. For many aspects of athletic performance, the ability of these metabolic systems to replenish ATP is the limiting factor in the level of performance. Two metabolic pathways are available to maintain the energy supply. The aerobic system relies on the availability of oxygen, and the anaerobic system can proceed in the absence of oxygen at the cellular level.

Aerobic Metabolism

When oxygen is available, aerobic metabolism is the primary source for replenishment of ATP. The aerobic system may use glucose or fatty acids to produce large quantities of ATP (Fig. 13). In aerobic metabolism, glucose is broken into two molecules of pyruvate, which then enter the Krebs (or TCA) cycle. Basically, in the Krebs cycle hydrogen atoms are removed from the pyruvate and combined with oxygen to produce water and liberate energy, which is made available to processes that transform low-energy phosphates into high-energy phosphates. In turn, these high-energy phosphates are coupled with ADP to produce ATP. In this manner, a molecule of glucose can be oxidized to result in 38 molecules of ATP by the overall reaction:

$$C_6H_{12}O_6 + 6O_2 + 38P + 38\ ADP \rightarrow 6CO_2 + 6H_2O + 38\ ATP$$

Glucose, considered the initial energy source, exists in the cell as a limited quantity of its phosphorylated form, glucose-6-phosphate. After the digestion of carbohydrates and sugars, glucose enters the bloodstream, from which it can enter the cell. Glucose not converted to glucose-6-phosphate can be stored in the form of glycogen. The quantity of stored glycogen is a product of the use and storage of glucose. Diets rich in carbohydrate may lead to a higher store of glycogen, which can prolong the cellular ability to continue energy production at a given rate. In addition, the use of glycogen could be diminished if there were other potential sources of energy for oxidative metabolism of muscle. Muscle glycogen levels, unlike those in liver, remain quite stable and usually do not decline during fasting. In cardiac muscle, glycogen levels may actually increase during fasting.

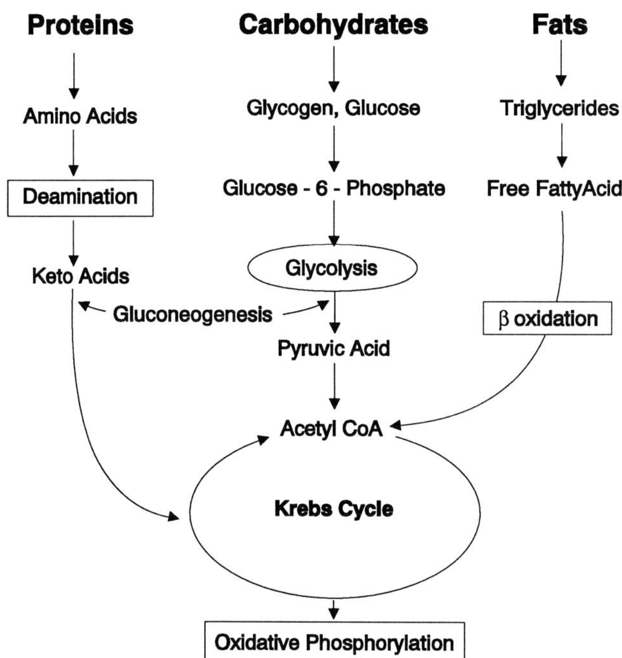

Figure 13
Foodstuffs (fats, carbohydrates, proteins) containing carbon and hydrogen for glycolysis, fatty acid oxidation, and the Krebs (or TCA) cycle in a muscle cell.

Anaerobic Metabolism

Anaerobic metabolism involves the hydrolysis of glucose molecules by a succession of steps to lactic acid; therefore, this system is sometimes referred to as lactic acid metabolism (Fig. 14). Glucose exists within the cell as either glucose-6-phosphate or as glycogen. By anaerobic metabolism, glucose can be rapidly transformed into two molecules of lactic acid plus sufficient energy to convert two molecules of ADP to ATP. However, the lactic acid produced is a relatively toxic substance, which causes acidosis and fatigue. Additionally, anaerobic metabolism uses the potential energy in a molecule of glucose very inefficiently. However, it is the energy system relied on by the muscle when a lot of energy is needed for a relatively short period of time.

Fat and Protein

Fat stores are abundant in the body and provide by far the largest potential source of energy. Fats usually are stored in the body as triglycerides, which consist of three separate fatty acids bound to the molecule glyceraldehyde. Triglycerides can be cleaved into free fatty acids, which can be cleaved by a process called beta-oxidation into successive

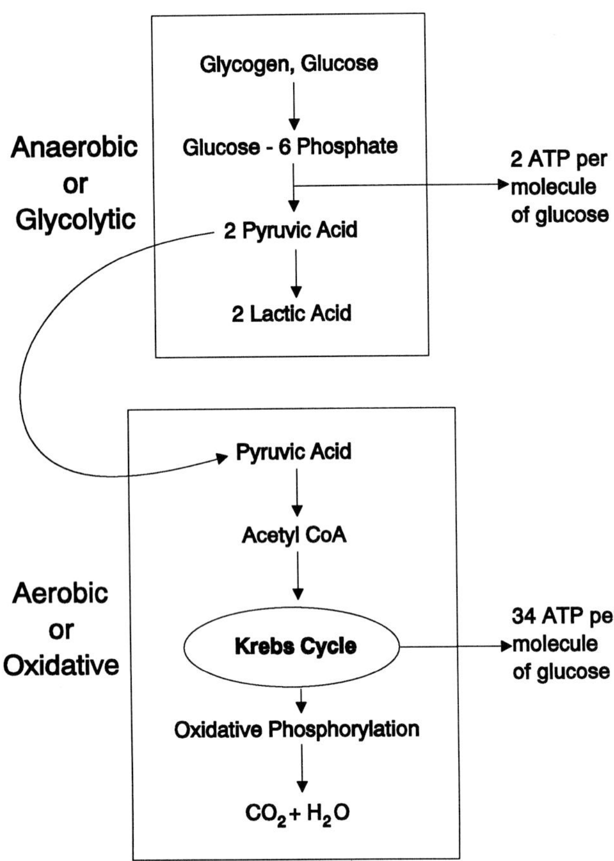

Figure 14
A summary of the ATP yield in the anaerobic and aerobic breakdown of carbohydrates. Glycolysis and anaerobic metabolism occur in the cytoplasm while oxidative phosphorylation occurs in the mitochondria.

two-carbon fragments called acetyl coenzyme A (acetyl CoA). Acetyl CoA can then enter the Krebs cycle, in which it is hydrolyzed, as are the products of glucose metabolism. The breakdown of a single free fatty acid molecule can yield sufficient energy to convert a variable amount of ADP to ATP, depending on the length of the carbon chain. For example, a fatty acid molecule with 16 carbon atoms can yield sufficient energy to convert as many as 129 molecules of ADP to ATP after complete oxidation.

Fatty acids can be stored within the muscle or supplied via the bloodstream. They can enter the bloodstream immediately after digestion or following mobilization from tissue sources such as adipose tissue. Their availability is quite unlikely to be a limiting factor in metabolism, except in unusual circumstances of malnutrition.

Under normal conditions, proteins never provide the primary fuel for metabolism, but they serve as an accessory source. Protein is hydrolyzed in the alimentary system into its constituent amino acids. Deamination of amino acids produces ketoacids, which can enter into the Krebs cycle for energy production. Ketoacids can also go through a process, called gluconeogenesis, by which they can be converted to glucose; this process occurs in conditions of severe glucose depletion when body proteins are hydrolyzed to provide energy substrate.

Use of Energy Sources

Aerobic and anaerobic metabolism take place simultaneously, and there is a well-ordered interaction between the two systems. It is not true that exercise of different intensity levels results in the use of one system exclusively; aerobic and anaerobic pathways are both used, and both carbohydrate and fat are used as energy sources for exercise of virtually any intensity. However, the two systems are quite distinct and can respond quite differently to stresses applied to muscle. Exercises designed to work the body at an intensity level that will not result in rapid fatigue because the energy demand can be met by the oxidative energy system are called aerobic exercises. Conversely, anaerobic exercise refers to exercise of high enough intensity and duration to cause the anaerobic system to produce enough by-products to cause fatigue and lead to cessation or reduction of exercise.

The different motor unit types have different levels of enzymes needed for the aerobic and anaerobic energy systems. Histochemical stains show that type I fibers have a higher concentration of the aerobic system enzymes and that type IIB fibers have a higher concentration of enzymes involved with anaerobic energy supply. Type IIA fibers generally have intermediate levels of both types of enzymes.

The intensity and duration of muscular activity greatly influence the use of the separate energy sources and metabolic systems. Brief exercises of high intensity, such as a short sprint, rely on stored phosphagens. As the intensity falls and the length of activity increases, the anaerobic system is more involved because it replenishes the supply of ATP. The production of acidosis induces fatigue and limits the duration of activity. As the exercise intensity falls further, such as in walking or jogging slowly, the metabolic demands can be met by aerobic metabolism. The level at which the body can meet its metabolic demands without developing acidosis is influenced by the rate at which the cardiovascular system can supply oxygen and by the metabolic capacity of the fibers. The metabolic pathways and energy sources are very much influenced by the state of training.

Aerobic metabolism uses either glucose derived from stored glycogen or fatty acids derived from stored triglycerides. An acute response during prolonged aerobic exercise is the shift to oxidation of fatty acids, which in turn conserves the limited carbohydrate stores in the body. That carbohydrates are the limiting factor is easily appreciated on realization that one pound of stored fat can produce more than enough energy to run a marathon.

Muscle Mechanics

The mechanical properties of muscle have in the past been subject to extensive investigation. The great majority of research in the field has concerned the study of isolated muscle or muscle fibers. Although some intricacies of muscle are not yet fully understood, the major properties of this tissue, both active and passive, are now clearly defined.

The forces produced by muscles will be considered, including their relationship to muscle length, shortening speed, time, and state of activation. Muscle can actively shorten, and it can resist lengthening by active or passive means. In classical mechanics, muscle has been considered to consist of contractile elements that respond to stimulation of the muscle and passive or elastic elements that can passively resist stretching, similarly to a spring. It was useful in previous models characterizing the load-deformation relationship of muscle to consider that there are elastic elements both in parallel and in series with the contractile element. Much of the pioneering work in this area was initiated by A.V. Hill and associates who proposed the famous three-element model of skeletal muscle (Fig. 15). This model consists of an active contractile element, which represents the muscle's response to stimulation, in series with an elastic element, the series elastic component. The series elastic component and the contractile element are in parallel with another elastic element, the parallel elastic component. The tension exerted by the parallel elastic component is independent of the contractile element and is felt to represent the tension in the connective tissue of the muscle. The series elastic component is located in the tendon as well as in the cross-bridges between the actin and myosin filaments. The dynamic performance of a muscle is dominated primarily by the properties of the muscle fibers and the aponeurosis; the tendon (another series elastic component) is probably too stiff.

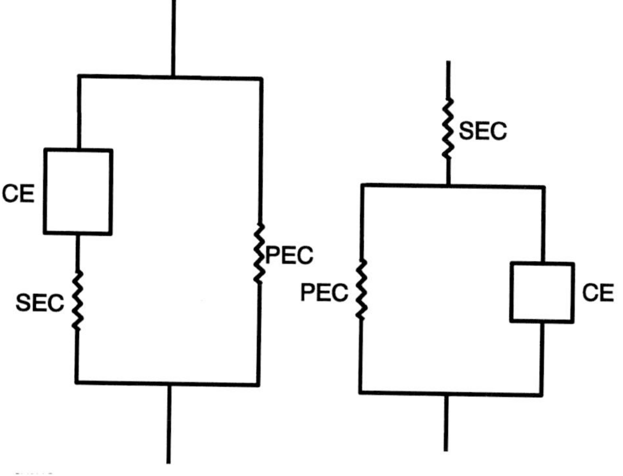

Figure 15
Hill's three-element model. Classical representations for the Hill model of muscle are CE = contractile element; SEC = series elements; PEC = parallel element.

It has been known for some time that muscle demonstrates nonlinear, time-dependent viscoelastic responses similar to those of other biologic tissues. Although Hill's model is useful in providing a general picture of muscle behavior, it must be treated as somewhat idealized. An accurate model of muscle would include a much more complex design describing its nonlinear and time-dependent functions. Because muscle consists of 75% water by weight and much of what remains is amorphous, long-chain polymer-like material, it is not surprising that this tissue demonstrates quite a bit of viscous behavior. Various mechanical models have been developed to account for these phenomena.

Length-Tension Relationship

Muscle can be stretched and its tension can be recorded mechanically. When this is done with unstimulated muscle, there is a period of length change before any tension is recorded. From that point there is a non-linear increase in tension, which is similar to the (toe-region) response of ligament and tendon. If the muscle is activated by tetanically stimulating the motor neuron, the tension produced is higher, especially at relatively small stretches in the muscle. At larger stretches, the tension in activated muscle approaches that in passively stretched muscle (Fig. 16).

Subtracting the tension in passively stretched muscle from the tension in actively stretched muscle at each length gives the portion of the tension that results from contractile muscle forces alone. Often, the onset of the rise in passive tension occurs near the peak of active tension production. There is considerable variability between muscles, but the active force is often high at muscle lengths that are not associated with significant passive tensions.

The tension in a passively stretched muscle can be quite significant at higher strains. In fact, the passive tension developed in muscle before mechanical failure occurs can be several times higher than that of the maximal active force of the muscle.

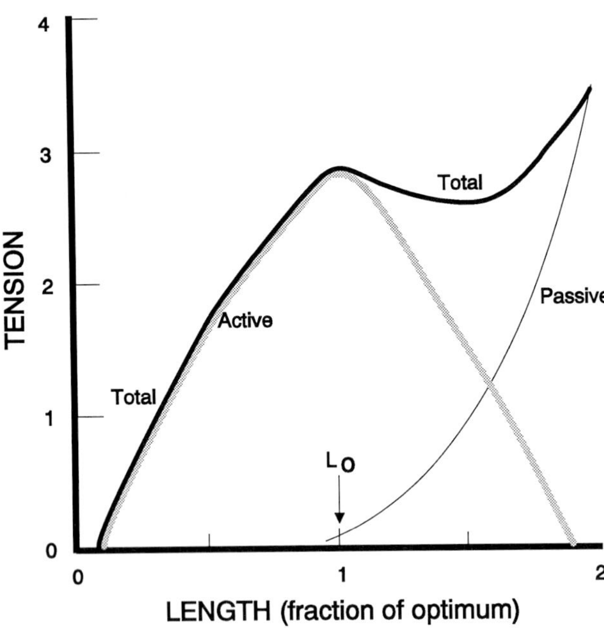

Figure 16
Representative isometric tension-length curve of skeletal muscle.

The viscoelastic properties of muscle are largely responsible for the tension in passively stretched muscle. This tension is due primarily to the connective tissue around muscle fibers and to the fascial components of the muscle belly. Recent studies indicate that some passive tension may come from the myofibrillar proteins themselves.

The passive stretch of a muscle can limit motions about joints, especially with muscles that span two joints and can be stretched by either. In most people, the hamstrings can easily limit knee extension with the hip flexed more than 90°. Similarly, the gastrocnemius can limit ankle dorsiflexion when the knee is extended. In both examples, the passive tension developed is sufficient to limit further muscle stretch without pain and high forces.

Myofibrillar ultrastructure provides an explanation for the length-tension relationship for active muscle. Force can be produced only when the cross-bridges of the thick filaments can interact with the thin filaments. Therefore, in the lengthened position the thick filaments are not overlapped by the thin filaments. As sarcomere length decreases, there is initially more overlap of thick and thin filaments. At more shortened positions the thick filaments of adjacent sarcomeres begin to abut the two lines and the tension begins to fall again. More shortening causes further collision of the filaments and successive loss of contractile force.

Blix Curve and Joint Torque

For a given degree of neurologic stimulus, the active force possible as a function of muscle length displays an ascending, then a descending, curve as noted above. Although the force that a muscle exerts may change with muscle length, human movement results primarily from the torques produced by this force. Thus, torque is defined as: $T = r \times F$, where T is torque, r is the moment arm or the perpendicular distance from the line of action of the muscle-force vector to the axis of rotation, and F is the applied force. Therefore, torque is a vector quantity having both a magnitude and a direction; it is measured in Newton·meters (N·m). The direction of a torque is along the axis of rotation and, thus, is perpendicular to the plane in which the twisting force is applied; it is given by the right-hand rule.

Variations in muscle torque represent the interaction of moment-arm and muscle-length effects. The torque produced by muscles around a joint is related both to the relationship of muscle tension versus length and to the moment arm determined by the perpendicular distance from the line of action of the muscle to the joint center of rotation. In many cases, torque can be predicted relatively well if joint mechanics are considered alone, and the neurologic stimulus to muscle force is considered to be a constant.

There are at least three strategies for altering torque production under this condition: changing the force produced by the muscle, changing the moment arm over which the muscle acts, and varying the angle between the line of force of the muscle and the joint access. In effect, the third strategy actually changes the length of the moment arm. At a constant neurologic stimulation, production of muscle force can be changed by altering the position on the length-tension curve at which the muscle is acting. Concentric action describes that situation in which the muscle, regardless of its length, is shortening and, hence, the muscle moment is in the same direction as the change in joint angle. In eccentric action, the muscle is lengthened, and the net muscle moment is in the opposite direction to the change in joint angle. The effect of changing the moment arm must be known to determine whether the torque produced will be greater in an eccentric contraction as compared with a concentric contraction. For example, in early swing, flexion is produced by a concentric action of the iliopsoas about the hip joint. This action produces an increasing torque with increasing flexion despite progressive shortening of the muscle because the moment arm is increasing. In contrast, at the end of swing as flexion of the hip and extension of the knee produces an eccentric action of the hamstrings, the moment arm of the iliopsoas about the knee joint is decreasing. The torque thus produced could be approximately the same throughout the muscle's action. For some muscles, such as the elbow flexors and extensors, the greatest torque seems to occur when the joint is in a mid-range position, and the torque falls when the joint is in full flexion or extension. At either extreme, the force of one of these two muscles may actually be maximal but the moment arm may be minimal. Such is the case of biceps action in resisting elbow moment from flexion to extension (eccentric) or in attempting to lift a weight with the elbow going from maximum extension to flexion (concentric). In both of these actions, the muscle changes its length and the moment arm continually changes. For some muscles, which have pulley systems for their tendons or retinacular sheaths maintaining the tendon close to or at a relatively constant distance from the joint access, the part that the moment arm plays in the changing torque as the muscle exerts its force may be less important.

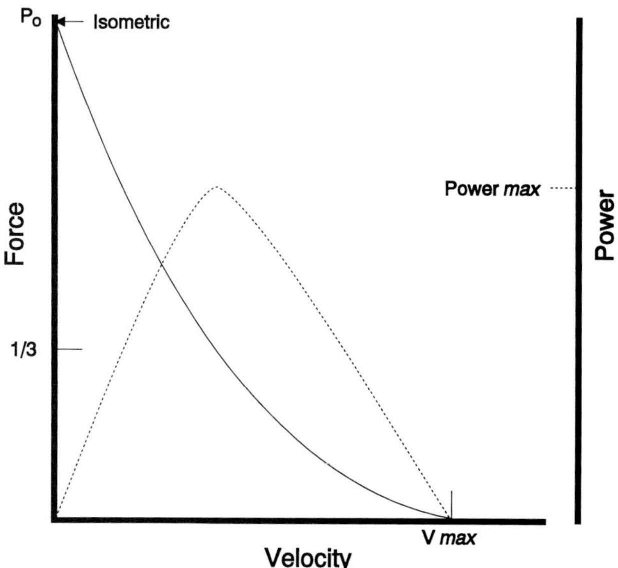

Figure 17
The classic force-velocity curve (dashed line) in an isolated muscle, showing the velocity of muscle contraction is maximal with zero load. The solid line gives the muscle power (muscle force X velocity of contraction).

Force-Velocity Relationship

Muscles are the primary tools for providing human motion; therefore, a consideration of muscle function and its relation to velocity can be valuable. When muscle is stimulated by its motor nerve, it generates force and attempts to shorten. Classic muscle physiology experiments have shown that the velocity at which a muscle can shorten is related to the load on the muscle. With low loads, muscle shortens at a higher velocity than with heavy loads. The relationship between force and velocity is hyperbolic and was described by A.V. Hill. Unlike the length-tension relationship, the force-velocity relationship does not have an anatomic basis. As the velocity of shortening approaches zero, muscle generates increasing force. Similarly, as the load approaches the maximal isometric force of the muscle, the velocity of shortening approaches zero. Based on this relationship, which applies only to tetanically-stimulated amphibian muscle, Hill developed the force-velocity relationship for the contractile elements as shown below.

$$(F + a)(v + b) = (F_{max} + a)b$$

where F is the muscle tensile force, V is the velocity of contraction, F_{max} is the maximum (tetanic) isometric force, and a and b are constants (usually about 0.25).

According to this equation, there is an inverse relationship between muscle force F and velocity of contraction (Fig. 17). This equation describes the force- velocity relationship of tetanically-stimulated skeletal muscle upon its immediate release from an isometric condition. It cannot describe the force-velocity relationship when a tetanically-stimulated muscle is slowly released. Furthermore, the theory described in this equation applies to the individual muscle fiber, thus limiting the direct extrapolation to clinical practice and the study of whole muscle systems.

Isokinetic dynamometers are popular in training and rehabilitation programs. These machines contain a servomechanism that permits motion with a constant angular velocity. The servomechanism regulates the joint torque to whatever torque is needed to maintain the joint velocity at the level selected. Because the resistance offered by the machine matches that of the individual, this type of exercise is also known as accommodating resistance exercise. Of course, constant angular velocity of the joint does not mean that the muscle itself is shortening at a constant velocity. However, it is apparent from the clinical application that there is an inverse relationship between velocity of movement and force production (as in Hill's equation). The muscles about the knee, for example, generate approximately 120% more joint torque at 60°/s than at an angular velocity of 360°/s.

Muscle that is activated eccentrically can produce more force and do more work (actually negative work) for the same velocity of movement than muscle that is activated concentrically. Kinesiology studies show that a very large portion of muscle activity occurs in an eccentric fashion. For example, gait studies show that many of the lower extremity muscle activities are eccentric and function to decelerate or control joint motion. The major portion of quadriceps activity occurs at heel strike while the knee is flexing rather than later during the gait cycle when the knee is extending. The potentially advantageous mechanisms of increased force production and diminished energy consumption are often at work as muscles function eccentrically.

The eccentric action of muscle can be contrasted to concentric action (Fig. 18). The shape of the force-velocity relationship is different; the velocity of lengthening is less than the velocity of shortening for a given increment of force. The muscle, therefore, acts as a stiffer material when it is resisting shortening. This changes abruptly near a force 50% greater than the maximal isometric force. The hyperbolic relationship between force and velocity is important clinically, because the force drops off rapidly as velocity increases.

Isokinetic dynamometers that can function in an eccentric fashion are now being used for training and rehabilitation routines. Of course, this requires a robotic capacity for the exercise device, because it must have power to generate motion of the lever arm in excess of what the muscle can resist.

The possibilities of eccentric training and rehabilitation, as long as they are performed properly and safely, are promising and are being investigated at present. Mechanical efficiency is higher and oxygen consumption lower with eccentric than with concentric action. This difference results in a lower energy cost during eccentric exercise and may make this training mode attractive in patients with low capacity to deliver energy to the muscles. Other favorable features of eccentric muscle action include submaximal neural activities during maximal voluntary activity and higher maximal torque values at the same corresponding velocity compared with concentric action. It also appears that repeated exposure to eccentric muscle action can result in adaptations leading to increased resistance to muscle soreness following exercise.

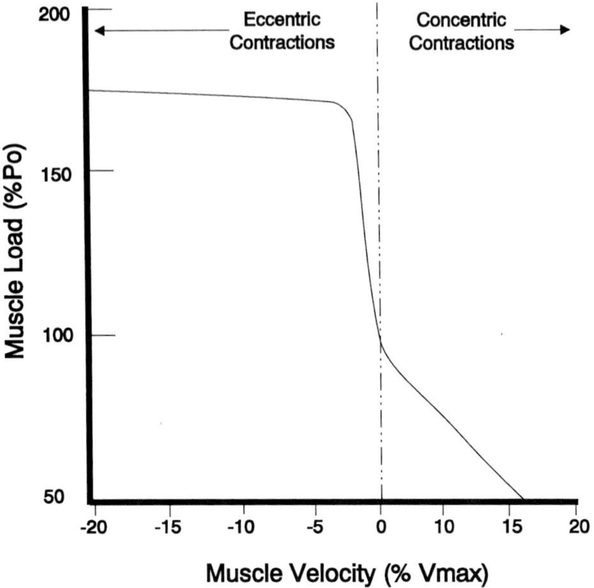

Figure 18
The highest force can be developed in a fast eccentric contraction and then declines to a minimum when the muscle is activated in a concentric contraction at high speeds. Note that force increases significantly in forced muscle lengthening (eccentric) contractions. P_o = isometric muscle force; V_{max} = maximum muscle velocity.

Training Effects on Muscle

Muscle is a tissue capable of significant adaptation as can be seen in the extremes of muscle capacity observed in the severely ill and the world-class athlete. The type and magnitude of the tissue response vary tremendously, based on the nature of the training. For example, it probably would not be difficult to distinguish the winners of the Olympic marathon from the Olympic shot-put champion. Muscle training can involve exercises aimed at increasing strength, endurance, and anaerobic fitness. Although most training regimens involve a mixture of these possibilities, it is instructive to consider them separately at first. Changes in muscle structure, function, and metabolism can thus be evaluated.

Strength Training

Observation of the muscles of competing power lifters and bodybuilders might lead to the idea that strength training results in relatively striking changes in muscle. High force, low repetition training results in an increase in muscle strength, which is proportional to the cross-sectional area of the fibers in the muscles. For years now the debate has been as to whether this increase in muscle size is a result of muscle hypertrophy, that is, an increase in the size of muscle fibers, or of hyperplasia, that is, an increase in the number of fibers. Experimental data exist in support of both arguments. Although the applicability to humans of data obtained using animals is somewhat limited, it appears likely that the majority of change that occurs with strength training is a result of hypertrophy. With an increase in fiber size, there is an increase in the amount of contractile proteins.

There also is a strong neurologic component to strength training. An accumulating body of evidence suggests that motor-unit recruitment provides an important contribution to the strength gains commonly seen following weight training. In an untrained person, it has been estimated that approximately 80% of the motor units can be stimulated voluntarily. Training is believed to result in an alteration of CNS firing of motor neurons to achieve better synchronization of muscle activation.

Metabolic changes in response to strength training are less remarkable than the changes in muscle size. There are increased amounts of phosphagens, the immediate source of muscle energy; however, there is little or no change in oxidative enzyme levels. In fact, the volume density of mitochondria may decrease with pure strength training. As the fiber size increases without a significant stimulus for an increase in mitochondrial density or size, the volume fraction of mitochondria decreases.

An increase in the force or tension on a muscle is needed to increase its strength over time. A technique called synergist ablation is often used in animal studies. It involves the surgical excision of a muscle with a function very similar to that of the muscle being tested. For example, if the gastrocnemius is removed, the remaining soleus has more work to do and it must resist more force.

In man, strength training involves increasing the resistance against which the muscle shortens. A resistance generally is chosen such that the muscle can move through a prescribed range of motion for only a few times (one to 15 repetitions) before being unable to repeat the movement. It is considered important to continue repeating until fatigue prevents continuing the exercise. A relatively high resistance and a low number of possible repetitions lead to increases in the strength and size of the muscle rather than an improved capacity for endurance, which would be the result of training against a resistance that could be repeated, for example, 20 times or more before fatigue. In general, strength training will involve several sets of repetitions to fatigue. Exercises are often arranged to work on separate muscle groups sequentially to allow the exercised muscle groups some recovery time before their next set. There are many different programs altering the number of sets and repetitions (or reps) to achieve the desired effect.

Strength training involves adaptations in all fiber types. These adaptations promote greater capacity of fibers to resist external loads, primarily through an increase in contractile protein content. Because the intensity of exercise is near maximal, all fiber types are recruited in the exercise. However, studies have shown that the type II fibers show a more pronounced hypertrophy than do the type I fibers. Type I fibers apparently can generate as much specific tension, or force per cross-sectional area, as type II fibers when tested under isometric conditions. Under high velocity conditions, individuals with a higher percentage of type II fibers may have an advantage. The overall result is the distribution of load across a greater muscle mass, which leads to a reduction of stress on these fibers. Again, there is a strong neurologic component to strength training; it is believed that in a poorly conditioned muscle as few as 60% of the fibers are firing simultaneously, whereas a well-conditioned muscle may have over 90% active fibers.

Endurance Training (Aerobic Training)

Training to increase muscle endurance and aerobic fitness involves a very different challenge to the muscle and an entirely different set of adaptations by the muscle and the cardiovascular system. Strength training involves presenting the muscles with a task they are not strong enough to perform; the adaptation is to get stronger, which involves getting larger. However, endurance training typically does not involve high forces or resistance type exercises. For example, distance running involves forces no higher than those required to take steps at a fast rate. The challenge presented to muscles during aerobic training is to take more and faster steps before fatigue. The adaptations, then, are those involved with the supply of energy rather than the size of the muscle. Therefore, the improvements in endurance as a result of aerobic training appear to result from changes in both central and peripheral circulation and muscle metabolism. Specifically, the contractile machinery of muscle adapts to use energy more efficiently.

Specific changes in the cardiovascular system occur with aerobic training; the body cannot rely exclusively on anaerobic processes for prolonged exercise. Aerobic training results in a greater reliance on oxidative metabolism to provide energy to skeletal muscle; therefore, the cardiovascular system must adapt to supply oxygen to the muscles at an increased rate. The heart develops a larger stroke volume and a larger ventricular size to accommodate this increase in stroke volume. More importantly, increases in pressure, work, and heart rate are minimized in favor of this increase in stroke volume. The heart rate at rest falls because the increased stroke volume means that fewer beats are required to deliver the same amount of blood. The circulatory system also adapts to improve blood flow to the muscles through control of the arterioles in the muscle. In addition, there is an increased number of capillaries within the muscle after endurance training. This is especially true for the type I fibers.

Changes in the muscle fiber itself are also noteworthy. Because oxidative metabolism involves the mitochondria, it is perhaps not surprising that mitochondrial size, number, and density are increased.

The physiologic significance of these changes has been debated. Some believe that the capillarization of skeletal muscle is not the limiting factor to whole body maximal aerobic power in humans. The enzyme systems of the Krebs cycle and the respiratory chain also show marked increases as do the enzyme systems involved with the supply and processing of fatty acids for use by the mitochondria. The increase in mitochondrial enzymes leads to a marked increase in the ability to oxidize pyruvic acid from glycogen and acetyl CoA from fats. There is also a decrease in glycolytic enzymes following aerobic training, which appears to be limited to fast-twitch muscles. These enzyme changes have not been found in humans.

With training, the metabolic pathways adapt to use a higher portion of fatty acids for fuel instead of glycogen. In long duration exercise, the supply of glycogen can limit endurance; this is particularly true for exercise lasting more than two hours. The relative use of different fuel sources can be estimated using indirect calorimetry. This technique monitors expired oxygen and carbon dioxide, thereby allowing determination of the ratio of oxygen consumed and carbon dioxide produced. The general formula for carbohydrate (glucose) use is $C_6H_{12}O_6 + 6O_2 \rightarrow 6CO_2 + 6H_2O$. The ratio of $CO_2/O_2 = 6/6 = 1.0$. For fats the general formula calls for the use of successive two-carbon fragments. An estimate of this formula is $3(CH_2\text{-}CH_2) + 9O_2 \rightarrow 6CO_2 + 6H_2O$. The ratio of $CO_2/O_2 = 6/9 = 0.7$. Respiratory gas measurements can be used to determine CO_2 production, O_2 consumption, and the CO_2/O_2 ratio during exercise. From this ratio it has been possible to demonstrate that aerobic training involves increased use of fat for energy.

Different muscle fiber types respond differently to endurance training. The oxidative capacity of all three fiber types increases. Very intense exercise in animals can lead to a conversion of type II to type I fibers; however, it has been more difficult to prove this conversion in man. Study results have generally indicated a change within type II fibers such that the percentage of more highly oxidative IIA fibers increases.

Specific responses are also possible in muscle as a result of dietary manipulations. The endurance capacity of muscle is related to the available stores of glycogen in the muscle fibers and in the liver. Glycogen, as the storage vehicle for glucose, is used extensively, especially in exercises of moderate to high intensity. Muscle and liver glycogen stores can be increased dietarily by the consumption of a diet high in carbohydrates and lower in fats for several days prior to competition or testing. In addition, exercise that effects a relative depletion of muscle glycogen prior to the high carbohydrate diet may increase the storage of glycogen in muscles. This routine of a high carbohydrate diet prior to an event involving endurance stresses is called carbohydrate loading.

Anaerobic (Sprint or Power) Training

Exercises of a high intensity that last for a few seconds to approximately two minutes require metabolic support primarily from anaerobic pathways. Such exercises rely primarily on the availability of ATP in the form of phosphagens and on the ability to supply energy through anaerobic glycolysis. The requirements for ATP use are higher than the ability of the aerobic system to supply ATP.

Although there have been far fewer investigations on the effects of anaerobic training, several adaptations have been documented. One of the primary adaptations is an increase in the level of stored phosphagens. In addition, there are elevations in some of the enzymes controlling glycolysis, such as phosphofructokinase and succinate dehydrogenase; however, these changes in enzyme levels are far less pronounced than with aerobic training. These changes appear to be confined primarily to fast-twitch muscle fibers.

Growth and Development of Muscle

Skeletal muscle cells develop from a mesodermal cell population arising from the somite. Muscle progenitor cells derive from mesoderm and are termed myoblasts early in the developmental period. These fusiform cells respond to molecular messengers in development to undergo mitosis. When sufficient numbers of cells exist, they undergo fusion to form long multinucleate cells that are called myotubes. These cells are the precursors of the eventual muscle fibers. The myotubes continue to differentiate into muscle fibers, which are large multinucleate cells. The fusion of myoblasts into myotubes is also a time of nearly synchronous differentiation of the muscle cells. Many of the contractile proteins appear synchronously; however, it appears that many of the specific genes coding for muscle proteins are regulated, coordinated, and influenced by a large number of factors. By the seventh week of gestation, distinct muscle and tendinous structures can be identified.

In addition, it is apparent that even embryonic muscle cells exhibit a number of isoforms of the myofibrillar proteins. Different isoforms may exist during different stages of development as well as in mature muscle. The further differentiation of the myotubes involves the production of structural proteins, the proteins and enzymes of the metabolic pathways, the association of the myotubes with the extracellular connective tissue matrix of muscle, and innervation.

Growth and Changes in Muscle Length

The development of muscle and hypertrophy associated with training or adaptation to stress have been discussed. There remains the question of how muscle grows in length. Bone, of course, has growth plates that increase its length. Muscles have no such specific structural adaptation, yet they are able to increase in length to accommodate for skeletal growth. The possibilities include increased tendon length, increased muscle length, or both. In immature animals it appears that both occur; muscle fibers and tendons increase in length. Elongation of the muscle fiber while the sarcomere length remains relatively stable can be explained by the addition of more sarcomeres to the muscle fibers during longitudinal growth. The region of the muscle-tendon junction shows a great deal of activity and adaptability during growth; fibers grow in length at this region rather than near the middle of the muscle fiber.

In mature animals, elongation of the muscle belly is the primary mechanism for changing the length of the muscle-tendon unit. Because, in mature animals, skeletal length is not increasing, studies have dealt with the response of muscle to immobilization in various positions that put the muscle-tendon unit under different degrees of stretch. Data from such studies are important because muscle growth may often be the limiting factor in surgical skeletal lengthening.

When muscle fibers are immobilized under stretch, the immediate effect is that the fibers are longer and the constituent myofibrils lengthen. The sarcomeres are longer initially as a result of the stretch that separates the A-bands and I-bands more than at normal rest length. After several weeks, the sarcomeres return to their normal rest lengths, although the whole muscle and fibers maintain their stretched length. This return to normal sarcomere length is effected by an increase in the number of sarcomeres in series in the myofibrils and, therefore, in the fiber. The additional sarcomeres are added at the region of the muscle-tendon junction.

Mechanically, the active portion of the length-tension diagram shifts so that the peak of force production occurs at a longer length. The addition of more sarcomeres in series implies an increase in the amount of skeletal muscle protein and an increase in muscle weight, even in the presence of immobilization. The increased weight comes from longer fibers rather than from an increase in cross-sectional area.

Adaptations also occur in the passive properties of muscle. If a muscle is held in a stretched position for as little as two weeks, the length-tension relation shifts to the right such that less passive force is generated in response to the same stretch. The opposite occurs for muscles immobilized in or restricted to a shortened position. After several weeks of being held shortened, muscles will generate more resistance for a given stretch or a given change in joint angle when the muscle length is increasing.

These concepts of changing muscle length in response to immobilization are not appreciated by many physicians who treat musculoskeletal conditions. The problem has not been widely studied in humans; however, data from animal studies make it clear that the muscle-tendon unit length is dynamic and can respond to length changes imposed by a growing skeleton or by external fixation of muscle length. In skeletally mature individuals, most of the length change occurs within the muscle tissue rather than in the tendon. A better understanding of the response of muscle to long-term length changes will improve results obtained from tendon and muscle transfers, limb length alterations, and even immobilization in muscle. Clinically, patients demonstrate reduced flexibility, decreased range of motion, and reduced tolerance to muscle work following immobilization. Although these findings appear to be consistent from patient to patient, it is only recently that the detrimental effects of total immobilization have been appreciated. Clearly, proper muscle function depends on a number of factors, including intact proprioceptive activity, motor innervation, mechanical load, and mobility of the joints. Interruption of any of the above can lead to reduced motion, and if severe enough, total immobilization.

Muscle Injury and Repair

Muscle injury can occur by a variety of mechanisms ranging from ischemia to direct injury by crush or laceration. Injured muscle undergoes processes of degeneration and regeneration; when muscle fibers undergo necrosis for any reason, the damaged fibers are removed by macrophages and other cells from the circulatory system. New muscle cells appear within the connective tissue framework of damaged muscle. These cells probably come from the population of relatively undifferentiated satellite cells that existed in a quiescent state beside the original muscle syncytium. Many progenitor cells begin to form myoblasts, which fuse to form myotubes. Myotubes coalesce and undergo a transition to muscle fibers. At the same time, a connective tissue basal lamina surrounding the muscle fiber and an extracellular matrix are formed. The muscle tissue regenerates simultaneously with the proliferation of fibrous connective tissue. The connective tissue proliferation may interfere with the ability of muscle to regenerate into normally functioning tissue. In rodents and other animals, regeneration of entire muscles may occur following revascularization. However, the regeneration process is generally less effective for muscles that weigh more than 1.5 g and, therefore, is unlikely to occur in a significant fashion in most human muscles. The response of human muscle varies with the nature and severity of the injury.

Recovery of muscle depends on revascularization from surrounding viable tissue. The regenerating myotubes and the neovascularization may influence one another's development. The process of reinnervation is also interesting from a cellular point of view. Part of the structural specialization of the synapse is the organization of the connective tissue basal lamina surrounding the muscle fibers. The specialized region of the basal lamina at the motor end plate may persist after death of the muscle fiber. Even without regeneration of the nerve, the site of the preexisting motor endplate region of basal lamina influences the development of muscle fibers regenerating within the basal lamina. Clearly, the regeneration of nerve fibers, muscle cells, and the connective tissue basal lamina have special and complex interrelationships in reinnervating muscle.

An important factor in regeneration of human muscle is the simultaneous and often more exuberant and predominant formation of connective tissue in the form of fibrosis or scar. The connective tissue regeneration can be extensive enough to interfere with muscle regeneration. A number of specific examples of muscle injury and the recovery processes are discussed below.

Muscle Laceration

Direct laceration of muscle is not uncommon in trauma. Several studies demonstrate the potential for recovery of lacerated muscle and the problems that often prevent recovery of normal tissue. Complete transection of a muscle can lead to a normal-appearing tissue only in very small muscles of animal models.

Lacerations in skeletal muscle usually result from direct trauma by a sharp object. Surgical exposures may require division of muscles. For normal function following lacerations, muscle must regenerate across the repair site, and tissue denervated by laceration of the muscle belly and separated from the intramuscular nerve supply must be reinnervated. Clinical experience has shown that functional recovery following muscle laceration is rarely complete, although partial recovery is usually possible.

Following complete laceration and suture repair of rabbit skeletal muscles, the muscle fragments healed primarily by dense connective tissue scar (Fig. 19). A small number of myotubes penetrated the scar tissue, but good regeneration of muscle tissue across the laceration was not seen. The muscle fragment isolated from the motor point had histologic findings of denervation. Recovery of muscle function was evaluated by measuring the isometric muscle tension following motor-nerve stimulation. Muscles lacerated near the mid-belly recovered approximately 50% of their ability to produce tension and could shorten about 80% of their normal amount. Recovery of muscle function after partial lacerations was proportional to the degree of laceration.

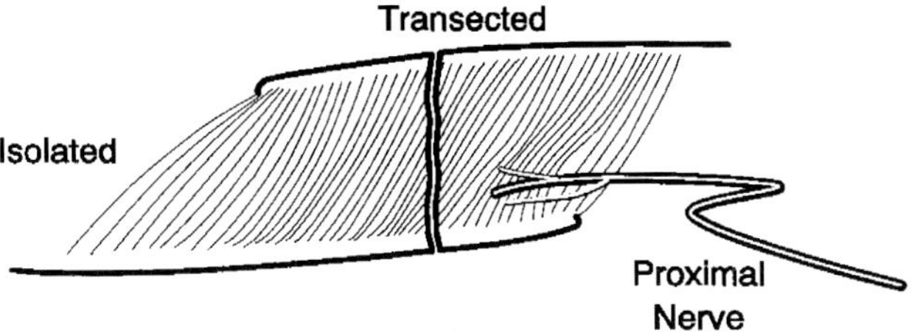

Figure 19
Schematic drawing of lacerated muscle. The laceration leaves fibers intact proximally and distally while dividing the central fibers. Scar tissue isolates the distal segment from its nerve supply. (Reproduced with permission from Garrett WE, Seaber AV, Boswick J, et al: Recovery of skeletal muscle following laceration and repair. *J Hand Surg* 1984;9A:683–692.)

A recent clinical study showed good correlation with these experiments. Muscle lacerations were repaired by connecting the proximal portion of the lacerated muscle to the distal portion by tendon grafts. At a mean follow-up period of 14 months, approximately 40% of the mean grip strength was recovered. Over half of the muscles achieved grade 4 or grade 5 strength by manual muscle testing.

Muscle Contusion

Muscle contusions usually result from nonpenetrating blunt injury. They occur frequently in accidents and sports and can cause significant disability and pain. The best method of treatment has not been clearly defined, but animal experiments provide some insight into the natural history of the injury. An inflammatory reaction and hematoma occurred soon after production of consistent lesions in rat gastrocnemius muscles. Later, scar formation consisting of dense connective tissue with variable amounts of muscle regeneration was seen. Mobilized muscle was compared to immobilized muscle in the recovery process. The inflammatory reaction in mobilized muscle was greater, but it disappeared more rapidly with more scar formation than in the immobilized muscle. The speed of tissue repair was related directly to vascular ingrowth during the repair process. Biomechanical testing showed faster recovery of tensile strength in mobilized muscles.

The quality of repair following blunt trauma varied with age; young rats demonstrated a more intense inflammatory reaction and hematoma formation than older rats. Incorporation of radioactively labeled proline demonstrated synthesis of extracellular connective tissue by two days following trauma, with most intensive synthesis occurring between days 5 and 21. The appearance and distribution of collagen types I, III, IV, and V and of fibronectin have also been studied using histologic and immunofluorescent techniques.

Severe blunt injury to muscle may result in bone formation within the muscle, referred to as myositis ossificans (Fig. 20). A prospective study of patients with quadriceps hematoma showed subsequent myositis ossificans in approximately 20% of cases. The new bone formed after blunt trauma can be contiguous with normal bone, periosteal, or completely free of any connection with existing bone, heterotopic. Experimentally, some animals, including rabbits, appear to develop primarily periosteal new bone. However, in other animals, such as sheep, both periosteal new bone and heterotopic bone occur. Periosteal reactive new bone developed in all sheep receiving blunt trauma to the anterior thigh muscles, whereas heterotopic bone occurred in 17% of the sheep. Multiple episodes of injury and hematoma formation increased the likelihood of formation of heterotopic bone.

Following direct injury, there is early swelling associated with bleeding and inflammation. The mass may enlarge or be symptomatic for several months before stabilizing. The mass may be associated with the possible appearance of heterotopic bone, if there is a history of a previous muscle contusion. This condition may also mimic osteogenic sarcoma with its mass effect and the appearance of irregular new bone. The histologic features may also be similar if a biopsy is performed early in the course of myositis ossificans. The heterotopic bone may absorb with time. Recovery of normal function is possible with the presence of myositis ossificans, but the recovery period is longer than that following an uncomplicated contusion. No specific treatment is recommended in addition to the treatment for contusions. Early surgery is to be avoided because it may exacerbate the heterotopic bone formation and prolong disability. Surgery should be considered only after the heterotopic bone is mature and no changes are occurring in both the clinical and radiologic evaluation of the patient.

Indirect Muscle Strain Injury

Indirect muscle injuries are caused by excessive force or stress on a muscle rather than by any direct trauma. This injury has been called a strain, muscle pull, muscle tear, and various other names. Indirect muscle injuries occur frequently, and are a major reason for time lost from athletic or occupational pursuits. Interest in the basic pathophysiologic characteristics of this injury has been relatively slow to develop despite its clinical significance.

Complete Muscle Tears

In one of the earliest studies of failure of the muscle-tendon unit in response to stretch, the gastrocnemius muscle-tendon unit of rabbits was strained to failure. The healthy tendon did not fail

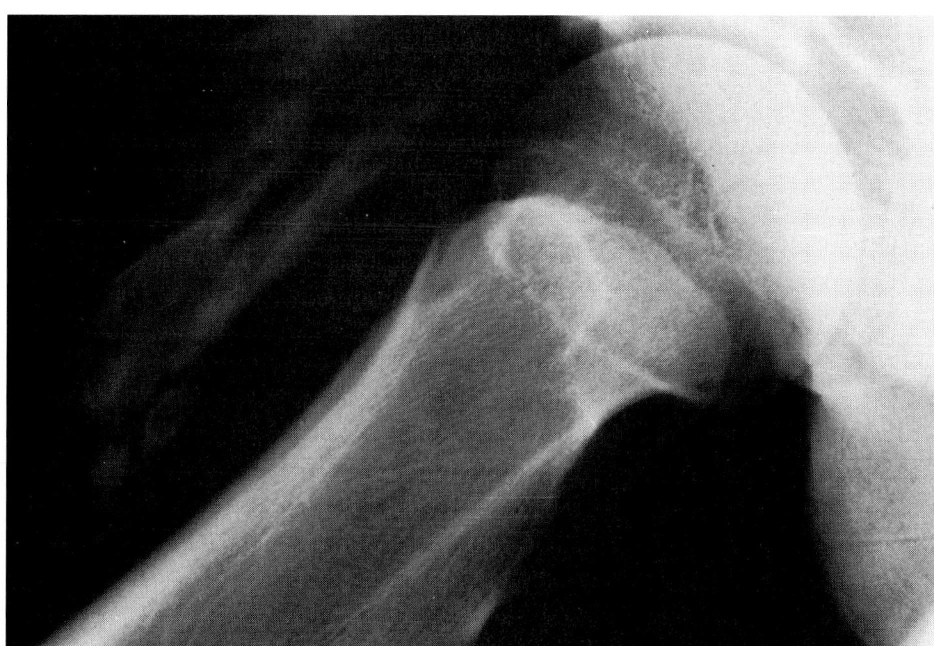

Figure 20
Radiograph of myositis ossificans of the rectus femoris. This 22-year-old patient suffered a quadriceps contusion which resulted in the above roentgenographic findings. The heterotopic bone gradually resorbed over time without consequence.

even after partial transection of the tendon. Failure occurred at the bone-tendon junction, the myotendinous junction, or within the muscle.

Rabbit muscle-tendon units stretched to failure consistently fail near the myotendinous junction. The tendons of origin and insertion of most muscles extend well into the length of the muscle, and the muscle fibers have an oblique angle of insertion into the tendons. The fiber architecture is quite variable in different muscles. Rabbit hind-limb muscles were strained to failure without any direct nerve or muscle activation. For all muscles and for a wide range of strain rates, failure consistently occurred near the myotendinous junction.

The exact site of failure has not been clearly determined. The muscle fiber can avulse from the tendon at the precise muscle-tendon junction; however, failure usually occurs within the muscle fiber within several millimeters of the junction. The terminal sarcomeres near the myotendinous junction are stiffer than the middle sarcomeres of a muscle fiber. The injury to muscle occurs within this region of relatively limited extensibility. There are structural differences in the region, but detailed studies of the region of injury are lacking.

The response of activated muscle to stretch has been investigated using rabbit muscles stretched to failure during activation by motor-nerve stimulation. Activated muscle tore at the same increase in length as submaximally stimulated or unstimulated muscle, but slightly greater forces were recorded at failure for the stimulated muscles. The ability of stimulated muscle to maintain a higher force during stretching allowed a stimulated muscle to absorb much more energy than an unstimulated muscle, suggesting that the active component of a muscle protects against injury through energy absorption (Fig. 21). This finding is significant in light of the ability of muscle to avoid injury to joints and to muscles themselves. Muscle often contracts eccentrically to absorb energy, as in the case of the quadriceps muscle in landing from a jump. Joint control and protection from injury may be better when muscles are able to absorb more kinetic energy.

Trainers and athletes have traditionally felt that weak or fatigued muscles were more likely to be injured. It might seem paradoxical that the lower force-generating capacity of weakened or fatigued muscle results in more injury; however, muscles often are activated as energy absorbers or motion controllers, actions requiring higher muscle forces. Clinically, muscle strains usually occur in the setting of powerful eccentric muscle activity. Weakened or fatigued muscles might absorb less energy or be less able to resist stretching.

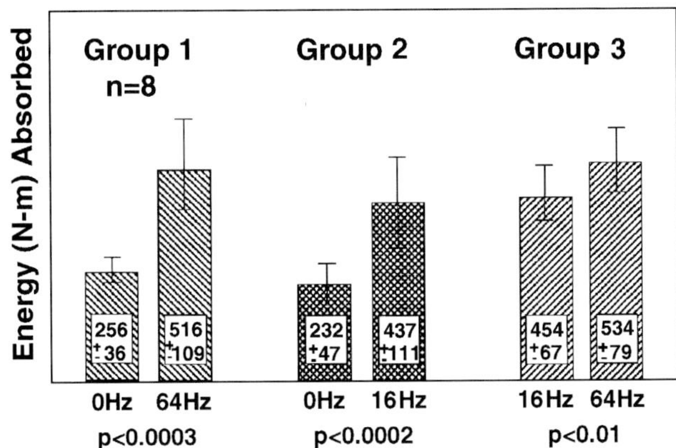

Figure 21
Energy absorbed by muscles strained to failure under varying conditions. In group 1, one rabbit extensor digitorum longus is strained to failure without muscle activation while the contralateral muscle is activated by nerve stimulation at 64 Hz. In group 2, one muscle is not activated and the other is activated by nerve stimulation at 16 Hz. In group 3, muscles are stimulated by the tetanic frequency (64 Hz) and by the submaximal frequency (16 Hz). (Adapted with permission from Garrett WE, Safran MR, Seaber AV, et al: Biomechanical comparison of stimulated and nonstimulated skeletal muscle pulled to failure. *Am J Sports Med* 1988;15:448–454.)

Incomplete Muscle Tears

Although complete muscle tears are seen clinically, incomplete injuries are much more common. Only a few studies have addressed the pathophysiologic features of incomplete muscle injury. Nondisruptive muscle injuries, produced by stretching rabbit anterior tibial muscles well into the elastic region of the load-deformation relation, resulted in a characteristic lesion near the myotendinous junction. Fiber disruption and a small amount of hemorrhage were initially present (Fig. 22). During the next one to four days, a cellular inflammatory response occurred with the appearance of edema and granulation tissue containing fibroblasts and inflammatory cells. After one week, a significant amount of scar tissue and repair were present. Physiologically, there was a consistent decrease in the ability of the injured muscles to produce active tension for the first few days. After seven days, the muscle approached normal tension production (Fig. 23).

Clinical studies of acute muscle strains reflect the changes seen in basic laboratory studies. Computed tomography and magnetic resonance imaging (MRI) demonstrate muscle abnormalities in the region of the muscle-tendon junction. Acute changes include evidence of inflammatory changes and edema at the site of injury. Among the frequently injured muscles are the hamstrings, the rectus femoris, and the gastrocnemius; all three cross at least

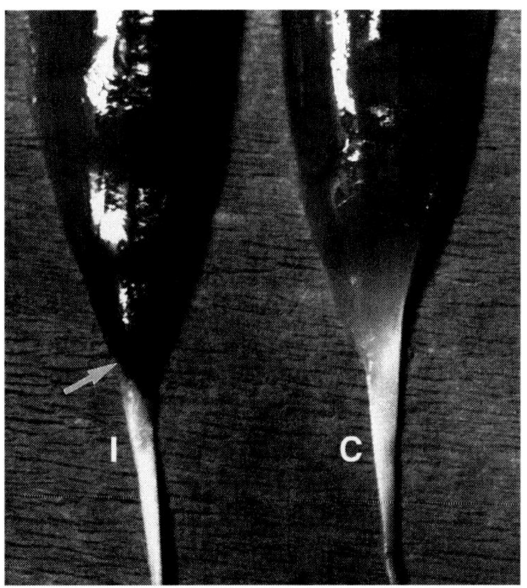

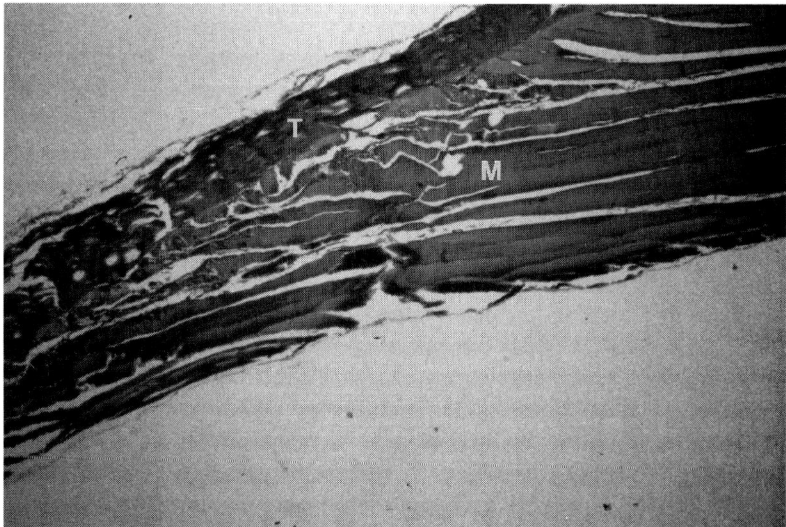

Figure 22
Left, Gross appearance of tibialis anterior (TA) muscle following controlled passive strain injury. A small hemorrhage (arrow) is visible at the distal tip of injured muscle at 24 hours. I = injured; C = control. **Right,** Histologic appearance of TA muscle immediately after passive strain injury. Note the rupture of fibers at the distal muscle-tendon junction, along with hemorrhage. T = tendon; M = intact muscle fibers (Masson's stain, X100).

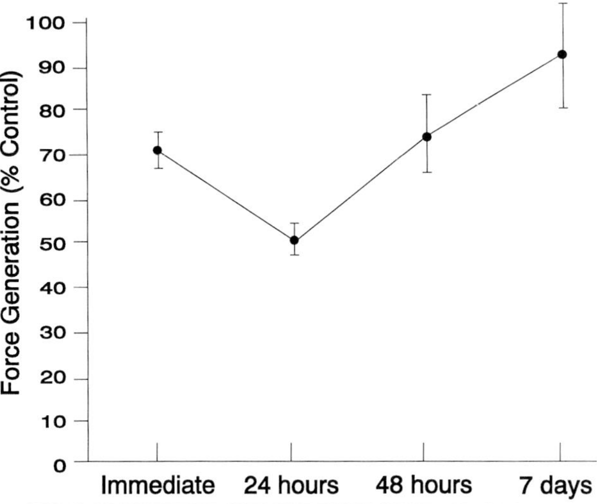

Figure 23
Percent of control force generation over range of frequencies versus time after controlled passive injury; immediately after injury (n = 30), 24 hours (n = 7), 48 hours (n = 8), 7 days (n = 8). All values ± SEM. (Reproduced with permission from Nikoloau PK, Macdonald BL, Clisson RR, et al: Biomechanical and histological evaluation of muscle after controlled injury. *Am J Sports Med* 1987;15:9–14.)

two joints and may be subject to more stretch. Studies of the muscle architecture demonstrate the extensive length of the muscle-tendon junction in these muscles. The region of the proximal or distal muscle-tendon junction extends the entire length of the muscle belly in the hamstring muscles.

Delayed Muscle Soreness

Delayed muscle soreness (DMS) is defined as muscular pain that generally occurs 24 to 72 hours after intense exercise. The damage is associated primarily with eccentric exercise and varies with both the intensity and duration of the exercise. DMS should be distinguished from discomfort during exercise that often is associated with muscle fatigue and from painful involuntary cramps caused by strong contractions of susceptible muscles, such as the gastrocnemius. DMS is characterized by a variable sense of discomfort in the muscle beginning several hours after exercise and reaching a maximum after one to three days. Clinically, patients usually demonstrate reduced activity and often display firm and swollen muscles. Peak swelling typically occurs one or more days following exercise. These findings strongly suggest that an increase in intramuscular pressure is present. Strength loss in the affected muscles is also common. In some cases, there can be up to a 50% loss in isometric strength immediately postexercise. This loss in strength usually lasts only a short time; however, measurable deficits can persist for up to ten days.

Many of the concepts of DMS were introduced by Hough at the beginning of this century. He showed that forceful jerky movements produced muscle discomfort 24 to 48 hours after exercise, particularly in someone unaccustomed to such exercise. Measurable muscle weakness accompanied the muscle soreness. Even after a brief conditioning period allowing for resolution of the soreness, the weakness persisted for several days. The soreness was considered the result of intramuscular damage to the structural elements of the muscle. This injury was readily reversible. Current studies in which muscle biopsies and animal models were used show that the original hypothesis of structural damage is indeed correct.

A number of theories have been proposed to explain the damage and subsequent repair that occur with DMS. Perhaps the most widely accepted is the hypothetical model that argues that mechanical factors are largely responsible for the initial events of the injury. This hypothesis is based on the assumption that high tensile stresses within the muscle result in structural injury. Sarcolemmal damage is accompanied by an influx of Ca^{2+}. The mitochondria accumulate this Ca^{2+}, leading to a reduction in cellular respiration. Further injury to the sarcolemma is accompanied by diffusion of intracellular components into the interstitium and plasma. Shortly thereafter, the phagocytic phase predominates as monocytes are converted to macrophages. Further accumulation of histamine and kinins as well as elevated pressure from tissue edema leads to an activation of receptors resulting in the painful sensation of DMS.

The structural abnormalities that accompany DMS are well documented and typically include Z-band streaming, A-band disruption, and myofibril misalignment. Soreness does not appear immediately after exercise despite muscle biopsies showing structural damage within one hour after exercise. These structural abnormalities are most severe two to three days after exercise and seem to occur primarily in the fast-twitch glycolytic (type IIB) fibers. Magnetic resonance images have demonstrated increased T_2 relaxation times lasting two to three months after the bout of exercise. Early changes in T_2 relaxation probably reflect changes in cell water resulting from edema and swelling. Recently, it has been suspected that muscle fiber disruption leads to a leakage of protein-bound ions, which in turn creates edema. Muscle soreness has been shown to be directly associated with swollen muscle fibers and elevated resting muscle pressures two days after a single bout of eccentric exercise.

Serology studies have shown that exhausting exercise may be associated with increased levels of intramuscular enzymes in the serum. The increased levels of common indicators of muscle damage, such as creatine kinase, myoglobin, and lactate dehydrogenase, may correlate with the presence of muscle soreness. In addition, there are indications that connective tissue breakdown is also a part of the syndrome of delayed muscle soreness. Increased levels of urinary hydroxyproline excretion, which are indicative of collagen or connective tissue breakdown, have been associated with delayed muscle soreness.

Recent studies have shown that the structural damage that occurs with eccentric exercise is repairable. Furthermore, it appears that change takes place, which allows the involved muscles to become more resistant to damage from a subsequent bout of eccentric exercise. The exact time course of these adaptations is not clear at this point.

Muscle Cramps

In spite of its frequency and impact on active exercise and work, the common muscle cramp is not well understood. Some muscles in certain individuals are susceptible to a very painful active contraction in a spasmodic fashion. The cramp begins when the susceptible muscle is in a shortened position and can usually be interrupted by stretch of the muscle by its antagonists or by external forces. For example, a cramp in the gastrocnemius can be stopped by active contraction of the ankle dorsiflexors and knee extensors or by standing on the toes and allowing the body weight and gravity to stretch the triceps surae. For many minutes after resolution of the cramp, the muscle shows evidence of altered excitability and fasciculations. Muscle cramps can occur after fatigue, prolonged muscle activity, dehydration, or even at night during sleep when the muscle remains in a shortened position. Cramping also occurs in clinical conditions such as renal failure, especially in the face of fluid and electrolyte disturbances. Susceptible muscles include the gastrocnemius, the hamstrings, the abdominal muscles, and a number of other muscle groups.

The electrical activity in the affected muscles is characteristic of that of motor units rather than that of individual muscle fibers, suggesting that the electrical activity responsible for cramps is coming from the nerve rather than from the mass action of individual muscle fibers. Specifically, it has been suggested that the active contractions of muscles are initiated from motor nerves once they have entered the belly of the muscles.

The etiology of abnormal action potentials is not well understood. Data from studies of athletes are ambiguous. Dehydration or loss of water and sodium are likely when cramps occur. Hydration and sodium replacement are frequently recommended for athletes. In studies of patients with renal failure it seems that the cramping condition can be ameliorated by correcting an abnormally low serum potassium. Lowered levels of serum Ca^{2+} and Mg^{2+} have also been implicated. However, data from these studies cannot be applied to cramps during athletic participation.

Immobilization and Disuse

When muscle is held immobilized for any significant length of time, there are a number of changes in its size and structure, physiologic properties, and metabolic properties. Disuse also can have many effects similar to those of immobilization. Disuse can occur without immobilization as a voluntary response to painful conditions or it can occur as a result of force deprivation by suspension, bed rest, or hypogravity states. In models of disuse or immobilization, muscle does not undergo its usual force production and its length changes because of lack of central nervous system drive, presence of motion restrictions, or deprivation of forces. For instance, disuse resulting from a painful condition may lead to motion limitation caused by voluntary CNS disuse. However, immobilization prohibits movement even though there may be near-normal activation of the muscle by the CNS. The muscle does not develop the normal stresses and strains but it may experience similar activation patterns, especially when a normal limb is temporarily immobilized.

Among the first changes occurring with immobilization is muscle atrophy; the weight of the entire muscle declines. The rate of loss of weight is not linear; it is more nearly exponential with more weight loss in the initial days than in subsequent days. The weight loss can be seen on a microscopic level as atrophy of individual muscle fibers. In general, all fibers demonstrate some atrophy. Depending on the experimental model, some muscles atrophy more than others; for example, the anti-gravity muscles from animals suspended and not allowed to bear weight atrophy more than other muscles.

Concomitant with loss of muscle mass is a loss of strength. Because strength or force production by muscle is a function of its cross-sectional area, it seems evident that loss of mass and cross-sectional area would result in strength decrements. When force production is normalized as strength per cross-sectional area, disuse and atrophy produce no change or a decrease in strength. Not only are mass and strength diminished by immobilization and disuse; the capacity of muscle to do prolonged work also decreases, or, as it is more commonly stated, the fatigability of muscle increases. Fatigability can be assessed by physiologic techniques, showing a decline in force with continued use. There are also biochemical correlates of fatigability, including lower energy supplies and increased amounts of lactic acid. The increased fatigability is associated with a diminished ability to use fats in aerobic metabolic pathways.

The changes that accompany immobilization of muscle are related to the lengths at which muscles are immobilized. Atrophy and strength loss are much more prominent in muscle immobilized under no tension than in muscles immobilized under some stretch. This factor may explain the clinical observation of quadriceps atrophy greater than hamstring atrophy in thigh musculature. Immobilization or even disuse occurring with the knee being held in extension results in shortened quadriceps with some degree of hamstring stretch. Immobilization in a stretched position leads to a decrease in strength and cross-sectional area, but a less pronounced change in mass because muscle fibers held under stretch synthesize new contractile proteins, and sarcomeres are added to the ends of the existing fibrils. Therefore, changes in cross-sectional area are somewhat offset by increasing numbers of sarcomeres in the length of the muscle. In addition to the fibrillar changes, muscle immobilized with some stretch of the fibers maintained its strength better without a decrement in force production per cross-sectional area.

There also are significant changes in the passive properties of immobilized muscle. Changes relating to muscle growth have been discussed above. The passive length-tension relationship of muscle varies with the position of immobilization. Muscle immobilized in a shortened position develops more tension in response to passive stretch to a given length than muscle held in a lengthened position. Muscle extensibility may be a significant cause of the limitation of joint motion after injury or immobilization.

Some research has been directed toward the cellular and molecular mechanisms of the changes seen with disuse or atrophy. The rate of protein synthesis in muscle decreases within hours of the initiation of immobilization. Hormonal effects also occur very early. The insulin sensitivity of immobilized muscle decreases relatively quickly, and it is, therefore, more difficult for glucose to enter the muscle. In addition, immobilization increases levels of corticosteroids, which should decrease muscle protein synthesis. A better understanding of these mechanisms may provide significant improvements in the clinical ability to prevent or reverse loss of muscular function accompanying disease or injury.

Hormonal Effects on Skeletal Muscle

The effects of insulin, growth hormone, and testosterone on skeletal muscle will be considered. In addition, the use of these agents as potential anabolic-androgenic agents by athletes will also be discussed.

Insulin

Insulin, a polypeptide hormone secreted by the islet cells of the pancreas, plays an important role in the regulation of the intermediary metabolism of carbohydrates, proteins, and fats. Its primary role in metabolism is anabolic, increasing the storage of glucose, fatty acids, and amino acids. Glucagon, which is also secreted by the islet cells, has an action reciprocal to that of insulin, causing glucose, fatty acids, and amino acids to be mobilized into the bloodstream.

The principal actions of insulin in muscle include increased glucose entry into the cell, increased glycogen synthesis, increased amino acid uptake, increased ribosomal protein synthesis, decreased protein catabolism, and decreased release of gluconeogenic amino acids. Therefore, insulin has a net anabolic effect on muscle as it promotes the storage of both carbohydrate and protein and leads to the use of glucose. Growth hormone and insulin have synergistic effects to increase protein stores within the body. These effects are counteracted by the glucocorticoids, which accelerate protein degradation and amino acid release and inhibit amino acid transport and conversion to protein.

In humans, insulin deficiency is a common and often pathologic state leading to diabetes mellitus, which can lead to polyuria, polydipsia, weight loss, hyperglycemia, glycosuria, ketosis, acidosis, and coma. It appears that regular physical exercise can have positive effects on individuals with diabetes mellitus. Exercise is typically recommended for persons who have type I diabetes, particularly if they do not suffer from complications such as proliferative retinopathy, nephropathy, or autonomic neuropathy. Adaptive effects occur in muscle because physical training in persons with diabetes can lead to increased hexokinase levels and decreased LDH (lactate dehydrogenase) activity. In persons with type II diabetes who engage in regular physical exercise, the activity of the oxidative enzymes can be increased similarly to that of healthy persons.

Growth Hormone (Somatotropin)

Growth hormone is a single-chain peptide hormone synthesized in the anterior segment of the pituitary gland. Its production is under both stimulatory and inhibitory hypothalamic control. Growth hormone exerts its anabolic effects on muscle by increasing amino acid transport into the cell and by incorporating these amino acids into proteins, resulting in an increase in skeletal muscle synthesis. The exact mechanism by which this increased protein synthesis occurs in muscle remains unknown. There is evidence that growth hormone may bind to receptors on the plasma membrane of muscle tissue and have a direct anabolic action. Other data suggest that these effects are indirect and result from the action of somatomedins or insulin-like growth factors (IGF). A number of these growth factors have been identified, and they differ in their growth-promoting activity. IGF-I, a peptide produced by the liver and other tissues, including skeletal muscle, is responsible for increased protein and mRNA synthesis, amino acid uptake, and growth of cartilage and muscle. It appears that the secretion of both IGF-I and IGF-II is influenced by growth hormone, because concentrations of both factors seem to fall with its deficiency.

The presence of growth hormone is crucial to the growth and development of various tissues including bone, connective, visceral, adipose, and skeletal muscle. Excessive production of growth hormone before closure of the epiphyses produces gigantism, whereas deficiency of the hormone leads to dwarfism. After epiphyseal closure, the main effect of growth hormone hypersecretion is cortical thickening and periosteal overgrowth leading to the well-known condition of acromegaly. Complications include increased mortality (50% by age 50), diabetes mellitus, atherosclerosis, neuropathy, and proximal myopathy of the hypertrophied muscles. These patients demonstrate selective type I fiber hypertrophy with atrophy of the type II fibers. Individuals often have skeletal muscle hypertrophy, but this is accompanied by weakness and fatigue, which probably is related to the atrophy of the type II fibers.

In addition to its growth-stimulating effects, growth hormone plays an important role in the regulation of metabolism. The general metabolic (lipolytic) effects are to reduce glucose and protein metabolism by shifting oxidative metabolism toward the use of fatty acids while sparing glucose and amino acids.

Testosterone

Androgens are synthesized primarily in the testicular interstitial cells of Leydig. Small amounts are produced by the ovaries and by the adrenal cortices of both sexes. Testosterone is the principal steroid hormone produced by the testes and has a considerable anabolic effect on muscle tissue. It is a 19-carbon steroid, which is synthesized from cholesterol in the Leydig cells and is also formed via progesterone and 17-hydroxyprogesterone. Small amounts are also formed in the adrenal cortex. The vast majority of this hormone is bound either to sex hormone-binding globulin or to albumin. Its plasma concentration is increased by estrogens and decreased by androgens. A small percentage (2%) exists in the unbound free form and exerts its anabolic effects by increasing protein synthesis and decreasing the rate of protein catabolism within the muscle fiber. The free, active hormone is used rapidly or is converted, primarily by the liver, into relatively inactive androgens that are excreted in the urine as neutral 17-ketosteroids, with small quantities also exiting through the bile (feces) and the skin.

Testosterone and other androgens exert a feedback inhibitory effect on pituitary gland secretion, develop and maintain the male secondary sex characteristics, and exert an important anabolic, growth-promoting action on both skeletal muscle and bone. This anabolic action of androgens has led to their use in counteracting effects of prolonged bed rest, disease, and surgical trauma. Androgen therapy can convert a mild negative nitrogen balance to a net retention of nitrogen. These effects are brought about by an increase in the synthesis and a decrease in the breakdown of protein. Androgens also promote physeal closure of the long bones.

Anabolic Steroids

It has been known for some time that the administration of testosterone to animals and humans can produce an increase in both muscle weight and strength. Testosterone has the effect of increasing body and muscle size (the "anabolic" effect) and the effect of virilization (the "androgenic" effect) or the expression of male sexual characteristics such as a lowered voice, increase in facial and body hair, and genital enlargement. A group of compounds have been developed in attempts to maintain the anabolic effects and avoid the virilizing effects. These compounds have been called anabolic steroids. None have ever really avoided the virilizing effects. These compounds have received a great deal of attention recently because of their use in sports. Although their use is considered both illegal and unethical, they are frequently used by athletes in particular sports and their effectiveness and risks are highly controversial.

Anabolic steroid use has become popular among athletes attempting to improve performance in events involving a large anaerobic energy requirement (for example, weightlifting and sprinting) as well as to increase strength and body weight. It has been reported that such athletes use 400% to 1,000% of the recommended medical dose of these agents. Whether or not these compounds are, in fact, effective remains controversial. The 1987 American College of Sports Medicine position statement on anabolic steroids concluded that "the gains in muscular strength achieved through high-intensity exercise and proper diet can be increased by the use of anabolic-androgenic steroids in some individuals." The 1991 American Academy of Orthopaedic Surgeons position statement emphasizes that the use of anabolic steroids "can cause serious harmful physiological, pathological, and psychological effects."

A number of investigations have been conducted to characterize the potential biochemical, physiologic, and performance-enhancing effects of anabolic steroids in animal models under both acute and chronic conditions. Perhaps because of the different forms of exercise and treatment protocols used, these studies have yielded conflicting evidence as to the potential performance-enhancing capability of these agents. Further studies are needed to critically evaluate the effects of anabolic steroids on muscle mass and strength. While the positive effects of anabolic steroids on muscle protein synthesis have been well documented, evidence relating exercise and steroid treatment to muscle fiber hypertrophy and enhanced performance needs to be more critically studied.

Although the long-term effects of high doses of anabolic-androgenic agents are not entirely clear, several facts have been well established. There are CNS effects that may include a sensation of well-being or euphoria and increased levels of aggression, which may lead to intense antisocial or psychotic behavior, in individuals taking large doses of these agents. Cardiovascular effects include decreased high-density-lipoprotein levels, stroke, and cardiomyopathy; myocardial infarctions have been documented in individuals administered large doses of anabolic steroids. Hepatic and endocrine dysfunction, negative reproductive effects (oligospermia; azospermia; testicular atrophy; reductions in testosterone and gonadotropic hormones; and decreased levels of luteinizing hormone, follicle-stimulating hormone, estrogens, and progesterone), and other adverse effects (renal dysfunction) have also been implicated as possible side effects of these agents. Premature epiphyseal closure has been reported in youths. Because of this irreversible halt in growth, these compounds are especially contraindicated prior to skeletal maturity.

The effects of these agents on skeletal muscle and tendon are less well documented. Changes in the morphology of the muscle-tendon unit have also been studied in animals. Anabolic agents used concurrently with swimming produced slow-twitch fiber hypertrophy in the rat. Exercise and steroid protocols by themselves increased the fast oxidative glycolytic fiber population and decreased the fast glycolytic subtype. Clinically, several cases of spontaneous tendon rupture have been reported in athletes taking large doses of anabolic steroids. Laboratory studies have shown that administration of large doses of anabolic steroids to rats produced inhibitory effects on collagen biosynthesis. None of these studies, however, conclusively confirm the use of these agents as the causative problem.

A relatively new ergogenic aid is human growth hormone. The development of synthetic agents has led to a dramatic increase in the use of these potentially anabolic agents. Similar to the use of other anabolic agents, the use of growth hormone is potentially widespread with serious side effects. These include diabetogenic effects, cardiomegaly, and acromegaly.

The physiologic mechanism responsible for exercise-induced muscle growth is unknown. Muscle hypertrophy can be induced by overload in castrated, hypophysectomized, and diabetic animals. Therefore, at least in some experimental animal models, the presence of testosterone, growth hormone, or insulin does not seem to be required to produce muscle hypertrophy. Maintenance of, as well as increases in, muscle size and strength can be achieved in actively exercising elderly humans and in aged animals in states of poor nutrition, although advanced age and malnutrition can decrease levels of certain growth factors.

Muscle Stretching and Viscoelasticity

Muscle stretching exercises or routines are frequently used by athletes before and during sports. They are also a part of many rehabilitation and fitness programs. Few scientific data address the efficacy of stretching in injury prevention and rehabilitation or in the enhancement of performance. Various reflexes involving the CNS and motor control of skeletal muscle are frequently mentioned as the scientific rationale for stretching. These reflexes are very important in the motor control of dynamic movement, but their effects on static stretching are unknown.

The effects of chronic stretching may be related to the previous discussions of longitudinal growth of muscle or to the effects of immobilization in extension. In these situations, the stretch is maintained long enough to allow time for biologic growth or rearrangement of muscle tissue. The acute effects of stretching have only recently been evaluated. Skeletal muscle exhibits the same viscoelastic effects seen in dense connective tissue and bone. These viscoelastic effects explain many of the effects of stretching.

Viscoelasticity, discussed in more detail in the chapter on biomechanics, describes the stress and strain relationship and its time-dependent nature. When muscle is stretched to a given length, it develops a certain tension. The tension does not remain constant with time. Instead the stress diminishes with time; this phenomenon is called stress relaxation. Muscle can lose more than 20% of the initial force in as little as 30 s. Muscle also exhibits creep behavior, meaning that when a given load is applied to a muscle it reaches an initial length and then will slowly stretch out with time. Viscoelastic phenomena can account for the diminished stiffness of muscle after stretching and for the increased range of motion allowed by stretching.

Another property of viscoelasticity that relates to muscle stretching is the dependence of stress developed in muscle to the rate of strain. Muscle stretched quickly is stiffer than muscle stretched slowly. Temperature effects also are important. Cold muscle is stiffer than warm muscle; therefore, warm muscle will develop less force than cold muscle when stretched to a given length. Viscoelasticity in muscle can certainly help to explain the common benefits attributed to stretching.

Common stretching routines usually advocate slow static stretching of the muscle-tendon unit. Under these conditions it appears that the electrical activity within muscle is minimal. This means that the resistance of muscle to stretch comes primarily from the mechanical properties of the muscle-tendon unit rather than from active contraction of the muscle. Therefore, the viscoelastic properties of muscle are probably more important to static muscle stretching than reflex-mediated relaxation controlled by the CNS.

Electromyography

Muscles and tendons can be thought of as the interface between the CNS and the skeleton. Communication between these effectors occurs through electrical activity. The electrical currents passing across the membranes of the muscle cells can be detected and measured by methods similar to those by which electrical currents in the heart are recorded as an electrocardiogram. The electromyographic (EMG) signal is the electrical representation of the neuromuscular activation associated with a contracting muscle. A number of uses for this technique have been developed to study normal muscle function and to assist in the diagnoses of muscle abnormalities.

Basically, the electrical signals within the muscle are detected by electrodes, amplified, and subsequently recorded or processed (Fig. 24). Surface electrodes are placed on the skin surface and can detect underlying muscle currents. These electrodes are simple and convenient for the study of large surface muscles. Needle electrodes, on the other hand, are inserted through the skin into the muscle. Insulated wire inside a needle-like cannula allows for the detection of a myoelectric signal from a smaller volume of muscle and may be used to study individual muscles and muscles not on the surface. Fine wire electrodes are very small and can be inserted into muscles and left for kinesiological studies. They are small enough and painless enough to cause little perturbation of the normal use of the

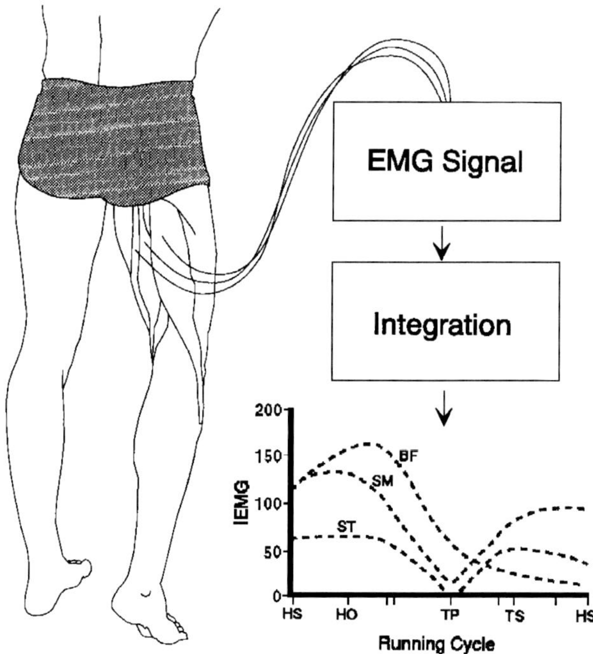

Figure 24
An averaged integrated electromyogram from biceps femoris (BF), semimembranosus (SM), and semitendinosus (ST). HS = Heel strike; HO = immediately prior to the heel lofting off treadmill; TP = thigh perpendicular to treadmill; TS = toe strike; IEMG = integrated electromyogram.

muscle. The signals detected by the electrodes are amplified and recorded with appropriate electrical considerations to ensure that the recorded signal most closely resembles the myoelectric signal generated within the muscle.

Central Nervous System Control

The study of electrical signals in the muscle has led to a tremendous insight into the nature of CNS control of muscle activity. Appropriate electrodes can actually evaluate the distribution and activity of single motor units. Sophisticated techniques of signal acquisition and decomposition have allowed researchers to analyze how the many motor units interact under conditions such as varying force and time of excitation. The CNS control depends on the type of muscle; small muscles and muscles needing fine control are somewhat different from the larger muscle groups. Small muscles are capable of higher frequencies of muscle activation with plateaus near 60 Hz compared to approximately 25 Hz for larger muscles. The smaller muscles, thus, have a larger range of control.

Data from EMG studies have provided information necessary to understand the control of force in muscle. Basically, force is increased in a muscle both by increasing the recruitment of motor units and by increasing the frequency of stimulation of recruited motor units. The changes in both recruitment and frequency are under the influence of a common drive from the CNS. The common drive allows the CNS to control motor units as a pool rather than as single units. The addition and subtraction of motor units is an orderly process based in large part on the size of the motor unit. The smallest motor units are recruited initially, followed by larger and larger motor units.

The recruitment pattern differs among muscles. In small muscles, the motor units are often fully recruited at force levels below 50% of a maximum contraction. Alterations in frequency provide additional control above this level. Larger muscles may not recruit all motor units until forces near maximum are achieved. The varying relationship between maximum force in a muscle and the mechanism of force control, that is, alterations in recruitment and stimulation frequency, might imply that there is not a strict relationship between muscle force output and the EMG signal. Although it is true that an increasing EMG signal is usually accompanied by increasing force, this relationship is not necessarily linear. In addition, the relationship varies among subjects and among different muscles. In general, the smaller muscles have a more linear relationship between force and the integrated EMG signal; larger muscles often demonstrate less linearity, with the signal increasing more than the force.

Electromyography has also been important in arriving at the present understanding of local muscle fatigue. An isometrically activated muscle might be expected to maintain a constant EMG signal; however, the EMG signal depends on time of activation, intensity of activation, and fatigue. In general, the integrated EMG signal increases with time when a constant force is achieved by a muscle. Although the amplitude of the signal increases, the mean and median frequencies of motor unit firing rates decrease. This shift in frequency begins very quickly after initiation of a sustained isometric contraction and continues with time. This measurable change provides an excellent parameter for studying the state of local muscle fatigue.

Clinical applications of the EMG signal to provide information regarding the state of muscle and its CNS control are increasing. EMG can provide an excellent measure of the degree of muscle activation; however, the EMG signal may not be a direct measure of the force output of the muscle. In addition, EMG may be able to provide information about the state of fatigue in muscle. Application of EMG techniques is increasing in the fields of athletic training and rehabilitation; these techniques are being applied to muscles of the limbs and of the axial skeleton.

EMG in Kinesiology

Kinesiology, or the study of movement, has benefited greatly from EMG techniques. Movement studies can be correlated with EMG studies to show when and to what extent the muscle is active in a particular movement. The use of EMG techniques to study gait has been invaluable. The combined effects of kinetic and potential energy, the interdependence of joint movements, and the influences of ground contact make it impossible to know about the state of muscle activity without a direct means of detection. Studies of gait in normal and pathologic states have benefited greatly from combining kinesiology and EMG.

EMG has been used in gait studies with increasing sophistication over the last 50 years. At present more applications are becoming apparent; complex motor activities such as throwing, swimming, and even a golf or tennis swing are being understood as never before. The data obtained are useful in understanding the movement and its disorders, and with time EMG techniques hold the promise of improving performance and of guiding and assessing rehabilitation. Implantable fine-wire electrodes and methods of telemetry have allowed increasing applications of these techniques.

EMG in Diagnosis of Neuromuscular Disease

Diagnostic EMG has made significant strides recently and is now a sophisticated tool in the diagnosis of neuromuscular pathology. Although primarily used by neurologists to study neurologic disease, EMG has significance for orthopaedics and the study of musculoskeletal problems. These applications specifically concern the presence and chronicity of injury to nerves and nerve roots.

Following injury to its motor nerve, the muscle is deprived of its normal control mechanism. In the case of a neurapraxia, the nerve distal to the site of injury does not undergo necrosis. However, the muscle is electrically silent even in response to efforts to activate the muscle. If the injury is an axonotmesis or a neurotmesis, the axon distal to the injury undergoes necrosis. The motor end plate eventually degenerates after several weeks, depending on the length of nerve between the injury and the synapse. After the synapse undergoes degeneration, changes occur within the membrane system of the muscle. The individual muscle fibers spontaneously depolarize and give rise to axonal action potentials. The spontaneous discharges are in single muscle fibers rather than in an entire motor unit; therefore, the potentials are smaller and occur intermittently. Needle electrodes detect these changes as fibrillations, which are indicative of denervation. If the nerve injury is due to an incomplete lesion to the nerve or to a single ventral root, as in a radiculopathy from the level of the spinal cord, apparently normal action potentials or action potentials of reduced magnitude exist, with fibrillations also evident when the muscle and nerve are at rest.

After denervation and distal axonal necrosis, reinnervation may occur. This may be due to regrowth of axons across the site of injury or it may be due to sprouting of collateral branches from axons reaching the muscles. The regrown axons and the sprouts give rise to large and atypical motor units. The action potentials of these motor units are large and complex in contrast to the normal motor unit action potential. These abnormal action potentials are called giant polyphasic action potentials and are a sign of reinnervation.

Selected Bibliography

Muscle Structure and Function

Burke RE: Motor unit properties and selective involvement in movement. *Exerc Sport Sci Rev* 1975;3:31–81.

Carlson FD, Wilkie DR (eds): *Muscle Physiology.* Englewood Cliffs, NJ, Prentice Hall Inc, 1974.

Huxley AF, Simmons RM: Proposed mechanism of force generation in striated muscle. *Nature* 1971;233:533–538.

Huxley AF: Muscle structure and theories of contraction. *Prog Biophys Biophys Chem* 1957;7:255–318.

Huxley HE: Electron microscope studies on the structure of natural and synthetic protein filaments from striated muscle. *J Mol Biol* 1963;7:281–308.

Huxley HE: The mechanism of muscular contraction. *Science* 1969;164:1356–1365.

Schaub MC, Watterson JG: Control of the contractile process in muscle. *Trends Pharmacol Sci* 1981;2:279–282.

Wickiewicz TL, Roy RR, Powell PL, et al: Muscle architecture of the human lower limb. *Clin Orthop* 1983;179:275–283.

Fiber Types and Adaptability of Muscle

Baldwin KM, Winder WW, Holloszy JO: Adaptation of actomyosin ATPase in different types of muscle to endurance exercise. *Am J Physiol* 1975;229:422–426.

Barany M, Close RI: The transformation of myosin in cross-innervated rat muscles. *J Physiol (Lond)* 1971;213:455–474.

Buchthal F, Schmalbruch H: Motor unit of mammalian muscle. *Physiol Rev* 1980;60:90–142.

Buller AJ, Eccles JC, Eccles RM: Interactions between motoneurones and muscles in respect of the characteristic speeds of their responses. *J Physiol (Lond)* 1960;150:417–439.

Close RI: Dynamic properties of mammalian skeletal muscles. *Physiol Rev* 1972;52:129–197.

Dubowitz V, Brooke MH (eds): *Muscle Biopsy: A Modern Approach.* London, WB Saunders, 1973, vol 2 in Major Problems in Neurology.

Gauthier GF: Skeletal muscle fiber types, in Engle AG, Banker BQ (eds): *Myology: Basic and Clinical.* New York, McGraw-Hill, vol 1, pp 255–283.

Henneman E: Relation between size of neurons and their susceptibility to discharge. *Science* 1957;126:1345–1347.

Johnson MA, Polgar J, Weightman D, et al: Data on the distribution of fibre types in thirty-six human muscles: An autopsy study. *J Neurol Sci* 1973;18:111–129.

Kugelberg E: Histochemical composition, contraction speed, and fatiguability of rat soleus motor units. *J Neurol Sci* 1973:20:177–198.

Lowey S, Risby D: Light chains from fast and slow muscle myosins. *Nature* 1971;234:81–85.

Martin WD, Romond EH: Effects of chronic rotation and hypergravity on muscle fibers of soleus and plantaris muscles of the rat. *Exp Neurol* 1975;49:758–771.

Pette D (ed): *Plasticity of Muscle.* Berlin, Walter de Gruyter, 1980.

Roy RR, Meadows ID, Baldwin KM, et al: Functional significance of compensatory overloaded rat fast muscle. *J Appl Physiol* 1982;52:473–478.

Salmons S, Sreter FA: Significance of impulse activity in the transformation of skeletal muscle type. *Nature* 1976; 263:30–34.

Samaha FJ, Guth L, Albers RW: Differences between slow and fast muscle myosin: Adenosine triphosphatase activity and release of associated proteins by p-chloromercuriphenylsulfonate. *J Biol Chem* 1970;245:219–224.

Sreter FA, Seidel JC, Gergely J: Studies on myosin from red and white skeletal muscles of the rabbit: I. Adenosine triphosphatase activity. *J Biol Chem* 1966;241:5772–5776.

Muscle Mechanics

Hill AV: The heat of shortening and the dynamic constants of muscle (1938): *Proc R Soc Lond (Biol)* 1938;126:136–195.

Huxley AF: Muscular contraction. *J Physiol (Lond)* 1974;243:1–43.

Kulig K, Andrews JG, Hay JG: Human strength curves. *Exerc Sport Sci Rev* 1984;12:417–466.

Woittiez RD, Huijing PA, Boom HB, et al: A three-dimensional muscle model: Quantified relation between form and function of skeletal muscles. *J Morphol* 1984;182:95–113.

Training Effects on Muscle

Gollnick PD, Armstrong RB, Saltin B, et al: Effect of training on enzyme activity and fiber composition of human skeletal muscle. *J Appl Physiol* 1973;34:107–111.

Gollnick PD, Matoba H: The muscle fiber composition of skeletal muscle as a predictor of athletic success: An overview. *Am J Sports Med* 1984;12:212–217.

Green HJ, Reichmann H, Pette D: Fibre type specific transformations in the enzyme activity pattern of rat vastus lateralis muscle by prolonged endurance training. *Pflugers Arch* 1983;399:216–222.

Holloszy JO: Biochemical adaptations in muscle: Effects of exercise on mitochondrial oxygen uptake and respiratory enzyme activity in skeletal muscle. *J Biol Chem* 1967;242:2278–2282.

Howald H, Hoppeler H, Claassen H, et al: Influences of endurance training on the ultrastructural composition of the different muscle fiber types in humans. *Pflugers Arch* 1985;403:369–376.

Komi PV, Rusko H, Vos J, et al: Anaerobic performance capacity in athletes. *Acta Physiol Scand* 1977;100:107–114.

Milner-Brown HS, Stein RB, Yemm R: Changes in firing rate of human motor units during linearly changing voluntary contractions. *J Physiol (Lond)* 1973;230:371–390.

Saltin B, Henriksson J, Nygaard E, et al: Fiber types and metabolic potentials of skeletal muscles in sedentary man and endurance runners. *Ann N Y Acad Sci* 1977;301:3–29.

Taylor NA, Wilkinson JG: Exercise-induced skeletal muscle growth: Hypertrophy or hyerplasia? *Sports Med* 1986;3:190–200.

Tesch P, Karlsson J: Isometric strength performance and muscle fibre type distribution in man. *Acta Physiol Scand* 1978;103:47–51.

Thorstensson A, Hulten B, von Dobeln W, et al: Effect of strength training on enzyme activities and fibre characteristics in human skeletal muscle. *Acta Physiol Scand* 1976;96:392–398.

Tipton CM, Schild RJ, Tomanek RJ: Influence of physical activity on the strength of knee ligaments in rats. *Am J Physiol* 1967;212:783–787.

Growth and Development of Muscle

Dix DJ, Eisenberg BR: Myosin mRNA accumulation and myofibrillogenesis at the myotendinous junction of stretched muscle fibers. *J Cell Biol* 1990;1:1885–1894.

Griffin GE, Williams PE, Goldspink G: Region of longitudinal growth in striated muscle fibres. *Nature* (New Biol) 1971;232:28–29.

Williams PE, Goldspink G: Changes in sarcomere length and physiological properties in immobilized muscle. *J Anat* 1978;127:459–468.

Williams PE, Goldspink G: Connective tissue changes in immobilised muscle. *J Anat* 1984;138:343–350.

Williams PE, Goldspink G: The effect of immobilization on the longitudinal growth of striated muscle fibres. *J Anat* 1973;116:45–55.

Muscle Injury and Repair

Armstrong RB: Mechanisms of exercise-induced delayed onset muscular soreness: A brief review. *Med Sci Sports Exerc* 1984;16:529–538.

Asmussen E: Observations on experimental muscular soreness. *Acta Rheum Scand* 1956;2:109–116.

Besson C, Rochcongar P, Beauverger Y, et al: Study of the valuations of serum muscular enzymes and myoglobin after maximal exercise test and during the next 24 hours. (author's translation) *Eur J Appl Physiol* 1981;47:47–56.

Byrnes WC, Clarkson PM, White JS, et al: Delayed onset muscle soreness following repeated bouts of downhill running. *J Appl Phys* 1985;59:710–715.

Denny-Brown D: Clinical problems in neuromuscular physiology. *Am J Med* 1953;15:368–390.

Friden J, Sjostrom M, Ekblom B: Myofibrillar damage following intense eccentric exercise in man. *Int J Sports Med* 1983;4:170–176.

Garrett WE Jr, Safran MR, Seaber AV, et al: Biomechanical comparison of stimulated and nonstimulated skeletal muscle pulled to failure. *Am J Sports Med* 1987;15:448–454.

Garrett WE Jr, Seaber AV, Boswick J, et al: Recovery of skeletal muscle after laceration and repair. *J Hand Surg* 1984;9A:683–692.

Hough T: Ergographic studies in muscular soreness. *Am J Physiol* 1902;7:76–92.

Hughston JC, Whatley GS, Stone MM: Myositis ossificans traumatica (myo-osteosis). *South Med J* 1962;55:1167–1170.

Jackson DW, Feagin JA: Quadriceps contusions in young athletes: Relation of severity of injury to treatment and prognosis. *J Bone Joint Surg* 1973;55A:95–105.

Lieber RL, Friden J: Selective damage of fast glycolytic muscle fibres with eccentric contraction of the rabbit tibialis anterior. *Acta Physiol Scand* 1988;133:587–588.

Lieber RL, Woodburn TM, Friden J: Muscle damage induced by eccentric contractions of 25% strain. *J Appl Physiol* 1991;70:2498–2507.

Maughan RJ: Exercise-induced muscle cramp: A prospective biochemical study in marathon runners. *J Sport Sci* 1986;4:31–34.

Moss HK, Herrmann LG: Night cramps in human extremities: Clinical study of physiologic action of quinine and prostigmine upon spontaneous contractions of resting muscles. *Am Heart J* 1948;35:403–408.

Nikolaou PK, Macdonald BL, Glisson RR, et al: Biomechanical and histological evaluation of muscle after controlled strain injury. *Am J Sports Med* 1987;15:9–14.

Parrow A, Samuelsson SM: Use of chloroquine phosphate—a new treatment for spontaneous leg cramps. *Acta Medica Scand* 1967;181:237–244.

Schwane JA, Johnson SR, Vandenakker CB, et al: Delayed-onset muscular soreness and plasma CPK and LDH activities after downhill running. *Med Sci Sports Exerc* 1983;15:51–56.

Shellock FG, Fukunaga T, Mink JH, et al: Exertional muscle injury: Evaluation of concentric versus eccentric actions with serial MR imaging. *Radiology* 1991;179:659–664.

Stauber WT: Eccentric action of muscles: Physiology, injury, and adaptation. *Exerc Sport Sci Rev* 1989;17:157–185.

Stewart WK, Fleming LW, Manuel MA: Muscle cramps during maintenance haemodialysis. *Lancet* 1972;1(759):1049–1051.

Tidball JG: Myotendinous junction: Morphological changes and mechanical failure associated with muscle cell atrophy. *Exp Mol Pathol* 1984;40:1–12.

Immobilization

Alford EK, Roy RR, Hodgson JA, et al: Electromyography of rat soleus, medial gastrocnemius, and tibialis anterior during hind limb suspension. *Exp Neurol* 1987;96:635–649.

Appell HJ: Morphology of immobilized skeletal muscle and the effects of a pre- and post-immobilization training program. *Int J Sports Med* 1986;7:6–12.

Booth FW: Physiologic and biochemical effects of immobilization on muscle. *Clin Orthop* 1987;219:15–20.

Booth FW, Seider MJ: Recovery of skeletal muscle after 3 months of hind limb immobilization in rats. *J Appl Physiol* 1979;47:435–439.

Jansson E, Sylven C, Arvidsson I, et al: Increase in myoglobin content and decrease in oxidative enzyme activities by leg muscle immobilization in man. *Acta Physiol Scand* 1988;132:515–517.

Lieber RL, Friden JO, Hargens AR, et al: Differential response of the dog quadriceps muscle to external skeletal fixation of the knee. *Muscle Nerve* 1988;11:193–201.

Lipschütz A, Audova A: The comparative atrophy of the skeletal muscle after cutting the nerve and after cutting the tendon. *J Physiol (Lond)* 1921;55:300–304.

MacDougall JD, Elder GC, Sale DG, et al: Effects of strength training and immobilization on human muscle fibres. *Eur J Appl Physiol* 1980;43:25–34.

Max SR: Disuse atrophy of skeletal muscle: Loss of functional activity of mitochondria. *Biochem Biophys Res Commun* 1972;46:1394–1398.

Roy RR, Bello MA, Bouissou P, et al: Size and metabolic properties of fibers in rat fast-twitch muscles after hind-limb suspension. *J Appl Physiol* 1987;62:2348–2357.

Sargeant AJ, Davies CT, Edwards RH, et al: Functional and structural changes after disuse of human muscle. *Clin Sci Mol Med* 1977;52:337–342.

Solandt DY, Partridge RC, Hunter J: The effect of skeletal fixation on skeletal muscle. *J Neurophysiol* 1943;6:17–22.

Thomason DB, Herrick RE, Surdyka D, et al: Time course of soleus muscle myosin expression during hindlimb suspension and recovery. *J Appl Physiol* 1987;63:130–137.

Tomanek RJ, Lund DD: Degeneration of different types of skeletal muscle fibres. II Immobilization. *J Anat* 1974;118:531–541.

Hormonal Effects

Alen M, Hakkinen K, Komi PV: Changes in neuromuscular performance and muscle fiber characteristics of elite power athletes self-administering androgenic and anabolic steroids. *Acta Physiol Scand* 1984;122:535–544.

AMA Council on Scientific Affairs. Drug abuse in athletes: Anabolic steroids and human growth hormone. *JAMA* 1988;259:1703–1705.

American College of Sports Medicine position stand on the use of anabolic-androgenic steroids in sports. *Med Sci Sports Exerc* 1987;19:534–539.

American Academy of Orthopaedic Surgeons Position Statement: Anabolic Steroids to Enhance Athletic Performance. Park Ridge, IL, American Academy of Orthopaedic Surgeons, 1991.

Apostolakis M, Deligiannis A, Madena-Pyrgaki A: The effects of human growth hormone administration on the functional status of rat atrophied muscle following immobilization. *Physiologist* 1980:23(suppl):S111–112.

Bach BR Jr, Warren RF, Wickiewicz TL: Triceps rupture: A case report and literature review. *Am J Sports Med* 1987;15:285–289.

Breuer CB, Florini JR: Amino acid incorporation into protein by cell-free systems from rat skeletal muscle: IV. Effects of animal age, androgens, and anabolic agents on activity of muscle ribosomes. *Biochemistry* 1965;4:1544–1550.

Dimauro J, Balnave RJ, Shorey CD: Effects of anabolic steroids and high intensity exercise on rat skeletal muscle fibres and capillarization: A morphometric study. *Eur J Appl Physiol* 1992;64:204–212.

Egginton S: Effects of an anabolic hormone on striated muscle growth and performance. *Pflugers Arch* 1987;410:349–355.

Exner GU, Staudte HW, Pette D: Isometric training of rats: Effects upon fast and slow muscle and modification by an anabolic hormone (nandrolone decanoate). I. Female rats. *Pflugers Arch* 1973;345:1–14.

Exner GU, Staudte HW, Pette D: Isometric training of rats: Effects upon fast and slow muscle and modification by an anabolic hormone (nandrolone decanoate). II. Male rats. *Pflugers Arch* 1973;345:15–22.

Florini J: Hormonal control of muscle growth. *J Anim Sci* 1985;61:21–37.

Goldberg AL, Goodman HM: Relationship between growth hormone and muscular work in determining muscle size. *J Physiol (Lond)* 1969;200:655–666.

Haupt HA, Rovere GD: Anabolic steroids: A review of the literature. *Am J Sports Med* 1984;12:469–484.

Herrick RT, Herrick S: Ruptured triceps in a powerlifter presenting as cubital tunnel syndrome: A case report. *Am J Sports Med* 1987;15:514–516.

Hill JA, Suker JR, Sachs K, et al: The athletic polydrug abuse phenomenon: A case report. *Am J Sports Med* 1983;11:269–271.

Kibble MW, Ross MB: Adverse effects of anabolic steroids in athletes. *Clin Pharm* 1987;6:686–692.

Michna H, Stang-Voss C: The predisposition to tendon rupture after doping with anabolic steroids. *Int J Sports Med* 1986;4:59.

Perlmutter G, Lowenthal DT: Use of anabolic steroids by athletes. *Am Fam Physician* 1985;32:208–210.

Muscle Stretching and Viscoelasticity

Dalton JD Jr, Seaber AV, Garrett WE Jr: Biomechanics of passively stretched muscle: Viscoelasticity vs. reflex effects. *Surg Forum* 1989;40:516–518.

Inman VT, Ralston HJ, de Saunder JB, et al: Relation of human electromyogram to muscular tension. *EEG Clin Neurophysiol* 1952;4:187–194.

Lippold OCJ: The relation between integrated action potentials in a human muscle and its isometric tension. *J Physiol (Lond)* 1952;117:492–499.

Taylor DC, Dalton JD Jr, Seaber AV, et al: Viscoelastic properties of muscle-tendon units: The biomechanical effects of stretching. *Am J Sports Med* 1990;18:300–309.

Chapter 4
Form and Function of Bone

Frederick S. Kaplan, MD
Wilson C. Hayes, PhD
Tony M. Keaveny, PhD
Adele Boskey, PhD
Thomas A. Einhorn, MD
Joseph P. Iannotti, MD, PhD

Chapter Outline

Introduction

Bone is an extremely well-organized tissue, from the modulation of the hydroxyapatite crystal arrangement at the molecular level to the strain pattern of the trabecular cascades at the organ level. The synergy of the molecular, cellular, and tissue arrangement provides a tensile strength nearly that of cast iron, with such an efficient use of material that the skeleton is of surprisingly low weight for such a supporting structure. At the microscopic level, bone consists of two forms: woven and lamellar (Fig. 1). Woven bone is considered immature bone, or primitive bone, and normally is found in the embryo and the newborn, in fracture callus, and in the metaphyseal region of growing bone. This type of bone also is found in tumors, osteogenesis imperfecta, and pagetic bone.

Woven, or primary, bone is coarse-fibered and contains no uniform orientation of the collagen fibers. It has more cells per unit volume than does lamellar bone, its mineral content varies, and its cells are randomly arranged. The relatively disoriented collagen fibers of woven bone give it isotropic mechanical characteristics; when tested, the mechanical behavior of woven bone is similar regardless of the orientation of the applied forces.

Lamellar bone begins to form one month after birth. By 1 year of age, it is actively replacing woven bone, as the latter is resorbed. By age 4, most normal bone is lamellar bone. Lamellar bone thus is a more mature bone that results from the remodeling of woven or previously existing bone. Lamellar bone is found in several structural and functional systems: trabecular lamellae; outer and inner circumferential lamellae; interstitial lamellae; and osteons with concentric lamellae. The highly organized, stress-oriented collagen of lamellar bone gives it anisotropic properties; that is, the mechanical behavior of lamellar bone differs depending on the orientation of the applied forces, with its greatest strength parallel to the longitudinal axis of the collagen fibers.

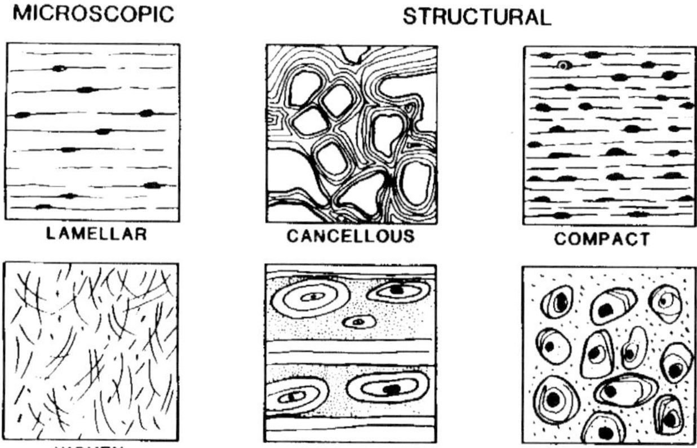

Figure 1
Diagrams of types of bone.

Woven and lamellar bone are structurally organized into trabecular (spongy or cancellous) bone and cortical (dense or compact) bone (Fig. 1). Cortical bone has four times the mass of trabecular (cancellous) bone, although the metabolic turnover of trabecular bone is eight times greater than that of cortical bone. Bone turnover is a surface event, and trabecular bone has a greater surface area than cortical bone.

Trabecular bone is found principally at the metaphysis and epiphysis of long bones and in cuboid bones such as the vertebrae. The internal beams or spicules of trabecular bone form a three-dimensional (3-D) branching lattice aligned along areas of stress. Trabecular bone is subjected to a complex set of stresses and strains, although compression seems to predominate. Figure 2 illustrates new woven bone in a trabecular pattern with no discernible matrix orientation (*left*) compared to lamellar bone arranged in a trabecular pattern (*right*) with a layered arrangement of matrix fibers.

Cortical bone is found as the "envelope" in cuboid bones, and it composes the diaphysis in long bones. Cortical bone is subject to bending and torsional forces as well as to compressive forces. In small animals, there is no special arrangement of the vascular network in cortical bone; it consists simply of layers of lamellar bone, called compact bone. In larger animals that experience rapid growth, cortical bone is made up of layers of lamellar bone and woven bone, with the vascular channels located mainly in the woven bone. This bone is termed plexiform bone (Fig. 1). Such an arrangement of bone allows rapid growth and the accumulation of large amounts of bone over a short time.

Haversian bone is the most complex type of cortical bone. It is composed of vascular channels circumferentially surrounded by lamellar bone. This complex arrangement of bone around the vascular channel is called the osteon. The osteon is an irregular, branching, and anastomosing cylinder composed of a more or less centrally placed neurovascular canal surrounded by cell-permeated layers of bone matrix. Osteons are usually oriented in the long axis of the bone and are the major structural units of cortical bone. Cortical bone is, therefore, a complex of many adjacent osteons and their interstitial and circumferential lamellae. Figure 3 illustrates a single osteon surrounded by interstitial lamellae. Figure 4 shows a photomicrograph of cortical bone from a femoral shaft with inner circumferential lamellae next to the marrow cavity (lower

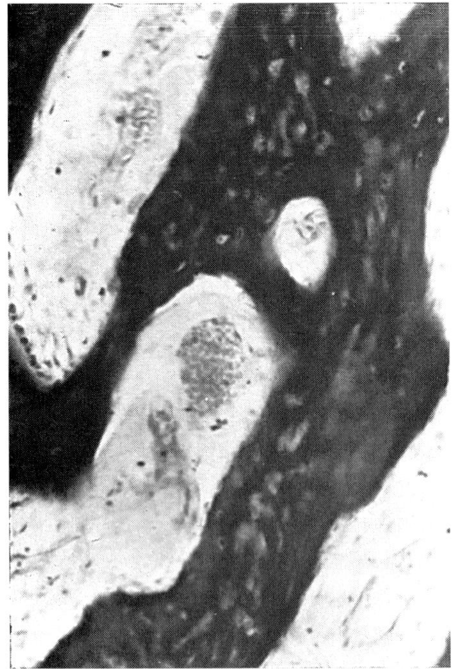
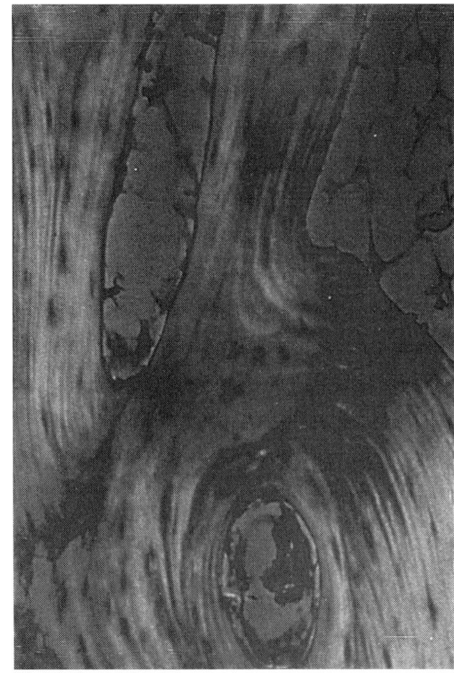

Figure 2
Photomicrographs of woven and lamellar bone.

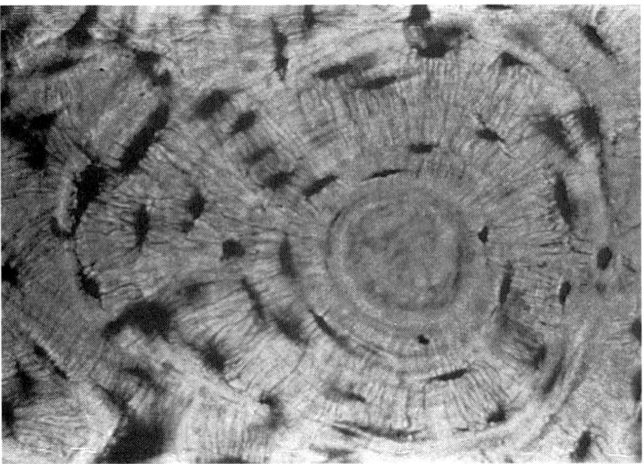

Figure 3
Photomicrograph of a bone osteon.

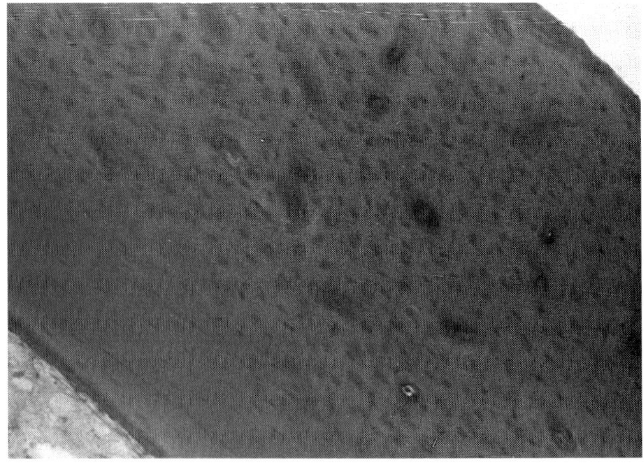

Figure 4
Photomicrograph of cortical bone.

left corner). Also shown are many osteons with their concentric lamellae, and the interstitial lamellae between osteons.

The central canal of an osteon, called the haversian canal, contains cells, vessels, and, occasionally, nerves. Most vessels in the haversian canals have the ultrastructural features of capillaries, although some smaller-sized vessels may resemble lymphatic vessels. When examined histologically, these smaller vessels contain only precipitated protein; their endothelial walls are not surrounded by a basement membrane. Such features are characteristic of lymphatic vessels. The basement membrane of capillary walls may function as a rate limiting or selective ion limiting transport barrier, because all material traversing the vessel wall must go through the basement membrane. The presence of this barrier is particularly important in calcium and phosphorus ion transport to and from bone, and is also important in explaining the response of bone to mechanical loads.

The capillaries in the central canals are derived from the principal nutrient arteries of the bone or the epiphyseal metaphyseal arteries. Figure 5, *left*, shows the nutrient artery of a long bone entering the shaft and branching to form the vascular network in cortical bone. Using lower magnification and injecting India ink (Fig. 5, *right*) provides a better picture of the complexity of this vascular network.

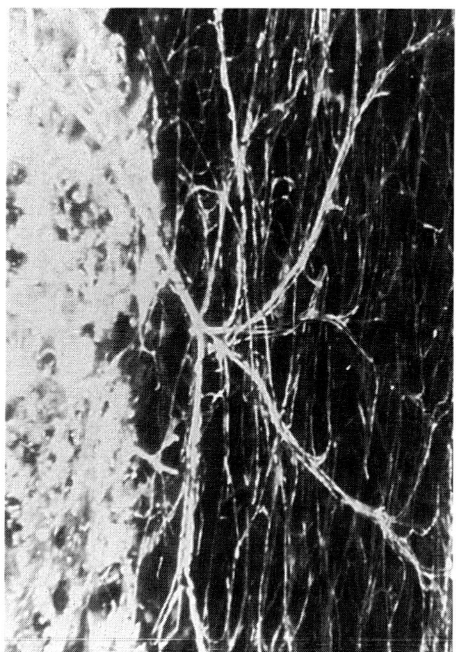

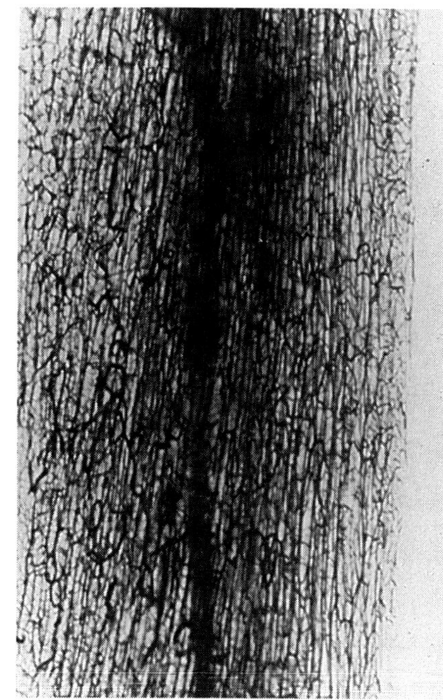

Figure 5
Photomicrograph showing vasculature of cortical bone.

Bone Cell Morphology

Osteoblasts

The major types of bone cells are the osteoblasts, osteocytes, and osteoclasts. The bone-forming cells are the osteoblasts and osteocytes; the principal difference between these cells is location. Osteoblasts line the surface of bone; osteocytes are osteoblasts encased in a mineralized matrix. Cells close to the osteoblast, but away from the bone surface, are sometimes referred to as preosteoblasts. All of these cells are derived from the same osteoprogenitor cell line. Factors that induce the process of bone cell differentiation are currently under active investigation, and these include the bone morphogenetic proteins along with other growth factors and cytokines. The interleukins, insulin-derived growth factor, and platelet-derived growth factor (PDGF), among others, all effect osteoblast differentiation in vitro.

The most distinctive features of the osteoblast are illustrated in the light and electron micrographs of osteoblasts adjacent to new bone (Fig. 6). At the light microscopic level (Fig. 6, *left*) the active osteoblast shows intense staining with basophilic stains, and appears to be polarized with the nucleus located at the end of the cell away from the bone surface. The apparent shape of the osteoblast is a function of the orientation of the section being examined. Some of the osteoblasts shown in the electron micrograph (Fig. 6, *right*) appear rectangular with their long axes perpendicular to the osteoid (bone surface). The cytoplasm of the cell is occupied by three major components; the nucleus, the Golgi apparatus, and the rough endoplasmic reticulum. The nucleus in the osteoblast is large relative to that in other cell types. The abundant rough endoplasmic reticulum is characteristic of cells that manufacture protein for export. The Golgi apparatus, adjacent to the nucleus, is responsible for the secretion of these proteins. Mitochondria and cytoskeletal elements are found throughout the cytoplasm.

Histochemical studies have demonstrated that alkaline phosphatase is distributed over the outer surface of the osteoblast cell membrane. As indicated by the electron photomicrograph, there is a layer of newly formed unmineralized bone matrix (osteoid) between the osteoblast cell membrane and the mineralized matrix of bone. An osteoblast is defined as a cell that produces type I collagen, is responsive to parathyroid hormone (PTH), and produces osteocalcin when stimulated by 1,25-dihydroxyvitamin D.

Osteocytes

Once an osteoblast becomes surrounded by bone matrix, which then becomes mineralized, the cell is characterized by a higher nucleus-to-cytoplasm ratio and contains fewer organelles. Such a cell is the osteocyte of bone, and although osteocytes are the most numerous of bone cells they seem to receive the least amount of attention. Light microscopy (Fig. 3) reveals osteocytes arranged concentrically around the central lumen of an osteon and between lamellae. They are uniformly oriented with respect to the longitudinal and radial axes of

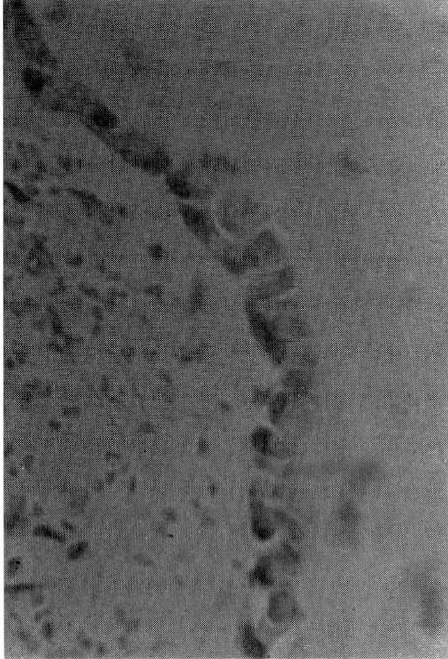

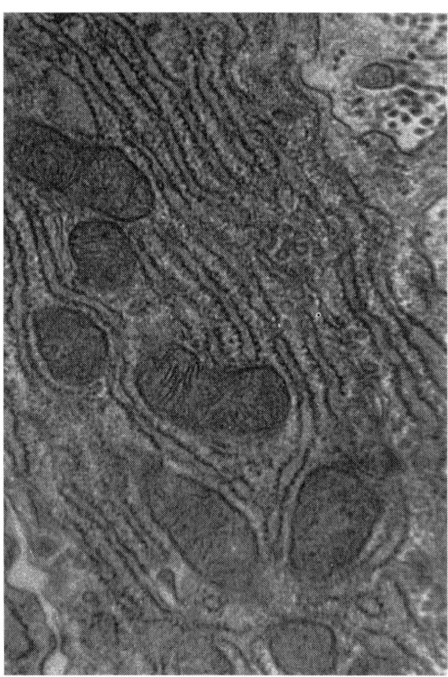

Figure 6
Light and electron photomicrographs of osteoblasts.

lamellae. Osteoblasts and osteocytes have extensive cell processes that project through the canaliculi, thereby establishing contact and "communication" between adjacent osteocytes and the central canals of osteons. The canaliculi are oriented in a radial fashion around the central haversian canal. Electron micrography of mature osteocytes shows a decreased organelle content, a greater nucleus-to-cytoplasm ratio, and numerous cell processes extending outward through the canaliculi (Fig. 7).

Osteocytes can metabolically manipulate their environment more or less independent of surface resorption and accretion. This ability is important to cellular regulation of calcium exchange. Bone crystals are extremely small and have a surface area of approximately 100 m^2/g or a total of 100 acres of surface area in the adult human body. Most of these crystals, buried away from the endosteal and periosteal bone surfaces, appear to be unavailable to effect the necessary exchange with extracellular fluid, making it difficult to explain the immediate exchange of bone mineral with the extracellular fluid. There is, however, a vast surface area on the haversian canal and lacunar walls and an even larger area on the canalicular walls, which in the adult totals about 300 m^2, or 3 acres, where bone mineral exchange with extracellular fluid can take place. The metabolic/structural role of osteocytes has not been identified, but their intricate 3-D distribution and their interconnecting cell processes (gap junctions) indicate that they are perfectly organized to serve as an intricate system to help communicate strain and stress signals and regulate the overall metabolism of the tissue.

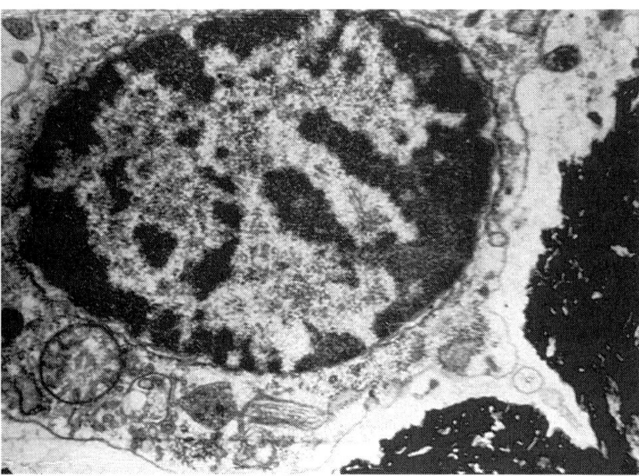

Figure 7
Electron photomicrograph of a mature osteocyte.

Osteoclasts

Osteoclasts are the major resorptive cells of bone and are characterized by their large size (20 to 100 μm in diameter) and their multiple nuclei. Osteoclasts are derived from pluripotent cells of the bone marrow, which are the hematopoietic precursors that also give rise to monocytes and macrophages. Whereas monocytes are mononuclear cells, macrophages and osteoclasts are formed from the fusion of monocytes. Osteoclasts differ from macrophages (foreign body giant cells) in that the osteoclasts produce tartrate-resistant acid phosphatase.

Osteoclasts are distinguished from macrophages by virtue of their ability to resorb bone and express certain cell surface markers as well as by their acid phosphatase activity. It is presumed that at some point during mononuclear cell development, the cell becomes committed to form either a macrophage or an osteoclast. The cellular origin of the osteoclast is underscored by recent clinical trials in which new osteoclast populations were found in patients with osteopetrosis who had received successful bone marrow allografts.

Osteoclasts lie in regions of bone resorption in pits called Howship's lacunae (Fig. 8). The electron photomicrograph (Fig. 8, *right*) demonstrates a strongly polarized cell with a paucity of rough-surfaced endoplasmic reticulum, a moderate number of ribosomes, numerous smooth vesicles, and well-developed mitochondria. As shown in the histologic section (Fig. 8, *left*), the other major feature of the osteoclasts is the ruffled (brush) border, which results from extensive infoldings of the cell membrane adjacent to the resorptive surface. Osteoclasts appearing some distance from the surface of bone do not have ruffled borders and are called "inactive" or "resting" osteoclasts. Direct observations show that the ruffled border of the osteoclasts sweeps across the surface of bone. The infolding of the ruffled border, which appears only over disrupted bone surfaces, greatly increases the surface area of the plasma membrane. The infolds of the ruffled border end in numerous channels and vesicles in the cell cytoplasm, within which lie numerous mineral crystals. Osteoclasts bind to the bone surface through cell attachment proteins called integrins, and they resorb bone by isolating an area of bone under the region of cell attachment. The osteoclasts then lower the pH of the local environment by production of hydrogen ions through the carbonic anhydrase system. The lowered pH increases the solubility of the hydroxyapatite crystals, and the organic components of the matrix are removed by acidic proteolytic digestion.

Cellular Mechanisms of Bone Modeling

All bone surfaces are continuous and typically are lined by resting osteoblasts called bone lining cells, with small intercellular gaps between the cells and their cytoplasmic processes. The endosteal surface is connected to the Volkmann's canals of the haversian systems via canaliculi. Although the cellular layer protects the bone from the extracellular fluid space, the osteoblasts on the bone surface are in direct chemical contact with the osteocytes within the mineralized bone by their cellular processes within the canaliculi. This organizational structure is consistent with the concept that bone cells are in intimate communication with each other and that osteoblasts receive the majority of local and systemic signals and then transmit them to other cells in bone. Conversely, strain-generated signals such as streaming potentials could be perceived by osteocytes, and their regulatory information passed on to the osteoblasts.

Depending on its functional activity, the osteoblast's structure or shape may change. The tall plump osteoblasts that line bone surfaces are metabolically active and dedicated to the process of bone matrix (osteoid) synthesis. Among the matrix ele-

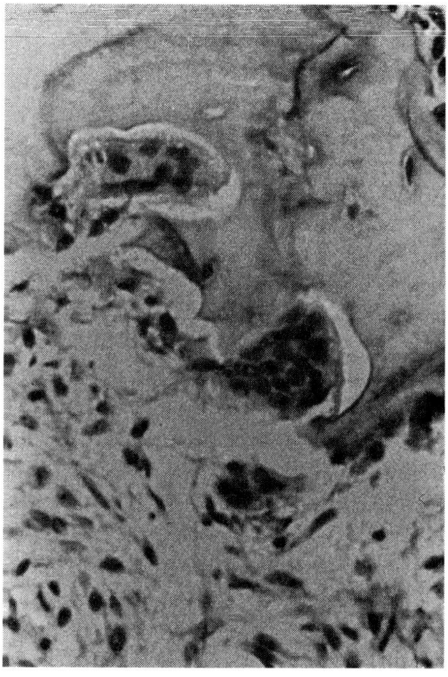

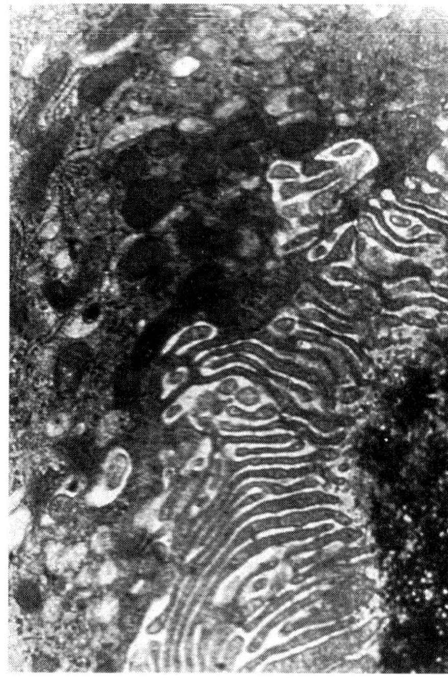

Figure 8
Light and electron photomicrographs of osteoclasts.

ments produced by osteoblasts are structural proteins, such as type I collagen; a variety of noncollagenous proteins, including osteocalcin and osteopontin, osteonectin, and proteoglycans (Table 1); and regulatory factors, such as cytokines, growth factors, and prostaglandins. On other bone surfaces, where bone is not being actively formed, the osteoblasts appear elongated and flat and are relatively quiescent metabolically. These osteoblasts are often called resting bone lining cells. Evidence suggests that these osteoblasts may be producing enzymes and enzyme-regulating proteins such as collagenase, collagenase inhibitor, and plasminogen activator, which are involved in the process of bone matrix degradation. In addition to the above synthetic products, osteoblasts produce neutral proteases, alkaline phosphatase, and other enzymes that degrade the extracellular matrix and prepare it for calcification. The lining osteoblasts are in communication with osteocytes through cell processes within the canaliculi that form gap junctions. Rapid fluxes of bone calcium across these junctions may be involved in the transmission of information between osteoblasts on the bone surface as well as to osteocytes within the structure of bone itself.

The specific receptor-effector interactions in osteoblasts are best illustrated by responses to PTH, prostaglandins, 1,25-dihydroxyvitamin D, and glucocorticoids. PTH and prostaglandins bind to cell surface-associated receptors and then trigger intracellular second messenger pathways to bring about the cellular response. These mechanisms include both the adenylate cyclase/cyclic adenosine monophosphate (cAMP) pathway and the phosphoinositol-calcium pathway. On the other hand, 1,25-dihydroxyvitamin D and glucocorticoids diffuse across the membrane and bind to cytosolic receptors, which then translocate to the nucleus of the cell and interact with nuclear DNA. Recent evidence suggests that osteoblasts also contain receptors for estrogen, and that these function like other steroid hormone receptors. How these estrogen receptors and the resultant osteoblastic responses function to regulate osteoclastic bone resorption remains unknown, although it is recognized that the actions of osteoblasts and osteoclasts are coupled.

Of the nonhormonal responses observed in bone, bioelectricity is among the most widely studied. Stress-generated electrical potentials experienced by bone are of two types: piezoelectric and

Table 1
The who's who of matrix proteins*

Protein*	Location**
Phosphorylated glycoproteins	
Bone sialoprotein I*/osteopontin/secreted sialophosphoprotein/bone phosphoprotein/2ar	B,C,N
Bone sialoprotein II*/bone sialoprotein/secreted sialoprotein II	B
Osteonectin/culture heat shock protein/SPARC	B,N
BAG-75*	B
Bone phosphoprotein	B
Phosphorylated proteins	
Dentin phosphophoryn/dentin phosphoprotein 24 kd-phosphoprotein/N-propeptide type I collagen	B
Proteins with γ-carboxyglutamic acid	
Osteocalcin/bone Gla protein/BGP	B
Matrix Gla protein*	B,C
Proteins with glycosaminoglycan side chains	
Cartilage proteoglycan (monomer & aggregate)	C
Bone proteoglycan I/biglycan/HAPG1	B,C,N
Bone proteoglycan II/decorin/HAPG2	B,C,N
Proteins derived from procollagen	
Chondrocalcin	C
24 kd bone phosphoprotein	B
Others	
Thrombospondin	B,C,N
SCAB 1-3	B,?

* Cell-binding proteins. Proteins separated by slashes (/) have extensive homology, or are identical proteins given different names by different researchers.
** B, found in bone and/or synthesized by osteoblasts; C, found in cartilage and/or synthesized by chondrocytes; N, found in other nonmineralizing tissues and synthesized by cells other than osteoblasts and chondrocytes; ?, unknown.
(Reproduced with permission from Boskey AL: Mineral matrix interactions in bone and cartilage. *Clin Orthop* 1992;281:244-274).

streaming potentials. In piezoelectric materials, the potentials are produced by strain in the organic components of the material; that is, collagens and proteoglycans, and do not depend on tissue viability. Streaming potentials result from electrolyte fluid flow produced by deformation of the material. In essence, these phenomena represent the direct conversion of mechanical energy to electrical energy using bone as the medium.

Cellular function generates bioelectric effects that are independent of stress. The ability of bone to act as a tissue that develops, produces, and transmits electrical signals depends on the function of its cells, matrix, and mineral phase. The role that these physiologic potentials play in the functional ability of bone to remodel is uncertain.

Osteoclasts at specific bone sites are activated only after disruption of the osteoid layer that covers the bone surfaces; an osteoblast-mediated effect. This exposure of the underlying mineralized matrix may be caused by the degradation of surface osteoid by collagenases elaborated by flat, elongated osteoblasts (resting bone lining cells), or by the contraction of osteoblasts in response to stimulation by PTH, 1,25-dihydroxyvitamin D, or prostaglandins of the E series. This contraction allows osteoclasts to gain access to the mineralized bone. What appears to be the degradation of the bone matrix also results in the activation of specific molecules buried within the bone matrix, for example, bone morphogenic proteins (BMP). These released signal molecules, which have mitogenic, differentiating, and chemoattracting properties, may be extremely important in the modulation of cellular events at specific regions in bone. Moreover, these molecules may be the key agents that regulate bone homeostasis by maintaining a coupling between bone formation and resorption. Other unreleased molecules in bone matrix may serve as anchoring molecules to which effector cells attach. Thus, as the bone is stimulated to resorb by a bone-resorbing hormone (PTH), it may release from its matrix a substance that stimulates bone formation—transforming growth factor beta (TGF-β) or BMP—thereby maintaining bone homeostasis. PTH mediates bone resorption by stimulation of PTH receptors on osteoblasts, which in turn mediate osteoclastic bone resorption; osteoclasts do not have PTH receptors.

As mentioned above, for an osteoclast to resorb bone, the osteoblast must first: (1) contract somewhat, so that the osteoclast can gain access to the bone surface, and (2) elaborate neutral proteases to degrade the thin layer of unmineralized osteoid covering the bone. Evidence suggests that osteoclasts must be exposed to a mineralized bone surface as well as to certain matrix components in order for them to become active.

Two intracellular areas of the osteoclast are important for its bone resorbing function. These are the clear zone and the ruffled border. The clear zone is that area of the osteoclast in which attachment of the cell to the bone surface takes place. Evidence suggests that attachment of the osteoclast to bone occurs through a receptor-mediated process (integrins). Once osteoclasts have attached to bone, the clear zone surrounds and seals off the area where bone is to be resorbed—much the same as a saucer placed upside-down on a table would seal off the area beneath it. This area of the bone is called the "subosteoclastic space." Bone resorption then takes place in this space in a concerted fashion in which intracellular carbonic anhydrase degrades carbonic acid to produce free protons (hydrogen ions). These protons are released from the cell by means of a hydrogen ion-adenosine triphosphatase (ATPase) pump. Because this area of the bone has been isolated beneath the osteoclast, these protons accumulate until the pH of this microenvironment reaches a low enough level (approximately pH 4) to dissolve the mineral phase of the bone and promote the activity of the matrix-degrading osteoclastic hydrolytic enzymes. These matrix-degrading lysosomal enzymes, including cathepsin B and acid phosphatase, are then released across the ruffled border, a complex of plasma membrane infoldings, and are the actual agents that degrade the organic matrix and continue to dissociate the mineral phase. Evidence suggests that some of the free mineral crystals and matrix components are phagocytized back into the cell, where they are degraded.

Because the remodeling of bone is a very specific spatial process, resorption must occur under close local control, possibly through the facility of other cells in bone and bone marrow. Because the predominant bone-resorbing hormones, such as PTH, 1,25-dihydroxyvitamin D, and prostaglandin E, do not have receptors on osteoclasts, their action to increase bone resorption must be mediated through another cell, such as the osteoblast, which does have receptors for these hormones. Other cells may also participate in the bone resorption process. For example, mast cells release heparin, an agent that enhances collagenase activity and may have a resorptive effect on bone matrix. Monocytes and lymphocytes may modulate bone remodeling through the release of local regulatory cytokines. At present, the specific cell and associated factors that regulate bone resorption are under active investigation.

Bone Matrix Composition

Bone is a composite material, consisting of mineral, proteins, water, cells, and other macromolecules (lipids, sugars, etc). Although bone cells are the principal regulators of bone metabolism, bone matrix and mineral participate in the control of cell-mediated processes. Therefore, the inorganic and organic components of bone have both structural and regulatory properties.

The composition of bone differs depending on site, animal age, dietary history, and the presence of disease. In general, however, the mineral or inorganic phase accounts for 60% to 70% of the tissue, water accounts for 5% to 8%, and the organic matrix makes up the remainder. Approximately 90% of the organic matrix is collagen; 5%, noncollagenous proteins. The mineral phase is an analogue of the naturally occurring mineral hydroxyapatite, $Ca_{10}(PO_4)_6(OH)_2$ (Fig. 9). The apatite crystals are small and contain abundant impurities (for example, carbonate, sodium, citrate), some of which reflect dietary history (for example, fluoride, strontium).

Inorganic Phase

The inorganic component of bone is principally composed of a calcium phosphate mineral analogous to crystalline calcium hydroxyapatite (Fig. 9). This apatite is present as a plate-like crystal, which is 20 to 80 nm long and 2 to 5 nm thick. The small amounts of impurities in hydroxyapatite, such as carbonate, which can replace the phosphate groups, or chloride and fluoride, which can replace the hydroxyl groups, may alter certain physical properties of the crystal, such as solubility. These altered properties may impart important biologic effects that are critical to normal function. Newly formed woven bone, which is not as well mineralized as mature lamellar bone, contains particles with a smaller average crystal size.

Organic Phase

The organic phase of the extracellular matrix of bone plays a wide variety of roles, determining the structure and the mechanical and biochemical properties of the bone. Approximately 90% of the organic matrix of bone is type I collagen; the remainder consists of noncollagenous matrix proteins, minor collagen types, lipids, and other macromolecules. Growth factors and cytokines, bone inductive proteins, and the more abundant matrix proteins such as osteonectin, osteopontin, bone sialoprotein, osteocalcin, bone proteoglycans, and other phosphoproteins and proteolipids make small contributions to the overall volume of bone and major contributions to its biologic function (Table 1).

Collagen is a ubiquitous protein of extremely low solubility, which consists of three polypeptide chains composed of approximately 1,000 amino acids each. It is the major structural component of the bone matrix. Bone collagen is constructed in the form of a triple helix of two identical α1(I) chains and one unique α2 chain stabilized by hydrogen bonding between hydroxyproline and other charged residues. This produces a fairly rigid linear molecule 300 nm long. Each molecule is aligned with the next in a parallel fashion in a quarter-staggered array to produce a collagen fibril (Fig. 10). The collagen fibrils are then grouped in bundles to form the collagen fiber (Fig. 11). Within the collagen fibril, gaps, called "hole zones," exist between the ends of the molecules. In addition, "pores" exist between the sides of parallel molecules. Noncollagenous proteins or mineral deposits can be found within these spaces (holes and pores). Mineralization of the matrix is thought to commence in the hole zones.

Collagen synthesis is completed within the cell, and processing continues in the extracellular ma-

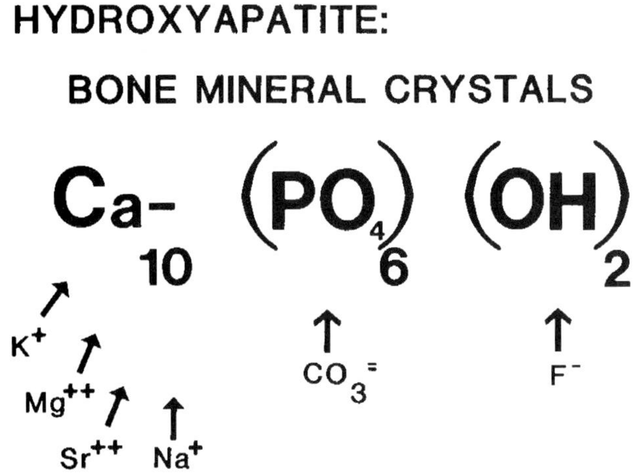

HYDROXYAPATITE:

BONE MINERAL CRYSTALS

$$Ca_{10}\,(PO_4)_6\,(OH)_2$$

K^+ → Ca; Mg^{++} → Ca; Sr^{++} → Ca; Na^+ → Ca

$CO_3^{=}$ → PO_4

F^- → OH

Figure 9
Hydroxyapatite crystals.

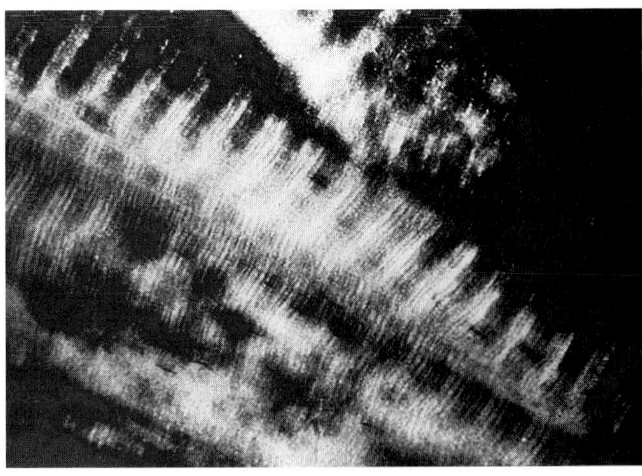

Figure 10
Electron photomicrograph of bone collagen.

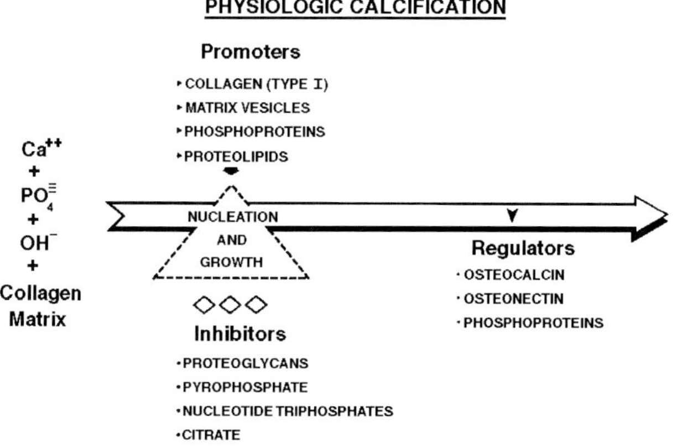

Figure 11
Scheme for initial calcification.

trix, and involves both posttranslational and postsecretory processing. In the cell, almost half of the proline and 15% to 20% of the lysine residues are hydroxylated on the individual α chains, and these hydroxylations are followed by the glycosylation of the hydroxylysine residues in an intracellular, posttranslational process. This step leads to the formation of the triple helical procollagen molecule, which is the secreted form. Once outside the cell, the terminal nontriple helical propeptides are enzymatically cleaved to form the collagen molecule. The collagen molecules are stabilized by cross-links formed between reactive aldehydes on different chains. The reactive aldehydes are formed by oxidative deamination of both lysine and hydroxylysine.

Several noncollagenous proteins have been described in Table 1. One of the more extensively studied noncollagenous proteins in bone is osteocalcin or bone γ-carboxyglutamic acid-containing protein (bone Gla protein). This is a small (5.8 kd) protein in which three glutamic acid residues are carboxylated as a result of the vitamin K-dependent posttranslational modification. The carboxylation of these residues converts this protein into a calcium and mineral binding protein. Osteocalcin accounts for 10% to 20% of the noncollagenous protein present in bone and is closely associated with the mineral phase. While the function of this bone-specific protein is not known, it is thought to play some role in attracting osteoclasts to sites of bone resorption. It may also regulate the rate of mineralization, or the final shape assumed by mineral crystals. The synthesis of osteocalcin is enhanced by 1,25-dihydroxyvitamin D and inhibited by PTH and corticosteroids. Osteocalcin is a synthetic product of osteoblasts, and the related dentin-forming cells, odontoblasts.

Animals treated with sodium warfarin (an agent that blocks the vitamin K-dependent carboxylation of glutamate residues in osteocalcin and other γ-carboxyglutamate containing proteins) have decreased amounts of carboxylated osteocalcin in their bones but few other significant changes in bone structure. Studies of patients who have been treated with sodium warfarin similarly show significant changes in osteocalcin biochemistry but no serious clinical effects. However, young animals treated with warfarin demonstrate premature epiphyseal closure, but no other long bone abnormalities. The appearance of warfarin embryopathy (nasal hypoplasia, stippled epiphyses, and distal extremity hypoplasia) in the offspring of women treated with warfarin during pregnancy suggests that osteocalcin, or more likely the γ-carboxylated matrix Gla protein, which is a component of both cartilage and bone, may play a role in bone development. It is interesting to note that a child with no history of pre- or postnatal exposure to warfarin was recently reported to have stippled epiphyses, a congenital deficiency of vitamin K-reducing enzymes, and defective posttranslational γ-carboxyl modification of osteocalcin. This suggests that the etiology of this disease may be related to the vitamin K-dependent synthesis of bone proteins.

Gamma carboxylated glutamic acid containing proteins (Gla proteins) such as osteocalcin have been shown to be elevated in the serum and urine of patients with Paget disease, primary hyperparathyroidism, renal osteodystrophy, and high turnover osteoporosis. Approximately 25% of urinary Gla proteins come from mineralized tissues. Most of the osteocalcin in bone is excreted in nonmetabolized form in the urine. Although osteocalcin has been touted as being potentially useful as a clinical marker in patients with osteoporosis, this application is limited because the presence of osteocalcin in the serum or urine could be caused either by extensive bone resorption or by increased bone formation. In fact, serum osteocalcin levels are believed to be indicative of bone formation. In conditions such as Paget disease, the extensive amount of newly formed woven bone with exposed mineral surfaces may serve as a "sink" for the deposition of circulating osteocalcin. This deposition would serve to lower the serum level of osteocalcin, masking both the bone resorptive and bone formative aspects of Paget disease, which would otherwise be reflected in high serum levels of osteocalcin. Recently, the presence of bone specific collagen cross-links has been shown to be a more sensitive marker of remodeling.

Other noncollagenous proteins found in bone may also be important in relation to their calcium and mineral binding properties. Osteonectin (SPARC), a 32-kd protein secreted by both osteoblasts and platelets, has been shown to bind both denatured collagen and hydroxyapatite. Although not entirely known, its role may be to regulate calcium concentrations or to potentiate nucleation or stabilization of calcium phosphate or the organization of mineral within the matrix framework. Phosphorylated sialoproteins, small proteoglycans, and other phosphoproteins synthesized by osteoblasts also play a role in matrix organization. Many of the phosphoproteins are believed to be localized in the "hole zones" of collagen fibrils. Their phosphate groups attract calcium to the area and may be responsible for the nucleation phenomena during the initial stages of mineralization.

Several of the bone matrix proteins (for example, osteopontin, bone sialoprotein, bone acidic glycoprotein, thrombospondin, and fibronectin) contain arginine-glycine-aspartic acid (RGD) sequences. Such sequences, characteristic of cell binding proteins, are recognized by a family of cell-membrane proteins known as integrins. The integrins span the cell membrane and provide a link between the extracellular matrix and the cytoskeleton of the cell. Integrins on osteoblasts, osteoclasts, and fibroblasts provide means for anchoring these cells to the extracellular matrix.

Present in very small amounts in the bone matrix are growth factors and cytokines such as transforming growth factor-beta (TGF-β), insulin-like growth factor (IGF), the interleukins (IL-1, IL-6), and bone morphogenic proteins (BMP1-6). These proteins bind to both the bone mineral and matrix, and are released during the process of osteoclastic bone resorption. Such proteins have important effects regulating bone cell differentiation, activation, growth, and turnover. It is likely that these growth factors serve as the coupling factors that link the processes of bone formation and bone remodeling. Growth factor and hormone interaction with cell receptors regulate the flux of calcium ions into and out of the cell, an event that may be key in controlling matrix mineralization.

Mineralization of the organic matrix of bone is a complicated process that is not fully understood. Osteoblasts regulate the concentrations of calcium ions in the matrix through the release of calcium from intercellular compartments. Osteoblasts also secrete the macromolecules which, as indicated above, determine the site and rate of initial calcification.

Bone Mineralization

Mineralization of skeletal tissues can be considered as having two distinct phases: (1) formation of the initial mineral deposit (initiation); and (2) proliferation or accretion of additional mineral crystals on the initial mineral deposits (growth). Of the total body mineral, only a small fraction represents the initial deposit. The bulk of the mineral comes from growth of the initial crystalline material.

Initiation of mineralization requires a combination of events, including increases in the local concentration of precipitating ions, formation or exposure of mineral nucleators, and removal or modification of mineralization inhibitors. The vast majority of mineral in the body is an analogue of the naturally occurring mineral, hydroxyapatite ($Ca_{10}(PO_4)_6(OH)_2$), shown in Figure 9. The apatite crystals in bone are extremely small (20 to 80 nm in the largest dimension) and contain numerous impurities that are adsorbed onto the surface or incorporated within the crystal. The increased solubility of bone mineral crystals, relative to geologic mineral or crystals in tooth enamel, results from both crystal size and impurities. The nature of the first mineral crystals deposited in bone and the site at which they are deposited is still unknown. Extracellular matrix vesicles, located at a distance from the collagen fibrils, have been identified as the site of initial mineral deposition in young, calcifying cartilage and in young bone; however, the bulk of the mineral in bone as well as much of the initial mineral is closely associated with collagen.

More energy is required to form the initial mineral crystals than is required to add ions or ion clusters to already existing crystals. Secondary nucleation, the growth of small crystallites in a branching manner from the surface of other small crystals, also requires less energy than does de novo initiation. To circumvent the large energy required of initial hydroxyapatite formation, a less stable (or metastable) precursor phase may form first, and later either be converted directly to hydroxyapatite or serve as a heterogenous nucleator of hydroxyapatite. A heterogenous apatite nucleator is a foreign material that has one or more surfaces on which apatite crystals can grow. Once primary nucleation has occurred, there is an early rapid increase in size from "crystal nuclei" to the first solid phase particles initially observed by electron microscopy. This process is termed "crystal growth." Operationally, the two processes, primary nucleation and crystal growth, have been defined as multiplication.

Of the connective tissue collagens, only type I (bone, tendon, skin) collagen can support hydroxyapatite deposition in vitro (Fig. 10). It has been shown that mineralized type I collagen contains cross-links that are chemically different from those in nonmineralized osteoid. Such collagen cross-linking may also affect the distribution of mineral within the collagen. What causes the orientation of matrix fibrils in lamellae is unknown; however, the pattern obviously forms prior to mineralization.

Some noncollagenous proteins, such as the phosphoproteins and osteonectin-collagen complexes, seem to promote collagen mineralization in vitro. In addition, certain proteolipids and calcium acidic phospholipid phosphate complexes also seem to promote hydroxyapatite deposition in vitro. Extracellular matrix vesicles may facilitate calcification by (1) concentrating ions; (2) providing a protective environment free of mineralization inhibitors; or (3) providing enzymes involved in matrix modification. Table 1 shows the noncollagenous proteins found to modulate bone mineralization.

Figure 11 shows that initial mineral deposition may be promoted both by the formation or exposure of nucleators and by the removal or modification of inhibitors. In vitro proteoglycans extracted from both calcifying and noncalcifying cartilage inhibit hydroxyapatite growth. Initial mineralization of collagen is still being investigated intensely.

After deposition of initial calcium phosphate crystals into collagen (mineral nucleation of osteoid), more and more hydroxyapatite must be added to give bone its rigidity. Although some of the new mineral added to osteoid is deposited by initial nucleation, most of the additional mineral is acquired by secondary nucleation, in which new crystals of apatite are deposited on nuclei of existing hydroxyapatite, and/or by crystal growth of hydroxyapatite already contained within the holes and pores of the collagen (Fig. 12). This accretion of new mineral continues until bone is fully mineralized; however, even fully mineralized mature bone is only 70% mineral, and the cells are always separated from the mineral by a thin layer of osteoid. Certain matrix proteins are believed to be involved both in limiting the size to which crystals grow and in preventing mineral deposition in certain areas.

In summary, from the physical chemical standpoint, mineral accretion in tissues arises by (1) primary or heterogenous nucleation; (2) crystal growth; and (3) secondary nucleation induced by previously formed crystals.

The increase in the number of mineral phase particles in the collagen fibrils, which accompanies mineral accretion, can, of course, occur in either the holes or the pores (Fig. 10). Electron microscope studies reveal that from the spatial point of view, mineralization proceeds as a discontinuous process. Discrete, physically separated loci within the osteoid fibrils become impregnated with mineral particles about the same time, forming a number of mineralization sites. It thus appears that initial mineralization takes place simultaneously at different locations within the collagen fibrils. Electron microscopy indicates that as crystal growth and secondary nucleation continue, the discrete growth areas enlarge and eventually coalesce. An understanding of how mineral accretion in bone as a whole proceeds, once nucleation begins in any one compartment, is integral to discussions of the influence of various metabolic and nutritional diseases on bone mineralization.

Bone Remodeling

Bone growth begins in utero and continues throughout adolescence until skeletal maturity. Long bones grow by two mechanisms. They grow in

MINERAL ACCRETION: ***BIOLOGICAL CONSIDERATIONS***
HETEROGENEITY WITHIN A COLLAGEN FIBRIL

PROGRESSIVELY INCREASING MINERAL MASS DUE TO:

1. INCREASED NUMBER OF NEW MINERAL PHASE PARTICLES (NUCLEATION)
   a. HETEROGENEOUS NUCLEATION BY MATRIX IN COLLAGEN HOLES (? PORES)
   b. 2° CRYSTAL INDUCED NUCLEATION IN HOLES AND PORES
2. INITIAL GROWTH OF PARTICLES TO ~ 400Å x 15–30Å x 50–75Å

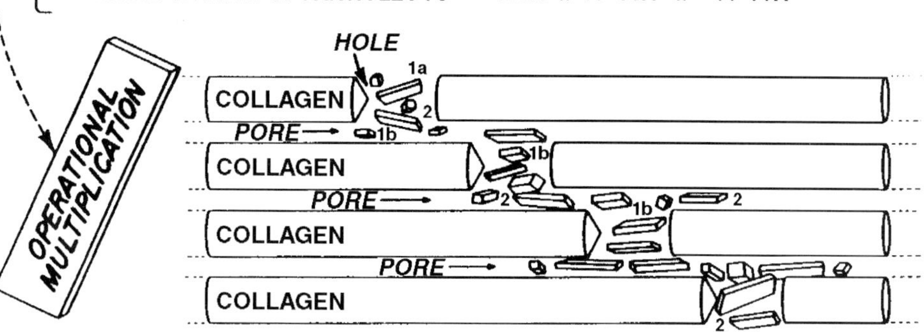

Figure 12
Diagram showing mineral accretion.

length by a process of endochondral ossification, and in width by a process of intramembranous or subperiosteal new bone formation. Even following skeletal maturity, bone continues to remodel throughout life and adapt its material properties to the mechanical demands placed on it. The cellular and molecular mechanisms by which bone responds to mechanical stress (Wolff's Law) are still poorly understood. These mechanisms are under intense investigation and may, in time, play an important role in the prevention and treatment of musculoskeletal disease. Investigation of the effects of biomechanics on bone remodeling is currently under way. See the chapter on biomechanics for a more detailed discussion of this subject.

Cortical bone constitutes approximately 80% of the skeletal mass, and trabecular bone approximately 20%. Bone surfaces may be undergoing formation or resorption, or they may be inactive. These processes occur throughout life in both cortical and trabecular bone. Bone remodeling is a surface phenomenon, and it occurs on periosteal, endosteal, haversian canal, and trabecular surfaces. The rate of cortical bone remodeling, which may be as high as 50% per year in the midshaft of the femur during the first two years of life, eventually declines to a rate of 2% to 5% per year in the elderly. Rates of remodeling in trabecular bone are proportionately higher throughout life and may normally be five to ten times higher than cortical bone remodeling rates in the adult (Fig. 13).

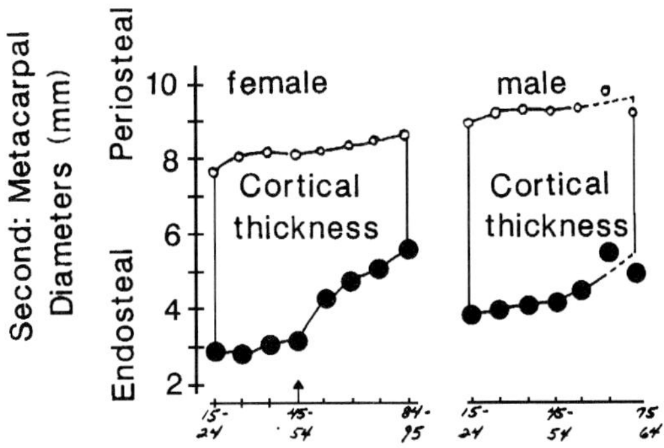

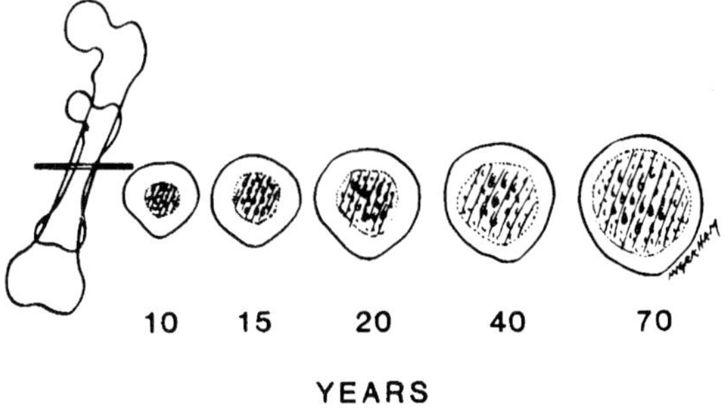

Figure 13
Effects of age on metacarpal cortex and femoral diaphysis.

Both cortical and trabecular bone are constantly remodeled by a specific cycle of cellular activity. Initially, bone is resorbed by osteoclasts both in the cortex and on the trabeculae (Fig. 14, 1). Bone formation by means of osteoblastic activity occurs on the site of the old resorbed bone (Fig. 14, 2). The osteoblasts themselves become incorporated into bone as osteocytes (Fig. 14, 3). Flattened cells line the surfaces of bone and probably have a function similar to that of osteocytes. Under normal circumstances, the remodeling process of resorption followed by formation is closely coupled and results in no net change in bone mass. A bone modeling unit (BMU) consists of a group of all the linked cells that participate in remodeling a certain area of bone through a sequence of cell activity consisting of activation, resorption, and formation. It was originally thought that all cells in a BMU originate from a single cell line. Recent work reveals that osteoclasts are derived from the monocyte macrophage cell line of bone marrow. The origin of the osteoblast is not well understood, but it may arise from a mesenchymal precursor or perivascular cell.

The dynamics of bone remodeling are illustrated in Figure 15. The left hand microradiograph shows a thin section of cortical bone after tetracycline double labeling. Tetracycline is incorporated at sites of active mineralization of the bone matrix (concentric circles); by measuring time and distance between deposits, mineralization rates in bone remodeling can be assessed. The peripheral darker areas represent quiescent areas of the osteon. In the right hand microradiograph, the most recently formed bone, which surrounds the haversian canal, is least mineralized and appears dark. The oldest bone, which is the most highly mineralized, but quiescent from the standpoint of remodeling, appears quite light. This figure demonstrates the heterogeneity of adjacent bone caused by age and the continual internal remodeling of cortical bone.

Cortical bone remodeling proceeds via cutting cones (Fig. 16) and is similar to processes in other hard biologic tissues. Cutting cones, or sheets of osteoclasts, bore holes through the hard bone, leaving tunnels that appear in a cross section as cavities. The head of the cutting cone consists of osteoclasts that resorb the bone. Closely following the osteoclast front is a capillary loop and a population of osteoblasts that actively lay down osteoid to refill the resorption cavity. By the end of the process, a new osteon has been formed, which is the substance of the cortical bone.

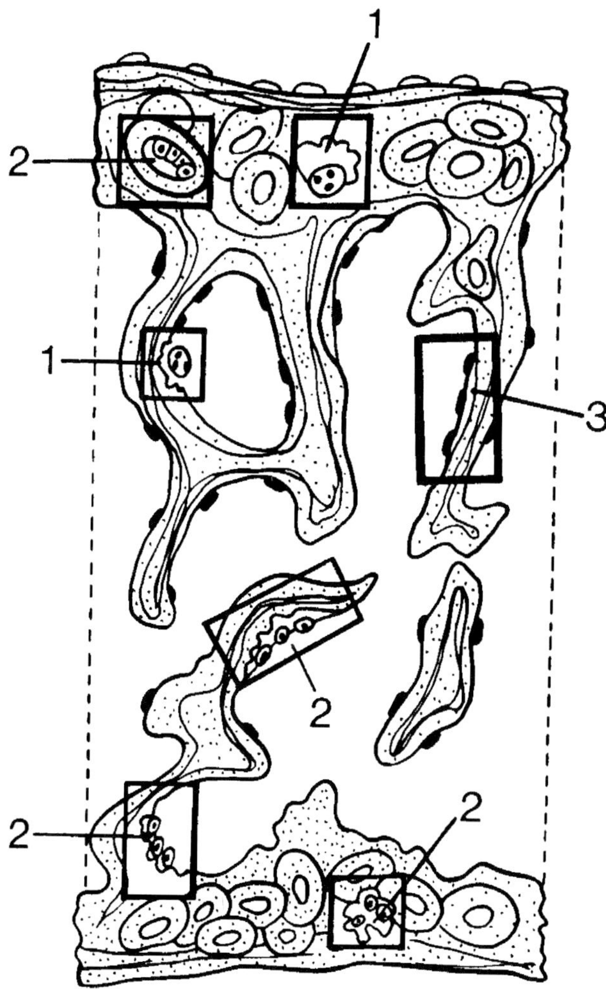

Figure 14
Schematic drawing showing principles of bone remodeling.

Bone Blood Flow

Anatomic Features

Bone has three separate but interactive circulatory systems, which are described using the long bone as a model. The nutrient supply originates from a major artery of the systemic circulation and enters the diaphysis through a foramen. The number of nutrient vessels differs for each long bone. Once in the medullary space, each nutrient vessel branches into ascending and descending medullary arteries and further subdivides into arterioles, which directly penetrate the endosteal surface and supply the diaphyseal regions. The metaphyseal complex is the second system that arises from the periarticular plexus (that is, the geniculate arteries); it penetrates the thin bone cortices to supply the metaphyseal regions. These vessels anastomose with the medullary arteries and with the epiphyseal system, of similar nature and origin, after closure of the growth plate. Finally, the periosteal capillaries supply the outer layers of cortical bone where there are muscular attachments. Brookes considers the periosteal capillary system where muscular attachments do not exist to be purely efferent from the cortex. Most researchers feel that the periosteal capillaries supply the outer 15% to 20% of the cortex (periosteal surface) even in the absence of muscular attachments. These three systems are interconnected; the watershed interconnections play a key role when the bone is injured. When the medullary system is taken away, for example, the periosteal system becomes dominant in the revascularization of the diaphyseal cortex.

The medullary arteries are thick walled near their origin from the nutrient system. The walls thin down to two flattened layers of cells as the artery moves toward the metaphysis. All along the endosteal surface, side branches exit into the haversian system capillaries, which ultimately return to venules in the medullary canal, which, in turn, drain into the central venous sinus and out the nutrient vein. The density of the venules is greater in the metaphyses and in areas where the hematopoietic marrow is active.

Clinical Relevance

Many clinical problems involving the musculoskeletal system have as their basis a disturbance of bone microcirculation. Osteomyelitis involves nonviable cortical or cancellous bone as the focus for bacterial adherence. Posttraumatic osteonecrosis involves an acute disruption of the arterial blood supply. Revascularization of these regions from metaphyseal sources, when the epiphyseal arteries cannot rapidly be recanalized, produces trabecular weakening and microfracture. Prosthetic joint devices generally devitalize endosteal surfaces; external fixation devices and bone plates affect both the endosteal supply (drilling into the medullary cavity) and the periosteal surface. The revascularization of these affected areas can produce pathologic bone resorption. Finally, fracture of bone, especially if it is a result of high-energy trauma, produces ischemic fragments that must be revitalized and are susceptible to infection. These topics are discussed in greater detail in future chapters.

Techniques for Study

Current knowledge of the vascular anatomy of bone is based on angiographic studies. Large vessel structure is studied using barium perfusate and standard radiographs; the microcirculation is studied using thin-section (200 to 400 mm), high-resolution microradiographs. By changing the character of the perfusate, the distal vascular tree can be defined. Specimens perfused with methylsalicylate

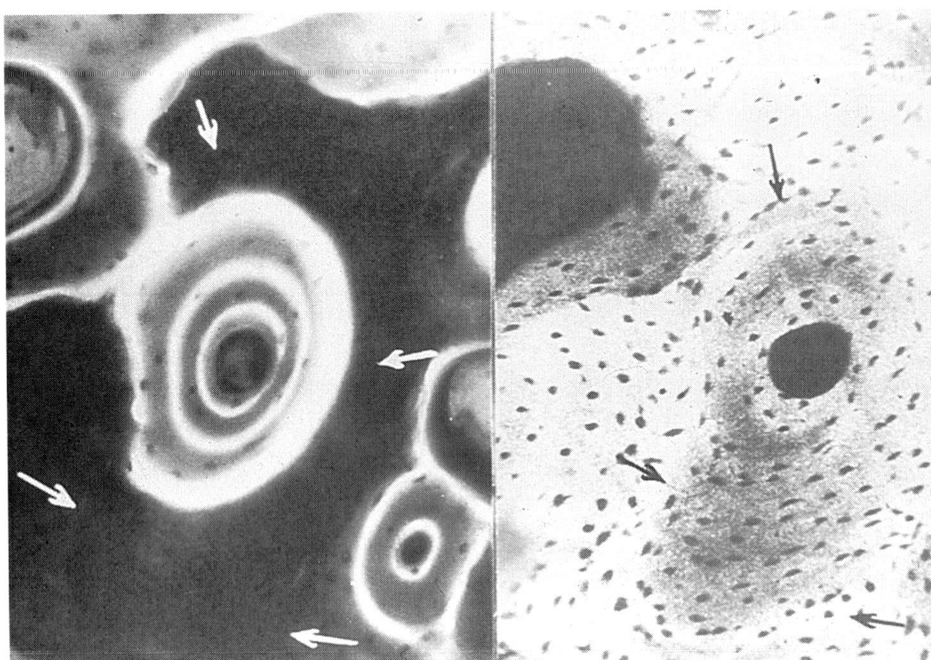

Figure 15
Microradiographs showing dynamics of bone remodeling.

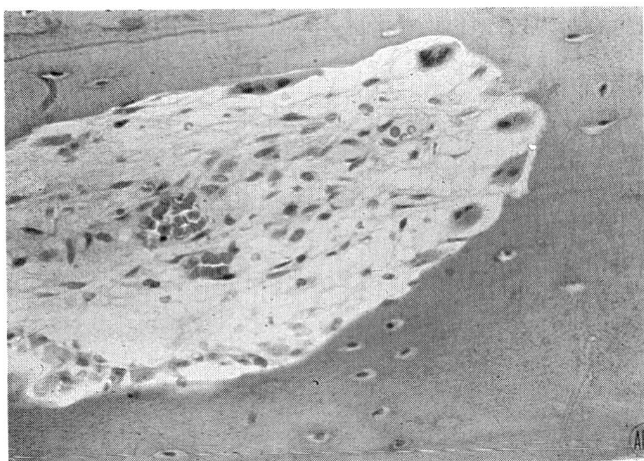

Figure 16
Photomicrograph showing cutting cones' mechanism.

or glycerin (Spalteholtz method) reveal 3-D structure. These techniques provide no information on the function of the microcirculation.

The Fick indicator dilution technique involves injecting bone-seeking isotopes such as those of strontium and measuring the relative counts in bone effluent referable to segments of bone removed. This method has inherent inaccuracies because the isotope is not extracted completely on the first pass through the bone.

Hydrogen washout involves measuring the concentration of hydrogen ion with a platinum electrode; the hydrogen is breathed and the electrode must be placed into the bone. The concentration of the hydrogen at the electrode is proportional to the blood flow in the region. Xenon washout uses the same basic principles with locally injected xenon gas. These methods are problematic because of the need to insert electrodes into the region of interest, which affects the local microcirculation.

Use of radiolabeled microspheres is generally accepted to be the most accurate method for the experimental measurement of bone blood flow. Fifteen-micrometer spheres are labeled with one of six isotopes; this size is optimum for distal arteriolar trapping. The spheres are injected into the central arterial circulation, and peripheral arterial sampling is preferred. After flushing with heparin-saline, the "reference organ" (peripheral arterial) sampling is stopped. Because of the limited number of isotopes, only six measurements can be obtained per animal. At sacrifice, the bone area of interest and blood extracted are counted, and the blood flow is calculated using standard equations. Because it requires removal of bone, the method is not appropriate for clinical studies.

Laser Doppler flowmetry assesses the number and velocity of moving blood cells under the probe, which must contact the region of interest. This method assesses only small areas of bone at depths of 2.9 mm for cortical bone and 3.5 mm for cancellous bone. The values, provided in milliVolts (mV), are proportional to flow. This method is applicable to the clinical setting but multiple measurements must be made.

Finally, vital microscopy enables direct study of the microcirculation within titanium hollow screws. Using pulsed labels and video cameras, quantitative data can be generated.

Assessment of bone blood flow with these methods has clarified several factors. There is great heterogeneity of flow within cortical and cancellous bone. Moreover, arteriovenous shunts within bone can produce a source of error for some of the methods of measurement. Values are generally reported as milliliters per minute per gram of tissue (ml/min/g of bone) and vary from 1.6 to 7.0 ml/min/g in cortical bone and 10.0 to 30.0 ml/min/g in cancellous bone. Vasomotion, or rhythmic dilation and contraction of precapillary beds, has been identified in bone. Bone has the ability to autoregulate flow. Arterial inflow stops when systemic arterial blood pressure falls below 80 mm Hg and the arterial oxygen tension falls below 75 mm Hg. Finally, within different regions of the bone hematocrit varies from 50% to 75% of the arterial hematocrit. The lowest hematocrits are found in regions with the highest perfusion rates.

Armed with these physiologic factors and the knowledge of how surgical manipulation influences bone flood flow, researchers can make progress in the development of new surgical techniques.

Biomechanics of Bone

Bone is the primary structural element of the human body. It serves to protect vital internal organs and provides a framework that allows skeletal motions. Bone differs from engineering structural materials in that it is self repairing and can alter its properties and geometry in response to changes in mechanical demand. While the hypertrophy that occurs in skeletal muscle in response to heavy exercise or the atrophy that occurs in response to disuse is obvious, it is less apparent that bone is also remarkably responsive to mechanical demands. Bone density reductions are known to occur with aging, disuse, and certain metabolic conditions. Increased bone density occurs with heavy exercise and after treatment with certain therapeutic agents. Moreover, changes in bone geometry are observed during fracture healing, with aging, with exercise, and after certain operative procedures. Understanding these phenomena, which appear to be adaptive, stress-related events, has been a central focus of bone physiology and biomechanics for over a century.

Many of these adaptive phenomena appear to be directed toward restoring and maintaining the structural integrity of the skeleton despite changes in the mechanical environment, a type of biomechanical homeostasis. Fracture healing and increased levels of bone density with severe exercise are obvious examples. Less obvious is the possibility that the cross-sectional geometry of long bones might change with aging in order to compensate for age-related reductions in bone density and mechanical properties. Epidemiologic evidence indicates that the reductions in bone density and strength known to occur in cortical bone with aging are not accompanied by dramatic increases in the incidence of shaft fractures among the elderly, suggesting that compensatory mechanisms are at work. However, such homeostatic, compensatory mechanisms do not appear to be sufficient to protect the aging skeleton against fracture at other skeletal sites such as the hip, spine, and distal radius.

In the United States alone, more than 250,000 hip fractures and 500,000 vertebral fractures occur each year among persons over age 45. As a result, there is an urgent need to improve our understanding of fracture etiology, to identify patients most at risk, and to develop cost-effective interventions aimed at fracture prevention. To do so, however, requires an understanding of such mechanical factors as the relative importance of bone loss and trauma in fracture etiology, the role of trabecular versus cortical bone in the strength of the hip and spine, the importance of fatigue damage accumulation in the etiology of spontaneous fractures, and the relationships between fracture risk and the different load regimes that occur both during the activities of daily living and in response to traumatic events, such as a fall from standing height.

To address these issues and to provide an objective basis for a number of common clinical decisions, current knowledge on the mechanical behavior of bone is summarized here. The review is divided into three main sections: (1) Bone tissue material properties; (2) whole bone structural properties; and (3) in vivo fracture prediction. By way of introduction, this text distinguishes between the behavior of bone tissue at the material level and the behavior of a whole bone at the structural level.

Material and Structural Behavior

The material behavior of bone describes how bone tissue behaves mechanically, regardless of where that tissue is located in any particular whole bone. To determine this fundamental material behavior, mechanical tests are performed on standardized specimens under controlled mechanical and environmental conditions. These tests are designed to eliminate any behavior associated with specimen geometry. The single requirement for the validity of the data obtained is that they be used only for bone with the same microstructure and in the same environment as the test specimens.

The simple equation for compression of a cylinder (Fig. 17, *top*) is:

$$F = (AE/l_o)\Delta l \qquad \textbf{(Eq. 1)}$$

where F is the force, Δl is the elongation of the cylinder, l_o is the original length, A is the cross-sectional area, and E is Young's modulus.

A plot of force against deformation (Fig. 17, *bottom left*) describes the structural behavior of the cylinder under axial loading. The slope of the force deformation plot, the axial structural stiffness, is directly proportional to both the cross-sectional area and the Young's modulus (quantity E), and is inversely proportional to the length. Thus, in a test of two cylinders made from the same material (E constant), and of equal lengths (l constant) but with different cross-sectional areas (A different), the slopes of the force-deformation curves, and thus the structural stiffnesses, would be different for the two cylinders. Similarly, two bones of equivalent tissue properties (same E), but with different geometries, will display different structural stiffnesses. Conversely, because whole bones have different cross-sectional areas and lengths, it is not possible to use force deformation plots of whole bones to compare the material behavior of the bone tissue within the bones.

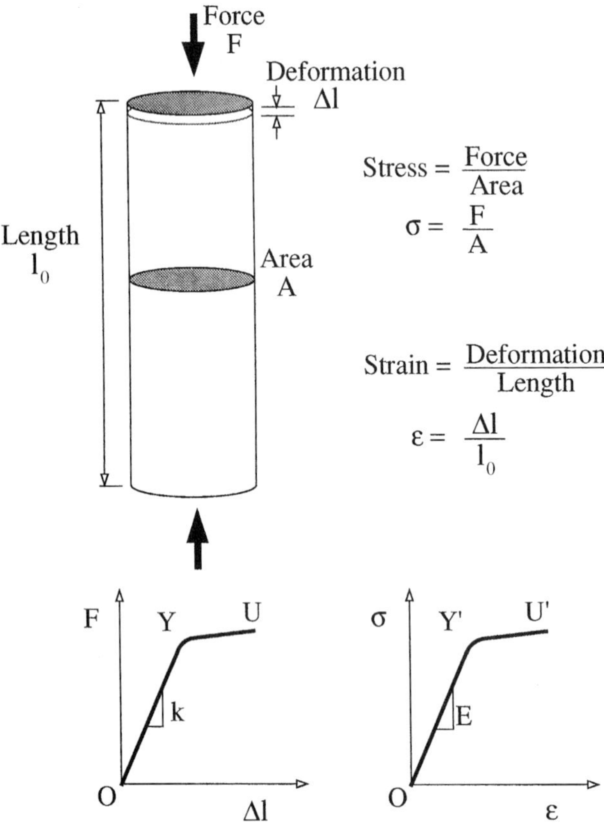

Figure 17
Top, Cylindrical specimen used in uniaxial compression tests of human bone. Stress and strain are calculated from the force, deformation, and dimensions of the specimen. **Bottom left,** The force-deformation plot describes the structural behavior of the specimen. The linear region (also known as the elastic region) is from O to Y. At Y, "yielding" occurs, with internal rearrangement of the structure, often involving damage to the material. In the region Y-U (also known as the postyield region), nonelastic deformation occurs until finally, at U, fracture occurs. **Bottom right,** The stress-strain plot describes the material behavior of the tissue which makes up the specimen. The elastic behavior occurs up to Y′, and the postyield behavior occurs after Y′. The yield strength is at Y′ and the ultimate strength is at U′ where fracture occurs. The Young's modulus E is the slope of the linear region of this plot. (Reproduced with permission from Keaveny TM, Hayes WC: Mechanical properties of cortical and trabecular bone, in Hall BK (ed): *Bone.* Boca Raton, FL, CRC Press, vol 7, pp 285–344.)

To eliminate these geometric effects, force is divided by cross-sectional area, F/A, and elongation is divided by original length, $\Delta l/l_o$, producing the geometrically normalized measures of force and elongation, known as stress s and strain e, respectively. Thus, the force deformation plot (Fig. 17, *bottom left*) is transformed to a stress-strain plot (Fig. 17, *bottom right*). Because the stress-strain relationship is independent of specimen geometry, this relationship describes only material behavior. The initial slope of the stress-strain plot is Young's modulus E. For example, the 316L stainless steel commonly used with bone plates has a Young's modulus of 200 GPa; polymethylmethacrylate bone cement (PMMA) has a Young's modulus of approximately 2.3 GPa; cortical bone and relatively stiff trabecular bone have Young's moduli of approximately 17 GPa and 1 GPa, respectively. These numbers indicate that the stainless steel is an order of magnitude stiffer than cortical bone.

A typical stress-strain curve for wet cortical bone obtained from the femoral diaphysis and tested in uniaxial tension is shown in Figure 18. This stress-strain curve can be broken into three regions: the initial linear region, the yield region, and the postyield region. The modulus is the slope of the linear region. In contrast, the strength properties are obtained from the yield and postyield regions. Yielding, the onset of permanent deformation, occurs at the junction of the linear and postyield regions. This junction defines the yield strength σ_y, which, for bone, represents the stress when microstructural damage starts to occur. Fracture occurs when the ultimate strength σ_{ult} is reached.

The most basic mechanical properties of bone are obtained from tests where standardized specimens are progressively loaded in one direction until fracture. Such tests (as shown schematically in Figure 17) are called uniaxial, monotonic tests. If the bone is stretched, the test is called a tension test; if the bone is compressed, the test is a compression

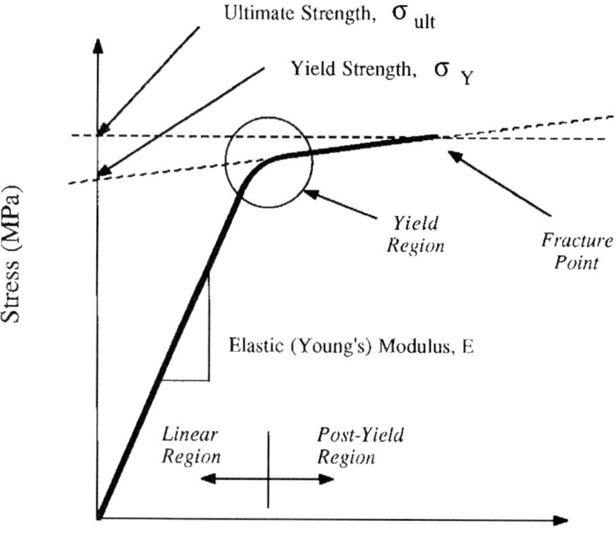

Figure 18
Typical stress-strain plot for cortical bone in tension, showing the linear, yield, and post-yield regions. Note that the yield and ultimate strengths are similar. (Reproduced with permission from Keaveny TM, Hayes WC: Mechanical properties of cortical and trabecular bone, in Hall BK (ed): *Bone.* Boca Raton, FL, CRC Press, 1993, vol 7, pp 285–344.)

test. If the bone is twisted, the test is a torsion test. For a torsion test, the bone specimen shown in Figure 17 would be twisted about its longitudinal axis (Fig. 19). By recording the values of torsion and angular twist of the bone, it is possible to plot a torsion twist diagram, exactly analogous to the force deformation plot for a compression or tension test. Similarly, if the torsion and angular twist were normalized by the appropriate geometric parameters, it would be possible to derive a stress-strain plot, where stress is called the shear stress, and strain is called the shear strain. The slope of the shear stress-strain plot is the shear modulus G. Thus, the shear modulus, in units of MPa, is directly analogous to the Young's modulus.

Other, more complicated loading configurations may sometimes be used where loads act simultaneously in different directions. These are called multiaxial tests. The strength properties of bone are different for multiaxial loading from those for the simpler, uniaxial loading cases. Furthermore, the material properties of bone under multiple low amplitude loading cycles (fatigue) are different from those for single, monotonic loads. Finally, all these properties depend on the rate of loading (its viscoelastic properties), the amount of time the loads act on the bone (creep), and the age of the bone tissue.

Review of the mechanical properties of materials (see the chapter on biomechanics) is suggested before continuing with examination of the material properties of bones.

Material Properties

Cortical and trabecular bone are distinguished from each other primarily by differences in porosity

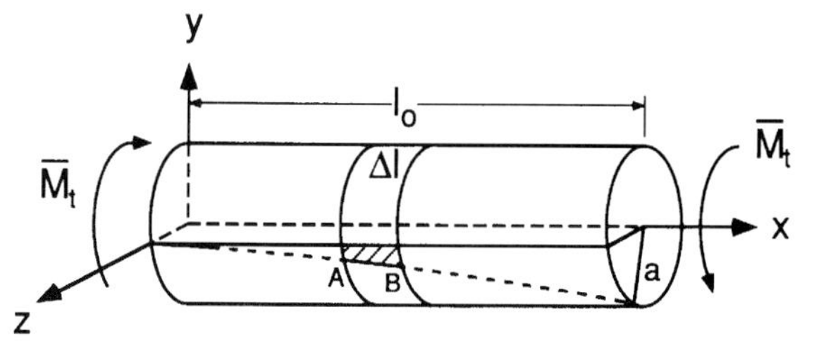

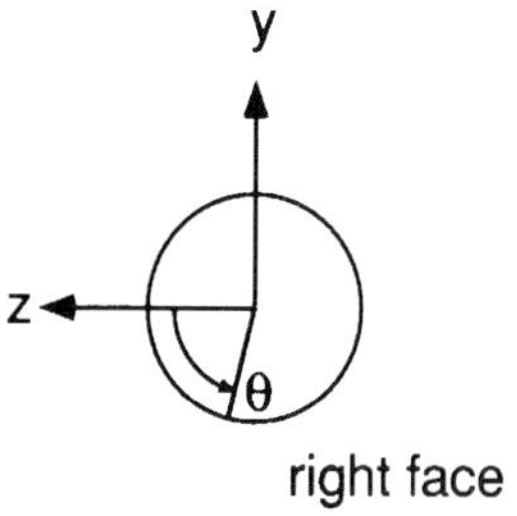

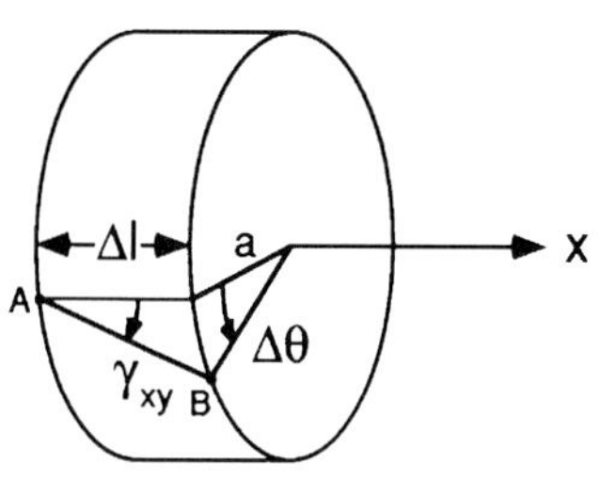

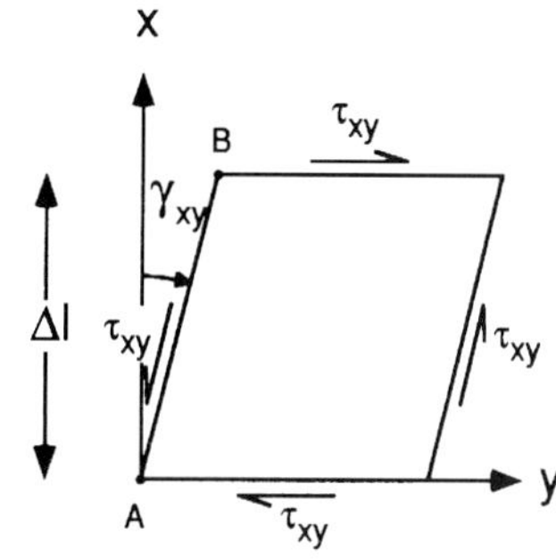

Figure 19
Top left, A circular shaft subject to twisting by a couple M_t at either end. The angle of twist θ between the right and left faces is given by $\theta = M_t l_o / G I_p$ **(top right). Bottom left,** The shear modulus G may be determined from the twist angle Δθ between two nearby surfaces separated by $G = (M_t \Delta l)/(\Delta\theta I_p)$. **Bottom right,** In the pure shear state, the shear stresses τ_{xy} act on each face.

and, consequently, apparent density. Apparent density is the ratio of the mass of bone tissue in a specimen to the bulk volume of the specimen (bone plus bone marrow spaces). Typically, mean values for the apparent density of hydrated human femoral cortical bone and proximal tibial trabecular bone are 1.85 g/cm^3 and 0.30 g/cm^3, respectively. The respective standard deviations are typically 0.06 g/cm^3 (± 3% of the mean value) and 0.10 g/cm^3 (± 30% of the mean value). This indicates that almost 70% of the apparent density values for femoral cortical bone are in the range 1.80 to 1.90 g/cm^3, while almost 70% of the values for tibial trabecular bone are in the range 0.20 to 0.40 g/cm^3. While the magnitudes of these ranges are similar, the percentage deviations are much larger for trabecular bone. This distinction is important because the material properties of trabecular bone are very sensitive to apparent density.

Because the densities of trabecular and cortical bone can overlap, cortical bone is usually defined as bone with less than approximately 30% porosity. However, porosity is not the only difference between cortical and trabecular bone. Trabecular bone can also be distinguished from cortical bone by differences in bone architecture (Fig. 20). Cortical bone can be described architecturally as a solid containing a series of voids: haversian and Volkmann's canals and, to a lesser extent, lacunae and canaliculi. The porosity of cortical bone tissue (typically 10%) is primarily a function of the density of these voids. However, trabecular bone can be described architecturally as a network of small, interconnected plates and rods of individual trabeculae with relatively large spaces between the trabeculae. Individual trabeculae contain only some of the voids (canaliculi and lacunae and, very seldom, haversian canals) that are contained in cortical bone. Therefore, the porosity of trabecular bone (typically 50% to 90%) is dominated by the spaces between individual trabeculae. It is the combination of differences in porosity and architecture that primarily differentiates cortical from trabecular bone and that accounts for their characteristic material properties.

Cortical Bone

Elastic behavior The elastic properties of isotropic materials do not depend on the orientation of the material with respect to the loading direction, and are characterized by a single modulus (Young's modulus). Most conventional engineering materials, such as 316L stainless steel, are isotropic. The other parameter necessary to fully characterize the elastic behavior of an isotropic material is Poisson's ratio. Poisson's ratio is a measure of how much a material bulges when compressed, or of how much a material

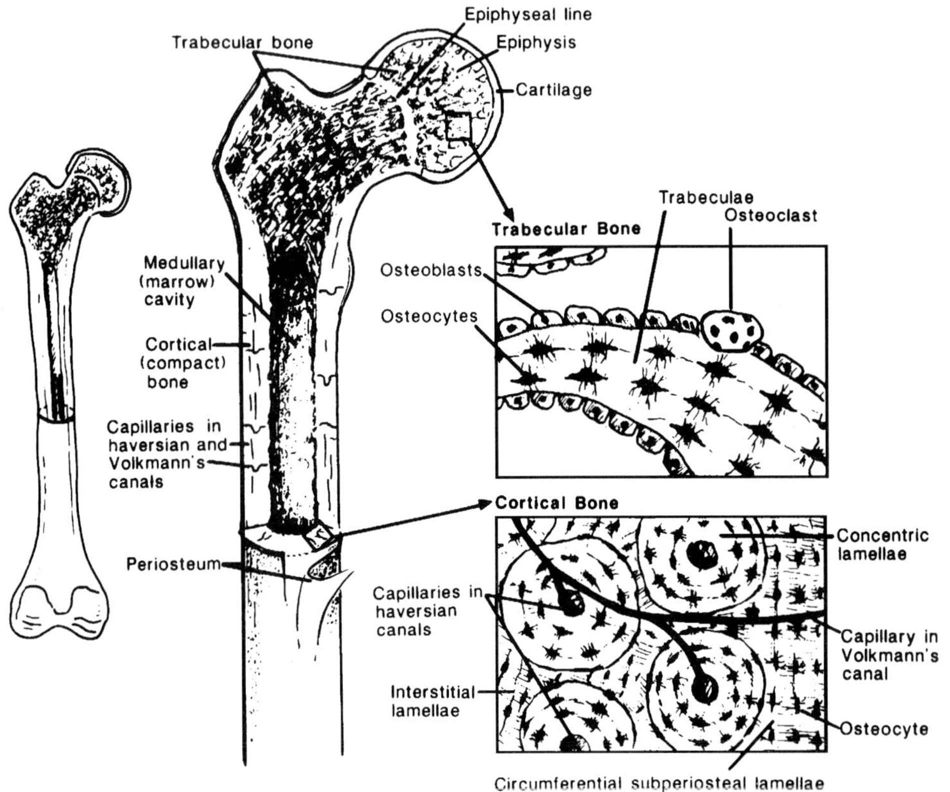

Figure 20
Schematic diagram of cortical and trabecular bone showing the different microstructures. (Reproduced with permission from Hayes WC: Biomechanics of cortical and trabecular bone: Implications for assessment of fracture risk, in *Basic Orthopaedic Biomechanics.* New York, NY, Raven Press, 1991, pp 93–142.)

contracts when stretched. This parameter, which typically is 0.3 for metals, also is found from a uniaxial test, and is the negative of the strain perpendicular to the loading direction divided by the strain along the loading direction.

The elastic properties of anisotropic materials depend on their orientation with respect to the loading direction. This is true for bone; however, the elastic properties of human cortical bone display a certain degree of symmetry, which reflects the bone's osteonal microstructure. The elastic properties of human cortical bone for loading in the plane transverse to the longitudinal axis are approximately isotropic and are substantially different from those for loading in the longitudinal direction, which is parallel to the axis of the osteons (along the longitudinal axis of the diaphysis). Therefore, human cortical bone usually is considered to be a transversely isotropic material. Transverse isotropy is a subset of anisotropy.

Two parameters, Young's modulus and Poisson's ratio, are used to describe the elastic properties of an isotropic material. Five parameters are needed to describe those of a transversely isotropic material: the longitudinal and transverse Young's moduli, the shear modulus, and two Poisson's ratios. The modulus of cortical bone in the longitudinal direction is approximately 1.5 times its modulus in the transverse direction and over five times its shear modulus. Its relatively high Poisson's ratios, with values up to 0.6, indicate that cortical bone bulges more than metals when subjected to uniaxial compression.

Strength The strength properties of cortical bone also depend on the loading direction, making it transversely isotropic from both modulus and strength perspectives. The strength of cortical bone also depends on whether it is loaded in tension, compression, or torsion. This represents an asymmetry in the strength properties, adding further complexity to the description of these properties. Consequently, it is not precise to specify the strength of cortical bone with a single number.

Typical stress-strain curves for uniaxial, monotonic tension and compression loading of cortical bone, both in the longitudinal and transverse directions, show that cortical bone is stronger in compression than in tension (Fig. 21). For example, the tensile strength in longitudinal loading is approximately 130 MPa, while the corresponding compressive strength is 190 MPa. For transverse loading, the tensile strength is very low (50 MPa), while the compressive strength (130 MPa) is comparable to the tensile strength in longitudinal loading. These data suggest that cortical bone has adapted to a situation in which compressive loading is greater than tensile loading. This situation is consistent with the combined bending and axial compressive loads that are thought to act on the femoral diaphysis during everyday activities such as walking. Under these loading conditions, maximum compressive stresses are larger than maximum tensile stresses.

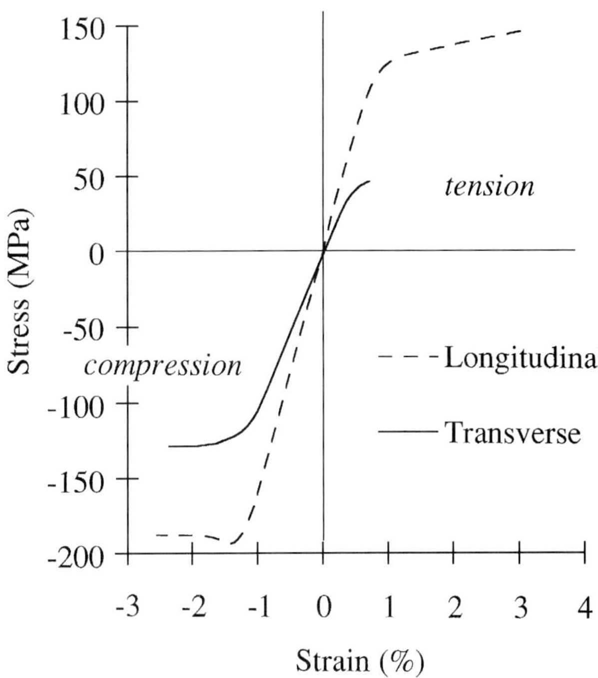

Figure 21
Stress-strain plots for human cortical bone for tensile and compressive loading. Data are shown for both longitudinal and transverse loading directions. (Adapted with permission from Gibson LJ, Ashby MF: *Cellular Solids: Structure and Properties.* Elmsford NY, Pergamon Press, 1988, based on curves and data from Reilly DT, Burstein AH: The elastic and ultimate properties of compact bone tissue *J Biomech* 1975; B:393–405 and Currey JD: *The Mechanical Adaptations of Bones* Princeton, NJ, Princeton University Press, 1984.)

Because the tensile and compressive yield strengths of cortical bone are approximately equal to the respective ultimate strengths (Fig. 21), the maximum stresses that bone can sustain are close to its yield strength. Thus, when cortical bone is loaded close to its yield point, it is also close to fracture. Furthermore, bone loaded by stresses that are just above its yield strength will deform by a relatively large amount compared to its elastic behavior. Therefore, cortical bone undergoes relatively large deformations just prior to fracture.

Energy absorption, ductility, and brittleness Materials that absorb substantial energy before failure are classified as tough materials. Biomechanically, toughness is important in traumatic events in which bone is forced to absorb energy, such as automobile accidents or falls. If the energy delivered to the bone is greater than the energy the bone can absorb, fracture occurs. Figure 21 indicates that, for both tensile and compressive loading in the longitudinal direction, the strains that occur in cortical bone at failure (ultimate strains) are much larger than those that occur at yielding (yield strains). Thus, for longitudinal loading, cortical bone is a tough material because it can absorb substantial energy before fracture. Furthermore, because the ultimate strain for longitudinal loading is substantially larger than the yield strain, cortical bone can be classified as a relatively ductile material for longitudinal loading.

The stress-strain curve for transverse loading (Fig. 21) shows that bone is tougher under compressive loads than under tensile loads. Consequently, bone has the lowest resistance to loading regimes that cause tensile stresses in the transverse direction; for example, those that can arise as "hoop" stresses when cementless hip prostheses are press fit into the diaphyses of long bones. Because the ultimate strain is close to the yield strain for tensile loading in the transverse direction, bone is relatively brittle for transverse loading. Thus, cortical bone can behave in a relatively ductile or brittle fashion, depending on the loading direction and on whether tensile or compressive forces are applied.

Viscoelastic behavior Cortical bone displays viscoelastic behavior because its mechanical properties are sensitive to both the strain rate and the duration of the applied loads.

Strain rate sensitivity The in vivo strain rate for bone can vary by more than an order of magnitude in the course of daily activities such as slow walking (strain rate ~ 0.001 per second), brisk walking (strain rate ~ 0.01 per second), and slow running (strain rate ~ 0.03 per second). Other activities, such as a jump from the height of two stairs or a fall from standing height, might result in strain rates as high as those encountered during slow and fast running, respectively. Generally, the strain rate increases as activity becomes more strenuous.

The mechanical properties of cortical bone are sensitive to strain rate. Figure 22 shows how the stress-strain behavior for longitudinal compression of bovine bone is sensitive to strain rate. The increase in the initial slope of the stress-strain plot as the strain rate increases indicates that cortical bone has a higher modulus at higher strain rates. However, for typical daily activities (strain rates from 0.001 to 0.01 per second), the modulus changes only by approximately 15%.

Over the complete range of strain rates, the yield and ultimate strengths of cortical bone increase as the strain rate increases (Fig. 22), thereby indicating that cortical bone is stronger for more strenuous activity. The same change in strain rate produces a relatively larger change in strength than in modulus (Fig. 23), indicating that ultimate tensile strength is slightly more sensitive to strain rate than is modulus. These data indicate that bone is approximately 20% stronger for brisk walking than for slow walking.

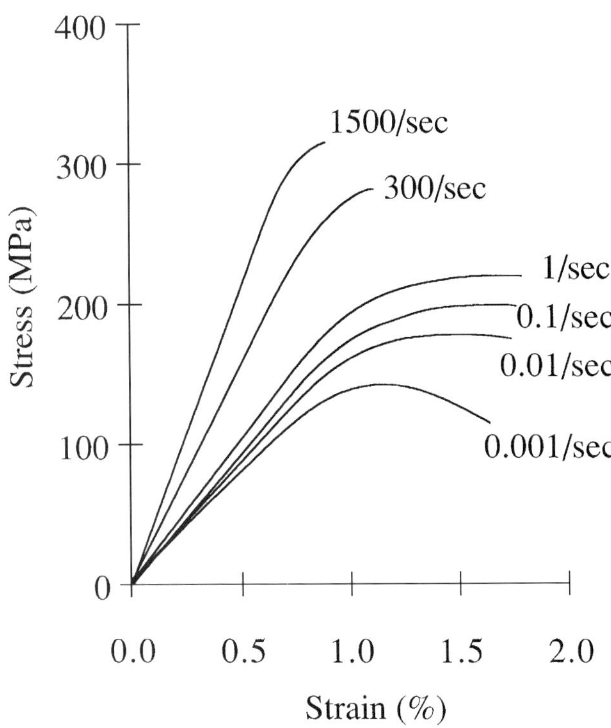

Figure 22
Strain rate dependence of cortical bone material behavior. Both modulus and strength increase for increased strain rates. (Reproduced with permission from McElhaney JH: Dynamic response of bone and muscle tissue. *J Appl Physiol* 1966; 21:1231–1236.)

At very high strain rates (greater than 0.1 per second) representing high impact trauma, cortical bone becomes more brittle (ultimate strain decreases) for loading in the longitudinal direction (Fig. 22). Thus, cortical bone exhibits a ductile to brittle transition as the strain rate increases. However, for the range of strain rates typical of more normal activity (less than 0.1 per second), ductility increases (ultimate strain increases) as the strain rate increases. Based on the shapes of these stress-strain plots and the fact that energy per unit volume is equal to the area below the stress-strain curve, the optimal range of strain rates for maximum energy absorption is 0.01 to 0.1 per second. This range suggests that bone has adapted to absorb energy from the impact that arises from relatively strenuous activities such as running.

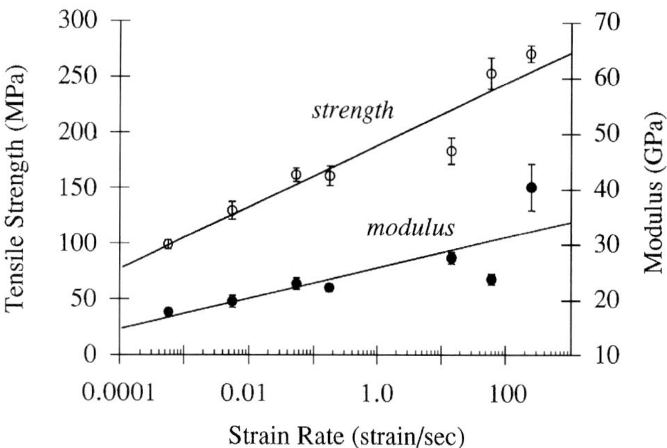

Figure 23
Comparison of strain rate sensitivities for modulus and ultimate tensile strength of human cortical bone for longitudinal loading. Over the full range of strain rates, strength increases by about a factor of three, and modulus by a factor of two. (Reproduced with permission from Wright TM, Hayes WC: Tensile testing of bone over a wide range of strain rates: Effect of strain rate, micro-structure and density. *Med Biol Eng Comput* 1976;14:671–680.)

Creep behavior If bone tissue is subjected to a constant stress for an extended period of time, it will continue to deform. This phenomenon is called creep. A typical creep curve for adult human cortical bone under tensile loading (Fig. 24) is a plot of strain as a function of time for a constant stress level. Cortical bone exhibits the same three characteristic stages of creep behavior as do many conventional engineering materials. In the primary stage, specimen strain continues after loading and the creep (increase in strain) rate gradually decreases. In the secondary stage, there is a lower, usually constant creep rate. Finally, in the tertiary stage, there is a marked increase in the creep rate just before creep fracture. If cortical bone is loaded at certain levels for enough time, creep fracture will occur, although the stress level is well below the yield and ultimate strengths (Fig. 24). As shown in Figure 25, the time required for creep failure (fracture) to occur decreases as the stress increases, and resistance to creep fracture is greater for compressive than for tensile loading.

If creep occurs without fracture, and the bone is fully unloaded, permanent deformation results. For example, if creep is a result of relatively high tensile stresses held for several minutes, and the specimen is unloaded before creep fracture occurs, the specimen will be permanently deformed such that it is longer than its original length. This behavior is referred to as viscoplastic: "visco" from the creep behavior during loading, and "plastic" from the permanent deformation after unloading. Furthermore, if the applied constant stress is above a threshold level (approximately 70 MPa, or 55% of its ultimate strength, for human cortical bone loaded in longitudinal tension), the rate at which creep deformation occurs and the magnitude of the per-

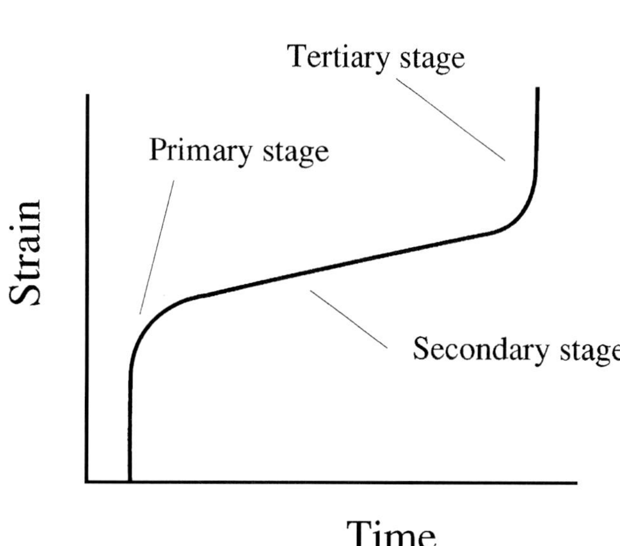

Figure 24
Schematic diagram showing the three stages of creep behavior of human cortical bone. (Reproduced with permission from Carter DR, Caler WE: A cumulative damage model for bone fracture. *J Orthop Res* 1985;3:84–90.)

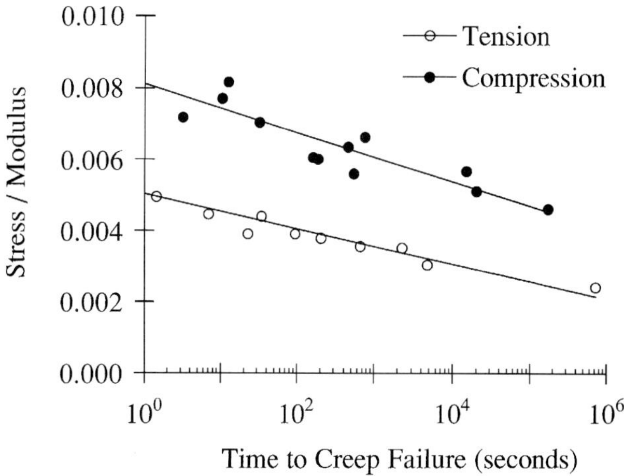

Figure 25
Creep fracture stress for human cortical bone as a function of the time to failure. To account for variations in modulus between specimens, stress values have been normalized (divided) by the initial modulus (measured at the beginning of the experiment). These data indicate that resistance to creep fracture is greater for compressive loading. (Reproduced with permission from Caler WE, Carter DR: Bone creep-fatigue damage accumulation. *J Biomech* 1989;22:625–635.)

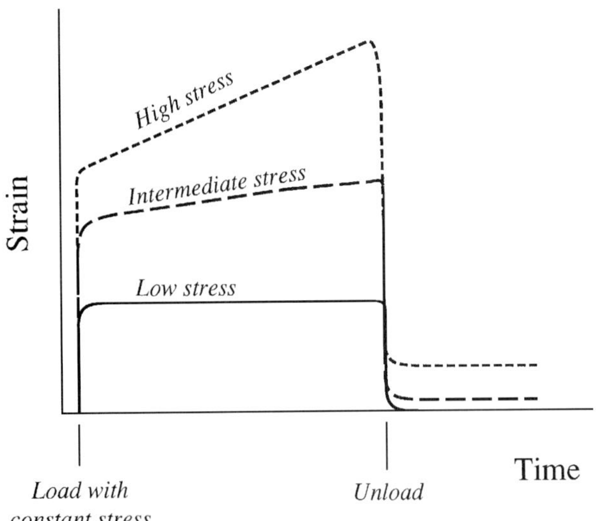

Figure 26
Schematic of typical strain-time curves, illustrating "viscoplastic" behavior of human cortical bone. In this experiment, the bone is loaded at a constant stress, and the strain is measured as a function of time. The specimen is then unloaded before creep fracture occurs. Typical behaviors are shown for different applied stresses. As the stress is increased, a creep threshold is reached, beyond which the creep rate (the slope in the second stage of creep behavior) increases. The permanent deformation (strain after unloading) also increases as the applied stress is increased. Interestingly, exactly similar behavior occurs for some chopped glass-fiber composite materials at elevated temperatures. (Reproduced with permission from Fondrk M, Bahniuk E, Davy DT, et al: Some viscoplastic characteristics of bovine and human cortical bone. *J Biomech* 1988;21:623–630.)

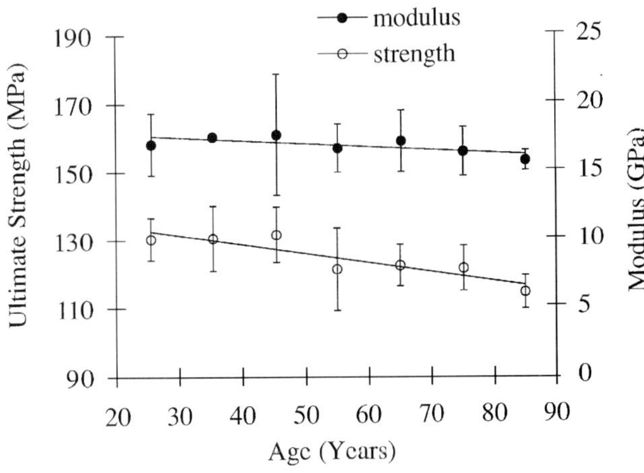

Figure 27
Age-related effects on longitudinal modulus and ultimate tensile strength of human femoral cortical bone. (Reproduced with permission from Burstein AH, Reilly DT, Martens M: Aging of bone tissue: Mechanical properties. *J Bone Joint Surg* 1976;58:82–86.)

manent deformation after unloading both increase sharply (Fig. 26). Creep studies have not yet been performed for loading in the transverse direction.

The mechanisms for creep behavior in cortical bone have not been determined. However, scanning electron micrographs of fractured surfaces have indicated that the creep mechanisms appear to be different for tensile and compressive loading. Osteon pullout is common for tensile loading, and fractures tend to cross through the osteons for compressive loading.

Age effects The modulus and strength properties of cortical bone progressively deteriorate with aging for both men and women. The longitudinal modulus and tensile yield strength of cortical bone taken from the femoral mid-diaphysis decrease by approximately 2% per decade after age 20 (Fig. 27). For example, from the third to ninth decades, respectively, the ultimate tensile strength of bone, for longitudinal loading, decreases from approximately 130 MPa to 110 MPa, and the corresponding elastic moduli change from approximately 17 GPa to 15.6 GPa. The slope of the stress-strain curve after yielding increases by 8% per decade. Probably the most significant change from a fracture risk perspective is the reduction in energy absorption (area under the stress-strain curve) that occurs with aging. The decrease in energy absorption by approximately 7% per decade results mainly from reductions in the ultimate strain. Taken together, these data indicate that cortical bone material in the human femur becomes less stiff, less strong, and more brittle with aging.

Microstructure and mechanical properties Age-related changes in material properties vary for different bones. For example, decreases in ultimate tensile strength and modulus are greater for the femur than for the tibia, although decreases in ultimate strain are similar for each bone. One explanation for this is that the rate of bone turnover may be greater in the tibia than in the femur, and the mechanism that reduces both modulus and strength is inhibited as new osteons are formed. However, many parameters affect the mechanical properties of cortical bone.

Parameters that have been investigated as determinants of the mechanical properties of cortical bone are apparent density (proportional to porosity), ash density (total mineral content divided by bulk volume), histology (number of osteons, primary versus secondary bone), collagen composition and content, orientation of the collagen fibers and mineral, composition of the cement lines, bonding between the mineral and collagen phases, and accumulation of microcracks in the bone matrix and around osteons.

It is difficult to correlate these parameters with the mechanical properties of cortical bone because the ranges of modulus and strength values for this tissue are relatively small. Consequently, many of these issues remain equivocal, and this discussion is limited to the less controversial findings. Modulus and ultimate strength have been positively correlated with apparent density using a power law in which the reported exponents for modulus are in the range of 1.5 to 7.5. Both monotonic and fatigue (see below) strengths were found to be sensitive to the relative number of osteons in the bone. Correlation of density and microstructure suggests that haversian remodeling of primary bone is accompanied by a reduction in density. Nevertheless, microstructure has been shown to affect some mechanical properties after these changes in density were taken into account. Probably the most important determinant of modulus and strength is the ash density or mineral content. In a study on properties of cortical bone from a wide range of species, multiple regression analysis demonstrated that almost 90% of the variance in modulus and strength can be explained using a power law model with both volume fraction (proportional to apparent density) and mineral content (proportional to ash density) as independent variables. Water content is also important in the mechanical properties of cortical bone. Wet bone, as found in situ, is less stiff, less strong, and less brittle than fully dried bone, although rewetting bone after it has been dried can almost fully restore its in situ behavior. Finally, collagen content has been shown to dominate the stiffness behavior after yielding has occurred.

Fatigue properties The strength properties described above characterize situations where there is a single application of force (monotonic loading). However, in vivo cortical bone is exposed primarily to repetitive, low intensity loading, which produces lower stress levels than those required to fracture a bone specimen during monotonic loading. This cyclic loading of bone can result in damage at the microstructural level. For example, during walking, the proximal femur is loaded cyclically with each step. The spine is loaded cyclically while a person is lifting objects, rising from a chair, and bending over. Not all loads result in damage to bone. If damage does occur, however, and if the damage accumulates over time, the strength of the bone is reduced. High levels of stress over shorter periods of time also may lead to fatigue damage, as shown by the relatively frequent incidence of stress fractures in military recruits, long distance runners, and race horses subjected to rigorous training programs. Thus, the major cause of these stress fractures appears to be fatigue damage accumulation. The mechanical properties of bone under the action of cyclic, repetitive loading are called the fatigue properties of bone.

Fatigue properties of cortical bone, besides being interesting for their role in stress fractures, are of interest as a potential stimulus for bone remodeling. Because the fatigue properties of cortical bone mainly have been measured in devitalized bone specimens, the effects of bone remodeling on the fatigue behavior of bone in vivo remain unknown. Physiologic levels of loading can induce fatigue damage and failure in vitro; therefore, bone remodeling, which occurs continuously in vivo, may repair the damage caused by relatively low intensity loading, such as occurs in walking. Studies have demonstrated that microcracks do occur in vivo. Thus, it has been hypothesized that bone remodeling occurs to repair microcracks that form in bone as a result of the repetitive loading of daily activity.

Up to 10% of age-related hip and over 50% of age-related spine fractures are classified as spontaneous because they occur without any obvious trauma. If fatigue cracks continue to occur in bone with continued repetitive loading, and there are age-related reductions in the rate of bone turnover to repair these cracks, bone monotonic strength may progressively be compromised with age. Thus, the fatigue behavior of bone may be a causative factor in spontaneous fractures.

To determine the fatigue properties of bone using traditional engineering techniques, standard specimens of bone are cyclically loaded to fracture in controlled environments at a fixed level of stress (or, sometimes strain). The number of load cycles at fracture is recorded as the fatigue life corresponding to the specified stress level. Testing is performed at different stress levels, and results usually are presented as a σ-n plot of stress level σ versus the logarithm of the fatigue life, or, number of cycles n (Fig. 28). This curve indicates that fatigue fracture will occur at any stress level above the endurance limit if the number of load cycles is large enough. The important concept is that fatigue fracture, like creep fracture, can occur at stress levels that are substantially lower than the monotonic strength.

The fatigue life of bone is better correlated with strains than with stresses, and in particular, with ranges of strains (defined as the difference between the maximum and minimum values of the applied cyclic strain). Figure 29 shows the in vitro fatigue life of human cortical bone for high cyclic strain ranges. Strain ranges representative of normal walking, mild exercise, and vigorous exercise are also

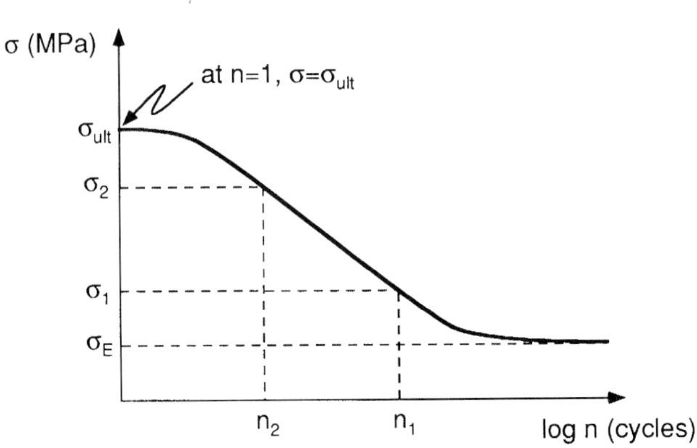

Figure 28
Idealized fatigue σ-n curve for cortical bone. Fatigue fracture occurs at stress level σ_1 in n_1 cycles, or at stress level σ_2 at n_2 cycles. Note that the fatigue life n is shown on a log scale.

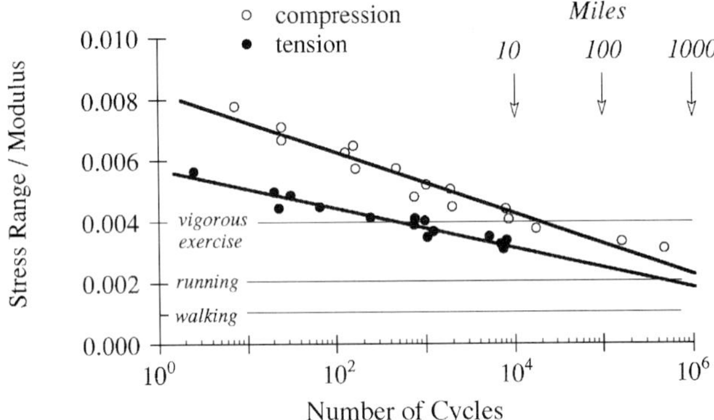

Figure 29
Fatigue life curve as a function of strain-range (stress range / modulus) for human femoral cortical bone for compressive and tensile loading. Typical strain-ranges for different activities are shown, and typical distances for walking and running are also shown. Behavior must be extrapolated for less strenuous activities. Note that, as with creep behavior, resistance to fatigue fracture is greater for compressive loading. (Reproduced with permission from Carter DR, Caler WE, Spengler DM, et al: Fatigue behavior of adult cortical bone: The influence of mean strain and strain range. *Acta Orthop Scand* 1981;52:481–490.)

shown. On average, approximately 5,000 cycles of loading correspond to the number of steps in 10 miles of running, while one million cycles correspond to 1,000 miles. The data in Figure 29 indicate that a total running distance of less than 1,000 miles could cause fracture of cortical bone tissue. This is consistent with stress fractures observed in military recruits who commonly undergo strenuous training programs of up to 1,000 miles of running over a six-week period.

The fatigue life of cortical bone also depends on temperature. Figure 30 shows the σ-n curve for bovine cortical bone for two different temperatures (21°C and 45°C). These data indicate that the fatigue life of cortical bone can be reduced considerably as the temperature increases from room temperature to body core temperature. Foot skin temperatures of up to 43°C have been recorded in subjects walking briskly in a warm environment. Because deep tissue temperatures in the extremities can be within 2°C of skin temperatures, bone temperatures in the foot may vary from less than room temperature to several degrees above body core temperature. The temperature dependence of fatigue properties may have physiologic consequences.

Increases in strain rate result in increases in the monotonic strength of cortical bone; however, for a fixed stress level, fatigue damage increases with increasing strain rate. Therefore, more fatigue damage occurs for more strenuous exercise. Furthermore, for a fixed stress level, the fatigue life of cortical bone in uniaxial tension is less than in uniaxial compression, indicating that regions of cortical bone loaded in tension are at a higher risk of fatigue failure than regions loaded in compression by the same magnitude force. Studies have shown that the damage patterns for tensile and compressive loading are different, with mostly osteon debonding for tension and oblique cracking for com-

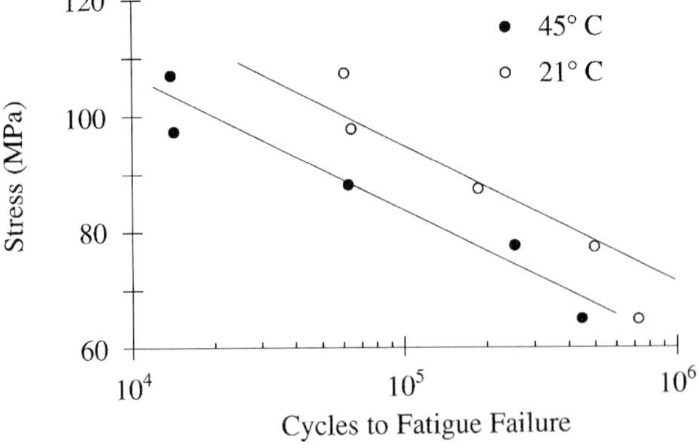

Figure 30
Temperature dependence of fatigue life for bovine femoral cortical bone. Each data point represents the mean value for six specimens tested at that stress level. Fatigue life is reduced by a factor of three when temperature is increased from 21°C to 45°C. (Reproduced with permission from Carter DR, Hayes WC: Fatigue life of compact bone: I. Effects of stress, amplitude, temperature and density. *J Biomech* 1976;9:27–34.)

pression. The curves shown in Figure 29 can be used to estimate the damage that accumulates in the bone as a result of a number of cycles of loading at a particular strain range level. One simple approach is to assume there is a linear rate of damage accumulation at each strain range level. Figure 29 indicates that the in vitro fatigue life at a strain range of 0.002 is approximately 10^6 cycles. Therefore, a linear damage model (known as Miner's Rule) implies that 10^4 cycles at a strain range of 0.002 (10 miles of running) uses up $10^4/10^6$ (0.01) of the fatigue life. In the absence of a biologic repair process, 100 of these ten-mile runs would use up all the fatigue life and cause fracture. Similarly, a few cycles at very high loads could substantially reduce the fatigue life, so that subsequent activities such as walking could cause fatigue fracture after, say, 10^6 cycles (approximately one year). Therefore, fatigue damage accumulation is probably an important causative factor in stress fractures.

Mechanisms of fatigue damage accumulation Because fatigue behavior is so important, much interest has developed in the actual mechanism of fatigue damage accumulation in cortical bone. The fatigue mechanism for cortical bone has been shown to be similar to the mechanism for artificial, oriented, short-fiber composite materials. There are three characteristic stages of fatigue fracture, corresponding to crack initiation, crack growth (propagation), and final fracture. Because the modulus of the bone decreases as cracks form, these three stages can be demonstrated by a plot of stiffness versus number of cycles (Fig. 31). In the primary stage of crack initiation within the bone, a small decrease in the stiffness and strength would be experienced. In the secondary stage, crack propagation results in a slow but steady further decrease in these values. Finally, in the tertiary stage, fracture is preceded by a rapid decrease in the ability to support load. The precise shape of these curves depends on the magnitude and sign (tension versus compression) of the applied load.

For cortical bone, haversian canals, lacunae, or canaliculi act as crack initiators because these discontinuities in the bone microstructure cause local increases in stress (stress concentrations). However, crack initiation, per se, is not necessarily detrimental to the structural integrity of cortical bone because cracks may induce bone remodeling. Cortical bone also has been shown to remodel such that stress concentrations about small holes are reduced. Bone not only repairs cracks, but also may remodel to reduce stresses about these cracks. What becomes important then, is how well bone can stop the growth of cracks so that they remain small enough to be repaired by remodeling.

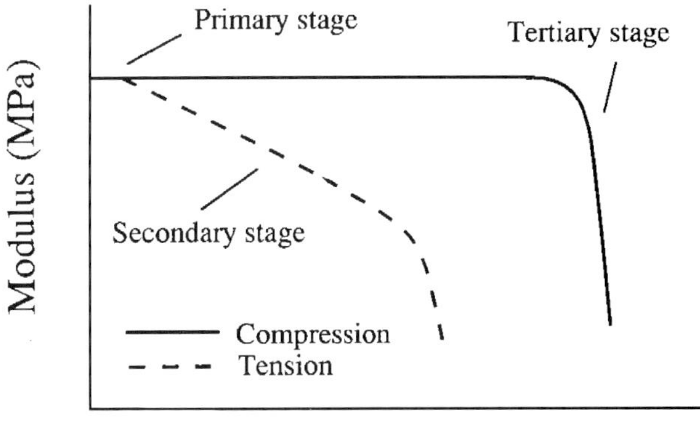

Figure 31
Schematic diagram of the modulus degradation which occurs for human cortical bone with fatigue loading. Note the different behaviors for tensile and compressive loading. The precise shape of these curves further depends on the magnitude of the applied stress. (Reproduced with permission from Pattin CAG: *Cyclic Mechanical Property Degradation in Bone During Fatigue Loading.* Palo Alto, CA, Stanford University, 1991. Thesis.)

The second and most important stage of fatigue failure is the slow propagation of these microcracks, which tend to join together once they progress beyond the initiation stage. The resulting larger cracks then run into weak material interfaces (cement lines) between the osteons in the secondary haversian systems, causing two things to occur. First, some osteons debond from the matrix, contributing to the "osteon pullout" phenomenon commonly observed on fractured surfaces of cortical bone. Second, the direction of crack propagation is changed from perpendicular to the loading direction to parallel to the loading direction. This change has the effect of producing a stress at the crack tip that, instead of opening the crack, is parallel to the crack and, therefore, harmless (does not open the crack).

These effects, and possibly others, tend to stop cracks from progressing across bone in the transverse direction, thereby increasing the bone's resistance to propagation of transverse cracks under longitudinal loading. Weak longitudinal interfaces in bone that stop the progression of transverse cracks include the interfaces between the osteons and the interstitial material, those between adjacent lamellae in the interstitial material, and those between the interfaces within single osteons. Therefore, even if cracks form easily because of bone's natural voids, other imperfections in the microstructure, namely the weak interfaces in the haversian system, tend to stop their progression under loads typical of normal activity.

This second stage of fatigue damage results in a slight reduction of modulus in bone; however, because damage accumulates, it reduces the fatigue life of bone. The final stage of fatigue fracture occurs because cracks coalesce and become so large that the weak interfaces can no longer absorb them. The specimen then fails as the final crack travels across the specimen, resulting in a sharp decrease in modulus followed by its fracture.

Trabecular Bone

There is a large variation in density for trabecular bone. Both spatial and temporal variations in trabecular bone density can occur as a result of changes in anatomic location and age, respectively. For example, trabecular bone material properties within the proximal tibia can vary by up to two orders of magnitude because of changes in density alone. Material properties for trabecular bone have been reported for most anatomic sites. In addition, noninvasive densitometric studies have shown that trabecular bone mineral density in the hip and spine decreases with age, reaching lower levels in women than men. Because in vitro biomechanical studies of cadaveric material have shown that the material properties of trabecular bone are very sensitive to apparent density, discussion of these properties requires reference to the anatomic location and the age of the tissue.

To further complicate matters, material properties of trabecular bone also depend on its architecture, which, like its density, depends on the anatomic site and, to a lesser extent, on age. While cortical bone is essentially a low porosity solid, trabecular bone is best described as an open-celled porous foam. Made up of a series of interconnecting trabeculae, trabecular bone can be idealized as a combination of rod-rod, rod-plate, or plate-plate basic cellular structures where rods and plates represent thin and thick trabeculae, respectively (Fig. 32). Depending on the type and orientation of these basic cellular structures, the mechanical properties can vary by at least an order of magnitude.

Elastic behavior In general, the modulus of trabecular bone can vary from approximately 10 MPa to 2,000 MPa, depending on the anatomic site and age. Trabecular bone is much less stiff than cortical bone, which has a modulus of approximately 17,000 MPa. However, there are regions in the skeleton, such as the cranium, the subchondral plate in the proximal tibia, the metaphyseal shell in the proximal femur, and the endplates in vertebral bodies, where the distinction between cortical and trabecular bone is less clear. Mean values of the modulus in these regions have been measured in the range of 1,150 MPa to 9,650 MPa. Because most research has focused on the material properties of the trabecular bone that is found in the metaphyses of long bones, attention is limited to these regions.

Dependence on Apparent Density As mentioned above, the material properties of trabecular bone are very sensitive to apparent density. In particular, it has been demonstrated that the modulus E of trabecular bone in any loading direction is related to its apparent density ρ by a power-law relationship of the form:

$$E = a + b\,\rho^{c} \qquad \textbf{(Eq. 2)}$$

where a, b, and c are constants that depend on the architecture of the tissue.

As with any power law, the most important parameter in this relationship is the exponent c, which directly affects how density affects the modulus. In general, the exponent has a value of approximately two (Fig. 33). Statistical analyses have shown that the best fit for the modulus of specimens pooled from a wide range of anatomic sites is obtained by a squared exponent. Consequently, a 25% reduction in density, as has been observed in elderly cadaveric vertebrae, results in a 56% decrease in modulus. Theoretical models that treat trabecular bone as a porous foam predict a squared power-law relationship when the idealized architecture is primarily open celled (a network of connecting rods, as most human trabecular bone appears to be). The main mechanism of deformation in these open-celled foams is bending of individual trabeculae, even though the bulk specimen is compressed without bending.

Dependence on architecture When the architecture is controlled, the variation in apparent density of trabecular bone can explain most of the variation in modulus. However, as can be seen from the scatter in modulus values for any particular value of apparent density (Fig. 33), other variables, namely the architecture, can also affect modulus. Scanning electron microscopes have been used successfully to illustrate the large variation in trabecular bone architecture over different anatomic sites.

The architecture of trabecular bone describes both the shape of the bone and its orientation. The basic structure describes the general connectivity of the trabeculae, the mean thickness of individual trabeculae, the mean spacing between trabeculae, and the number of trabeculae. There is a clear relationship between the density of the bulk trabecular bone and both the number and mean thickness of individual trabeculae. For the lumbar spine, there is a strong linear relationship between density and these variables (Fig. 34). In the subcapital region of the proximal femur, however, the relationship be-

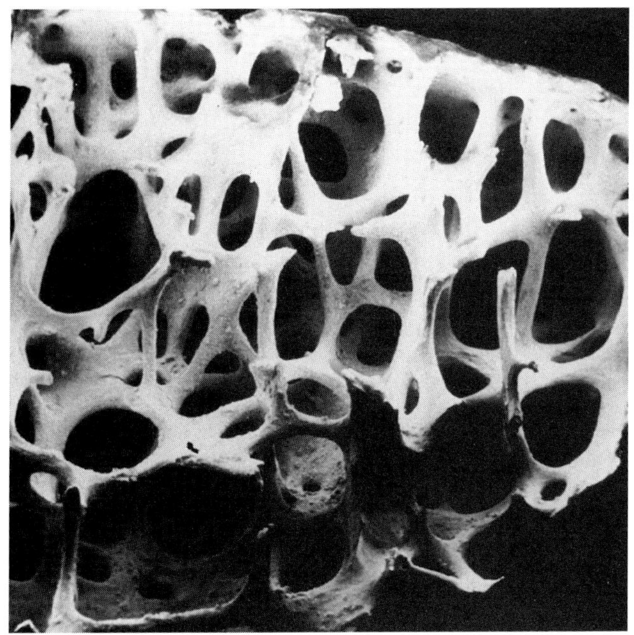

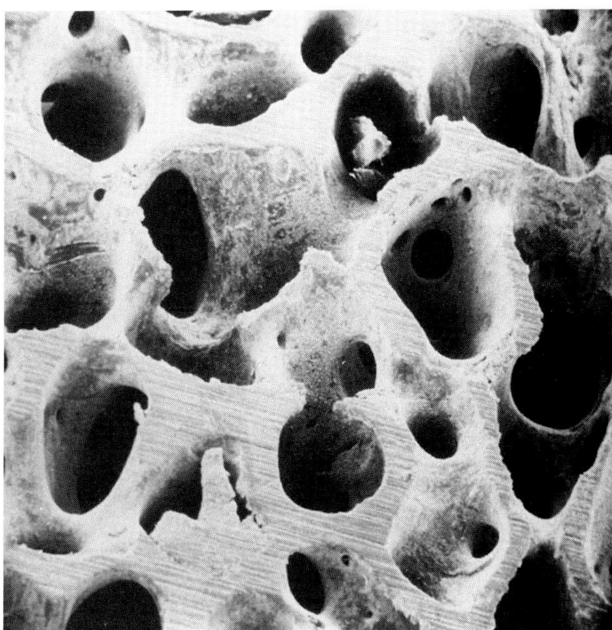

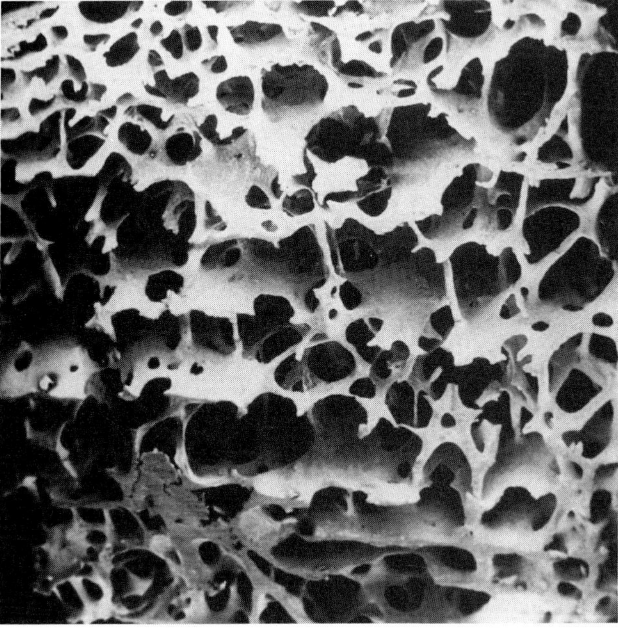

Figure 32
Scanning electron micrographs showing the various basic cellular structures of human trabecular bone: **top left,** the rod-rod basic cellular structure, from the femoral head; **top right,** the more dense plate-plate cellular structure, also from the femoral head; **bottom,** the plate-rod cellular structure, from the femoral condyle. (Reproduced with permission from Gibson LJ: The mechanical behavior of cancellous bone. *J Biomech* 1985;18:317–328.)

tween mean trabecular thickness and density is highly nonlinear (Fig. 34).

Apart from affecting its modulus, the shape of the basic cellular structure can also affect the Poisson's ratio of trabecular bone. For isotropic metals, Poisson's ratio must fall between 0 and 0.5. However, theoretical values of Poisson's ratio for open-celled foam materials such as trabecular bone may be negative (the material contracts when compressed) or well above unity, depending on the cell structure. For example, the Poisson's ratio for cork is approximately zero, allowing a cork to be pushed into a wine bottle without breaking the bottle. Mean values (± standard deviation) of Poisson's ratio for trabecular bone have been reported in the range 0.06 ± 0.03 to 0.95 ± 1.29.

The other factor that relates to the bone's architecture is the orientation of the basic cellular structures, reflected as the mean orientation of the trabeculae. The orientation of individual trabeculae is controlled mainly by the direction of the forces applied to the skeleton, according to the widely cited, but still qualitative Wolff's Law. Figure 35 shows modulus as a function of apparent density for

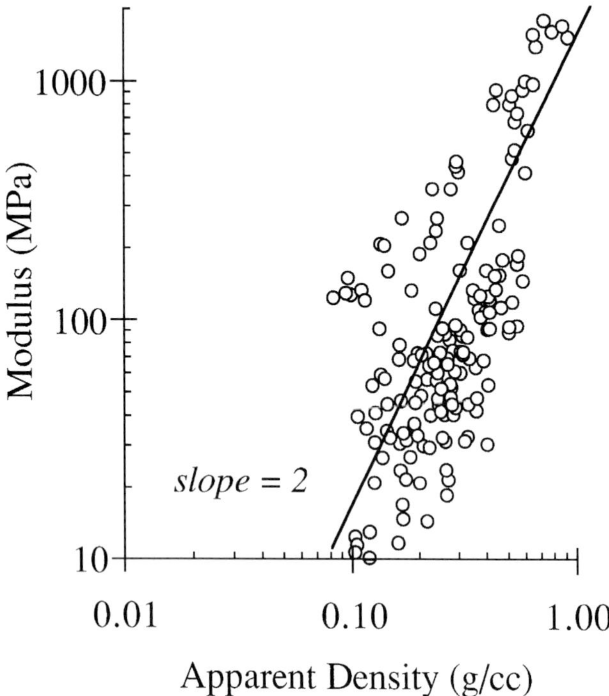

Figure 33
Compressive modulus as a function of apparent density for trabecular bone. The orientation of the specimen is not controlled. In general, the modulus of trabecular bone, when taken from a wide range of species and anatomic locations, varies as a power-law function of density with an exponent of approximately two. (Reproduced with permission from Keaveny TM, Hayes WC: Mechanical properties of cortical and trabecular bone, in Hall BK (ed): *Bone*. Boca Raton, FL, CRC Press, 1993, vol 7, pp 285–344.)

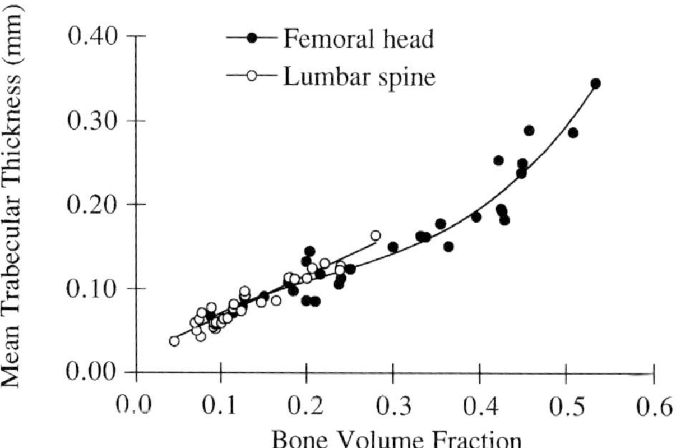

Figure 34
Mean thickness of the trabeculae in the lumbar spine and the subcapital region of the proximal femur as a function of bone volume fraction, which is proportional to apparent density. (Reproduced with permission from Snyder BD, Hayes WC: Multiaxial structure-property relations in trabecular bone, in Mow VC, Ratcliffe A, Woo SL-Y (eds): *Biomechanics of Diarthrodial Joints*. New York, NY, Springer-Verlag, 1990, pp 31–59.)

bovine trabecular bone in different orientations. These data indicate that there can be a 10-fold difference in modulus.

The different architectures that exist for trabecular bone result in an anisotropy of elastic properties. In contrast to cortical bone, trabecular bone is nearly isotropic at some anatomic sites (proximal humerus), and highly anisotropic at others (elderly lumbar spine). Because trabecular bone is both anisotropic and heterogeneous, it is difficult to generalize about its elastic properties. In order to understand structure-anisotropy relations for trabecular bone, stereologic methods recently have been developed to quantify the architecture (sometimes called the morphology). To develop structure-anisotropy relations, the measured anisotropic mechanical properties of specimens of trabecular bone must be correlated with the stereologic descriptions of their architecture. The results from these studies indicate that there are excellent correlations between architecture and mechanical properties, and that multivariate regressions that include both architecture and density provide modestly improved correlations with mechanical properties compared to the use of density alone. However, because these experiments are so difficult to perform, the results are sparse and cannot yet be generalized.

Uniaxial strength Much research has focused on the compressive strength of trabecular bone because its in vivo failure is believed to be dominated by compressive loads. Figure 36 shows typical stress strain plots for specimens of trabecular bone with different apparent densities under uniaxial compressive loading. Both the elastic and postyield behaviors are sensitive to apparent density. These characteristics are also displayed by artificial and natural porous foam materials such as aluminum honeycombs, cork, and balsa wood.

The stress strain plots in Figure 36 have three regions that represent distinct phases of material behavior. In the first stage, the material is in the linear region, in which individual trabeculae bend and compress as the bulk tissue is compressed. In the second stage, failure occurs by fracture of some trabeculae and buckling of others. As more and more trabeculae fail, the strain increases until broken trabeculae begin to fill the pores, causing the specimen to stiffen in stage three. Lower density specimens can deform more before the final stiffening phase than can higher density specimens (Fig. 36). This ability to deform to compressive strains of over 50% highlights a unique feature of trabecular bone: it can absorb considerable energy (area under the stress-strain curve) for large compressive loads while maintaining a minimum mass.

The compressive strength of trabecular bone also is related to its apparent density by a squared

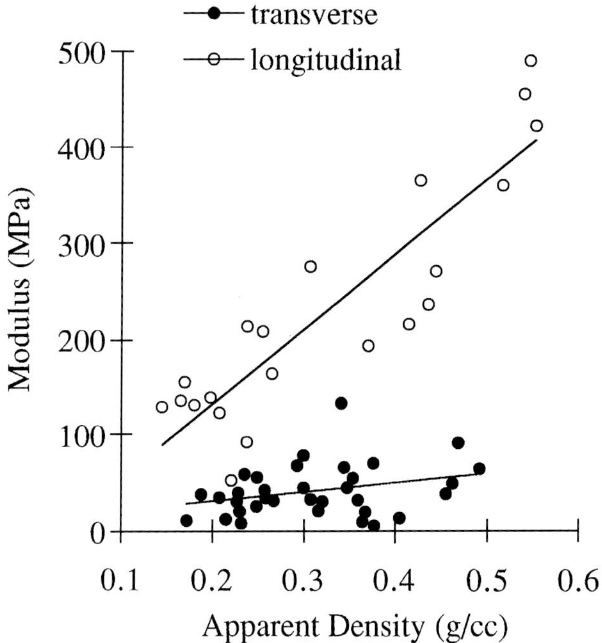

Figure 35
Compressive modulus as a function of apparent density and loading direction for trabecular bone. Data are presented for specimens loaded in longitudinal and transverse directions, demonstrating the sensitivity of modulus to loading direction. (Reproduced with permission from Williams JL, Lewis JL: Properties of an anisotropic model of cancellous bone from the proximal tibial epiphysis. *J Biomech Eng* 1982;104:50–56.)

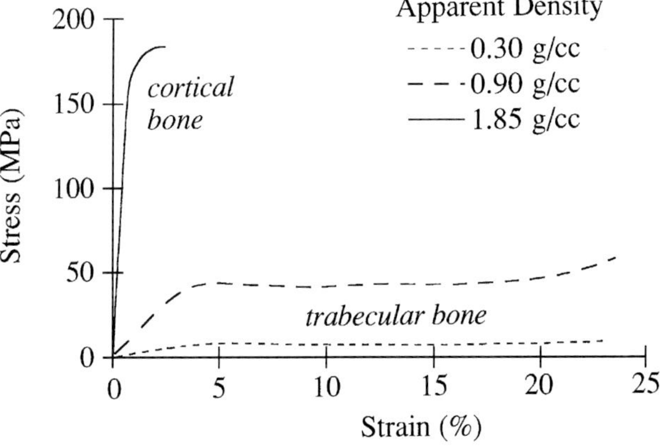

Figure 36
Example of typical compressive stress-strain behaviors of trabecular and cortical bone for different apparent densities. (Reproduced with permission from Keaveny TM, Hayes WC: Mechanical properties of cortical and trabecular bone, in Hall BK (ed): *Bone.* Boca Raton, FL, CRC Press, 1993, vol 7, pp 285–344.)

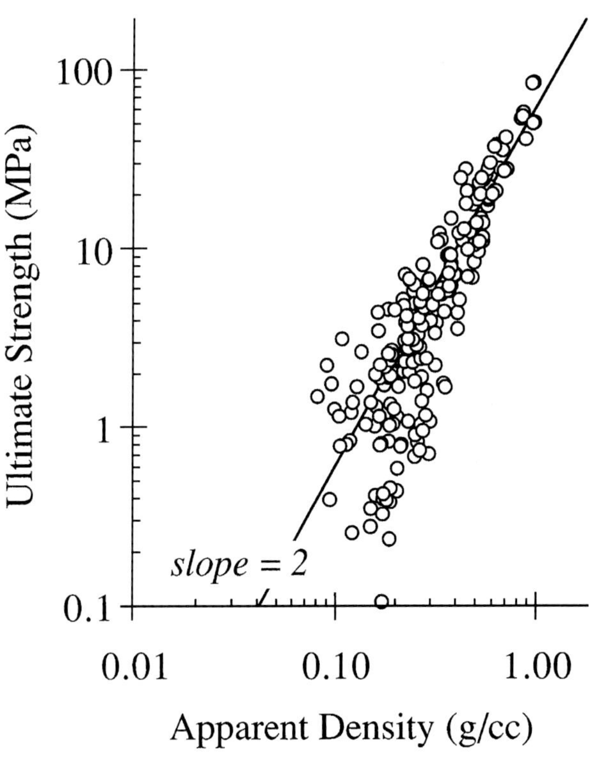

Figure 37
Ultimate compressive strength as a function of apparent density for trabecular bone. In general, compressive strength varies as a power-law function of density with an exponent of approximately two. (Reproduced with permission from Keaveny TM, Hayes WC: Mechanical properties of cortical and trabecular bone, in Hall BK (ed): *Bone.* Boca Raton, FL, CRC Press, 1993, vol 7, pp 285–344.)

power-law relationship (Fig. 37). Many studies have demonstrated strong linear relationships between compressive strength and modulus. Thus, stiffer trabecular bone is proportionally stronger, which suggests that the main parameter that may control failure in trabecular bone is not the maximum level of stress, but the maximum level of strain (strain = stress divided by modulus). This supposition is supported by the evidence that trabecular bone yields at strains in the range of 1% to 4%, with only a weak dependence on density.

These relationships between apparent density and both modulus and strength have important physiologic and clinical consequences. First, bone can easily regulate its strength and stiffness by adjusting its apparent density. Second, subtle changes in bone apparent density result in large changes in strength and modulus, indicating that an order of magnitude reduction in both trabecular bone strength and modulus can occur by the time density reductions of 30% to 50% are visible radiographically. Thus, conventional radiographic techniques used to assess fracture risk of whole bones are poor indicators of bone tissue strength.

The tensile behavior of a block of trabecular bone is much different from its compressive behavior (Fig. 38). While the linear behavior is similar to that for compressive loading, the postyield behavior

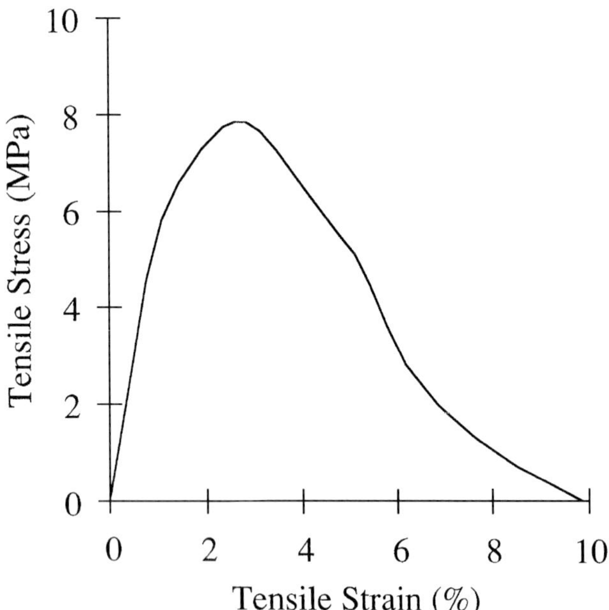

Figure 38
Tensile stress-strain behavior of trabecular bone. Compare this with the compressive behavior shown in Figure 36. (Reproduced with permission from Carter DR, Schwab GH, Spengler DM: Tensile fracture of cancellous bone. *Acta Orthop Scand* 1980;51:733–741.)

is completely different. For tensile loading, failure occurs by fracture of the individual trabeculae. As more trabeculae fracture, the specimen can take less and less load, until finally complete fracture occurs. This behavior is similar to that for fiber-reinforced concrete, and is typical of engineering materials designed to resist primarily compressive forces.

Comparison of the compressive and tensile behaviors of trabecular bone (Figs. 36 and 38) indicates that the postyield load-carrying capacity of trabecular bone is high for compression and almost negligible for tension. Thus, trabecular bone loaded beyond the ultimate strength in compression can still carry substantial load; it will not significantly overload surrounding trabecular bone, and failure will not spread to the surrounding tissue. However, for tension loading beyond the ultimate strength, no load can be carried by the tissue because it fractures. In this case, the surrounding tissue must carry the full load, and thus may be overloaded. If subsequent failure of that material occurs, a cascade effect could result in which a crack could propagate across a whole bone causing fracture. Although local failure of trabecular bone in compression is not likely to lead to failure of a whole bone, local failure in tension could have catastrophic consequences.

Viscoelastic behavior Because very few experiments have been performed in which constant loads have been held on trabecular bone for extended periods of time, its creep behavior is poorly understood. However, both modulus and strength of trabecular bone have been shown to be weakly dependent on strain rate. For most activities, the relationship between apparent density ρ and both modulus E and strength σ_{ult} can be expressed as a function of strain rate g by the following power-law relationships:

$$E = a + h\gamma^{0.06}\rho^{c} \quad \textbf{(Eq. 3a)}$$

$$\sigma_{ult} = m + n\,\gamma^{0.06}\rho^{d}, \quad \textbf{(Eq. 3b)}$$

where a, h, c, m, n, and d are constants. A squared exponent, c = d = 2, on ρ is a good representation of the general behavior of trabecular bone, and the small exponent on γ implies that the sensitivities of both modulus and strength to strain rate are weak. For example, a 100-fold increase in strain rate from 0.001 (slow walking) to 0.1 (very strenuous exercise) would result in increases of approximately 30% in both modulus and strength. As indicated by the exponent on γ, the strength and modulus adjust equally to changes in strain rate, as they do for changes in density.

Bone marrow may also play a role in trabecular bone's load-carrying capacity, but only at very high strain rates (for example, above 10 per second, as in gunshot wounds). Restricting the bone marrow from flowing through the intertrabecular spaces, as for very high strain rates, can further enhance the mechanical properties (Fig. 39). Therefore, trabecular

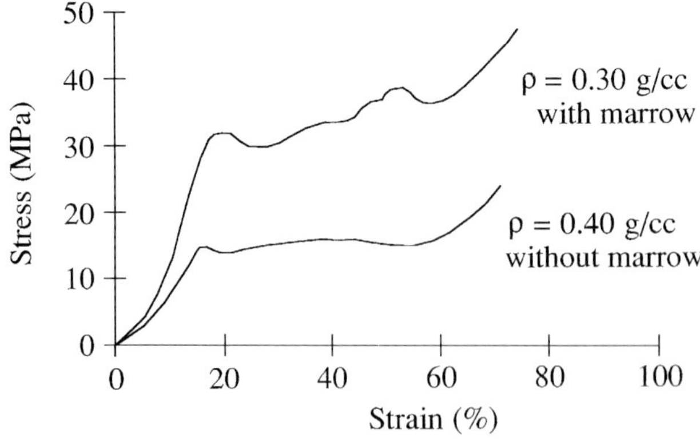

Figure 39
Stress-strain curves for two specimens of trabecular bone, one with bone marrow, the other without marrow. The strain rate for this test was very high (10/s), representative of severe traumatic loading. The modulus and strength are significantly higher for specimens with bone marrow. However, bone marrow only affects mechanical behavior at these high loading rates. (Reproduced with permission from Carter DR, Hayes WC: The compressive behavior of bone as a two-phase porous structure. *J Bone Joint Surg* 1977;59:954–962.)

bone becomes stiffer and stronger for severe, traumatic compressive loading, and can absorb more energy than for physiologic loading. However, at physiologic rates, the marrow plays a negligible role in the viscous behavior of trabecular bone.

Age effects Age-related fractures are an enormous clinical and social problem in the United States, particularly for the spine, distal radius, and proximal femur, which are largely trabecular bone structures. The ways in which both density and architecture can affect the material properties of trabecular bone have been discussed. Both of these parameters change with aging, resulting in age-related trabecular bone fragility, which has been associated with the large incidence of hip, spine, and radial fractures in the elderly. Although absolute bone density is not a particularly good predictor of hip and spine fracture risk, changes (decreasing) in bone density and the resulting increase in bone fragility are good predictors of spine fracture. Thus, a major research area in trabecular bone biomechanics is quantification of age-related changes in trabecular bone density and architecture, particularly for the spine.

Figure 40 shows typical age-related changes in human trabecular bone from the lumbar spine. As the bone loses mass, its density diminishes and its architecture changes. The reductions in density depend on a number of factors, including gender and anatomic site. In general, bone mineral "density" (which reflects the areal density of both trabecular and cortical bone for a particular cross-section) declines with age, reaching lower levels in females than males. To reflect these gender-specific bone mineral "density" reductions, osteoporosis has been categorized as senile or postmenopausal. Senile osteoporosis affects both females and males, resulting in equal reductions in cortical and trabecular bone mass. Postmenopausal osteoporosis is thought to affect a relatively small subset of females, and it is characterized by excessive and disproportionate trabecular bone loss. In the lumbar spine, direct measurements have shown a decrease in trabecular bone density of approximately 50% from ages 20 to 80 years.

Results of histomorphometric studies also have shown that aging results in changes in trabecular bone architecture. These studies have demonstrated that, with decreasing density, the number and thickness of the trabeculae decrease, while the size of the intertrabecular spaces increases. Data from 3-D stereologic studies have demonstrated that, regardless of density, the number of horizontal trabeculae in the lumbar spine is less than the number of vertical

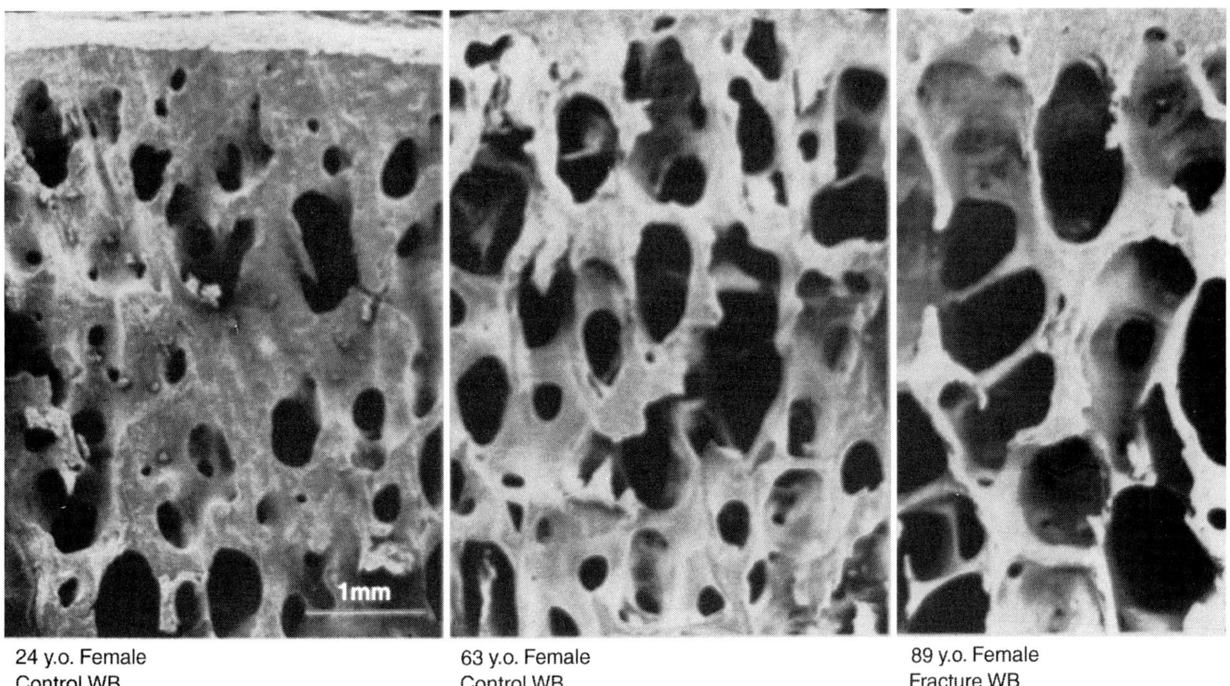

Figure 40
Photographs showing age-related changes in apparent density and architecture of human trabecular bone from the femoral head. (Courtesy of Marc D. Grynpas, PhD.)

trabeculae, and that the number of vertical trabeculae decreases with decreasing density at twice the rate of the horizontal trabeculae (Fig. 41). Thus, contrary to the evidence from earlier two-dimensional (2-D) histomorphometric studies, vertical trabeculae do not become thicker with aging, and preferential loss of horizontal trabeculae does not appear to occur in the lumbar spine. In fact, these data from 3-D studies suggest that preferential loss of vertical trabeculae occurs with increasing age. This loss of trabeculae may be more damaging to the structural integrity of trabecular bone than mere thinning because lamellar new bone can be formed only on existing surfaces, making complete loss of a single trabecula irreversible.

Because the strength of trabecular bone depends on both apparent density and architecture, these age-related changes can substantially weaken it. For example, failure caused by buckling of individual trabeculae is more likely when trabeculae become fewer, thinner, and longer. This reduced resistance to failure caused by buckling of individual trabeculae has been referred to as a "triple jeopardy," because three independent factors—reduction in number, decrease in thickness, and increase in length—contribute to the weakening mechanism. In addition, failure of individual trabeculae may occur by fracture. The weakening mechanism for fracture is reduction in the number and thickness of the trabeculae, which might be referred to as a "double jeopardy."

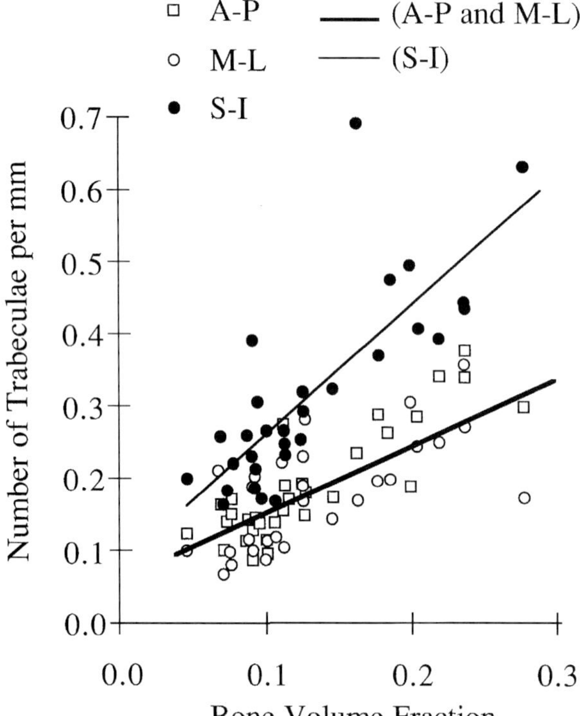

Figure 41

Decrease in the number of vertical (S-I) and horizontal (M-L, A-P) trabeculae with decreasing bone volume fraction (proportional to apparent density) for the human lumbar spine. The rate of loss of vertical trabeculae is twice that of the horizontal trabeculae. Even so, there are always more vertical than horizontal trabeculae (M-L, medial-lateral direction; S-I, superior-inferior direction; A-P, anteroposterior direction). (Reproduced with permission from Snyder BD, Hayes WC: Multiaxial structure-property relations in trabecular bone, in Mow VC, Ratcliffe A, Woo SL-Y (eds): *Biomechanics of Diarthrodial Joints*. New York, NY, Springer-Verlag, 1990, pp 31–59.)

The observed reductions in trabecular bone density are manifested as changes in the architecture, which can be quite subtle. Because of the double and triple jeopardy mechanisms, the accompanying reductions in strength may be greater than those suggested by reductions in density alone. Obviously, the accelerated bone loss that occurs with postmenopausal osteoporosis further reduces the strength of trabecular bone. Thus, normal, age-related changes, coupled with pathologic processes, can produce substantial changes in the strength of trabecular bone. This weakening must play a significant role in the etiology of age-related fractures of the hip and, particularly, of the spine. Although the material properties of trabecular bone are significantly influenced by bone density as defined by equations 3a and 3b, the influence of the 3-D architecture and connectivity of trabecular bone have not been included in these equations. However, the density, 3-D architecture, and connectivity of trabecular bone are significantly altered in pathologic states such as osteoporosis.

Fatigue properties Fractures of individual trabeculae have been observed in the lumbar spine, acetabulum, femoral head, and proximal tibia of postmortem human specimens. Tiny cracks within individual trabeculae can be repaired by callus formation, which is similar to that in fractures of long bones, resulting in the appearance of a "node" of new woven or lamellar bone about the original crack. It has been suggested that these cracks are caused by fatigue loading and that such cracks may play a role in bone remodeling, age-related fractures, subchondral collapse after aseptic necrosis of the femoral head, degenerative joint disease, and other bone disorders.

The only fatigue data available for trabecular bone are for bovine bone. Preliminary data suggest that the uniaxial compressive strength of trabecular bone can be reduced by an order of magnitude by 10^6 cycles of loading (Fig. 42). Furthermore, the resistance of trabecular bone to fatigue failure appears to be similar to that of cortical bone. The

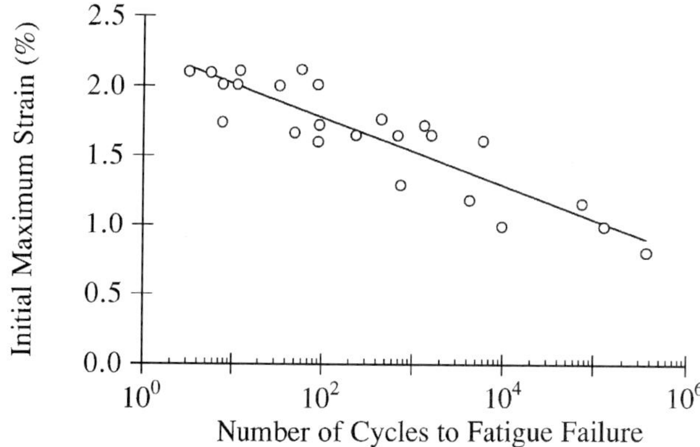

Figure 42
Fatigue, strain-life curve for bovine distal femoral trabecular bone. This experiment was performed by cyclically compressing the bone specimens between upper and lower stress levels. For each specimen, this stress range was constant so that the specimen was always in compression. The upper load level was varied for different specimens while the lower stress level was held constant. To account for variations in density, the loading is described here by dividing the upper stress level by the specimen modulus (obtained at the start of the experiment). (Reproduced with permission from Keaveny TM, Hayes WC: Mechanical properties of cortical and trabecular bone, in Hall BK (ed): *Bone*. Boca Raton, FL, CRC Press, 1993, vol 7, pp 285–344.)

mechanism for fatigue damage in trabecular bone involves fracture and buckling of individual trabeculae and, as such, differs from that of cortical bone in which cracks accumulate within the bone matrix.

Structural Properties

Bones of the appendicular skeleton are long, slender, and slightly curved. They are loaded primarily by compressive contact forces applied at the joint surfaces and by tensile muscle forces applied about the articulating surfaces. The contact forces are generally larger in magnitude than the muscle forces. The diaphysis, therefore, is loaded by a net compressive force. The combined action of the compressive and tensile forces about the joint result in a net bending moment acting on the diaphysis. This bending moment also can exist in the absence of muscle forces because of the curvature of the bone. Moreover, torque about the longitudinal axis can result in a net torsional moment about the diaphyseal axis. Therefore, long bones are subjected to a combination of axial compressive forces, bending moments, and torsion. Review of the behavior of simple structures (see the chapter on biomechanics) is suggested before continuing with examination of the structural properties of bones.

Bending of Bone

A bone can be subjected to bending loads in a number of ways, including the application of two sets of forces near the ends (Fig. 43). This loading configuration, known as four-point bending, often is used in the laboratory for studying the biomechanics of bone, and it subjects the central section of the bone to a constant bending moment M.

The mid-span deflection δ of a beam in four-point bending (Fig. 43) is given by:

$$\delta = Fa(3L^2 - 4a^2)/24EI \quad \textbf{(Eq. 4)}$$

where E is the modulus of the beam material, Fa is the resultant bending moment over the mid portion of the beam, L is the length of the beam, and I is the second moment of area (also known as the areal moment of inertia). Increasing the moment of inertia and modulus will increase the bending (structural) stiffness of a bone; increasing the length will decrease the stiffness.

While the cross-sectional area is the most important geometric parameter for axial loading, the moment of inertia is the most important geometric parameter for bending. The moment of inertia describes how the material is distributed with respect

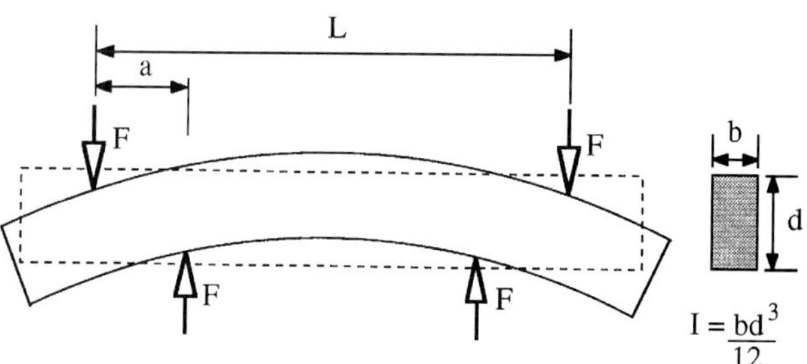

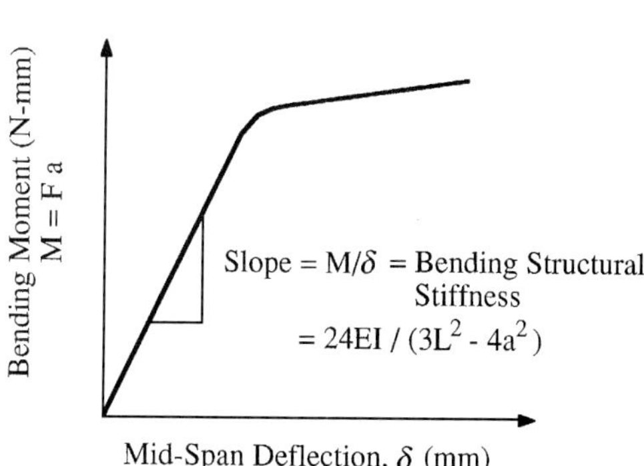

Figure 43
Beam in four-point bending, showing the undeformed shape in dashed lines and the deformed shape in solid lines. The midspan deflection δ depends on the applied bending moment, M = Fa; the geometry, L and I; and the material properties, E. The quantity I is called the areal moment of inertia.

to a specified reference axis, called the neutral axis. A region of material that is at a greater distance from the neutral axis is much more efficient in resisting bending about that axis than a region of material coincident with it. For example, consider the bending behavior of a long slender meterstick. The bending stiffness is lower when the meterstick is bent on the flat surface than when it is bent on the narrow edge because more of the material is located coincident with the neutral axis for the former case.

Long bones are hollow, with most bone tissue located away from the neutral axis, which is the centroid of the cross section. The long bone's hollow tubular structure has a physiologic role, which includes providing a bone marrow reservoir and a medullar blood supply. However, from a mechanical perspective, this geometry represents an excellent design to resist primarily bending loads in both frontal and sagittal planes and torsional loads about the diaphyseal axis.

Combined Axial and Bending Loads on Bone

The stress in the femur resulting from a combination of axial and bending loads is simply the sum of the stresses caused by each loading mode. In mathematical terms, this can be written

$$\sigma = - F/A \pm M_b t/2I \qquad \text{(Eq. 5)}$$

where F is the net axial load resulting from the joint contact and muscle forces, A is the cross-sectional area, M_b is the bending moment at the cross-section, t is the distance between the point at which the stress is calculated and the neutral axis, and I is the moment of inertia. The negative sign indicates compressive stresses, and the positive sign indicates tensile stresses.

The femur behaves as follows under combined axial and bending loads. Bending in the frontal plane causes tensile stresses along the lateral aspect and compressive stresses along the medial aspect. From Equation 5, the maximum tensile stress, which occurs on the lateral periosteal surface, is

$$\sigma_t = -F/A + M_b R/I \qquad \text{(Eq. 6a)}$$

The maximum compressive stress, which occurs on the medial periosteal surface, is

$$\sigma_c = -F/A - M_b R/I \qquad \text{(Eq. 6b)}$$

where t = R is the outside radius of the diaphysis (assumed to be circular). The medial compressive stresses from axial loading and bending are of the same sign; that is, they are additive. This property implies that there always will be compressive stresses on the medial side. On the lateral side, by contrast, the stresses resulting from axial loading and bending are of opposite signs. Either tensile or compressive stresses could occur here, depending on the relative magnitudes of the axial and bending stresses. Because bending stresses at the periosteal surfaces in the femoral diaphysis are generally much greater than axial stresses, tensile stresses occur on the lateral aspect of the femur.

Bending of the femur in the sagittal plane as a result of posteriorly directed loads also results in tensile and compressive stresses in the anterior and posterior aspects, respectively. Similar situations occur in most long bones. In general, compressive stresses are higher than tensile stresses throughout the appendicular skeleton. The compressive strength of cortical bone is greater than the tensile strength, indicating that cortical bone tissue has adapted to the higher compressive stresses that occur in long bones because of the combined compressive and bending loads commonly encountered during daily activities.

Age-Related Remodeling of the Diaphysis

Age-related remodeling of cortical bone can result in large changes in the areal moment of inertia. These geometric changes also can influence the bending stresses and, therefore, the strength of a long bone. For simplicity, assume that the femoral diaphysis can be idealized as a circular cylinder with inner and outer diameters R_i and R_o, respectively. Figure 44 shows three such cylinders with different dimensions. Cylinder A (solid; R_o = 0.94 cm) is a hypothetical solid diaphysis. Tubes B (hollow; R_o = 1.09 cm, R_i = 0.53 cm) and C (hollow; R_o = 1.25 cm, R_i = 0.76 cm) are based on typical cross-sectional geometric properties for young (B) and elderly (C) adults. These cylinders can be used to estimate how the strength of the diaphysis changes as the geometric and material properties change over time.

Recall that axial stresses are proportional to the applied axial force, and inversely proportional to the cross-sectional area $\sigma = F/A$. The cross-sectional areas are 2.77 cm^2, 2.85 cm^2, and 3.09 cm^2 for A, B, and C, respectively. Thus, if the axial loads are assumed to be constant, the axial stresses for A and B are similar because their cross-sectional areas are similar. Axial stresses in C are approximately 11% lower than in A. Recall also that bending stresses are directly proportional to the quantity R_o/I, where I is the moment of inertia, $\sigma = M_b R_o/I$. The values of R_o/I are 1.54 cm^{-3}, 1.03 cm^{-3}, and 0.75 cm^{-3} for A, B, and C, respectively. Assuming again that the applied bending moment is constant for each cylinder, the bending stresses are therefore maximum in the solid cylinder (A) and are progressively reduced in the hollow tubes (B and C).

These simple calculations indicate that axial stresses are relatively insensitive to age-related geo-

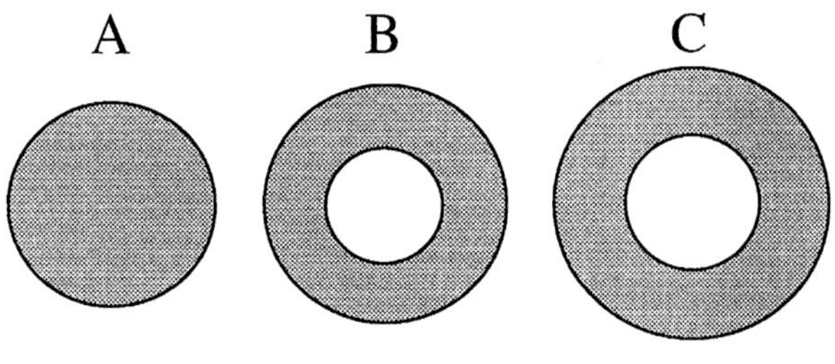

	A	B	C
Area (cm^2)	2.77	2.85	3.09
Relative Axial Strength	1.00	1.03	1.11
Moment of Inertia (cm^4)	0.61	1.06	1.67
Relative Bending Strength	1.00	1.49	2.05

Figure 44
Relative axial and bending strengths for cylinders B and C with respect to a solid cylinder A. Cylinder B represents a young diaphysis; cylinder C represents an elderly diaphysis, with enlarged endosteal and periosteal diameters. Axial strengths are relatively similar. Bending strengths, however, are progressively higher for cylinders B and C, respectively. This indicates that age-related diaphyseal expansions increase the strength of the diaphysis, which, in turn, may offset the age-related decreases in tissue strength that are known to occur for cortical bone.

metric changes, but bending stresses are quite sensitive. Age-related endosteal and periosteal expansions of the diaphysis, therefore, can reduce bending stresses (if the external loads are identical) by over 25% with respect to younger bones. Because age-related changes also result in reductions in the strength of cortical bone tissue, the age-related geometric remodeling process may serve to compensate for these tissue-level strength reductions. Evidence in support of this mechanism comes from the lack of an exponential increase in diaphyseal fracture incidence in the elderly. This is in contrast to the high rate of fracture in the proximal femur and spine, where this age-related compensatory geometric remodeling does not occur.

Torsion of Bones

If a bone is subjected to torques applied at its ends (Fig. 19), the cross section at one end rotates with respect to the cross section at the other end. The total angle of twist θ between the two ends of the bone is given by

$$\theta = M_t l_0 / G I p \quad \textbf{(Eq. 7)}$$

where θ is the angle of twist (in radians, 2π radians = 360°), M_t is the torque (in Newton-meters, N·m), l_0 is the length of the bone, G is the shear modulus (in MPa), and Ip is the polar moment of inertia (in m^4). The shear modulus G measures the resistance of a material to shearing deformations. For most materials, the shear modulus is about one-half the Young's modulus. The polar moment of inertia Ip like the areal moment of inertia I expresses how the material in a cross section is distributed with respect to a specified axis. In the case of the areal moment of inertia, this specified axis (the neutral axis) is in the plane of the cross section. In the case of torsion, the polar moment of inertia describes the distribution of the cross-sectional area with respect to an axis perpendicular to the cross section and corresponding to the longitudinal, centroid axis of the bar. For a solid, cylindrical bar of diameter D, the polar moment of inertia Ip is given by

$$Ip = \pi D^4/32 \quad \textbf{(Eq. 8)}$$

Torsional loads cause shear stress τ, which can be calculated for a circular cylinder as follows

$$\tau = M_t r / Ip \quad \textbf{(Eq. 9)}$$

where r is the distance from the axis of torsion and M_t is the torque. Equation 9 indicates that shear stresses are zero at the center of the circular cross section where r = 0 and maximum at the surface where r = D/2.

Combined Axial, Bending, and Torsional Loads

Stresses resulting from axial loading and bending can be combined by simple addition when the stresses act in the same direction. When shear stresses resulting from torsion are superimposed, the axial, bending, and shear stresses are combined in a more complex manner to give a tensile or compressive stress, called a principal stress, which acts in the principal direction. When there is no torsion, the principal stress is the sum of the axial and bending stresses, and the principal direction is in the direction of the axial and bending stresses. For combined axial, bending, and shear stresses, the principal stress will be greater than the sum of the axial and bending stresses, and the principal direction will differ from the direction of the axial and bending stresses. Thus, the effect of imposing a torsional load on combined axial and bending loads is to increase the principal stress and change the principal direction.

The principal stress resulting from combined axial, bending, and torsional loads is derived by calculating the normal stress caused by combined axial and bending loads, then calculating the shear stress caused by torsion, and, finally, using standard engineering formulae to calculate the principal stress from the normal and shear stresses. If the mid-diaphysis of an elderly femur is assumed to be circular and to have inner and outer radii of 0.76 cm and 1.25 cm, respectively, then the areal and polar moments of inertia are 1.66 cm^4 and 3.32 cm^4, respectively, and the cross-sectional area is 3.09 cm^2. Typical axial, bending, and torsional loads on the femoral diaphysis of an elderly male (70 kg) during normal gait are approximately 800 N, 90 N·m, and 35 N·m, respectively. Using Equations 6a and 9, the combined axial (-2.6 MPa) and tensile bending (67.8 MPa) stress is 65.2 MPa; the shear stress is 13.2 MPa. The corresponding tensile principal stress is 67.8 MPa. These stresses would act on the lateral aspect of the diaphysis. For the medial aspect, there are compressive bending stresses, and the compressive principal stress is -72.8 MPa. Thus, for normal gait in an elderly male, the superposition of the torsional load on the combined axial and bending loads increases the magnitude of the maximum tensile and compressive stresses in the diaphysis by approximately 3.9% and 3.4%, respectively. Consequently, torsional loading of the diaphysis does not contribute much to its fracture by either tensile or compressive failure of cortical bone tissue. However, if shear stresses become greater than the shear strength of cortical bone (70 MPa), failure could occur by shear failure of the cortical bone tissue.

Bone Metabolism and Mineral Homeostasis

Bone-mineral homeostasis is tightly controlled by the synchronized action of the vitamin D_3 metabolites, parathyroid hormone (PTH), and calcitonin. Together these hormones regulate the dietary absorption of calcium, bone mineral resorption and deposition, and renal secretion and resorption of calcium and phosphorus. In this way, the control of bone mineral homeostasis is an integral part of the control of the serum calcium concentration.

Vitamin D Pathways

Vitamin D is a potent calcitropic hormone. Its primary function is to enhance calcium and phosphorus absorption across the lumen of the small intestine and to enhance calcium and phosphorus resorption from bone. Ultraviolet light acting on the skin transforms 7-dehydrocholesterol into Vitamin D_3 (cholecalciferol). One hour of direct sunlight on a Caucasian face produces the daily requirement of 400 units of vitamin D. Dark skinned individuals require more direct sunlight. Vitamin D occurs rarely in natural foods (cod-liver oil) and, consequently, is added to some foods as vitamin D_2 (radiated ergosterol). Vitamin D (D_2 or D_3) is hydroxylated in the liver to 25-hydroxyvitamin D (25(OH)vitamin D_3). Both vitamin D_3 and 25(OH)vitamin D_3 are inactive precursor vitamins. A serum 25(OH)vitamin D_3 level is the best indication of body stores of vitamin D_3. In the presence of PTH, or hypocalcemia or hypophosphatemia, an enzyme in the mitochondria of the kidney's proximal tubules hydroxylates the 25(OH)vitamin D_3 into the active hormone metabolite 1,25-dihydroxyvitamin D_3 (1,25$(OH)_2$ vitamin D_3). Figures 45 and 46 illustrate the metabolic pathways of vitamin D.

Calcium Homeostasis: Vitamin D, PTH, and Calcitonin

The maintenance of a stable calcium gradient between the extracellular and intracellular environments is essential for life. Normally, extracellular concentration of calcium is about five orders of magnitude (10^5) greater than the intracellular concentration. A number of complex intracellular systems are responsible for the microregulation of intracellular calcium homeostasis. Of total body calcium, 99% is sequestered in the skeleton, leaving approximately 1% to circulate in the extracellular fluid. It is this 1% that is so assiduously controlled and regulated by the PTH-vitamin D-calcitonin endocrine system. These three calcitropic hormones, in conjunction with other paracrine factors, not only modulate the concentration of serum calcium in the extracellular fluid, they control the fluctuation of the calcium from the outside to the inside of the cell. The endocrine control of cytosolic and extracellular calcium and associated phosphorus metabolism are outlined in Table 2.

Calcium Nutritional Requirements

Proper calcium nutrition is critical to bone maintenance. Chronic mild deficiency will lead to a negative calcium balance and gradual loss of bone

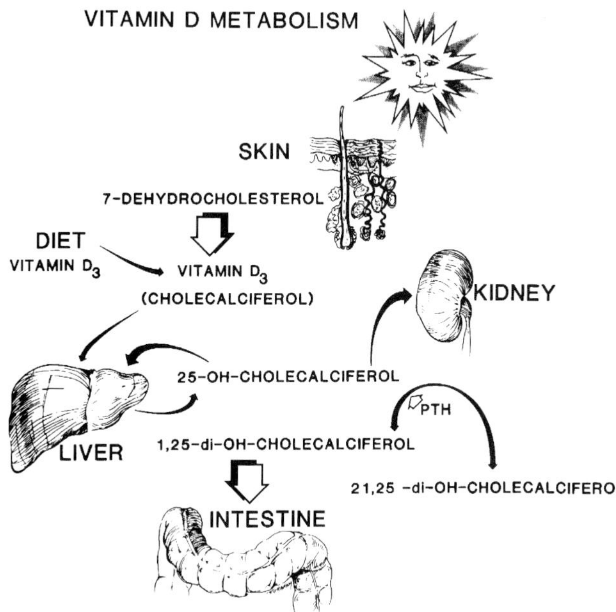

Figure 45
Diagram showing the metabolic pathways of vitamin D.

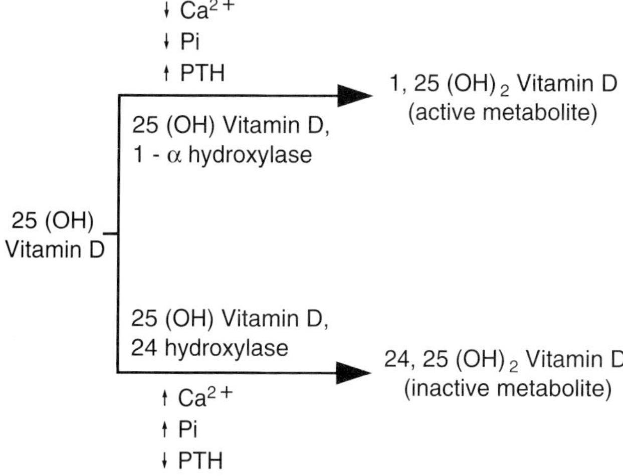

Figure 46
Vitamin D metabolism in renal tubular cell.

mass. In young individuals, approximately 15% to 25% of ingested calcium is absorbed. In elderly persons, this percentage declines; consequently, the elderly require more dietary calcium to achieve the same net calcium transport across the intestinal lumen. Augmented dietary calcium also may be necessary during the adolescent growth spurt, during early adulthood when maximum bone mass is being achieved, during pregnancy, and, especially, during lactation.

Table 3 provides guidelines for minimum daily calcium requirement by age and activity level.

Elaborate endocrine feedback loops exist to prevent dangerous and life-threatening hypocalcemia. A reduction in ionized serum calcium levels engenders a host of protective mechanisms, which serve to restore the serum calcium level to normal through more efficient absorption from the gastrointestinal tract, reabsorption from the kidney, and resorption from bone. Primary disorders of this regulatory system may lead to chronic hypocalcemia or hypercalcemia and promote symptomatic clinical disease. The major metabolic pathways involved in the maintenance of a normal concentration of calcium in the extracellular fluid are outlined in Figure 47.

Age-Related Changes in Bone Mass and Morphology

Figure 48 illustrates the relationship between age, bone mass, and gender. Much anabolic skeletal activity occurs during the adolescent growth spurt. Early in adolescence, the skeleton undergoes rapid longitudinal growth with only moderate increase in mineral content. The addition of layers of bone at the periosteum and endosteum is balanced by an increase in the porosity of the bone. Increased bone turnover provides some of the minerals needed for the new bone. Not until late adolescence, when longitudinal growth slows, does bone mineral content rapidly increase. Bone mass peaks after skeletal maturity some time during the third decade.

In the period between the onset of adolescence and skeletal maturity, dietary habits and hereditary factors play a large role in determining the ultimate size of the bone mineral bank. The size of this bank stays nearly constant throughout most of adult life, with the body redistributing its assets according to structural needs. Until adolescence, bone mass is equal for blacks and whites; thereafter, bone mass increases to a greater level in blacks. The factors responsible for this are unknown. By the fifth decade, bone mass begins to decline, with dramatic gender differences in bone loss. Both men and women lose cortical bone at the same rate; however, trabecular bone mass decreases more rapidly in women with the onset of menopause and thereafter. Local bone loss is variable throughout the skeleton. Evidence from kinetic studies indicates that after age 40, formation rates remain constant while resorption rates increase. Over several decades, the skeletal mass may be reduced to 50% of original trabecular and 25% of cortical mass.

In the decade after age 40, men lose only about 0.5% to 0.75% of bone mass yearly, while women lose bone at more than twice that rate (1.5% to 2% a year).

Table 2
Regulation of calcium and phosphate metabolism

	Parathyroid hormone (PTH) (peptide)	1,25 $(OH)_2$ D* (steroid)	Calcitonin (peptide)
Origin	Chief cells of parathyroid glands	Proximal tubule of kidney	Parafollicular cells of thyroid gland
Factors stimulating production	Decreased serum Ca^{2+}	Elevated PTH Decreased serum Ca^{2+} Decreased serum P_i	Elevated serum Ca^{2+}
Factors inhibiting production	Elevated serum Ca^{2+} Elevated 1,25 $(OH)_2$ D	Decreased PTH Elevated serum Ca^{2+} Elevated serum P_i	Decreased serum Ca^{2+}
Effect on end organs for hormone action			
Intestine	No direct effect Acts indirectly on bowel by stimulating production of 1,25 $(OH)_2$ D in kidney	Strongly stimulates intestinal absorption of Ca^{2+} and P_i	?
Kidney	Stimulates 25 (OH) D - 1α - OH_{ase} in mitochondria of proximal tubular cells to convert 25 (OH) D to 1,25 $(OH)_2$ D Increases fractional resorption of filtered Ca^{2+} Promotes urinary excretion of P_i	?	?
Bone	Stimulates osteoclastic resorption of bone Stimulates recruitment of preosteoclasts	Strongly stimulates osteoclastic resorption of bone	Inhibits osteoclastic resorption of bone ? Role in normal human physiology
Net effect on calcium and phosphate concentrations in extracellular fluid and serum	Increased serum calcium Decreased serum phosphate	Increased serum calcium Increased serum phosphate	Decreased serum calcium (transient)

* 1,25 $(OH)_2$ D = 1,25-dihydroxyvitamin D; PTH = parathyroid hormone; 25 (OH) D = 25-hydroxyvitamin D.
(Adapted from an original painting by Frank H. Netter, MD from the CIBA COLLECTION OF MEDICAL ILLUSTRATIONS, copyright by CIBA-GEIGY Corporation.)

Table 3
Guidelines for calcium requirements

Group	Daily Elemental Calcium Requirements*
Children	500-700 mg
Growth spurt to young adult (10–25 years)	1,300 mg
Adult male (25–65 years)	750 mg
Adult female (25–55 years)	
Postmenopausal	1,500 mg
Elderly	1,200 mg
Pregnancy	1,500 mg
Lactation	2,000 mg
Healing long bone fracture	1,500 mg

*One daily equivalent of calcium is equal to 250 mg of elemental calcium. One equivalent is equal to an 8 oz glass of milk.

The rate of bone loss following menopause may temporarily approach 3% a year in some women.

Figure 49 depicts the four major mechanisms of bone mass regulation. In the healthy young adult skeleton, bone formation and resorption are tightly coupled. Uncoupling leads to changes in bone density in adults. Increased bone formation without elevated resorption will result in increased bone mass; an unchecked increase in osteoclast activity will cause an overall loss of bone mass.

Metabolic Bone Disease

Metabolic bone diseases are generalized disorders of skeletal homeostasis and comprise some of the most common and some of the most esoteric disorders seen by the orthopaedist. Although, over the past decade, great progress has been made in the understanding of metabolic bone disease, diagnostic

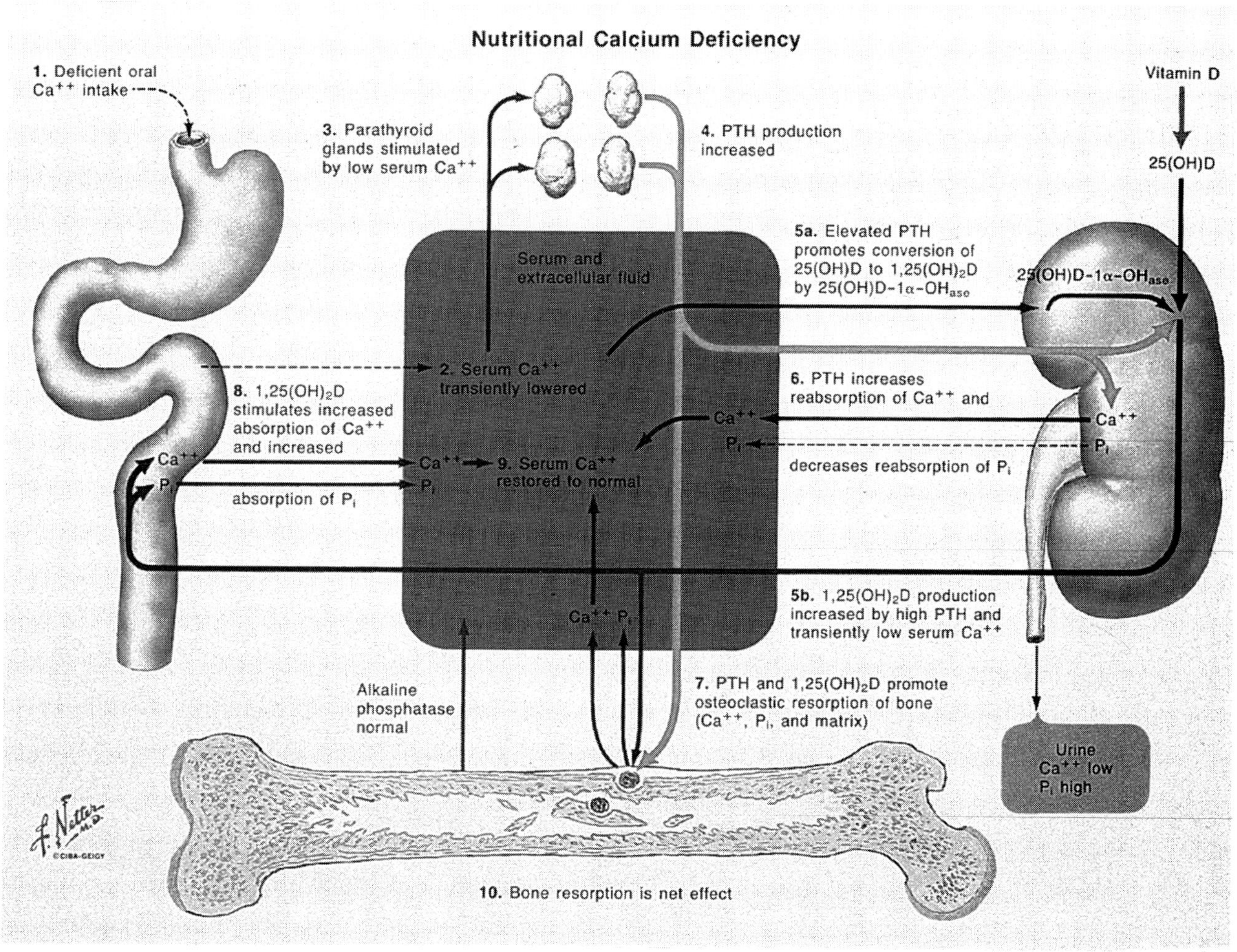

Nutritional Calcium Deficiency

1. Deficient oral Ca^{++} intake

3. Parathyroid glands stimulated by low serum Ca^{++}

4. PTH production increased

Vitamin D

25(OH)D

Serum and extracellular fluid

5a. Elevated PTH promotes conversion of 25(OH)D to $1,25(OH)_2D$ by 25(OH)D-1α-OH_{ase}

25(OH)D-1α-OH_{ase}

2. Serum Ca^{++} transiently lowered

6. PTH increases reabsorption of Ca^{++} and

8. $1,25(OH)_2D$ stimulates increased absorption of Ca^{++} and increased

absorption of P_i

9. Serum Ca^{++} restored to normal

decreases reabsorption of P_i

5b. $1,25(OH)_2D$ production increased by high PTH and transiently low serum Ca^{++}

Alkaline phosphatase normal

7. PTH and $1,25(OH)_2D$ promote osteoclastic resorption of bone (Ca^{++}, P_i, and matrix)

Urine Ca^{++} low P_i high

10. Bone resorption is net effect

Figure 47
Nutritional calcium deficiency. (© Copyright 1987 CIBA-GEIGY Corporation. Reprinted with permission from the CIBA COLLECTION OF MEDICAL ILLUSTRATIONS, illustrated by Frank H. Netter, MD. All rights reserved.)

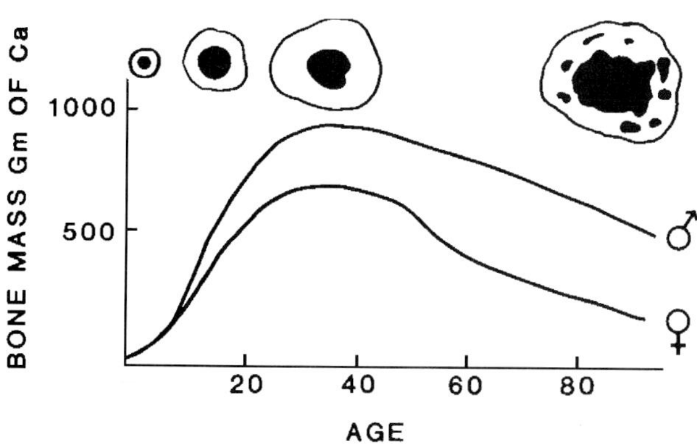

Figure 48
Graph showing the relationship among bone mass, age, and sex.

difficulty has resulted in great confusion, making basic definitions essential. Osteopenia is a generic word used to describe the radiographic picture of decreased bone density. Osteopenia is neither a disease nor a diagnosis and conveys no information about the underlying etiology of the condition. Osteoporosis, on the other hand, is a more specific term referring to a state of decreased mass per unit volume (density) of normally mineralized bone matrix (Fig. 50, *top center*). When this decrease leads to increased skeletal fragility, a pathologic state of osteoporosis exists. Osteomalacia refers to an increased, normal, or decreased mass of insufficiently mineralized bone matrix (Fig. 50, *top right*). Figure 50, *bottom*, is a photomicrograph of a transcortical bone biopsy specimen, which demonstrates sparse trabeculae with cortical resorption.

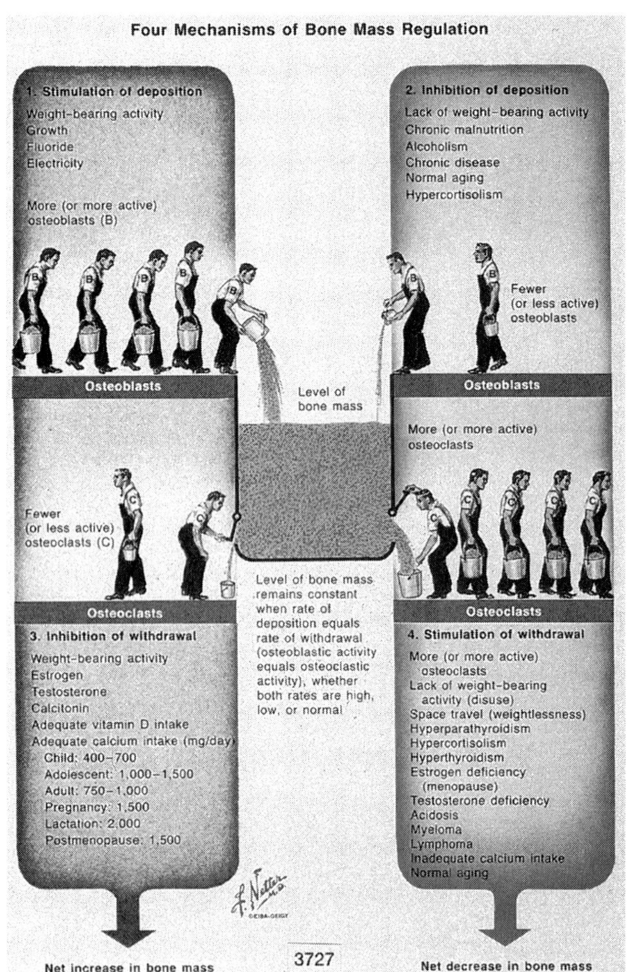

Figure 49
Four mechanisms of bone mass regulation. (© Copyright 1987 CIBA-GEIGY Corporation. Reprinted with permission from the CIBA COLLECTION OF MEDICAL ILLUSTRATIONS, illustrated by Frank H. Netter, MD. All rights reserved.)

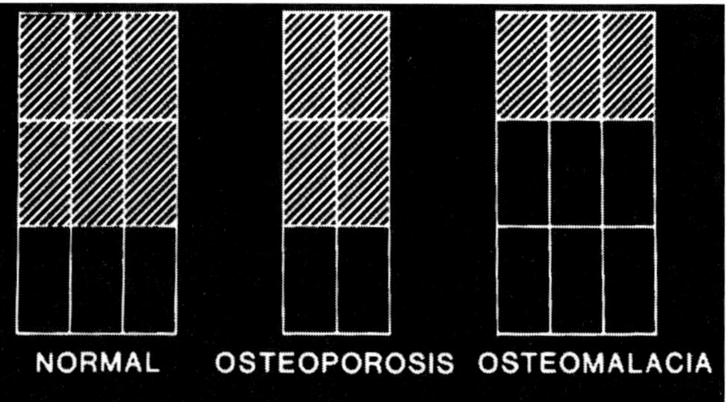

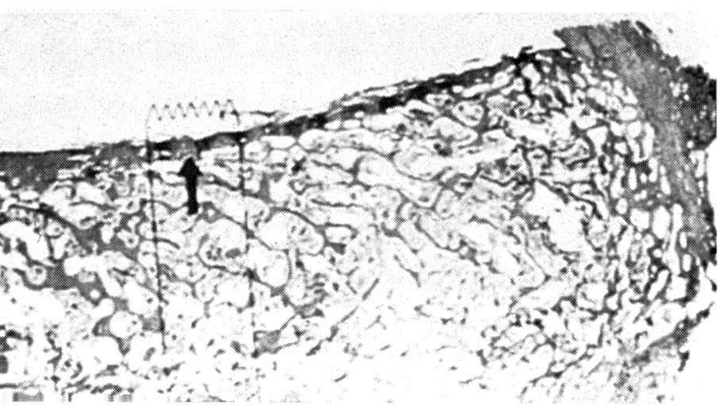

Figure 50
Top, Diagram showing amount (number of sections) of normally mineralized (cross-hatched sections) and insufficiently mineralized (blank sections) bone matrix. **Bottom,** Photomicrograph of transcortical bone biopsy specimen.

Osteomalacia

Deficient or impaired mineralization of bone matrix (osteoid) is the diagnostic feature of all osteomalacic syndromes, regardless of etiology. Rickets, the juvenile counterpart of osteomalacia, refers to the impaired mineralization of cartilage matrix (chondroid) and a resultant arrest in formation of primary spongiosa. Osteomalacia can be present at any age, once lamellar bone has formed. Rickets is exclusively a disorder of children.

The single most important causative factor in the development of osteomalacia is the failure to maintain a serum calcium-phosphorus level sufficient to promote mineralization of newly-formed osteoid. The etiologies of osteomalacia are numerous but easily may be classified into five major categories (Outline 1). The serum, urine, and bone biopsy findings in the various metabolic bone diseases are detailed in Table 4.

The management of the individual osteomalacic condition depends on the specific pathophysiology. The unifying theme in the treatment of all rachitic and osteomalacic conditions is the restoration of the serum calcium-phosphorus level to normal so that normal mineralization of cartilage and bone matrix can occur. Vitamin-D deficiency states may be treated by providing the vitamin, which is a fat-soluble sterol that has a long half-life, or providing its metabolites, 25(OH) vitamin D or $1,25(OH)_2$ vitamin D, just distal to any metabolic block. Vitamin D-resistant conditions are treated by providing phosphorus, and possibly other nutrients, and suppressing the excess of PTH, which will arise with phosphate treatment alone, with the administration of calcitriol (1,25-dihydroxyvitamin D). All therapy must be carefully monitored to prevent hypercalcemia or an excess of vitamin D. Calcitriol therapy should be stopped 24 hours prior to corrective osteotomies, and may be resumed following surgery when the patient is ambulatory.

Outline 1:
Causes of rickets and osteomalacia

Nutritional Deficiency
- Vitamin D deficiency
- Dietary chelators (rare) of calcium
  - Phytates
  - Oxalates (spinach)
- Phosphorus deficiency (unusual)
  - Antacid (aluminum-containing) abuse leading to severe dietary phosphate binding

Gastrointestinal absorption defects
- Post-gastrectomy (rare today)
- Biliary disease (interference with absorption of fat-soluble vitamin D)
- Enteric absorption defects
  - Short bowel syndrome
  - Rapid-transit (gluten-sensitive enteropathy) syndromes
  - Inflammatory bowel disease
    - Crohn's disease
    - Celiac disease

Renal tubular defects (renal phosphate leak)
- X-linked dominant hypophosphatemic vitamin D-resistant rickets (VDRR) or osteomalacia
- Classic Albright's syndrome or Fanconi's syndrome-type I
- Fanconi's syndrome-type II
- Phosphaturia and glycosuria
- Fanconi's syndrome-type III
- Phosphaturia, glycosuria, and aminoaciduria.
- Vitamin D-dependent rickets (or osteomalacia)-type I. A genetic or acquired deficiency of renal tubular 25-hydroxyvitamin D 1-alpha hydroxylase enzyme prevents conversion of 25 hydroxyvitamin D to active polar metabolite 1,25 dihydroxyvitamin D.
- Vitamin D-dependent rickets (or osteomalacia)-type II. This represents enteric end organ insensitivity to 1,25 dihydroxyvitamin D and is probably caused by an abnormality in the 1,25 dihydroxyvitamin D nuclear receptor.
- Renal Tubular Acidosis
  - Acquired—associated with many systemic diseases
  - Genetic:
    - Debre-De Toni-Fanconi syndrome
    - Lignac-Fanconi syndrome (cysteinosis)
    - Lowe's syndrome

Renal Osteodystrophy

Miscellaneous Causes
- Soft-tissue tumors secreting putative factors
  - Fibrous dysplasia
  - Neurofibromatosis
  - Other soft-tissue and vascular mesenchymal tumors
- Anticonvulsant medication. Induction of hepatic P450 microsomal enzyme system by some anticonvulsants (phenytoin, phenobarbital, mysoline) causes increased degradation of Vitamin D metabolites.
- Heavy metal intoxication
- Hypophosphatasia
- High dose diphosphonates
- Sodium fluoride

Renal Osteodystrophy

Renal osteodystrophy is a common complication of chronic renal failure and is one of the most common causes of osteomalacia. Chronic glomerular disease leads to renal insufficiency, azotemia, and acidosis. The resulting metabolic changes often produce profound skeletal effects. These skeletal changes can include rickets or osteomalacia (Fig. 51, *left*), osteitis fibrosa (Fig. 51, *right*), osteoporosis, osteosclerosis, and metastatic calcification.

The mechanism of the bone changes in renal osteodystrophy is complex (Fig. 52). The major abnormalities are phosphate retention secondary to uremia and insufficient renal synthesis of $1{,}25(OH)_2$ vitamin D. These two abnormalities result in hypocalcemia leading to secondary hyperparathyroidism, with bone changes of osteitis fibrosa. In some cases of secondary hyperparathyroidism, the solubility of serum calcium and phosphorus is exceeded, and ectopic calcification may occur in the conjunctivae, blood vessels, periarticular tissues,

Table 4
Serum and urine findings in various metabolic bone diseases

Disorder	[Ca]*	[Pi]	AP	PTH	25 (OH) Vitamin D	1,25 $(OH)_2$ Vitamin D	Urinary Calcium	Bone Biopsy Findings	Associated Findings
Postmenopausal osteoporosis (type I)	N	N	N	N,↓	N	N	↑,N	Variable	Osteopenia
Age-related osteoporosis (type II)	N	N	N	↑,N	N	N	N	Variable	Osteopenia
Chronic glucocorticoid associated osteoporosis	N	N	N	↑,N	N	N	↑,N	Inactive turnover	Severe osteopenia
Primary hyperparathyroidism	↑	N,↓	N,↑	↑	N	↑,N	↑	Active turnover; peritrabecular fibrosis	Variable, depending on degree of hypercalcemia
Cancer with bony metastases	↑	↑,N	↑,N	N,↓	N	N,↓	↑↑	Tumor	History of primary tumor; bony destruction; + bone scan
Multiple myeloma; lymphoma	↑	↑,N	↑,N	N,↓	N	N,↓	↑↑	Confirmatory for tumor	Destructive lesions on radiographs; abnormal protein electrophoresis
Primary carcinoma not involving bone	↑	↓	↑,N	↓	N	↓	↑↑	Variable	Osteopenia, ↑ PTH-related peptide
Sarcoidosis	↑	↑,N	↑,N	N,↓	N	↑	↑	Active turnover	Hilar adenopathy
Hyperthyroidism	↑	N	N	N,↓	N	N	↑	Active turnover	↑ FTI; ↓ TSH; Osteopenia; tachycardia, tremor, systemic hyperthyroid changes
Vitamin D intoxication	↑	↑,N	↑,N	N,↓	↑↑↑	N	↑	Active turnover	History of excessive vitamin D intake
Milk-alkali syndrome	↑	↑,N	↑,N	N,↓	N	N,↓	↑	Variable	History of excessive calcium and alkalai ingestion (antacids).
Severe generalized immobilization	↑	↑,N	↑,N	N,↓	N	N,↓	↑↑	Active turnover	Osteopenia; multiple fractures; neurologic dysfunction
Vitamin D deficiency (dietary; gastrointestinal)	N,↓	↓	↑	↑	↓	↓	↓	Osteomalacia	
Dietary phosphate deficiency (Rare)	N	↓	↑	N	N	↑	N	Osteomalacia; absence of hyperparathyroid changes	Phosphate-binding antacid abuse with normal renal function
Mesenchymal tumor producing phosphaturic factor	N	↓	↑	N	N	N	N	Osteomalacia; absence of hyperparathyroid changes	Normal 1,25$(OH)_2$ vitamin D level but inappropriately low considering degree of phosphaturia
vitamin-D resistance (X-Linked dominant-Albright's syndrome)	N	↓	↑	N	N	N	N	Osteomalacia; absence of hyperparathyroid changes	Normal 1,25$(OH)_2$ vitamin D level but inappropriately low considering degree of phosphaturia
Fanconi-type II	N	↓	↑	N	N	N	N	Osteomalacia; absence of hyperparathyroid changes	Normal 1,25$(OH)_2$ vitamin D level but inappropriately low considering degree of phosphaturia; glycosuria
Fanconi-type III	N	↓	↑	N	N	N	N	Osteomalacia; absence of hyperparathyroid changes	Normal 1,25$(OH)_2$ vitamin D level but inappropriately low considering degree of phosphaturia; aminoaciduria
Vitamin D dependent rickets (type I) rare	↓	↓	↑	↑	N	↓↓	↓	Osteomalacia; hyperparathyroid changes	Defect in renal converting enzyme from 25(OH) vitamin D to 1,25 $(OH)_2$ vitamin D
Vitamin D dependent rickets (type II) rare	↓	↓	↑	↑	N	↑↑	↓	Osteomalacia; hyperparathyroid changes	Probable 1,25$(OH)_2$ vitamin D receptor defect
Renal tubular acidosis	↓	↓	↑	↑	N	↑,N	↑	Osteomalacia; hyperparathyroid changes	Elevated blood urea nitrogen and creatinine
Renal osteodystrophy (mixed)	N,↓	↑↑	↑	↑↑	N	↓↓	–	Pure osteomalacia; aluminum at mineralization front	Elevated blood urea nitrogen and creatinine
Renal osteodystrophy (predominant aluminum-associated osteomalacia)	↑,N	↑,N	↑	↑	N	↓↓	–	Pure osteomalacia; aluminum at mineralization	Elevated blood urea nitrogen and creatinine
Hypophosphatasia	↑	↑	↓↓	N	N	N	↑	Pure osteomalacia	Elevated urinary phosphoethanolamine; early loss of teeth

*Ca, calcium; Pi, phosphate; AP, alkaline phosphatase; PTH, parathyroid hormone; 25(OH) Vitamin D, 25 hydroxyvitamin D; 1,25$(OH)_2$ vitamin D, 1,25 dihydroxyvitamin D.

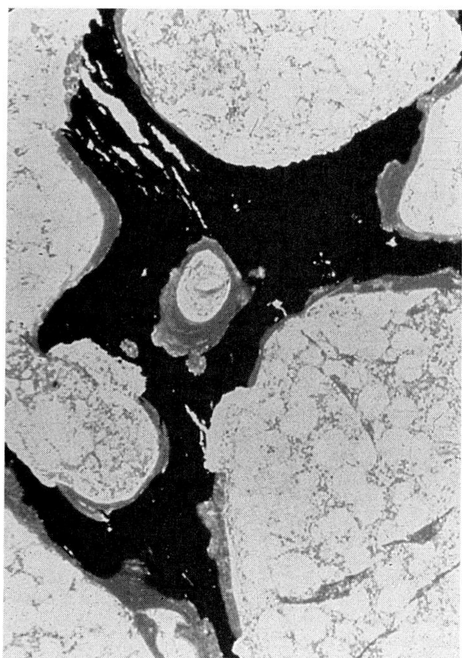

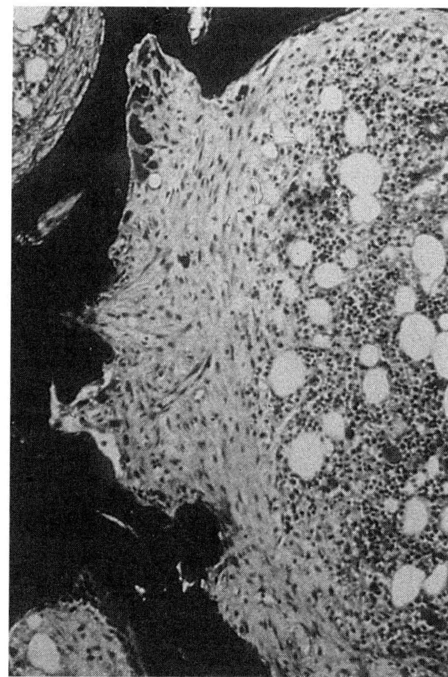

Figure 51
Photomicrographs showing hyperparathyroidism.

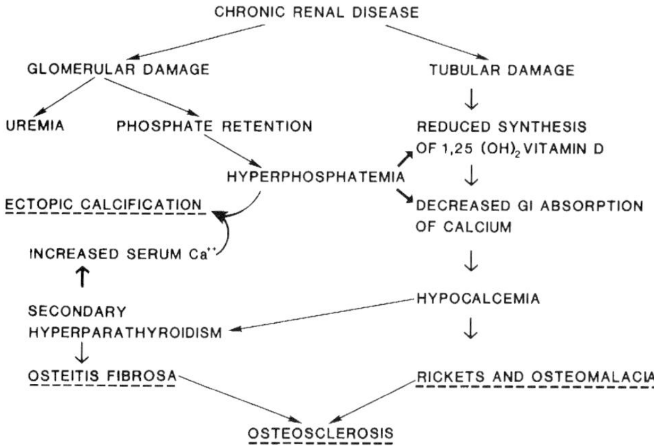

Figure 52
Pathogenesis of bone changes in renal osteodystrophy.

and skin. As the renal failure progresses and the glomerular filtration rate falls below 20 ml/min, the persistent acidosis further aggravates the negative calcium balance.

During the past decade, a form of renal osteodystrophy has been identified, which is characterized by pure osteomalacia. The commonly accepted cause is aluminum from the aluminum-containing phosphate binders that are prescribed for the treatment of hyperphosphatemia in renal failure. Aluminum is readily absorbed in the gastrointestinal tract and normally is excreted by the kidneys. However, in the presence of renal failure, aluminum may accumulate and preferentially be deposited in the brain, leading to dementia, and in the bone, leading to osteomalacia. The mechanism by which aluminum deposition causes osteomalacia is unclear, but evidence suggests that the aluminum inhibits mineralization either by inhibiting calcium (cation) deposition or by toxicity to osteoblastic mitochondrial function. Attempts to eradicate this problem have included the investigational substitution of calcium carbonate, an alternate phosphate binder.

The skeletal manifestations of renal osteodystrophy are similar to those of other forms of rickets/osteomalacia. Most patients have severe bone pain and tenderness and may have pathologic fractures. The radiographic findings of renal osteodystrophy reflect the clinical and biochemical changes seen and vary widely, with most patients exhibiting a mixed disease pattern (Fig. 53).

Osteosclerosis may be present in 20% of renal osteodystrophy patients; it may be eccentrically located in the long bones or seen as dense and lucent bands in the spine ("rugger-jersey" spine). Hyperparathyroidism can result in osteosclerosis through an increase in osteoid deposition and osteoblastic activity. Slipped capital femoral epiphyses may be indicative of renal osteodystrophy in children (Fig. 54).

Laboratory findings include elevated blood urea nitrogen and creatinine levels, normal or low serum calcium, and a serum inorganic phosphate that is

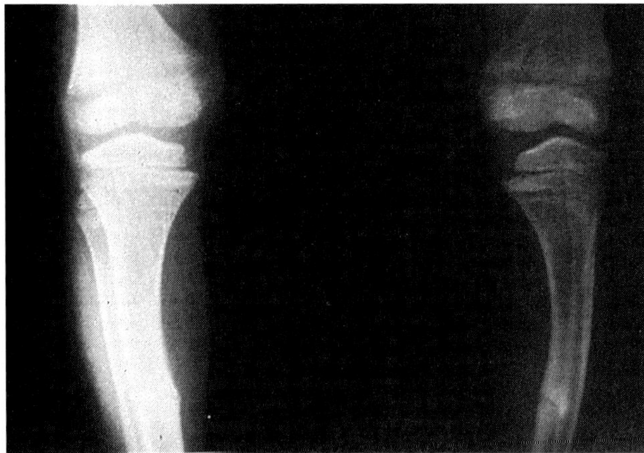

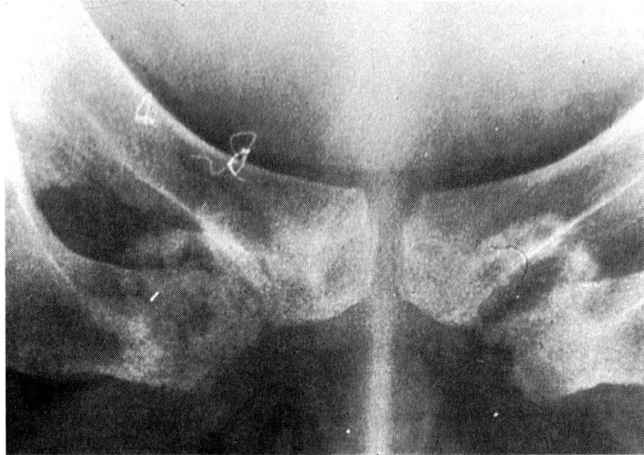

Figure 53
Radiographs showing osteomalacia.

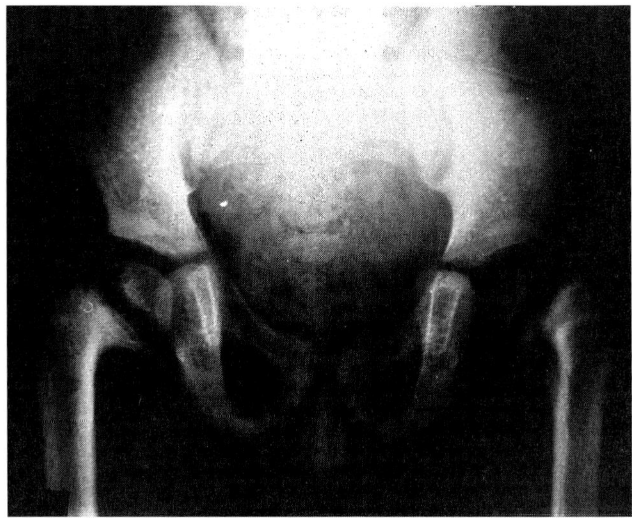

Figure 54
Radiograph of renal osteodystrophy.

usually over 5.5 mg%. The alkaline phosphatase and PTH levels are almost invariably elevated. Approximately 20% of patients with renal osteodystrophy have relatively normal calcium and phosphorus levels, have only slightly increased PTH levels, and suffer from profound osteomalacia. These findings probably are related to extremely high levels of phosphate-binder related aluminum deposits in the bone of some of these patients.

Although the diagnosis of renal osteodystrophy is usually obvious, a tetracycline-labeled bone biopsy is used for the best evaluation of the individual components of this disease. Analysis of a bone biopsy currently is the only reliable means of determining bone aluminum deposition. This evaluation is needed to guide treatment of the variable components (that is, osteomalacia, hyperparathyroidism, and aluminum deposition).

Medical treatments for renal osteodystrophy include (1) adjusting the serum calcium and phosphorus levels to normal; (2) suppressing secondary hyperparathyroidism; (3) preventing extraskeletal deposits of calcium and phosphorus by normalization of the calcium-phosphorus level; and (4) chelating bone aluminum in patients with aluminum-associated osteomalacia. Overall management of the renal disease includes chronic dialysis or renal transplantation. Additional measures include administration of calcium carbonate to diminish hyperphosphatemia, administration of 1,25$(OH)_2$ vitamin D to increase calcium absorption and to decrease PTH secretion, and parathyroidectomy to control the occasional autonomous hyperparathyroidism. Because, in the presence of bone aluminum deposition, parathyroidectomy may actually worsen bone change by decreasing bone remodeling rates, a bone biopsy is suggested in patients who have renal osteodystrophy before consideration of parathyroidectomy. Desferoxamine, a chelator of trivalent cations, has proven to be an effective chelator of aluminum in patients in whom a biopsy has documented aluminum-associated osteomalacia.

Endocrinopathies Affecting Bone

A large number of endocrinopathies affect bone formation or resorption and lead to impaired bone metabolism. Some of these are PTH excess, thyroid hormone excess, glucocorticoid excess (Cushing's disease), juvenile onset diabetes mellitus (type I), and estrogen deficiency (Fig. 55). PTH enhances both bone resorption (osteoclastic activity) and bone formation (osteoblastic activity). With continuous production or administration of PTH, overall metabolism is enhanced and resorption surpasses formation leading to net bone loss. However, recent studies indicate that pulsed administration of PTH may enhance formation over resorption. Thyroid

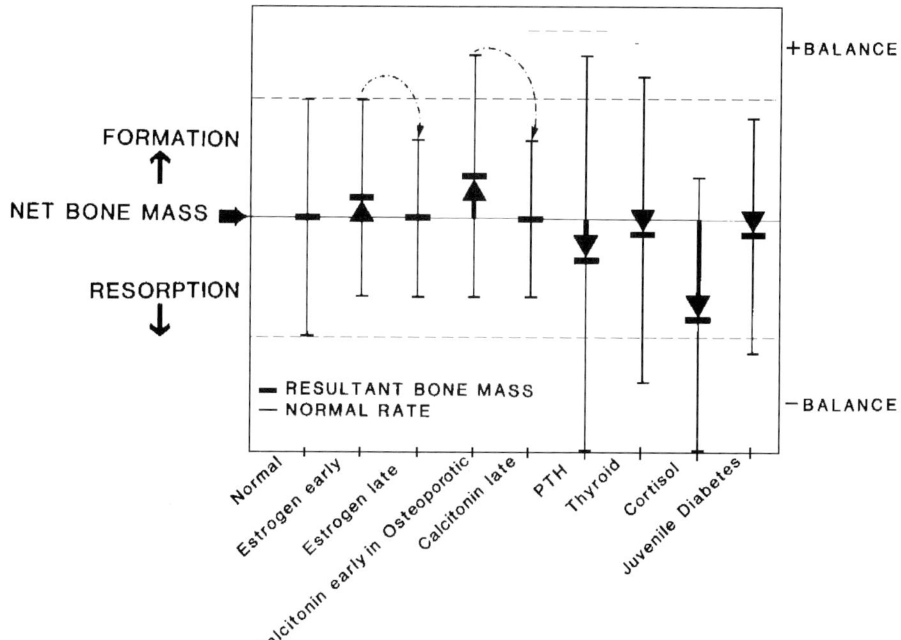

Figure 55
Bone mass regulation by hormones.

hormone excess leads to excessive bone turnover and results in gradual net bone loss. Thyroid hormone immunoradiometric assay (TSH-IRMA) is the best assay for monitoring thyroid replacement to prevent iatrogenic hyperthyroidism.

Excessive cortisol, either endogenous or exogenous, is most deleterious to bone mass. This corticosteroid decreases calcium absorption across the intestinal lumen, enhances calcium loss from the kidney, inhibits bone formation (especially collagen synthesis), and causes secondary hyperparathyroidism with concurrent enhancement of bone resorption, resulting in marked loss of bone mass. An alternate-day treatment regimen with one day at physiologic levels may be less damaging. Administration of calcium, vitamin D, hydrochlorothiazide (to prevent renal calcium loss), and calcitonin (to prevent bone resorption) may counter some of the deleterious effects of cortisol administration.

Juvenile onset diabetes mellitus (type I) may lead to bone loss. Poorly controlled diabetes mellitus leads to diuresis of calcium. Bone formation is decreased and secondary hyperparathyroidism compensating for urinary calcium loss leads to net bone loss.

Clinically, estrogen supplementation decreases bone loss but does not appreciably alter formation. Consequently, the primary effect of estrogen therapy is the maintenance of bone mass. Calcitonin decreases osteoclastic and osteocytic bone resorption and, for the short term, enhances bone formation, leading to slight net bone accretion. In long-term treatment, osteoblastic activity slows and bone mass becomes stabilized.

Osteoporosis

With advancing age everyone loses bone mass, but not everyone has osteoporosis. The two most important determinants in the development of osteoporosis are peak bone mass and the rapidity of bone loss thereafter.

Peak bone mass generally is achieved in the early part of the third decade of life. Thereafter, bone is lost at a rate that depends on several factors. These factors include (1) the normal aging process; (2) the accelerated bone loss associated with menopause; and (3) genetic, environmental, and nutritional conditions and chronic disease states.

The mechanism of bone loss resulting from normal aging is poorly understood. Based solely on normal aging, the rate of bone loss in women is twice that of men. This bone loss is independent of menopausal bone mass loss. Factors that contribute to bone loss include decreased activity; a calcium-deficient diet; inherited characteristics; and factors related to childbirth, premature menopause, and alcoholism.

Estrogen deficiency is directly implicated in the etiology of osteoporosis. Although postmenopausal women produce estrogen, the levels are below those of premenopausal women and age-matched men. Twenty percent of postmenopausal women have a marked paucity of estrogen. In addition, smoking enhances estrogen degradation and low body fat results in insufficient estrogen production.

The primary consequences of postmenopausal bone loss are hip, distal radius, and vertebral fractures. Calcium intake and absorption have been identified as key factors in fracture incidence. Individuals ingesting physiologic levels of calcium have one fourth to one third the rate of hip fractures experienced by individuals with low calcium intake. Excess calcium intake may be harmful and is less effective than estrogen in preventing osteoporosis.

Treatments of osteoporosis have had variable success because of inaccurate diagnosis and insufficient understanding of the disease process. Calcium, physiologic vitamin D, calcitonin plus calcium, estrogen plus calcium, and mild exercise appear to decrease bone resorption and to mineralize osteoid, but do not increase total bone mass (Fig. 56). Although estrogen receptors recently have been found in bone-forming cells, the exact mechanism of estrogen's effect on bone remains elusive. Although low levels of activity can decrease bone loss, extensive exercise can augment bone mass in highly stressed bone. Recently, the management of osteoporosis has been directed at prevention.

Differential Diagnosis of Osteoporosis and Osteomalacia

These two osteopenic conditions seen in adults are commonly confused. Osteoporosis is characterized by a decreased density of normally mineralized bone matrix. Osteomalacia refers to an increased, normal, or (most commonly) decreased mass of insufficiently mineralized bone matrix (Fig. 57). Insufficient mineralization includes unmineralized osteoid and delayed mineralization of osteoid.

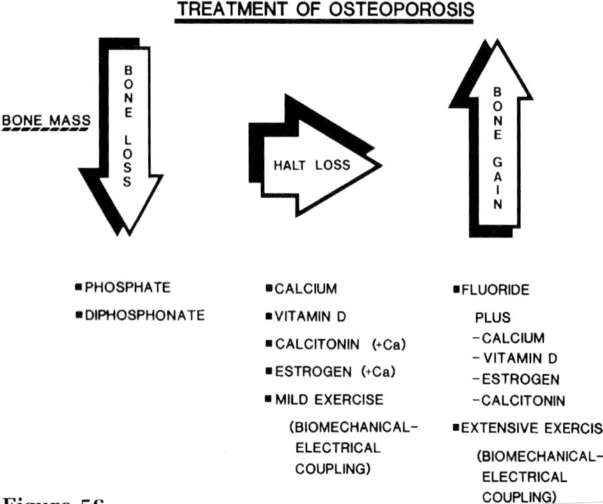

Figure 56
Recommended treatments for osteoporosis.

Osteoporosis, which is much more common than osteomalacia, is age-related and occurs most often in the elderly. Occasionally, onset may result from rare genetic and less common determinants such as hyperglucocorticoidism, hyperthyroidism, hyperparathyroidism, alcohol abuse, tumors, immobilization, and chronic disease.

Unlike its more easily diagnosed childhood counterpart, rickets, adult osteomalacia may be difficult to diagnose clinically. Incidence is evenly distributed throughout all age groups. The most common causes are chronic renal failure, vitamin D deficiency (found in approximately 30% of institutionalized elderly persons), abnormalities of the vitamin D pathway, and hypophosphatemic syndromes. Rarer causes are renal tubular acidosis, aluminum intoxication, hypophosphatasia, and tumors.

Symptoms of osteoporosis are not usually evident until spontaneous fractures occur, when pain is felt at the fracture site. The most common sites for symptomatic osteoporosis are the spine, ribs, hips, and wrists. Osteomalacia, in contrast, may cause generalized bone pain and bone tenderness, predominantly in the appendicular skeleton.

The radiographic features of the two diseases are often similar, but axial changes predominate in osteoporosis and appendicular changes in osteomalacia. Osteomalacia should be suspected in anyone with symmetric pathologic features, atraumatic fractures, or pseudofractures (Looser's zones), which are small, incomplete cortical fractures perpendicular to the long axis of a bone and often bilaterally symmetric. Common areas of involvement include the medial borders of the scapulae, ribs, ischiopubic rami, femoral necks, lateral borders of the femurs, and distal radii.

Results of routine laboratory studies are normal in osteoporosis but may be abnormal in osteomalacia. Osteomalacia should be suspected when the product of the serum calcium level multiplied by the serum phosphate level is chronically below 30, especially if accompanied by an elevated bone-specific alkaline phosphatase level and a 24-hour urinary calcium excretion of less than 50 mg. Osteomalacia caused by vitamin D deficiency should be suspected both in a person who has bone pain or pathologic fracture and is taking anticonvulsants or has a history of malabsorption syndrome, and in an elderly person who has a fracture of the femoral neck. The serum level of 25(OH)vitamin D is an excellent indicator of total body reserves of vitamin D.

Because these two diseases are very similar, a diagnosis of osteomalacia should be excluded by means of a transiliac bone biopsy following a two-course administration of tetracycline. In 50% of patients, osteomalacia cannot be diagnosed by labo-

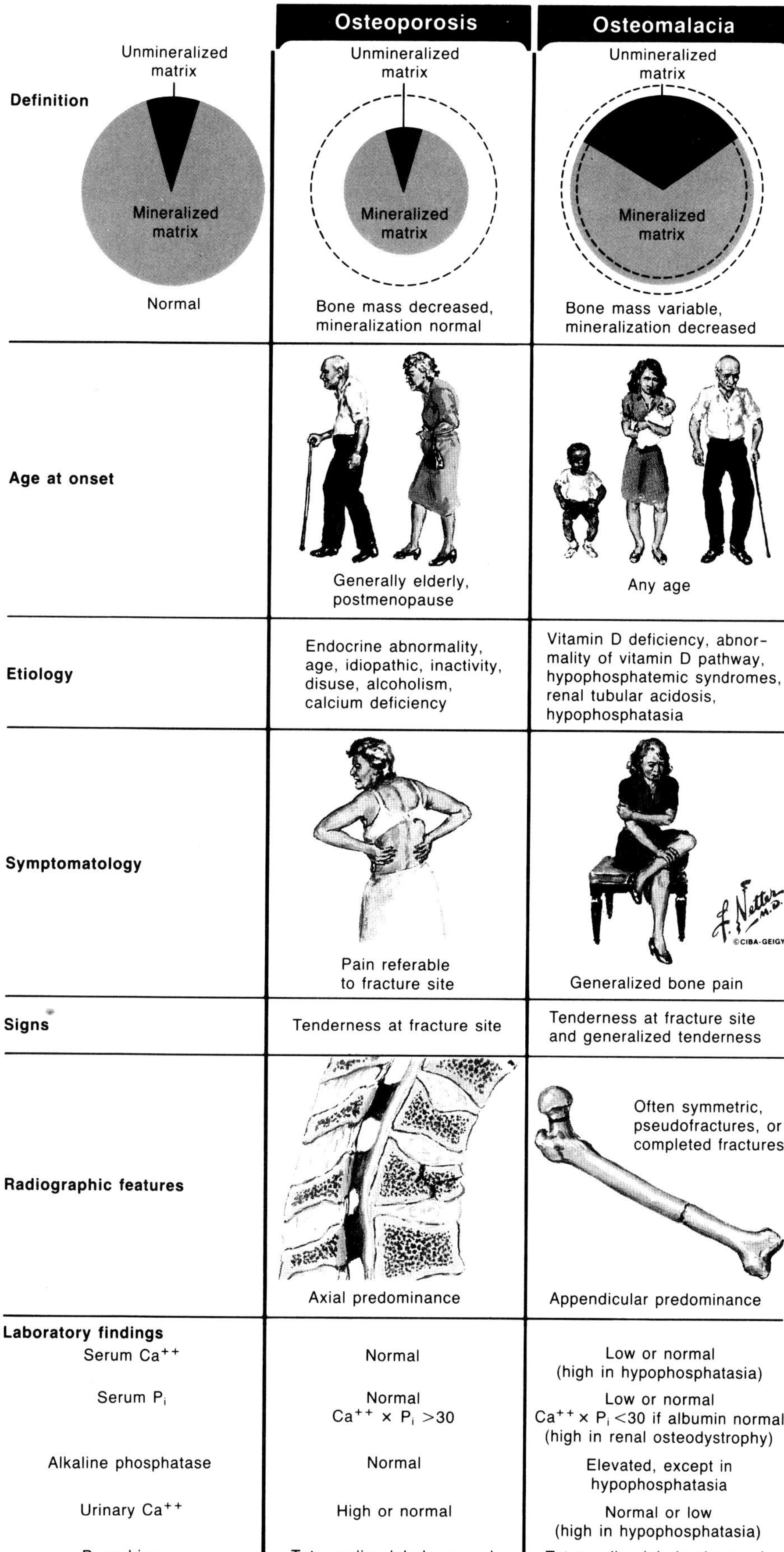

Comparison of Osteoporosis and Osteomalacia

	Osteoporosis	Osteomalacia
Definition (Normal: Unmineralized matrix / Mineralized matrix)	Unmineralized matrix / Mineralized matrix. Bone mass decreased, mineralization normal	Unmineralized matrix / Mineralized matrix. Bone mass variable, mineralization decreased
Age at onset	Generally elderly, postmenopause	Any age
Etiology	Endocrine abnormality, age, idiopathic, inactivity, disuse, alcoholism, calcium deficiency	Vitamin D deficiency, abnormality of vitamin D pathway, hypophosphatemic syndromes, renal tubular acidosis, hypophosphatasia
Symptomatology	Pain referable to fracture site	Generalized bone pain
Signs	Tenderness at fracture site	Tenderness at fracture site and generalized tenderness
Radiographic features	Axial predominance	Often symmetric, pseudofractures, or completed fractures. Appendicular predominance
Laboratory findings		
Serum Ca^{++}	Normal	Low or normal (high in hypophosphatasia)
Serum P_i	Normal $Ca^{++} \times P_i > 30$	Low or normal $Ca^{++} \times P_i < 30$ if albumin normal (high in renal osteodystrophy)
Alkaline phosphatase	Normal	Elevated, except in hypophosphatasia
Urinary Ca^{++}	High or normal	Normal or low (high in hypophosphatasia)
Bone biopsy	Tetracycline labels normal	Tetracycline labels abnormal

Figure 57
Comparison of osteoporosis and osteomalacia. (© Copyright 1987 CIBA-GEIGY Corporation. Reprinted with permission from the CIBA COLLECTION OF MEDICAL ILLUSTRATIONS, illustrated by Frank H. Netter, MD. All rights reserved.)

ratory values and can be distinguished from osteoporosis only by bone biopsy. However, the diagnosis of osteomalacia will be expedited if the physician is familiar with the causes and has a high index of suspicion.

Noninvasive Bone Density Measurement

Although plain radiographs are useful in the initial evaluation of osteopenia, they are the least accurate, least precise method of assessing bone density. In general, a decrease in bone mass of at least 30% is necessary to be detected on plain films. Other noninvasive radiographic and radioisotope techniques have been developed to determine skeletal mass. These methods are more precise, sensitive, and safe.

Noninvasive bone densitometry provides information about the density of bone at a specific site being measured. Density measurements of the lumbar spine have correlated relatively well with the incidence of spontaneous vertebral fractures (R = 0.6 to 0.8). However, bone densitometry does not provide information about current rates of bone remodeling, and it offers no predictive information on future bone loss rates. Current rates of bone remodeling can be determined using various indirect serum and urine biochemical determinations in conjunction with an evaluation of dynamic bone remodeling parameters on an undecalcified transiliac bone biopsy, if indicated. Baseline and serial bone density measurements are useful in monitoring the progress of therapeutic regimens.

Although bone mass is a major determinant of fracture threshold, other factors, such as cardiovascular status, medications, neuromuscular disorders, body habitus, and falls, may play an important role in the incidence of fractures.

Presently, three methods are widely available for bone densitometry: Single photon absorptiometry (SPA) for measurement of bone mineral in the appendicular skeleton; dual energy X-ray absorptiometry (DEXA) for assessment of integral (cortical and trabecular) bone mineral in the spine, hip, or total body; and quantitative computed tomography (QCT) for the assessment of trabecular bone mineral in the lumbar vertebral bodies and proximal femur. The two most useful techniques for assessing the mineral status of the axial skeleton are DEXA and QCT.

Single Photon Absorptiometry (SPA)

The principle behind SPA is that the density of the cortical bone is inversely proportional to the quantity of photons passing through.

In SPA, the radioisotope iodine 125 emits a single-energy beam of photons that passes through the bones of the forearm. A sodium iodide scintillation counter is moved systematically across the opposite side of the forearm to detect transmitted photons. With denser bone, there is more attenuation of the photon beam, and fewer photons pass through to the counter.

The examination is performed most commonly to detect the bone mineral content of the radius at the middiaphysis, which is predominantly cortical bone, or at the distal metaphysis, which normally contains abundant trabecular bone. The distal site is irregular in shape and reproducibility is more difficult. However, SPA of the midradius is reproducible and provides an accurate determination (± 3% to 4%) of the density of cortical bone at that site. Although the radiation dose is minimal (10 mrem), the cost is low, and patient acceptance is high, this method cannot be used for the accurate prediction of changes in the axial skeleton because of alterations in signal caused by the thick tissues in these anatomic areas.

Dual Photon (DPA) and Dual-Energy X-ray Absorptiometry (DEXA)

DPA allows for the measurement of axial skeletal bone mineral density by accounting for the attenuation of the signal by the soft tissues. In the last five years, an X-ray-based, rather than isotope-based, dual-energy projectional system (DEXA) has been developed. This technology initially was applied to measurement of bone density in the proximal femur, and it has shown excellent correlation with DPA in the spine. According to preliminary results, DEXA has significant advantages over the old DPA techniques, including superior precision, lower radiation dose, shorter examination time, higher image resolution, and greater technical ease. The method is safe, quick, and readily available. DEXA can be used to assess baseline bone density in a patient at risk for osteoporosis, and it can be used safely and accurately to follow prevention regimens or the course of therapy.

Quantitative Computed Tomography

QCT generates a cross-sectional image of the vertebral body. This image allows preferential measurement of trabecular bone density. Because the rate of turnover in trabecular bone is nearly eight times that in cortical bone, QCT provides a uniquely sensitive indicator of bone density in a region of the skeleton that is highly vulnerable to early metabolic changes. This technique, developed by Cann and Genant, involves the simultaneous scanning of a phantom composed of tubes containing standard solutions of a bone mineral equivalent. This phantom is used to calculate a standard calibration curve from which the vertebral trabecular bone density can be extrapolated. Measurements taken from the centers of vertebral bodies T-12 to L-4 are averaged to yield a mean bone density. Because the central portion of the vertebral body (trabecular bone) can be measured selectively, osteophytes and aortic calcifications are excluded. As with DEXA, precision is excellent, but it may be reduced in severely osteopenic and kyphotic individuals as a result of difficulty in relocating the exact sites of previous measurements. Accuracy is within 5% to 10%. A further decrease is possible because of the variable fat content of the bone marrow, especially in older patients. The radiation dose is higher than with the DEXA techniques.

Transiliac Bone Biopsy

Accurate information concerning rates of bone turnover and mineralization can be determined only from direct sampling of bone. The iliac crest is a readily accessible biopsy site and reflects changes at other clinically relevant sites. A 5- to 8-mm diameter core is obtained through a small 1-cm biopsy incision under local anesthesia.

Time-spaced dynamic tetracycline labeling permits the determination of mineralization rates in specimens that have not been decalcified. Tetracycline binds to newly mineralized osteoid. Two weeks before a bone biopsy, the tetracycline is administered twice each day for three days; this procedure is then repeated in the three days immediately prior to the bone biopsy. The mean distance between the tetracycline labels, as seen and measured using fluorescent microscopy, is divided by the number of days between the two courses of tetracycline to determine the mineral apposition rate. Abnormal patterns of fluorescent label deposition are the diagnostic hallmark of osteomalacia. When normal mineralization is present, as in osteoporosis, two distinct bands will result from the two doses of tetracycline. When mineralization is impaired, as in the case of osteomalacia, a single band of fluorescence will result.

Bone histomorphometry involves the quantitative analysis of undecalcified bone in which the parameters of skeletal remodeling are expressed in terms of volumes, surfaces, and cell numbers. Clinical and biochemical studies often fail to predict histologic changes. In addition, histologic changes vary regionally and are strongly influenced by local factors, including weightbearing stress (magnitude and direction), blood supply, marrow environment, and type of bone (cortical versus trabecular).

Bone biopsy is not necessary for evaluation of most patients with metabolic bone disease. However, biopsy is an important diagnostic tool in men and women younger than age 50 who have idiopathic osteopenia, in any patient in whom osteomalacia is highly suspected, and in patients with chronic renal failure with skeletal symptoms. Because of the inherent problem of regional sample error, bone biopsy should not be used to establish the diagnosis of osteoporosis; rather, it should be used to exclude a diagnosis of osteomalacia in a patient with osteopenia. In the evaluation of a patient with renal failure, bone biopsy can provide information to distinguish osteomalacia from osteitis fibrosa from aluminum-associated bone disease.

In Vivo Fracture Prediction

Because QCT presents a number of significant advantages in the development of objective fracture risk predictors for the hip and spine, this section provides a summary of knowledge on the development and in vitro validation of regional fracture risk predictors for these two sites. The results are discussed in light of available evidence on in vivo loads associated both with the activities of daily living and with trauma. The findings are then compared against comparable estimates of fracture risk for diaphyseal regions.

Factor of Risk

In engineering, the design of failure-resistant structures requires three important pieces of information: (1) the geometry of the structure; (2) the mechanical properties of the materials from which the structure is made; and (3) the location and direction of the loads to which the structure is subjected. Engineering theories based on this information can be used to estimate the stresses in the structure for various imposed loads. These stresses then can be compared against the known strengths of the materials within the structure to test for failure. The ratio of the material strength to the imposed stress at each point is called the safety factor. An alternative definition of the safety factor is expressed in terms of forces, and is the ratio of the force required to cause failure of the entire structure to the imposed force.

The inverse of the safety factor, called the risk factor, also provides a convenient measure of fracture risk for a structure under a particular set of loading conditions. The risk factor r is given by

$$r = F_{service}/F_{failure} \quad \textbf{(Eq. 10)}$$

where $F_{service}$ is the imposed load and $F_{failure}$ is the magnitude of the imposed load that would cause failure for the structure. When the risk factor is low (for example, much less than one), the force required to cause failure is much greater than the imposed force, and the structure can be expected to be at low risk of failure under the imposed loads. Conversely, when the risk factor is high (for example, close to or greater than one), the structure is at high risk of failure. In engineering design, it often is possible to decrease the risk factor by increasing the size of the structure, using a stronger material, or, in some cases, reducing the magnitude of the imposed loads. Most engineering structures operate with risk factors in the range of approximately 0.15 to 0.20.

Fracture prediction in the human skeleton is complicated because there is considerable uncertainty about the magnitudes and directions of the imposed loads at the hip and spine during typical daily activities. Even less is known about the forces generated as a result of a traumatic event such as a fall. Skeletal regions at high risk of age-related fractures exhibit far more complex geometries than most engineering structures, and these geometries can change with bone remodeling. As a consequence, it is difficult to estimate in vivo skeletal stresses caused by normal or traumatic loads. In addition, bone density, microstructure, and morphology not only exhibit marked spatial heterogeneity but also change dramatically as a consequence of aging and disease. In view of these complexities, it is not surprising that very little is known regarding the risk factors that exist in skeletal regions such as the hip and spine under the imposed loads associated with either normal daily activity or traumatic events.

QCT and Material Properties of Trabecular and Cortical Bone

Because of the potential influence of age-related reductions in cortical and trabecular density in hip and spine fractures, many attempts have been made to use noninvasive radiographic techniques to estimate bone density and thereby predict material properties. In this regard, for quantitation of small geographically discrete values of bone, QCT presents a number of significant advantages over other densitometric techniques such as SPA and DPA, DEXA, and conventional radiography. With the information available in QCT scans, it is possible to isolate densitometric and geometric changes in both cortical and trabecular compartments, whereas other radiographic methods present combined densitometric and geometric variations along the scan path in both cortical and trabecular compartments. In addition, the QCT densitometric data can be calibrated, using appropriate phantoms, so that direct correlations can be made between QCT density and bone density, and thereby to mechanical properties of the bone tissue. This is not possible with most other densitometric techniques, which measure only the structural behaviors of the combined cortical and trabecular bone compartments. The value of QCT for measurement of small volumetric areas of bone, however, is offset by its requiring a radiation dose 20 times greater than DEXA.

To establish correlations between QCT data and the compressive material properties of trabecular bone, scans are taken at defined locations and then small specimens are removed and tested in vitro to determine elastic modulus and uniaxial compressive strength. Experiments have shown relatively strong correlations between the QCT density and modulus ($R^2 \approx 0.70$) and compressive strength ($R^2 \approx 0.70$, Fig. 58). Thus, QCT can be used to estimate the modulus and strength of trabecular bone tissue. However, only poor correlations have been found between QCT data and both modulus and strength of cortical bone tissue. Presumably, this lack of correlation is due to the very narrow range in cortical bone densities coupled with the inability of QCT to differentiate between these densities (poor resolution). Research in this area is still in progress.

QCT and Vertebral Body Failure

Numerous studies have been performed to correlate the load required to fracture an isolated lumbar vertebral body (posterior elements removed) in

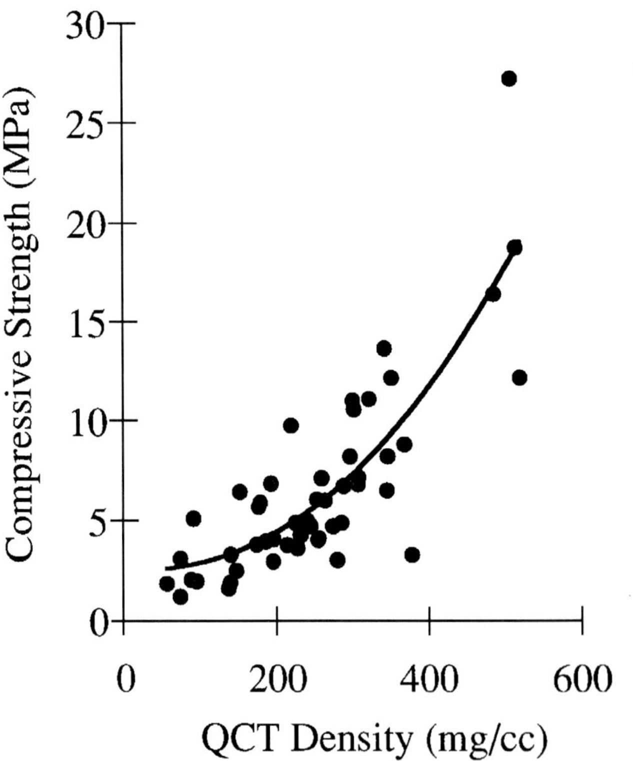

Figure 58
Ultimate compressive strength of femoral subcapital trabecular bone and QCT equivalent density. $Y = 8.9 \times 10^{-6} X^{2.31} + 2.78$; $R^2 = 0.70$. (Reproduced with permission from Lotz JC, Gerhart TN, Hayes WC: Mechanical properties of trabecular bone from the proximal femur: A quantitative study. *J Comput Assist Tomogr* 1990;14:107–114.)

vitro and some integral measure of its QCT density as measured in a typical clinical scan. Strong correlations have been found between the fracture load and the (directly measured apparent) density of trabecular bone within the vertebral body ($R^2 \approx 0.80$), but correlations between the fracture load and the mean QCT density ($R^2 \approx 0.50$, Fig. 59) are only moderate. The mean value of the fracture loads for uniaxial compression of intact, elderly lumbar vertebrae is approximately 3,100 to 3,400 N. To calculate risk factors, these mean values must be compared against estimates of the in vivo loads imposed on the lumbar spine during normal daily activities. Using a variety of experimental and theoretical techniques, in vivo lumbar spine compressive loads have been predicted, which range from 440 to 700 N for relaxed standing, 1,100 N for coughing, 1,800 N for sit-up exercises, 1,850 N for forward flexion of 20° while lifting a 20-kg mass, and 3,400 N for lifting 20 kg with the back bent and knees straight. Some mathematical models have predicted lumbar forces as high as 5,400 N during lifting of a 50-kg mass with the legs straight. Predictions have also been made of lumbar compressive loads in the range 18,800 to 36,400 N during power lifting by highly trained athletes.

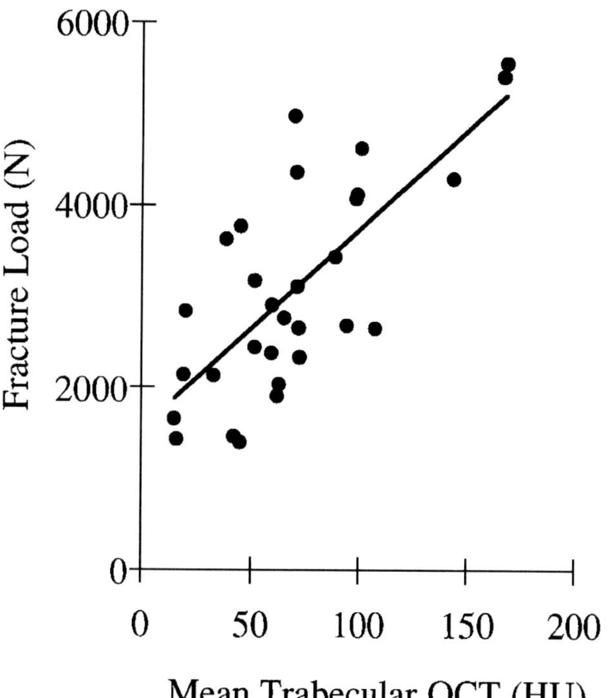

Figure 59
Failure load for an isolated lumbar vertebral body (posterior elements and endplates removed) under uniaxial compression and mean QCT value (in Hounsfield units, HU) of the trabecular bone within the vertebral body. Y = 21.5 X + 1540; $R^2 = 0.54$. (Reproduced with permission from Mosekildel L, Bentzen SM, Ørtoft G, et al: The predictive value of quantitative computed tomography for vertebral body compressive strength and density. *Bone* 1989;10:465–470.)

Fracture Risk Factors for the Spine

While such large forces would be unlikely to occur in the elderly subjects who might be candidates for fracture risk prediction, they indicate that dynamic activities and the lifting of heavy objects are likely to increase spinal forces well above the average vertebral fracture loads measured in vitro using elderly cadaveric subjects. Note that all in vitro failure experiments have been conducted using isolated vertebral bodies (for example, with the posterior elements removed and without the potential of load carrying by intra-abdominal pressure). Current evidence suggests, however, that intra-abdominal pressure reduces spinal compressive forces only by about 15% and that the facet joints carry only between 3% to 25% of lumbar spine loads. Thus, even if additive maximum contributions (40%) from intra-abdominal pressure and the facet joints are assumed, estimated lumbar spine loads from common daily activities (such as forward flexion of 20° with a 10-kg mass in each hand) are about 1,100 N. For lifting a 50-kg mass with the knees straight, estimated forces are 3,200 N. Based on the in vitro failure data for elderly spines, these two loading cases would involve risk factors of about 0.33 for forward flexion with 20 kg in each hand to about 1 for lifting 50 kg with the knees straight. With reported in vitro fracture loads for lumbar vertebrae ranging from less than 2,000 N to over 5,000 N (Fig. 59), it is not surprising that vertebral compression fractures are such a common occurrence among the elderly.

QCT and Proximal Femur Failure

To investigate relationships between QCT densitometric parameters and spontaneous fractures of the proximal femur, proximal femora have been scanned with QCT and then mechanically loaded in vitro using forces typical of single-legged stance. In one such study, fracture forces were in the range of approximately 2,000 to 8,500 N. Work to fracture (area under the force-deformation curve, which is a measure of the energy absorbed during the fracture process) was in the range of approximately 20 to 100 joules (J). In these experiments, moderate positive correlations were observed between the force required to cause in vitro fracture and the mean QCT number (reported in Hounsfield units, HU) from the trabecular bone within the subcapital region ($R^2 \approx 0.60$, Fig. 60). Slightly improved correlations were obtained using the sum of the intertrochanteric trabecular and cortical HU values multiplied by their respective cross-sectional areas. Fracture forces for simulated normal gait measured in various other

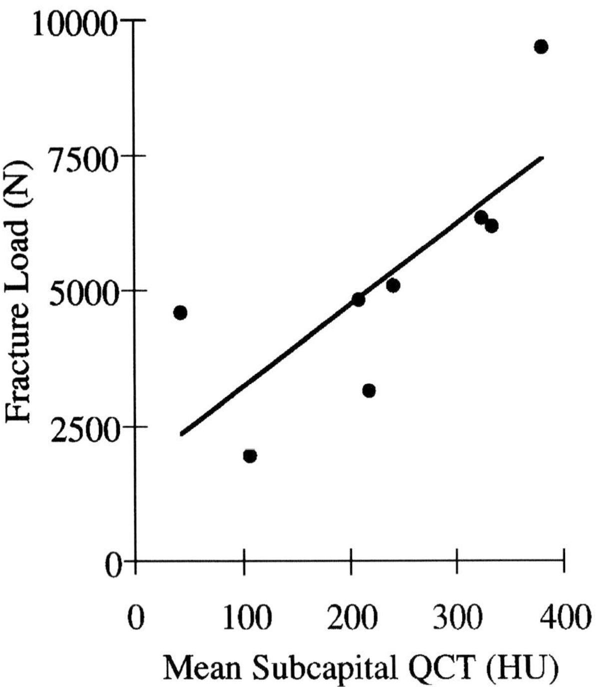

Figure 60
Force required to fracture the proximal femur under single-legged stance loading conditions and mean QCT value (in HU) of the trabecular bone within the subcapital region of the proximal femur. These data relate to prediction of spontaneous hip fractures. Y = 15.0 X + 1750; R^2 = 0.59. (Reproduced with permission from Esses SI, Lotz JC, Hayes WC: Biomechanical properties of the proximal femur determined in vitro by single-energy quantitative computed tomography. *J Bone Miner Res* 1989;4:5715–5722.)

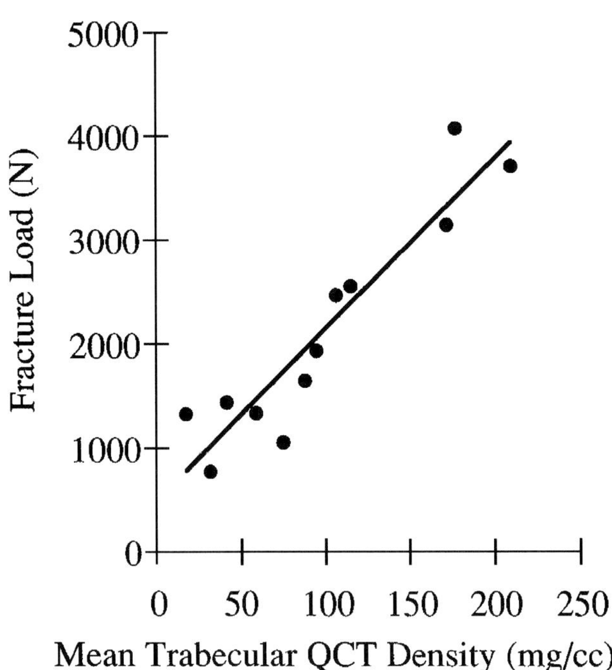

Figure 61
Force required to fracture the proximal femur under loading conditions representative of a fall to the side of the hip and mean QCT value (in equivalent density, mg/cc) of the intertrochanteric trabecular bone. These data relate to prediction of traumatic hip fractures. Note that the range of forces required to cause fracture is much lower for traumatic fractures than for spontaneous fractures (see Figure 60). Y = 16.2 X + 495; R^2 = 0.87. (Reproduced with permission from Lotz JC, Hayes WC: The use of quantitative computed tomography to estimate risk of fracture of the hip from falls. *J Bone Joint Surg* 1990;72A:689–700.)

in vitro experiments were in the range 1,000 to 12,750 N.

All these data relate to loading conditions for normal gait, and, therefore, are applicable only to hip fractures that occur during activities such as single-legged stance and normal gait. Spontaneous hip fractures associated with these activities represent less than 10% of the more than 250,000 hip fractures that occur annually in the United States. More than 90% of all hip fractures are associated with trauma caused by a fall, usually from standing height or lower. Under such traumatic conditions, the magnitudes and directions of the forces applied to the hip are probably much different from those that occur during normal gait. To investigate the ability of QCT data to predict fracture for these traumatic conditions, mechanical tests must be performed in vitro using loads typical of such trauma as a fall from standing height directly onto the side of the greater trochanter. For these experiments, fracture loads range from approximately 800 to 4,000 N. These loads are much lower than those required to fracture the femur in vitro for simulated gait loads (1,000 to 12,750 N). Similarly, work to fracture values range from approximately 5 to 500 J for a simulated fall from standing height, and are relatively low compared to gait values (20 to 100 J). The most significant relationships between the magnitude of the traumatic fracture loads and QCT indices of bone strength occur in the intertrochanteric region. Very significant positive correlations have been found between mean intertrochanteric trabecular QCT value and whole bone strength ($R^2 \approx 0.90$, Fig. 61). Even stronger correlations have been observed between whole bone strength and the mean intertrochanteric trabecular QCT value multiplied by the total intertrochanteric cross-sectional area. These findings indicate that QCT can provide an excellent predictor of the strength of the proximal femur whole bone as measured in vitro for certain assumed traumatic loading conditions.

These studies on whole bone strength and QCT, although preliminary, provide first-order estimates of the strength of the proximal femur for loads representing normal gait and one type of fall. In elderly cadaver specimens, both the upper end of the range and the mean values for fracture load were about twice as high for gait loads as for loads representing a fall. These differences are probably the consequence of differences in whole bone strength when the approximately elliptical femoral neck is loaded against its geometrically weak axis (relatively low areal moment of inertia) for a fall instead of against its strong axis (relatively high areal moment of inertia) for normal gait. Lower cortical and trabecular bone tissue strengths for transverse loading may also account for lower whole bone strengths for loading to the side of the hip.

Fracture Risk Factors for the Hip

To estimate fracture risk factors for the hip, the in vitro measurements of whole bone strength must be compared with estimates of in vivo loading on the proximal femur for different activities. A variety of mathematical models for single-legged stance have predicted in vivo forces that range from as low as 1.8 times body weight (BW) to six times BW. During normal gait, predictions are in the range of approximately three to eight times BW. Hip joint forces of seven to eight times BW have been predicted for stair ascent and of approximately three times BW for rising from a chair. In vivo forces at the hip joint for total hip arthroplasty patients have been measured directly using instrumented prostheses. For normal, quiet gait, various studies have consistently reported in vivo hip joint forces of approximately three times BW; forces as high as 5.5 times BW have been reported for dynamic loading associated with periods of instability during single-legged stance.

For the 55 kg individual typical of elderly populations at high risk of hip fracture, forces of three times BW for single-legged stance correspond to values of about 1,600 N. Forces of six times BW (representative of stair ascent and more dynamic activities) correspond to values of about 3,200 N. A typical mean value for in vitro failure load (5,250 N, for example) would then indicate risk factors of approximately 0.30 and 0.60 for single-legged stance and more dynamic activities, respectively. Using the entire range of reported in vitro failure loads (1,000 to 12,750 N) would suggest a range of risk factors of 0.13 to 1.6 for single-legged stance and 0.25 to 3.2 for stair ascent. These predictions suggest that some spontaneous fractures of the hip are to be expected in response to habitual activities such as single-legged stance, normal gait, and stair ascent.

It is far more difficult to estimate risk factors for falls because in vivo forces on the hip during impact from a fall have not yet been measured. However, it is possible to compare the work to fracture values for femora tested in vitro against the potential energy available during a fall from standing height. Epidemiologic studies have indicated that the available potential energy for individuals who fall and fracture a hip (500 J) significantly exceeds the energy for individuals who fall and do not fracture (450 J). These energies are an order of magnitude greater than the maximum work to fracture in the in vitro experiments simulating a fall to the side of the hip, and nearly 20 times the reported mean work to fracture. Therefore, much less energy is needed to fracture the proximal femur than is available in a simple fall from standing height. It follows that a fall to the side of the hip from standing height involves substantial trauma to the skeleton.

Other potentially important factors that can influence the force delivered to the proximal femur during impact from a fall include energy absorption processes in soft tissues overlying the greater trochanter, the state of muscle contraction, and the position of the trunk and extremities at impact. Preliminary experiments have predicted peak impact forces ranging from approximately 5,000 to 9,000 N in the muscle-relaxed state and from approximately 7,000 to 15,500 N in the muscle-active state. In females, threefold increases in soft-tissue thickness cause a 20% reduction in predicted peak impact force. More significantly, falling in a muscle-relaxed state reduces peak forces by more than half. Comparing these estimates of fall impact force with the average in vitro failure load data described above indicates risk factors in the range of 2.5 to 7.1. The inescapable conclusion is that in elderly individuals, any fall with direct impact to the greater trochanter has a high probability of fracturing the hip. This is true regardless of the thickness of the soft tissue overlying the hip, the state of muscle activity at impact, or, more interestingly, the fragility of the bone within the proximal femur.

In Vivo Fracture Risk Prediction

A final step toward the development of clinical fracture risk predictors is to test their discriminatory and predictive power in clinical populations. Women with vertebral fractures generally have lower spinal bone mass than controls. Approximately 90% of women with vertebral fractures have spinal bone mineral density values (as measured by DPA) of less than 0.97 g/cm^2. In older women, however, there is substantial overlap in QCT equivalent mineral density between individuals with atraumatic vertebral fractures and age-matched controls. This overlap reduces the predictive power of spinal QCT for an individual patient; it also is consistent with the concept that loading conditions are important in spine fracture etiology. For the hip, densitometric evidence suggests that the frequency of femoral neck fractures increases as bone mineral density declines below a densitometric threshold (using DPA or DEXA) of about 0.95 g/cm^2. However, for those over age 70 (who represent 90% of hip fracture patients), there is considerable overlap in densitometric measures between hip fracture patients and controls. Thus, as with the spine, densitometric estimates of proximal femoral strength are not good predictors of fracture risk.

For both the spine and hip, loading histories such as repeated bending and lifting of objects, chronic coughing, frequent stair ascent, or the single incidence of a fall are not accounted for in simple densitometric comparisons to fracture thresholds or in approaches that rely on densitometric comparisons with age- and gender-matched controls. Without data on the activity (and thus the force) precipitating a spontaneous fracture, little can be said about the relative importance of loading factors and bone fragility in the etiology of these fractures. A comparable situation exists for hip fractures that result from falls, although in this case it appears that for elderly individuals at greatest risk, factors related to the mechanics of the fall dominate the etiology, while factors related to densitometric measures alone have much less significance. Until better data are available on the activities and loading parameters that cause fracture, it will be difficult to establish and reliably test densitometric fracture risk predictors.

Paget Disease

In 1877, Sir James Paget described a bone disease that he called "osteitis deformans." Autopsy studies have yielded a 3% prevalence in a population age 40 and older and a 10% prevalence in those patients over 90 years old. The disease is more common in North America, England, Australia, New Zealand, and Germany than elsewhere; it is rare in Scandinavia. In 15% to 25% of cases, a familial incidence has been clearly documented. Clinically, a large number of patients are asymptomatic.

The radiographic features of Paget disease are illustrated in Figure 62. The distal tibia demonstrates the advancing osteolytic front, whereas thickening of the cortices with loss of normal architectural configuration and deformity is seen in the proximal portion of the tibia.

In the initial phase of Paget disease, the dominant feature is osteoclasis (Fig. 62). Pagetic bone is remodeled at a higher rate than that required by the mechanical forces applied to it. In the active phase, both osteoclastic destruction and osteoblastic formation (the two phases of bone remodeling) occur in the same area of the bone. The inactive or "burnt out" phase is characterized by a dense mosaic bone pattern and little cellular activity. Often all three phases of Paget disease may be seen in the same bone biopsy specimen. Although the remodeling of pagetic bone is abnormal, the process of mineralization is normal.

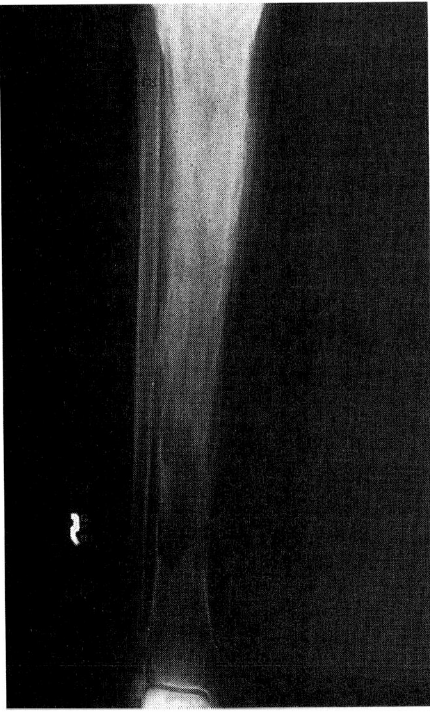

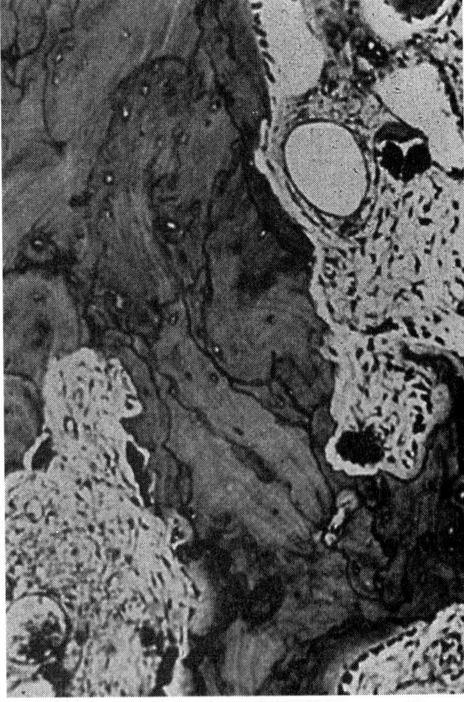

Figure 62
Radiographic features **(left)** and osteoclasis **(right)** in Paget disease.

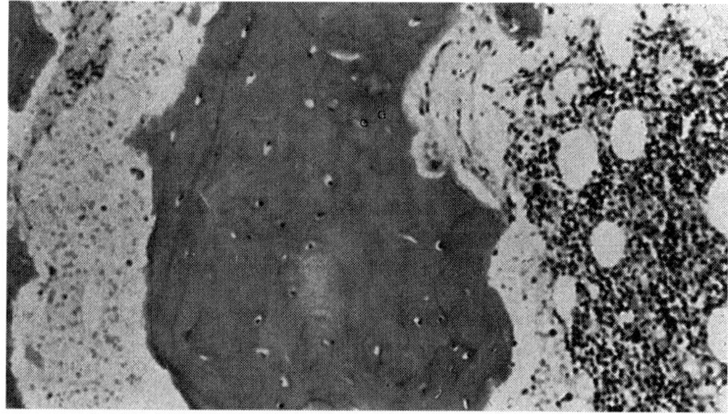

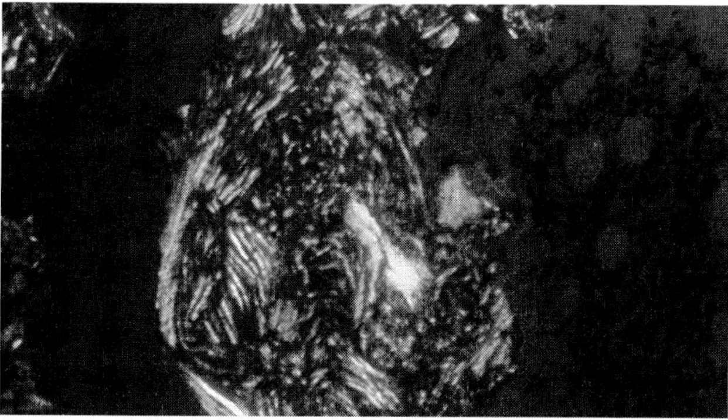

Figure 63
Photomicrograph showing biopsy of a pagetic vertebral body viewed under normal (**top**) and polarized (**bottom**) light.

Multiple resorbing and forming surfaces are characteristic of pagetic bone. This chaotic process leads to reorganization of the large plates of oriented lamellar bone into small areas of disorganized bone segments (Fig. 62).

In a biopsy of a pagetic vertebral body (Fig. 63), multiple resorbing lacunae are visualized. When the same slide is viewed under polarized light, there is evidence for disorganization of the collagen fibrils. The consequence of disorganization of the matrix is the enhanced brittle nature of the pagetic matrix and the high incidence of pathologic fracture and deformity. Fractures heal in pagetic bone at a slower rate than normal, and the remodeling process never restores the strength of the fracture site to that of normal bone.

Besides the classic radiographic and morphologic characteristics of Paget disease, the hypermetabolic state gives rise to scintiphotographic and chemical abnormalities. Alkaline phosphatase, a hallmark of bone formation, and urinary hydroxyproline, an indicator of bone resorption, are both elevated in active Paget disease. The coupling that exists between osteoblastic bone formation and osteoclastic bone resorption causes this elevation.

Although the etiology of Paget disease is unknown, recent evidence points to a possible slow viral infection as the cause of the disease. Measles and paramyxovirus-like inclusion bodies have been found in the nuclei of pagetic osteoclasts. Current treatment is directed at controlling osteoclast activity.

The indications for pharmacologic intervention in Paget disease are: (1) bone pain; (2) preparation for orthopaedic surgery; (3) treatment of spinal stenosis; (4) prevention of fractures or skeletal deformity in patients with rapidly progressive osteolytic lesions or in young patients; and (5) treatment of high output congestive heart failure.

Calcitonin decreases bone resorption by a direct effect on osteoclastic activity and morphology. The mechanism of diphosphonates on bone metabolism is unknown. At low dosage, diphosphonate curtails the resorption of bone. With chronic use of diphosphonates, bone formation is also inhibited. Unlike calcitonin, which enhances fracture repair, diphosphonate impairs mineralization, which produces osteoid accumulation. Following long-term therapy, diphosphonate may impair fracture union. Mithramycin is a chemotherapeutic agent that can rapidly decrease osteoclastic activity. Although the risk of toxicity is greater compared to that of calcitonin and diphosphonate administration, mithramycin is very effective in treating pending paraplegia and forms of Paget disease recalcitrant to the other agents.

Selected Bibliography

Bone Cell Morphology

Bone: *The Osteoblast and Osteocyte,* Hall BK (ed). Caldwell, NJ, The Telford Press, 1990, vol 1.

Bone: *The Osteoclast,* Hall BK (ed). Boca Raton, FL, CRC Press, 1991, vol 2.

Bone Matrix Composition

Bone: *Bone Matrix and Bone Specific Products,* Hall BK (ed). Boca Raton, FL, CRC Press, 1991, vol 3.

Boskey AL: Mineral-matrix interactions in bone and cartilage. *Clin Orthop* 1992;281:244-274.

Eyre DR: The collagens of musculoskeletal soft tissues, in Leadbetter WB, Buckwalter JA, Gordon SL (eds): *Sports-Induced Inflammation.* Park Ridge, IL, American Academy of Orthopaedic Surgeons, 1990, pp 161–170.

Heinegard D, Oldberg A: Structure and biology of cartilage and bone matrix noncollagenous macromolecules *FASEB J* 1989;3:2042–2051.

Poole AR, Matsui Y, Hinek A, et al: Cartilage macromolecules and the calcification of cartilage matrix. *Anat Rec* 1989;224:167–179.

Bone Mineralization

Bone: *Bone Metabolism and Mineralization,* Hall BK (ed). Boca Raton, FL, CRC Press, 1992, vol 4.

Boskey AL: Noncollagenous matrix proteins and their role in mineralization. *Bone Miner* 1989;6:111–123.

Bone Remodeling

Bone: *Fracture Repair and Regeneration,* Hall BK (ed). Boca Raton, FL, CRC Press 1992, vol 5.

Bone Blood Flow

Brookes M: *The Blood Supply of Bone: An Approach to Bone Biology.* London, Butterworth and Company, 1971.

Hellem S, Jacobsson LS, Nilsson GE, et al: Measurement of microvascular blood flow in cancellous bone using laser Doppler flowmetry and ^{133}Xc-clearance. *Int J Oral Surg* 1983;12:165–177.

Rhinelander FW: Tibial blood supply in relation to fracture healing. *Clin Orthop* 1974;105:34–81.

Tøndevold E: Haemodynamics of long bones: An experimental study on dogs. *Acta Orthop Scand Suppl* 1983;205:9–48.

Tothill P: Bone blood flow measurement. *J Biomed Eng* 1984;6:251–256.

Bone Metabolism and Mineral Homeostasis

Boden SD, Kaplan FS: Calcium homeostasis. *Orthop Clin North Am* 1990;21:31–42.

Einhorn TA, Levine B, Michel P: Nutrition and bone. *Orthop Clin North Am* 1990;21:43–50.

Eriksen EF, Colvard DS, Berg NJ, et al: Evidence of estrogen receptors in normal human osteoblast-like cells. *Science* 1988;241:84–86.

Ettinger B, Genant HK, Cann CE: Postmenopausal bone loss is prevented by treatment with low-dosage estrogen with calcium. *Ann Intern Med* 1987;106:40–45.

Reichel H, Koeffler HP, Norman AW: The role of the vitamin D endocrine system in health and disease. *N Engl J Med* 1989;320:980–991.

Metabolic Bone Disease

Bockman RS, Weinerman SA: Steroid-induced osteoporosis. *Orthop Clin North Am* 1990;21:97–107.

Bullough PG, Bansal M, DiCarlo EF: The tissue diagnosis of metabolic bone disease: Role of histomorphometry. *Orthop Clin North Am* 1990;21:65–79.

Cann CE, Genant HK, Kolb FO, et al: Quantitative computed tomography for prediction of vertebral fracture risk. *Bone* 1985;6:1–7.

Genant HK, Block JE, Steiger P, et al: Appropriate use of bone densitometry. *Radiology* 1989;170:817–822.

Kaplan FS, Fallon MD, Boden SD, et al: Estrogen receptors in bone in a patient with polyostotic fibrous dysplasia (McCune Albright syndrome). *N Engl J Med* 1988;319:421–425.

Kelly TL, Slovik DM, Schoenfeld DA, et al: Quantitative digital radiography versus dual photon absorptiometry of the lumbar spine. *J Clin Endocrinol Metab* 1988;67:839–844.

Kelsey JL, Hoffman S: Risk factors for hip fractures. *N Engl J Med* 1987;316:404–406.

Komm BS, Terpening CM, Benz DJ, et al: Estrogen binding, receptor mRNA, and biologic response in osteoblast-like osteosarcoma cells. *Science* 1988;241:81–84.

Lukert BP, Raisz LG: Glucocorticoid-induced osteoporosis: Pathogenesis and management. *Ann Intern Med* 1990;112:352–364.

Mankin HJ: Rickets, osteomalacia, and renal osteodystrophy: An update. *Orthop Clin North Am* 1990;21:81–96.

Mazess RB: Bone densitometry of the axial skeleton. *Orthop Clin North Am* 1990;21:51–63.

Mazess RB: Bone density in diagnosis of osteoporosis: Thresholds and breakpoints. *Calcif Tissue Int* 1987;41:117–118.

Merkow RL, Lane JM: Paget's disease of bone. *Orthop Clin North Am* 1990;21:171–189.

Riggs BL, Melton LJ III: Involutional osteoporosis. *N Engl J Med* 1986;314:1676–1686.

Singer FR, Schiller AL, Pyle EB, et al: Paget's disease of bone, in Avioli LV, Krane SM, (eds): *Metabolic Bone Disease.* New York, Academic Press, 1978, vol 2, pp 490–575.

Weinerman SA, Bockman RS: Medical therapy of osteoporosis. *Orthop Clin North Am* 1990;21:109–124.

Chapter 5
Growth Plate and Bone Development

Joseph P. Iannotti, MD, PhD
Steven Goldstein, PhD
Janet Kuhn, PhD
Louis Lipiello, MD
Frederick S. Kaplan, MD

Chapter Outline

Introduction

An understanding of bone formation, growth, and maturation is fundamental to orthopaedics. Bone formation and skeletal growth constitute a fascinating process of unique morphologic and biochemical changes that occur during fetal development and are capitulated on a daily basis throughout adolescent development. Growth plate cartilage is unlike hyaline or articular cartilage because of its unique blood supply, zonal structure, biochemistry, and process of matrix mineralization. This chapter will review bone formation, growth, and maturation in health and disease.

The bony skeleton is formed by two distinct processes: intramembranous and endochondral bone formation. Intramembranous bone formation occurs at the periosteal surfaces of all bones and in parts of the pelvis, scapula, clavicles, and skull, when osteoblasts form a calcified osteoid matrix within a collagenous framework; this process begins with differentiation of primitive mesenchymal cells. Endochondral bone formation occurs at the growth plates and within fracture callus when osteoblasts form osteoid on a cartilaginous framework. The growth plates are formed within a cartilaginous mass of mesenchymal cells during embryonic and fetal development. After fetal development the process of bone formation continues throughout growth.

Bone Development

During the sixth week of human embryonic development mesenchymal cells differentiate, condense, and transform into chondrocytes that form a cartilaginous model of the future skeleton. In the central portion of the cartilaginous anlage, the chondrocytes hypertrophy and the matrix begins to calcify. During the seventh embryonic week, a periosteal sleeve of bone is formed around the periphery of the anlage (Fig. 1). This bone is formed directly in a collagenous matrix by osteoblasts in a process called intramembranous bone formation. At the end of the eighth week, capillary buds invade the central portion of the hypertrophied and calcified cartilaginous anlage. Vascular invasion into the cartilaginous anlage signals the transition of embryonic to fetal development and brings to the cartilaginous anlage mesenchymal cells that differentiate into osteoblasts and osteoclasts. The osteoblasts produce an osteoid matrix on the surfaces of the calcified cartilaginous bars and form the primary trabeculae; this process is called endochondral (or enchondral) bone formation. The osteoclasts remove the primary trabecular bone to form a medullary canal. From the process of endochondral bone formation and osteoclastic resorption, a growth plate is formed at either end of the bone. Once the growth plate has been formed, longitudinal growth of the bone occurs by appositional growth of cells from within the growth plate, and new bone is formed on the metaphyseal side of each growth plate through a process that recapitulates the stages that occurred in the central portion of the original cartilaginous anlage. This process continues until closure of the growth plates at skeletal maturity.

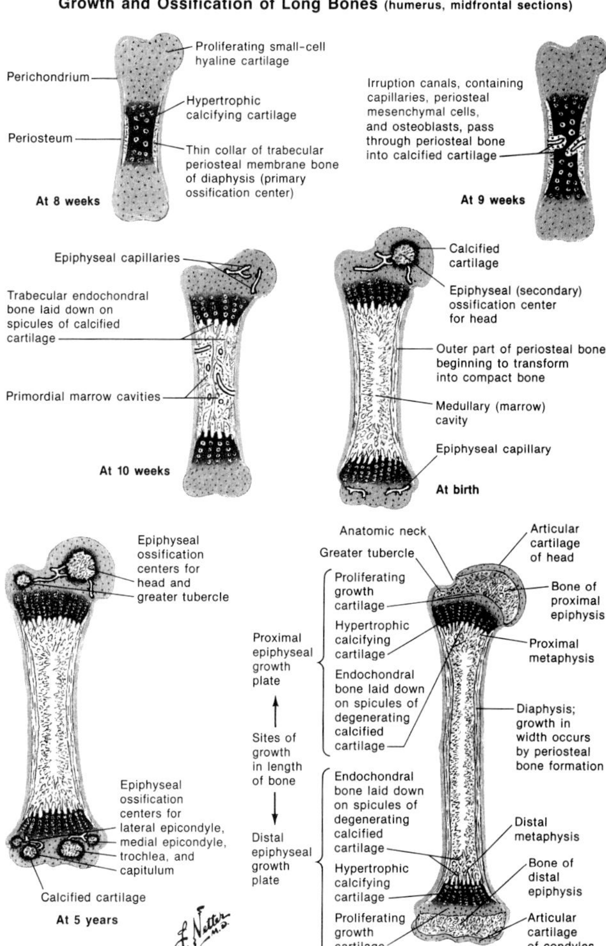

Figure 1
Development of a typical long bone. Formation of the growth plate and secondary centers of ossification. (© Copyright 1987 CIBA-GEIGY Corporation. Reprinted with permission from THE CIBA COLLECTION OF MEDICAL ILLUSTRATIONS, illustrated by Frank H. Netter, MD. All rights reserved.)

At specific times in the development of each long bone, a secondary center of ossification forms at the end of each bone. The development of the secondary center of ossification is the mechanism through which the shape and form of the joint surface are determined in diarthrodial joints. The secondary ossification center, being a growth plate, is also influenced by genetic, mechanical, and hormonal factors. Therefore, the processes of chondrocyte cell division, cell hypertrophy, matrix calcification, vascular invasion, and osteoblastic new bone formation occur in the same sequence as in the primary growth plate. However, unlike the growth plates associated with the primary ossification center, the epiphyseal end of the long bone enlarges as a result of radial apposition of cells around the secondary ossification center. The rate of growth around the secondary center is much slower than that in the vicinity of the primary growth plate.

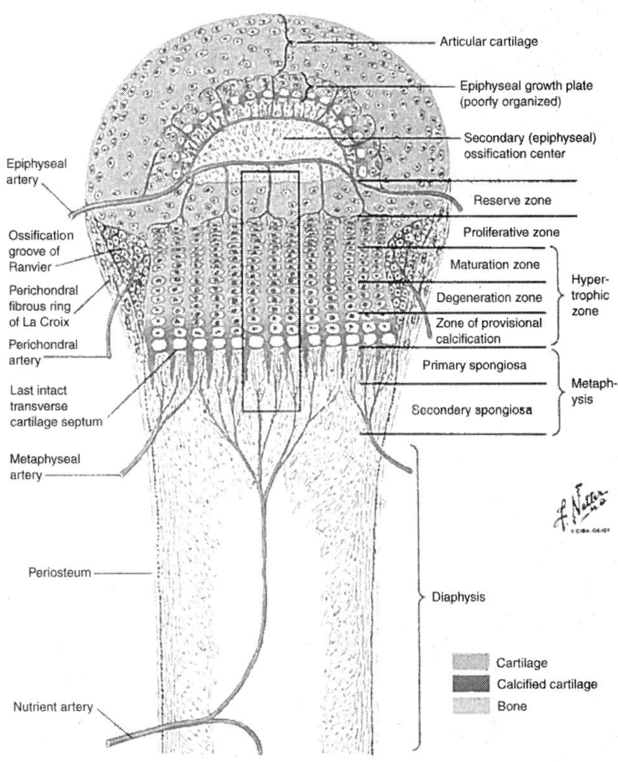

Figure 2
Structure and blood supply of a typical growth plate. (© Copyright 1987 CIBA-GEIGY Corporation. Reprinted with permission from THE CIBA COLLECTION OF MEDICAL ILLUSTRATIONS, illustrated by Frank H. Netter, MD. All rights reserved.)

Structure, Function, and Biochemistry of the Normal Growth Plate

Introduction

The process of endochondral bone formation, which occurs in all growth plates, is unique to the immature skeleton. This process comprises a series of events that occur on a daily basis in a well-defined regular sequence.

The function of the growth plate is related to its structure as an organ, which depends on the integrated function of three distinct tissue types. The growth plate is composed of a cartilaginous component that has three histologically distinct zones: reserve, proliferative, and hypertrophic; surrounded by a fibrous component; and bounded by a bony metaphyseal component. Each component has a unique structure, biochemistry, and function; together, these result in longitudinal and latitudinal growth and remodeling of the developing skeleton. The vascular supply of the growth plate results in unique biochemical properties and is integral to normal function.

Vascular Supply to the Growth Plate

There are three major vascular supplies of the growth plate (Fig. 2). The epiphyseal artery enters the secondary center of ossification. The terminal branches of this artery pass through the reserve zone cartilage of the upper growth plate, terminate at the uppermost cell of the proliferative zone, and supply oxygen and nutrients to the proliferative zone chondrocytes. These vessels do not penetrate into the proliferative or hypertrophic zones. The main nutrient artery of the long bone enters the metaphysis. Its capillary loops end at the last cartilaginous transverse septum of the bone-cartilage interface of the growth plate. These vessels turn back on themselves to form a venous return. This is an area of venous stasis and low blood flow; the vessels do not penetrate the hypertrophic zone of the growth plate. The structure of this vascular supply results in an avascular lower proliferative and hypertrophic zone, which is a major factor influencing growth plate chondrocyte physiology. The periphery of the growth plate is supplied by metaphyseal arteries and a perichondral artery to the perichondral ring of LaCroix.

The Cartilaginous Component of the Growth Plate

The cartilaginous component of the growth plate is divided histologically into three zones: the reserve zone, the proliferative zone, and the hypertrophic zone. Each zone has characteristic histologic and biochemical features that define its formation (Figs. 2 and 3).

Reserve Zone

The reserve zone, located just below the secondary center of ossification, is histologically characterized by a sparse distribution of single or paired round cells in an abundant matrix. These cells contain an abundant amount of endoplasmic reticulum characteristic of active protein synthesis. How-

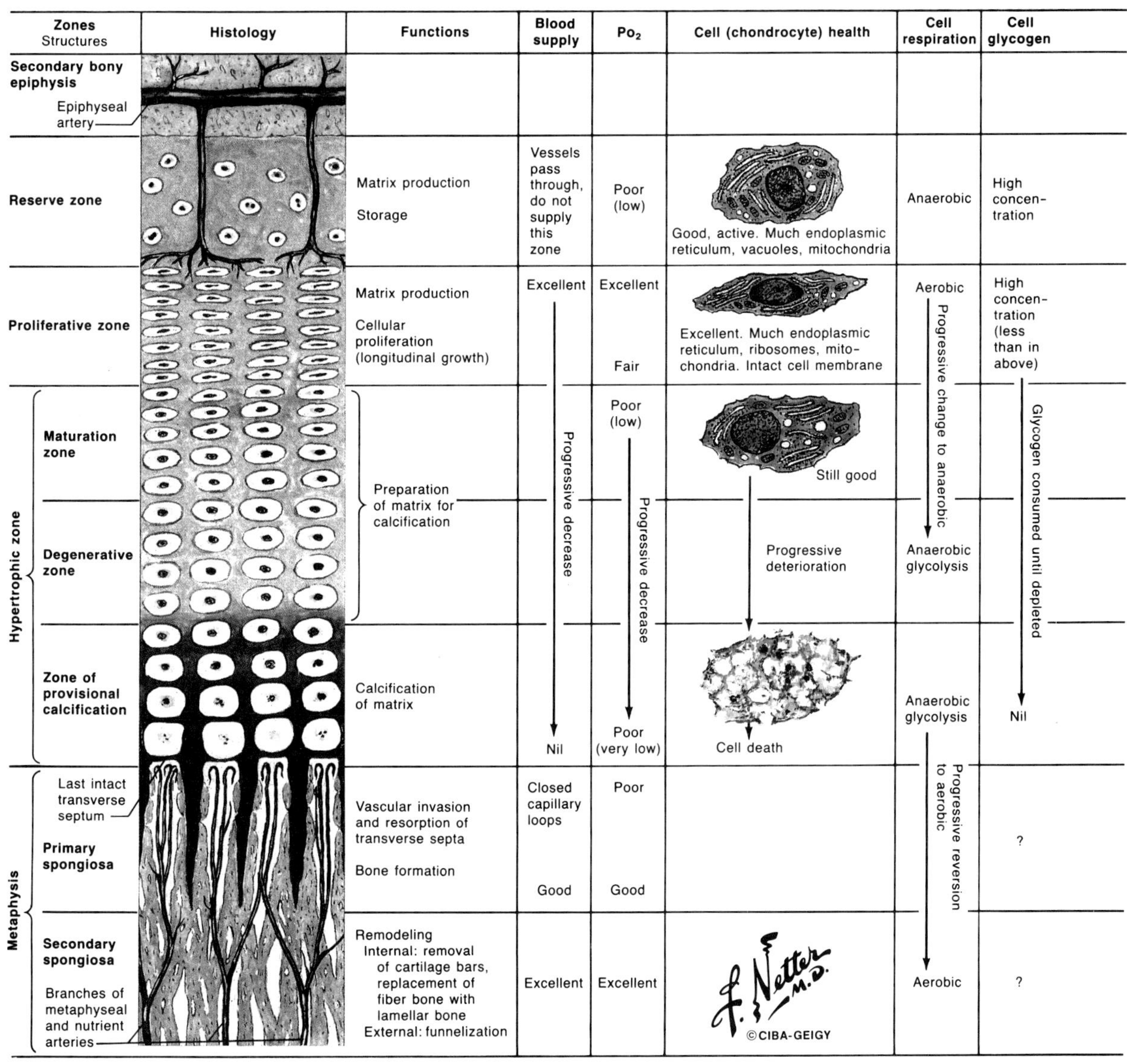

Zones
Structures
Histology
Functions
Blood supply
Po2
Cell (chondrocyte) health
Cell respiration
Cell glycogen
Secondary bony epiphysis
Epiphyseal artery
Reserve zone
Matrix production
Storage
Vessels pass through, do not supply this zone
Poor (low)
Good, active. Much endoplasmic reticulum, vacuoles, mitochondria
Anaerobic
High concen-tration
Proliferative zone
Matrix production
Cellular proliferation (longitudinal growth)
Excellent
Excellent
Fair
Excellent. Much endoplasmic reticulum, ribosomes, mito-chondria. Intact cell membrane
Aerobic
High concen-tration (less than in above)
Progressive change to anaerobic
Hypertrophic zone
Maturation zone
Degenerative zone
Preparation of matrix for calcification
Progressive decrease
Poor (low)
Progressive decrease
Still good
Progressive deterioration
Anaerobic glycolysis
Glycogen consumed until depleted
Zone of provisional calcification
Calcification of matrix
Nil
Poor (very low)
Cell death
Anaerobic glycolysis
Nil
Metaphysis
Last intact transverse septum
Primary spongiosa
Vascular invasion and resorption of transverse septa
Bone formation
Closed capillary loops
Good
Poor
Good
Progressive reversion to aerobic
?
Secondary spongiosa
Branches of metaphyseal and nutrient arteries
Remodeling
Internal: removal of cartilage bars, replacement of fiber bone with lamellar bone
External: funnelization
Excellent
Excellent
Aerobic
?
F. Netter M.D.
©CIBA-GEIGY

Figure 3

Zonal structure, function, and physiology of the growth plate. (© Copyright 1987 CIBA-GEIGY Corporation. Modified with permission from THE CIBA COLLECTION OF MEDICAL ILLUSTRATIONS, illustrated by Frank H. Netter, MD. All rights reserved.)

ever, cellular proliferation in the reserve zone is sporadic. The reserve zone chondrocytes have the lowest intracellular and ionized calcium content, and they do not contribute to longitudinal growth.

The collagen content (type II collagen) is highest in the matrix of the reserve zone, and the collagen fibers are in a nondirectional pattern. There is a large number of matrix vesicles in the reserve zone matrix, but they do not participate directly in mineralization. The matrix proteoglycans are in an aggregate form, which is inhibitory to matrix mineralization. Although vascular channels pass through the reserve zone, they do not supply it with oxygen, and as a result the oxygen tension is low (20.5 ± 2.1 mm Hg).

These data indicate that the reserve zone has the capacity to produce a cartilaginous matrix, but is relatively inactive in cell or matrix turnover. Its role in growth plate function is not clear. The reserve zone does not actively participate in longitudinal growth through cell proliferation, matrix synthesis, or calcification. Although most growth plate abnormalities affect the reserve zone, no known disease state primarily affects this zone.

The Proliferative Zone

The proliferative zone is characterized histologically by longitudinal columns of flattened cells. The cytoplasm contains glycogen stores and is rich in endoplasmic reticulum, suggesting a rich source of nutrients for aerobic glycolysis and a high capacity for protein synthesis. Of the three zones, this zone has the highest rate of proteoglycan synthesis and turnover. The total intracellular calcium content is approximately equal to that of the reserve zone, but the ionized calcium concentration is significantly greater, suggesting that the proliferative zone chondrocyte is not actively accumulating calcium for matrix mineralization.

The uppermost cell in each column is the progenitor cell for longitudinal growth of the cell column. This cell is not derived from the reserve zone cells. Longitudinal growth in the growth plate is equal to the number of cell divisions multiplied by the maximum size of the last hypertrophic zone cell. In addition, total longitudinal growth for the life span of the growth plate depends on the total number of progenitor cell divisions and on the number of reiterative divisions of each daughter cell derived from each progenitor cell division. The rate of cell division is influenced by hormonal and mechanical factors, but the total number of progenitor cell divisions is determined genetically for each growth plate.

The distribution of collagen fibrils and matrix vesicles in the matrix of the proliferative zone is nonuniform. The highest volume fraction and number of matrix vesicles is in the interterritorial matrix of the lower proliferative and upper hypertrophic zones. These matrix vesicles participate in matrix mineralization in the lower hypertrophic zone. The proteoglycans of the proliferative zone are in an aggregated form and, in this zone, they inhibit matrix mineralization. The oxygen tension is higher in the proliferative zone than in any other zone (57.0 ± 5.8 mm Hg). This high oxygen tension appears to be secondary to the rich vascular supply of the proliferative zone. The presence of rich glycogen stores and a high oxygen tension supports aerobic metabolism in the proliferative zone chondrocyte.

The functions of the proliferative zone—matrix production and cellular division—together contribute to longitudinal growth.

The Hypertrophic Zone

The hypertrophic zone is characterized by cells that are five to ten times the size of the proliferative zone cells. In early electron microscopy studies in which aqueous fixation techniques were used, the lowest cells of the hypertrophic zone were found to be fragmented and nonviable. Results of more recent morphologic studies, in which anhydrous fixation techniques were used, suggest that all of the hypertrophic zone cells maintain cellular morphology compatible with active synthetic cellular functions. Data from many biochemical studies support the active role of the hypertrophic zone chondrocyte in synthesis of novel matrix proteins. Although the hypertrophic zone chondrocyte is metabolically active, the data do not suggest or support the concept that the hypertrophic zone cell survives the process of vascular invasion or transforms to another cell type in the metaphysis. The ultimate fate of the hypertrophic zone cell is cell death.

Biochemical analysis shows that the hypertrophic zone cells are very metabolically active. Of all the zones, the hypertrophic has the highest content of glycolytic enzymes. The hypertrophic zone chondrocyte synthesizes alkaline phosphatase, neutral proteases, and type x collagen, thereby participating in matrix mineralization.

The hypertrophic zone is avascular and, as a result, the oxygen tension is quite low (29.3 ± 2.4 mm Hg). In the normally mineralized hypertrophic zone the diffusion coefficient is very high, resulting in a high barrier to the diffusion of oxygen and nutrients from the metaphysis.

Metabolic activity in the hypertrophic zone cells differs from that in most animal cells. In most cell types, glucose is oxidized to pyruvate in the cytoplasm, and the pyruvate is then further oxidized in the mitochondria by the Krebs cycle enzymes (tricarboxylic acid cycle). The Krebs cycle is an important additional energy source for most cells. In most animal cells, pyruvate enters the mitochondria by the glycerol phosphate shuttle. On the other hand, the metabolic activity, poor diffusion of nutrients, and avascularity of the hypertrophic cell zone result in a catabolic energy state. The major energy source for production of adenosine triphosphate (ATP) in the hypertrophic zone chondrocytes is aerobic glycolysis of glucose from endogenous glycogen stores. In the growth plate, pyruvate continues to enter the mitochondria but at a much reduced rate, and glucose 3 phosphate does not enter the mitochondria because the growth plate zone lacks the glycerol phosphate shuttle. Because of this lack, the growth plate's major ATP energy source from glucose stores is cytoplasmic anaerobic glycolysis. During maturation of the hypertrophic zone cell, its cytoplasm is depleted of endogenous glycogen stores, which further compromises energy production.

In the hypertrophic zone chondrocyte, the energy derived from mitochondrial electron transport is used primarily in the accumulation, storage, and release of calcium rather than for ATP production. The hypertrophic zone chondrocytes contain the largest amount of total cellular calcium and the greatest labile pool of stored calcium in their mitochondria. This zone also has the highest concentration of cytosolic ionized calcium. The primary functions of the hypertrophic zone are to prepare the matrix for calcification and then to calcify it.

Cartilage Matrix Turnover

Various genetic, humoral, and mechanical factors stimulate macromolecule and matrix vesicle biosynthesis in the growth plate. These factors are discussed later in this chapter. Several enzymes are synthesized by the chondrocyte along with tissue enzyme inhibitors and activators that regulate matrix degradation. The degradative enzymes found in the growth plate include a class of metalloproteinases that depend on zinc and calcium for enzyme activity. The enzymes found in the growth plate are collagenase, gelatinase, and stromelysin. The growth plate chondrocytes produce these enzymes in a latent (inactive) form, but the enzymes can be activated by interleukin-1 and plasmin. When activated, these enzymes, singularly or in combination, can degrade both the collagenous and proteoglycan components of the matrix. Their activity also is regulated by a locally produced tissue inhibitor, tissue inhibitor of metalloproteinases (TIMP), which can bind irreversibly to these enzymes to make them inactive. The presence and amount of metalloproteinases and their inhibitor (TIMP) vary among different zones of the growth plate. In addition, the factors produced in one zone can act at more distant sites within the growth plate. The activation of the enzymes is differentially regulated by interleukin-1 (IL-1) and TIMP. The coordinated effects of these factors within the growth plate, therefore, are complex and, at this point, remain poorly understood.

The Metaphysis

The metaphysis functions in the removal of the mineralized cartilaginous matrix of the hypertrophic zone, the formation of bone, and the histologic remodeling of the cancellous trabeculae. It is characterized by anaerobic metabolism, vascular stasis, and low oxygen tension (19.8 ± 3.2 mm Hg). The vascular stasis and low oxygen tension result from the arteriovenous loops at the cartilage-bone junction and low blood flow. The metaphysis begins distal to the last intact transverse septum of each cartilaginous cell column of the hypertrophic zone (Fig. 2). The unmineralized last transverse septum is removed by lysosomal enzymes, the cartilaginous lacunae are invaded by endothelial and perivascular cells, and the hypertrophic zone cell is removed. The factors that induce vascular invasion of the last hypertrophic zone cell are poorly understood. Traditional thought has suggested that mineralization of the cartilage matrix is a prerequisite step in vascular invasion. After the last transverse septum is removed, osteoblasts from the metaphysis line the calcified longitudinal bars of cartilage. Between the capillaries and the osteoblasts lie polymorphic osteoprogenitor cells. The osteoblasts produce a bone matrix on the calcified cartilage bars. This area of sparse bone formed on a central core of calcified cartilage is termed the primary trabecular bone or primary spongiosa. The osteoblasts progressively lay down bone on the cartilage template and more distally in the metaphysis. The initial woven bone and cartilage bars of the primary trabeculae are resorbed by osteoclasts and are replaced by lamellar bone to produce the secondary trabecular bone or secondary spongiosa in a process termed histologic, or internal, remodeling.

The remodeling process at the metaphyseal-diaphyseal junction requires the synchronized functions of osteoclastic bone resorption and osteoblastic new bone formation. This process of external or anatomic remodeling occurs around the periphery and subperiosteal regions of the metaphysis, and results in narrowing of the diameter of the metaphysis to meet the diaphysis of the bone; the process is called funnelization. In the process of anatomic remodeling, osteoclasts remove bone from the periphery of the metaphysis, and new bone is formed at the endosteal surfaces.

The Fibrous Structure

Surrounding the periphery of the growth plate are a wedge-shaped groove of cells, the ossification groove of Ranvier, and a ring of fibrous tissue, the perichondral ring of LaCroix (Figs. 2 and 3). The cells in the groove of Ranvier are active in cell division and contribute to an increase in the diameter, or latitudinal growth, of the physis. Three cell types constitute the groove of Ranvier. An osteoblast-type cell forms the bony portion of the perichondral ring at the metaphysis, a chondrocyte-type cell contributes to latitudinal growth, and a fibroblast-type cell covers the groove and anchors it to the perichondrium above the growth plate. The structure of the perichondral ring of LaCroix varies greatly among species, among different growth plates in the same species, or with the age of the animal. The basic structure is a fibrous collagenous network that is continuous with the fibrous portion of the groove of Ranvier and the periosteum of the metaphysis. The perichondral ring functions as a strong mechanical support at the bone-cartilage junction of the growth plate.

Growth Plate Mineralization

The mineralization of growth plate cartilage is unique and significantly different from the mineralization of bone (osteoid). The difference is based on the unique handling of intracellular calcium stores by the growth plate chondrocytes; the hypoxic environment, which results from the growth plate's unique blood supply; the growth plate's unique energy metabolism; the presence of matrix vesicles as the initial site of mineralization; and the coordinated functions of several unique matrix macromolecules.

The many factors that play a role in growth plate mineralization (Fig. 4) may be divided into four major groups: intracellular calcium homeostasis, microenvironmental factors, the systemic hormonal milieu, and the extracellular matrix vesicles and macromolecules. The growth plate chondrocyte plays a central role in the process of matrix mineralization through intracellular calcium transport; the synthesis, secretion, and postsecretion modification of the matrix macromolecules that participate in mineralization; the ability to respond to systemic and microenvironmental factors; and the biogenesis of matrix vesicles.

Intracellular calcium apparently plays a significant role in matrix calcification. In fact, the growth plate chondrocyte mitochondria seem to be specifically adapted for calcium transport. Electron-dense granules of calcium phosphate appear in hypertrophic zone mitochondria. Localization of mitochondrial calcium shows accumulation in the upper two thirds of the hypertrophic zone and depletion in the lowest chondrocytes. The loss of mitochondrial calcium in the lower hypertrophic zone is associated with matrix vesicle hydroxyapatite crystal nucleation (Fig. 5). These data suggest a transfer of intracellular calcium to extracellular sites during the process of hydroxyapatite crystal formation.

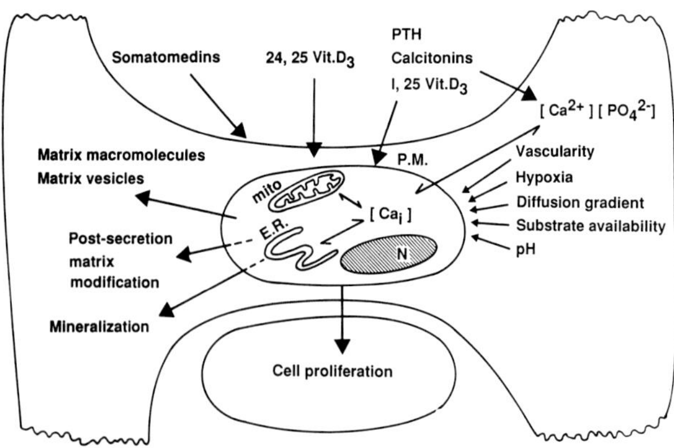

Figure 4
The factors influencing growth plate chondrocyte function and matrix mineralization. (Reproduced with permission from Iannotti JP: Growth plate physiology and pathology. *Orthop Clin North Am* 1990;21:1–17.)

In isolated growth plate chondrocytes and mitochondria, there is a metabolic specialization for calcium transport. In comparison with nonmineralizing cells, the chondrocyte mitochondria have a greater capacity for calcium accumulation and a greater ability to maintain these stores in a labile form for calcium release. In cells where the endogenous calcium stores are low, the endoplasmic reticulum is the major intracellular regulator of the cytosolic (cytoplasmic) ionized calcium concentration. This is the situation in all nonmineralizing cells as well as in the reserve and proliferative zone chondrocytes. As the hypertrophic zone chondrocytes accumulate calcium, the capacity of the endoplasmic reticulum to accumulate calcium is saturated, and the mitochondria become the major source of calcium accumulation and regulation. Under high calcium-loading conditions, the mitochondria buffer the cytosolic ionized calcium concentration at an increased level. This ionized calcium pool is a major regulator of cellular metabolic function, and changes in the labile calcium pool have a profound effect on cellular functions. The high concentration of intracellular ionized calcium in the hypertrophic zone chondrocytes is correlated with matrix vesicle secretion from the plasma membrane of the isolated growth plate chondrocytes.

In summary, in the proliferative zone the oxygen tension and glycogen stores stay high, the cells have a low ionized and total calcium content, and the mitochondria are primarily involved in ATP production. The cells are actively involved in division and matrix production. In the hypertrophic zone the oxygen tension and nutrients are low, the mitochondria are initially active in calcium accumulation, and the cells secrete matrix vesicles. In the lower hypertrophic zone, mitochondrial calcium is released and matrix mineralization occurs (Fig. 6). The factors that initiate mitochondrial calcium accumulation and induce calcium release are poorly understood at this time.

Several other factors within the matrix affect mineralization. Histochemical stains of the growth plate indicate that the hypertrophic zone matrix contains disaggregated proteoglycan. Electron microscopy reveals that the length of the proteoglycan aggregates and the number of subunits of the aggregate decrease from the reserve zone through the hypertrophic zone (Fig. 7). It is suggested that in vivo the disaggregated form of proteoglycan participates in matrix mineralization by binding and localizing calcium to the matrix. In vitro, aggregated proteoglycan inhibits calcium phosphate crystal formation. The disaggregation of proteoglycan in vivo results from the enzymatic degradation by lysozyme or neutral protease.

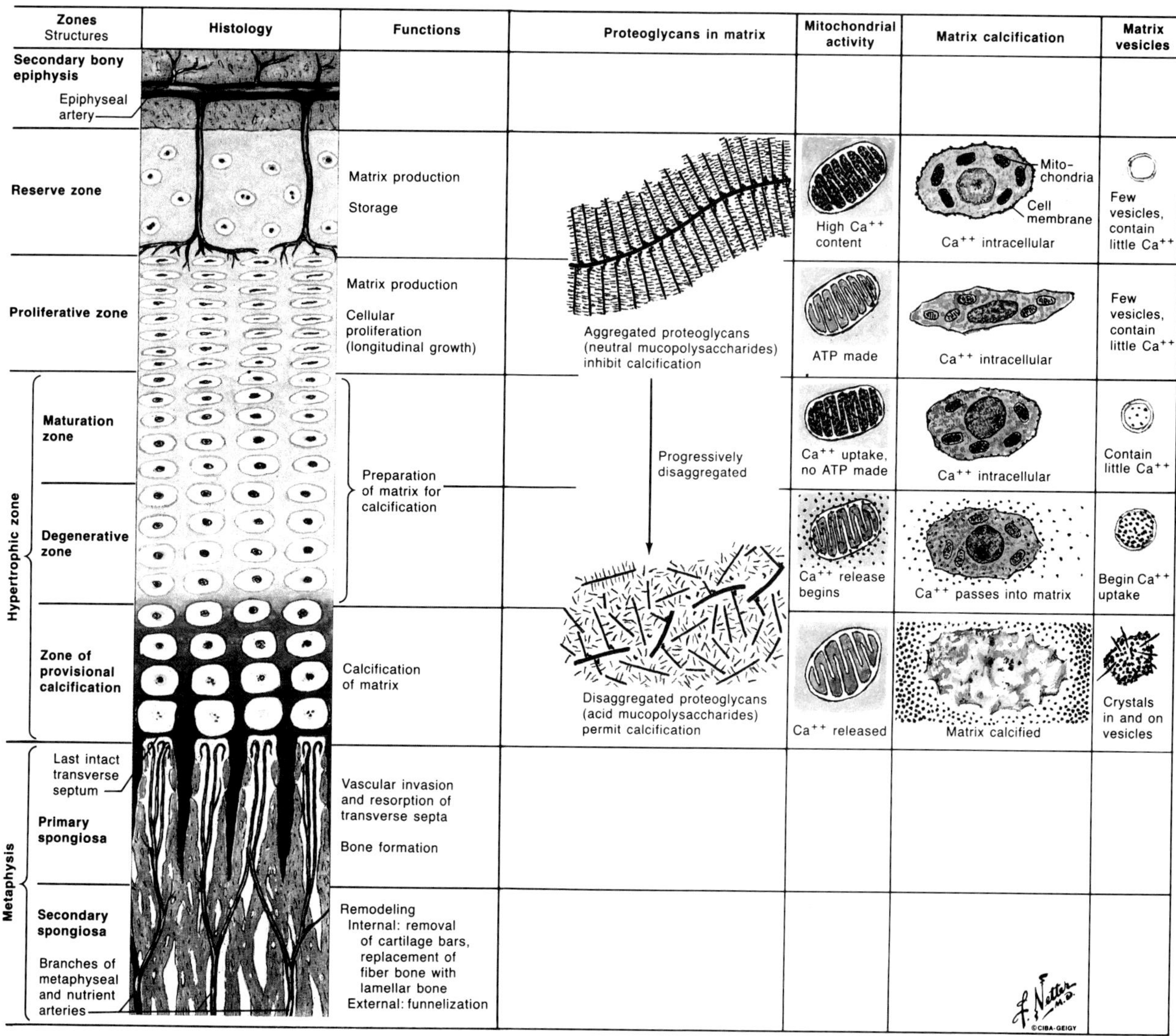

Zones
Structures
Histology
Functions
Proteoglycans in matrix
Mitochondrial activity
Matrix calcification
Matrix vesicles
Secondary bony epiphysis
Epiphyseal artery
Reserve zone
Matrix production
Storage
Mito-chondria
Cell membrane
High Ca++ content
Ca++ intracellular
Few vesicles, contain little Ca++
Proliferative zone
Matrix production
Cellular proliferation (longitudinal growth)
Aggregated proteoglycans (neutral mucopolysaccharides) inhibit calcification
ATP made
Ca++ intracellular
Few vesicles, contain little Ca++
Hypertrophic zone
Maturation zone
Progressively disaggregated
Ca++ uptake, no ATP made
Ca++ intracellular
Contain little Ca++
Preparation of matrix for calcification
Degenerative zone
Ca++ release begins
Ca++ passes into matrix
Begin Ca++ uptake
Zone of provisional calcification
Calcification of matrix
Disaggregated proteoglycans (acid mucopolysaccharides) permit calcification
Ca++ released
Matrix calcified
Crystals in and on vesicles
Metaphysis
Last intact transverse septum
Primary spongiosa
Vascular invasion and resorption of transverse septa
Bone formation
Secondary spongiosa
Branches of metaphyseal and nutrient arteries
Remodeling
Internal: removal of cartilage bars, replacement of fiber bone with lamellar bone
External: funnelization
F. Netter M.D.
©CIBA-GEIGY

Figure 5
Zonal structure, function, and intracellular calcium transfer in the growth plate. (© Copyright 1987 CIBA-GEIGY Corporation. Modified with permission from THE CIBA COLLECTION OF MEDICAL ILLUSTRATIONS, illustrated by Frank H. Netter, MD. All rights reserved.)

Although the major collagen in the hypertrophic zone is type II, the hypertrophic zone chondrocytes also produce and secrete type X collagen into the matrix. Results of some studies suggest that type X collagen is associated with matrix vesicles and may play a supportive role in matrix mineralization. Ascorbate (Vitamin C) may play a role in mineralization by stimulating matrix vesicle formation and type X collagen synthesis. (For more information on collagen types refer back to the chapter on articular cartilage.)

The initial nucleation site for matrix calcification is currently controversial, although most data would support the primary role of the matrix vesicle in this process. Matrix vesicles are 100- to 150-mm trilamellar membrane structures produced by the chondrocyte plasma membrane; they are rich in alkaline phosphatase and neutral proteases. Alkaline phosphatase may participate in mineralization by hydrolysis of pyrophosphate, a mineralization inhibitor. Hydrolysis of pyrophosphate, ATP, and other phosphodiesterases results in a local increase in phosphate. The neutral proteases of the matrix vesicles help degrade aggregated proteoglycans, producing disaggregated proteoglycans, which promote mineralization. The matrix vesicles can actively accumulate calcium by energy-dependent transport and are rich in calcium-binding phospholipids. The

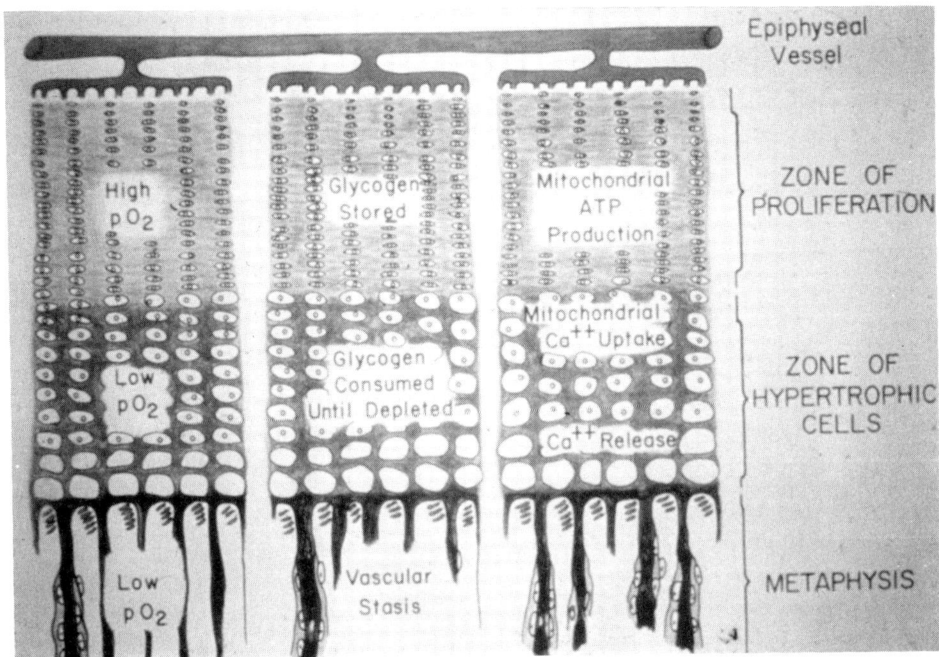

Figure 6
Metabolic events in the growth plate.

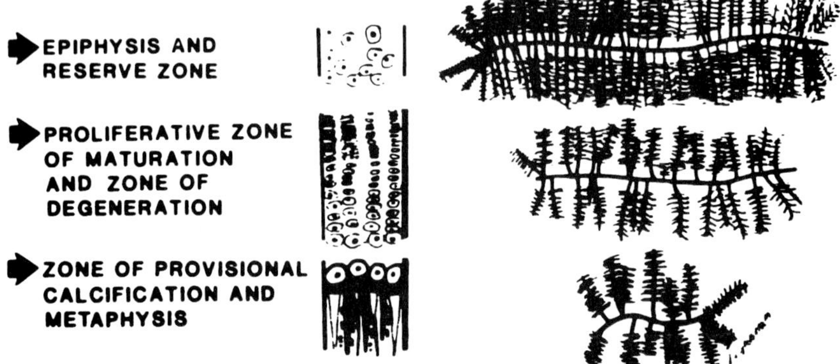

Figure 7
Proteoglycan aggregates: zonal variation.

accumulation of calcium in the vesicle and the local increase in phosphate contribute to a local increase in the calcium phosphate product and, thereby, participate in the process of mineralization.

Other proposed sites of initial mineralization are associated with proteoglycans and a calcium-binding protein, chondrocalcin (C-propeptide of type II collagen). Chondrocalcin has been shown to be associated with the initial site of calcification, and is produced by the hypertrophic zone chondrocyte in response to stimulation by the vitamin D metabolite, 24,25 dihydroxy vitamin D. The precise relationship among these factors, mineralization, and matrix vesicles is not clear. The initial form of mineral deposition is also not clearly established although it has been studied extensively.

Effect of Hormones and Growth Factors on the Growth Plate

Introduction

Many hormones, vitamins, and growth factors affect the growth plate by influencing chondrocyte proliferation, maturation, macromolecule synthesis, intracellular calcium homeostasis, or matrix mineralization. Research in this area of growth plate physiology recently has led to new information and development of many new concepts. Although many more factors influencing the growth plate have been defined, the integrated view of all of these factors in the overall function of the growth plate and of their sites and mechanisms of action is presently incomplete. Some of the factors (systemic hormones, vitamins, and growth factors) are produced at a site distant from the growth plate and, therefore, act on the chondrocytes through a classic endocrine mechanism. Other factors both are produced and act within the growth plate and, therefore, function as paracrine or autocrine factors. Paracrine factors are produced by one cell within a tissue and affect a different cell in that tissue. Autocrine factors are produced by and affect the same cell in the tissue.

In the differentiation zones of the growth plate, cells are distinguished by their involvement in the processes of differentiation, proliferation, maturation, and hypertrophy. Therefore, some factors have a specific effect on a particular zone (Table 1). In addition, the sensitivity of each zone of the growth plate to hormone stimulation can vary with the age of the animal. Some hormone effects may qualitatively or quantitatively depend on the species. To make matters even more complex, a combination of factors, acting in concert, influence the function of individual cells. Available evidence strongly suggests that each growth plate zone may be specifically targeted by one or more agents to effect a particular stage in the cell maturation phenomena (Fig. 8). This differential hormonal or growth factor sensitivity provides for a continuum of maturational events, culminating in bone growth.

Systemic Hormones and Vitamins

Thyroxine

The thyroid hormones thyroxine (T_4) and 3,5,3′ triiodothyronine (T_3) are peptide hormones produced by the thyroid gland and transported to the target site on server proteins. T_4 is the primary secretory product of the thyroid, and 80% of T_3 is formed from deiodination of T_4 in the liver and kidney. Although there is less T_3 in the circulation, it has three to four times greater biologic activity than T_4. The thyroid hormones act on the proliferative and upper hypertrophic zone chondrocytes through a systemic endocrine mechanism (Fig. 8).

Thyroxine is essential for cartilage growth; it increases DNA synthesis in cells from the proliferative zone. Thyroxine has a second and entirely independent effect on cell maturation, increasing glycosaminoglycan and collagen synthesis and alkaline phosphatase activity. Its effect on cartilage growth is mediated by a synergy between thyroxine and insulin-like growth factor/somatomedin-C (IGF-I/SM-C). For example, anti IGF-I antibodies inhibit cartilage growth stimulation by T_3 but do not inhibit chondrocyte maturation as monitored by alkaline phosphatase activity. Administration of T_4 alone to thyroidectomized and parathyroidectomized animals results in hypertrophic chondrocyte maturation, but little growth; administration of growth hormone alone does not affect maturation, but generates normal cellular proliferation. The two agents together restore both growth and maturation. T_3 does not stimulate IGF-I synthesis by chondrocytes; it simply enhances the growth effects of IGF-I. Excess T_4 results in protein catabolism, and a deficiency results in growth retardation, cretinism, and abnormal degradation of mucopolysaccharides.

Parathyroid Hormone

Parathyroid hormone (PTH), an 84-amino-acid protein produced by the parathyroids, acts primarily on the proliferative and upper hypertrophic zone chondrocytes (Fig. 8). Although PTH is found primarily bound to cells in the hypertrophic zone, it has the same qualitative effect on cells from different zones. This hormone has a direct mitogenic effect on epiphyseal chondrocytes and stimulates proteoglycan synthesis. Its effect on proteoglycan synthesis is mediated by an increase in the intracellular ionized calcium concentration and stimulation of protein kinase C. PTH has a synergistic effect that enhances the mitogenic effect of local growth factors.

Calcitonin

Calcitonin (CT), a peptide hormone produced by the parafollicular cells of the thyroid, acts primarily in the lower hypertrophic zone (Fig. 8). It has been documented to accelerate growth plate calcification and cellular maturation.

Glucocorticoids

Adrenal corticoids (glucocorticoids), 4-ring steroid hormones produced by the adrenal cortex, primarily affect the zones of cellular differentiation and proliferation. Supraphysiologic amounts of glucocorticoids adversely affect growth and regeneration of epiphyseal cartilage, resulting in growth retardation. Excessive amounts of glucocorticoid from either endogenous or exogenous sources inhibit both

Table 1
Effect of hormones and growth factors on the growth plate

Hormone/Factor	Systemic/Local Derivation	Biologic Effect: Proliferation	Biologic Effect: Macromolecule Biosynthesis	Biologic Effect: Maturation Degradation	Biologic Effect: Matrix Calcification	Zone Primarily Affected
Thyroxine	Systemic (thyroid)	+ (T_3 with IGF-I)	0	+ (T_3 alone)	0	Proliferative zone and upper hypertrophic zone
Parathyroid	Systemic (parathyroid)	+	++ (proteoglycan)	0	0	Entire growth plate
Calcitonin	Systemic (thyroid)	0	0	+	+	Hypertrophic zone and metaphysis
Excess corticosteroids	Systemic (adrenals)	-	-	-	0	Entire growth plate
Growth Hormone	Systemic (pituitary)	+ (through IGF-I locally)	+ (slight)	0	0	Proliferative zone
Somatomedins	Systemic Local paracrine (liver, chondrocytes)	+	+ (slight)	0	0	Proliferative zone
Insulin	Systemic (pancreas)	+ (through IGF-1 receptor)	0	0	0	Proliferative zone
1,25 $(OH)_2D_3$	Systemic (liver, kidney)	0	0	+ (indirect effect serum [Ca] × [PO])		Hypertrophic zone
24,25 $(OH)_2D_3$	Systemic (liver, kidney)	+	+ (collagen II)	0	0	Proliferative zone and hypertrophic zone
Vitamin A	Systemic (diet)	0	0	-	0	Hypertrophic zone
Vitamin C	Systemic (diet)	0	+ (collagen)	0	+ (matrix vesicles)	Proliferative zone and hypertrophic zone
EGF	Local paracrine (endothelial cells)	+	- (collagen)	0	0	Metaphysis
FGF	Local paracrine (endothelial cells)	+	0	0	0	Proliferative zone
PDGF	Local paracrine (platelets)	+	+ (noncollagenous proteins)	0	0	Proliferative zone
TGF-β	Local paracrine (platelets, chondrocytes)	±	±	0	0	Proliferative zone and hypertrophic zone
BDGF	Local paracrine (bone matrix)	0	+ (collagen)	0	0	Upper hypertrophic zone
IL-1	Local paracrine (inflammatory cells, synoviocytes)	0	-	++ activates tissue metallo-proteinases	0	Entire growth plate
Prostaglandin	Local autocrine	±	+ (proteoglycan) - (collagen and alkaline phosphatase)	0	Bone resorption with osteoclasts	Hypertrophic zone and metaphysis

Effects are (+) increase stimulation; (0) no known effect; (-) inhibitory; (±) depending on the local hormonal milieu.
Hormones/factors are (EGF) epidermal growth factor; (FGF) fibroblast growth factor; (PDGF) platelet-derived growth factor; (TGF-β) transforming growth factor-beta; (BDGF) bone-derived growth factor; (IL-1) interleukin-1.

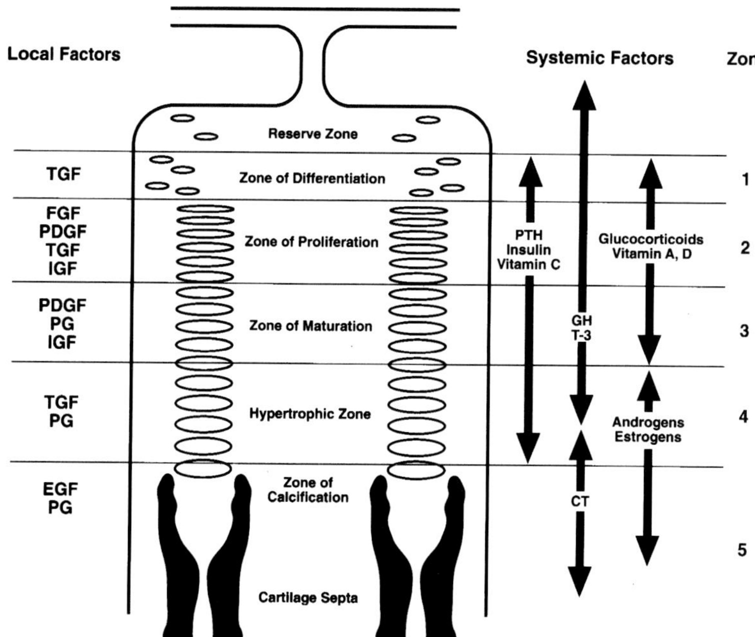

Figure 8
Schematic representation of the growth plate demonstrating the proposed site of action of local and systemic hormones, growth factors, and vitamins.

the mitotic and the synthetic activity of chondrocytes. This catabolic effect of glucocorticoids has been documented at high concentrations where the growth rate of long bones is inversely correlated with hormone concentration. This metabolic suppression is attributed to a depression of glycolysis and a reduction of energy stores. The primary influence of glucocorticoids is a decrease in proliferation of chondroprogenitor cells in the zone of differentiation. An adverse effect of corticosteroids, apparent in the growth apparatus of young growing animals, is suppression of longitudinal growth and skeletal maturity.

Sex Steroids

Androgens (C_{19} steroids) function primarily in the lower portion of the growth plate to stimulate mineralization. Androgens are considered to be anabolic factors, and they stimulate proteoglycan synthesis in epiphyseal chondrocytes in vitro. This effect is age-dependent insofar as animals do not respond after reaching skeletal maturity. The androgens' anabolic effect also is manifested as an increased deposition of glycogen and lipids in cells and an increase in proteoglycans in cartilage matrix. Supraphysiologic doses of androgens depress growth and accelerate growth plate closure. According to results of recent studies, testosterone and dihydrotestosterone can stimulate DNA synthesis in chondrocytes of male growth plate tissue, whereas only dihydrostestosterone is active in female tissue. In both tissues, receptors were found only for the dihydrotestosterone metabolite, suggesting that this is the primary active androgen metabolite.

Estrogens (C_{18} steroids) decrease tibial length by specific inhibition of metaphyseal bone resorption and, thus, endochondral growth, increasing the thickness of the growth plate. It has been suggested that the acceleration of cell hypertrophy induced by estrogens may be interference in proteoglycan processing for extracellular transport.

Growth Hormone

Growth hormone (GH) is a peptide hormone produced by the pituitary. Growth hormone and its mediators, the somatomedins, act throughout the growth plate and primarily affect cellular proliferation. Hypophysectomy results in delayed or reduced osteogenesis, a decrease in mineralization, reduction in cartilage differentiation, and cessation of growth. GH is essential for growth plate function, but its mechanism of action remains unclear. The effects of GH are mediated by the production of a group of peptide growth factors termed somatomedins or, in current terminology, insulin-like growth factors (IGF). It is uncertain whether the effects of GH are indirect and result from the production of serum-derived IGF by the liver or whether there is a direct GH effect to induce chondrocytes to produce IGF locally (paracrine or autocrine effect). Earlier work suggested that GH effects were indirect, and were mediated only by the GH-dependent serum IGF. However, when GH binds to epiphyseal chondrocytes there is a local synthesis of IGF. Hence, the direct effect of GH creates target cells in which IGF-I induces a selective multiplication (clonal expansion) of differentiated cells.

Receptors for two members of the somatomedin family, IGF-I (somatomedin C or SM-C) and IGF-II (multiplication stimulatory activity), have been found in the growth plate. A complex pattern of graded specificity of receptors for each exists; cells in the zone of differentiation bind IGF-I, but the greatest binding is in the proliferative zone. GH regulates both the number of cells containing IGF receptors and the local synthesis of IGF-I by the chondrocytes in all zones of the growth plate. A "functional heterogeneity" exists in chondrocytes in the proliferative and hypertrophic zones, in that the cellular response to IGF-I declines with maturation and hypertrophy of the cells. IGF-II appears to be a more potent clonal growth effector during fetal life, and IGF-I has a greater effect during postnatal life. The somatomedins' structure and function are described in the chapter on articular cartilage.

Insulin

Juvenile diabetics may exhibit a decrease in growth despite elevated levels of GH and normal IGF-I and IGF-II levels. It has been suggested that there is a decrease in a circulating growth plate factor, which contributes to growth retardation. Insulin can cross-react with IGF-I receptors and, therefore, may have some minor anabolic or permissive effect at physiologic insulin levels.

Vitamin D Metabolites

The active metabolites of vitamin D are the 1,25 and 24,25 dihydroxylated forms of vitamin D_3, both of which are produced by the liver and kidney. Vitamin D deficiency results in an elongation of the cell columns of the growth plate. This effect is considered to be secondary to a vitamin D-induced decrease in systemic calcium and phosphorus and the subsequent inhibition of mineralization. A direct mitogenic effect of vitamin D has been reported with 24,25 dihydroxy vitamin D (24,25 $(OH)_2$ D_3), but not with 1,25 $(OH)_2$ D_3. The 24,25 $(OH)_2$ D_3 metabolite significantly increases DNA (deoxyribonucleic acid) synthesis as well as inhibiting chondrocyte proteoglycan synthesis. The 1,25 $(OH)_2$ D_3 inhibits the proteoglycan synthetic response to local growth factors. The vitamin D metabolites are bound to cells in all growth plate zones except the hypertrophic zone. The highest levels are found in the zone of proliferation. Vitamin D excess is associated with atrophic changes mediated by an effect on the normal differentiation pattern. The pathologic effects of vitamin D excess and deficiency are discussed later in this chapter.

Vitamin A

The carotenes are essential for epiphyseal cartilage cell metabolism. A deficiency state results in impairment of the cell maturation phenomena of the growth apparatus. This deficiency culminates in suppression of growth and in abnormal bone shape. Excessive vitamin A leads to bone weakness resulting from increases in lysosomal body membrane fragility.

Vitamin C

Ascorbic acid primarily influences the growth apparatus by virtue of its requirement as a cofactor in the enzymatic synthesis of collagen. Ascorbate has been shown to stimulate matrix mineralization in in vitro cultures of growth plate chondrocytes, through its stimulation of matrix vesicle formation and the synthesis of alkaline phosphatase and types II and X collagen.

Growth Factors

Not all of the known growth factors have been tested specifically on epiphyseal chondrocytes. Epidermal growth factor polypeptide (EGF), generally found at high levels in platelets and glandular tissue, has been shown to influence the growth plate. It is found in endothelial lining cells in the growth plate, lying between invading capillaries and calcifying cartilage septa. EGF induces cell replication and inhibits collagen synthesis and alkaline phosphatase activity in calvarial cultures. Fibroblast growth factor (FGF) is a family of polypeptides derived from multiple areas, including endothelial cell growth factor, that stimulates cell replication of chondrocytes. Platelet-derived growth factor (PDGF) stimulates DNA synthesis and cell replication as well as protein synthesis. Transforming growth factor-beta (TGF-β), a constituent of bone matrix, is a multifunctional peptide that controls cell replication and differentiation. It is involved in cartilage formation during the first step of endochondral bone formation. Release of TGF-β is stimulated by PTH, but the overall effect of TGF-β appears to depend on constituent growth factors in the cell. Therefore, its effects may be stimulatory or inhibitory depending on the hormonal environment when TGF-β is introduced to the chondrocytes. A positive effect on synthesis of cartilage matrix has been described. Significantly, TGF-β is a potent inhibitor of a lymphocyte-activating factor called interleukin-1 (IL-1), which induces degradation in growth plate chondrocytes. Bone-derived growth factor or B2-macroglobulin (BDGF) has been isolated from bone matrix. BDGF stimulates collagen synthesis and has been found in serum and on the surface of all cell types. It apparently interacts with receptors for hormones and is thought to be a modulator of binding of other growth factors or circulating hormones to such receptors.

Prostaglandins

These ubiquitous biologically active agents are present in nanomolar levels in growth plate cells and affect cellular processes by altering intracellular cAMP levels. An acceleration in DNA synthesis has been observed in epiphyseal chondrocytes, as well as inhibition of alkaline phosphatase activity and collagen synthesis and stimulation of proteoglycan synthesis. An alteration in types of prostaglandins is seen during the various stages of endochondral ossification. Some evidence indicates that, at elevated levels, these factors delay proliferation and maturation of cells and inhibit bone elongation and cell production rate.

Biomechanics of the Growth Plate

Introduction

As the weakest structure in the developing ends of long bones, the growth plate is a common site for injury. Given that the growth plate is solely responsible for longitudinal growth of the skeleton, the importance of understanding both the characteristics and consequences of growth plate injuries is clear. All injury is associated with failure, whether physiologic failure of systems or processes or mechanical failure of tissues. Mechanical disruption of the growth plate can lead to physiologic failure; appropriate treatment depends on comprehension of the mechanical properties of the growth plate, of the mechanical conditions that cause injury, and of the ultimate effect on the adjacent bone.

When an injury actually leads to growth abnormalities and bone deformities, treatment is required to correct them. In such cases, an understanding of the growth plate's response to mechanical stimuli would be of significant benefit, creating the potential for controlling bone growth through strategic surgical interventions.

The Mechanical Properties of Growth Plate Cartilage

Unlike those of many biologic tissues such as bone, articular cartilage, tendon, and ligament, the mechanical properties of growth plate cartilage have infrequently been investigated. Characterization of these properties is essential for a fundamental understanding of the tissue, both as an organ of growth and as a structural element. In addition, analytic mechanical models of the growth plate depend on several input parameters, including material properties.

The equilibrium compressive modulus (see section on the biphasic nature of articular cartilage) has been measured from cartilaginous materials that are similar to the growth plate. Equilibrium moduli for articular cartilage, chondroepiphyseal cartilage, and reserve zone cartilage have been reported to be between 0.4 and 1.5 MPa, 0.7 MPa, and about 0.35 MPa, respectively. In recent studies, values for the equilibrium compressive moduli of bovine growth plate and rabbit growth plate have been found to be approximately 0.17 to 0.9 MPa and 0.044 MPa, respectively. Presently, no data exist to describe the failure, tensile, or shear properties of growth plate cartilage.

Although differences in mechanical test parameters, anatomic position, age, or species of test specimens may account for some of the large variation in modulus values, the intimate relationship between morphology and mechanical properties, or structure and function, must certainly play a significant role. Though the constituent materials of the growth plate are similar to these other cartilaginous tissues, differences exist with respect to the amount, composition, and organization of the matrix, as well as the cellular architecture and density. The relationship between growth plate morphology and tensile failure has been investigated using the proximal tibiae of growing rats. The weakest portion of the growth plate was found to be the hypertrophic zone, in which the matrix volume is low and the cellular content is high. At the onset of sexual maturation in the rat, the hypertrophic zone of the growth plate increases in width, and the tensile strength decreases. Consistent cleavage through the hypertrophic zone at failure reinforces the concept that mechanical properties depend on regional morphology.

Factors Affecting Growth Plate Fracture and Failure Strength

Growth plate injuries occur when the mechanical demands placed on a bone exceed the mechanical strength of the epiphysis-growth plate-metaphysis complex. Two of the factors that determine the incidence of injury are (1) the ability of the growth plate to resist failure (that is, the mechanical properties of the growth plate as discussed above), and (2) the forces applied to the bone or the stresses induced in the growth plate. The characteristics of the fracture have great clinical significance for treatment options and predicted outcomes. The Salter-Harris classification system for growth plate injuries was proposed in an effort to relate the mechanisms, characteristics, and prognoses of these fractures.

As originally proposed, Salter-Harris type I injuries involve complete separation of the epiphysis from the metaphysis with no associated bone fracture, and are produced by shear or tensile forces

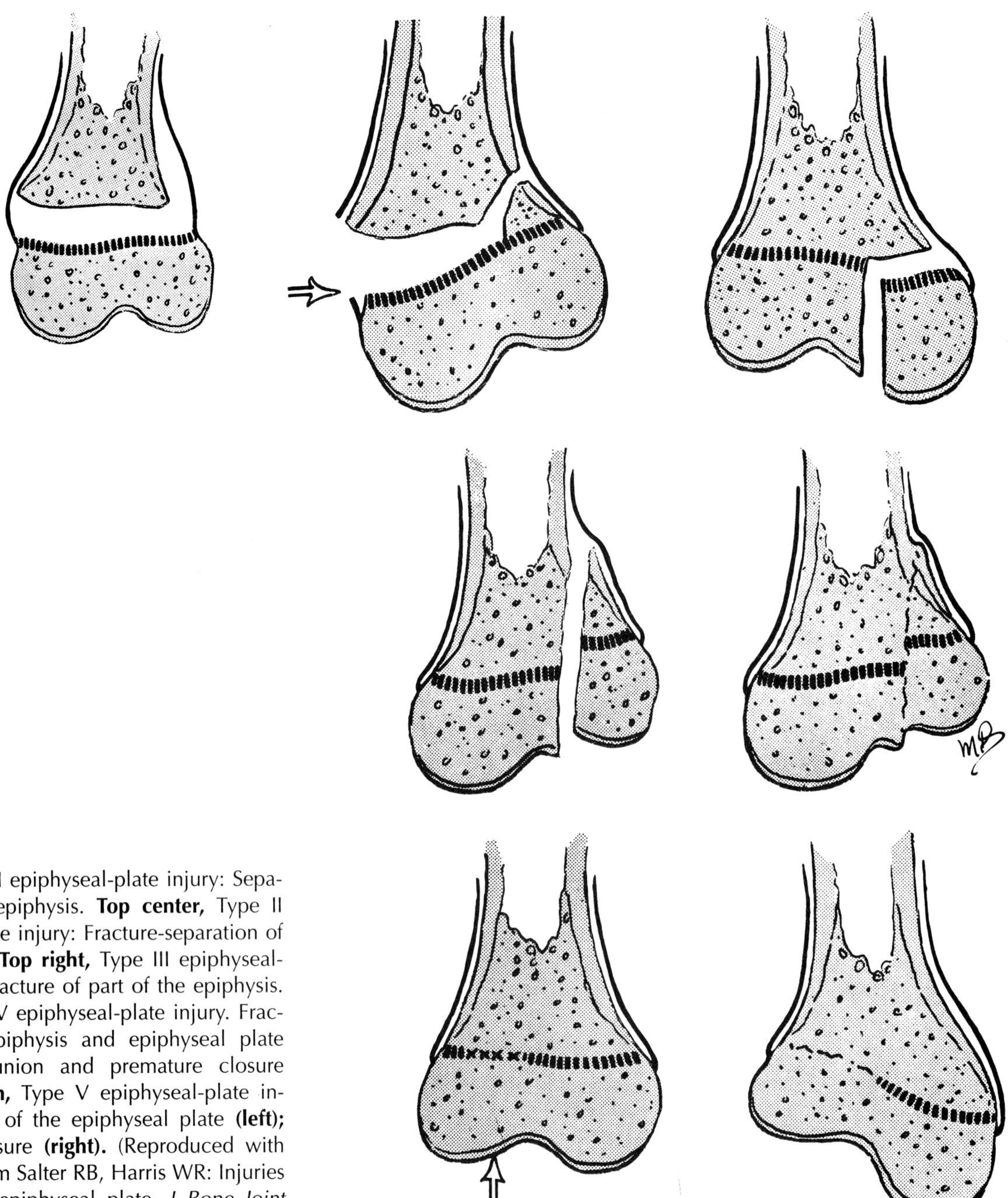

Figure 9
Top left, Type I epiphyseal-plate injury: Separation of the epiphysis. **Top center,** Type II epiphyseal-plate injury: Fracture-separation of the epiphysis. **Top right,** Type III epiphyseal-plate injury: Fracture of part of the epiphysis. **Center,** Type IV epiphyseal-plate injury. Fracture of the epiphysis and epiphyseal plate **(left).** Bone union and premature closure **(right). Bottom,** Type V epiphyseal-plate injury. Crushing of the epiphyseal plate **(left);** Premature closure **(right).** (Reproduced with permission from Salter RB, Harris WR: Injuries involving the epiphyseal plate. *J Bone Joint Surg* 1963;45A:587–622.)

(Fig. 9, *top left*). This type of injury is most common in early childhood when the growth plate is relatively thick. The fracture line propagates principally through the lower hypertrophic zone, leaving the reserve and proliferative zones attached to the epiphysis. In this situation, the cells responsible for interstitial growth of the growth plate and the epiphyseal blood supply are undisturbed, and the prognosis for continued normal growth is excellent.

A type II injury (Fig. 9, *top center*) is also thought to be produced by shear or tensile forces and is the most common injury. It consists of fracture along the growth plate with an attached metaphyseal bone fragment. The anatomic position of the metaphyseal fragment depends on load direction. With a bending or angulation force, the metaphyseal fragment is normally located on the compressive or concave side, while the periosteum is torn on the tensile or convex side. The reserve and proliferative zones remain with the epiphysis, the circulation is usually preserved, and the prognosis for further growth is excellent.

The type III injury (Fig 9, *top right*) is intra-articular and attributed to shear forces at the joint.

The fracture passes from the joint surface to the growth plate and out toward the periphery along the lower hypertrophic zone. As long as the epiphyseal blood supply is left intact, prognosis is good.

The type IV fracture (Fig. 9, *center*) is similar to type III, except that the fracture continues across the full thickness of the growth plate to include a metaphyseal fragment, thereby producing a complete split of the bone end. Accurate realignment is essential to prevent formation of a bony bridge and growth arrest.

A type V injury (Fig 9, *bottom*) results from a large compressive force that crushes the cells of the "germinal" or reserve zone. The prognosis is poor.

Although the Salter-Harris classification system is useful clinically, growth plate fractures are actually much more complex. Accurate assessment of the detailed histologic pattern of fracture is important because the location of damage determines the fate of proliferative cell activity, epiphyseal blood supply, and, therefore, future growth. Although a consistent plane of separation through the hypertrophic zone has been seen in several experiments, other studies have revealed a more variable histologic pattern of fracture. It has been demonstrated that transphyseal fractures of the lower extremities of rats and rabbits did not exclusively produce damage to the hypertrophic zone. Although the greater proportion of each fracture involved the hypertrophic zone, damage was also noted in the proliferative and reserve zones. Only 15% of rat proximal tibiae tested in a separate study failed uniformly at the level of the growth plate-metaphysis junction, while 85% of the specimens displayed crack propagation through the upper proliferative and reserve zones. The type of load applied to a bone also affects the fracture pattern. It has been shown that tensile forces applied to the rat proximal tibiae produce separation through the reserve zone, while shear forces produce fractures through both the proliferative and hypertrophic zones. Even with application of the same type of load, both the gross fracture pattern and the histologic fracture pattern (zones involved) can vary depending on the load direction.

It is important to realize that, unlike controlled laboratory tests, clinical fractures occur under multiaxial loading conditions and failure is ultimately determined by the internally induced stresses in the bone and growth plate. These stresses must be distinguished from the externally applied load type. An externally applied compressive, tensile, or shear load cannot be expected to have the same effect on bones of different geometry and growth plate curvature, because these loads, singly or in combination, induce a complex three-dimensional stress state within the structures. Any one of these loading modes can induce all types of stresses (compressive, tensile, and shear) throughout the entire growth plate (Fig. 10) and, therefore, cause variable fracture patterns. In short, it is difficult to correlate fracture patterns to externally applied loads without consideration of other factors, including regional geometry and local material properties. Thus the mechanism of injury can also be deduced based on the Salter-Harris classification system.

The majority of studies on the biomechanics of growth plate injuries have been conducted on a macrostructural whole bone level, in which the observed fracture or failure properties reflect the combined effects of the bone geometry and size, the growth plate topology, and the bone and growth plate cartilage mechanical properties. Experiments on isolated specimens of growth plate cartilage control for differences in the geometric and structural variables and reveal a relationship between mechanical stress and fracture pattern for growth plate cartilage alone. Isolated rectangular specimens of bone-growth plate-bone from the bovine femur and tibia have been tested, and the correlation between stress and histologic fracture pattern reported (Fig. 11). Tensile stresses cause the greatest damage in the upper proliferative zone. Shear stresses induce failure between the upper proliferative zone and the

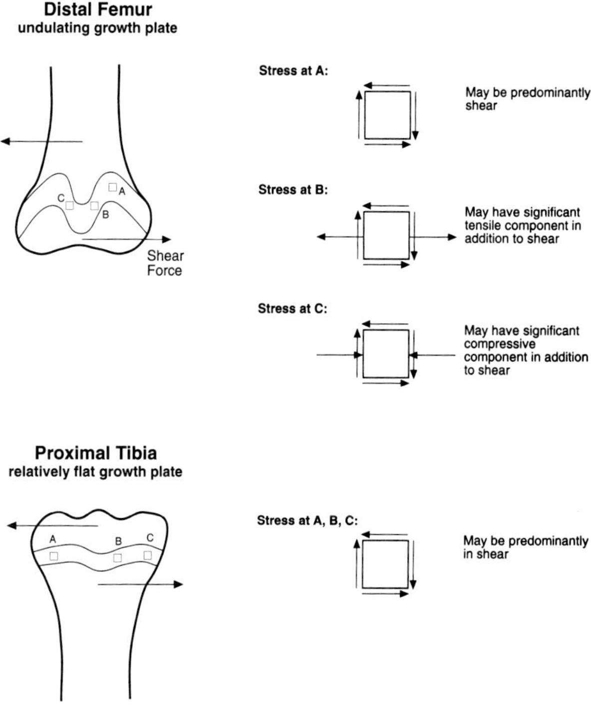

Figure 10
If the type of externally applied force is differentiated from the internally induced stresses, it can be better understood why different failure patterns can easily result when the same type of force is applied to different bones and growth plates.

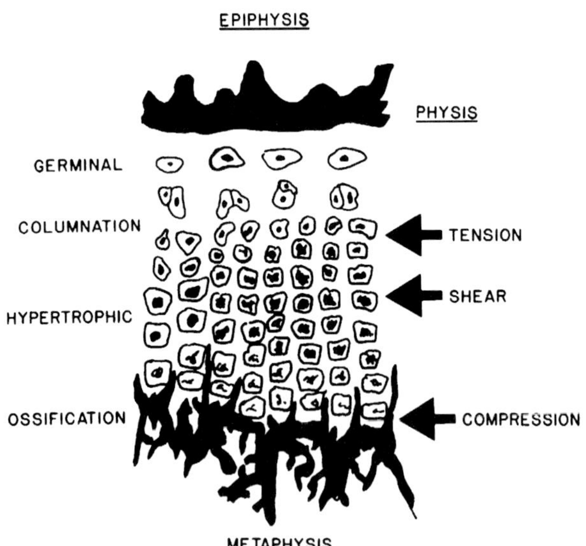

Figure 11
The histologic zone of failure varies with the type of loading applied to the specimens. (Reproduced with permission from Moen CT, Pelker RR: Biomechanical and histological correlations in growth plate failure. *J Pediatr Orthop* 1984;4:180–184.)

lower hypertrophic zone. Such damage may be deleterious to the activity of the dividing cells of the growth plate and can affect future growth. Under compressive stress, damage is found primarily in the metaphyseal trabeculae, with little damage to the growth plate cartilage itself. This finding contradicts the concept of a crushing injury to the growth plate as a cause for growth arrest (Salter-Harris type V). An important point, however, is that damage to the growth mechanism may occur without visible evidence of fracture.

Experimental studies have shown that growth plate failure strength and fracture patterns are influenced by other factors in addition to the type and direction of force. These include morphology, age, the support of surrounding structures, and tensile and compressive factors.

Morphology

The growth plate adapts its form to follow the contours of principal tensile stresses. These contours allow the growth plate to be subjected mostly to compressive stress. The avoidance of shear stresses provides an optimal geometry for strength of the mechanical interface.

The gross morphology of the distal bovine physis was studied and found to exhibit three-dimensional (3-D) undulations. The primary contours correspond to the four ridges and valleys. The distance between the apices is about 50 mm, and the amplitude is 10 mm. The secondary contours are a finer pattern of undulations within the primary contours, with a spatial periodicity of 5 mm and amplitude of 1 mm. The tertiary contours have an even smaller spatial periodicity (0.5 mm) and amplitude (0.1 mm). The primary and secondary contours are the same on the epiphyseal and metaphyseal sides of the physes. The tertiary contours, however, are unrelated on either side and appear to reflect the randomness of physeal growth. Radiographically a layer of dense trabecular bone is adjacent to and parallel to the primary contour of the growth plate on the metaphyseal side (Fig. 12).

The Effect of Age on Failure Strength and Fracture Patterns

Mechanical tests on human cadaveric femoral heads of various ages (from less than 13 months to greater than 15 years) have shown that the shear strength of the capital femoral epiphysis increases with age. This increase in strength can be attributed both to the increasing overall size of the femoral head and to the developmental changes to the growth plate topology (Fig. 13). With increasing age, the growth plate becomes thinner and exhibits an increased number of mamillary processes and curves, thereby creating an undulating surface that imparts an increased resistance to shear. This general finding of increased failure strength with age has been reported consistently regardless of the type of applied force (shear or tension), the type of bone, or the species.

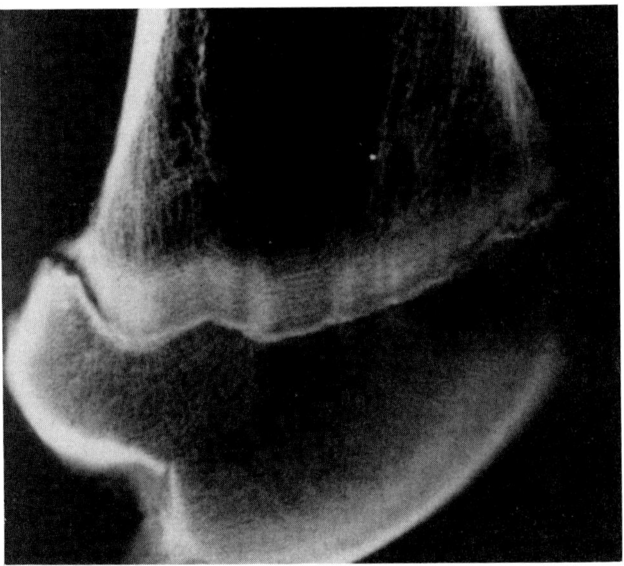

Figure 12
Radiograph of plate and trabecular bone structure in parasagittal section. (Reproduced with permission from Cohen B, Chorney GS, Phillips DP, et al: The microstructural tensile properties and biochemical composition of the bovine distal femoral growth plate. *J Orthop Res* 1992;10:263–275.)

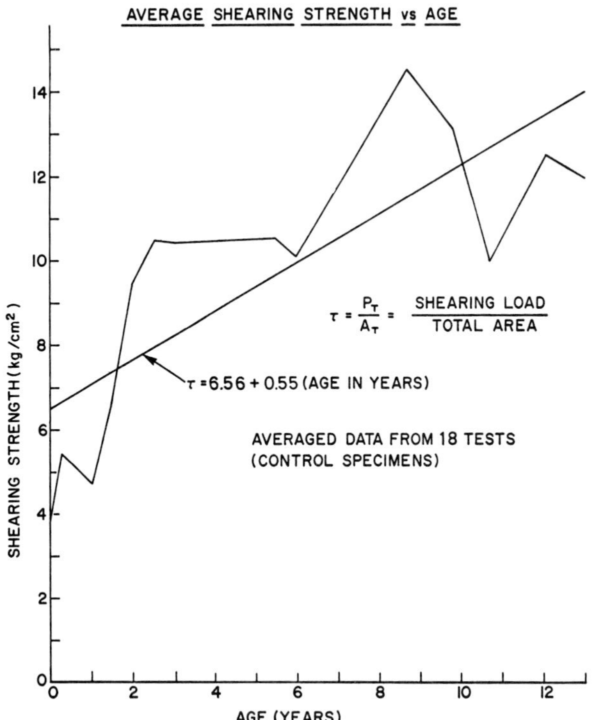

Figure 13
Shear stress (τ) for 18 control specimens versus age. The straight line represents a least-squares fit of the data. (Reproduced with permission from Chung SM, Batterman SC, Brighton CT, et al: Shear strength of the human capital epiphyseal plate. *J Bone Joint Surg* 1976;58A:94–103.)

Experimental data have also been presented to support the fact that age or stage of skeletal development influences the growth plate fracture pattern. Under controlled shear tests on human and rabbit proximal femurs, it has been shown that the transphyseal fracture (type I) occurs most frequently in the very young as proposed by Salter and Harris; however, it may not pass exclusively through the lower hypertrophic zone. In older bones, fractures tend to pass through both the growth plate and the metaphysis or epiphysis (types II-IV).

The Effect of Surrounding Structures on Failure Strength

The growth plate is surrounded circumferentially by the perichondral region, which is composed of a dense cell layer, a loosely packed cell layer, an overlying fibrous tissue, and in some cases, an inner bony ring. The strongly oriented collagen fibers of the perichondral region are firmly anchored to the epiphysis and metaphysis, immediately adjacent to the growth plate. These characteristics of location and microstructure suggest a function of mechanical support, in which the perichondral region serves as a limiting membrane, providing lateral constraint to the growth plate cartilage. The perichondral region is included in Ogden's classification scheme for growth plate and epiphyseal injuries; an Ogden type VI injury describes the potential for osseous bridge formation and angular deformity as a result of damage to these peripheral structures.

In tension and shear tests on the proximal tibiae of rats, an intact periosteum/perichondral region has been shown to increase the failure strength significantly. It has also been demonstrated, using human cadaveric femoral heads, that an intact perichondral region can improve shear strength.

As a result of continued skeletal development, the significance of the perichondral region diminishes with age. As its thickness and size decrease, other topologic and histomorphometric characteristics of the growth plate begin to dominate the biomechanical properties. The role of the perichondral region in the mechanical support of the growth plate under joint compression has not been studied, nor has the effect of its presence on fracture patterns.

Tensile and Compressive Properties

The microstructural tensile properties of the bovine femoral growth plate have been determined by controlled uniaxial tension tests. The tensile properties obtained from such tests' stress strain curves are shown in Table 2. The ultimate strain at failure (average 13.8%) has been noted to be fairly uniform throughout the growth plate. However, a significant difference has been noted among the anatomic sites for ultimate stress and tangent modulus. The anterior region of the growth plate seems stronger and stiffer than the other sites. The growth plate is also stronger and stiffer in the periphery than in the interior. These findings correlate with biochemical studies showing that the collagen content is also highest in the anterior regions.

Compression studies on uniform cylindric specimens also have been performed on similar bovine distal femoral specimens. The boundary conditions on fluid flow through the bony interfaces on either side of the growth plate are unknown; therefore, no assumptions on the boundary conditions have been made. Three models representing the different possibilities of boundary conditions have been used to analyze the experimental data. The three models are: (1) both sides are completely permeable; (2) the metaphyseal side is free draining and the epiphyseal side is impermeable; and (3) both sides are impermeable.

The compressive modulus (equilibrium stress/applied strain) of growth plate has been found to be higher for the interior sites (0.90 MPa) than for the periphery (0.71 MPa). This difference between the interior and the periphery has been found to be independent of the boundary conditions.

Table 2
Tensile properties by various anatomic groupings (mean ± SD)

Region	Ultimate Stress[a] (MPa)	Ultimate Strain[b]	Tangent Modulus[a]
Anterior (n=20)	4.10 ± 0.97	0.137 ± 0.05	48.6 ± 25.1
Posterior/lateral (n=30)	3.05 ± 0.80	0.123 ± 0.04	37.9 ± 16.7
Posterior/medial (n=29)	2.30 ± 0.68	0.160 ± 0.06	23.5 ± 14.9
Center (n=7)	2.16 ± 0.79	0.1117 ± 0.06	27.0 ± 11.8
Average	2.97 ± 0.80	0.138 ± 0.06	34.6 ± 17.7
Periphery (n=30)	3.50 ± 1.06	0.132 ± 0.06	44.5 ± 26.1
Interior (n=56)	2.68 ± 0.96	0.141 ± 0.06	29.3 ± 14.2

[a]Significantly different, $p < 0.01$
[b]Not significantly different, $p > 0.1$
(Reproduced with permission from Cohen B, Ghorney GS, Phillips DP, et al: The microstructural tensile properties and biochemical composition of the bovine distal femoral growth plate. *J Orthop Res* 1992;10:263–275.)

The Response of the Growth Plate to Mechanical Stimuli

It has long been recognized that mechanical forces can influence the shape and length of growing bones. Both in vitro and in vivo studies on embryonic tissue have confirmed that mechanical factors can influence bone development during the earliest stages of endochondral ossification. As the primary ossification center expands toward the epiphyses, the specific shapes and contours of the ossification front begin to define the topology of the developing growth plate. This topology may, in part, be determined by the mechanical stresses of daily function. Experiments have suggested that growth plates develop in a way that reduces shear stress at the bone-growth plate interfaces. Such a condition is attained by a growth plate contour that runs perpendicular to lines of principal compression or tension. These same studies further implied that growth plates composed of hyaline cartilage are subjected predominantly to compressive stresses, while growth plates or portions of growth plates composed of fibrocartilage primarily experience tensile stresses. These latter growth plates have often been referred to as apophyses.

The influence of mechanical factors continues to be exhibited during subsequent stages of bone development; in particular, the development of the secondary ossification center. Finite element modeling techniques have been used to evaluate the stress patterns in immature human bones. Specific functions of the calculated stresses have been found to correlate with the propensity for cartilage to be replaced by bone. One hypothesis proposes that intermittent shear stresses tend to accelerate, and intermittent hydrostatic compressive stresses tend to inhibit, the process of endochondral ossification. This hypothesis was used, along with a series of geometric and analytical assumptions, to predict formation of the secondary ossification center. With further experimental verification, this theory has the potential to be a powerful tool.

The concept that mechanical factors can influence bone growth in length is embodied in the Hueter-Volkmann Law. This law simply states that compression forces inhibit growth, and tensile forces stimulate growth. Although some clinical treatments for bone deformities in children are predicated on it, this description of the interaction between mechanics and bone growth is insufficient and lacks quantification. No bounds or ranges on the magnitudes of these forces have been identified, and because both compressive and tensile forces exist simultaneously in bones of the human skeleton, it is doubtful that all compressive forces inhibit growth and all tensile forces stimulate it.

Despite these shortcomings, experimental evidence for the general theme of the Hueter-Volkmann Law is abundant. Many animal studies have been performed in which some alteration is made to the "normal" mechanical environment of a growing bone, and the resultant changes in bone growth measured. Metal staples or wires applied across the growth plate can slow or arrest growth, resulting in the production or treatment of nonuniform growth rates and angular deformities. However, the control of growth by use of staples or wires is unpredictable and often irreversible. Casting is another method that can inhibit growth or cause an abnormal angulation. Periosteal stripping has been attempted as a means of stimulating growth by releasing the presumed compressive force on the growth plate caused by the dense longitudinal fibers of the periosteum. The increases in length obtained from this procedure, although sometimes statistically significant, have been small and may not be sufficient to be practical for correction of large limb length discrepancies. In addition, periosteal division may compromise the structural failure strength of the growth plate. External fixator devices have been applied across growth plates to produce static or dynamic tension or distraction and, thereby, stimulate growth. Chondrodiastasis is an example of such a procedure. Experimental results have been mixed. Although growth plate widening and increased growth are seen in some cases, no significant differences in length are observed in others.

An alternative principle has been proposed in which certain increases in both tension and compression can stimulate growth, while certain decreases in tension and increases in compression can inhibit growth. This chondral modeling theory is described graphically by a chondral growth-force response curve (Fig. 14). It is an attractive theory because of its ability to explain many clinical findings such as congenital dysplastic hip, congenital metatarsus varus, and other deformities. However, as in the case of the Hueter-Volkmann Law, the relationship between the specific character of the loads and the growth response is unknown.

The variability seen in outcomes from clinical attempts to alter growth and the lack of conclusive experimental data might be explained by a limited understanding of the mechanics that control the response. In vitro experiments on the effects of mechanical stress on the biosynthetic and mitotic activity of chondrocytes may aid in elucidating these mechanisms. Although no definitive conclusions have been reached, data from recent studies indicate that high static compressive stresses decrease the biosynthesis of extracellular macromolecules, whereas low intermittent compressive stresses increase matrix synthesis.

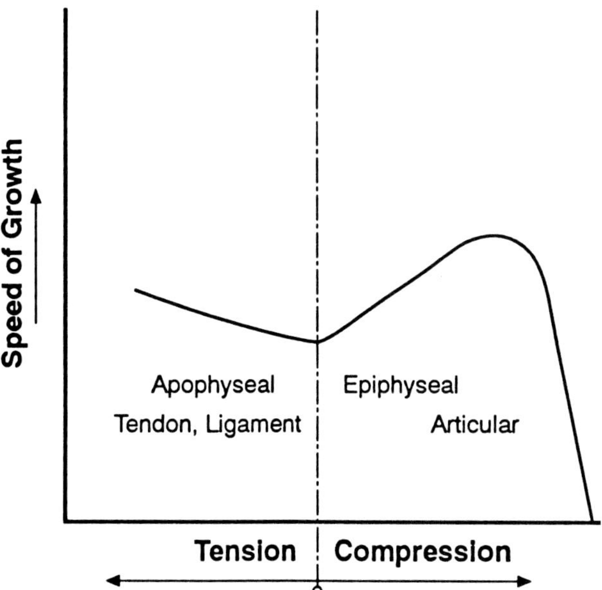

Figure 14
Growth response of cartilage types to physiologic loads. (Reproduced with permission from Frost HM: A chondral modeling theory. *Calcif Tissue Int* 1979;28:181–200.)

In summary, both the function of the growth plate and its susceptibility to failure depend on a complex interaction between external influences and the growth plate's constituent morphology. Continuing research efforts directed towards characterizing its material properties, structural morphology, and biosynthetic and metabolic activity are needed to support clinical diagnosis and treatment.

Pathologic States Primarily Affecting the Growth Plate

The primary function of the growth plate is longitudinal growth, which is accomplished through cellular proliferation and maturation, matrix production and mineralization, endochondral ossification, and resorption (remodeling). Defects in this function may be secondary to environmental, nutritional, hormonal, or genetic factors that primarily affect one or more of these processes.

Environmental Factors

Irradiation

Irradiation primarily affects longitudinal chondroblastic proliferation, but does not affect latitudinal bone growth. It results in a shortened bone of normal width, and may radiographically resemble achondroplasia.

Bacterial Infection

The metaphyseal portion of the growth plate is affected by bacterial invasion. Bacteria lodge in the vascular sinusoids and soon produce one or more small abscesses. Explanations given for bacterial infection in the metaphysis include sluggish circulation, low oxygen tension, and deficiency of the reticuloendothelial system. Extension of the infection through the haversian canals results in osteomyelitis of cortical bone and subperiosteal abscess formation. In most long bones, the joint capsule and growth plate are natural barriers to intra-articular extension of the osteomyelitis or subperiosteal abscess. In the proximal femur, the metaphysis is intra-articular, and pyarthrosis often is associated with hematogenous osteomyelitis. Pyarthrosis can result in femoral avascular necrosis and proteolytic degeneration of the articular cartilage.

The cartilaginous portion of the growth plate is usually a barrier to bacterial infection. Severe infection may result in local or total cessation of growth, which will lead to angular deformity or stunted growth. Mild infection may result in growth stimulation. This phenomenon traditionally had been attributed to local hyperemia. Papain, which is a proteolytic enzyme released from bacteria, has been shown, in small quantity, to stimulate growth; however, a larger amount will depress chondroblastic proliferation and result in proteolytic matrix degradation.

Nutritional Disorders

Malnutrition or protracted illness, if severe enough, will result in depressed chondrogenesis and stunted growth. In these states, metaphyseal bone formation continues until complete occlusion of the marrow space at the cartilage-bone junction occurs and a seal is formed. When normal growth resumes, the bone seal remains as a permanent marker of growth arrest; it is seen on radiographs as a dense line known as a Harris growth arrest line.

Rickets

Rickets results from a deficiency of the vitamin D metabolite 1,25 dihydroxycholecalciferol and may be caused by nutritional factors or renal disease. Vitamin D-deficient states result in a decrease in serum calcium and depression of cartilage matrix calcification. In this disease, a calcifiable cartilage matrix is produced, but the calcium/phosphate product is inadequate to support mineralization. Histologically, the reserve and proliferative zones are normal, but the hypertrophic zone is greatly expanded, which results in widening of the growth plate. The radiographic findings in rickets include no zone of provision calcification, increased separation between the epiphysis and the diaphysis, and flaring of the metaphysis (Fig. 15, *top*). Cartilage bars extend into the metaphysis (Fig. 15, *bottom left*). Unmineralized osteoid is formed on uncalcified bars of cartilage and a primary spongiosa is absent (Fig. 15, *bottom right*). In the rachitic growth plate, the hypertrophic chondrocyte mitochondria retain large amounts of calcium. These mitochondria do not demonstrate loss of calcium until reversal of the pathologic state and mineralization of the matrix. In addition, because the cartilage matrix is not mineralized, the ability of nutrients to diffuse into the hypertrophic zone is greater than in normally mineralized growth plate tissue, and this situation may play a role in the expansion of the hypertrophic zone. In rickets, metaphyseal vascular invasion of the cartilage does not occur (Fig. 16). Normally, the last transverse septum is invaded by capillary buds, but it has been postulated that this cannot occur in the mineral-deficient matrix. Vascular invasion may depend on the production of cartilage-derived growth factor.

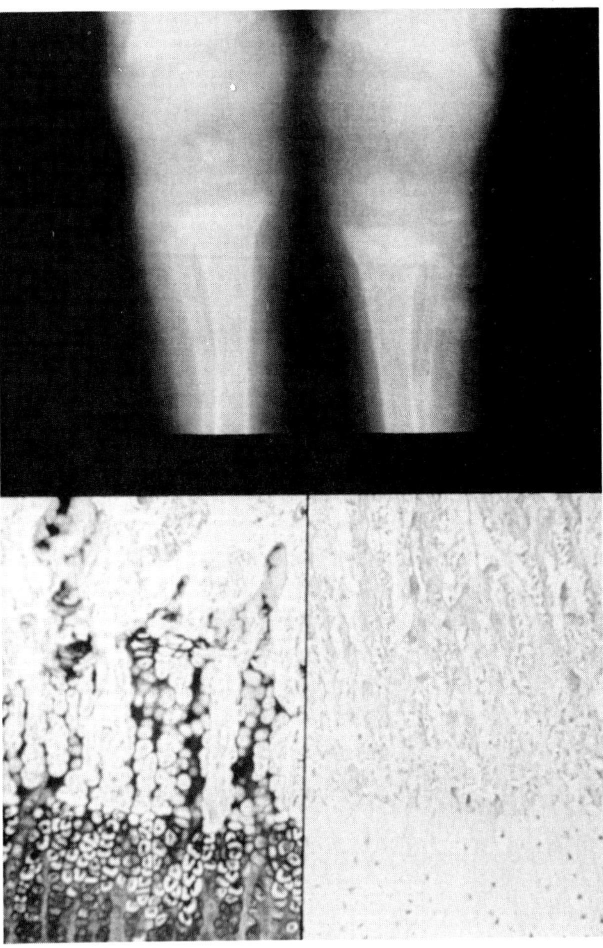

Figure 15
Histologic and radiographic features of rickets.

Scurvy

Scurvy results from vitamin C deficiency. Metabolically, vitamin C deficiency produces a decrease in chondroitin sulfate synthesis (enzymatic impairment of the conversion of glucose to galactosamine) and a deficiency in collagen synthesis (impaired hydroxylation of proline). The greatest deficiency in collagen synthesis is seen in the metaphysis. The microscopic appearance of the cartilaginous portion of the growth plate is normal, but that of the metaphysis is quite abnormal. The metaphysis is primarily affected because of the large amount of type I collagen present in that region of the growth plate. The calcified cartilage bars have a scant amount of osteoid, and they extend deep into the metaphysis. The accumulation of calcified cartilage at the metaphysis-growth plate junction results in a white line on the radiograph (line of Fraenkel). The bony trabeculae are sparse and thin and a generalized osteoporosis exists. The metaphyseal bone is weakened, and microfractures, hemorrhage,

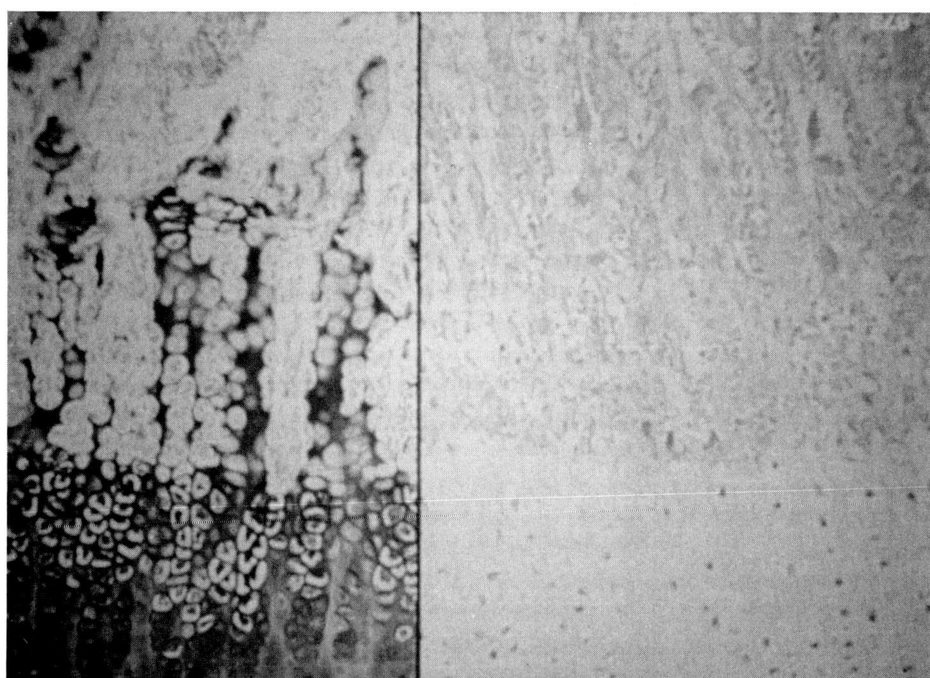

Figure 16
Vascular loops in rickets.

debris, and fibrous tissue accumulate. This region of detritus is called the zone of Trummerfeld. Collapse of the metaphysis along with continued latitudinal growth result in the formation of Pelkin's lateral spurs. Dislocation of the growth plate may occur.

Inheritable Disorders

Defects in Matrix Synthesis: Chondrocytes

In all disorders that affect chondrocyte proliferation there is, by definition, a quantitative decrease in matrix production. In some disorders the matrix is qualitatively changed. Figure 17 demonstrates the various abnormalities of the growth plate. All produce severe skeletal dysplasia, short stature, and severe deformity. In diastrophic dwarfism there is a defect in type II collagen synthesis. In pseudoachondroplastic dwarfism there is an abnormal accumulation of alternating electron-dense and electron-lucent layers of rough-surfaced endoplasmic reticulum. This ultrastructural abnormality results from an abnormal processing and transport of a defective proteoglycan core protein from the endoplasmic reticulum to the Golgi apparatus. In Kniest syndrome there is an autosomal dominant inheritance of a defect in processing of proteoglycans.

The six classes of mucopolysaccharidosis are characterized by lysosomal storage of undegraded glycosaminoglycans and, therefore, by large accumulations of these glycoproteins within the cell (Table 3). As a group the clinical presentation of the mucopolysaccharidoses is somewhat varied by the specific enzyme defect and the glycoprotein accumulated. Each type of mucopolysaccharide has a varied toxic effect on the central nervous system, skeleton, ocular, or visceral organ systems (Table 3).

The general clinical characteristics of this group of diseases may not be specific for any one type, but the pattern should suggest the presence of the disease. All children have stunted growth, facial abnormalities (gargoyle features), and deafness. Some have corneal clouding and mental retardation. Skull films may show thickening of the diploe and occasionally a "slipper-shaped" sella turcica. The chest radiographs may demonstrate paddle-shaped ribs. The pelvis films frequently show coxa vara with variable degrees of femoral capital dysplasia. The long bones typically demonstrate diaphyseal shortening and widening. The metacarpals demonstrate a "pencil sharpened" proximal epiphysis, and Madelung wrist deformity may be present.

Defects in Matrix Synthesis: Osteoblasts

Osteogenesis imperfecta is the result of a defect in type I collagen metabolism. The typical histologic and radiographic features are depicted in Figure 18. In this disorder, the collagen fiber does not mature beyond the reticulum fiber stage. Collagen maturation in the connective tissues throughout the body is affected. Endochondral bone formation in the metaphysis and intramembranous bone formation are severely affected. The cartilaginous portion of the growth plate is normal as is cartilage calcification. The mineralized osteoid is scant; the trabeculae are thin and few in number; and the cortices

Zones Structures	Histology	Functions	Exemplary diseases	Defect (if known)
Secondary bony epiphysis Epiphyseal artery	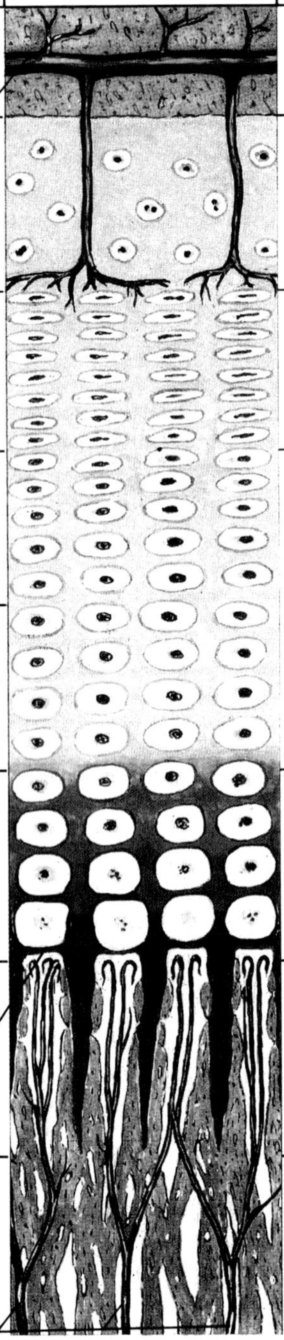			
Reserve zone		Matrix production Storage	Diastrophic dwarfism (also, defects in other zones)	Defective type II collagen synthesis
			Pseudoachondroplasia (also, defects in other zones)	Defective processing and transport of proteoglycans
			Kneist syndrome (also, defects in other zones)	Defective processing of proteoglycans
Proliferative zone		Matrix production Cellular proliferation (longitudinal growth)	Gigantism	Increased cell proliferation (growth hormone increased)
			Achondroplasia	Deficiency of cell proliferation
			Hypochondroplasia	Less severe deficiency of cell proliferation
			Malnutrition, irradiation injury, glucocorticoid excess	Decreased cell proliferation and/or matrix synthesis
Hypertrophic zone				
Maturation zone		Preparation of matrix for calcification	Mucopolysaccharidosis (Morquio's syndrome, Hurler's syndrome)	Deficiencies of specific lysosomal acid hydrolases, with lysosomal storage of mucopolysaccharides
Degenerative zone				
Zone of provisional calcification		Calcification of matrix	Rickets, osteomalacia (also, defects in metaphysis)	Insufficiency of Ca^{++} and/or P_i for normal calcification of matrix
Metaphysis				
Last intact transverse septum **Primary spongiosa**		Vascular invasion and resorption of transverse septa Bone formation	Metaphyseal chondrodysplasia (Jansen and Schmid types)	Extension of hypertrophic cells into metaphysis
			Acute hematogenous osteomyelitis	Flourishing of bacteria due to sluggish circulation, low Po_2, reticuloendothelial deficiency
Secondary spongiosa Branches of metaphyseal and nutrient arteries		Remodeling Internal: removal of cartilage bars, replacement of fiber bone with lamellar bone External: funnelization	Osteopetrosis	Abnormality of osteoclasts (internal remodeling)
			Osteogenesis imperfecta	Abnormality of osteoblasts and collagen synthesis
			Scurvy	Inadequate collagen formation
			Metaphyseal dysplasia (Pyle disease)	Abnormality of funnelization (external remodeling)

F. Netter M.D.

Figure 17
Zonal structure and pathologic defects of cellular metabolism. (© Copyright 1987 CIBA-GEIGY Corporation. Modified with permission from THE CIBA COLLECTION OF MEDICAL ILLUSTRATIONS, illustrated by Frank H. Netter, MD. All rights reserved.)

are thin and osteoporotic. Radiographs show fractures in various stages of healing.

Defects in Calcification

Jensen's disease is characterized by persistence of hypertrophic cells in the metaphysis. The failure of the hypertrophic cells to degenerate and to be invaded by the metaphyseal vessels may be caused by a deficiency in glycolytic enzymes. Calcification of the cartilage matrix is sparse and irregular and does not support normal osteoid or the formation of primary bony trabeculae. The end result is stunted

Table 3
Toxic effects of mucopolysaccharidoses

Syndrome	Skeletal Dysplasia	Mental Retardation	Corneal Clouding	Deafness	Inheritance	Glycoproteins Accumulated	Enzyme Defect
Hurlers (MPS-1H)	++	++	++	+	Autosomal recessive	Chondroitin sulfate B	α-L-iduronidase
Hunters (MPS-II)	+	+	-	++	Sex-linked recessive	Chondroitin sulfate B + heparitin sulfate	Sulfoiduronate sulfatase
Sanfilippo (MPS-III)	+-	++	-	+	Autosomal recessive	Heparitin sulfate	4 types - each a different enzyme
Morquio (MPS-IV)	++	-	+	+	Autosomal recessive	Keratan sulfate	Glucosamine-6 sulfatase
Scheie (MPS-IS)	+	-	+	+	Autosomal recessive	Chondroitin sulfate B	α-L-iduronidase
Maroteaux-Lamy (MPS-VI)	++	-	+	+	Autosomal recessive	Dermatan sulfate	Arylsulfatase β

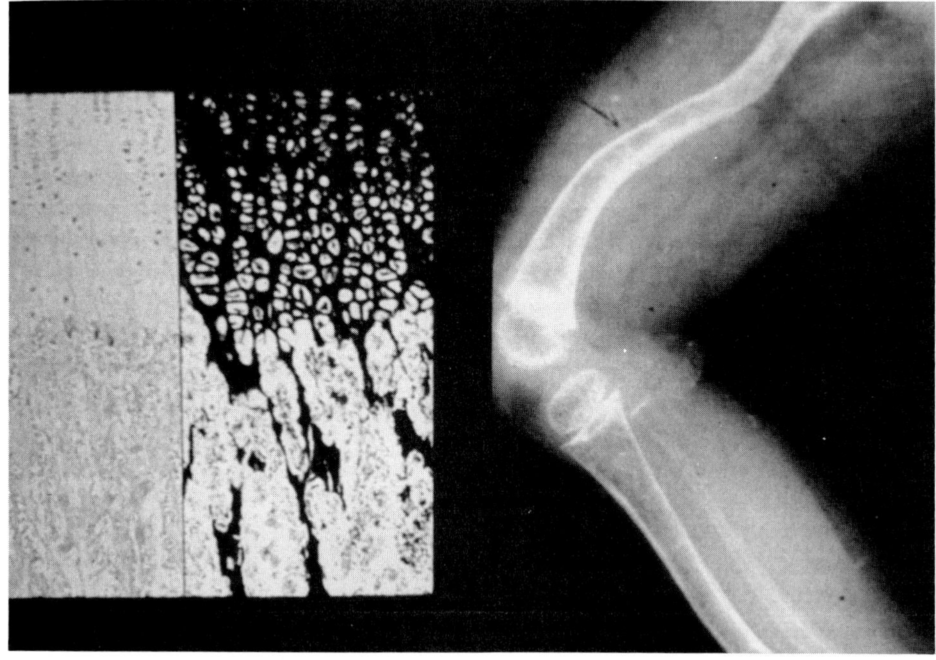

Figure 18
Histologic and radiographic features of osteogenesis imperfecta.

growth. The lower extremities are affected to a greater extent than the upper extremities. Radiographs show a normal epiphysis with a flared, irregularly shaped metaphysis, which contains cystic radiolucencies with central punctate calcification.

Hypophosphatasia is an inherited autosomal recessive defect in alkaline phosphatase, an enzyme that degrades phosphate esters in cartilage in bone (for example, ATP and pyrophosphate). These phosphate esters inhibit cartilage calcification. In hypophosphatasia, the serum calcium/phosphate product is normal but the matrix does not calcify. The hypertrophic zone widens, and the osteoid formed on the cartilage bars does not mineralize. The histologic and radiographic findings in hypophosphatasia and rickets are very similar. The growth plate is widened because of an increase in the hypertrophic zone, but the proliferative and reserve zones are normal. The hypertrophic zone cells persist into the metaphysis. The zone of provisional calcification and the primary spongiosa do not form. Radiographically, the growth plate is widened and there is flaring of the metaphysis. The end result is stunted growth.

Hypophosphatemic familial rickets (vitamin D-resistant rickets) results in the typical skeletal changes seen in vitamin D-deficiency rickets. This disorder is a sex-linked dominant disorder characterized by low calcium and phosphorus, a high alkaline phosphatase activity, and abnormal conversion of vitamin D to its active metabolites.

Defects in Cell Proliferation

Although achondroplasia is the most common form of short stature, little is known about its pathogenesis. The inheritance pattern is autosomal dominant. Most cases are spontaneous mutations and result in rhizomelic (primarily affecting the proximal aspect of the limb) disproportionate short stature. The typical radiographic and histologic characteristics are depicted in Figure 19. Achondroplasia is a germ plasm defect in which the proliferation and maturation of chondrocytes are severely inhibited. The cell columns are very short, and the hypertrophic zone is narrow. The metaphysis shows few calcified cores of cartilage and scanty new bone formation. Because periosteal new bone formation is normal, the width of the diaphysis is, therefore, normal. The metaphysis of the bone is widened as a result of normal latitudinal growth. The metabolic defect is thought to be deficient cell proliferation, which may be secondary to a deficiency in oxidative phosphorylation. Study of cartilage proteoglycans in achondroplasia did not demonstrate any major abnormalities.

Defects in Bone Remodeling

Osteopetrosis is characterized by abnormal internal or histologic remodeling. The typical radiographic and histologic characteristics are depicted in Figure 20. Osteopetrosis is also termed marble bone disease or Albers-Schönberg disease. It occurs in two forms: an autosomal recessive malignant form, which usually results in intrauterine death, and a relatively benign autosomal dominant form. In this disorder, there is an abnormality of osteoclast function and a defect in resorption of the primary spongiosa. The disease is characterized histologically by persistence of calcified cartilage bars in the diaphysis of the bone, and absence of a medullary cavity and marrow space. The interior of the bone is filled with chondro-osseous material. The defect in osteoclast function appears to be caused by an absence of marrow-derived osteoclast precursor cells, a deficiency in the production of specific growth factors necessary for osteoclastic differentiation, or a functional abnormality of the mature osteoclasts. This defect can be corrected with bone marrow transplant, which reverses the histologic, clinical, and radiographic signs of the disease. Radiographically, osteopetrosis is characterized by uniform opacity of the bones with no discernible internal architecture. In some less severely affected individuals, transverse radio-dense banding may be seen in the metaphysis.

Osteochondromas (exostosis, multiple exostoses, diaphyseal aclasis) are a result of a defect in

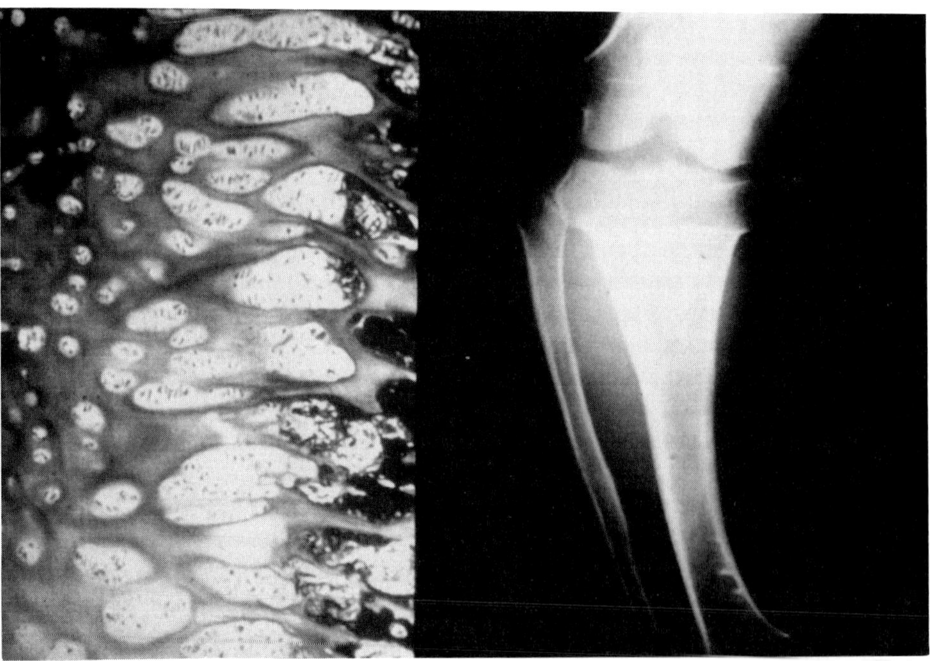

Figure 19
Histologic and radiographic features of achondroplasia.

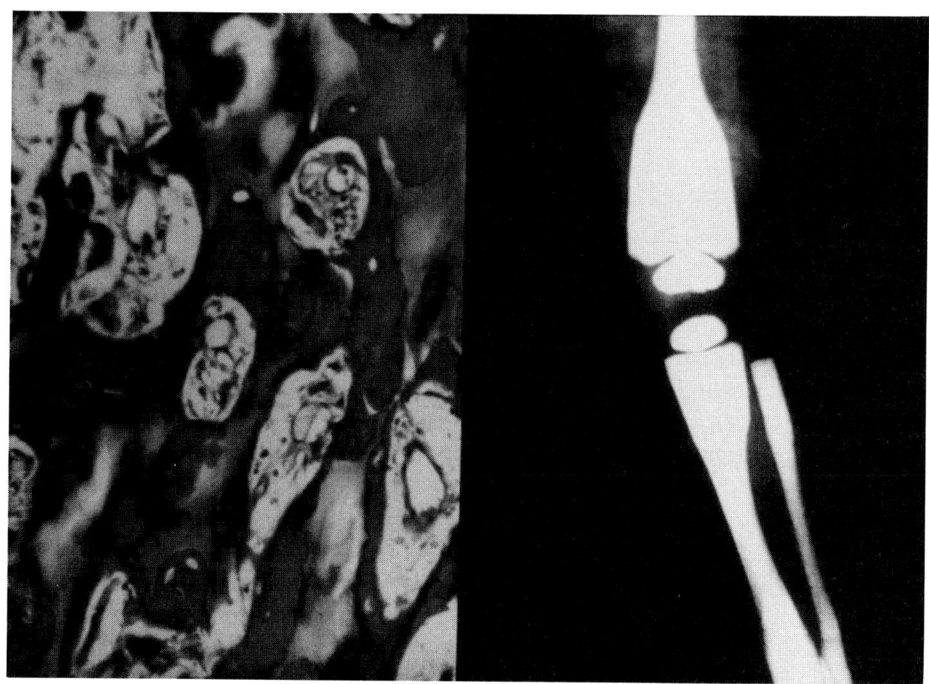

Figure 20
Histologic and radiographic features of osteopetrosis.

the perichondral ring of LaCroix and the groove of Ranvier. In this disorder, a bony protuberance arises from the periphery of the metaphysis. This structure has all growth plate zones represented and closes at skeletal maturity. Experimental evidence shows that an exostosis results from a mechanical defect in the perichondral ring. The etiology of multiple familial exostoses is unclear. Angular deformity can occur in severely affected individuals. The exostosis has a cartilaginous cap, which can undergo neoplastic degeneration, particularly in axial locations in patients with multiple lesions.

Pyle's disease or familial metaphyseal dysplasia is failure of external remodeling in the distal end of the metaphysis. The normal funnelization that narrows the metaphysis to meet the diaphysis is delayed. This defect produces a splayed, or Erlenmeyer-flask, deformity of the metaphysis. The major clinical manifestation is genu varum. Histologically the fiber bone of the secondary spongiosa is not resorbed or remodeled to lamellar bone until far down in the diaphysis.

Genetically Controlled Musculoskeletal Disorders

Biochemical reactions directing growth and development, as well as many structural variations and many degenerative processes treated by orthopaedists, are under genetic control. Present estimates suggest that genetic and environmental factors are nearly equal as causes of anomalies in the roughly 5% of babies born with some congenital defect.

There are three major types of genetic control: Mendelian inheritance; polygenic inheritance; and chromosomal imbalance. Many genetic diseases are not present or apparent at birth; they may be encountered at any age (Table 4).

The classic and basic tool of genetics is construction of a pedigree, which is well within the expertise of orthopaedists. Patients with genetic disease sometimes know that it "runs in the family," but often have peculiar notions as to the mechanisms. Sometimes family members are unaware of obvious genetic transmission. It is not enough to ask if other family members have a similar condition. A

Table 4
Age of manifestation of exemplary genetic diseases

Age	Disorder
Conception	Chromosomal rearrangements (miscarriage)
Birth	Clubfeet Dislocated hip Skeletal dysplasias
Childhood	Morquio's syndrome Multiple exostoses Vitamin D-resistant rickets Duchenne's muscular dystrophy
Adolescence	Scoliosis Ankylosing spondylitis
Middle Age	Dupuytren's contracture

minimum routine involves three steps: (1) draw the pedigree to include third-degree relatives; (2) name all individuals and inquire about their health; (3) review the pedigree on a subsequent visit. Mendelian and polygenic inheritance and chromosomal rearrangements will be briefly reviewed with particular emphasis on orthopaedic disease.

Mendelian Inheritance

In 1866, Gregor Mendel described the basis of what we now know as Mendelian inheritance. These patterns control the transmission of many conditions of the musculoskeletal system. The controlling gene may be on a chromosome unrelated to gender determination (an autosome) or may be on the chromosome controlling gender (gender-linked or x-linked). Four inheritance patterns occur: autosomal dominant; autosomal recessive; gender-linked dominant; and gender-linked recessive.

Autosomal Dominant Conditions

In Figure 21, typical examples of an autosomal dominant pedigree are given. Note the following genetic features: (1) the heterozygote state manifests the condition; (2) 50% of offspring are affected with no gender preference; (3) normal offspring do not transmit the condition; and (4) male-to-male transmission is required to confirm this pattern of inheritance. Autosomal dominant conditions often arise as spontaneous mutations, and they are typically nonlethal structural abnormalities. A condition is dominant when it is expressed clinically although only one of the two alleles for that gene is abnormal. For example, if half of the structural protein coded by a particular gene is abnormal, then any tissue composed of that protein is likely to be clinically abnormal. The presence of an abnormal gene is an all-or-none phenomenon called "penetrance"; the severity of manifestation of the gene in a particular individual is called "expressivity." There may be much variation in the expressivity of an abnormal gene in any particular family; that is, members of the family who have the abnormal gene may have a range of manifestations. Certain members may have manifestations more severe or less severe than other family members who also have the abnormal gene.

On the right side of Figure 21 is a young man with achondroplasia, a typical example of an autosomal dominant condition and the most common of the skeletal dysplasias. Other examples of autosomal dominant conditions include Marfan syndrome, osteogenesis imperfecta (types I and IV), multiple exostoses, multiple epiphyseal dysplasia, and fibrodysplasia ossificans progressiva.

Autosomal Recessive Conditions

In Figure 22 a typical example of an autosomal recessive pedigree is shown. Note the following clinical features: (1) the homozygote state manifests the condition; (2) parents are unaffected, but may be related; and (3) 25% of offspring are affected with no sex preference.

Autosomal recessive conditions are classically enzyme defects, "inborn errors of metabolism." "Recessive" means that both of the alleles for that gene must be abnormal to be expressed clinically. If, for example, only one of the alleles that codes for an enzyme is abnormal, then 50% of the enzyme produced will be normal and 50% abnormal. Under most conditions there will still be enough normal enzyme (50%) to catalyze the particular reaction in question, so the disease will not be expressed clinically. This situation is referred to as the heterozygote or carrier state. Single affected persons in a pedigree are common. Parents need not be related to possess common genes. There is little variability in expressivity.

Figure 22 also shows three children with diastrophic dwarfism, an example of an autosomal recessive condition and a severe chondrodysplasia characterized by short limbs, short stature, severe

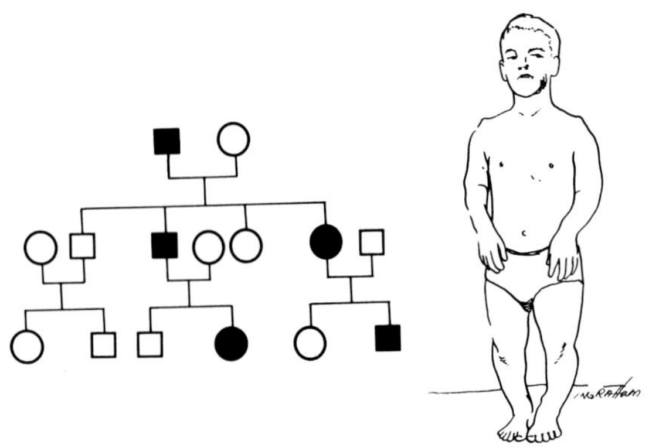

Figure 21
Pedigree chart—autosomal dominant inheritance pattern.

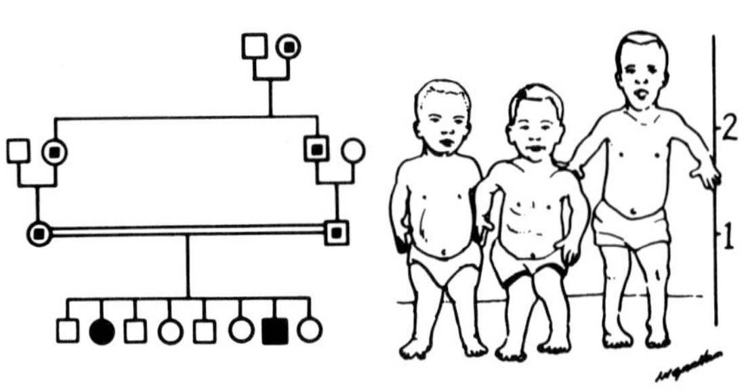

Figure 22
Pedigree chart—autosomal recessive inheritance pattern.

kyphoscoliosis, joint contractures, hip dysplasia, ear malformation, genu valgum, hitchhiker's thumb, and clubfeet. A specific enzyme defect has not yet been identified in this condition.

Other autosomal recessive conditions are: (1) most mucopolysaccharidoses, including the Hurler and Scheie syndromes, the Sanfilippo syndromes, the Morquio syndromes, and the Maroteaux-Lamy syndrome; (2) homocystinuria; (3) ochronosis; (4) the Ehlers-Danlos syndrome (type V). Specific enzyme defects have been identified for most of these conditions. The mucopolysaccharidoses can be identified chemically, for example, by the presence of specific mucopolysaccharides that appear in the urine because of the absence or inactivity of a specific degradative enzyme. The clinical manifestations of most mucopolysaccharidoses are caused by abnormal accumulation and storage of mucopolysaccharide in lysosomes of numerous tissues including liver, spleen, skin, cartilage, bone, and brain.

Gender-Linked Dominant Conditions

A typical example of a gender-linked dominant pedigree is seen in Figure 23. Note the following clinical features: (1) the heterozygote manifests the condition; (2) affected females transmit the x-linked gene to half their daughters and half their sons; (3) affected males transmit the x-linked gene to all daughters and to none of their sons; (4) father-to-son transmission does not occur; and (5) males tend to be more severely affected than females. The right side of Figure 23 shows family members afflicted with hypophosphatemic vitamin D-resistant rickets (VDRR) and osteomalacia, the classic gender-linked dominant orthopaedic condition.

Gender-Linked Recessive Conditions

A representative gender-linked recessive pedigree is shown in Figure 24. Note the following clinical features: (1) the heterozygote male is clinically affected, but the heterozygote female is not; (2) the affected male transmits the gene to all daughters, who are carriers, and to none of his sons; and

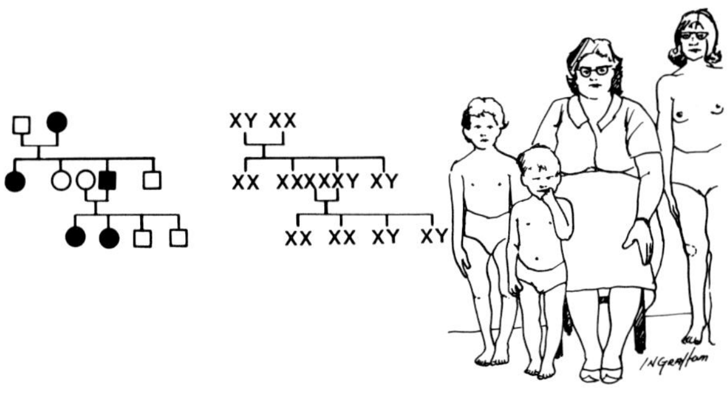

Figure 23
Pedigree chart—gender-linked dominant inheritance pattern.

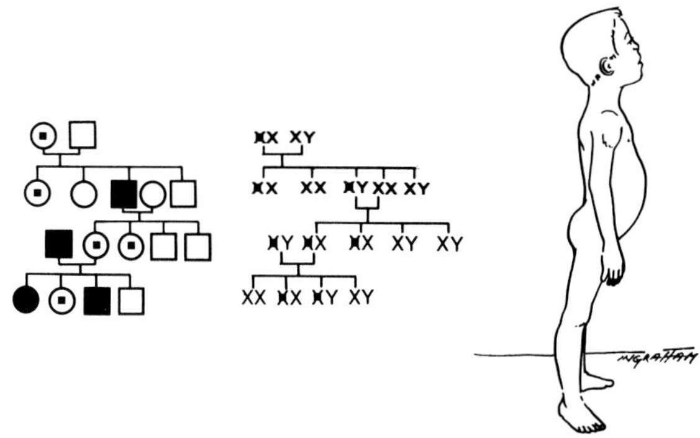

Figure 24
Pedigree chart—gender-linked recessive inheritance pattern.

(3) the carrier female transmits the gene to one-half of her daughters, who are carriers, and to one-half of her sons, who are affected.

On the right side of Figure 24 is a child with Duchenne's muscular dystrophy, the prototype of all muscular dystrophies inherited as a gender-linked (x-linked) recessive condition. Classically, this form of dystrophy affects only males who have inherited the condition from their carrier mothers. A high mutation rate exists, with up to one-third of cases believed to represent mutation. Duchenne's muscular dystrophy typically presents at 3 to 5 years of age with signs of proximal weakness. Independent ambulation is lost, usually by 11 to 13 years of age. Death occurs in the early 20s from cardiomyopathy, or earlier from pulmonary insufficiency. Creatine phosphokinase elevation and abnormalities detected by electromyography and muscle biopsy confirm the diagnosis. Many of the carriers can be identified by enzymatic abnormalities. Two additional examples of x-linked recessive inheritance include classic hemophilia and Hunter's syndrome (mucopolysaccharidosis II).

Chromosome Abnormalities

The last major category of genetic abnormalities comprises chromosomal abnormalities, which are common but often result in miscarriage. About 20% of spontaneous abortions exhibit chromosome abnormalities. About 1% of live births have chromosome abnormalities. The left-hand side of Figure 25 shows the normal human male karyotype. The normal male has 22 pairs of chromosomes called autosomes and one "X" and one "Y" chromosome. Chromosomes are divided into seven groups according to morphologic characteristics and are numbered. Chromosome rearrangements that occur in nature are varied and complex. The classic mechanism of producing an extra chromosome (trisomy) or loss of a chromosome (deletion) is failure of separation during reduction division.

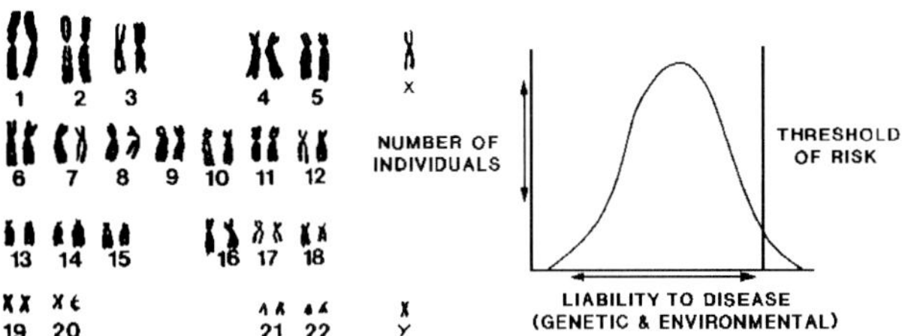

Figure 25
Composite diagram—polygenic inheritance.

Other types of errors include mosaics (more than one line of cells); translocation (fragmentation of a chromosome with transfer of genetic material to another chromosome); and deletions of parts of chromosomes. Regularity in these accidents allows the delineation of various syndromes, and recent banding techniques have led to increased sophistication in identifying the chromosomes involved. Even so, it is important to realize that large fragments of genetic material are involved, and the clinical syndromes produced are not uniform. The indications for chromosome studies are not precise, but a karyotype analysis should be considered in infants who exhibit the triad of multiple anomalies (especially facial), failure to thrive, and mental retardation. Characteristic associations of chromosome abnormalities that may be seen by orthopaedists include polydactyly in the trisomy-13 syndrome, radioulnar synostosis in the multiple-x syndromes, vertical tali in trisomy-18, and clubfeet in several of the deletion syndromes. The most common chromosome abnormalities with skeletal changes are Down and Turner's syndromes.

Polygenic Inheritance

A second major type of inheritance is polygenic inheritance, which refers to the effects of multiple genes and alleles interacting with environmental factors to influence form and function and incidence of disease. For example, genetic factors appear to control the time of growth-plate closure, but a large number of nutritional and endocrine health factors influence metabolism of the growth plate as well. Height is, therefore, a polygenic trait. Clubfeet, congenital dislocation of the hip, and idiopathic scoliosis are examples of polygenic traits. There are important clinical features of polygenic inheritance, some of which are illustrated on the right side of Figure 25.

The likelihood of a condition's occurring in the population can be depicted by a normal Gaussian curve. There is a "threshold" at which a portion of the population may be affected. The threshold reflects both genetic and permissive environmental factors. The level of risk is low. The frequency of recurrence of the same polygenic trait in offspring of unaffected parents is usually in the range of 2% to 6%. There is an increased risk in relatives of those affected, with the increase proportional to the genetic similarity. This relationship can be depicted as a shift of the curve on the threshold. The increased risk in relatives is illustrated by idiopathic scoliosis. Thus, scoliosis occurs in approximately 11% of first-degree relatives, 2% of second-degree relatives, and 1% to 2% of third-degree relatives. The threshold of risk is affected by race, sex, and geography. The varying proportions of males to females in polygenic traits illustrate modification by gender.

Risk and severity relate to intrafamily patterns of involvement. Thus, if a parent and child are affected, the odds of subsequent children being affected are greatly increased. The greater the severity, the greater the odds of subsequent children being affected. If the affected individual is of the least-likely affected sex, the odds of subsequent children being affected are generally increased. The inheritance of clubfoot will be used as a specific example: idiopathic clubfoot occurs in the United States in about one of every 1,000 births and has a two to one male-to-female ratio. It is bilateral in half the children affected. In order to define the recurrence risk for a family, examination must exclude phenocopies (look-alikes), syndromes, Mendelian inherited conditions, and chromosomal rearrangements associated with clubfeet.

Selected Bibliography

Introduction

Boskey AL: Current concepts of the physiology and biochemistry of calcification. *Clin Orthop* 1981;157:225–257.

Brighton CT: Clinical problems in epiphyseal plate growth and development, in American Academy of Orthopaedic Surgeons *Instructional Course Lectures, XXIII.* St. Louis, CV Mosby, 1974, pp 105–122.

Heinegård D, Oldberg A: Structure and biology of cartilage and bone matrix non-collagenous macromolecules. *FASEB J* 1989;3:2042–2051.

Hunter GK: Role of proteoglycan in the provisional calcification of cartilage: A review and reinterpretation. *Clin Orthop* 1991;262:256–280.

Iannotti JP: Growth plate physiology and pathology. *Orthop Clin North Am* 1990;21:1–17.

Poole AR, Matsui Y, Hinek A, et al: Cartilage macromolecules and the calcification of cartilage matrix. *Anat Rec* 1989;224:167–179.

Trippel SB: Basic science of the growth plate. *Curr Opin Orthop* 1990;1:279–288.

Structure, Function, and Biochemistry of the Normal Growth Plate

Brown CC, Hembry RM, Reynolds JJ: Immunolocalization of metalloproteinases and their inhibitor in the rabbit growth plate. *J Bone Joint Surg* 1989;71A:580–593.

Hunziker EB, Schenk RK, Cruz-Orive LM: Quantitation of chondrocyte performance in growth-plate cartilage during longitudinal bone growth. *J Bone Joint Surg* 1987;69A:162–173.

Growth Plate Mineralization

Brighton CT, Hunt RM: Mitochondrial calcium and its role in calcification: Histochemical localization of calcium in electron micrographs of the epiphyseal growth-plate with K-pyroantimonate. *Clin Orthop* 1974;100:406–416.

Buckwalter JA: Proteoglycan structure in calcifying cartilage. *Clin Orthop* 1983;172:207–232.

Poole AR, Pidoux I, Reiner A, et al: Association of an extracellular protein (chondrocalcin) with the calcification of cartilage in endochondral bone formation. *J Cell Biol* 1984;98:54–65.

Effect of Hormones and Growth Factors on the Growth Plate

Atkin I, Pita JC, Ornoy A, et al: Effects of vitamin D metabolites on healing of low phosphate, vitamin D-deficient induced rickets in rats. *Bone* 1985;6:113–123.

Balogh K Jr, Kunin AS: The effect of cortisone on the metabolism of epiphyseal cartilage: A histochemical study. *Clin Orthop* 1971;80:208–215.

Barling PM, Bibby NJ: Study of the localization of [3H]-bovine parathyroid hormone in bone by light microscope autoradiography. *Calcif Tissue Int* 1985;37:441–446.

Bauer GC, Carlson A, Linquist B: Evaluation of accretion, resorption and exchange reactions in the skeleton. *Kungl Fysiogr Sallskap Lund Forhandl* 1955;25:1–16.

Burch WM, Corda G : Calcitonin stimulates maturation of mammalian growth plate cartilage. *Endocrinology* 1985;116:1724–1728.

Burch WM, Van Wyk JJ: Triiodothyronine stimulates cartilage growth and maturation by different mechanisms. *Am J Physiol* 1987;252(2 pt 1):E176–E182.

Canalis E: Effect of growth factors on bone cell replication and differentiation. *Clin Orthop* 1985;193:246–263.

Canalis E, McCarthy T, Centrella M: Growth factors and the regulation of bone remodeling. *J Clin Invest* 1988;81:277–281.

Carrascosa A, Audi L, Ferrandez MA, et al: Biological effects of androgens and identification of specific dihydrotestosterone-binding sites in cultured human fetal epiphyseal chondrocytes. *J Clin Endocrinol Metab* 1990;70:134–140.

Chandrasekhar S, Harvey AK: Transforming growth factor-beta is a potent inhibitor of IL-1 induced protease activity and cartilage proteoglycan degradation. *Biochem Biophys Res Commun* 1988;157:1352–1359.

Corvol MT, Carrascosa A, Tsagris L, et al: Evidence for a direct in vitro action of sex steroids on rabbit cartilage cells during skeletal growth: Influence of age and sex. *Endocrinology* 1987;120:1422–1429.

Crabb ID, O'Keefe RJ, Puzas JE, et al: PTH effects on chondrocytes from different maturational stages of the growth plate. *Trans Orthop Res Soc* 1989;14:84.

Crabb ID, O'Keefe RJ, Puzas JE, et al: Direct effects of PTH and vitamin D on chondrocytes and modulation of local growth factor sensitivity. *Trans Orthop Res Soc* 1989;14:521.

Dearden LC, Mosier HD Jr, Brundage M, et al: The effects of different steroids on costal and epiphyseal cartilage of fetal and adult rats. *Cell Tissue Res* 1986;246:401–412.

Dorfman A, Schiller S: Effects of hormones on the metabolism of acid mucopolysaccharides of connective tissue. *Recent Prog Horm Res* 1958;14:427–453.

Fahmy A, Talley P, Frazier HM, et al: Ultrastructural effects of estrogen on epiphyseal cartilage. *Calcif Tiss Res* 1971;7:139–149.

Fine N, Binderman I, Somjen D, et al: Autoradiographic localization of 24R,25 dihydro D 3 in epiphyseal cartilage. *Bone* 1985;6:99–104.

Goldstein S, Unterman TG, Phillips LS: Nutrition and somatomedin. XV. Growth plate, growth factor and biologically active somatomedins in rats with streptozotocin-induced diabetes. *Ann Nutr Metab* 1987;31:367–377.

Iannotti JP, Brighton CP, Iannotti V, et al: Mechanism of action of parathyroid hormone-induced proteoglycan synthesis in the growth plate chondrocyte. *J Orthop Res* 1990;8:136–145.

Isaksson O, Binder C, Hall K, et al (eds): *Growth Hormone: Basic and Clinical Aspects.* Amsterdam, Excerpta Medica, 1987.

Kapur SP, Reddi AH: Influence of testosterone and dihydrotestosterone on bone-matrix induced endochondral bone formation. *Calcif Tissue Int* 1989;44:108–113.

Maor G, Silbermann M: In vitro effects of glucocorticoid hormones on the synthesis of DNA in cartilage of neonatal mice. *FEBS Lett* 1981;129:256–260.

Martineau-Doize B, Lai WH, Warshawsky H, et al: In vivo demonstration of cell types in bone that harbor epidermal growth factor receptors. *Endocrinology* 1988;123:841–858.

Nilsson A, Isgaard J, Lindahl A, et al: Regulation by growth hormone of number of chondrocytes containing IGF-I in rat growth plate. *Science* 1986;233:571–574.

Ogden JA, Southwick WO: Endocrine dysfunction and slipped capital femoral epiphysis. *Yale J Biol Med* 1977;50:1–16.

O'Keefe RJ, Crabb ID, Puzas JE, et al: The influence of prostaglandins on DNA and matrix synthesis by growth plate chondrocytes. *Trans Orthop Res Soc* 1989;14:535.

O'Keefe RJ, Puzas JE, Brand JS, et al: Effect of transforming growth factor-beta on matrix synthesis by chick growth plate chondrocytes. *Endocrinology* 1988;122:2953–2961.

Preece MA: The effect of administered corticosteroids on the growth of children. *Postgrad Med J* 1976;52:625–630.

Ray RD, Asling CW, Walker DG, et al: Growth and differentiation of the skeleton in thyroidectomized-hypophysectomized rats treated with thyroxin, growth hormone and the combination. *J Bone Joint Surg* 1954;36A:94–103.

Salmon WD Jr, Daughaday WH: A hormonally controlled serum factor which stimulates sulfate incorporation by cartilage in vitro. *J Lab Clin Med* 1957;49:825–836.

Simon MR, Cooke PS: Cellular heterogeneity and insulin-like growth factor I immunoreactivity among epiphyseal growth plate chondrocytes in the pig. *Acta Anat (Basel)* 1988;133:66–69.

Tapp E: The effects of hormones on bone in growing rats. *J Bone Joint Surg* 1966;48B:526–531.

Trippel SB, Chernausek SD, Van Wyk JJ, et al: Demonstration of type I and type II somatomedin receptors on bovine growth plate chondrocytes. *J Orthop Res* 1988;6:817–826.

Ueno K, Haba T, Woodbury D, et al: The effects of prostaglandin E2 in rapidly growing rats: Depressed longitudinal and radial growth and increased metaphyseal hard tissue mass. *Bone* 1985;6:79–86.

Uhthoff HK, Wiley JJ (eds): *Behavior of the Growth Plate.* New York, Raven Press, 1988.

Vetter U, Zapf J, Heit W, et al: Human fetal and adult chondrocytes: Effect of insulin like growth factors I and II, insulin and growth hormone on clonal growth. *J Clin Invest* 1986;77:1903–1908.

Wientroub S, Wahl LM, Feuerstein N, et al: Changes in tissue concentration of prostaglandins during endochondral bone differentiation. *Biochem Biophys Res Commun* 1983;117:746–750.

Wu LN, Sauer GR, Genge BR, et al: Induction of mineral deposition by primary cultures of chicken growth plate chondrocytes in ascorbate-containing media: Evidence of an association between matrix vesicles and collagen. *J Biol Chem* 1989;264:21346–21355.

Sporn MB, Roberts AB (eds): *Handbook of Experimental Pharmacology: Peptide Growth Factors and Their Receptors, Parts I and II.* Berlin, Springer Verlag, vol 95, 1990.

The Mechanical Properties of the Growth Plate and its Response to Mechanical Stimuli

Amamilo SC, Bader DL, Houghton GR: The periosteum in growth plate failure. *Clin Orthop* 1985;194:293–305.

Arkin AM, Katz JF: The effects of pressure on epiphyseal growth: Mechanism of plasticity of growing bone. *J Bone Joint Surg* 1956;38A:1056–1076.

Blount WP, Clarke GR: Control of bone growth by epiphyseal stapling: A preliminary report. *J Bone Joint Surg* 1949;31A:464–478.

Bonnell F, Peruchon E, Baldet P, et al: Effects of compression on growth plates in the rabbit. *Acta Orthop Scand* 1983;54:730–733.

Brashear HR Jr: Epiphyseal fractures: A microscopic study of the healing process in rats. *J Bone Joint Surg* 1959;41A:1055–1064.

Bright RW, Elmore SM: Physical properties of epiphyseal plate cartilage. *Surg Forum* 1968;19:463–464.

Bright RW, Burstein AH, Elmore SM: Epiphyseal-plate cartilage: A biomechanical and histological analysis of failure modes. *J Bone Joint Surg* 1974;56A:688–703.

Brown TD, Singerman RJ: Experimental determination of the linear biphasic constitutive coefficients of human fetal proximal femoral chondroepiphysis. *J Biomech* 1986;19:597–605.

Carter DR: Mechanical loading history and skeletal biology. *J Biomech* 1987;20:1095–1109.

Carter DR, Orr TE, Fyhrie DP, et al: Influences of mechanical stress on prenatal and postnatal skeletal development. *Clin Orthop* 1987;219:237–250.

Carter DR, Wong M: Mechanical stresses and endochondral ossification in the chondroepiphysis. *J Orthop Res* 1988;6:148–154.

Chung SM, Batterman SC, Brighton CT: Shear strength of the human femoral capital epiphyseal plate. *J Bone Joint Surg* 1976;58A:94–103.

Cohen B, Chorney GS, Phillips DP, et al: The microstructural tensile properties and biochemical composition of the bovine distal femoral growth plate. *J Orthop Res* 1992;10:263–275.

Frost HM: A chondral modeling theory. *Calcif Tissue Int* 1979;28:181–200.

Glücksmann A: The role of mechanical stresses in bone formation in vitro. *J Anat* 1942;76:231–239.

Glücksmann A: Studies on bone mechanics in vitro: II. The role of tension and pressure in chondrogenesis. *Anat Rec* 1939;73:39–55.

Gray ML, Pizzanelli AM, Grodzinsky AJ, et al: Mechanical and physiochemical determinants of the chondrocyte biosynthetic response. *J Orthop Res* 1988;6:777–792.

Gray ML, Pizzanelli AM, Lee RC, et al: Kinetics of the chondrocyte biosynthetic response to compressive load and release. *Biochim Biophys Acta* 1989;991:415–425.

Greco F, de Palma L, Speccia N, et al: Growth-plate cartilage metabolic response to mechanical stress. *J Pediatr Orthop* 1989;9:520–524.

Haas SL: Retardation of bone growth by a wire loop. *J Bone Joint Surg* 1945;27:25–36.

Haas SL: The localization of the growing point in the epiphyseal cartilage plate of bones. *Am J Orthop Surg* 1973;15:563–586.

Hall BK: In vitro studies on the mechanical evocation of adventitious cartilage in the chick. *J Exp Zool* 1968;168:283–306.

Hall BK: Immobilization and cartilage transformation into bone in the embryonic chick. *Anat Rec* 1972;173:391–403.

Houghton GR, Rooker GD: The role of the periosteum in the growth of long bones: An experimental study in the rabbit. *J Bone Joint Surg* 1979;61B:218–220.

Jenkins DH, Cheng DH, Hodgson AR: Stimulation of bone growth by periosteal stripping: A clinical study. *J Bone Joint Surg* 1975;57B:482–484.

Jones IL, Klämfeldt A, Sandström T: The effect of continuous mechanical pressure upon the turnover of articular cartilage proteoglycans in vitro. *Clin Orthop* 1982;165:283–289.

Klein-Nulend J, Veldhuijzen JP, Burger EH: Increased calcification of growth plate cartilage as a result of compressive force in vitro. *Arthritis Rheum* 1986;29:1002–1009.

Lee KE, Pelker RR, Rudicel SA, et al: Histologic patterns of capital femoral growth plate fracture in the rabbit: The effect of shear direction. *J Pediatr Orthop* 1985;5:32–39.

Moen CT, Pelker RR: Biomechanical and histological correlations in growth plate failure. *J Pediatr Orthop* 1984;4:180–184.

Morscher E: Strength and morphology of growth cartilage under hormonal influence of puberty: Animal experiments and clinical study on the etiology of local growth disorders during puberty. *Reconstr Surg Traumatol* 1968;10:3–104.

Morscher E, Desaulles PA, Schenk R: Experimental studies on tensile strength and morphology of the epiphyseal cartilage at puberty. *Ann Pediatr Basel* 1965;205:112–130.

Mow VC, Proctor CS, Kelly MA: Biomechanics of articular cartilage, in Nordin M, Frankel BH, Forssén K, et al (eds): *Basic Biomechanics of the Musculoskeletal System,* ed 2. Philadelphia, Lea & Febiger, 1989, pp 31–58.

Ogden JA: Injury to the growth mechanisms of the immature skeleton. *Skeletal Radiol* 1981;6:237–253.

Porter RW: The effect of tension across a growing epiphysis. *J Bone Joint Surg* 1978;60B:252–255.

Rudicel S, Pelker RR, Lee KE, et al: Shear fractures through the capital femoral physis of the skeletally immature rabbit. *J Pediatr Orthop* 1985;5:27–31.

Ryöppy S, Karaharju EO: Alteration of epiphyseal growth by an experimentally produced angular deformity. *Acta Orthop Scand* 1974;45:490–498.

Salter RB, Harris WR: Injuries involving the epiphyseal plate. *J Bone Joint Surg* 1963;45A:587–622.

Shapiro F, Holtrop ME, Glimcher MJ: Organization and cellular biology of the perichondrial ossification groove of Ranvier: A morphological study in rabbits. *J Bone Joint Surg* 1977;59A:703–723.

Siffert RS: The effect of staples and longitudinal wires on epiphyseal growth: An experimental study. *J Bone Joint Surg* 1956:28A:1077–1088.

Simon MR, Holmes KR: The effects of simulated increases in body weight on the developing rat tibia: A histologic study. *Acta Anat (Basel)* 1985;122:105–109.

Smith WS, Cunningham JB: The effect of alternating distracting forces on the epiphyseal plates of calves: A preliminary report. *Clin Orthop* 1957;10:125–130.

Smith JW: The relationship of epiphysial plates to stress in some bones of the lower limb. *J Anat* 1962;96:58–78.

Smith JW: The structure and stress relations of fibrous epiphysial plates. *J Anat* 1962;96:209–225.

van Kampen GP, Veldhuijzen JP, Kuijer R, et al: Cartilage response to mechanical force in high-density chondrocyte cultures. *Arthritis Rheum* 1985;28:419–424.

Warrell E, Taylor JF: The role of periosteal tension in the growth of long bones. *J Anat* 1979;128:179–184.

Pathologic States Primarily Affecting the Growth Plate

Maynard JA, Ippolito EG, Ponseti IV, et al: Histochemistry and ultrastructure of the growth plate in achondroplasia. *J Bone Joint Surg* 1981;63A:969–979.

Stanescu V, Stanescu R, Maroteaux P: Pathogenic mechanisms in osteochondrodysplasias. *J Bone Joint Surg* 1984;66A:817–836.

Genetically Controlled Musculoskeletal Disorders

Antonarakis SE: Diagnosis of genetic disorders at the DNA level. *N Engl J Med* 1989;320:151–163.

Botstein D, White RL, Skolnick M, et al: Construction of a genetic linkage map in man using restriction fragment length polymorphisms. *Am J Hum Genet* 1980;32:314–331.

Donis-Keller H, Green P, Helms C, et al: A genetic linkage map of the human genome. *Cell* 1987;51:319–337.

McKusick VA: Mapping and sequencing the human genome. *N Engl J Med* 1989;320:910–915.

Chapter 6
Molecular and Cellular Biology of Inflammation and Neoplasia

Dempsey S. Springfield, MD
Mark E. Bolander, MD
Gary E. Friedlaender, MD
Nancy Lane, MD

Chapter Outline

Molecular Biology

Normal and abnormal physiologic processes involve complex interactions among several different types of molecules. These interactions are controlled and directed by DNA (deoxyribonucleic acid) in the cell's nucleus. The nuclear DNA contains all the genetic information needed to direct protein synthesis, and proteins are the compounds used to regulate all cellular functions. The analysis of these cellular processes, including the flow of genetic information among DNA, RNA (ribonucleic acid), and protein is the province of molecular biology. The techniques of molecular biology are being applied to every field in medicine including orthopaedics. The increase in understanding afforded by the application of molecular biology has initiated a dramatic and extensive advance in the treatment of disorders related to the musculoskeletal system.

The human genome is contained in the 23 pairs of chromosomes located in the nucleus of each cell. At least 150,000 different genes are carried on the chromosomes. Chromosomes contain DNA, some RNA, and protein bound to the DNA. Although every cell contains all 46 chromosomes, only a limited number of genes are expressed by any differentiated cell. The regulation of gene expression, therefore, determines the functional qualities of each cell.

Beginning with William Harvey's work on circulation in the 17th century, physicians have tried to relate their knowledge of structures in the human body to normal physiology and the pathology of disease. Gregor Mendel's 1865 work on plants was the first to relate the characteristics of an organism, or phenotype, to bits of genetic information or genes inside the cell. For the 40 to 50 years after Mendel's work, the identity of the gene was shrouded in mystery. Genes were described only in terms of their outward manifestations; nothing was known about their structure or how they function in biologic organisms.

In 1894, Oswald Avery and his colleagues focused attention on DNA as the molecule of heredity, but it was not until 1952 that Alfred Hershey and Martha Chase performed the experiments that proved that the cell's genes were contained in the DNA molecules. The subsequent delineation of the physical arrangement of the DNA molecule was made possible by two achievements. The first was elucidation of the basis for anatomic arrangements formulated by Linus Pauling in his theory on the nature of the chemical bond, published in 1935. The second was the analysis of the DNA structure by X-ray diffraction completed by Rosalind Franklin in 1951. In that same year, James Watson and Francis Crick proposed what since has been accepted as the model for the DNA structure (Fig. 1).

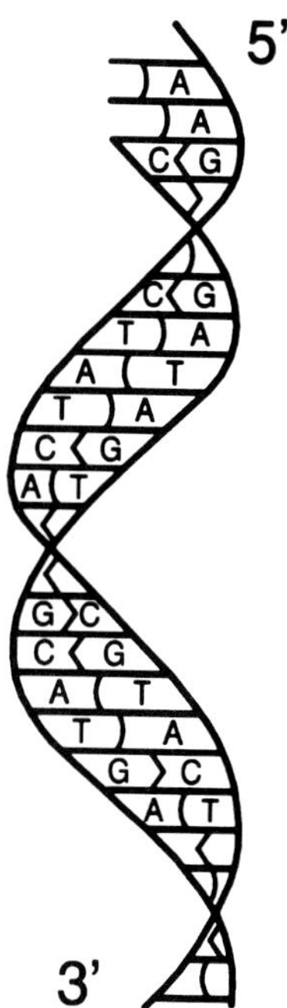

Figure 1
A model for the structure of DNA. Two strands of DNA run in opposite directions forming an alpha helix that resembles a twisted ladder. Deoxyriboses linked by phosphodiester bridges make up the backbone of DNA. The two strands of DNA are connected by a pair of nucleotides (the rungs of the ladder) held together by hydrogen bonds. A = adenine; T = thymine; C = cytosine; G = guanine.

DNA has two backbone spans made up of two alternating five-carbon sugar molecules (d-ribose and d-2-deoxyribose). Each sugar molecule has one of four nitrogenous bases (adenine, guanine, cytosine, and thymine). These two molecules are joined to each other by a phosphate bond between carbons 3 and 5. The complex of a sugar molecule with its phosphate and nitrogenous base is called a nucleotide. The two backbone strands twist around each other with the nitrogenous bases of each strand pointed toward one another. The nitrogenous bands of one strand are joined to those of the other strand by hydrogen bonds; adenine is always joined to thymine and guanine to cytosine. Thus, the nucleotide alphabet (sequence) in one half of the DNA helix determines the sequence in the other half. All of the nuclear DNA is contained in the 23 pairs of chromosomes.

DNA is necessary for three critical cellular functions: (1) accurate DNA self-replication during the process of cell division; (2) production (or transcription) of messenger RNA (mRNA); and (3) regulation of cell division and mRNA production.

DNA self-replication is now known to require that the two strands of DNA separate one from the other and a new complementary strand be made for each of the original strands. DNA polymerase is the enzyme that is needed for synthesizing a DNA chain complimentary to an existing template strand of DNA. This process occurs during cell division and accounts for the increase in nuclear DNA during the cell cycle.

DNA controls cellular function by making the proteins that produce cellular functions. A gene is that portion of the DNA that codes for a specific protein and adjacent noncoding portions of that DNA. To create one of these proteins, the DNA of the gene coding for that protein is first transcribed to an mRNA with the assistance of RNA polymerase. Messenger RNA then builds proteins from amino acids through a process called translation (Fig. 2). The mRNA molecule is translated into a protein by joining amino acids together in a specific sequence. The sequence of the amino acids and, therefore, the type of protein produced is determined by the sequence of nucleotides in the mRNA. The control of protein production, both type and rate, is a function of DNA.

This relationship between DNA and specific protein production was first supported by the demonstration that mutations in the gene (changes in the nucleotide sequence in the DNA) produced changes in the amino acid sequence of that gene's protein product. Final proof came in 1966, when Marshall Nurenberg and his colleagues cracked the genetic code and determined which nucleotides coded for specific amino acids. This work completed the genetic dictionary for the translation of mRNA into amino acids (Fig. 3).

Genes account for as little as 5% of the total DNA molecule. Between functional genes are vast regions of noncoding, often repetitive, DNA sequences. The regulation information for gene transcription and mRNA synthesis resides in these untranslated (noncoding) regions of DNA. The most important region of regulatory DNA, called the gene promoter, is located directly adjacent to the protein coding region of the gene (Fig. 4). The promoter contains binding sites for the RNA polymerase and other proteins required for initiating transcription. Promoters for a large number of genes have been analyzed and their sequences compared. This comparison has identified several common regions of DNA sequence, called consensus sequences. Each of these consensus sequences is named for its specific nucleotide sequence, and each sequence functions as the binding site for specific proteins involved in

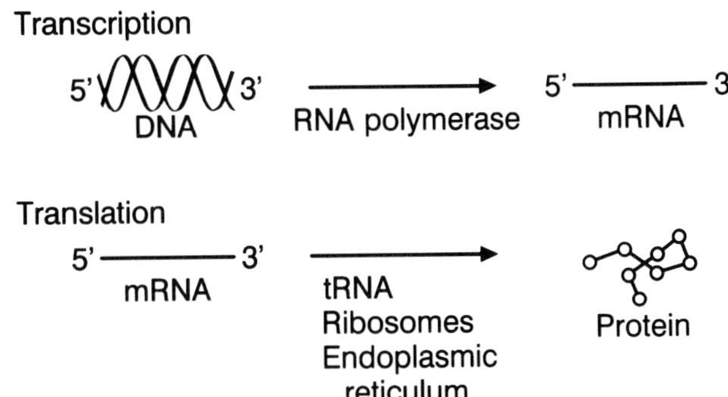

Figure 2
Genetic information stored in DNA flows into RNA and then into proteins through the processes of transcription and translation. Transcription of DNA into an RNA occurs in the nucleus. mRNA is transported to the cytoplasm. Translation of mRNA into proteins occurs in the endoplasmic reticulum. DNA = deoxyribonucleic acid; RNA = ribonucleic acid; mRNA = messenger RNA; tRNA = transfer RNA.

Codon	Amino acid	Codon	Amino acid	Codon	Amino acid	Codon	Amino acid
A A G	Lys	C A G	Gln	G A G	Glu	T A G	Stop
A A A		C A A		G A A		T A A	
A A C	Asn	C A C	His	G A C	Asp	T A C	Tyr
A A T		C A T		G A T		T A T	
A C G	Thr	C C G	Pro	G C G	Ala	T C G	Ser
A C A		C C A		G C A		T C A	
A C C		C C C		G C C		T C C	
A C T		C C T		G C T		T C T	
A G G	Arg	C G G	Arg	G G G	Gly	T G G	Trp
A G A		C G A		G G A		T G A	Stop
A G C	Ser	C G C		G G C		T G C	Cys
A G T		C G T		G G T		T G T	
A T G	Met	C T G	Leu	G T G	Val	T T G	Leu
A T A	Ile	C T A		G T A		T T A	
A T C		C T C		G T C		T T C	Phe
A T T		C T T		G T T		T T T	

Figure 3
Genetic dictionary for the translation of messenger ribonucleic acid into amino acids. A = adenine; T = thymine; C = cytosine; G = guanine.

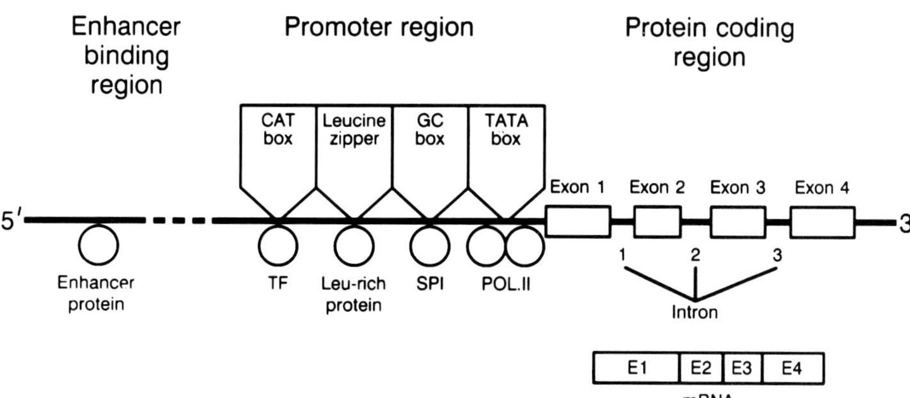

Figure 4
Diagrammatic representation of gene structure showing protein coding and regulator regions. Regulatory elements shown include enhancer and promoter binding regions (CAT, TATA, and GC boxes). Promoter and enhancer proteins stimulate gene transcription by binding to these sites. mRNA = messenger ribonucleic acid; TF = transcription factor; POL. II = RNA polymerase II; SPI = serum promoter.

gene regulation. A sequence called the TATA box is the binding site for RNA polymerase II, a CG box is the binding site for a serum promoter (SP-1), and a CAT box is the binding site for transcription factors (TF). Binding of proteins specific to a consensus sequence activates the gene and initiates transcription of mRNA. In addition to consensus sequences, other promoter regions stabilized by a zinc atom are called zinc fingers. Another promoter region, which is notable because it binds to multiple leucine amino acids in proteins, is called a leucine zipper. Although the exact sequences of these promoter elements vary from gene to gene, they are present in virtually every eukaryotic cell.

A different region of DNA contains regulatory elements called gene enhancers. Enhancers are binding sites for proteins or riboprotein complexes that are important in regulating transcription. Like promotors, enhancers stimulate mRNA synthesis, but unlike promoters, they are not absolutely required for transcription and their function is independent of their position in the gene. The activity of many enhancers is tissue specific, suggesting that enhancer activation of gene expression is an important mechanism for regulating differentiated cell function. However, the specific mechanisms of enhancer function have not been elucidated. The presumed importance of enhancers has led to their currently being the subject of intense investigations.

After transcription of mRNA and before its transport into the cytoplasm for translation, the mRNA undergoes two important modifications. Guanine residue with an added methyl group (a guanine cap) is attached to the five prime (5′) end of the mRNA. This guanine cap maintains orientation and protects mRNA from degradation. The second modification is the cleavage of mRNA at the three prime (3′) end and the addition of a tail of approximately 200 adenine residues (poly-A tail). Like the guanine cap, the poly-A tail enhances mRNA stability.

The mRNA transcribed from the DNA contains two types of DNA sequences called introns and exons. Exons are the coding blocks of the protein sequences; the function of the introns is not completely understood, but it is believed that they are responsible for or participate in regulation of protein synthesis. Introns and exons are interspersed along the transcribed mRNA. Before translation, the intron blocks are removed from the RNA by a process called splicing (Fig. 5). The rate at which introns are excised controls mRNA processes and, in turn, the rate of protein synthesis. Different mRNA transcripts can be created from the same gene by splicing some of the exons with the introns while leaving others. This process is called alternative splicing and can produce several isoforms of a protein from the same gene. These protein isoforms have subtle but potentially important differences in function. Cell function is a reflection of the action of its proteins; therefore, any alteration in the DNA can result in an altered function of the cell (Fig. 6).

Tools and Techniques of Molecular Biology

An understanding of DNA and the basic mechanisms of molecular biology has to be supplemented with a familiarity with the common tools used in molecular studies. This section briefly defines some of the more commonly used molecular biology techniques.

Restriction Enzymes

Restriction endonucleases (restriction enzymes) are used as molecular scalpels to cut DNA in a precise and predictable manner. Restriction enzymes break the DNA backbone at locations identified by a specific sequence of the nucleotides in the DNA (Fig. 7). Restriction enzymes were initially isolated from bacteria and are named by a convention that identifies the bacteria of origin and the order of discovery of the enzyme from that bacteria. For example, *Eco*RI

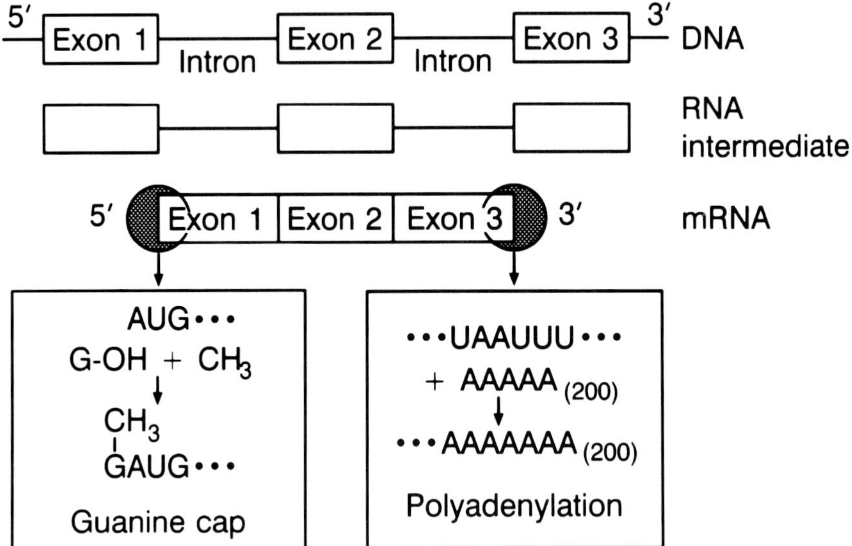

Figure 5
Modification of mRNA in the cell nucleus.

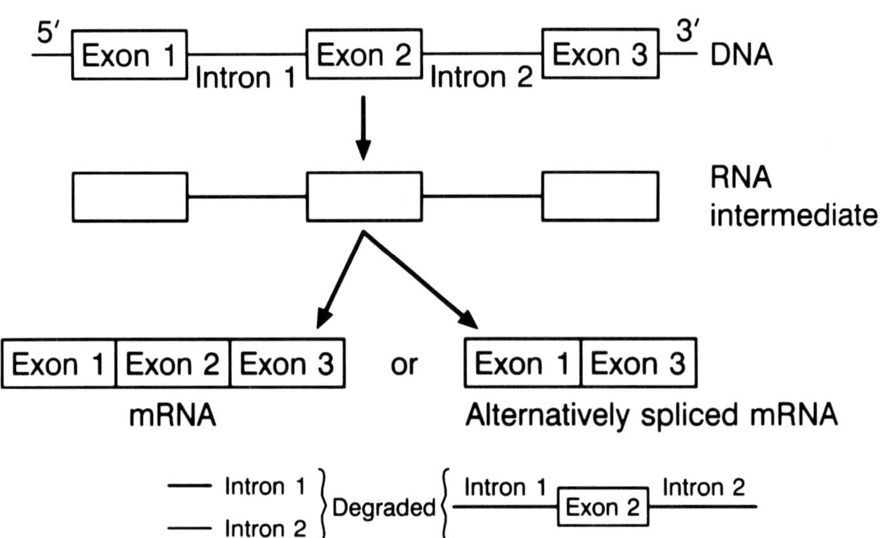

Figure 6
Alternative splicing of mRNA. By including or excluding exons, different proteins can be transcribed from the same gene.

was the first restriction enzyme isolated from the *Escherichia coli* bacteria strain Ry13, and Hind III was the third enzyme isolated from *Haemophilus influenzae* bacteria strain Rd. Some restriction enzymes cut cleanly through the DNA helix on both strands at the same position, leaving flush or blunt-ended fragments. Other restriction enzymes cleave each strand at different levels, at positions two or four nucleotides apart. This creates fragments with exposed ends of short, single-stranded sequences. These single-stranded sequences are called cohesive ends or sticky ends and can serve as a template for realignment of the cut DNA.

To date, more than 1,200 restriction enzymes have been isolated. More than 130 unique nucleotide sequences located randomly along the length of DNA are recognized by one or more of these enzymes. The use of different enzymes with known cleavage locations allows the DNA to be cut into fragments of different sizes. Fragments of DNA cut with restriction enzymes are frequently called restriction fragments.

Agarose Gel Electrophoresis

Agarose gel electrophoresis is used to separate DNA fragments of different sizes (Fig. 8). It takes

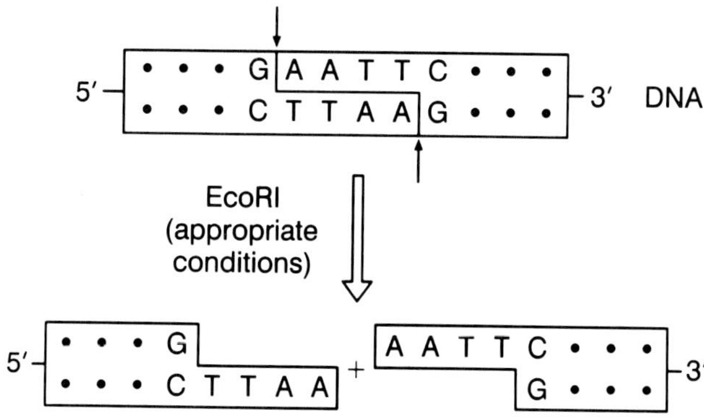

Figure 7
Restriction enzyme cutting of DNA by the *Eco*RI enzyme occurs at sequence-specific sites. Restriction by *Eco*RI results in DNA fragments with 5′ overhangs ("sticky ends"). Other enzymes cut DNA at other sequences. A = adenine; T = thymine; C = cytosine; G = guanine.

advantage of the fact that DNA is negatively charged. When placed in an electric field, DNA molecules are attracted toward the positive pole and repelled from the negative pole. Agarose, a highly purified form of agar, forms a gelatin-like network of cross-linked molecules with large pores. Under the influence of an electric field, DNA moves into and through the agarose gel. The porous agarose gel acts as a sieve through which smaller molecules move more easily than larger ones; consequently, the distance a DNA fragment moves under the influence of the electric field is inversely proportional to its size or molecular weight. In a given period of time, smaller DNA molecules migrate further from the original point than larger ones.

This technique is commonly used in conjunction with restriction enzymes. Restriction enzymes cut DNA samples, generating restriction fragments that then are electrophoresed in agarose gel to separate the fragments on the basis of size. When stained with a fluorescent dye (ethidium bromide), the DNA fragments can be seen under an ultraviolet (UV) light.

DNA Ligation

The extremely large size of DNA from the human chromosome makes study of a specific gene difficult, if not impossible. To facilitate analysis, genes are removed from DNA and attached to independent pieces of nonhuman DNA called plasmids. Ligation is the process of attaching these genes to the plasmids.

Ligation can be thought of as a reverse of restriction enzyme cutting. A gene or fragment of DNA can be cut out of a large DNA fragment or chromosome by using two different restriction enzymes that leave sticky ends at the end of the DNA. The restriction fragments that contain the gene can be identified by agarose gel electrophoresis, isolated by eluting the fragment from the agarose gel, and ligated into a plasmid. In ligation, the single-stranded overhangs of the sticky ends form hydrogen bonds with complimentary nucleotides in the overhangs of other fragments generated by the same restriction enzyme. Hydrogen bonding between nucleotides in the sticky ends holds the DNA together long enough for an enzyme (DNA ligase) to reform the intermolecular bonds of the DNA backbone that were broken by the restriction enzyme. This covalently links the two fragments of DNA into a stable, single strand of DNA. DNA fragments that are ligated together in this fashion are called recombinant DNA.

Plasmid Vectors

Plasmids are self-replicating, functioning strands of extrachromosomal DNA found in bacteria. Plasmids can be used as carriers (vectors) for recombinant DNA (Fig. 9). A gene of interest can be ligated into a plasmid; this plasmid, now called a recombinant plasmid, is inserted into a bacteria. The process of inserting a plasmid into a bacteria is called transformation. Once inside the bacterial cell wall, the inserted plasmid will replicate and increase, or amplify, the number of copies of recombinant DNA in the bacteria. In some bacterial systems, the plasmid will also direct the synthesis of a protein from the recombinant DNA plasmid, and this protein is called a recombinant protein.

As mentioned, recombinant DNA usually must be placed inside a living bacterial cell for replication and further study. A suitable bacterial cell must be found to take up the DNA for replication and expression of the protein. The bacteria *Escherichia coli (E coli)* is the organism most widely used in molecular biology for these purposes. *E coli* will readily take up recombinant DNA plasmids, and these plasmids will replicate extensively. The mechanisms for DNA transcription and protein synthesis are the same in *E coli* as in mammalian cells. This permits human proteins not found in the bacteria to be expressed by these bacteria. The strain of *E coli* used in the laboratory has been genetically modified in a way that prevents it from becoming a human pathogen, thus eliminating the risk of accidental passage of a recombinant DNA into a human.

Genomic Library

Ligating a gene into a plasmid vector and transforming *E coli* provides a simple solution for analyzing a specific gene once it has been isolated. There are over 150,000 genes, however, and the initial

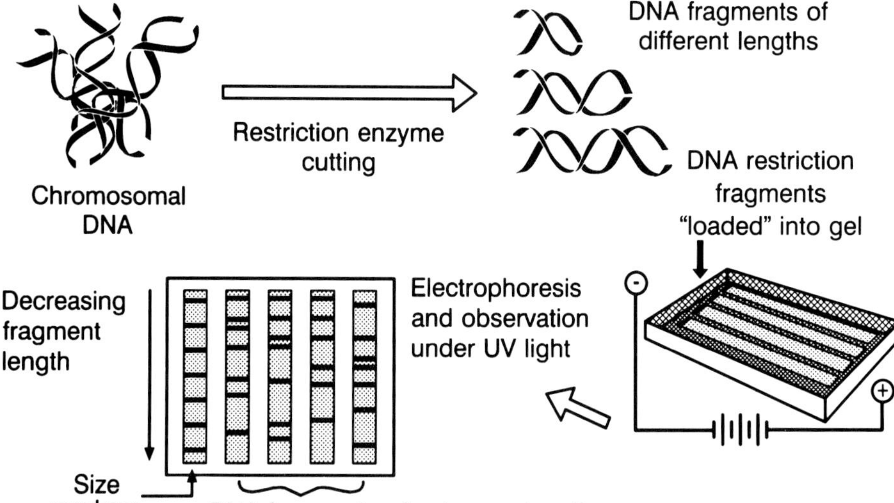

Figure 8
Agarose gel electrophoresis separates DNA fragments based on size. Different fragments are visualized in ultraviolet (UV) light after staining with ethidium bromide, a fluorescent dye that binds to DNA or RNA.

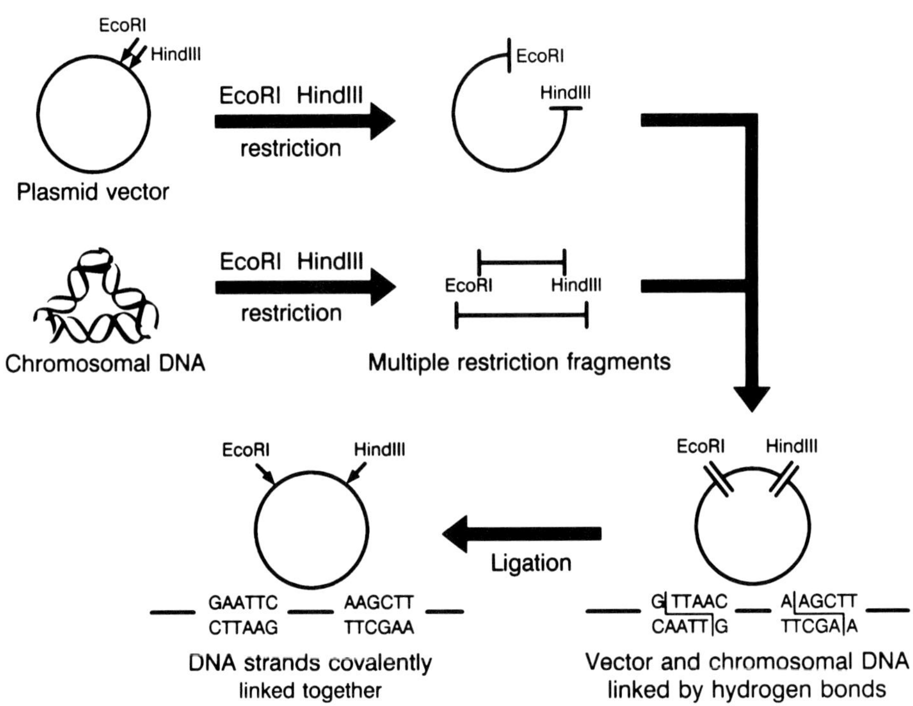

Figure 9
DNA ligation.

problem of isolating a gene is difficult. Their isolation has been addressed through the formation of a genomic DNA library. A sample of human genomic DNA is cut with restriction enzymes to generate many (typically more than 10^6) DNA fragments. The restriction fragments are mixed with plasmid molecules that have been digested with the same restriction enzymes and then covalently joined by DNA ligase. This collection of recombinant plasmids, containing all the genes in the genome, is the genomic library.

Recombinant plasmids are transformed into *E coli* cells. Each cell takes a different plasmid, carrying a different fragment of human DNA. Techniques have been developed for the isolation and purification of a single colony of bacterial cells and the recovery of the single recombinant plasmid that the bacterial cell colony contains. The process of isolating a single recombinant DNA fragment or gene from the genomic library is called screening (Fig.10, *top*).

Using similar techniques, a library can be made from DNA derived from mRNA. This DNA library,

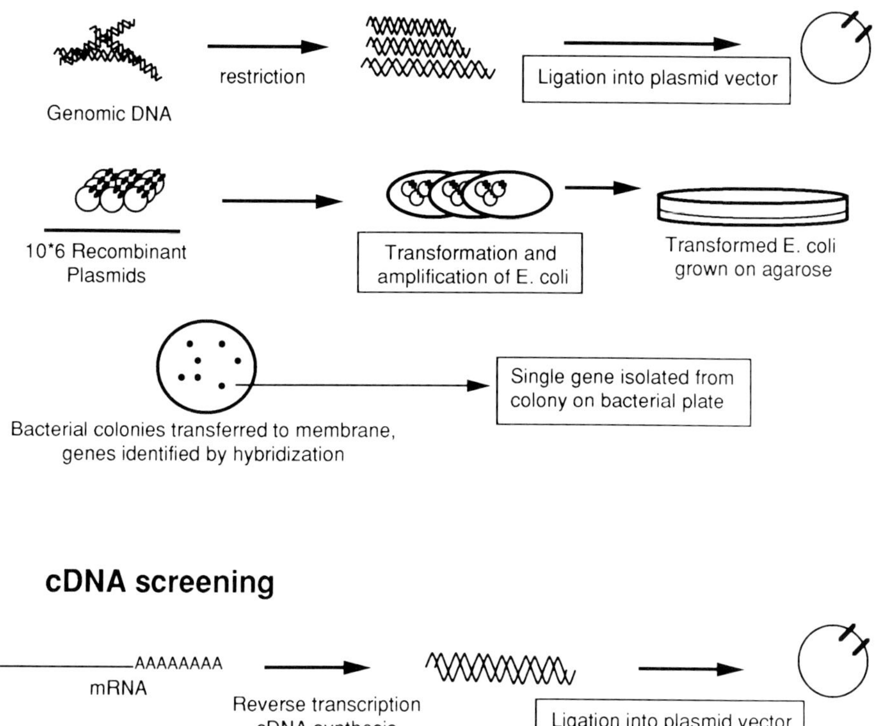

Figure 10
Construction of a genomic library. A genomic library is the mixture of recombinant plasmids that contains fragments of all the DNA in the chromosome. The entire genome, restricted into small fragments, is ligated into plasmid vectors restricted by the same enzymes. These recombinant plasmids transform bacteria, which can be screened to isolate specific genes of interest.

called a complementary DNA (cDNA) library because the DNA is complementary to the mRNA, contains only DNA coding for proteins made by the cells (that is, the source of the mRNA) (Fig. 10, *bottom*). A cDNA library eliminates DNA that codes for other proteins and DNA that is in regulatory regions of the chromosome. Consequently, cDNA libraries have the advantage of containing DNA that is specific for genes expressed by particular cells or tissues. These libraries can be constructed so that the bacteria will synthesize the proteins coded by these genes. These libraries, called expression libraries, greatly facilitate the process of identifying and isolating genes of interest.

Sequencing of DNA

After a gene has been isolated by screening either a genomic or cDNA library, the next step is to determine the nucleotide sequence of the gene. The most frequent method used is the chain-termination method developed by Fred Sanger, called the dideoxy sequencing method (Fig. 11). In DNA replication, DNA polymerase I synthesizes a new strand of DNA from a DNA template using the four nucleotides: adenine (A), cytosine (C), guanine (G), and thymine (T), to reconstruct the DNA backbone. A chemically altered nucleotide, a dideoxynucleotide, will interrupt the synthesis of the backbone because it cannot link with the next adjacent nucleotide. Synthesizing a DNA strand with a mixture of nucleotides and a single dideoxynucleotide (a, c, g, or t) results in a family of truncated DNA fragments whose length corresponds to the position of the dideoxynucleotides. High-resolution electrophoresis determines the lengths of these fragments. If this process is repeated in four reactions, each containing a different dideoxynucleotide, a truncated DNA fragment is synthesized for each base in the DNA sequence. By comparing the length of DNA fragments in each reaction, the DNA sequence can be deduced. After the DNA sequence is obtained, the protein sequence can be determined by translating the genetic code.

Transgenic Animals

The techniques for inserting foreign DNA into *E coli* bacteria have been extended to mammalian cells, making it possible to study cloned genes in cultured cells or in whole organisms. A transgenic animal is created by inserting a foreign gene, called a transgene, into a single-cell embryo. The transgene then is carried by repeated series of cell duplications into every cell of the organism (Fig. 12).

This novel technique has been used in several different ways to study the function of cloned genes and the regulation of the expression of these genes.

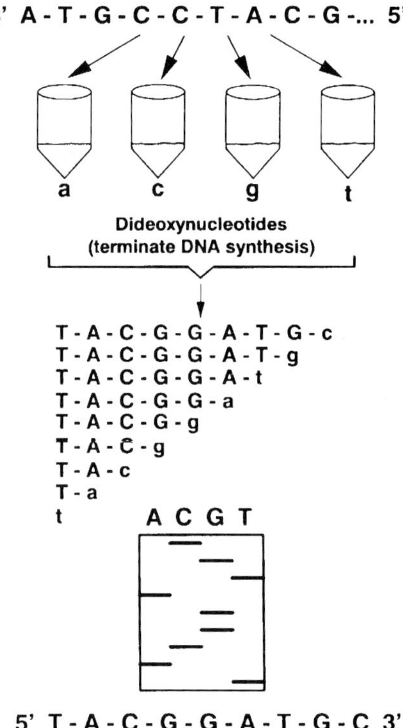

Figure 11
Sanger DNA sequencing. Four simultaneous reactions, each with a different dideoxynucleotide, will generate a family of DNA fragments that can be separated by high-resolution electrophoresis. The relative size of these fragments indicates the DNA sequence. By using the genetic code, the protein sequence can be predicted from the cDNA sequence. A = adenine; T = thymine; C = cytosine; G = guanine.

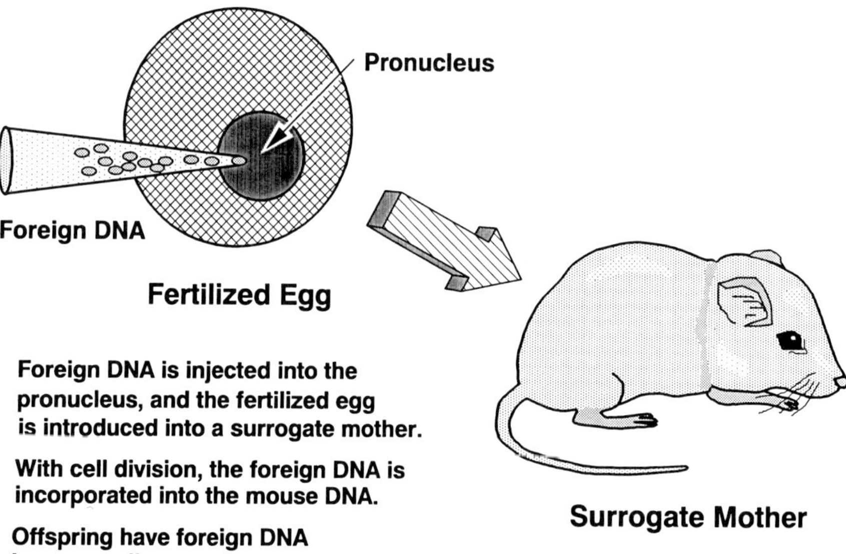

Pronucleus
Foreign DNA
Fertilized Egg
Foreign DNA is injected into the pronucleus, and the fertilized egg is introduced into a surrogate mother.
With cell division, the foreign DNA is incorporated into the mouse DNA.
Offspring have foreign DNA in every cell.
Surrogate Mother

Figure 12
Transgenic mice. Recombinant DNA is injected into a fertilized mouse egg. With cell division, the foreign DNA will incorporate into the chromosome. As the egg develops into an embryo, every cell in the animal contains the foreign DNA.

In the first transgenic animal study, the promoter region that controls expression of the insulin gene was ligated to a marker gene and injected into a single-cell mouse embryo. Analysis of tissues from embryonic mice demonstrated that the marker gene was expressed only in the beta cells of the pancreas, indicating that expression of a transgene in transgenic animals is normally regulated. In more recent studies, techniques have been developed to artificially control the expression of the transgene, allowing for a very sophisticated analysis of gene expression and protein function. Undoubtedly, this will be a very powerful tool for determining the function of isolated genes.

Southern and Northern Hybridization

This is also referred to as Southern or Northern blotting. It is often important to determine if a particular DNA or RNA sequence is present in an extract of DNA or RNA. For example, the presence of a DNA sequence could indicate that a particular gene is expressed, whereas lack of a particular DNA sequence could indicate the presence of a mutation or allelic deletion that interferes with gene expression. The techniques that identify a DNA or RNA sequence in a mixture of different DNA and RNA species are called Southern and Northern hybridization, respectively. Southern hybridization identifies DNA and Northern hybridization identifies RNA.

Heating DNA to temperatures of about 90°C or incubation in solutions with a pH > 10.5 disrupts the hydrogen bonds between base pairs and causes the complementary strands to dissociate. This process is called denaturation. If the temperature is allowed to slowly cool, or if the pH decreases, the complementary strands realign and hydrogen bonds reform, a process called hybridization. Hybridization does not necessarily occur between the two DNA strands that were originally associated, but can occur between any two complementary sequences of either RNA or DNA. To identify a particular RNA or DNA, called a target sequence, the sequence is hybridized to a small complementary fragment of radiolabeled DNA, called a probe. Detection of the probe by autoradiography identifies the presence of the complementary DNA or RNA target.

The application of this technology to the detection of DNA is called Southern hybridization after its discoverer, Edward Southern. DNA from cells or tissue is size-separated by gel electrophoresis and then blotted, or transferred, to a nylon or nitrocellulose membrane. Heating or exposure to UV light fixes the DNA to the membrane. DNA on the membrane and the radiolabeled DNA probe are denatured by heating, and then incubated together under conditions where hybridization will occur. The hybridization conditions are critical to the outcome of these experiments: stringent conditions (high temperature and low sodium concentrations) permit hybridization of exact complementary sequence matches, and nonstringent conditions allow hybridization of sequences that have mismatches between the bases. At the conclusion of the incubation, probe that has not hybridized to the DNA is removed from the membrane by washing, and hybridized probe is identified by autoradiography. Southern hybridization is commonly used to detect restriction fragment length polymorphisms (RFLPs) or to identify the presence of genomic DNA fragments.

If the radiolabeled DNA probe is hybridized to RNA rather than to DNA, then the process is called Northern hybridization. Northern hybridization is similar technically to Southern hybridization; the major difference is that the RNA is single-stranded and does not need to be denatured. Hydrogen bonding between internal complementary RNA sequences forms secondary structures, however, and RNA is electrophoresed in denaturing gels to prevent these secondary structures from interfering with separation. Northern hybridization is used most frequently to evaluate mRNA levels in cells or tissue because it gives an indication of the level of gene expression.

Polymerase Chain Reaction (PCR) Amplification

PCR amplification is a method for the repetitive synthesis of specific DNA sequences in vitro. Starting with two short DNA primers that hybridize to opposite DNA strands flanking a DNA region of interest, a PCR cycle results in the synthesis of the DNA fragment defined by the primers (Fig. 13). Because the DNA products of one cycle serve as templates for synthesis in subsequent cycles, the number of DNA copies doubles at each cycle. Repeated

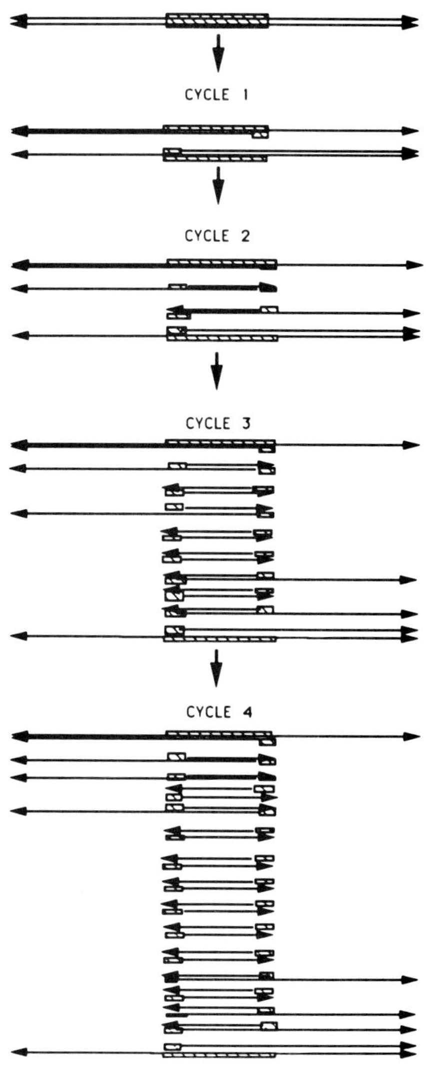

Figure 13
Polymerase chain reaction amplification cycles.

cycles of synthesis result in the exponential amplification of the target DNA. The use of thermostable DNA polymerase (Taq polymerase, isolated from the *Thermus aquaticus* bacteria found in Old Faithful geyser at Yellowstone Park) allows the reaction to be automated in a thermocycler device.

Initially, PCR amplification was considered to be a method for producing copies of a specific DNA or RNA sequence, and early applications included the prenatal diagnosis of sickle-cell anemia and the identification of estrogen receptor gene expression in fracture repair. Further experience has resulted in broader applications, however, and in addition to detecting DNA or RNA sequences, current use includes screening genomic DNA for mutations in known genes and the detection of new genes. Development and application of PCR technology continues at a rapid pace. PCR amplification has proven to be such a powerful technique that it has begun to transform the way biologists think about studying basic problems. The impact of PCR in clinical medicine is only beginning to be realized.

Genetic Diseases

Armed with the basic understanding of the mechanisms by which genetic information stored in DNA in the nucleus regulates protein synthesis and cell function, medical scientists have attempted to define how abnormalities in this process are responsible for causing disease. The tools described above are presently being used in the study of genetic or inherited diseases.

More than 3,000 inherited disorders have been identified. The specific pattern of inheritance, dominant versus recessive or autosomal versus sex-linked, reveals that inherited diseases are caused by abnormalities limited to a specific gene. The causative genes have been identified for only a fraction of these inherited or genetic diseases (Table 1). The immediate challenge to understanding genetic diseases is to isolate the genes responsible for these illnesses and to analyze the genes for their specific mutations. Over the past decade, there has been rapid progress in the development of techniques to characterize the specific molecular defects that cause genetic diseases. The most direct technique is the identification of the abnormal protein that causes the disease. Once the abnormal protein is identified, the gene for this protein can be isolated and sequenced and the specific genetic mutation identified. Studies using this approach have resulted in identification of the underlying genetic mechanism in several diseases of the musculoskeletal system. For example, an abnormality in type I collagen was found to produce osteogenesis imperfecta, and since this was discovered, a mutation in both of the genes for type I collagen has been found (Fig. 14). The identification of collagen abnormalities in cartilage disease has prompted investigation of the type II collagen gene, and recent reports indicate that mutations of the type II collagen gene have been found in chondrodystrophies and osteoarthritis. More recently, mutations in the gene for a newly identified protein, fibrillin, have been identified in patients with Marfan's syndrome.

Table 1
Genetic mutations known to cause musculoskeletal diseases

Genetic Disease	Abnormal Gene
Osteogenesis imperfecta	Type I collagen
Marfan's syndrome	Fibrillin gene
Selected chondrodystrophies	Type II collagen
Vitamin D-resistant rickets	Vitamin D receptor
Familial aortic aneurysm	Type III collagen

If an abnormal protein has not or cannot be identified, a second approach, called linkage analysis, can be used to identify the abnormal gene. In order to use linkage analysis, the inheritance pattern of the disorder of interest must be known. Linkage analysis uses marker genes, genes with a known location, to find the abnormal gene. This technique has been used to identify a number of skeletal diseases associated with the type II collagen gene.

Linkage analysis works like this: DNA is polymorphic, meaning that it varies slightly from one individual to the next. Restriction enzymes are enzymes that cleave DNA at specific nucleotides (marker genes) and produce fragments of DNA. When a cleavage point is altered because the DNA is polymorphic, the length of the fragment of DNA produced is altered. This is called a restriction fragment length polymorphism (RFLP). Polymorphic DNA sequences that alter restriction fragment length can be identified by restriction analysis and Southern hybridization (Southern blotting).

Linkage analysis looks for a marker gene, recognized by an RFLP, associated with an abnormality. If a marker gene, with an abnormal position, in a family with a genetic disease follows the inheritance pattern of that disease, the marker gene is said to be linked to the abnormal gene producing the disease (Fig. 15). The more closely alike the two patterns are, the closer the linkage and the closer the two genes are in the genome. A marker gene can be closely linked with a disease gene without being identical. Obviously, the more closely a polymorphic marker gene follows the inheritance pattern of an abnormal gene, the greater the probability that the marker gene itself is the abnormal gene.

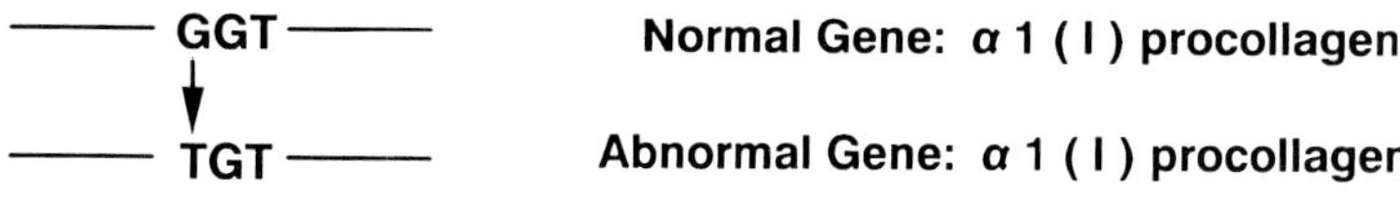

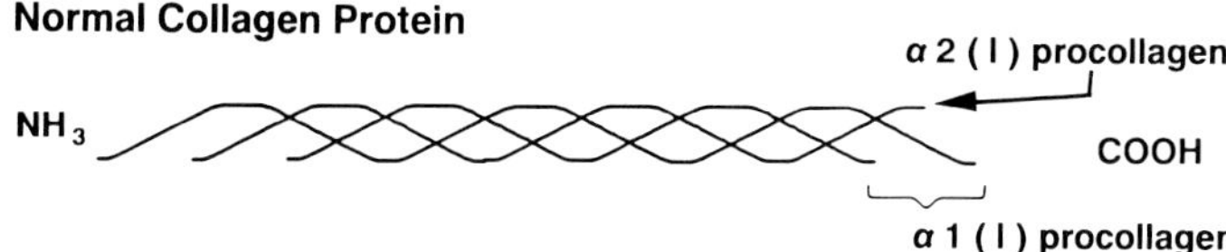

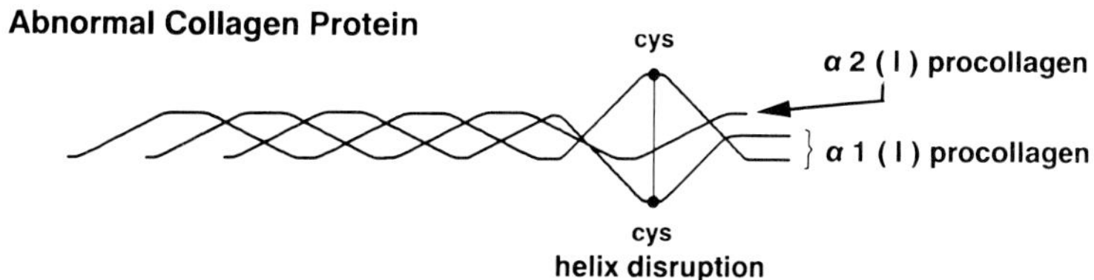

Figure 14
Mutations in collagen I gene cause abnormalities in the collagen protein and are responsible for osteogenesis imperfecta. **Top,** Mutations in the gene cause changes in the protein sequence. In this example, a G to C mutation causes a *cys* to substitute for a *gly* in the helical portion of the collagen I molecule. **Bottom,** Abnormal fiber formation changes the protein properties as demonstrated by a change in the temperature sensitivity of the collagen triple helix.

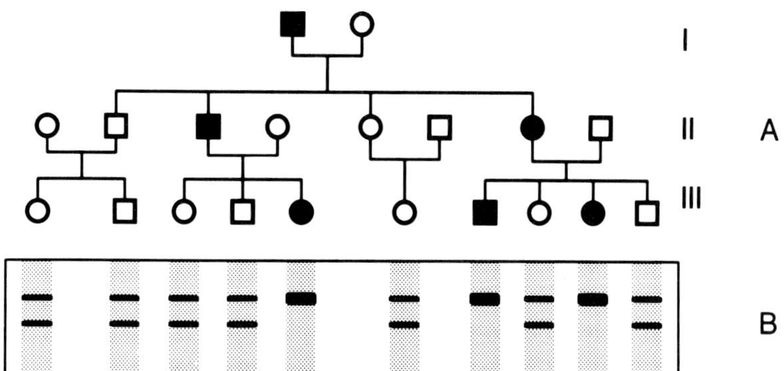

Figure 15
Linkage analysis.

Linkage analysis has been used to study Stickler's syndrome (ophthalmoarthropathy), a disease that affects the eyes and joints. Because type II collagen is found in both of these tissues, the collagen type II gene is a candidate for the abnormal gene causing this disease. Using the type II collagen gene as a marker, a polymorphism has been identified that is strongly linked to the disease in one family. This finding suggests that the type II collagen gene is the gene causing this disease. In another family with Stickler's syndrome, however, there is no linkage with the collagen II gene, suggesting other genetic abnormalities can also cause this disease.

Linkage analysis is a powerful tool, but it has obvious limitations. The first limitation is the requirement that large families or a number of large families must be studied to obtain meaningful information. The second limitation is the small number of known polymorphic markers in the chromosome. The greater the number of RFLPs, the greater the likelihood of establishing linkage. Areas of the genome in which there are few markers are difficult to analyze. Finally, linkage does not always localize the gene; it may only place the disease gene within a broad genetic neighborhood. Nonetheless, for a genetic disease without an abnormal candidate protein, linkage analysis provides an organized technique for characterizing the abnormal gene. The field of linkage analysis continues to evolve as additional polymorphic markers become available. The long-term goal is to have evenly spaced polymorphic markers available for all chromosomes so that investigators can quickly determine the chromosomal locus of a disease gene. Another aspect of this research is the greater understanding of diseases in general. Increasingly, it is becoming obvious that many diseases are genetic or, at least, a person's genetic make-up is extremely important in determining what diseases that person will develop.

The identification of mutations responsible for genetically transmitted diseases should benefit accurate prenatal diagnosis and counseling. Additionally, identification and study of abnormal genes should eventually lead to a more complete understanding of the function of normal genes. The prospect of gene therapy, now in its infancy, raises the hope that in the future genetic diseases can not only be diagnosed, but also treated.

Basics of Neoplasia

Tumors are clones of cells induced to aberrancy by mutations in genes controlling cell growth. Evolution from normal growth to malignancy is paralleled by a process of progressive damage to DNA and genes that is driven by enhanced tumor cell survival. Neoplastic cells become increasingly resistant to external regulatory signals. The normal controls on cell proliferation, which act throughout the cell cycle, no longer function to precisely orchestrate cell, tissue, and organ function or development.

Current investigations of colon cancers and other tumors indicate that tumorigenesis, for a cell to develop a malignant phenotype, requires that two highly complex pathways be affected and uncoupled. The first pathway, involving the stimulation of DNA transcription, translation, and replication, must be inappropriately turned on. The second pathway, involved in the control or suppression of growth, must be made ineffective.

The hundreds of genes involved in the growth of a cell, when quantitatively or qualitatively abnormal or hyperfunctional, are termed oncogenes. Their products are active in signal reception by the cell, signal transduction, and a cascade of events that regulate events in the cell nucleus. A mutation in one of the two alleles of an oncogene is dominant in leading to cell transformation.

The second pathway involved in tumorigenesis, growth suppression, involves mutations in genes that can inhibit cell proliferation. For example, the first well established growth-suppressing protein, retinoblastoma protein (pRB-1), can act as a negative regulator of gene expression. Mutations in this protein lead to unrestricted proliferation. Mutations in pRB are seen in retinoblastomas and in some osteosarcomas. The function of another tumor suppressor protein, p53, is to prevent entrance into S-phase of the cell cycle. Mutation of the p53 gene and subsequent loss of function are seen in many advanced tumors, including osteosarcomas and chondrosarcomas.

Tumor suppressor genes act in a recessive fashion. Both alleles must be mutated before the tumor phenotype will be seen. Inheritance of mutated tumor suppressor genes has been clearly shown in the familial retinoblastoma syndrome (RB-1 gene) and the Li-Fraumeni syndrome (p53 gene). In these families, mutations in one allele are inherited from one parent. Tumorigenesis begins if a mutation subsequently develops in the allele inherited from the other parent.

In humans, the degree or extent of differentiation of cells varies, although in the adult human there are probably no cells that retain the ability to differentiate into any and all types of cells. Primitive mesenchymal cells in the connective tissues, also called stem cells, retain the ability to differentiate into specific cell types when called on to do so by regulatory conditions. Multipotential stem cells in the bone marrow, blood, and periosteum can become osteoblasts, fibroblasts, or chondroblasts depending on local and systemic stimuli. The fact that all of the DNA is available introduces an additional mechanism of neoplasia. If a differentiated cell begins to express a portion of its DNA that is not normally expressed by that cell, the cell may be stimulated to begin and continue its cycle of replication. This mechanism of neoplasia is called epigenesis, in contrast to mutagenesis, in which the sequence of DNA in the cell is altered. If the daughter cells continue to read this usually restricted area of DNA, the neoplastic cell line is sustained, and a tumor is produced. Clinically, this mechanism probably explains the cause of benign, noninvasive tumors and is probably not a common means of producing a malignant tumor. It is not uncommon, however, for a malignancy to produce proteins and enzymes that have functions not usually associated with the normal function of the neoplasm's cell of origin. It is likely that epigenetic behavior explains the production of these normal or near normal proteins by malignant cells (Fig. 16).

This condition of tumor cells producing proteins is known as the paraneoplastic syndrome. There are a number of well recognized paraneoplastic syndromes (Table 2). In the more common ones, the neoplastic cells produce a polypetide hormone (for example, adrenocorticotrophin, ACTH, or par-

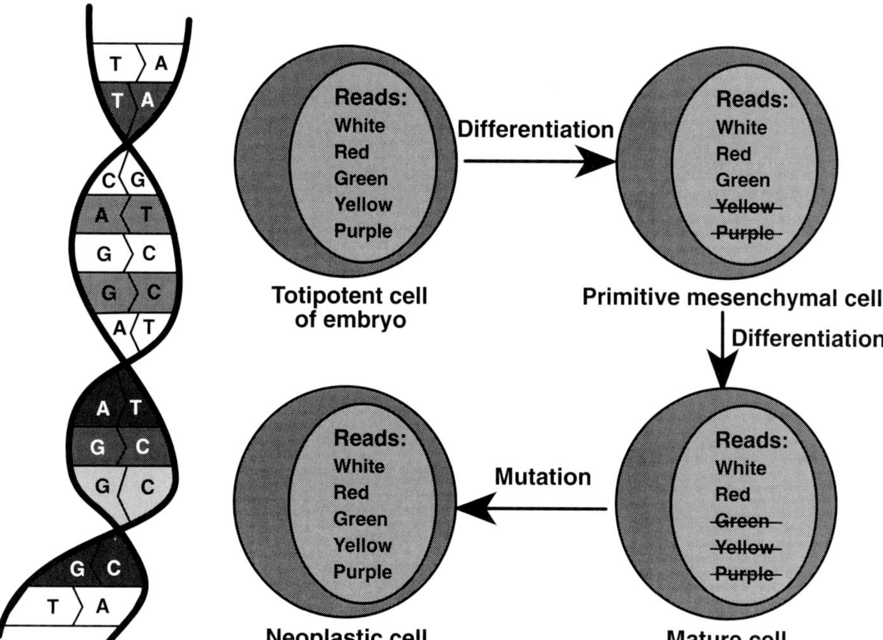

Figure 16
Pathologic cell differentiation.

athormone, PTH), which functions like the normal hormone but is not responsive to normal feedback or other modulating mechanisms. The enzyme is normal enough to produce its usual effect on the patient and results in the patient having clinical symptoms associated with overproduction of that enzyme. The most common example is the production of parathormone from a lung or breast cancer giving rise to hypercalcemia and other clinical findings of hyperparathyroidism. Numerous other paraneoplastic syndromes have been described. They are not common, but they can be significant in the management of patients who have neoplasms.

Cell Cycle and Controls

The normal cell cycle is divided into five phases (Fig. 17), starting with the resting cell (G_0 phase). As the G_0 cells begin the active process of cell division, but before there is an appreciable increase in nuclear DNA, they are said to be in G_1 phase. When the amount of DNA is increased a measurable amount, but before all the DNA has been replicated, the cells are said to be in S phase. They remain in S phase until the amount of DNA is twice normal, and then the cells are said to be in G_2 phase. As the nucleus begins to divide into two separate nuclei (mitosis) they are said to be in M phase, and as they complete their division and separate into two cells, these cells return to G_0 phase and do not replicate again or they return to G_1 phase and repeat the cell cycle.

By convention, the amount of DNA is measured in reference to the amount of DNA in an egg and sperm. This is half the amount of DNA in a normal cell and is called haploid. A normal cell has twice that amount and is therefore called diploid. Cells in G_2 and M phases have four times the haploid amount and are called tetraploid.

Cells enter and complete the cell cycle under strict controls. The normal initiating factors are extracellular stimuli, which signal the cells that additional cells of their type are needed. It is not clear what these signals are. The signals are read by the nuclear DNA, which then produces cyclins, kinases, and possibly other agents (proteins and enzymes) that stimulate cell division. When no more cells are needed, the information is transmitted back to the cell via the DNA, and cell division is stopped.

This process of cell division occurs continuously in every organ in the body. However, when an increase is needed, for example, when a bone breaks, the number of osteoblasts must be increased, and their production is increased dramatically until the fracture is healed. Once the increased numbers of osteoblasts are not needed, the normal osteoblasts begin to reduce their reproduction rate, and cell division returns to a steady state.

In order for a neoplasm to develop, the cells that make up that neoplasm must lose control of their normally closely controlled cell division. The one abnormal function that all neoplasia has in common is uncontrolled or pathologic cell division. This is true of benign and malignant neoplasms. While normal cells divide under strict controls,

Table 2
Paraneoplastic syndromes

System	Syndrome
Endocrine	ACTH/Cushing's syndrome
	Syndrome of inappropriate secretion of antidiuretic hormone (SIADH)
	Tumoral or oncogenic osteomalacia
	Hypercalcemia
	Hypoglycemia
	Miscellaneous agents—
	calcitonin
	gonadotropins
	human placental lactogen (HPL)
	growth hormone (GH)
	prolactin
	thyrotropic substances
Neurologic	Central nervous system
	Spinal cord
	Peripheral nerves
	Neuromotor end plate
Hematologic	Anemia
	Erythrocytosis
	Granulocytosis
	Eosinophilia/basophilia
	Thrombocytopenia
	Thrombocytosis
	Disseminated intravascular coagulation (DIC)
Renal	Nephrotic syndrome
Skin	Acanthosis nigricans
	Leser-Trélat
Gastrointestinal	Protein-losing enteropathies
Miscellaneous	Fever
	Lactic acidosis
	Hyperlipidemia
	Hypertension
	Hypotension
	Amylase
	Hypertrophic pulmonary osteoarthropathy (HPO)
	Amyloidosis

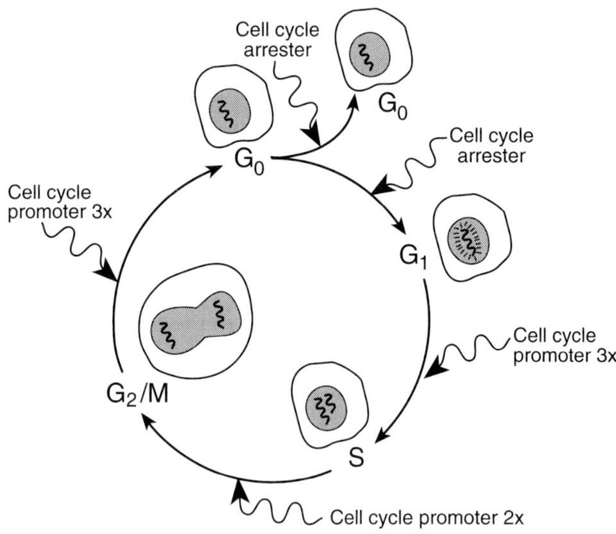

Figure 17
Normal cell cycle.

reproducing themselves only as needed, neoplastic cells reproduce irrespective of need. The loss of normal control of cell division can result from abnormal stimuli that produce cell division (oncogenes) or from the loss of normal proteins responsible for restricting cell division (tumor suppressor genes).

This loss of control can be the result of malfunction within that portion of the DNA responsible for cell replication, or it can be the result of a malfunction in a portion of the DNA that produces a factor that stimulates cell division (growth factor). Whether one mechanism is more often the cause of a tumor's development or whether both are equally important is not clear. However, most believe that the common cause of a cell losing control of its division process is a malfunction of the normal controls of the cell cycle and not simply the continued stimulus for cell division from an abnormally produced cellular protein. It is thought that the changes in the nuclear DNA that lead to the production of a tumor are usually alterations (mutations) in that DNA.

The term oncogene has been given to any abnormality in the DNA that leads to the production of a neoplasm in a dominant fashion (Fig. 18). The alterations in the DNA are usually minor, just one or a few changes in the nucleotide sequence (a point mutation), and it has only been during the last decade that these alterations have been identified. Since their discovery, the understanding of oncogenes and how they function has rapidly increased, but there remains considerable knowledge to be learned. A number of oncogenes have been identified and more will certainly be found (Table 3).

At least some oncogenes are located in that portion of the DNA responsible for controlling the cell cycle, others may be located in a portion of the DNA responsible for the production of the numerous proteins that have the capability to stimulate cell division (growth factors), and still others may work in some as yet undefined way. The action of the oncogene may take place at a cell membrane receptor, at an intracellular transducer, or directly on a nuclear transcription factor. However, if the oncogene is to produce a clinical neoplasm, the observed effect of that oncogene must include uncontrolled cell division.

Recent work suggests that tumor suppressor genes act directly on the mechanisms that control the cell cycle. Proteins called cyclins and enzymes called kinases directly control the cell cycle, and although only three cyclins have been found, more

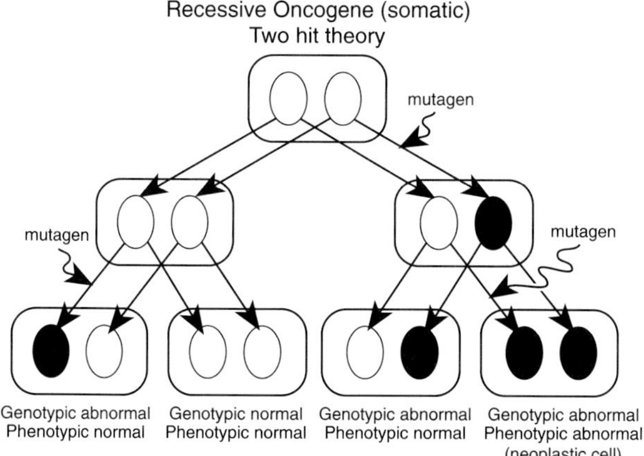

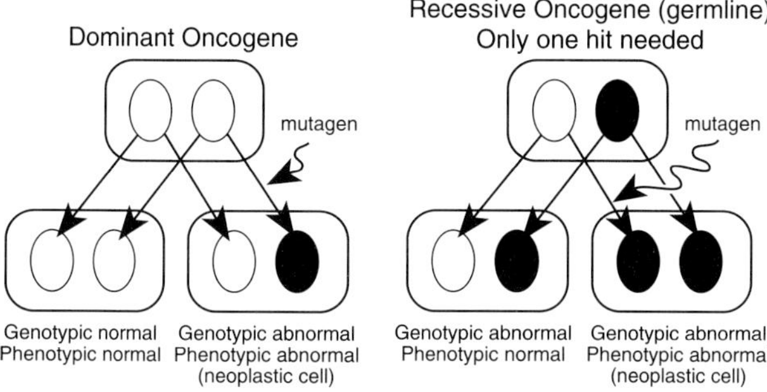

Figure 18
Formation of oncogenes and recessive oncogenes.

must exist. The cyclins and kinases act at various times during the cell cycle, not only to get a cell to begin its cycle but also to continue it through the entire cycle. Some tumor suppressor genes are known to act on the cyclins or kinases as their method of participating in the control of the cell cycle. It is thought that p53, for instance, normally suppresses cell division by blocking the cell cycle through its actions on the cyclins, but if it is absent or abnormal, the cell-cycle suppressing effect of p53 is absent and the cell cycle continues unrestrained. As more is learned, it is likely that other oncogenes and tumor suppressor genes will be found to influence the cell cycle in similar ways.

When the oncogene or mutated tumor suppressor gene is present only in the cells of the neoplasm, it is called a somatic defect. Somatic defects are thought to be the most common type of DNA alteration leading to a neoplasm. A somatic defect occurs during DNA replication when an error in replication occurs and altered DNA is produced (a mutation). Carcinogenic agents and irradiation are thought to cause tumors by increasing the frequency of mutation in cells. It is the alteration of the cell's DNA that leads to the production of a neoplastic daughter cell. Consequently, the DNA mutation must be passed on to subsequent cells if a neoplasm is to develop. Alterations to DNA during cell division probably occur frequently, but most of these alterations either (1) do not produce changes in the cell's behavior, (2) prevent the cell from reproducing, or (3) are repaired by DNA repair mechanisms.

When oncogenes or other mutated tumor suppressor genes are present in every cell in the individual, they are called germline defects. Germline defects are not common, or at least are not commonly recognized. Germline mutations are usually tumor suppressor genes (recessive); consequently, there is no neoplasm unless there is a mutation of the other (second) allele. A germline defect increases the probability that an individual will develop a neoplasm by reducing the DNA mutations that must take place before a neoplasm will develop.

The most studied tumor suppressor gene mutation of significance for the musculoskeletal system is the retinoblastoma or RB-1 gene. This mutation was originally found in patients with familial retinoblastoma and was thought to be specific for this uncommon malignancy. Subsequently, it has been found to be associated with a number of seemingly unrelated malignant tumors, including osteosarcomas.

Retinoblastoma can occur sporadically or in families. The familial type of retinoblastoma is associated with alterations in chromosome 13. Germline defects, like the RB gene in patients with familial retinoblastoma, do not produce a neoplasm by themselves. They require the addition of another alteration, a somatic defect, to produce a neoplastic cell. Familial retinoblastoma is an example of a somatic and germline defect working together to produce a neoplasm (Fig. 19). The patient inherits the altered DNA (germline defect) with the RB oncogene from one parent and a normal DNA from the other parent. As long as one of the two strands of DNA is normal, tumor suppressor activity is present and the cell will behave normally. If there is mutation of the other allele during DNA duplication (a somatic defect), one of the daughter cells will have two abnormal genes for the tumor suppressor gene. This cell will become the initial cell of the malignant retinoblastoma. In nonfamilial, spontaneously occurring retinoblastoma, the two alleles for the RB gene are mutated sporadically. The incidence of sporadic retinoblastoma is much less than that of familial retinoblastoma.

Patients with familial retinoblastoma had been known to have an increased incidence of subsequent osteosarcoma, and it was discovered in the mid 1980s that osteosarcoma cells often had the same RB gene abnormality. The altered gene, which actually is only near the RB gene and is not the same one that leads to retinoblastoma, has been found in only a few osteosarcomas, but it is suspected that this oncogene is at least part of the genetic mechanism

Table 3
Oncogenes and anti-oncogenes associated with human tumors

Oncogene	Tumor	Anti-oncogene	Tumor
*erb*B1	Squamous cell carcinoma	RB	Retinoblastoma, breast cancer, small cell lung cancer, osteosarcoma
c-*myc*	Burkitt's lymphoma		
GL1	Glioblastoma		
Neu/*erb*B2	Carcinoma of breast, salivary gland, and stomach	p53	Diverse (colon carcinoma, Li-Fraumeni syndrome)
L-*myc*	Carcinoma of lung	MCC	Colon carcinoma
N-*myc*	Neuroblastoma	DCC	Colon carcinoma
int-2	Carcinoma of breast	WT	Wilms' tumor
bcl-1	Follicular lymphoma	NF	Neurofibromatosis
abl	Chronic myelocytic leukemia	*erb*A	Erythroleukemia
Ras	Lung cancer		
c-*fos*	Osteosarcoma		
c-*Src*	Colon cancer		

Many other oncogenes are known (eg, c-*kit*, c-*fms*, *fig*, *bok*, c-*jun*, *met*, *trk*, *ret*, *pim*, *lck*, *sis*, etc.) and the list is increasing. The same is true for the anti-oncogenes.

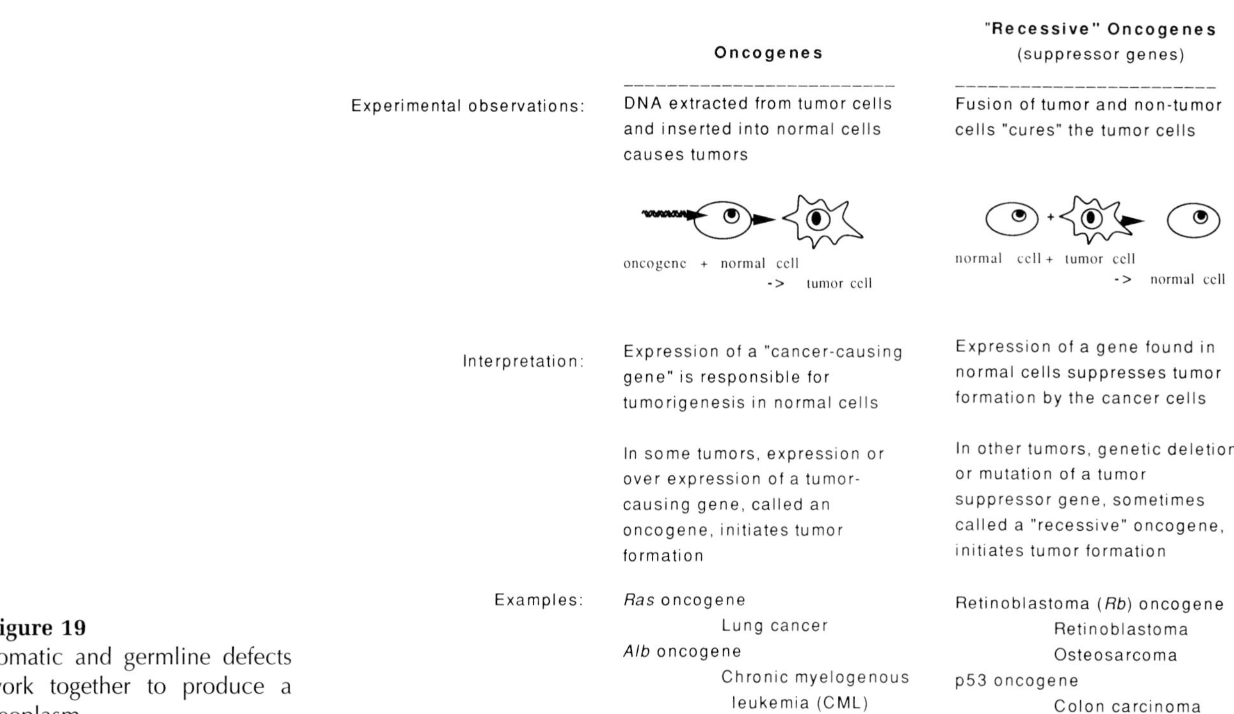

Figure 19
Somatic and germline defects work together to produce a neoplasm.

that produces an osteosarcoma. Although recent work in familial malignancies has revealed a higher than suspected incidence of malignancies in some families, the oncogenes associated with musculoskeletal tumors are thought to be somatic mutations more often than germline.

Wilms' tumor and neuroblastoma also occur with a familial pattern. To produce a neoplastic cell, the familial type of neoplasms must have a germline defect to which a somatic defect is added. Most somatic defects that occur during DNA duplication seem to be spontaneous, and they are probably not uncommon. However, there are agents associated with an increase in the occurrence of somatic defects; these agents are called mutagens. Recognized mutagens include ionizing radiation, nitrogen mustard, some polycyclic aromatic hydrocarbons, and alkylating agents. Carcinogens are agents that have been associated with an increase in cancers. As carcinogens are studied more closely, they are usually found to work through a gene defect; therefore, all carcinogens are probably mutagens.

Since the discovery of the RB gene, another mutated tumor suppressor gene important for musculoskeletal neoplasms has been identified. The p53 oncogene, which is located on chromosome 17, has been found to be abnormal in a number of malignant tumors including chondrosarcomas and osteosarcomas. The p53 oncogene is also commonly abnormal in breast, colon, and lung cancers. As was previously mentioned, p53 is thought to act directly on the cell cycle mechanism. Normally, p53 is responsible for stopping cell division of a cell that has been damaged. This normal mechanism probably exists to allow the damaged cell to repair its DNA before the cell divides and passes the abnormality to the next generation. When the p53 gene is missing or altered, a cell with damaged DNA may continue to divide, reproduce the defective DNA, continue to divide, and, if the alteration in DNA allows uncontrolled cell division, eventually produce a neoplasm.

Oncogenes are classified as either a proto-oncogene or an antioncogene (Fig. 18). Proto-oncogenes are also called dominant oncogenes. This type of oncogene can be thought of as an oncogene that produces a neoplasm by its presence. The proto-oncogenes occur as the result of alterations in that portion of the DNA that normally controls cell division and growth. The normal DNA mutates or malfunctions in some way, and this results in uncontrolled stimulation of cell division. Retroviruses that produce tumors act as proto-oncogenes by providing the necessary stimulants for continued cell division. Antioncogenes are also called recessive oncogenes or tumor suppressor genes. This type of oncogene can be thought of as an oncogene that produces a neoplasm by its absence. The antioncogenes, like proto-oncogenes, result from an alteration in nuclear DNA that is normally present, but the function of the normal recessive oncogene is to suppress cell division. Therefore, when this part of the DNA functions improperly, the normal suppression of cell division is lost, and the cells lose their normal cell division restraints. Both the RB gene and the p53 gene are antioncogenes (recessive or tumor suppressor genes).

The number of known oncogenes and tumor suppressor genes has increased dramatically in the past few years. More than 25 have been identified, and it is expected that many more will be found.

Chromosomal Abnormalities

The RB and p53 oncogenes are most commonly produced by point mutation alterations in the DNA; alteration of the chromosome's appearance is not necessary to produce their effect. However, there are gross alterations in chromosomes that contain the DNA portion, including the RB or p53 oncogenes, which will have similar effects. In all likelihood, the gross chromosomal alterations result in damage to the DNA in similar ways to point mutations, but on a larger scale. As a means of illustration, suppose that a doctor's office is on the fourth floor of the hospital. If a working crew comes along and guts that office, that doctor cannot take care of any patients, but the overall structure of the building is unchanged. That change is like a point mutation; it would be difficult to be aware of the alteration without looking very closely. If the same working crew destroyed the entire hospital, the results for the doctor would be the same. That doctor would not be able to take care of any patients, but an observer would need only limited knowledge of the doctor's city to see the damage. This change is like single translocations between chromosomes. If the working crew dropped a nuclear bomb on the hospital, that doctor still would not be able to take care of patients, but this alteration would be obvious to anyone. It is like a multiple chromosomal alteration (Fig. 20).

A number of chromosomes are important in the development of musculoskeletal tumors. As mentioned, the RB gene is located on chromosome 13, although the gross appearance of the chromosome is not altered in most patients with familial retinoblastoma or in most osteosarcomas. In Ewing's sarcoma, a characteristic translocation between chromosomes 11 and 22 has been identified, and it is indicated by

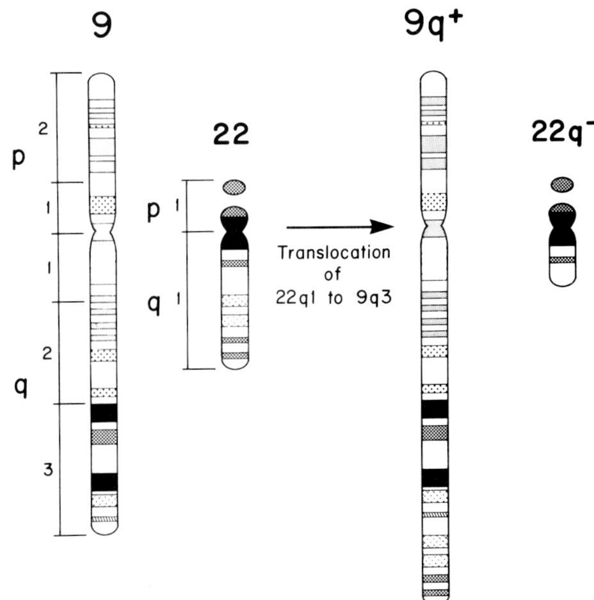

Figure 20
A translocation that involves the *abl* cellular oncogene.

the notation [t(11;22),(q24;q12)]. The notation is universal, and it indicates the exact location of the translocation. The t indicates that it is a translocation. The numbers in the first set of parentheses are the two chromosomes involved in the translocation. The next set of letters and numbers indicate the breakpoint for the chromosomes. A q indicates that the break is on the long arm of the chromosome, and a p indicates it is on the short arm. The numbers with these letters indicate the position on the arm of the chromosome. Reading the chromosomal abnormality involved with Ewing's sarcoma [t(11;22),(q24;q12)] reveals that there is a reciprocal translocation between chromosomes 11 and 22, with the breakpoints on the long arms at positions 24 and 12. Translocations are the most common chromosomal alterations found to be associated with neoplasia, but they are found only in the neoplastic cells, not in the patient's normal cells. They are, therefore, somatic chromosomal defects and not germline chromosomal defects.

Another musculoskeletal tumor with a known frequent chromosomal abnormality is liposarcoma. The chromosomal abnormality associated with liposarcoma is indicated by [t(12;16),(q13;p11)]. Therefore it is a translocation between chromosomes 12 and 16 with the breakpoints on the long arm at position 13 and the short arm at position 11, respectively.

Chromosomal abnormalities have not been routinely looked for in musculoskeletal tumors, and there is much to be learned about their frequency and importance. Although chromosomal abnormalities may be more or less frequent, their relative importance is difficult to establish. The chromosomes do not need to be abnormal for the DNA to malfunction enough to produce a neoplasm, and, in all likelihood, future research should concentrate on the oncogene point mutations rather than on the gross chromosomal defects.

One of the interesting recent developments in understanding how neoplasms develop and behave has been the realization that neoplastic cells develop additional somatic gene defects as they replicate their DNA. These additional gene alterations can change the behavior and capabilities of the subsequent daughter neoplastic cells, compared to the parent neoplastic cell. In some cases this explains how a benign tumor, for example a neurofibroma, can be transformed into a malignant one, a neurofibrosarcoma. Continued alterations in the genetic structure also probably explain the uncommon phenomenon of spontaneous remission. The most common spontaneous remission of a malignant tumor is the change of a neuroblastoma to a benign ganglioneuroma. This does not seem to be simply a case of a cell line dying, but rather of cells losing their malignant potential with further DNA replication. It is as if the daughter cells had their DNA altered such that they are no longer capable of metastasizing. Another explanation would be that the malignant cells die off, leaving only benign cells behind. In any event, continued alterations in cellular DNA may add or subtract from a neoplasm's behavioral characteristics.

Growth Factors

The group of proteins that control and influence cell growth and division are called growth factors. Alterations in growth factors or inappropriate response to growth factors may lead to the growth of a neoplasm, and it is likely that growth factors play a pivotal role in tumor production (Fig. 21). Growth factors are polypeptides that bind to specific cell membrane receptors to stimulate certain functions within the cell. Usually more than one acts on a cell at a time to regulate that cell's activity. The polypeptides are produced under the direction of nuclear DNA. By attaching to the cell surface, they activate the intracellular mechanisms (their cell of origin and adjacent cells) and lead to cell division. As investigations into the behavior of the growth factors increase, it is apparent that their functions are crucial to cellular activity and an understanding of them should improve understanding of how cell growth, activities, and division are controlled.

Growth factors are named after their origin or apparent action. Platelet-derived growth factor (PDGF) was first found in platelets, but is now known to be present in transformed mesenchymal cells and large vascular endothelial cells. It is a strong mitogen, meaning it can stimulate both DNA production and cell division. Transforming growth factor type beta (TGF-β) is one of a number of transforming growth factors; the other common one is called transforming growth factor type α. These growth factors transform fibroblastic cells in monolayer culture and stimulate colony formation in soft agar. TGF-β is one of the most important growth factors in the musculoskeletal system because its major effect is to stimulate mesenchymal cells to divide. It is an unusual growth factor in that it has both stimulatory and inhibitory properties. Bone morphogenic proteins (BMPs) are members of the TGF-β family of growth factors. Insulin-like growth factors (IGF-I, IGF-II) are another type of growth factor, and they have some of the properties of insulin. Somatomedin C is another name given to IGF-I. Interleukin 2 (IL-2), another growth factor, was originally called T-cell growth factor because it stimulates T cells (T lymphocytes). T cells are thought to be important as host defenders against malignant cells, and IL-2 has been used in experi-

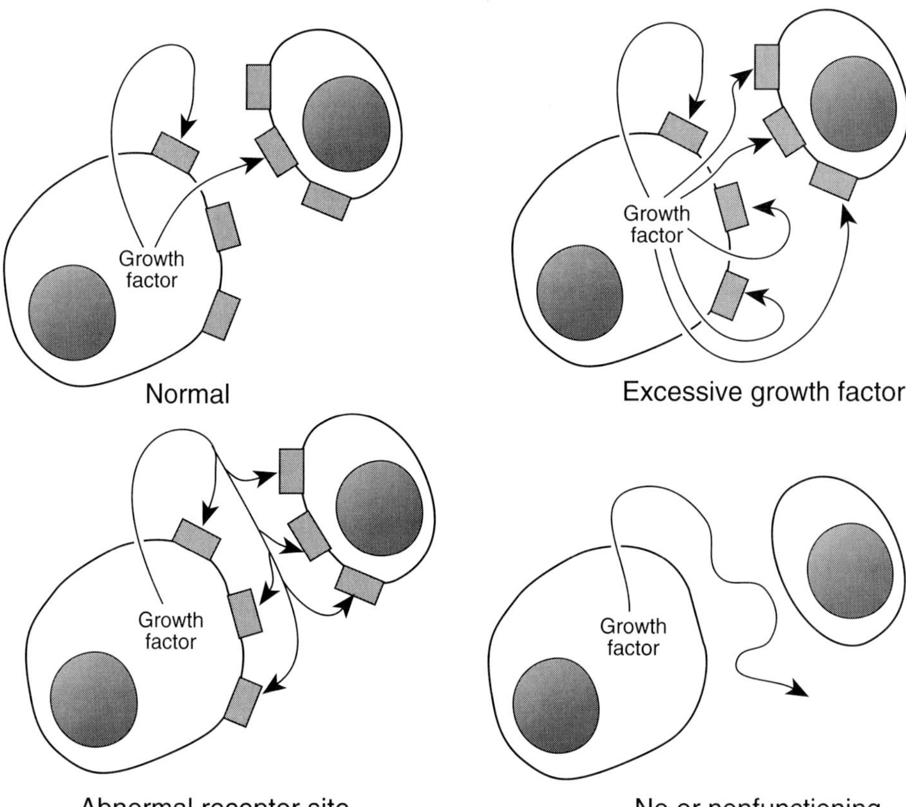

Figure 21
Growth factors in tumor production.

mental and clinical trials in an attempt to stimulate the host's own T cells to eradicate sarcomas. Although some of these experimental trials have looked promising, IL-2 has not yet proven to be of sufficient benefit to be routinely used as an antineoplastic agent. Other growth factors include endothelial cell growth factor, fibroblast growth factor, nerve growth factor, and the colony-stimulating growth factors. Additional growth factors are certain to be identified in the future. Manipulation of growth factors offers a potential means of treating neoplasia, but this is in the future.

The current understanding of these growth factors is that they are produced by the cell, released by that cell, and then act on that same cell, adjacent cells, and maybe distant cells. Their most common function is to stimulate DNA production and cell division. The growth factor proteins are quickly produced and released but short acting, and they are able to modulate behavior of the cell quite rapidly. The cells are continuously monitored, and changes are made, through the action of growth factors, as needed. Cells can be quickly stimulated to reproduce or make a certain product as necessary. When normal tissue sustains an injury, growth factors are released (for example, TGF-β, a growth factor responsible for regulating cell repair activity), which increase the reparative capabilities of the mesenchymal cells. As soon as the tissue has been repaired, growth factor production is reduced to normal, and the cells decrease their level of activity back to the normal baseline level.

It is likely that some of the point mutation DNA defects and the chromosomal alterations that lead to the production of a neoplasm do so through alterations in growth factor or growth factor-like proteins. The DNA defect could alter the growth factor, the ability of the cell to transport the growth factor, the cell membrane receptor, or the response of the cell to the growth factor's message after it is bound to the cell membrane. Pathologic function at any and all of these steps could lead to the production of a tumor.

Growth factors must play a role in some, if not all, neoplasms. The cell membranes of some tumor cells have been shown not to have abnormal growth factor receptors and many do not need growth factor stimulation for growth. These neoplastic cells are not controlled by the normal growth factors and, therefore, are free to divide as they please. In other tumors, there is an increase in growth factor production and c-sis (a proto-oncogene) codes for PDGF.

Neoplastic cells that overexpress c-sis may not need other growth factors for continued growth and cell division. Probably some of the other oncogenes also produce normal or near-normal growth factors, which provide just the additional stimulus needed for a cell to become neoplastic. In any event, growth factors are important in normal cell growth and division, and under pathologic situations they can abnormally stimulate continued cell division and, therefore, the production of a tumor.

In summary, the prerequisites for a tumor to develop are (1) the cell loses its normal cell division regulatory mechanisms so that cell division continues unrestrained, and (2) the cells produced have sufficient machinery to survive. When these cells are not capable of infiltrating the local normal tissues, a benign noninvasive tumor is produced. When the cells can invade locally but cannot spread to a distant site, the tumor is still benign but is locally invasive. When the neoplastic cells, in addition to having the ability to continually divide, can leave the initial colony, survive a trip to a distant site, and form a colony at this distant site (a metastasis), the tumor is malignant.

Drug Resistance

Recently another interesting and important somatic genetic alteration, unrelated to cell division, has been found in some tumors. The protein made by this gene is thought to be a normal protective cellular mechanism that rids toxins from the cell. Normal cells protect themselves from harmful substances by being able to selectively pump these substances out of their cytoplasm through their cell wall membranes. The pump, present in the cell wall membrane, is called p-glycoprotein (Fig. 22). In addition to pumping other natural toxins from the cytoplasm, this pump eliminates doxorubicin hydrochloride and other chemotherapeutic agents from the cell, keeping the intracellular concentrations low and preventing any toxic effect on the tumor cells. Consequently, the cell is "resistant" to doxorubicin hydrochloride. This mechanism allows normal and neoplastic cells to develop resistance to this and other chemotherapeutic agents.

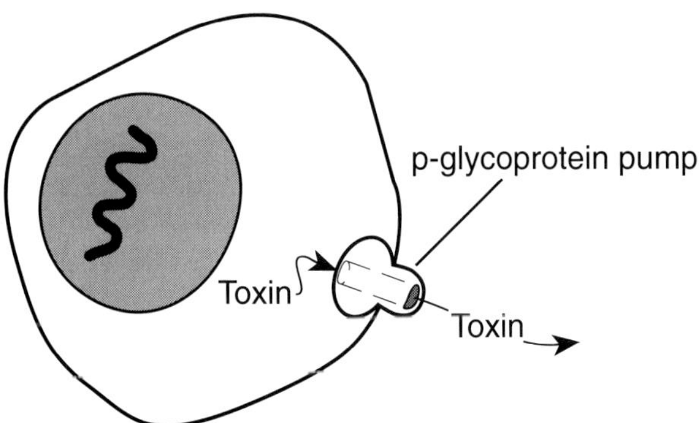

Figure 22
The p-glycoprotein pump.

Recently, two genes have been found that are believed to confer resistance to chemotherapeutic agents. They have been called multidrug resistance gene 1 and multidrug resistance protein (MDR1 and MRP). MDR1 and MRP are responsible for the production of p-glycoprotein-like proteins. The mechanism of drug resistance is not fully understood, but it is thought that when the cell is challenged by a toxic agent like doxorubicin hydrochloride, the MDR1 or MRP genes are stimulated to activate and produce increased amounts of p-glycoproteins, which then pump out the toxic agent.

Molecular biology is a new field that has considerable promise in helping both understanding and treatment of musculoskeletal disorders, including neoplasia. This field of biology should grow rapidly and change the practice of medicine.

Mechanism of Metastasis

A neoplasm is considered malignant if at least one of its cells can escape from the primary site, travel to a distant site, survive at that distant site, reproduce to produce daughter neoplastic cells at the new site, and attract sufficient blood supply to be able to continue multiplying. This is not an easy task, and most cells that escape the primary neoplasm do not survive. It has been predicted that less than one in every ten thousand neoplastic cells that escape the primary site is able to complete the process of producing a metastatic focus. The most difficult part of the process is thought to be during the time that the cell or a small group of cells is isolated from the primary neoplasm and before the cells lodge at a distant site. However, during every step of the metastatic process the neoplastic cells must do things they do not ordinarily do. These new functions are either the result of altered DNA resulting from mutagenesis or of the cell reading part of the DNA not ordinarily read (epigenesis) (Fig. 23).

The metastatic cell must be mobile so that it can escape from the primary neoplasm. It must produce and excrete degradative enzymes that break down the collagenous structures surrounding the tumor to get to the capillary system of the lymphatics and blood vessels. Locally aggressive, nonmetastasizing neoplasms must produce a number of degradative enzymes to invade local tissues, whereas metastasizing tumors must produce the same or similar degradative enzymes as well as others. The degradative enzymes produced include collagenases, hydrolases, cathepsin D, and proteases. These enzymes allow the neoplastic cell to break down tissues that otherwise would prevent movement. The metasta-

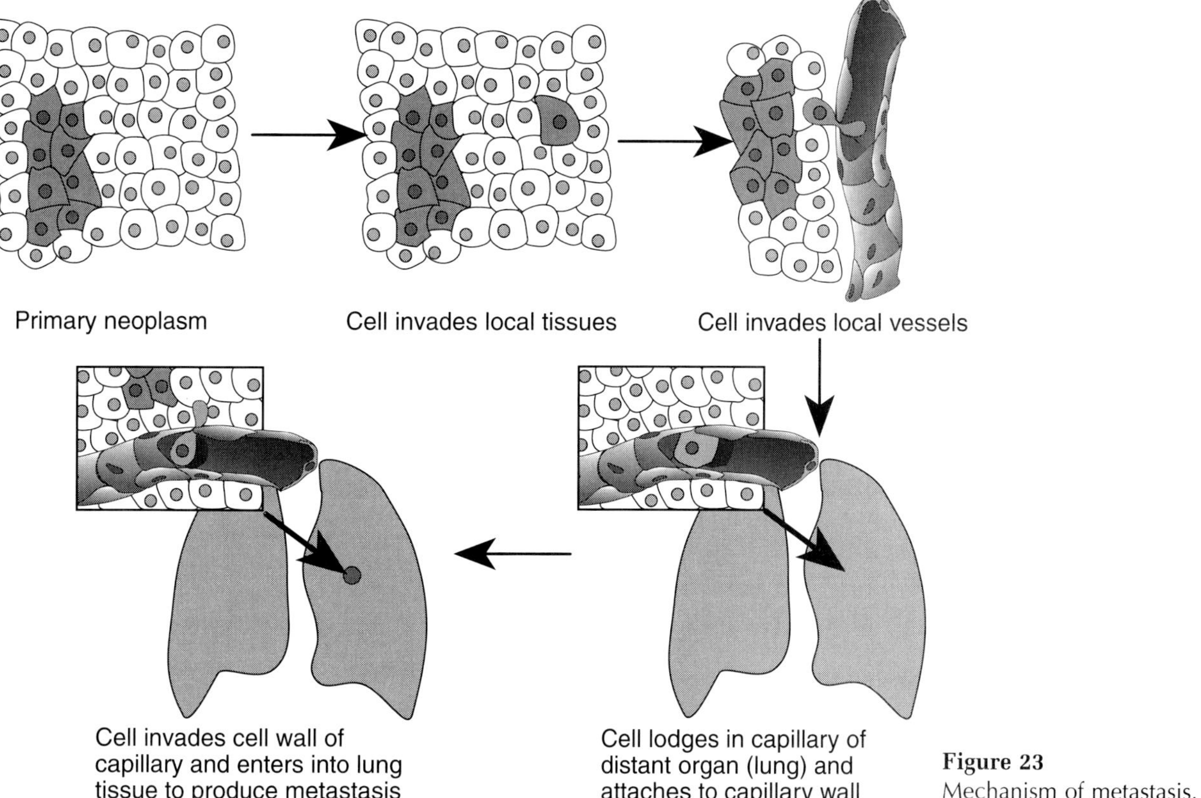
Primary neoplasm
Cell invades local tissues
Cell invades local vessels
Cell invades cell wall of capillary and enters into lung tissue to produce metastasis
Cell lodges in capillary of distant organ (lung) and attaches to capillary wall

Figure 23
Mechanism of metastasis.

sizing cell must migrate through the tissues to gain access to an efferent vessel. It is not clear what directs the cell's movement in a specific direction. It may be a random process or there may be electrical signals or a chemical process. The metastasizing cell finds an efferent vessel and passes through that vessel's wall to enter the vessel's lumen. It is commonly said that carcinomas metastasize via both lymphatics and vascular channels, but that sarcoma only metastasizes via vascular channels. Clinically, this seems to be true, based on the infrequent incidence of lymphatic metastasis of a sarcoma, but it is not. The infrequency of sarcoma metastasis to a lymph node is more likely a factor of the metastatic sarcoma not being able to grow in lymph nodes, not of how the metastasizing cell leaves its site of origin. Both carcinoma and sarcoma cells exit the primary site via lymphatic and vascular capillaries.

Passage through the vessel wall is not difficult. The neoplasm is surrounded by lymphatic and vascular capillaries that have large holes in their endothelium and basement membrane; these holes are large enough for the metastasizing cell to pass through. It is not necessary to postulate other methods for the cell to gain access to the vessel's lumen, but it is possible that the metastasizing cell uses its degradative enzymes to break down the vessel's wall to enter into the lumen.

To this point in the metastatic process there has been little difficulty for the neoplastic cell, and many malignant cells are capable of accomplishing these steps. They even are able to float through the vascular system and remain viable, but very few are able to divide or begin a new focus of the tumor. It is likely that every patient with a malignant tumor has circulating malignant cells very early in the course of the disease, probably before having a clinically apparent neoplasm. It has been predicted that in patients with carcinoma of the breast, malignant cells have already escaped and are circulating in the vascular and lymphatic systems even when the primary neoplasm is only 0.125 cm in diameter. Whether the patient develops a clinical metastasis is determined more by whether these circulating neoplastic cells have the mechanisms capable of starting a new colony of malignancy cells than by their ability to gain access to the vessel's lumen.

The trip within the vascular or lymphatic system is the first aspect of the metastatic process that limits the number of surviving cells. It is not clear what causes the death of these circulating cells, but few are able to survive within the circulatory system. Host defenses must play a role, but the exact mechanism remains unclear. Macrophages are important in killing the neoplastic cells in the circulation and may be the principal method of limiting the number of viable malignant cells in circulation. One of the ways neoplastic cells are protected during their travels through the vascular system is to be surrounded by a fibrin-platelet clot. The fibrin-platelet clot with a central nidus of neoplastic cell(s) isolates the metastasizing cell from the hostile environment and prevents the macrophages from getting to the neoplastic cells. The fibrin-platelet clot also helps the metastasizing cell to lodge at a distant site. Lodging must happen before the malignant cell can enter a distant organ. The observation of this clot and the realization of its importance has lead to the suggestion that prevention of the clot would make the metastasizing cell more vulnerable. Experimental studies supported this suggestion, but in clinical trials the use of heparin as a method of preventing the fibrin-platelet clot has not reduced the incidence of metastasis. Despite current inability to show a clinical benefit, anticoagulation still may prove to be a way of reducing the development of metastatic disease.

These metastatic cell-fibrin-platelet clots must become trapped in capillary beds in a variety of organs, but most neoplasms have a predilection for a specific site of metastasis and a site selection process must take place. In 1889, Paget suggested his seed and soil hypothesis to explain why metastatic disease was more common in certain sites. Paget's hypothesis was that the metastatic cells were distributed evenly over the body, but that only certain organs provided the proper environment (soil) for the growth of the neoplastic cell. In 1928, Ewing offered another hypothesis. He suggested that the metastatic cells were not distributed evenly throughout the body, but were filtered out by the first capillary bed they encountered. For Ewing's theory to explain the low incidence of metastasis from sarcoma to lymph nodes, it was necessary to say that sarcoma cells do not invade lymphatics, which is known not to be true. In all likelihood, both hypotheses are partly true, but the selection process is much more complicated than either suggests. It is increasingly obvious that local factors are important and that although metastasizing cells may be filtered out in capillary systems, their growth to produce a clinical metastasis depends on a variety of factors. One of the more important variables is probably local growth factors that must play an important role in helping the metastatic cell to survive and divide in its new environment.

Once the metastatic cell-fibrin-platelet clot has lodged in a capillary, the metastatic cell must exit the vessel lumen and enter the local tissue. This may be the most difficult step in the development of a metastatic focus. The metastatic cell must attach to the endothelium of the vessel wall before it can pass through the wall. A large family of cell-surface molecules called integrins plays an important, but not fully understood, role in the process of attachment. These integrins are thought to be important in the transport of cells through the basement membrane of normal vessels. The vessels at the site of metastatic spread, unlike those at the primary tumor, are normal, do not have holes in them, and are not easily transgressed. The integrins seem to act as facilitators to the passage of cells through the vessel wall. A possible explanation for the site-specific nature of metastasis could be that the neoplastic cell-integrin match must be specific. It is possible that for the integrin to help the neoplastic cell through the vessel wall, it must first recognize that cell, and this recognition may be a rare event. There is evidence that the metastasizing neoplastic cell also produces type IV collagenase. Type IV collagen is the predominant collagen of the basement membrane, and a specific collagenase for type IV collagen must be produced for the cell to exit the vascular tree.

Once the metastatic cell is outside the vessel and in the local tissues, one of three events may happen. The first possibility is that the cell does not survive or that if it survives, it does not or cannot divide and, therefore, no further evidence of its metastasis is present. The second possibility is that the cell survives and may even be able to divide, but it cannot obtain its own blood supply. Such cells live through diffusion of nutrients with their cell divisions limited, and they do not represent an immediate threat to the host. This is an in situ neoplasm. It is possible that these dormant foci of tumor explain the very late clinical metastatic disease. They remain present but dormant for years as an in-situ focus of neoplasm but then, for some reason, finally obtain their own blood supply and begin to grow and produce a clinical metastasis. The third possibility is that the metastatic cell is able from the outset to attract its own blood supply, and this blood supply permits unlimited cell division.

The ingrowth of new blood vessels into any tissue is called angiogenesis. Angiogenesis must occur for the metastatic focus to become a clinically important metastasis. A diffusible substance has been found in neoplastic tissue, which stimulates the production of new vessels and has been called tumor angiogenesis factor (TAF). Another, more purified factor, which also stimulates vessel formation, is called angiogenin. These factors are probably excreted by the neoplastic cells to stimulate the production of vessels that will grow into the in-situ metastatic focus so it can continue to grow.

There is much to be learned about the process of metastasis, and a better understanding may provide keys to eliminating the ability of neoplasms to metastasize. The details of neoplastic cell invasion through normal tissue, how the metastasizing cell survives the trip within the vascular circulation, how the cell attaches to the endothelium of a normal vessel and gets through the vessel wall, and, finally, how the metastatic cell attracts its own blood supply all need to be understood more thoroughly. Then methods of preventing one or more of these steps to clinical metastatic disease could be accomplished.

Classification

Tumors are classified in a variety of ways in an attempt to group together those that will behave in a similar fashion. The classification systems used are generally agreed upon, but are often modified as new information is found. The current systems were developed before molecular biology was established and, for the most part, use histologic criteria to separate the different tumors from one another. In the near future, it is possible that an entirely new system will be developed based on the molecular biologic similarities between neoplasms, but for now histologic criteria continue to be used.

The first major division in the classification of neoplasms is between those that are malignant and those that are benign. Malignant tumors are those that have the ability to spread to a distant site and grow at this distant site, to metastasize. A benign tumor does not have this ability. However, in the musculoskeletal system there are exceptions to the rule that benign tumors do not metastasize. Giant cell tumor of bone is the most common bone tumor to spread to a distant site and still be called benign; up to 5% of benign giant cell tumors metastasize. Osteoblastoma and chondroblastoma have done the same thing, but do so much less frequently. These tumors are still called benign because of the rarity of metastasis and because the metastatic foci rarely represent a threat to the patient's life.

The second major division in the classification of tumors is confined to the malignant tumors, and separates them into those called carcinoma and those called sarcoma. Carcinomas are malignant tumors that arise from cells of endothelial or epithelial origins, and sarcomas are malignant tumors that arise from cells of mesenchymal origins. Benign tumors are not formally separated as arising from endothelial/epithelial or mesenchymal origins, but the separation is recognized.

Another division in the classification of neoplasms is based on their microscopic appearance, which is thought to indicate their cell of origin. As mentioned, the classification system was devised when molecular biology was not available, and the microscope was the most sophisticated tool used to study these tumors. The pathologists looked at the tumors through their microscopes and decided that those that looked alike should be grouped together, with the assumption that they would behave in a similar fashion because of their like appearance and suspected similar cells of origin. This has been a reasonable assumption, but in the future it may be supplanted by a more accurate method of judging neoplastic cell behavior. Biologic behavior of tumors can be predicted to a degree by their microscopic appearance, but variations are often great, even between two tumors that look alike. As more is learned about molecular biology, the mechanisms used by neoplastic cells will be better understood, and it will be possible to group those tumors with similar molecular biologic characteristics, irrespective of their microscopic appearance.

Any neoplasm classified as arising from bone should be composed of cells whose normal ancestors would have been in bone. Those neoplasms that look as if they are made up of bone-forming cells (that is, osteoblasts) are grouped together. The benign ones include osteomas, osteoblastomas, and osteoid osteomas; the malignant ones are all osteosarcomas. Neoplasms that are made of cartilage cells are grouped together, too. The benign ones include enchondromas, osteochondromas, and chondroblastomas; the malignant ones are all chondrosarcomas. This is repeated for all the tissues of the body. Some neoplasms arise from cells whose normal cell counterpart is still not known, and these are usually grouped individually. Ewing's sarcoma is an example of a tumor whose cell of origin remains undetermined.

Malignant neoplasms are grouped further, based on more subtle microscopic characteristics. Within each major category, there are subcategories based on specific features of a type of tumor. For example, malignant fibrohistiocytoma is a major category of sarcomas, and it has at least five subgroups including myxoid, inflammatory, giant cell, storiform-pleomorphic, and angiomatoid. An additional grouping of malignancies, based on the subjective assessment of the neoplasm's risk of metastasis, is their histologic grade.

The benign neoplasms of all types are subgrouped, but not histologically graded. Benign neoplasms, for the most part, do not have histologic criteria that indicate whether they have the capability to act aggressively or whether they are latent. Benign neoplasms of the same type can be separated further based on their clinical behavior. Despite similar or identical histologic appearance, benign tumors can act quite differently and may need very different treatment. Recognizing these differences is important, and it cannot be assumed that the specific diagnosis indicates the biologic activity of the tumor. This is especially true of giant cell tumor of bone but is true of all benign tumors. It is important when planning treatment to remember that the natural history of the specific lesion is a critical variable in the management of benign musculoskeletal neoplasms.

Staging

Benign Tumors

Few authors have tried to separate benign tumors into stages according to their clinical behavior, but Enneking has and his system is useful. Enneking recommends separating all benign tumors into one of three stages: 1, 2, or 3. The stage is determined by the biologic behavior of the tumor as expressed by either its character on presentation or its ability to recur. Usually the plain radiograph is the best predictor of a specific tumor's behavior, but the clinical history is also useful. The more aggressive the tumor appears on the radiograph and the more rapidly it is growing based on the patient's history, the higher the stage. Usually, the higher the stage, the more aggressive the treatment needs to be if local control is to be achieved.

Stage 1 lesions are the least active benign neoplasms. Enneking calls these latent or inactive lesions. They often will spontaneously resolve or remain unchanged, causing the patient no problems (Fig. 24). These patients come to the physician complaining of an unrelated problem, and the lesion is found when a radiograph is taken or the patient sustains a pathologic fracture through the lesion. The patient should not have symptoms before the fracture. On the radiograph, the lesion is completely intraosseous and has a well developed rim of reactive bone around it, there is no evidence of cortical destruction, and there is no periosteal or endosteal reaction. Common examples include unicameral or simple bone cysts, nonossifying fibroma, and enchondroma. These neoplasms do not require treatment.

Stage 2 lesions are the medium active lesions. Enneking calls these active lesions (Fig. 25). These are benign tumors that do not spontaneously resolve. However, they grow slowly, do not invade normal tissues, expand by "pushing" the surrounding tissues aside, and have a true capsule. The patient usually has a mild ache or reports having had a dull ache before sustaining a pathologic fracture through the lesion. Not uncommonly, the patient reports that the symptoms have been present for months to years without significant change or only a gradual increase in intensity. These lesions are reasonably well outlined on the radiograph, although they will not have a well developed reactive rim around them. There may be cortical destruction, but the periosteum has been able to continue to contain these lesions, and there is no soft tissue extension. There may be a minimal amount of active periosteal reaction but this should be limited. Common examples include most giant cell tumors of bone, chondroblastoma, osteoblastoma, and chondromyxofibroma. These lesions require surgical removal, which can be successfully done with an intralesional curettage.

Stage 3 lesions are the most aggressive benign tumors. Enneking calls these lesions aggressive lesions (Fig. 26). These lesions have all the characteristics of a malignant tumor, except they do not metastasize. They penetrate the cortex, invade the adjacent local tissues, and have a pseudocapsule,

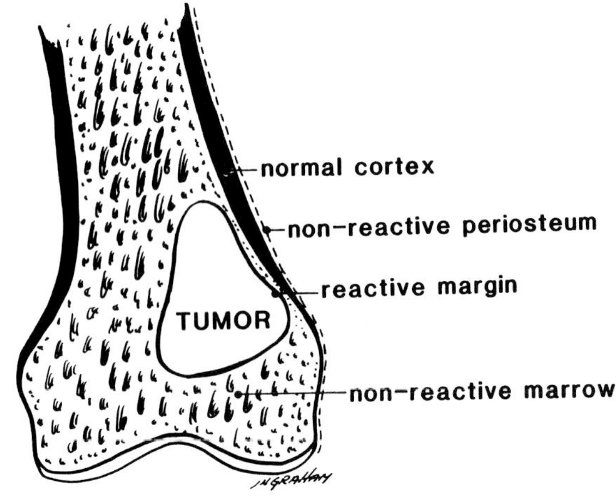

Figure 24
Stage 1 lesion.

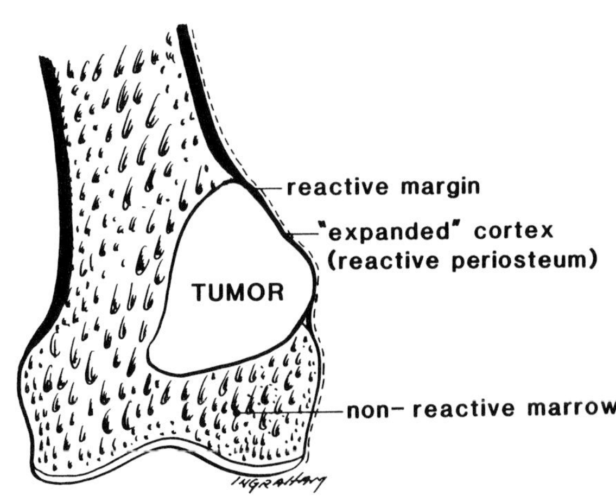

Figure 25
Stage 2 lesion.

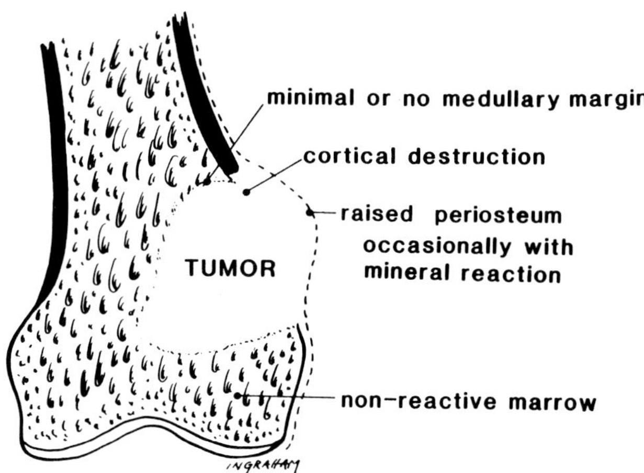

Figure 26
Stage 3 lesion.

just like a malignancy. The patient complains of progressive symptoms, usually pain, of a short duration (a few weeks at most). On the radiograph these are ominous looking lesions. There is an ill-defined border with destruction of the cortex, invasion of adjacent soft tissues, and an active periosteal reaction. This active periosteal reaction can include the type of periosteal reactions that are associated with malignant tumors, including onion skinning, hair-on-end, sunburst, and a Codman's triangle. Some giant cell tumors of bone present as stage 3 lesions, and many aneurysmal bone cysts are stage 3 lesions. The only other common example of a stage 3 lesion is a variant of osteoblastoma, sometimes called malignant osteoblastoma although the lesions do not metastasize.

The stage cannot be predicted by the histologic appearance. Usually the appearance of the lesion through the microscope is the same for stages 2 and 3, although there may be a slight increase in cellularity and mitotic figures in the stage 3 tumors.

Malignant Tumors

The staging of malignant tumors is common; there are numerous staging systems, depending on the neoplasm in question, and for some neoplasms there is more than one staging system. Most malignancies are staged using four variables: histologic grade of the tumor (G), its size or anatomic location (T), the presence of metastasis to local lymph nodes (N), and the presence of other distant metastatic foci of the disease (M). This is often referred to as the GTN&M system. For malignant neoplasms of the musculoskeletal system, the significance of metastatic disease to lymph nodes and of that to a distant organ, usually the lung, is the same; therefore, a distinction between these two types of metastasis is not necessary. Thus, the staging of musculoskeletal malignant tumors does not include separate categories for spread to a lymph node and spread to a distant organ, but instead puts both of these in the same category. Patients with a lymph node or distant organ metastasis have a poor prognosis regardless of all other variables, but for the patient with a musculoskeletal malignant tumor without clinically apparent metastatic disease, the histologic grade of the tumor is the single most important prognostic variable. The size of the tumor is important as well, but it is not as important as histologic grade; it is better to have a large low grade tumor than a small high grade one.

Histologic grade is a subjective assessment of the neoplasm using its microscopic characteristics. In all the grading systems used, tumors with a higher histologic grade have a higher incidence of metastasis. Although some grading systems use two grades, others use three and still others four.

Numerous variables are subjectively assessed, and based on their presence and degree a histologic grade is assigned to the tumor. Although the variables are agreed on, the interpretation of their degree varies among pathologists. Therefore, it is common for different pathologists to assign different grades to the same neoplasm.

The variables used to assign a histologic grade include the ratio of cells to matrix, the number of mitoses, the presence of abnormal mitoses, variation in cell size and shape (pleomorphism), the degree of differentiation of the cells, and the presence of necrosis. The more the tumor looks like its normal counterpart, the fewer mitoses, the fewer cells per visual field, the less necrosis, and the more the neoplastic cells look alike, the less likely the tumor is to metastasize and, therefore, the lower its grade. A tumor that has few mitoses, no necrosis, and little cellular variation is a grade 1 malignancy with a limited risk of metastasis (Fig. 27). The risk of distant spread would be from 10% to 25%. The higher the number of mitoses and the number of cells per field, the greater the variance in size and shape, and the more necrosis that is present, the higher the grade. Tumors with the highest grade are thought to have somewhere around an 80% risk of metastatic spread. Because histologic grading systems vary slightly depending on the histologic type, the exact risk of metastatic disease depends on the histologic type.

There are a few exceptions among musculoskeletal tumors to the rules of histologic grading. The most notable is Ewing's sarcoma. These highly malignant tumors may have areas of necrosis, but their mitotic rate is usually low and the cells are almost identical in appearance. If the usual criteria were used, Ewing's sarcoma would not be graded as high

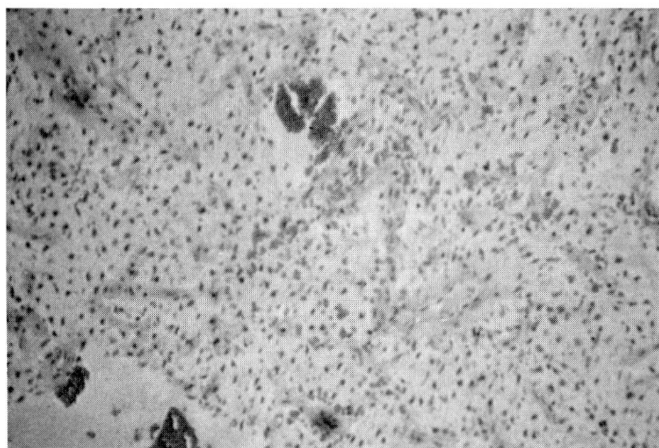

Figure 27
Low-grade sarcoma (grade 1, myxoid liposarcoma, 40X). Low-grade sarcomas have few, if any, mitoses, no necrosis, uniform cells, and recognizable matrix. This tumor has approximately a 25% risk of metastasizing.

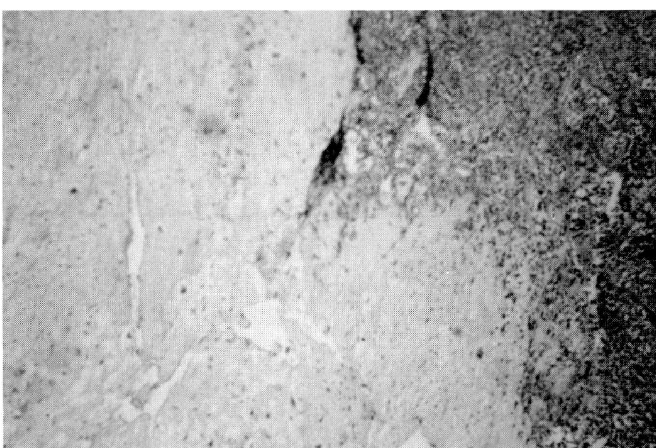

Figure 28
Chondrosarcoma (10X). This is a low power histologic view of a dedifferenIated chondrosarcoma. The tissue on the left is low-grade chondrosarcoma and the tissue on the right is high-grade spindle-cell sarcoma. It is only because of its association with the chondrosarcoma that the high-grade spindle component can be recognized as chondrosarcoma. Dedifferentiated sarcomas have an especially high incidence of metastasis.

as its natural history indicates. For this reason, Ewing's sarcoma is not graded and all are considered to be a histologically high grade. Chondrosarcoma is another musculoskeletal tumor that is graded slightly differently. Chondrosarcoma is, in general, less malignant than most musculoskeletal tumors, and the highest grade chondrosarcoma, excluding dedifferentiated chondrosarcoma, does not have the same risk of metastasis as the highest grade osteosarcoma. Grading of tumors is subjective and it is always helpful to know the pathologist and the grading system used.

In the musculoskeletal system, there is a type of tumor that is more dangerous than those with the highest grade. These higher than high grade neoplasms are said to have dedifferentiated (Fig. 28). This is seen most commonly in chondrosarcoma, and patients with one of these tumors have an especially high risk of metastasis. The histologic appearance of the neoplasm may be so undifferentiated that the only way to know its cell of origin is that a portion of the more differentiated tumor remains.

As previously mentioned, any neoplasm that has metastasized has the highest risk of taking the patient's life, regardless of all other factors. Every staging system has a separate category for the patients with metastatic disease. Depending on the number of histologic grades used, the staging system may have two major groups, three major groups, or four major groups. Within each of these histologic groups the tumors are separated again depending on size or degree of local involvement (compartment). These staging systems are accurate enough to separate tumors into groups with reasonably similar prognosis. It is important to remember, however, that these groupings are not 100% accurate, and it is not uncommon to observe a neoplasm in one stage behave more like a tumor from another stage. For example, occasionally a typical low grade parosteal osteosarcoma will metastasize and take a patient's life.

The most widely used staging system for musculoskeletal tumors is the one proposed by Enneking and associates. It is often called the Enneking system (Table 4). It is also known as the Musculoskeletal Tumor Society (MSTS) System because it was adopted by the Musculoskeletal Tumor Society.

Table 4
Enneking system

Stage	Description
Stage I	Low histologic grade A. Intracompartmental B. Extracompartmental
Stage II	High histologic grade A. Intracompartmental B. Extracompartmental
Stage III	Metastatic disease A. Intracompartmental B. Extracompartmental

The Enneking system has five major categories, and some have elected to make it six by dividing the patients with metastatic disease by compartmental location.

This is a surgical staging system and, as such, was designed for the surgeon. There are two large categories (stages) based on histologic grade, with a third stage for all patients with metastatic disease at presentation either to a lymph node or other organ. The patients are separated first by whether their neoplasm is high histologic grade or low histologic grade. The low histologic grade neoplasms are predicted to have not more than a 25% chance of metastasizing. All other tumors are considered high grade. The low grade tumors are designated as being I and the high grade are II. Within each of these two groupings, the tumors are separated based on whether they are within a single compartment (intracompartmental) designated as A or in more than one compartment (extracompartmental) designated as B. Intracompartmental tumors are almost always smaller than extracompartmental tumors, and, because this is a surgical staging system, compartments were used to groups tumors because these give the surgeon a better concept of what type of surgical resection will be needed.

The body is divided into meaningful anatomic compartments with fascial boundaries between the compartments. The fascial boundaries are barriers to growth of the neoplasms, and when a neoplasm has crossed one of these barriers, the neoplasia is thought to be more aggressive and require more aggressive treatment (Table 5).

In the article reporting the Enneking staging system, the authors suggested a nomenclature to be used to describe oncologic surgical margins. The terms proposed have improved the classification of oncologic procedures so that surgeons can communicate better. These terms have gained widespread acceptance and are used throughout the world to define all types of surgical margins. The terms refer to the relationship between the tumor with its reactive rim (pseudocapsule) and the closest resection margin made by the surgeon. The four terms are intralesional, marginal, wide, and radical (Fig. 29).

Intralesional surgical margin refers to a margin in which the surgeon operates within the lesion and removes a portion, scrapes, or curettes out the lesion from within the pseudocapsule. This operation leaves macroscopic neoplasia in the patient. An incisional biopsy is an intralesional operation, as is a curettage. This type of margin is sufficient for tumors that do not require surgical removal, such as latent benign tumors. Some active benign tumors can be controlled with an extended intralesional margin, which is a curettage that removes the tumor, pseudocapsule, and a small portion of the surrounding normal tissues.

Marginal surgical margin refers to a margin through the pseudocapsule of the tumor. If the neoplasia has infiltrated the pseudocapsule, this margin will leave microscopic foci of tumor in the patient. Latent and most active benign lesions usually do not infiltrate their pseudocapsule; therefore, a marginal margin is adequate for these types of tumors. However, all aggressive benign and malignant tumors require more than a marginal margin. A tumor shelled out is removed with a marginal margin.

Wide surgical margin is the margin obtained when the lesion, its pseudocapsule, and a portion of normal surrounding tissue are removed as a single

Table 5
Surgical sites (T)

Intracompartmental (T_1)	Extracompartmental (T_2)
Intraosseous	Soft-tissue extension
Intra-articular	Soft-tissue extension
Superficial to deep fascia	Deep fascial extension
Paraosseous	Intraosseous or extrafascial
Intrafascial compartments	Extrafascial planes or spaces
Ray of hand or foot	Midfoot and hindfoot
Posterior calf	Popliteal space
Anterolateral leg	Groin—femoral triangle
Anterolateral thigh	Intrapelvic
Medial thigh	Midhand
Posterior thigh	Antecubital fossae
Buttocks	Axilla
Volar forearm	Periclavicular
Dorsal forearm	Paraspinal
Anterior arm	Head and neck
Posterior arm	
Periscapular	

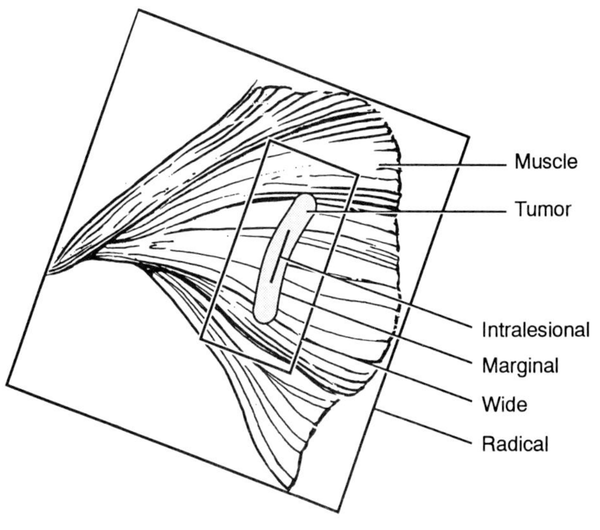

Figure 29
Oncologic surgical margins.

specimen. This is often called an en bloc resection. The thickness of the normal tissue required for the margin to be classified as wide is not specified and can be extremely thin, even a few millimeters, if the surgeon is sure that there is normal tissue beyond the pseudocapsule. In practice, it is safer to have one or more centimeters of normal tissue surrounding a tumor that requires a wide surgical margin. This margin removes all of the neoplastic tissue including those cells that have infiltrated the pseudocapsule, the so-called satellite lesions. This is an adequate surgical margin for almost all nonrecurrent neoplasia, including the most malignant. Recurrent tumors almost always have such poorly defined margins that they require a greater surgical margin to insure a complete resection.

Radical surgical margin is obtained when the tumor is removed with the entire compartment or compartments that are involved by the tumor. This margin was once thought to be necessary for the highest grade malignant tumors because of the finding of nodules of malignant cells beyond the confines of the pseudocapsule. These nodules are called skip lesions and were initially thought to be a reflection of a locally aggressive tumor. However, these nodules are better thought of as metastasis, and they have the same significance as a metastasis. Recurrent malignant tumor that is to be treated with surgery alone should usually be treated with radical surgical margin.

In 1977 the American Joint Commission on Staging and End Results Studies (AJC) developed a staging system for soft-tissue sarcomas, but were unable to do the same for sarcomas of bone. The soft-tissue sarcoma staging system was revised in 1988 (Table 6). This staging system uses the traditional GTN&M system. In the AJC staging system, there are three histologic grades—G1, G2, and G3. The tumors are separated with regard to size between those that are five centimeters in diameter or less, T1, and those that are larger, T2. The presence of lymph node involvement and distant metastasis are indicated with an N0 or N1 and an M0 or M1, respectively.

This staging system has four major groupings with two subdivisions in each group. Because the most important prognostic factor for all tumors that are not already metastatic is their histologic grade, that is the determinant of the primary grouping. Size is the other major prognostic factor, and it is, therefore, the determinant of a subdivision for each histologic grade. For those patients that have a metastasis at their initial presentation, a fourth category is provided.

Table 6
AJC staging system

Stage	Description
1A - G1, T1, N0, M0	low grade, 5 cm or less, no lymph node or distant metastasis
1B - G1, T2, N0, M0	low grade, larger than 5 cm, no lymph node or distant metastasis
2A - G2, T1, N0, M0	medium grade, 5 cm or less, no lymph node or distant metastasis
2B - G2, T2, N0, M0	medium grade, larger than 5 cm, no lymph node or distant metastasis
3A - G3, T1, N0, M0	high grade, 5 cm or less, no lymph node or distant metastasis
3B - G3, T2, N0, M0	high grade, larger than 5 cm, no lymph node or distant metastasis
4A - Gany, Tany, N1, M0	any grade, any size, with lymph node metastasis but no distant metastasis
4B - Gany, Tany, Nany, M1	any grade, any size with or without lymph node metastasis, but with distant metastasis

Flow Cytometry and Cytofluorometry

Although histologic grade is currently the single most prognostic factor available, it is too subjective and not sufficiently accurate. There are many patients with high-grade sarcomas who do not develop metastasis and some with low-grade sarcomas who do. This may be a reflection of the lack of quantification of histologic grading or, more likely, a reflection of the lack of correlation between histologic appearance and ability to spread to a distant site. The desire to have better predictors of the ability of a neoplasia to develop metastasis has stimulated a search for indicators or markers of this ability. DNA content of tumor cells may be such a marker. Flow cytometry and cytofluorometry are currently being used to measure DNA content of tumor cells but, as yet, it is not known if they are predictive.

Flow cytometry and cytofluorometry are methods by which the amount of DNA in cells is quantified. The theoretical basis to use these tools to predict the degree of malignancy is that the more normal the amount of DNA, the more normal the cell and vice versa. In some neoplasia (breast, colon) these methods have shown promise but so far they have had limited usefulness in musculoskeletal neoplasia. Additional work is being done, and many aspects of these techniques need to be examined.

In flow cytometry thousands of cell nuclei, usually normal and neoplastic together, are passed through the machine and every cell's DNA is measured; in cytofluorometry, each cell is examined under the microscope and only those that are neoplastic have their DNA measured. The two methods provide similar information, but cytofluorometry has the advantage of allowing direct observation of each cell measured. Both techniques use a DNA-specific fluorescent dye (propidium iodide or ethidium bromide) as a marker of the DNA content and measure the emitted fluorescent signal when the nucleus is exposed to light in the excitation spectrum for that dye. The intensity of the emitted signal is directly related to the amount of DNA present in the nucleus, and the amount of DNA may be an indication of the degree of alteration in the cell's genetic information as it relates to cell replication, but not necessarily to function.

The amount of DNA in the nucleus of a cell varies throughout the cell cycle in a defined manner. By convention, the amount of DNA in an ovum and sperm is called haploid or C. A normal resting cell in G0 phase of the cell cycle will have twice that amount, referred to as diploid or 2C. As the cell increases its DNA in preparation for division and is in S phase, the amount of DNA increases; then, when the cell is ready to divide in G2 and M phases, it will have twice the normal amount of DNA, referred to as tetraploid or 4C. Any concentration of DNA in a cell that does not fit this pattern is pathologic. Most cells are in G0 or G1 phase, and the DNA histogram (obtained with flow cytometry or cytofluorometry) is a peak of cells with 2C amount of DNA. There are always some cells in the process of dividing, so some will have twice the amount of DNA or 4C. Fewer cells will be in S phase and have an amount between 2C and 4C. When the normal distribution of DNA content of a group of cells is measured and plotted on a graph, a pattern is produced with a large peak at the 2C position, a smaller peak at the 4C position, and an even smaller number of cells between these two peaks (Fig. 30, *left*). This distribution pattern of DNA/cell in a group of normal cells is called a diploid or euploid pattern. When there are more than the normal number of cells in G2 or M phase (more than 15%), the peak at the tetraploid position will be abnormally large (Fig. 30, *center*). This is called a euploid-polyploid pattern and is considered pathologic. When there are abnormal cells, their concentration of DNA may be abnormal and they will produce an abnormal peak on the graph, which is not at the 2C or 4C position (Fig. 30, *right*). This pattern is called aneuploid and is considered an indicator of malignancy.

Examination of benign and malignant tumors of the musculoskeletal system has shown that the ploidy or pattern of the tumor's DNA content is only a relative indicator of its ability to metastasize. Benign tumors have a normal (diploid) DNA pattern, or, occasionally, a euploid-polyploid pattern. Sarcomas may display all three patterns and, to date, there has been no clear correlation between ploidy and degree of malignancy. This may be related to how well the quantitative increase in DNA reflects the qualitative change in the function of the oncogenes, which in benign tumors may not be high. Recent data suggest that ploidy is predictive for osteosarcoma and chondrosarcoma.

Cytofluorometry offers additional insight into a cell's behavior. After the cells have been stained and as the fluorescent light is passed through them, the cells are examined with a microscope and the signal measured as each cell is observed. This limits the cells whose DNA is measured to those cells specifically selected rather than measuring the DNA content of all the cells in a suspension as is done with flow cytometry. In addition and probably more importantly, any manipulation of cells can be directly observed, and it is possible to confirm which cells have been affected. Quantitative assessment of abnormal DNA here is only as good as the fluoro-

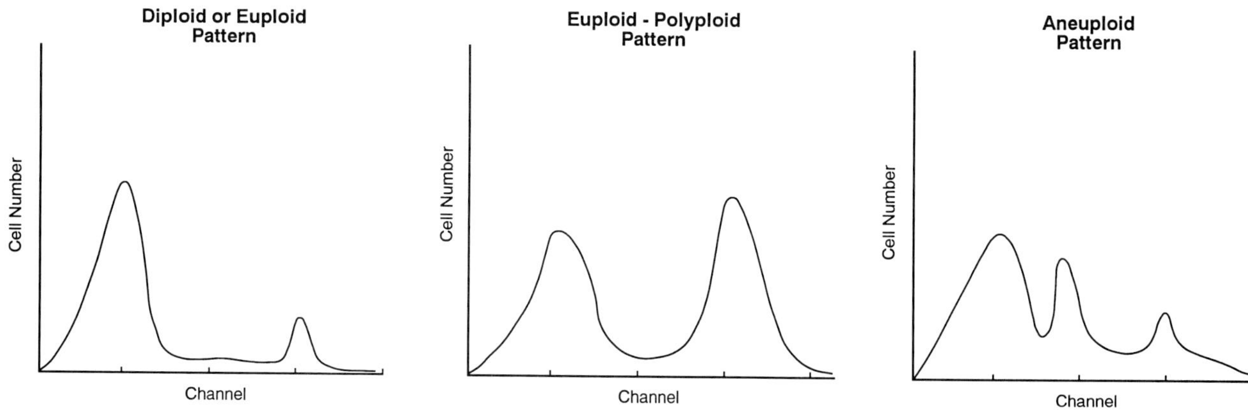

Figure 30
DNA histograms showing diploid or euploid pattern (**left**), euploid-polyploid pattern (**center**), and aneuploid pattern (**right**).

chrome dyes available to detect these abnormalities. This may also offer the opportunity to discover more about how the cells work.

A fluorochrome can be tagged to a protein or other substance; this fluorochrome can then be observed as it acts with the cell in question. An example of this technique is the examination of the p-glycoprotein previously mentioned. To determine whether a specific cell has p-glycoprotein in its cell wall, a monoclonal antibody is made to p-glycoprotein, a fluorochrome is attached to the antibody, and the fluorochrome-antibody molecule is mixed with the cells. The cells are then examined using cytofluorometry, and the amount of the fluorochrome in the cells is measured. Because the fluorochrome-antibody attaches to p-glycoprotein, the amount of fluorochrome is directly related to the amount of p-glycoprotein. There is no limitation to the examinations that can be done.

One of the more interesting examinations done using cytofluorometry is testing a neoplastic cell's ability to handle doxorubicin hydrochloride, a chemotherapeutic agent used to treat patients with a variety of sarcomas. Doxorubicin hydrochloride is a natural fluorochrome, and it can be seen when examined under ultraviolet light. When living neoplastic cells are exposed to doxorubicin hydrochloride, the doxorubicin enters the cells passively and is then pumped out of the cell, probably through the p-glycoprotein pump. The more efficient the cell is at eliminating the doxorubicin hydrochloride, the less likely it will be damaged by the drug. The intracellular concentration of doxorubicin hydrochloride can be measured using the cytofluorometer and the sensitivity of the cell to the drug determined. Further work in this area may provide a means of selecting the most effective chemotherapeutic agent for each neoplasm.

Additional means of predicting a tumor's ability to metastasize are needed, because current methods may still be considered crude and need improvement. Based on the principles described in this chapter, there should be a means of accurately determining if a specific neoplasm is able to spread to a distant site. Considerable research is being done to find new techniques.

Immunobiology

The immune system is a complex interaction of cells and their molecular products for the purposes of defense against foreign substances, homeostasis of endogenous cellular activity (removal of dead, damaged, or altered cells), and surveillance against mutations or malignant transformation. Infection, transplantation, oncology, and autoimmunity, including rheumatoid arthritis, are topics in immunobiology of particular relevance to orthopaedics. There is also growing evidence that immunocompetent cells are responsible for the production of cytokines, messengers, and other factors that control or participate in bone remodeling.

The immune system is capable of initiating two broad categories of response. The nonspecific immune response, or inflammatory reaction, begins when an antigen is recognized as foreign and is followed by a relatively homogenous and predictable sequence of events. The specific immune response involves not only recognizing an antigen as foreign, but also considerable heterogeneity of cellular and humoral activity and memory for specific antigens. The latter results in a more rapid and increasingly vigorous response to that same stimulus on reexposure.

The Nonspecific Immune (Inflammatory) Response

The inflammatory reaction to physical injury, such as fracture, soft tissue trauma, or a foreign body, or to a chemical stimulus begins with the release of histamine. Histamine causes a local increase in blood flow and vascular permeability, resulting in an exudate and infiltrate of phagocytic cells that phagocytize and enzymatically digest offending materials. The efficiency of this inflammatory reaction may be enhanced by factors associated with activation of the complement system or abrogated by antiinflammatory drugs including aspirin, steroids, and nonsteroidal antiinflammatory agents.

The Specific Immune Response

The specific immune response has traditionally been divided into its cell-mediated and humoral components. Macrophages, B lymphocytes, and T lymphocytes contribute to the initiation and generation of humoral and cell-mediated immunity. All of these are of bone marrow origin (Fig. 31).

Antigens

Antigens are capable of evoking an immune response and specifically reacting with the humoral or cellular products of that response. The most potent antigens are large, complex molecules, such as proteins and polysaccharides; lipids and low-molecular-weight substances tend to be weakly immunogenic. There is generally a selective portion of the antigenic molecule, termed its reactive site or antigenic determinant, that is responsible for the antigen's ability to evoke a response.

Macrophages

Macrophages process antigen, rendering it capable of stimulating other immunocompetent cells (lymphocytes). Macrophages also elaborate media-

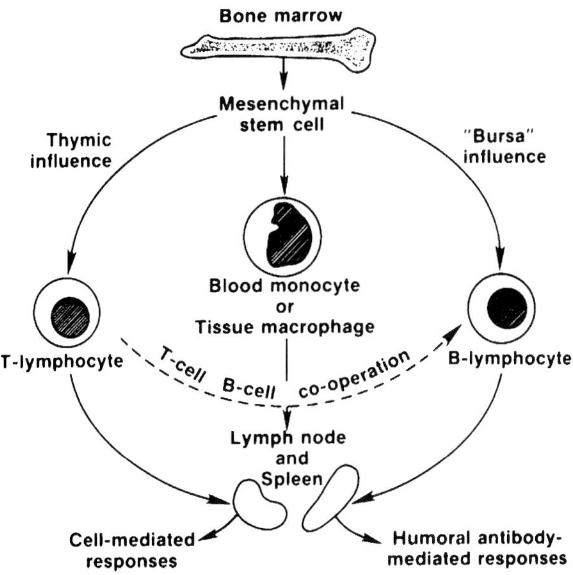

Figure 31
Primitive mesenchymal cells residing in the bone marrow differentiate into T lymphocytes, B lymphocytes, and macrophages. These cells populate the primary lymphoid structures, lymph nodes, and the spleen and cooperate in producing cell-mediated and humoral responses. (Reproduced with permission from Friedlaender GE: Immunology, in Albright JA, Brand RA (eds): *The Scientific Basis of Orthopaedics,* ed 2. Norwalk, CT, Appleton & Lange, 1987, p 484.)

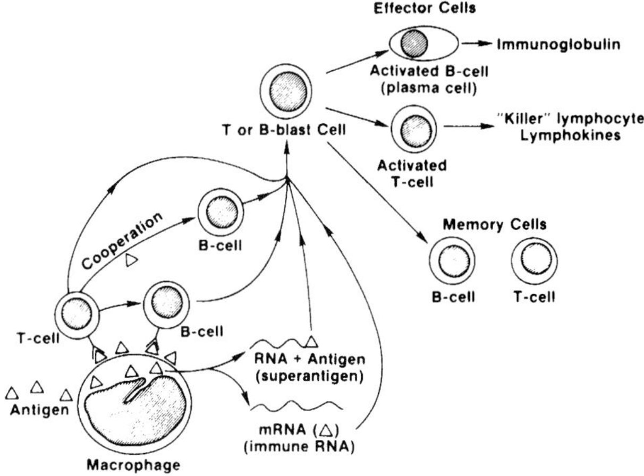

Figure 32
Antigen processing by macrophages. (Reproduced with permission from Friedlaender GE: Immunology, in Albright JA, Brand RA (eds): *The Scientific Basis of Orthopaedics,* ed 2. Norwalk, CT, Appleton & Lange, 1987, p 491.)

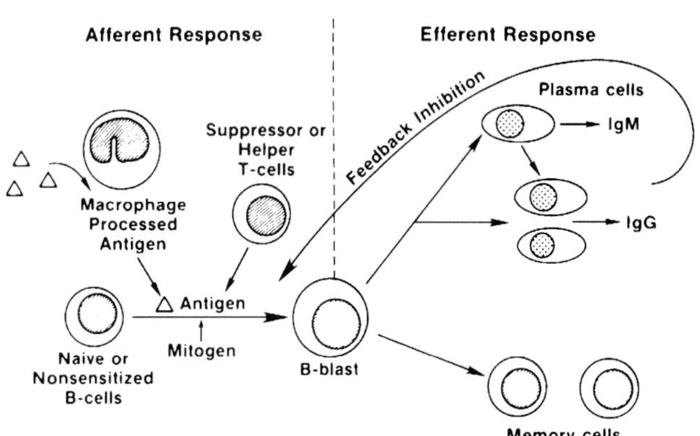

Figure 33
The humoral antibody response; activation of B cells and immunoglobin production. (Reproduced with permission from Friedlaender GE: Immunology, in Albright JA, Brand RA (eds): *The Scientific Basis of Orthopaedics,* ed 2. Norwalk, CT, Appleton & Lange, 1987, p 492.)

tors that influence other cells and may themselves function as effector cells (Fig. 32).

B Lymphocytes

The B lymphocytes (B cells) are named for the bursa of Fabricius, an organ in the chicken first discovered to influence their functional evolution. When stimulated, B lymphoblasts enlarge and differentiate into plasma cells, and they produce a specific class of immunoglobulins (Ig antibodies) directed against a specific antigen (Fig. 33). Furthermore, subsets of activated B lymphocytes develop memory for the initiating antigen and persist in anticipation of rechallenge by that same antigen. Although they are morphologically indistinguishable from T lymphocytes by routine light microscopy, B lymphocytes can be identified by the presence of immunoglobulins, the alloantigens of the major histocompatibility complex (HLA system in humans), and a variety of other receptor sites and markers on the cell-surface membrane.

Immunoglobulins

Immunoglobulins, or antibodies, are the products of B-cell (plasma cell) activation. The basic structure of these molecules includes two identical light and two identical heavy chains that are held together by disulfide bonds in a Y-configuration (Fig. 34). Within each chain are constant portions (sequences of amino acids) and variable regions, the latter containing the antigen binding site that is responsible for the diversity and specificity of antibody molecules.

Five classes of immunoglobulins have been described, each with distinct categories of function. The most common immunoglobulin, IgG, is a 150,000 molecular-weight-monomer of the basic molecule (Fig. 35). It can cross the placenta, thereby providing early protection for the fetus and neonate,

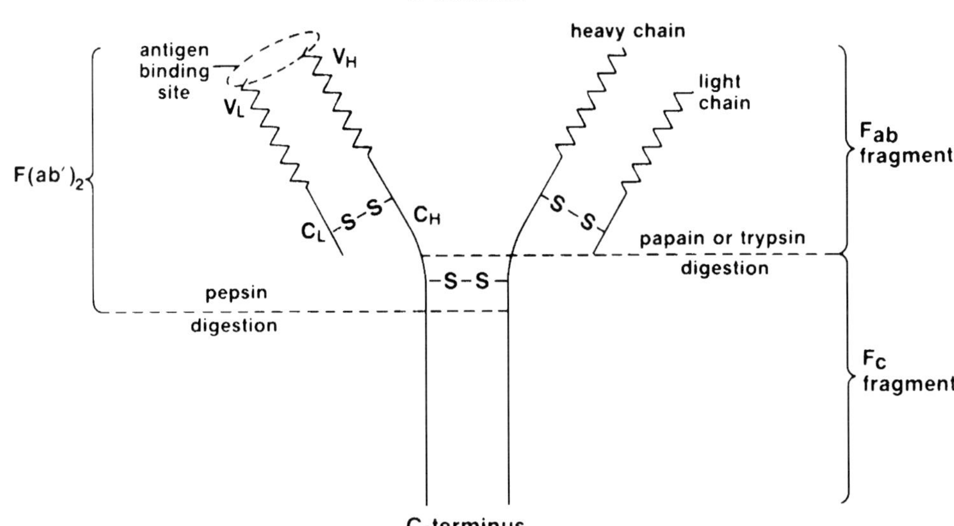

Figure 34
The basic subunit structure of the immunoglobulin molecule. (Reproduced with permission from Friedlaender GE: Immunology, in Albright JA, Brand RA (eds): *The Scientific Basis of Orthopaedics,* ed 2. Norwalk, CT, Appleton & Lange, 1987, p 486.)

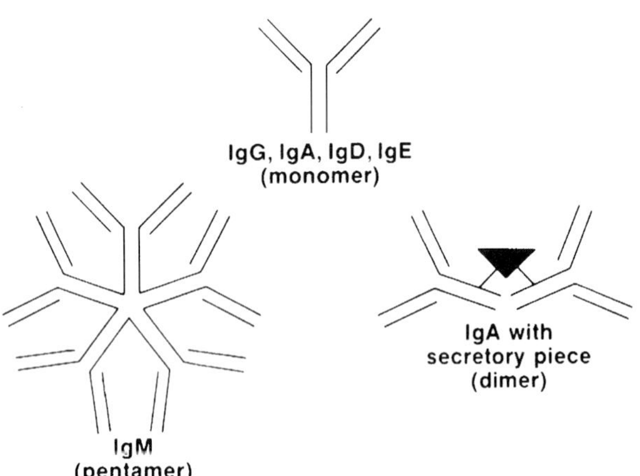

Figure 35
Structural configurations of basic immunoglobulin subunits. (Reproduced with permission from Friedlaender GE: Immunology, in Albright JA, Brand RA (eds): *The Scientific Basis of Orthopaedics,* ed 2. Norwalk, CT, Appleton & Lange, 1987, p 487.)

it fixes complement, and it occurs in response to most infectious organisms. IgM is a pentamer with a molecular weight of 750,000. It is incapable of crossing the placenta, but is the first immunoglobulin produced by the fetus and the first to appear following B-lymphoblast stimulation. IgA, often a dimer with an associated secretory piece, is found predominantly on mucosal surfaces; it possesses antimicrobial activity. IgE, or reagin, is primarily a mediator of hypersensitivity (allergic) responses. IgD, the least well-characterized immunoglobulin, apparently serves as a receptor molecule on the surface membranes of lymphocytes.

While plasma cells may produce more than one class of immunoglobulin over time or contain more than one type of immunoglobulin surface membrane marker, the cell manufactures only a single class, or specific molecule, at a time. The specificity of immunoglobulin production by normal, activated B lymphocytes has been combined with the immortality of myeloma cells in vitro to form hybridomas capable of producing large quantities of pure monoclonal antibody. In a potentially tedious, but highly rewarding manner, spleen cells (lymphocytes) from animals challenged with crude or heterogeneous antigen sources can be combined with myeloma cells to develop a spectrum of monoclonal antibodies that must then be tested for their specificity. These purified immunoglobulins have proven to be very valuable research tools, assay reagents, and potentially efficacious therapeutic agents.

T Lymphocytes

T lymphocytes (T cells) originate in the bone marrow and mature in the thymus. When appropriately stimulated, T cells may produce cytokines that influence themselves and other cells (Fig. 36). T cells can be placed in subsets according to function and distinguished by cell-surface marker (for example, CD4, CD8). $CD8^+$ cells are either "killer" cells that can directly lyse appropriate antigen-bearing target cells or suppressor cells that inhibit either antibody synthesis or other T cell responses (Fig. 33). Indeed, this suppressor activity may be responsible for the persistence of tolerance, the inactivity of the immune system to some exogenous (foreign) antigens,

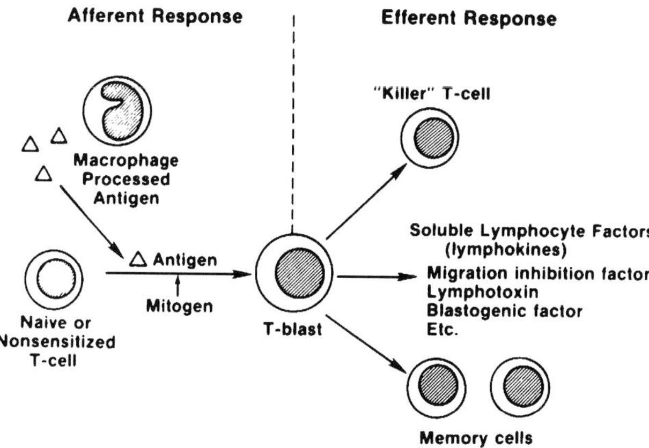

Figure 36

The cell-mediated immune response. (Reproduced with permission from Friedlaender GE: Immunology, in Albright JA, Brand RA (eds): *The Scientific Basis of Orthopaedics,* ed 2. Norwalk, CT, Appleton & Lange, 1987, p 493.)

or the definition of the nature of self versus nonself as the fetus matures and establishes its molecular identity. $CD4^+$ cells are helper T cells that play an important role in generating $CD8^+$ cells as well as facilitating B cell responses, including the production of immunoglobulin (Fig. 33). Both of these subsets can form memory cells that respond in an accelerated fashion when they encounter the same antigen a second time.

Cytokines

Cytokines are soluble proteins or glycoprotein molecules secreted by a variety of cells in response to a challenge by a foreign antigen or other stimulant. They are primarily involved in regulating immune and inflammatory responses, but can also be responsible for tissue injury in response to some infections and autoimmune diseases. They have been grouped into a variety of functional categories including interferons, growth factors, and colony-stimulating factors (CSF), as well as interleukins. The CSFs promote the growth and differentiation of bone marrow progenitor cells. Interleukins were so named because they were originally considered to be produced by leukocytes and to communicate regulatory signals to other such cells. It is now known that T cells produce cytokines other than interleukins, that they are not the only cells that produce interleukins, and that the function of interleukins includes regulating the growth and differentiation of leukocytes and promoting hematopoiesis. There are at least 13 types of interleukins. Many of these cytokines play important roles in the bone remodeling cycle, including bone homeostasis, fracture repair, and graft incorporation.

The Complement System

The complement system is a group of 20 plasma and five cell membrane proteins that work in a cascading sequence to amplify various phases or manifestations of the immune response and to interface with other organized systems of the body such as the coagulation system (Fig. 37). Immune complexes composed of antigens and immunoglobulins, particularly IgG and IgM classes, when bound to cell membranes, have the ability to "fix" and activate the C1 component of the complement system and the entire pathway. Sequential events lead to a new complex, membrane damage, and a variety of other inflammatory events. These result from other complexes and increase vascular permeability, enhance phagocytosis, act as chemotactic molecules, or cause membranolysis of target cells. Consequently, this system represents an important immunologic effector mechanism.

Immunogenetics

Human leukocyte antigen (HLA) molecules are the essential and central molecular contributors to the specificity of immune recognition. The HLA genes located on the short arm of chromosome 6 govern the production of these antigens and compose the major histocompatibility complex (MHC) in humans. At one end of this complex are at least six loci encoding for proteins known as class I histocompatibility antigens. These include the loci for the transcription of HLA-A, B, and C proteins, the three classically considered major histocompatibility barriers to allogeneic transplantation. Each locus is highly polymorphic, with more than 80 variants described for HLA-A and B. HLA-E, F, and G are also located here. At the other end of the HLA region lie approximately 14 loci labeled HLA class II genes; these encode either for α polypeptides or for β polypeptides. These loci, together considered the D region, may be considered to be divided into three major subregions known as DR, DQ, and DP. Between the class I and class II regions lie a cluster of genes encoding complement components C2, C4, and Bf.

Tolerance and Autoimmunity

The immune system is under genetic control and is governed by a limited set of genes. These genes vary among different individuals and are a key element in allowing the immune system to discriminate self from nonself. Tolerance is the lack of reactivity to antigen, whether endogenous (self) or exogenous. Once thought to represent an unresponsiveness learned by the immune system after exposure to antigens during fetal development, it is now clear that tolerance is a more dynamic state, prob-

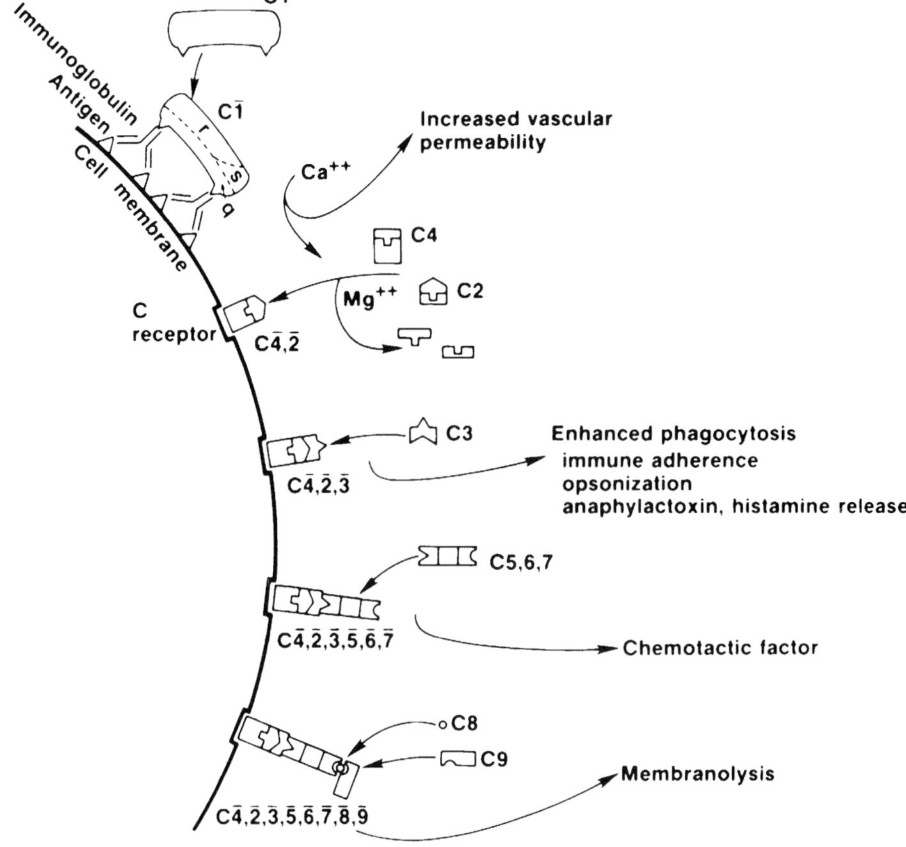

Figure 37
Complement cascade. (Reproduced with permission from Friedlaender GE: Immunology, in Albright JA, Brand RA (eds): *The Scientific Basis of Orthopaedics,* ed 2. Norwalk, CT, Appleton & Lange, 1987, p 491.)

ably perpetuated by the presence of suppressor T cells. Consequently, if these suppressor mechanisms are deleted, previously nonantigenic molecules will elicit a reaction. When this process occurs with antigens intrinsic to the host, the response is termed autoimmunity. In the autoimmune disorders, variation among genes in different individuals is a prime determinant of disease susceptibility. Developmental and environmental factors act in concert with this immunogenetic contribution to trigger the disease process. Examples include systemic lupus erythematosus, ankylosing spondylitis, psoriatic arthritis, and Sjögren's syndrome. Table 7 illustrates the distribution of the gene variant found in patients who have these diseases as compared to the normal population. Hashimoto's thyroiditis and rheumatoid arthritis are also often considered autoimmune disorders. An earlier suggested scenario for the production of an autoimmune response was the release of a previously sequestered or recently altered self molecule. It is most likely, however, that autoimmune diseases represent an alteration in the normal balance between induction and suppression mechanisms of immunologic control.

Transplantation

Intraspecies tissue transplantation in genetically nonidentical members is called allogeneic grafting (previously called homogeneic). Tissues transplanted across species are called xenografts (formerly called heterografts). Immunoglobulin and cellular immune responses can be detected following transplantation of fresh allogeneic or xenogeneic bone. These responses are directed most notably against those cell surface glycoproteins determined by the MHC or histocompatibility antigens (HLA). Such responses are diminished if the graft is frozen prior to implantation and nearly undetectable if the tissue has been freeze-dried (lyophilized). Even where a detectable immune response occurs, the biologic and clinical fates of bone allografts have been remarkably good, albeit with room for improvement. This fact suggests that the immune response plays an important but perhaps not crucial role in allograft incorporation.

Oncology

Malignant cells may possess unique cell-surface antigens that have escaped the surveillance func-

Table 7
Associations between human leukocyte antigen alleles and susceptibility to some rheumatic diseases

Disease	HLA Marker	Frequency (%) in Patients (Whites)	Frequency (%) in Controls (Whites)	Relative Risk
Ankylosing spondylitis	B27	90	9	87
Reiter's syndrome	B27	79	9	37
Psoriatic arthritis	B27	48	9	10
Inflammatory bowel disease with spondylitis	B27	52	9	10
Adult rheumatoid arthritis	DR4	70	30	6
Polyarticular juvenile rheumatoid arthritis	DR4	75	30	7
Pauciarticular juvenile rheumatoid arthritis	DR8	30	5	5
	DR5	50	20	4.5
	DR2.1	55	20	4
Systemic lupus erythematosus	DR2	46	22	3.5
	DR3	50	25	3
Sjögren's syndrome	DR3	70	25	6

(Reproduced with permission from Nepom BS, Nepom GT: Immunogenetics and the rheumatic diseases, in McCarty DJ (ed): *Arthritis and Allied Conditions: A Textbook of Rheumatology*, ed 10. Philadelphia, Lea & Febiger, 1985, p 99.)

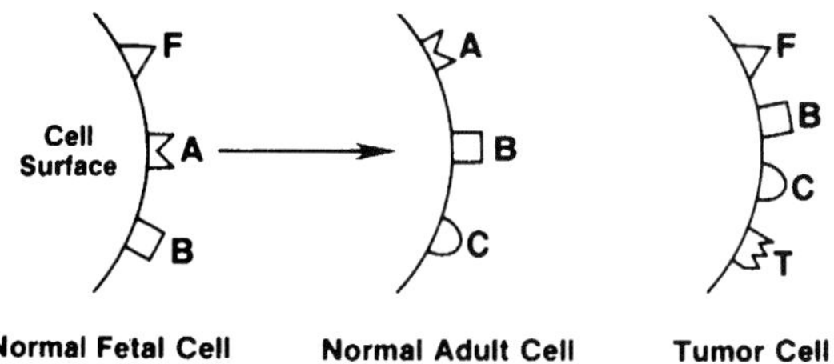

Figure 38
Tumor cells have cell-surface antigens common to other normal cells, which reflect the tissue of origin (B,C). They may also demonstrate antigens normally only present on fetal cells (F) and loose antigens common to the cell type of origin (A); they certainly acquire new tumor-associated antigens (T). (Reproduced with permission from Friedlaender GE: Immunology, in Albright JA, Brand RA (eds): *The Scientific Basis of Orthopaedics*, ed 2, Norwalk, CT, Appleton & Lange, 1987, p 502.)

tion of an individual's immune system (Fig. 38). These proteins, however, may still be detectable by immunologic techniques (including tumor markers of diagnostic and prognostic significance, such as prostate-specific antigen) and be available for targeted delivery of antibody-coupled therapeutic agents (drugs, isotopes). Tumor immunobiology has remained extremely complex, reflecting tumor cell heterogeneity and the technical difficulties of developing specific reagents, including monoclonal antibodies to these antigens. As such, it represents a fertile and worthwhile area for continued investigation.

Inflammatory and Autoimmune Diseases

Rheumatoid Arthritis

Rheumatoid arthritis (RA) is an example of a clinical disease that is felt to be secondary to pathology within the immunobiologic processes, demonstrating features of both specific inflammatory processes. Clinical, radiographic, and some histologic findings are similar to those found in patients who have one of the other common inflammatory arthritides. RA, however, is the most common of the inflammatory arthritides. It affects about 1% of the population worldwide, with a ratio of three women to one man. Adult RA is typically a symmetric polyarthritis, which involves the small joints before large joints, and the patient usually has serum rheumatoid factors. The frequency of the disease increases from the third decade on, reaching 5% or more of the population aged 70 years and above.

Studies of the class II gene products (HLA-DR, HLA-DQ, and HLA-DP) of the major histocompatibility complex provide convincing evidence that there is a genetic predisposition for the disease. Susceptibility to a number of diseases, including RA, seems to be determined by these D-region immune response genes. In patients who have seropositive RA, the primary susceptibility haplotype in most ethnic groups is HLA-DR4. Although the relative risk of developing RA is several times greater in DR4 individuals, only a minority of them are affected. Because class II molecules are involved in antigen presentation to T lymphocytes, it is hoped that further analysis of these molecules will lead to an identification of the infectious or chemical agents responsible for RA.

Pathogenesis

The earliest events in RA are difficult to document; however, available evidence suggests that microvascular injury and mild synovial cell proliferation are the first lesions. Only mild perivascular lymphocytes are found in synovial biopsies from patients seen in the initial phase of RA. Polymorphonuclear leukocytes (PMNs) are seen in the superficial synovium; plasma cells are rarely seen. The small blood vessels are obliterated by inflammatory cells and organized thrombi. Electron-microscopic examination discloses the presence of gaps between vascular endothelial cells and of cell injury. These microvascular changes suggest that the etiologic factor may be carried to the joint by the circulation.

As the disease progresses, a chronic synovitis ensues. Light-microscopic examination discloses a number of histologic changes (Fig. 39). These include hyperplastic synovial lining cells layered to a depth of six to ten cells, venous distention resulting from swollen endothelial cells, and capillary obstruction. In addition, walls of venules and arterioles are infiltrated with neutrophils, areas of thrombosis and perivascular hemorrhage are seen, and the synovium is filled with mononuclear cells. Chronic inflammatory cells are seen only occasionally in the later stages of the disease, and many have the HLA antigens on their surface, which is a measure of activation. Although plasma cells and B lymphocytes are few in number, the rheumatoid synovium makes and contains large amounts of immunoglobulin. Immunofluorescent analysis of the plasma cells located in the subsynovium shows IgG to be the predominant class of cytoplasmic immunoglobulin, occurring in 30% to 60% of cells; IgM, occurring in 10% to 30% of cells, is less common. Excessive production of synovial immunoglobulin might be secondary to B-cell hyperactivity caused by a polyclonal B-cell activator, or B cells may be driven by unrestrained T-helper-inducer cells, or a lack of suppressor T-cells could account for the unbridled antibody production.

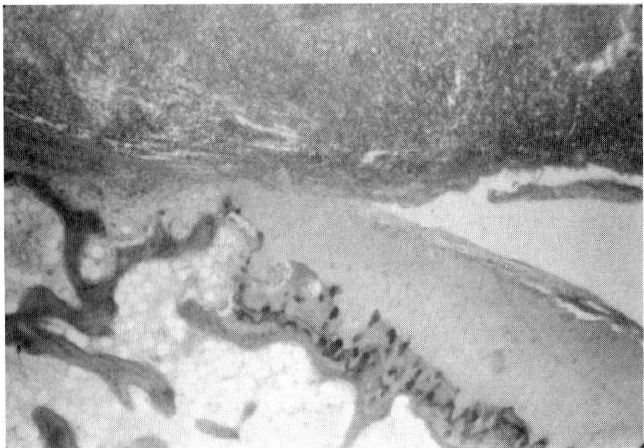

Figure 39
Photomicrograph showing rheumatoid arthritis.

Rheumatoid factors are autoantibodies that are specific for antigenic determination in the C-γ2 and C-γ3 homology regions of the Fc fragment of human IgG. This molecule is a detectable marker of the disease and a participant in the development of immune complexes that activate the complement system. Rheumatoid factors in RA serum also cross-react with IgG from other species. The usual clinical tests for rheumatoid factor are agglutination procedures that use either sheep red blood cells sensitized with rabbit anti-sheep cell antibodies or inert latex or bentonite particles that have human IgG absorbed onto their surface. The latex agglutination or bentonite flocculation tests are commonly used in clinical practice. These systems detect primarily 19S IgM rheumatoid factors. More sensitive and specific immunoassays can demonstrate antigamma globulins (rheumatoid factors of the IgG, IgA, and IgE classes) in a large percentage of rheumatoid sera, and occasionally even in the absence of IgM rheumatoid factor.

Standard flocculation tests detect IgM rheumatoid factors in the serum of approximately three fourths of adult patients who have RA, primarily those with the HLA-DR4 haplotype. A positive test is by no means diagnostic of this disorder, because rheumatoid factors are also found in 1% to 5% of normal subjects. The incidence increases with advancing age and in a variety of disease states. RA patients usually have rheumatoid factor in higher concentrations than normal subjects or those with nonrheumatologic disease. The exact biologic role of rheumatoid factors is unknown. Under certain circumstances, these factors can protect the host by enhancing the clearance of immune complexes from the bloodstream. In other circumstances, rheumatoid factors can augment the inflammatory response by increasing complement fixation, altering properties such as size or solubility of the immune complexes, or making the immune complexes more susceptible to ingestion by phagocytic cells. These characteristics are probably important in synovial tissues and fluids.

The cells present in typical rheumatoid joint effusion differ from those in the synovial membrane. The joint fluid usually has a decreased viscosity; approximately 20,000 white cells per cc, of which 75% are polymorphonuclear forms; rare red blood cells; and no crystals or bacteria. Mononuclear cells, although present with surface characteristics similar to their counterparts in the synovium, are in the minority. The effusions have less hemolytic complement than serum from the same patients and show evidence of activation of both the classic and alternate pathways. Complement components and biologically active fragments of the complement sequence, anaphylotoxins (C5A and C3A), and chemotactic factors, have been identified in synovial fluid immune complex levels. The dominant immune complexes contain anti-IgGs of both the IgM (conventional rheumatoid factor) and IgG classes.

Although the inciting factors in RA remain undefined, the mechanisms leading to chronic joint inflammation have been defined to some extent. The important interaction is between macrophage-type cells and T lymphocytes. These cells, acting with B cells, cause local production of antibody. Immune complexes formed within the joint activate the complement. These complexes then are phagocytized by PMNs and the macrophage-like cells in the synovial tissues, resulting in the release of a variety of mediators and giving rise to inflammation. Leukocytes adherent to cartilage can degrade proteoglycan and collagen in their attempts to eliminate the sequestered immune complexes. Simultaneously, the macrophages and T cells communicate with dendritic cells in the synovial lining through soluble substances to stimulate the release of molecules capable of causing bone and cartilage erosion. The erosion results in the characteristic rheumatoid deformities and functional disability. How the synovial cells are stimulated and by what are not completely defined, but stimulators probably include IL-1, fibroblast activating factor, prostaglandins, and PDGF. The reactive synovium and enzymes released from the damaged synovial cells and PMNs damage the articular cartilage. The released proteases break down the collagen fragments. These fragments are then further broken down by other proteolytic enzymes, resulting in the destruction of articular cartilage not covered by the pannus of synovium.

Extra-articular Manifestations

Although characteristically a joint disease, RA can affect a number of other tissues. Low grade fever, mild lymphadenopathy, anorexia, muscle atrophy, and weight loss are all evidence of the systemic nature of the disease. Subcutaneous nodules occur at some time in over 20% of RA patients and almost always are associated with the rheumatoid factor in the blood. On histologic examination, the nodules show a core of degenerating connective tissue surrounded by a palisade of epithelial cells and chronic inflammatory cells. Nodules usually appear in areas subjected to mechanical pressure, especially the olecranon, the extensor surfaces of the forearms, the Achilles tendon, and periarticular structures. Unusual locations include the pleura, meninges, back of the head, pinna of the ears, and bridge of the nose. The nodules, which are not tender, are firm oval or round masses in the subcutaneous or deeper tissues.

A spectrum of vascular lesions accompanies RA. Inflamed capillaries and small venules participate in the development of both rheumatoid nodules and synovitis. Other lesions include a bland intimal proliferation commonly affecting digital and mesenteric vessels; subacute lesions of arterioles and venules; and, occasionally, a widespread necrotizing arteritis of small and medium sized arteries, which may be indistinguishable from polyarteritis nodosa. This form of rheumatoid vasculitis characteristically produces polyneuropathy, skin necrosis and ulceration, digital gangrene, perforation of the nasal septum, and visceral infarction. The prognosis for this fulminant vasculitis was exceedingly poor before the advent of immunosuppressive (cyclophosphamide) treatment. Circulating immune complexes are implicated in the pathogenesis of most vascular lesions. Involvement of viscera, such as the eyes, heart, lungs, and the peripheral nervous system, results in a basic lesion that is a mixture of granulomatous response, analogous to the rheumatoid nodule, and some form of vascular injury. For instance, an inflammatory microvasculopathy can be found throughout the myocardium in almost 40% of autopsied RA patients. Less common are granulomatous lesions involving the epicardium, myocardium, and valves. Interstitial pulmonary disease likely results from vascular abnormalities mediated by the immune complex, and intrapulmonary nodules reflect granulomatous responses. About 15% of RA patients experience dryness of mucous membranes, particularly of the eyes and mouth, caused by chronic inflammation of exocrine glands.

Gout

Gout has been afflicting humans for centuries. The clinical syndrome of gout often is associated with a purine-rich diet and ethanol use, both of which increase the level of uric acid. In the patient who already is overproducing purines, these dietary factors may lead to the shifts in uric acid concentration necessary for an acute attack. The enzyme deficiency probably is due to a single dominant gene abnormality, but this has not yet been definitively shown (Fig. 40).

Hyperuricemia leads to urate crystal deposits in tissues; the presence of these tissue deposits is

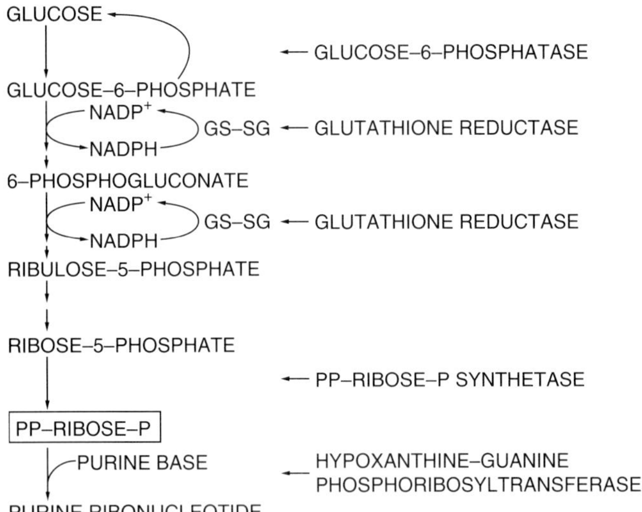

Figure 40
Enzymatic effects that may result in increased phosphoribosylpyrophosphate. NADP = nicotinamide-adenine dinucleotide phosphate; NADPH = reduced NADP. (Reproduced with permission from Levinson DJ: Clinical gout and the pathogenesis of hyperuricemia, in McCarty DJ (ed): *Arthritis and Allied Conditions: A Textbook of Rheumatology,* ed 11. Philadelphia, Lea & Febiger, 1989, p 1659.)

required for a diagnosis of gout. Sodium urate solubility is about 6.8 mg/dl, and urate crystals may form at concentrations greater than this value. Because the solubility of sodium urate is reduced as the temperature of the tissue is lowered, crystals are more common in the extremities. This behavior explains why acute attacks are most common in the first metatarsophalangeal joint. Other common locations of urate deposits, so-called tophi, are the helix of the ear, olecranon and prepatellar bursae, and Achilles tendons.

Acute attacks are caused by a rapid increase or decrease in the concentration of uric acid. Common causes of a rapid change include ethanol ingestion, trauma, exercise, and surgery. Ethanol increases urate production, and metabolism of ethanol causes an increase in the concentration of blood lactate. Like a number of other small organic acids, lactic acid blocks the renal excretion of uric acid, probably through inhibition of tubular secretion. If the blood lactate level remains above 20 to 25 mg/dl for a sufficient time, uric acid output by the kidney is reduced sharply. When a large purine- and protein-rich meal is accompanied by large amounts of ethanol, the lactic acid produced in the metabolism of the ethanol temporarily blocks the disposal of uric acid by the kidneys, leading to a greater rise in serum urate concentration than that produced by the same meal taken without ethanol ingestion.

The demonstration of monosodium urate monohydrate (MSU) crystals is mandatory for establishing the diagnosis of gout because high serum urate levels alone can be misleading as an indication for this condition. The MSU crystals are long, thin, needle-shaped structures that are strongly negatively birefringent. (Crystals of calcium pyrophosphate dihydrate, which are indicative of another crystal deposition disease, are weakly positively birefringent.) (Fig. 41). The MSU crystals are ingested by inflammatory cells, and the presence of these intracellular MSU crystals is diagnostic of gout. The MSU and calcium pyrophosphate crystals are water soluble and, if the tissue or joint fluids are placed in water, the crystal dissolves and cannot be seen.

The inflammatory response to the crystals is produced by a variety of mechanisms, including activation of the classic complement pathway, activation of Hageman factor, and stimulation of PMNs. It probably is mainly the interaction of the MSU crystals and PMNs that produces the histologic findings of gout and its clinical symptoms.

The PMNs phagocytize the MSU crystals and release lysosomal proteases, oxygen-derived free radicals, lipoxygenase-derived products of arachidonic acid, and neutral proteases including collagenase. The PMNs also secrete a low molecular-weight chemotactic glycoprotein called crystal-induced chemotactic factor. Mononuclear inflammatory cells also phagocytize MSU crystals and release prostaglandin E2, lysosomal enzymes, and tumor necrosis factor-alpha (TNF-α). In addition, there is an increased release of IL-1 associated with MSU crystal phagocytosis. These factors contribute to the inflammation of the tissues, particularly synovium, and produce the effects of gout.

An acute attack is associated with all the typical findings of an acute inflammatory event. There is pain, swelling, and erythema of the joint. The synovial fluid leukocyte counts are elevated from 2,000

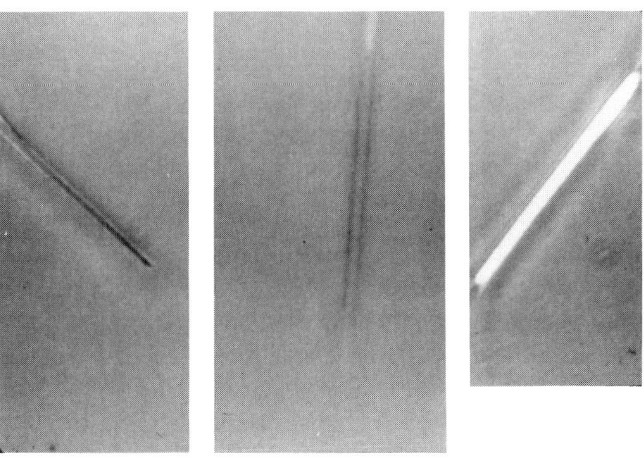

Figure 41
Polarized light photomicrograph of a urate crystal.

to 100,000 cells/mm^3 in acute gouty arthritis and consist predominantly of PMNs. Effusions appear cloudy as a result of the high concentration of cells, and negatively birefringent crystals are present. Occasionally, masses of crystals produce a thick, pasty white joint fluid. Because infection can coexist with urate crystals, joint fluid cultures should be obtained if the diagnosis is in question. The acute process can be relieved by reducing the reaction of the PMNs to the crystals; this is done with anti-inflammatory agents. Colchicine or indomethacin are the agents most commonly used.

Early attacks tend to subside spontaneously over three to ten days, even without treatment. Desquamation of the skin overlying the affected joint may occur when the inflammation subsides. After an acute attack the patient is often completely symptom free until the next episode, which may not occur for months or years. Over time, attacks tend to occur more frequently, to involve more joints, and to persist longer. Some mild arthralgias between attacks may be caused by gout, but other causes should be sought as well.

The more chronic aspects of gout, sometimes called tophaceous gout, are the results of the more prolonged deposition of urate crystals in tissues and of the damage caused by these deposits (Fig. 42). These deposits commonly are seen in the helix of the ear, olecranon and prepatellar bursae, and Achilles tendon. The tophi are composed of large deposits of MSU crystals and an associated chronic inflammatory response (Fig. 43). The material is a creamy white and may ulcerate the skin, leading to a secondary infection. The deposits and inflammatory response, when present in a joint, lead to destruction of the joint by direct damage from both the tophus and the reactive synovium. Such chronic joint findings are currently uncommon because of the availability of agents that can control the uric acid levels of patients with hyperuricemia.

The kidneys are the second most frequently affected organ, after the joints. Parenchymal compromise and renal stones may occur in patients with gout. Proteinuria and mild hypertension have been reported in 20% to 40% of patients with gout, but both are usually benign in idiopathic gout. In the parenchymal disease of gout, the kidneys are usually small and equally affected. The cortical area is reduced in width. Histologic examination of kidneys from patients with gouty nephropathy reveals that urate crystals are located primarily in the medullary interstitium, papillae, and pyramids. Like other tophi, they may be surrounded by a chronic inflammatory reaction with foreign body giant cells. Nephrosclerosis and other evidence of hypertensive disease are also common. This risk of urolithiasis clearly is increased in patients with gout. Stone formation rates increase from 11% in patients whose urinary uric acid excretion is under 300 mg/day to 50% in patients whose excretion is 1,100 mg/day. Uric acid stones are radiolucent, small, and round, but sometimes contain calcium salts, which are radiopaque. An increase in calcium stones has been reported in patients with gout.

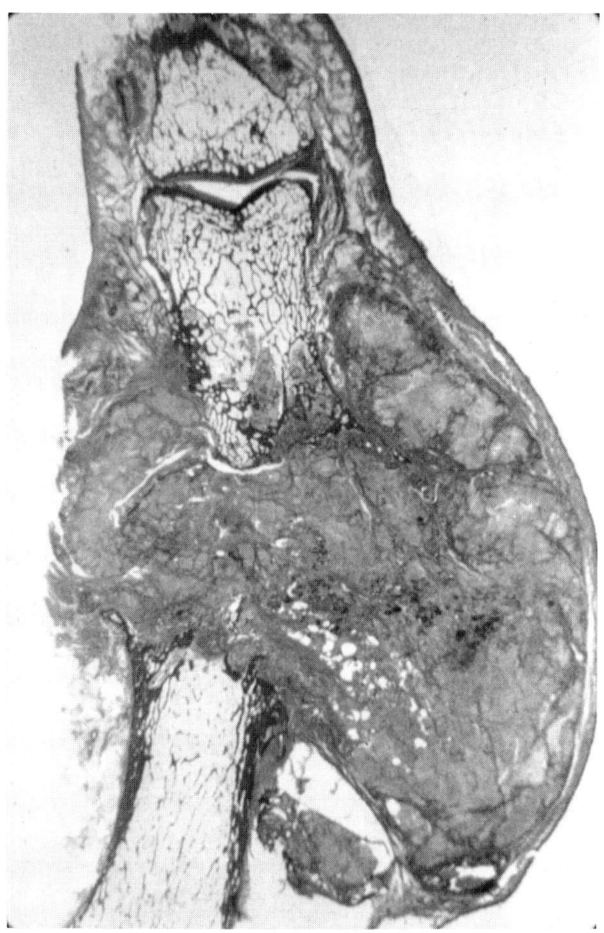

Figure 42
Photomicrograph showing gout; tophus, joint destruction, and marrow invasion by the reactive tissue are visible.

Calcium Pyrophosphate Deposition (CPPD) Disease

Calcium pyrophosphate crystal deposition (CPPD) disease initially was called pseudogout because of its similarity to clinical gout; however, a better understanding of this disorder has led to the selection of CPPD disease as the proper name.

The reason for CPPD is not known, although there are a number of theories. The deposits are thought to develop initially in articular cartilage. The earliest deposits are seen at the periphery of the

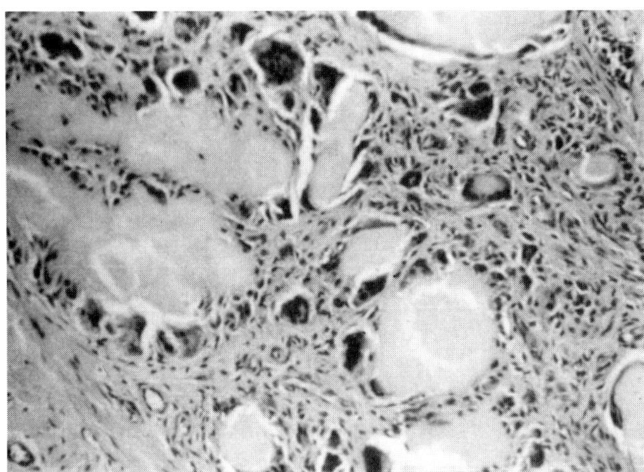

Figure 43
Photomicrograph showing gouty synovitis.

chondrocytes, with larger deposits of up to 0.5 cm seen. These larger deposits have the same white chalky appearance as gouty tophi. Although the causative factor is unknown, an increase of either calcium or inorganic pyrophosphate in the cartilage is presumed to lead to crystal formation within the cartilage and, thus, the clinical syndrome of CPPD.

The arthritis of CPPD can be classified as hereditary, sporadic (idiopathic), or associated with trauma and various metabolic diseases, including hyperparathyroidism, familial hypocalciuric hypercalcemia, hemochromatosis, hemosiderosis, hypothyroidism, gout, hypomagnesemia, hypophosphatasia, amyloidosis, osteoarthritis, diabetes mellitus, acromegaly, and Wilson's disease. Most patients with the familial disease show an autosomal dominant pattern of inheritance and have not had any of the associated metabolic diseases. In about 5% of patients who have CPPD, the disease has a pseudorheumatoid arthritis pattern with multiple joint involvement, usually symmetric. This pattern also involves low-grade inflammation lasting for weeks or months. Morning stiffness, fatigue, synovial thickening, flexion contractures, and elevated sedimentation rate often lead to a misdiagnosis of rheumatoid arthritis. The negative association of rheumatoid arthritis with urate gout does not hold for CPPD; about 1% of patients who have CPPD also have fully expressed rheumatoid arthritis. Other patients who have CPPD develop pseudo-osteoarthritis symptoms or pseudoneurotrophic symptoms.

The acute attack of pseudogout is thought to represent an inflammatory response to CPPD crystals that are shed from cartilage. Phagocytosis of crystals by PMNs results in release of lysosomal enzymes and a cell-derived chemotactic factor. The crystals have rhomboid structures that are weakly positively birefringent (Fig. 44). (MSU crystals are strongly negatively birefringent.)

The crystals often can be seen on a radiograph (Fig. 45). The deposits are punctate and linear in appearance, and are seen in articular cartilage, fibrocartilage, ligaments, and joint capsules. The menisci of the knee are the structures most commonly involved, and usually both menisci in both knees are involved. The fibrocartilage of the distal radioulnar meniscus is another commonly involved structure. The deposits in articular cartilage are in the middle of the cartilage and parallel to the joint surface. Large joints are more commonly involved.

Other Calcium Crystal Deposition Diseases

Calcium phosphates, including hydroxyapatite, are the main constituents of most extraskeletal calcific deposits, as well as of normal bone and tooth mineral. Articular and periarticular calcifications are often of no consequence, because most deposits remain inert. Crystal shedding can result in acute inflammation, however, and crystals have been associated with osteoarthritis and destructive arthropathies.

Calcification at or near a tendon insertion is common. The supraspinatus tendon is involved most frequently, but other sites include tendons around the hip, knee, wrist, and other joints. Some patients have several sites involved, and familial cases have been described. Very large deposits or multiple sites should raise the suspicion of a metabolic cause, although most cases are idiopathic. Acute calcific periarthritis, an attack of inflammation apparently caused by the release of crystals from these deposits, can occur at any age and in either sex. The onset is usually abrupt; it may follow

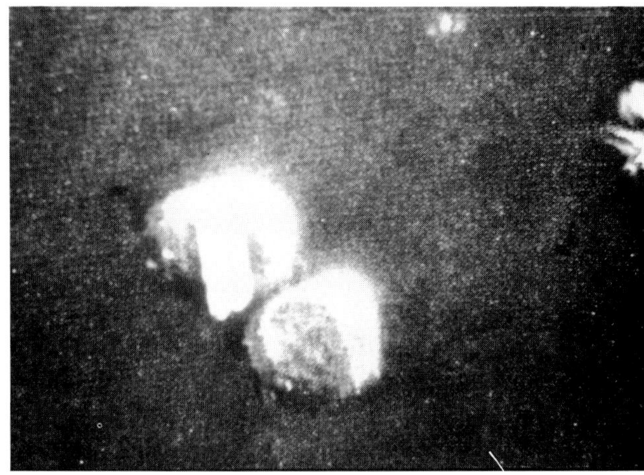

Figure 44
Photomicrograph showing weakly positive birefringent calcium pyrophosphate crystal.

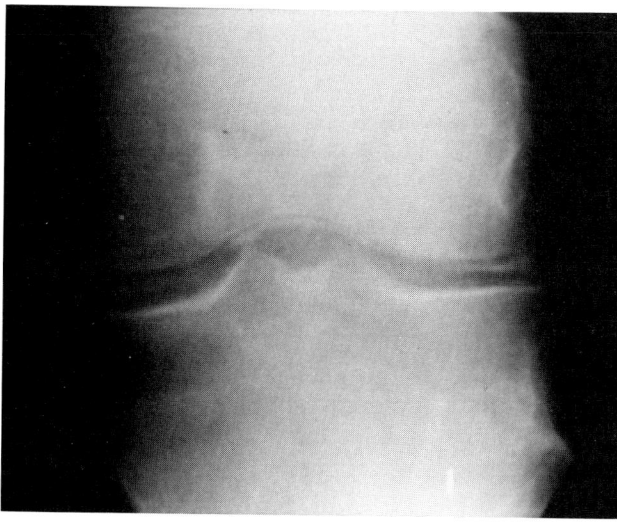

Figure 45
Radiograph showing deposition of calcium pyrophosphate crystals.

trauma but is often spontaneous. About 70% of the attacks occur in the shoulder, with inflammation that generally involves the subacromial bursa as well as the tendons. Radiographs show a change from the normally distinct clear deposit to a fluffy, diffuse area of radiodensity, often followed by disappearance of calcification, presumably due to shedding of crystals and their removal by phagocytosis.

If synovial fluid is removed during an attack, the calcific deposits can be identified by examining the fluid under a light microscope; these deposits may reveal glossy nonbirefringent globules of aggregated apatite-like crystals. Brushite or calcium oxalate are birefringent in polarized light microscopy. Alizarin red S staining of the fluid, although nonspecific, will reveal calcium-containing material as red globules and has been recommended as a screening technique. In clinical practice a plain radiograph followed by light microscopy of synovial fluid, perhaps with alizarin red S staining, and then electron microscopy of selected samples in a reference laboratory is probably the best approach to the detection of apatites.

Seronegative Spondyloarthropathies

The prototype of this disease is ankylosing spondylitis, a chronic systemic inflammatory disorder of undetermined etiology that primarily affects the sacroiliac joints and the axial spine. There are few studies of early pathologic changes in the sacroiliac joints and the axial skeleton because of the obvious difficulty in obtaining such specimens; moreover, early cases rarely come to autopsy. Ankylosing spondylitis differs from rheumatoid arthritis not so much in the specific histologic findings observed in the early stages of the disease as in the distribution of these lesions, their subsequent course, and inflammation at the bone-ligament junction (enthesis), including the sacroiliac joints and the vertebral column.

Studies from open biopsies of the sacroiliac joints of patients with early ankylosing spondylitis have shown that the most constant finding is subchondral osteitis, sometimes with marked proliferation of capillaries and fibrous tissue. This granulation tissue invades the overlying cartilage and is accompanied by cartilage metaplasia and ossification. The inflammatory cells are sparse or absent in the tissue, and there is no evidence of pannus formation. Electron-microscopic examination of the granulation tissue indicates the presence of numerous mast cells, often in contact with lymphocytes. Mast cell degranulation has been observed in areas of localized cartilage destruction. The sequence of events that follows this early stage of subchondral inflammation appears to be fibrous tissue proliferation and reactive cartilaginous and osseous changes that ultimately result in fibrous and then bony ankylosis.

A common site of inflammation in spondyloarthropathies is at the insertions of tendons, ligaments, and articular capsules into bone. This focal inflammatory lesion is called enthesopathy because the enthesis is defined as the part where tendons, ligaments, and capsule are attached to bone. Enthesopathies are quite characteristic of the spondyloarthropathies, although they can occur in other diseases as well.

The inflammatory process occasionally may affect some extra-articular areas, such as the eyes and the aortic root. Active iritis (anterior uveitis) is typically unilateral in onset. If it is not properly treated, there is a risk of scarring of the iris, posterior synechiae, secondary glaucoma, and cataract formation, which can result in visual impairment. A focal inflammatory process at the root of the aorta and adjacent aortic ring, as well as at the ascending aorta, may occur in some patients. In the involved area, there is perivascular infiltration of the vasa vasorum with lymphocytes and plasma cells. There is resultant scarring of the aorta and weakening of the elastic tissue, which may lead to dilatation of the aortic ring and resultant aortic valve incompetence. Patients also may develop chronic infiltrative and fibrotic changes in the upper lung fields that mimic tuberculosis and amyloidosis.

Mucocutaneous lesions are frequently seen in patients with psoriatic arthritis, Reiter's syndrome, and enteropathic arthropathy. The primary skin lesions of psoriasis are papules or macropapules covered with grayish white scales that tend to slough off when gently rubbed. Patients with Reiter's syndrome develop small shallow painless ulcers on the glans penis and urethral meatus (balanitis circinata), painless oral ulcers, and skin lesions called keratoderma blenorrhagica that are very similar to psoriatic plaques.

Laboratory findings in these patients are significant for the presence of the HLA-B27 antigen. It is positive in 90% of white subjects with ankylosing spondylitis, 48% of those with Reiter's syndrome, and 70% of those with rheumatoid arthritis, as compared to 9% of white adults without these diseases. Synovial fluid analysis shows leukocyte counts ranging from 500 to 75,000 cells/mm^3, and a majority of those cells are PMNs. Synovial fluid complement levels can be increased; the serum erythrocyte sedimentation rate is elevated; but tests for rheumatoid factor and antinuclear antibodies are negative.

Neoplastic Diseases

In the last section of this chapter, a brief description of the major tumors of the musculoskeletal system is presented to provide the reader with a general clinical picture with which the basic science understanding of neoplasia can be integrated.

Bone-Forming Tumors

Osteoid Osteoma

Osteoid osteoma was originally described in the mid-1930s, when it was recognized that this abnormality was a neoplasm and was separate from sterile abscesses that are now called Brodie's abscesses and from osteomyelitis of Garre. Osteoid osteoma is a benign tumor and accounts for 10% of all benign bone tumors. Males are affected at a ratio of 3:1 over females, and 80% of the patients are between 5 and 24 years of age.. The patient invariably complains of an intense pain at the site of the lesion. The pain is an unrelenting, sharp, boring pain that is worse at night and is usually completely relieved by aspirin. Half of all osteoid osteomas are found in either the femur (usually proximal) or the tibia, and the other half are distributed throughout the remainder of the skeleton. An osteoid osteoma is one of the few lesions that may occur in the posterior elements of the spine. Patients with an osteoid osteoma of the spine may come to the physician with an occult lesion and a painful scoliosis. The appearance of an osteoid osteoma on a plain radiograph is diagnostic. It consists of dense reactive bone with a central radiolucent nidus. The lesion itself (the nidus) may not be seen on the plain radiograph because of the intense reaction that surrounds it. A computed tomography (CT) scan is useful when trying to see the nidus (Fig. 46, *left*). There is intense uptake of technetium on the nuclear scan. On gross inspection the nidus of an osteoid osteoma is red and is surrounded by dense white bone. The nidus is small, less than 1 cm in diameter, and it is composed of vascular channels, osteoblasts, and a thin, lace-like osteoid seam. Multinucleated giant cells can be seen, but are not common (Fig. 46, *right*). This lesion will spontaneously involute over time, usually years, but most patients have too much pain to wait and elect to have a curettage or excision.

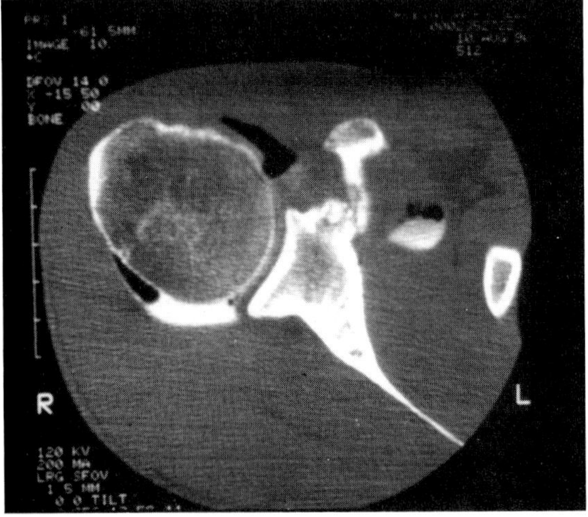

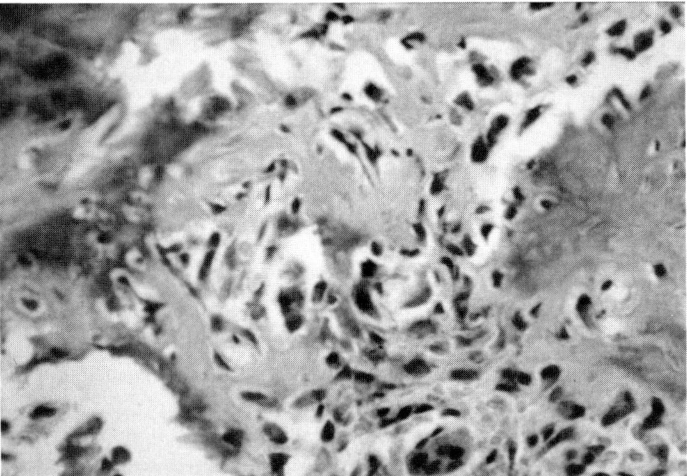

Figure 46
Osteoid osteoma. **Left,** The osteoid osteoma could not be seen on the plain radiograph, but it is easily seen at the base of the coracoid on the CT scan of a patient who complained of shoulder pain. Thin cuts (3 mm) may be needed to see these small lesions. **Right,** Medium power (40X) microscopic view of the nidus of an osteoid osteoma. Osteoblastoma has the identical histologic appearance but is larger. The tissue is composed of plump osteoblast, osteoid, vessels, and, usually, multinucleated giant cells.

Osteoblastoma

Osteoblastoma is a benign, primary bone tumor sometimes called a giant osteoid osteoma because it is histologically identical to an osteoid osteoma. The distinguishing characteristic is that osteoblastoma is larger than osteoid osteoma, usually measuring more than 2 cm in diameter. It is significantly less common than osteoid osteoma. Males are affected twice as often as females, and 50% of the patients are between 10 and 20 years of age. The patient comes in most often complaining of pain, but the pain is not as intense as that of an osteoid osteoma and it is not relieved by aspirin. Ten percent of the lesions are in the posterior elements of the spine, whereas the remainder arise throughout the skeleton. When osteoblastoma involves a long bone, it is usually in the diaphysis and is primarily a radiolucent lesion with minimal amounts of irregular radiodensities (Fig. 47). There is minimal surrounding reactive bone. Osteoblastoma is a progressive lesion that is usually managed successfully with a curettage; however, occasionally a locally aggressive lesion recurs after curettage and will require a resection.

Osteosarcoma

Osteosarcoma is a malignant primary bone tumor, second in frequency only to myeloma. The classic high-grade osteosarcoma is the most frequent subtype of this tumor, and there are approximately 200 new cases each year in the United States. Of these patients, half are in the second decade of life and 75% will be between the ages of 8 and 25 years. Half of these tumors are located in either the distal femur or proximal tibia, with the proximal humerus, proximal femur, and pelvis being the next most common sites. Males and females are affected with equal frequency. The patient usually complains of mild pain and has a palpable firm mass. Half of the patients will have an elevated serum alkaline phosphatase. The plain radiograph of an osteosarcoma is usually diagnostic (Fig. 48, *left*). The typical lesion is located in the metaphysis, involves the medullary canal, has an extraosseous component, is both lytic (radiolucent), and blastic (radiodense), and has a periosteal reaction suggestive of rapid growth, such as Codman's triangle or sunburst pattern. Many lesions will have a soft tissue component with a fluffy density suggestive of neoplastic bone. Classic high-grade osteosarcoma is subdivided into chondroblastic, fibroblastic, osteoblastic, mixed, and telangiectatic osteosarcomas. This histology of classic high-grade osteosarcoma varies considerably, but all the subdivisions have an area where malignant spindle cells make osteoids (Fig. 48, *right*). Approximately 80% of the patients with a classic high-grade osteosarcoma will have at least micrometastases (subclinical) at the time of presentation. Adjuvant chemotherapy and surgical resection is the treatment of choice.

A second type of osteosarcoma is called juxtacortical osteosarcoma. These osteosarcomas arise from or are adjacent to the external surface of the bone and usually do not involve the medullary canal. They tend to be less aggressive locally and have less potential for distant metastasis. Some subclassify juxtacortical osteosarcomas into those that are periosteal and those that are parosteal. Patients with a juxtacortical osteosarcoma usually are treated with surgery alone unless there is medullary involvement and a histologic high-grade component. Outline 1 lists the types of osteosarcoma.

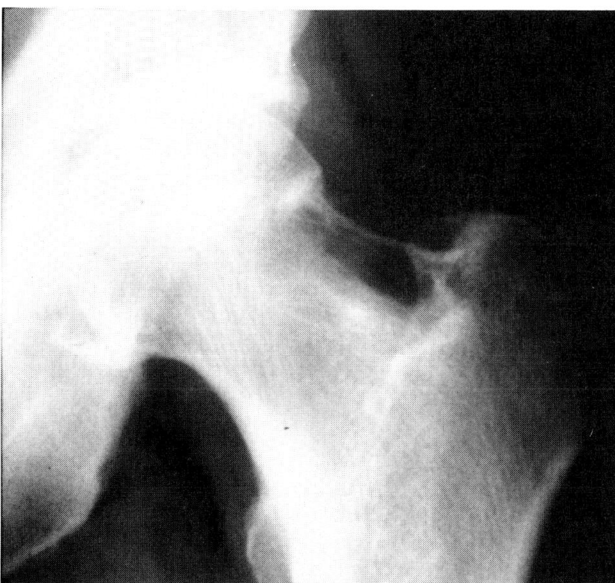

Figure 47
Osteoblastoma. This osteoblastoma is in the metaphysis of the proximal femur (femoral neck). As may be the case, this lesion is radiolucent, but osteoblastoma may have areas with bone formation. The bone in the lesion is minimally mineralized and much of the tissue is unmineralized bone. This lesion was treated with a curettage.

Cartilage-Forming Tumors

Enchondroma

Enchondroma may be the result of epiphyseal growth cartilage that does not remodel and persists in the metaphysis, or it may be persistence of the original cartilaginous anlage of the bone. Both have been suggested as explanations of the origin of this common benign tumor. Enchondromas account for 10% of benign bone tumors. They do not produce symptoms. Forty percent of them are found in bones of the hand or feet, with the femur and proximal humerus being the next most common sites. They are typically located in the metaphysis and are central within the medullary canal. In the pediatric

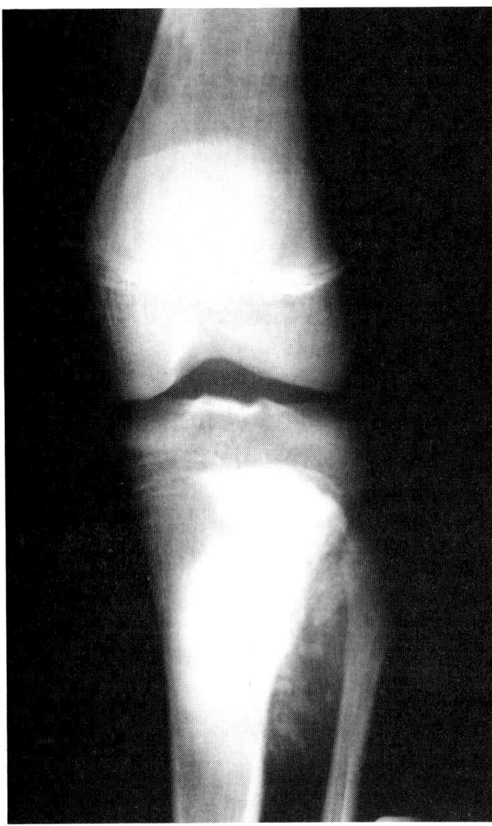

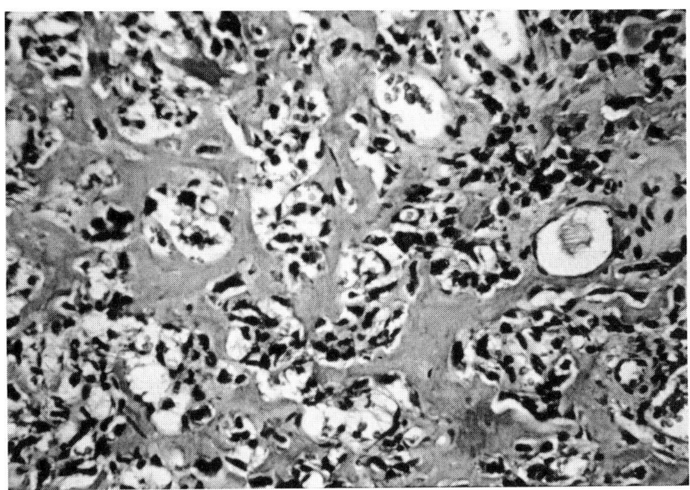

Figure 48
Osteosarcoma. **Left,** Because all the characteristics findings of this osteosarcoma are on the plain radiograph, it can be used to make the diagnosis. The patient is a teenager (the growth plates are just closing). The lesion is in the metaphysis (tibia) and is making bone that is both intraosseous and extraosseous. **Right,** This osteosarcoma (40X) is an osteoblastic variant composed only of malignant cells and bone. The cells are irregularly shaped with larger and darker than normal nuclei. The bone is poorly organized and varies in size and shape. Fracture callus can look like osteosarcoma to the unwary; therefore, the clinical presentation should always be considered when evaluating the histology of a potential osteosarcoma.

Outline 1
Types of osteosarcoma

- Juxtacortical
  - Parosteal
  - Periosteal
- Paget's sarcoma
- Radiation associated
- Craniofacial
- Low grade, intraosseous
- High grade, classic
  - Osteoblastic
  - Fibroblastic
  - Chondroblastic
  - Telangiectatic

age group the lesions are usually radiolucent, but in adults there commonly are intralesional calcifications (Fig. 49). Patients with multiple enchondromas are said to have Ollier's disease; these patients have an approximately 15% risk of developing a chondrosarcoma sometime during their life span. Patients with multiple enchondromas and soft-tissue hemangiomas are said to have Maffucci's disease. These patients have an even greater risk of developing chondrosarcoma or, more commonly, a carcinoma. The enchondromas of all of these disorders are histologically normal but have slightly hypercellular hyaline cartilage (Fig. 50). Treatment is not required, but if it is elected a thorough curettage should be done.

Exostoses (Osteocartilaginous Exostoses, Osteochondroma)

Exostoses are common and account for approximately 40% of all benign bone tumors. They do not produce symptoms other than the presence of a mass unless they press directly on a nerve or artery. Occasionally, a patient will develop an inflamed bursa overlying the exostosis and have acute pain, but a plain radiograph is diagnostic with the cortex of the bone blending into the cortex of the exostosis (Fig. 51). There is a varying amount of calcification in the cartilaginous cap. The base of an exostosis may either be broad (sessile exostosis) or narrow (pedunculated exostosis). Exostoses usually grow until late in the third decade of life. Their growth appearance is that of a cauliflower. The cap is covered with cartilage, which is usually less than 1 cm thick. The cartilage appears to be normal hyaline cartilage that is undergoing normal enchondral ossification. Patients with multiple exostoses are said to have multiple inheritable exostoses, which is an autosomal dominant genetic trait with variable penetrance. Symptomatic exostoses can be surgically excised.

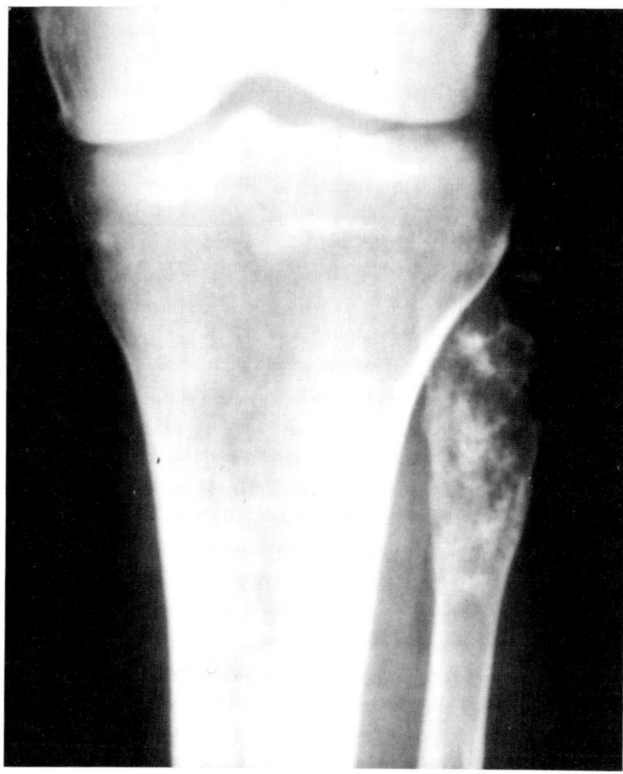

Figure 49
Enchondroma. Radiograph of the proximal tibia and fibula of an adult patient who had had a minor injury to the knee and no symptoms referable to the fibular lesion. The intramedullary calcifications are typical of an inactive cartilaginous lesion (enchondroma). Medullary infarctions can have calcification and should be on the differential diagnosis. As long as the pattern of calcification is uniform and there is no endosteal resorption or periosteal reaction, the lesion can be considered inactive and benign; if there are any signs of activity the lesion should be considered malignant, and further investigation is warranted.

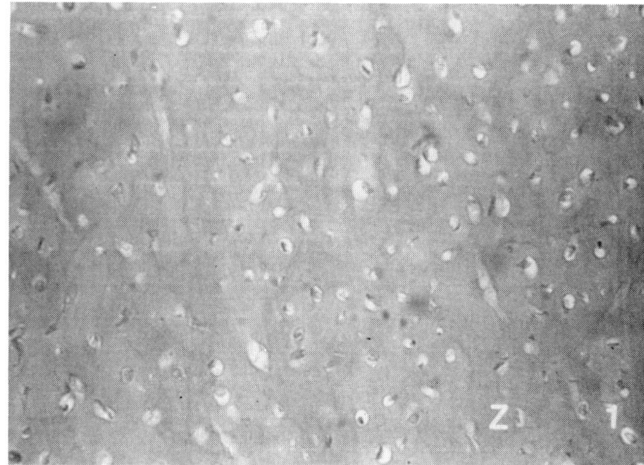

Figure 50
Enchondroma (10X). Typical microscopic appearance of an enchondroma; the lesion looks like normal hyaline cartilage except that it is hypercellular. There is no calcification on this photograph.

Chondromyxofibroma

Chondromyxofibroma is benign and uncommon. Males are affected more frequently than females (2:1), and the lesion is usually discovered in the second or third decade of life. Approximately one third of the chondromyxofibromas occur in the tibia, usually in the proximal tibia. Chondromyxofibroma is a radiolucent lesion that involves the medullary canal but is eccentric and erodes the cortex. It is usually contained by the periosteum, which is raised, and on the plain radiograph has the appearance of an aneurysmal bone cyst. The tumor is composed of cartilage, myxomatous tissue, and fibrous tissue in varying amounts. Most chondromyxofibromas can be adequately treated with a thorough curettage.

Chondroblastoma (Codman's tumor)

Chondroblastoma is an uncommon, benign bone tumor arising from the secondary ossification center. It accounts for approximately 1% of all benign bone tumors. The patient is usually in the second decade of life and still has open growth plates. The patient complains of pain in the adjacent joint and will have loss of motion and an effusion. The plain radiograph is usually diagnostic because there is a radiolucent lesion within the secondary ossification center with small foci of calcification that may be seen better on plain tomograms or a CT scan (Fig. 52, *left*). The tumor consists of chondroblasts, which are cuboidal shaped cells with a distinct nucleus and pink cytoplasm, that are arranged in a so-called cobblestone appearance. There is usually calcification within the matrix and multinucleated giant cells are common (Fig. 52, *right*). Chondroblastomas are treated with an intralesional curettage.

Chondrosarcoma

Chondrosarcoma is a primary malignant tumor of bone, which is composed of malignant chondrocytes within a cartilage matrix. It is a relatively common tumor, accounting for 20% of all bone tumors. Usually it is found in patients between 50 and 70 years of age, and it arises most often in the metaphysis of the proximal femur or in the pelvis. Chondrosarcoma may arise from a preexisting enchondroma or exostosis. The patient usually complains of a gradually increasing dull, persistent, deep pain. On the plain radiograph, the lesion is principally radiolucent; there is a varying amount of intralesional calcification and radiographic evi-

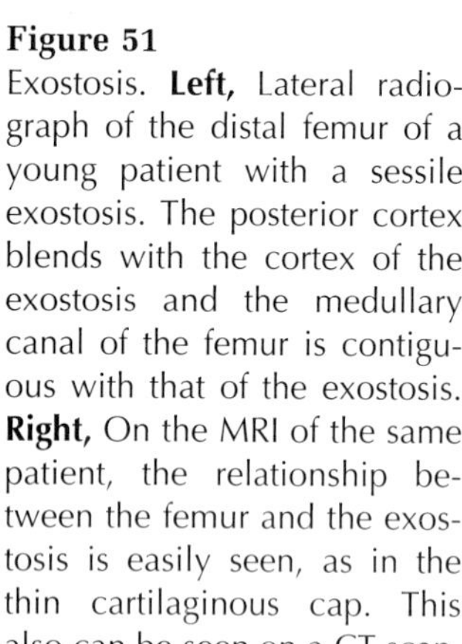

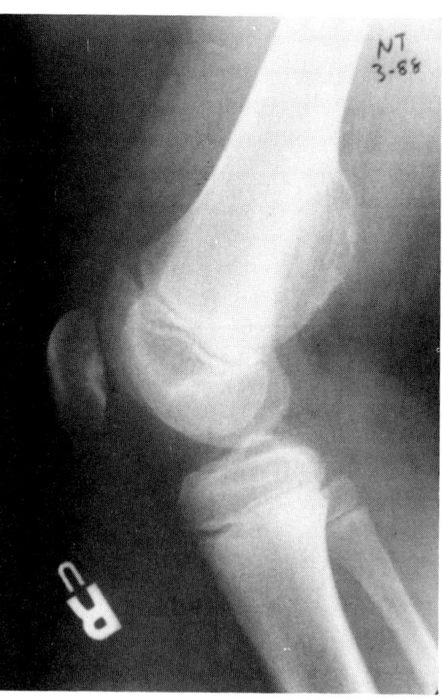

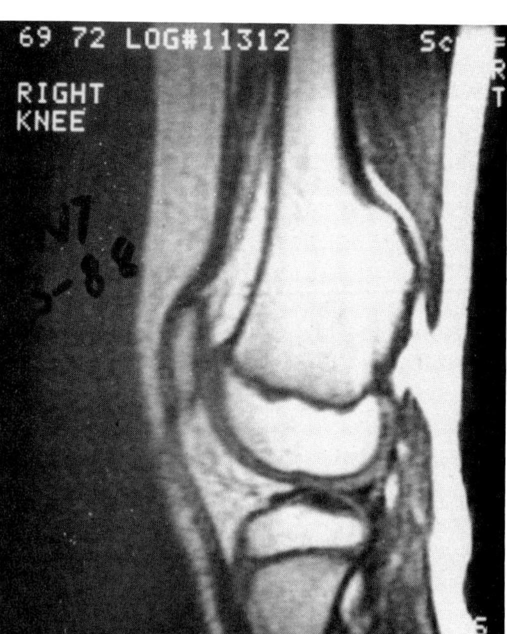

Figure 51
Exostosis. **Left,** Lateral radiograph of the distal femur of a young patient with a sessile exostosis. The posterior cortex blends with the cortex of the exostosis and the medullary canal of the femur is contiguous with that of the exostosis. **Right,** On the MRI of the same patient, the relationship between the femur and the exostosis is easily seen, as in the thin cartilaginous cap. This also can be seen on a CT scan.

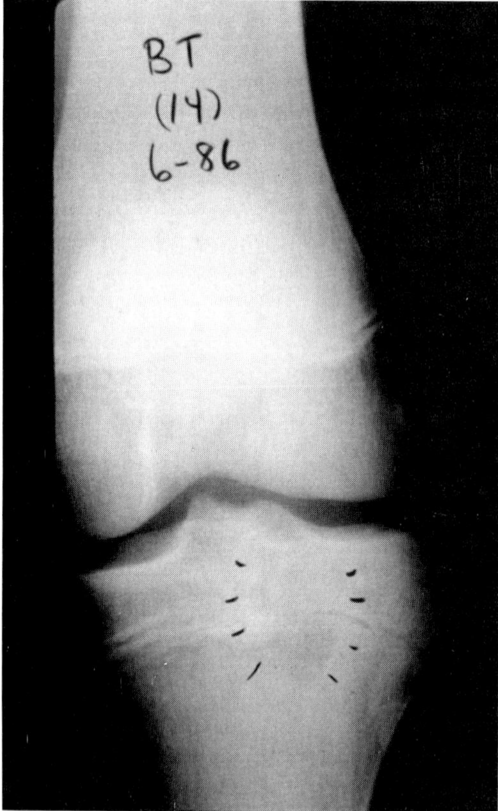

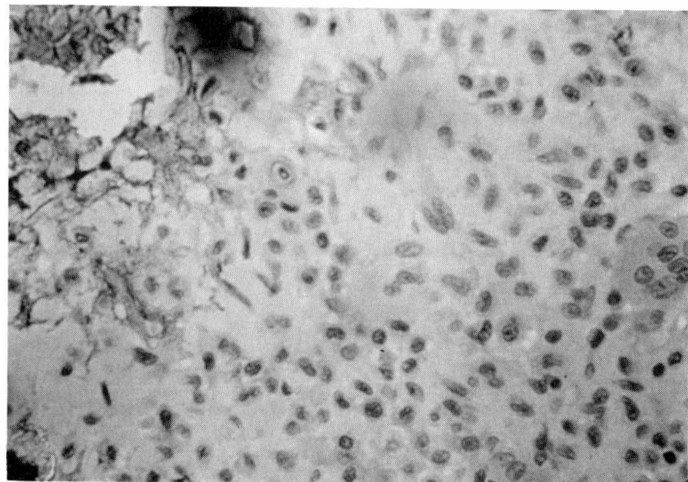

Figure 52
Chondroblastoma. **Left,** Radiograph of a patient who complained of pain in the knee and had an effusion in the knee. The radiolucent lesion in the secondary ossification center is subtle and is outlined by the waxed pencil marks. The intralesional calcifications are not seen on this plain radiograph but were seen on a CT scan. **Right,** Chondroblastomas (40X) are composed of chondroblasts, areas of chondroid matrix, and flicks of calcification.

dence of bone destruction with endosteal and periosteal reaction (Fig. 53, *left*). Chondrosarcomas can have a similar appearance to metastatic carcinoma. The nuclei of the chondrocytes are abnormally large, and there are frequently double nuclei within a single chondrocyte (Fig. 53, *right*). Chondrosarcoma is usually treated with surgical resection alone.

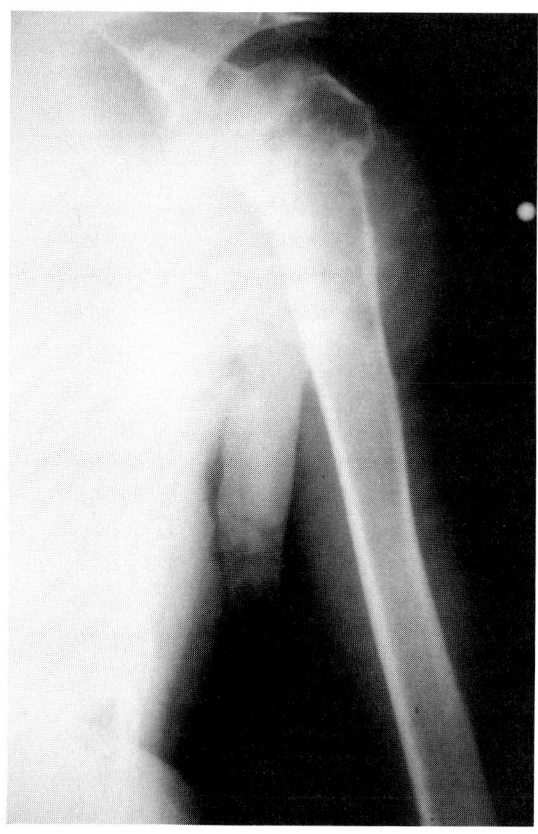

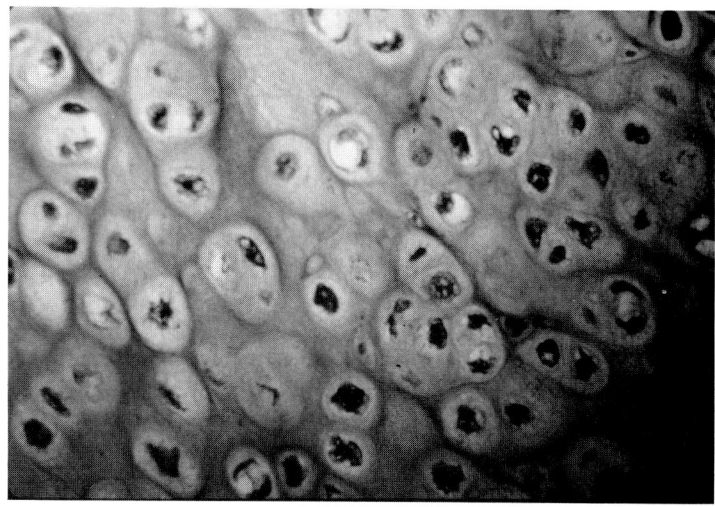

Figure 53
Chondrosarcoma. **Left,** Radiograph of a 50-year-old man's left humerus. He had had increasingly severe pain in the shoulder for three months, and a palpable mass was found under the deltoid upon examination. There is destruction of bone in the proximal humerus with cortical erosion and an extraosseous mass. There is less intralesional calcification than is usually seen with a chondrosarcoma. **Right,** (40X). Low grade lesions can be difficult to distinguish from benign, active cartilage. Medium grade lesions, as shown here, are more cellular than normal cartilage and often have chondrocytes with two nuclei but still are recognized easily as cartilage. High-grade lesions have minimal cartilage matrix, the chondrocytes may look like undifferentiated spindle cells, and there are numerous mitoses.

Lesions of Fibrous Origin

Nonossifying Fibroma (NOF)

Nonossifying fibroma, also called fibroma of bone, nonosteogenic fibroma, metaphyseal fibrous defects, or fibrous cortical defects, is a benign tumor that is the single most common tumor of bone. Up to 40% of children will have this lesion, which is found most often between the ages of 4 and 8 years. Ninety percent of these lesions are located within the distal femur; they produce no symptoms. The lesion may be either a small (less than 0.5 cm) radiolucent lesion within the cortex or a larger lesion within the medullary canal, which is located eccentrically and surrounded by a reactive rim of bone (Fig. 54). There should be no periosteal reaction unless there has been a pathologic fracture. Nonossifying fibroma consists of benign, spindle fibroblastic cells arranged in a storiform pattern. Multinucleated giant cells are common, and, often, areas of large lipid laden macrophages are seen. Hemosiderin within the fibroblastic stroma cells and multinucleated giant cells is usual. Most of these lesions do not require treatment and will spontaneously resolve, but if treatment is elected, intralesional curettage is adequate.

Fibrous Dysplasia

Fibrous dysplasia is a benign condition that is probably a developmental abnormality and not a neoplasm. It is a common disorder and produces a variety of complaints and physical findings. The majority of patients (85%) have a single skeletal lesion (monostotic fibrous dysplasia), whereas the remainder have multiple lesions (polyostotic fibrous dysplasia). The patients with polyostotic fibrous dysplasia may have only two or three small areas of involvement, or they may have extensive skeletal abnormalities with grossly deformed bones. The patient usually has no symptoms but may complain

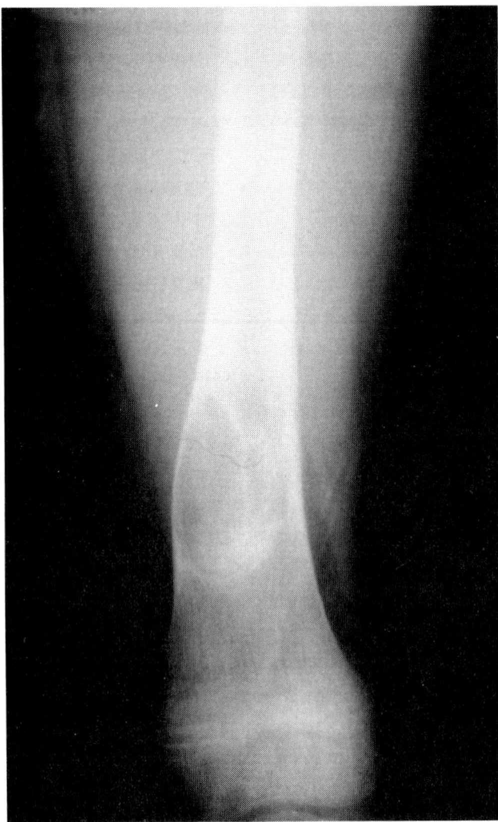

Figure 54
Nonossifying fibroma. Typical nonossifying fibroma as seen on the anterior-posterior radiograph of a 16-year-old girl's femur. It is located in the metaphysis of a long bone, is eccentric, and the cortex "bulges" around it. The extent of the lesion is easily seen and is marked by a thin shell of reactive bone.

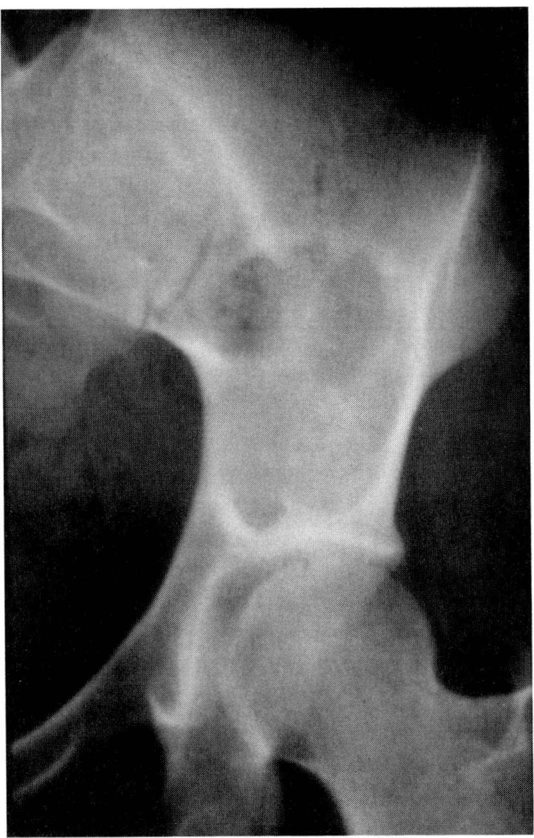

Figure 55
Fibrous dysplasia. Typical fibrous dysplasia of the ilium. This bone is not deformed, but fibrous dysplasia may lead to deformity of the bone. The extent of this lesion is easily seen, but often fibrous dysplasia seems to blend into the adjacent normal bone and it can be difficult to see its extent on plain radiographs. This patient only had one lesion; therefore, this is monostotic fibrous dysplasia. Multiple lesions are not uncommon; when this occurs, it is said to be polyostotic.

of pain suggestive of a weakened bone or an impending pathologic fracture. Albright described a triad of fibrous dysplasia, café-au-lait spots, and precocious puberty, and this syndrome bears his name. The plain radiograph is usually diagnostic although variable (Fig. 55). Fibrous dysplasia involves the medullary canal and produces the so-called ground glass appearance on the radiograph. The involvement is usually diaphyseal, the diaphysis is usually larger, and it is difficult to define the endosteal border or the cortex. Occasionally, there is a dense reactive rim around a small area of fibrous dysplasia. Fibrous dysplasia is composed of fibrous tissue with normal-appearing nuclei in irregularly-shaped strands of osteoid and bone (Fig. 56). There are few if any osteoblasts present, and the osteoid seems to arise directly from the background fibrous stroma. Multinucleated giant cells are rare but occasionally there will be nodules of benign hyaline cartilage. Fibrous dysplasia does not require treatment unless there is deformity of the bone or pathologic fracture.

Osteofibrous Dysplasia (Ossifying Fibroma)

Osteofibrous dysplasia is an uncommon lesion that arises almost exclusively within the tibia and can be confused with fibrous dysplasia and adamantinoma. It is benign, but locally aggressive. It tends to be located within the anterior cortex of the tibia and may be associated with a progressive angular deformity. The management of this lesion is controversial.

Miscellaneous Lesions

Unicameral Bone Cyst, Simple Bone Cyst

Unicameral bone cysts are not always unicameral. These are common benign lesions found in the metaphyses of children. The proximal humerus and proximal femur account for 90% of all unicameral bone cysts. Patients with unicameral bone cysts do not have symptoms unless the bone is fractured or near fracture (Fig. 57). The cysts seem to arise from

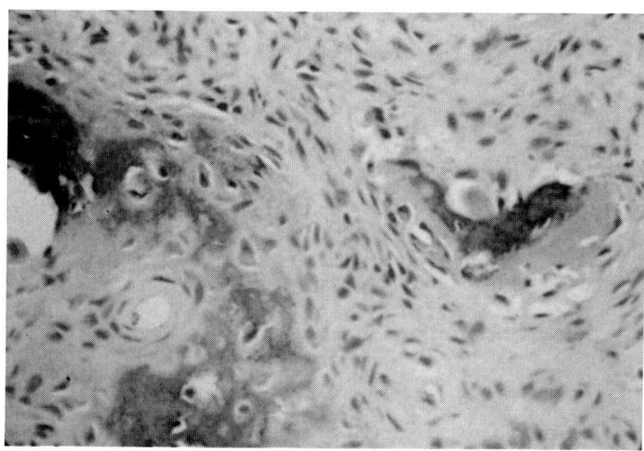

Figure 56
Fibrous dysplasia (40X). Fibrous dysplasia is composed of a stroma with benign fibroblasts with interspersed foci of osteoid and bone. The bone is unorganized and has few surface osteoblasts.

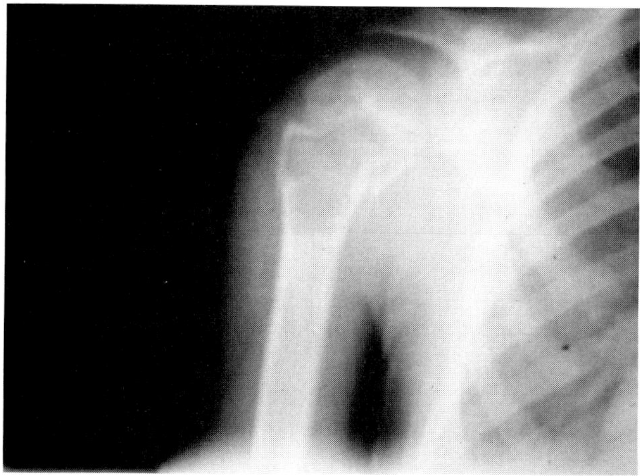

Figure 57
Unicameral or simple bone cyst. These common lesions seem to arise from the metaphyseal side of the growth plate. This patient sustained a pathologic fracture. The radiolucent defect of a unicameral bone cyst should be centrally located; the cortex does not remodel normally and, therefore, is broader than normal but should not be wider than the growth plate.

the epiphyseal plate and initially are immediately adjacent to the growth plate, extending into the metaphysis. The metaphyseal bone does not remodel normally, and the metaphysis is broader than normal. A thin rim of bone borders the unicameral bone cyst. When the cyst becomes mature (latent), usually after the patient reaches the age of 10 years, the epiphysis grows away from the lesion. Unicameral bone cysts will spontaneously heal. The cysts contain a synovial-like fluid, and the lining of the cyst wall is composed of synovial-like cuboidal cells. Intralesional injection of cortical steroids is the most common current treatment.

Aneurysmal Bone Cyst

Aneurysmal bone cyst is a controversial lesion. Some authors believe that this lesion occurs only in association with other bone tumors, whereas many authors believe aneurysmal bone cyst can be a primary diagnosis. It does occur in association with giant cell tumor, chondroblastoma, and osteoblastoma, but the majority of aneurysmal bone cysts do not have a recognizable, underlying associated diagnosis. Aneursymal bone cyst is a benign condition that occurs most commonly in teenagers; 80% of patients are between the ages of 10 and 20 years. The patient complains of mild pain. More than 50% of these cysts arise in large tubular bones and another 30% arise within the spine. On the plain radiograph, an aneurysmal bone cyst is a radiolucent lesion arising within the medullary canal of the metaphysis, resorbing the cortex and elevating the periosteum to produce the aneurysmal appearance (Fig. 58, *left*). Usually, there is a thin shell of reactive periosteal bone containing the lesion, which may or may not be seen on the radiograph. Not uncommonly, the periosteal reaction is quite active, and an aneurysmal bone cyst can have the radiographic appearance of a malignant lesion. When an aneurysmal bone cyst arises from the spine, it usually originates in the posterior elements but often will extend into the vertebral body. Aneurysmal bone cyst is a cavitary lesion with a villous lining. Microscopic examination reveals the lining to be composed of hemosiderin-laden macrophages, multinucleated giant cells, a fibrostroma, and, usually, small amounts of osteoid (Fig. 58, *right*). The appearance is very similar to that of a giant cell tumor. Curettage is adequate treatment although, occasionally, this lesion will recur.

Giant Cell Tumor of Bone

Giant cell tumor of bone is a benign tumor that occurs predominantly in the third and fourth decades of life, is common, and represents 20% of all benign tumors of bone. The patient complains of pain that is usually mild to moderate. When the lesion involves the distal femur or proximal tibia, the symptoms may mimic an internal derangement of the knee. The tumor is a radiolucent lesion involving the metaphysis and epiphysis of the long bone (Fig. 59, *left*). It invariably extends to and sometimes through the subchondral bone. There are no intralesional densities. The lesion is usually eccentric, and the cortex may be eroded. Giant cell

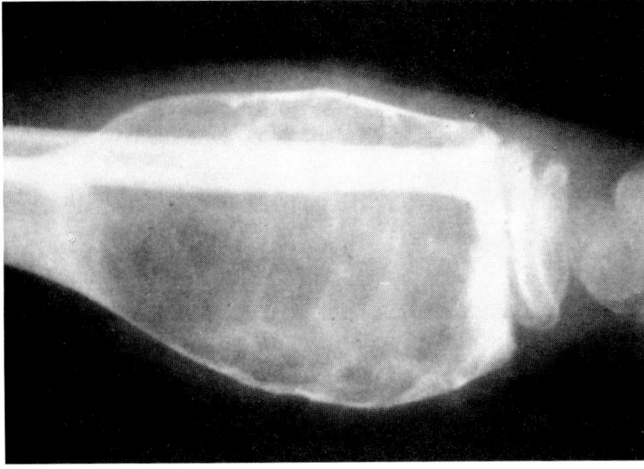

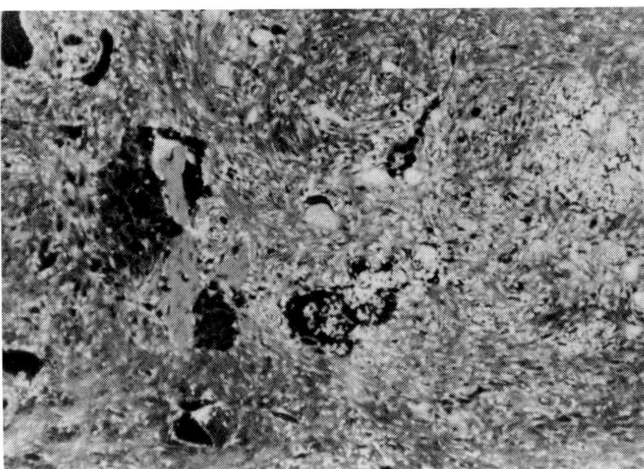

Figure 58
Aneurysmal bone cyst. **Left,** Radiolucent lesions are usually located in the metaphysis; cysts may occur in any location and are common in the posterior elements of the spine. The periosteum usually contains the lesion, and the thin shell of bone can usually be seen as an expansion of the cortex. **Right,** (10X). Blood-filled cavity with a shaggy lining made up of benign stroma cells and multinucleated giant cells. There is often hemorrhage within the lesion and areas of reactive bone.

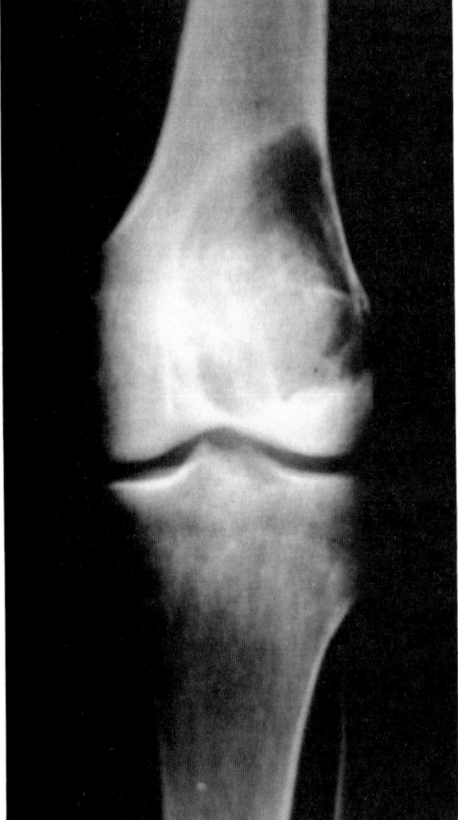

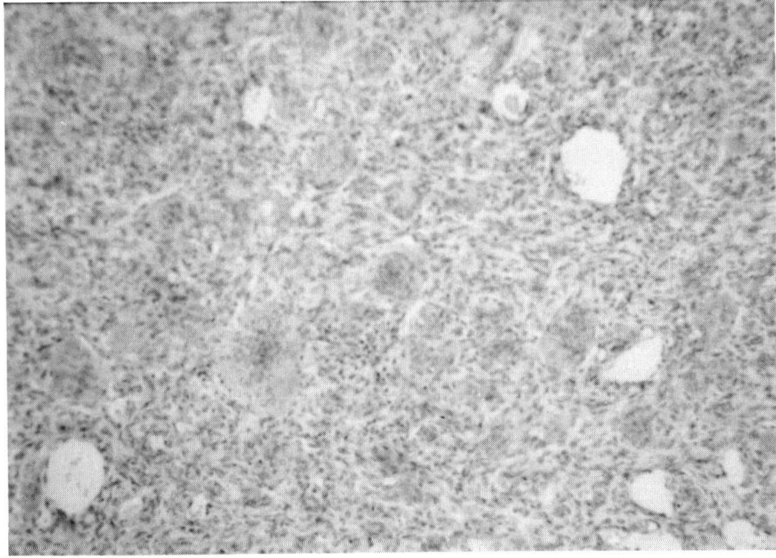

Figure 59
Giant cell tumor of bone. **Left,** The lesion can usually be diagnosed from the clinical presentation and appearance on the plain radiograph. It has a well defined border, but usually no reactive rim of bone. There can be cortical erosion and even an extraosseous component. **Right,** (10X). Tumor of bone is composed of multinucleated giant cells with a background stroma of mononuclear cells that have nuclei that look identical to those of the multinucleated giant cells.

tumor of bone is composed of multinucleated giant cells, a background of fibrous tissue, and small, single nucleated cells whose nuclei appear identical to the nuclei of the multinucleated giant cells (Fig. 59, *right*). Mitoses are common but normal. Giant cell tumor of bone is one of the few benign bone tumors that commonly has areas of spontaneous necrosis. The patient should be treated with an extended intralesional curettage or marginal resection. Approximately 5% of patients with giant cell tumor of bone develop pulmonary metastases. These metastases are usually benign lesions that are managed successfully with surgical resection.

Ewing's Sarcoma

Ewing's sarcoma is a malignant tumor and, prior to the use of routine adjuvant chemotherapy, was the most lethal primary bone tumor, with a five-year survival of less than 15%. Recently, the five-year disease-free survival has increased to approximately 65%. Ewing's sarcoma makes up 5% of all primary malignant bone tumors. Males are affected more commonly (3:2), and most patients are between the ages of 5 and 30 years. The femur is the single most common site of origin (20%) with other common sites being the pelvis (12%) and the humerus (11%). Black people rarely have Ewing's sarcoma. The patient usually complains of pain at the location of the primary tumor, but may have systemic signs and symptoms of fever and weight loss. The typical plain radiograph of a Ewing's sarcoma reveals diffuse destruction of bone, extension of the tumor through the cortex, a soft tissue component, and a periosteal reaction (Fig. 60, *left*). The periosteal reaction may produce a Codman's triangle, onion skinning, or sunburst appearance. Ewing's sarcomas are most common in the metaphysis, as are all bone tumors, but unlike other bone tumors they also are not uncommon in the diaphysis. This tumor has the ability to permeate the cortex of a bone (with limited changes on the radiograph), raise the periosteum (which reacts), and extend into the adjacent soft tissues. Ewing's sarcoma is composed of monotonous sheets of small, round cells (Fig. 60, *right*). These cells have distinct nuclei with a nuclear border but an indistinct cytoplastic border. Mitoses are uncommon, but areas of spontaneous necrosis are usually seen. The cells have cytoplastic glycogen granules, and the glycogen produces the positive periodic acid-Schiff (PAS) stain. The glycogen of a Ewing's sarcoma is dissolved by diastases, and, therefore, the PAS stain is diastases sensitive. Glycogen granules can be seen with the electron microscope. The nuclear DNA of a Ewing's tumor has a characteristic abnormal karyotype, t(11;22)(q24;q12).

Soft-Tissue Tumors

Lipoma

Lipoma is a common, benign tumor that occurs most often in the subcutaneous tissue of adults, but lipomas may arise within a muscle. The subcutaneous lipomas do not cause symptoms, are soft and moveable, may grow slowly, and are often removed for cosmetic reasons. The intramuscular lipomas

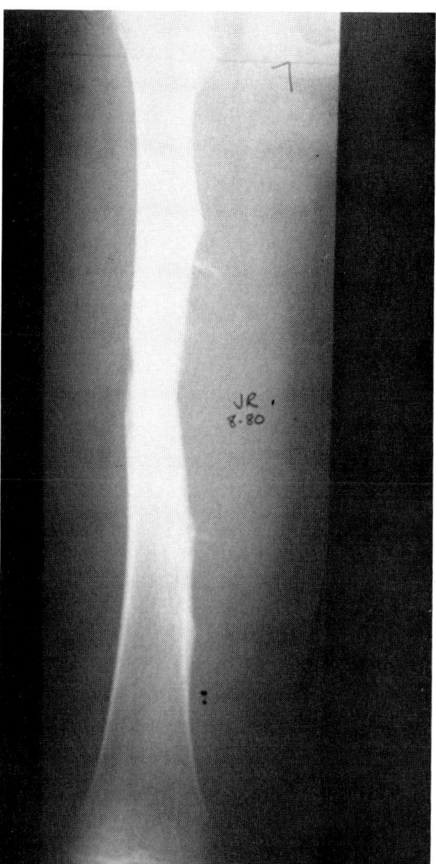

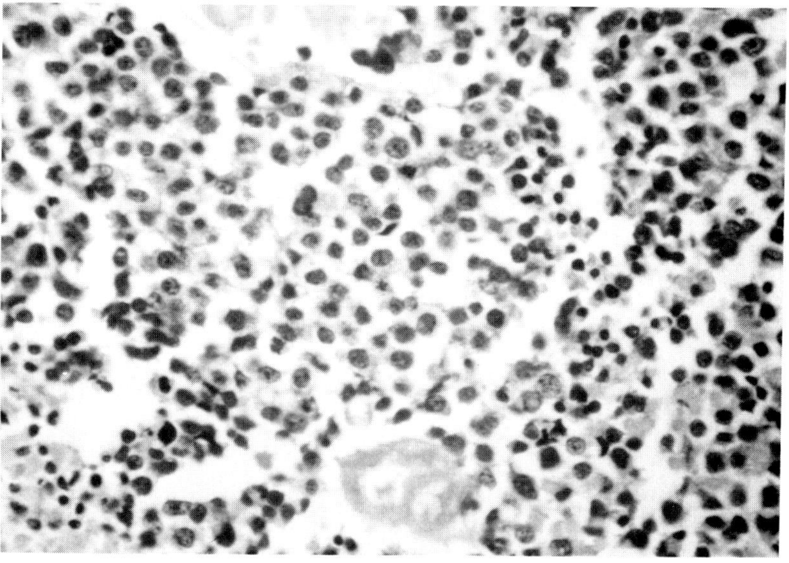

Figure 60
Ewing's sarcoma. **Left,** Anterior-posterior radiograph of a typical Ewing's sarcoma of the diaphysis of the femur. The apparent circumferential appearance of this lesion is almost diagnostic of the condition. **Right,** (40X). Ewing's sarcoma is composed of small dark blue cells that are identical in appearance; the nuclei and cytoplasm are easily seen but the cell membranes are ill defined. Necrosis is common and pseudorosettes formed with viable cells are clustered around a small area of necrosis.

may produce a mild, achy discomfort, but even large ones can be asymptomatic. These benign tumors can grow to be greater than 10 cm, and removal is indicated to relieve symptoms or for cosmetic reasons. The incidence of lipomas becoming liposarcoma is extremely low. Lipomas can be diagnosed with a CT scan or MRI (Fig. 61). They have the density and signal of normal fat. They are composed of normal, mature, adult fat cells and are encapsulated.

Hemangioma

A hemangioma may be a true, benign neoplasm, a hematoma, or an arteriovenous malformation. Their origin is controversial. Hemangiomas are the most common tumors in infancy and childhood and account for 7% of benign soft-tissue tumors in all age groups. They are most common in the head and neck. Capillary hemangiomas constitute the largest group of benign vascular tumors. The juvenile hemangioma variant of capillary hemangioma occurs every 200 live births. These may be cutaneous or deep and usually are seen within the first few weeks of life. They often enlarge for the first six months but then regress, and 95% completely disappear by the age of 7 years. They do not require treatment. Cavernous hemangiomas are not as common as the capillary type, but they do not spontaneously regress and may require treatment. They most commonly arise within muscle and invade tissue planes extensively. The patient usually complains of mild pain. On the plain radiographs small, smooth, round calcifications are often seen. These are phleboliths. The cavernous hemangioma has an indirect communication with a major vascular tree and is not easily filled with contrast on an angiogram or venogram. The MRI signal has a characteristic mixed pattern. The histologic appearance of hemangioma is of benign but abnormal vascular channels of varying size with normal fibrous tissue between the vascular spaces (Fig. 62). Capillary hemangiomas are composed of predominantly small arterial vessels, while cavernous hemangiomas are composed of venous vessels. Surgical resection or embolization is the treatment of choice for cavernous hemangioma.

Fibromatosis

There are a variety of fibrous lesions that occur within the musculoskeletal system, but aggressive fibromatosis (extra-abdominal desmoid) is the most common and troublesome. Aggressive fibromatosis is an infiltrative benign fibrous lesion. It can occur in any location within the musculoskeletal system and at any age. It is composed of dense collagen and fibroblasts. The histologic appearance is identical to that of Dupuytren's and plantar's fibromatosis. Surgical resection is recommended.

Benign Tumors of Nerve Origin

There are two common benign tumors that arise from nerves: neurilemomas and neurofibromas.

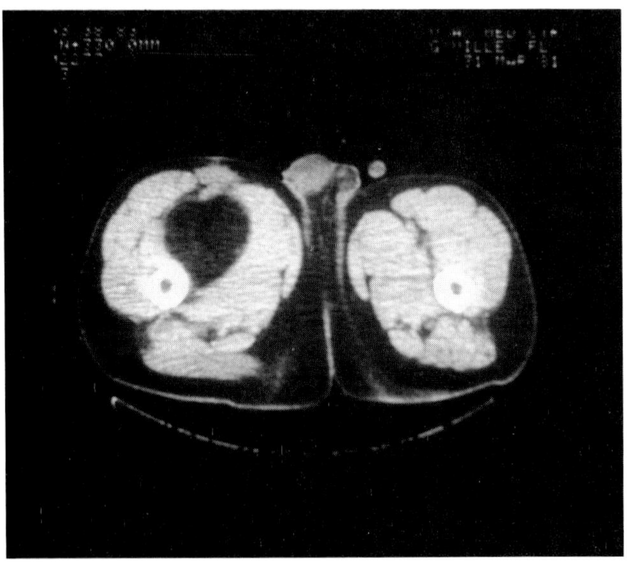

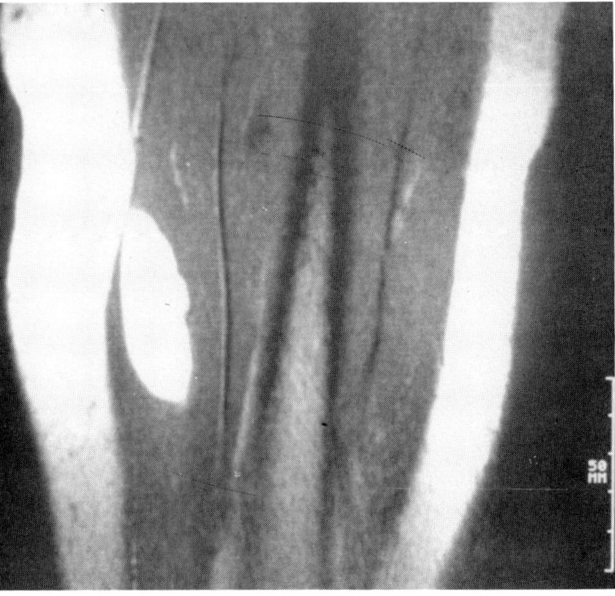

Figure 61
Lipoma. **Left,** On the CT scan the entire lesion has the density of fat (approximately -70 Hounsfield units). **Right,** On an MRI a lipoma has all the signal characteristics of normal fat regardless of the TR and TE settings. This lipoma is easily seen and has the same signal as the subcutaneous fat on this T1-weighted image.

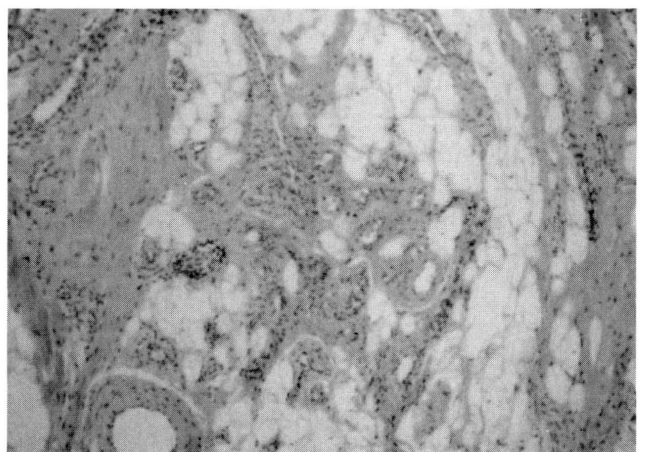

Figure 62
Hemangioma (10X). These benign lesions, also called arteriovenous malformations, are composed of numerous vessels (venous, arterial, or a combination) and fat.

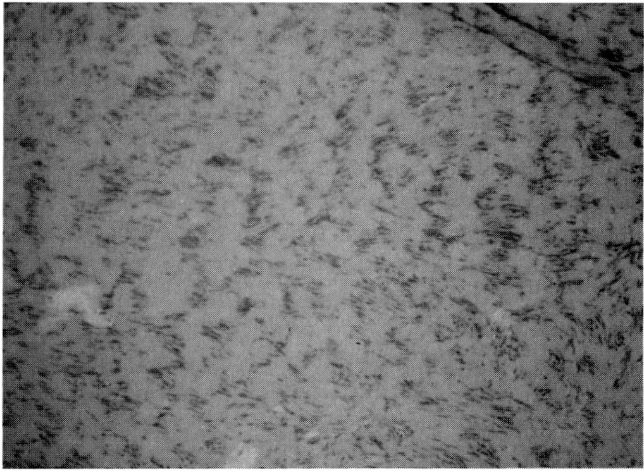

Figure 63
Neurilemoma (10X). This benign tumor of the nerve sheath, also called Schwannoma, has a classic Antoni A type appearance with the nuclei palisaded one on top of the other.

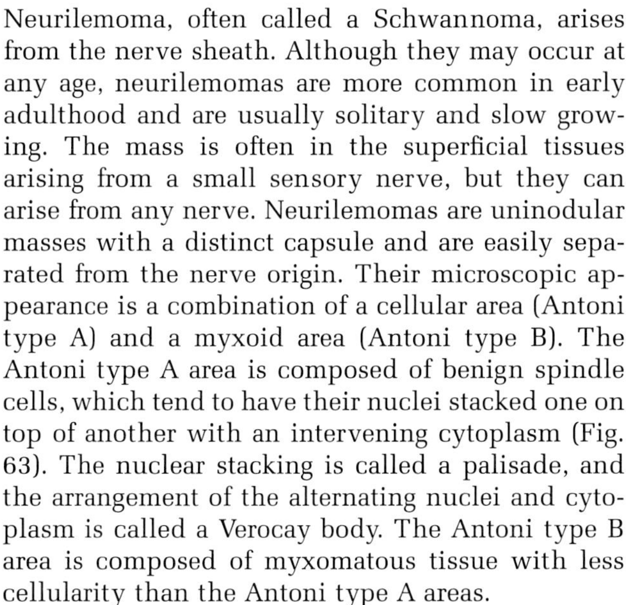

Neurilemoma, often called a Schwannoma, arises from the nerve sheath. Although they may occur at any age, neurilemomas are more common in early adulthood and are usually solitary and slow growing. The mass is often in the superficial tissues arising from a small sensory nerve, but they can arise from any nerve. Neurilemomas are uninodular masses with a distinct capsule and are easily separated from the nerve origin. Their microscopic appearance is a combination of a cellular area (Antoni type A) and a myxoid area (Antoni type B). The Antoni type A area is composed of benign spindle cells, which tend to have their nuclei stacked one on top of another with an intervening cytoplasm (Fig. 63). The nuclear stacking is called a palisade, and the arrangement of the alternating nuclei and cytoplasm is called a Verocay body. The Antoni type B area is composed of myxomatous tissue with less cellularity than the Antoni type A areas.

Neurofibromas may be solitary or multiple. Patients with multiple neurofibromas are said to have von Recklinghausen's disease. The majority of patients, 90% or more, have a solitary lesion. The lesion may arise in the skin, from a small sensory nerve, or from a major peripheral nerve. Unlike neurilemomas, neurofibromas tend to be intimately associated with the nerve fibers and are often difficult to separate from the nerve of origin. Neurofibromas are not encapsulated and are composed of elongated wavy cells with dark nuclei. Patients with solitary neurilemomas and neurofibromas have an insignificant incidence of malignant degeneration; however, patients with von Recklinghausen's disease have a significant incidence of developing a neurofibroma.

Rhabdomyosarcoma

Rhabdomyosarcoma is a malignant tumor of muscle. Once rhabdomyosarcoma was thought to occur in adults, but the majority of those lesions identified as rhabdomyosarcoma in adults have been reclassified as malignant fibrous histiocytoma. Rhabdomyosarcoma occurs almost exclusively in patients younger than 15 years of age. It accounts for approximately 3.5% of childhood malignancies, with approximately 350 new cases per year in the United States. There are four histologic subtypes: embryonal, botryoid, alveolar, and pleomorphic. Botryoid type is histologically identical to embryonal type, but its gross appearance is different because it arises in a hollow viscus. Pleomorphic rhabdomyosarcoma is the least common histologic type, is most common in extremities, and occurs principally in young adults. Embryonal rhabdomyosarcoma is the most common type; it usually arises in the head, neck, genitourinary tract, or retroperitoneum; it occurs in the first decade of life. Alveolar rhabdomyosarcoma occurs in the extremity. The patients, who are usually between 10 and 25 years of age, complain of the presence of a mass. Rhabdomyosarcoma consists of poorly differentiated rhabdomyoblasts with a limited collagen matrix. Rhabdomyoblasts are small, round cells with dark-staining nuclei and a limited amount of eosinophilic cytoplasm (Fig. 64). Alveolar rhabdomyosarcoma is composed of small round tumor cells loosely arranged together in groups by dense collagen bundles, producing an alveolar appearance. Patients with rhabdomyosarcoma are treated initially with chemotherapy and then with either irradiation or a surgical resection.

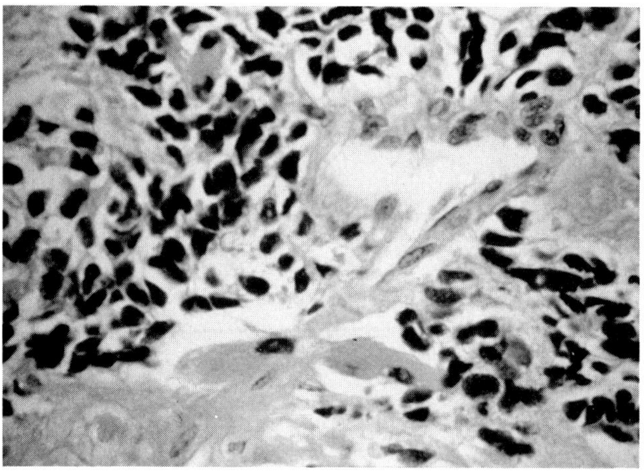

Figure 64
Rhabdomyosarcoma (40X). This most common malignant solid tumor of children is distinctly rare in adults. It commonly involves the head and neck regions or genitourinary system. The tumor is composed of small dark blue cells that invade the local soft tissues.

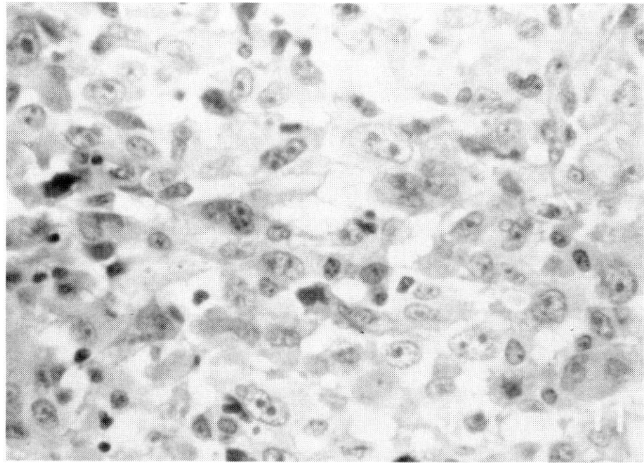

Figure 65
Malignant fibrous histiocytoma (40X). Common features include large bizarre malignant cells, a storiform pattern, necrosis, and abnormal mitotic figures. Large malignant cells with double nucleoli and abnormal mitoses are seen on this high-power photomicrograph.

Malignant Fibrous Histiocytoma

Malignant fibrous histiocytoma is the most common malignant soft-tissue tumor in adults. There is a similar, but less common, lesion that occurs within bone. Malignant fibrous histiocytoma of soft tissue is more common in patients over 50 years of age, and it may involve the subcutaneous tissue or deep structures. White males are the most commonly affected group. Histologic subtypes include storiform pleomorphic (the most common), myxoid, giant cell, and inflammatory. The lower extremity is the most common location, as it is for all soft tissue sarcomas. The patients complain of a mass. The tumor contains a mixture of collagen arranged in a storiform pattern with pleomorphic malignant cells (Fig. 65). The variation in cell morphology is great, and large, bizarre cells are the hallmark of malignant fibrous histiocytoma. Surgical resection is the treatment of choice.

Liposarcoma

Liposarcoma is a malignant soft-tissue tumor arising from lipoblasts. Liposarcoma and malignant fibrous histiocytoma account for the majority of soft-tissue sarcomas, each being approximately 20% of all soft-tissue sarcomas. Patients with liposarcoma are most often between 40 and 60 years of age. Liposarcomas are usually deep tumors, located most commonly in the thigh or retroperitoneum. It is rare for them to arise in a preexisting lipoma. Subtypes include myxoid, round cell, well differentiated, and pleomorphic. Myxoid liposarcoma is the most common subtype (up to 50%), and consists of lipoblasts of varying maturity, a plexiform capillary system, and a myxoid matrix (Fig. 66). Surgical resection is the treatment of choice.

Synovial Cell Sarcoma

Synovial cell sarcoma is a malignant tumor of soft tissue, the cellular characteristics of which suggest that it arises from primitive synovial cells. However, the tumor rarely occurs within a joint; it is usually located in the deep soft tissues near the joint. It accounts for 10% of all soft-tissue sarcomas. Most patients are between 15 and 35 years of age, and males predominate slightly. Synovial cell sarcoma has a higher than usual incidence of spread to

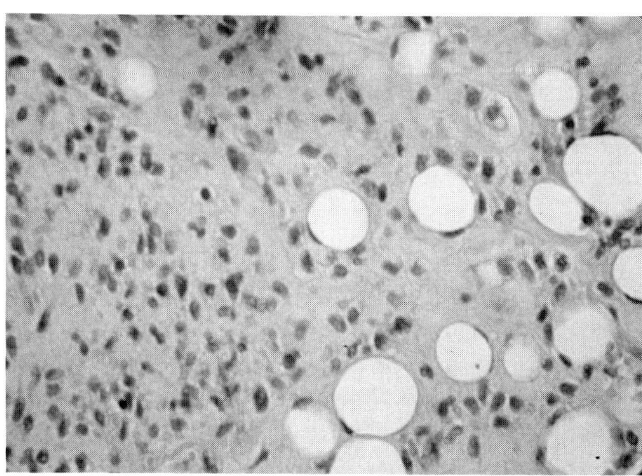

Figure 66
Liposarcoma (40X). Photomicrograph shows a few almost normal fat cells combined with nondescript small round cells with a myxoid extracellular ground substance.

regional lymphatic structures when compared to other soft-tissue sarcomas, and up to 25% of these tumors will have lymph node metastasis. The head, neck, and trunk account for 15% of lesions, and the upper and lower extremities account for over half. Almost 10% arise in the hands or feet. Synovial cell sarcoma may have calcification or ossification within the tumor, which may be seen on a radiograph. The characteristic histologic findings are a biphasic tumor with epithelioid cells (resembling a carcinoma) and spindle cells. Usually, the spindle cell component predominates. Surgical resection is the treatment of choice.

Fibrosarcoma

Fibrosarcoma is a malignant soft-tissue tumor of fibroblastic origin. It is clinically indistinguishable from other malignant soft-tissue tumors. It is most common between the ages of 30 and 55 and is found most often in the thigh. Fibrosarcomas are composed of uniform spindle cells and a collagenous matrix arranged in a herringbone pattern. Surgical resection is the treatment of choice.

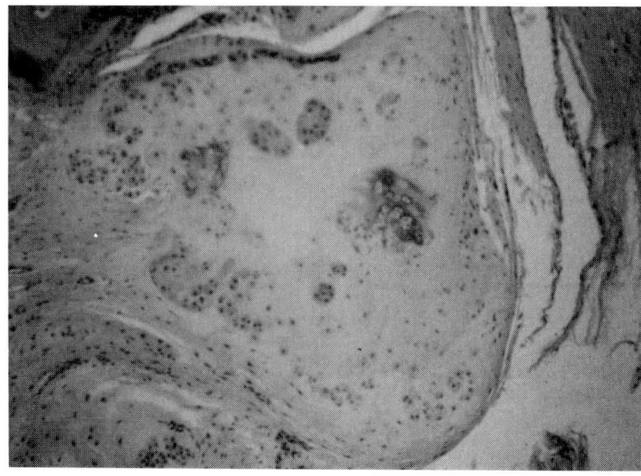

Figure 67
Synovial chondromatosis (10X). Nodules of cartilage protrude into the joint and often become detached to become loose bodies; a typical nodule of cartilage is seen on this low-power photomicrograph.

Primary Synovial Tumors

Synovial Chondromatosis

Synovial chondromatosis is a disorder of the subsynovial cell. These cells produce nodules of cartilage, which are extruded into the joint and become loose bodies (Fig. 67). The cartilaginous loose bodies can enlarge while free within the joint because they continue to receive nutrition from the synovial fluid. They may develop central calcification or, if reattached to the synovial surface and vascularized, undergo enchondral ossification. Whether calcified or ossified the cartilaginous loose bodies are visible on plain radiographs. The knee is the most commonly involved joint, accounting for approximately 75% of cases. Synovial chondromatosis occurs in both sexes and all age groups; the patient complains of mild joint pain and effusion, and often locking. Management of the disorder should be symptomatic. Most patients with swelling, pain, and locking are improved by removal of the loose bodies and excision of all grossly abnormal synovium.

Pigmented Villonodular Synovitis

Pigmented villonodular synovitis is a process involving the synovium, which is characterized by hypertrophic synovium with areas of brown or yellow villi and nodules. The synovium contains a fibrous stroma, histiocytes, mutinucleated giant cells, and hemosiderin. These findings are seen in joints, tendon sheaths, or bursae. Three-quarters of the cases involve the knee, with the hip, shoulder, and elbow accounting for most of the other cases. The patients may be any age. They have chronic effusion and mild pain. Aspiration of the joint reveals a blood- or hemosiderin-stained fluid. The diagnosis can usually be made from the characteristic irregular surface of the synovium on an arthrogram. The hypertrophic synovium can invade the bone. Surgical synovectomy is the treatment of choice. The incidence of recurrence is up to 40%, and intra-articular injection of radioactive materials has been used to treat recurrent disease.

Suggested Reading List

Molecular Biology

Alberts B, Bray D, Lewis J, et al (eds): *Molecular Biology of the Cell,* ed 2. New York, Garland Publishing, 1989.

Erlich HA: *PCR Technology: Principles and Applications for DNA Amplification.* New York, Stockton Press, 1989.

Lewin B: *Genes,* ed 3. New York, John Wiley & Sons, 1987.

Sambrook J, Fritsch EF, Maniatis T: *Molecular Cloning: A Laboratory Manual,* ed 2. Cold Spring Harbor, NY, Cold Spring Harbor Laboratory Press, 1989, vols 1, 2, and 3.

Watson JD, Hopkins NH, Roberts JW, et al: *Molecular Biology of the Gene,* ed 4. Menlo Park, CA, Benjamin/Cummings Publishing Company, 1987, vols 1 and 2.

Watson JD, Tooze J, Kurtz DT: *Recombinant DNA: A Short Course.* New York, Scientific American Books, 1983.

Weinberg RA: Finding the anti-oncogene. *Sci Am* 1988;259:44–51.

White R, Lalouel J-M: Chromosome mapping with DNA markers. *Sci Am* 1988;258:40–48.

Immunobiology

Goldberg VM: The immunology of articular cartilage, in Moskowitz RW, Howell DS, Goldberg VM, et al: *Osteoarthritis Diagnosis and Management.* Philadelphia, WB Saunders, 1984, pp 81–92.

Goldberg VM, Powell A, Schaffer JW, et al: Bone Grafting: Role of histocompatibility in transplantation. *J Orthop Res* 1985;3:389–404.

Horowitz MC, Friedlaender GE: Induction of specific T-cell responsiveness to allogeneic bone. *J Bone Joint Surg* 1991;73A:1157–1168.

Stevenson S: The immune response to osteochondral allografts in dogs. *J Bone Joint Surg* 1987;69A:573–582.

Rheumatoid Arthritis

Scott DG, Bacon PA, Tribe CR: Systemic rheumatoid vasculitis: A clinical and laboratory study of 50 cases. *Medicine (Baltimore)* 1981;60:288–297.

Weisman M, Zvaifler N: Cryoimmunoglobulinemia in rheumatoid arthritis: Significance in serum of patients with rheumatoid vasculitis. *J Clin Invest* 1975;56:725–739.

Zvaifler NJ: Rheumatoid arthritis, in Schumacher HR, Klippel JH, Robinson DR (eds): *Primer on the Rheumatic Diseases,* ed 9. Atlanta, Arthritis Foundation, 1988, pp 83–87.

Zvaifler NJ: Etiology and pathogenesis of rheumatoid arthritis, in McCarty DJ (ed): *Arthritis and Allied Conditions: A Textbook of Rheumatology,* ed 10. Philadelphia, Lea & Febiger, 1985, pp 557–570.

Gout

Holmes EW: Clinical gout and the pathogenesis of hyperuricemia, in McCarty DJ (ed): *Arthritis and Allied Conditions: A Textbook of Rheumatology,* ed 10. Philadelphia, Lea & Febiger, 1985, pp 1445–1480.

McCarty DJ: Crystal identification in human synovial fluids: Methods and interpretation. *Rheum Dis Clin North Am* 1988;14:253–267.

Palmer DG, Highton J, Hessian PA: Development of the gout tophus: An hypothesis. *Am J Clin Pathol* 1989;91:190–195.

Puig JG, Michan AD, Jimenez ML, et al: Female gout: Clinical spectrum and uric acid metabolism. *Arch Intern Med* 1991;151:726–732.

Resnick D: Common disorders of synovium-lined joints: Pathogenesis, imaging abnormalities, and complications. *AJR* 1988;151:1079–1093.

Schumacher HR Jr: Pathology of crystal deposition diseases. *Rheum Dis Clin North Am* 1988;14:269–288.

Terkeltaub RA, Ginsberg MH: The inflammatory reaction to crystals. *Rheum Dis Clin North Am* 1988;14:353–364.

Calcium Pyrophosphate Deposition Disease

Doherty M: Calcium pyrophosphate deposition disease and other crystal deposition diseases. *Curr Opin Rheumatol* 1990;2:789–796.

McCarty DJ: Calcium pyrophosphate dehydrate crystal deposition disease, in Schumacher HR, Klippel JH, Robinson DR (eds): *Primer on the Rheumatic Diseases,* ed 9. Atlanta, Arthritis Foundation, 1988, pp 207–210.

Calcium Crystal Deposition Diseases

Dieppe PA: Apatite and other miscellaneous calcium crystal deposition diseases, in Schumacher HR, Klippel JH, Robinson DR (eds): *Primer on the Rheumatic Diseases,* ed 9. Atlanta, Arthritis Foundation, 1988, pp 211–213.

Seronegative Spondyloarthropathies

Khan MA, Skosey JL: Ankylosing spondylitis and related spondyloarthropathies, in Samter M, Talmage DW, Frank MM, et al (eds): *Immunological Diseases,* ed 4. Boston, Little, Brown and Company, 1988, pp 1509–1538.

Neoplastic Diseases

Beauchamp CP, Duncan CP, Dzus AK, et al: Osteoblastoma: Experience with 23 patients. *Can J Surg* 1992;35:199–202.

Campanacci M, Capanna R, Picci P: Unicameral and aneurysmal bone cysts. *Clin Orthop* 1986;204:25–36.

Eckardt JJ (ed): Newest knowledge of osteosarcoma. *Clin Orthop* 1991;270:2–312.

Goldenberg RR, Campbell CJ, Bonfiglio M: Giant-cell tumor of bone: An analysis of two hundred and eighteen cases. *J Bone Joint Surg* 1970;52A:619–664.

Harris WH, Dudley HR Jr, Barry RJ: The natural history of fibrous dysplasia: An orthopaedic, pathological, and roentgenographic study. *J Bone Joint Surg* 1962;44A:207–233.

Healey JH, Ghelman B: Osteoid osteoma and osteoblastoma: Current concepts and recent advances. *Clin Orthop* 1986;204:76–85.

O'Connor MI, Pritchard DJ: Ewing's sarcoma: Prognostic factors, disease control, and the reemerging role of surgical treatment. *Clin Orthop* 1991;262:78–87.

Szendroi M, Cser I, Konya A, et al: Aneurysmal bone cyst: A review of 52 primary and 16 secondary cases. *Arch Orthop Trauma Surg* 1992;116:318–322.

Chapter 7
Bone Injury, Regeneration, and Repair

Robert F. Ostrum, MD
Edmund Y.S. Chao, PhD
C. Andrew L. Bassett, MD, ScD, LHD
Carl T. Brighton, MD
Thomas A. Einhorn, MD
Tyler S. Lucas, MD
Hannu T. Aro, MD
Myron Spector, PhD

Chapter Outline

Injury to bone can have a multitude of causes. Infection, tumor, genetic disorders, and many others can all produce changes in bone that could be considered injurious to this tissue. Bone injury from any cause must be viewed in terms of its effect on the cellular content of bone, the ability of such cells to produce extracellular matrix, and the structure and organization of the organic and inorganic components of bone itself. This chapter describes those injuries to bone caused by circulatory loss and physical injury, because such injuries jeopardize cell viability and structural integrity. Injury to one affects the other; loss of cell viability will directly and indirectly affect the structural organization of bone. Similarly structural repair necessitates cellular changes. In the strictest sense, bone repair is a regenerative process that brings about changes in all aspects of the organ system. In this chapter, each type of bone injury is discussed along with the ways in which the system as a whole responds to injury. Depending on the nature of the injury and the proposed method of repair, certain aspects of the process play a predominant role, but the underlying reactions and principles remain the same and need to be understood if normal functioning bone is to be maintained.

Osteonecrosis

Osteonecrosis can arise from a variety of disorders. The term itself, defined as the in situ death of a segment of bone, actually refers to the death of the cells within bone from lack of circulation, not from disease. Unless secondary effects occur, the organic and inorganic matrix of the structural components of bone are not affected; dead bone refers to dead cells. Such cells include osteocytes, whether they are in cortical or cancellous bone, and usually include the cells of the hematopoietic and fatty marrow contents as well. The term osteonecrosis is preferred to such commonly used terms as avascular necrosis and aseptic necrosis because (1) it is the most appropriate description of the histopathologic process seen, and (2) it doesn't suggest any specific etiology.

Etiology

Osteonecrotic bone is not avascular; the vessels are still present. However, in all causative mechanisms of osteonecrosis, the circulation within the vessels is compromised. Such compromise may be grouped into four mechanisms: (1) mechanical disruption of the vessels, (2) occlusion of the arterial vessels, (3) injury to or pressure on the arterial wall, and (4) occlusion to the venous outflow vessels. Mechanical vascular disruption may result from a fracture or dislocation, or from such atraumatic events as stress, fatigue fractures, or similar events. Arterial occlusion can arise from thromboses, embolism, circulating fat, nitrogen bubbles, or abnormally shaped cells (sickle cell crises). Temporary or permanent damage to an intact vessel wall can arise from within the wall as in vasculitis or radiation injury, from within the vessel as in the release of materials that can cause angiospasm, or from external pressure or chemical reaction on the wall as in extravasated blood, fat, or cellular elements in the marrow cavity. In a closed system, if the circulation in the venous outflow is compromised by any of these mechanisms so that venous pressure exceeds arterial pressure, circulation to the cells supplied by this source will be compromised. If a sufficient collateral circulation is present at any site where such compromise occurs, cells remain viable. Because bone has a rich blood supply that varies widely from site to site, only cells in certain locations seem susceptible to becoming nonviable.

Osteonecrosis can be the result of trauma. A displaced fractured femoral neck, dislocation of the femoral head, displaced fracture of the scaphoid, displaced fracture of the talar neck, and a four-part fracture of the humeral head are the most common traumatic injuries leading to osteonecrosis and its clinically significant secondary complications of collapse of the subchondral bone and adjacent articular surface. The osteonecrosis associated with infection (osteomyelitis or pyarthrosis) is thought to be produced by the combination of increased intramedullary pressure and arterial occlusion. In cases in which osteonecrosis is associated with Gaucher's disease, the marrow cavity is packed with Gaucher's cells (macrophages filled with cerebroside). In cases in which it is associated with sickle-cell disease, the marrow cavity is packed with sickled red blood cells. The osteonecrosis in these last two diseases seems to result from direct occlusion of the intraosseous arteries. The osteonecrosis associated with decompression sickness, so-called caisson's disease, probably is caused by vascular occlusion by nitrogen bubbles that come out of solution with the rapid drop in barometric pressure. Osteonecrosis after irradiation of bone probably occurs as a result of radiation damage to the capillaries. It also occurs in association with ethanol abuse, corticosteroid administration, hyperlipidemia, pancreatitis, and, very often, in otherwise normal individuals (idiopathic osteonecrosis).

Idiopathic osteonecrosis and osteonecrosis associated with ethanol or corticosteroids account for the vast majority of cases of nontraumatic osteonecrosis. The mechanism(s) that cause osteonecrosis in these patients are unknown. In fact, there is some evidence to suggest that the use of corticosteroids in renal transplant subjects may not be the causative agent related to the osteonecrosis associated with them. One proposed mechanism is arterial occlusion by fat emboli (Fig. 1); it is postulated that the fat emboli arise from a fatty liver, from plasma lipoproteins, or directly from marrow fat. There is experimental evidence supporting this mechanism, but whether it is the cause of osteonecrosis in a significant percent of humans is not known. A popular explanation for idiopathic osteonecrosis, especially that seen in the femoral head, is intraosseous hypertension. The theory is that the intraosseous vessels are occluded secondary to excessive pressure within the medullary canal. The cause of the suspected intraosseous hypertension is not known. Although measurement of the intraosseous pressure of bones with early osteonecrosis reveals increased pressure, it is not clear whether this pressure is a cause or an effect or, as some believe, an artifact of the measuring devices. The only conclusion that should be made is that the cause of osteonecrosis in the majority of cases still is not adequately understood.

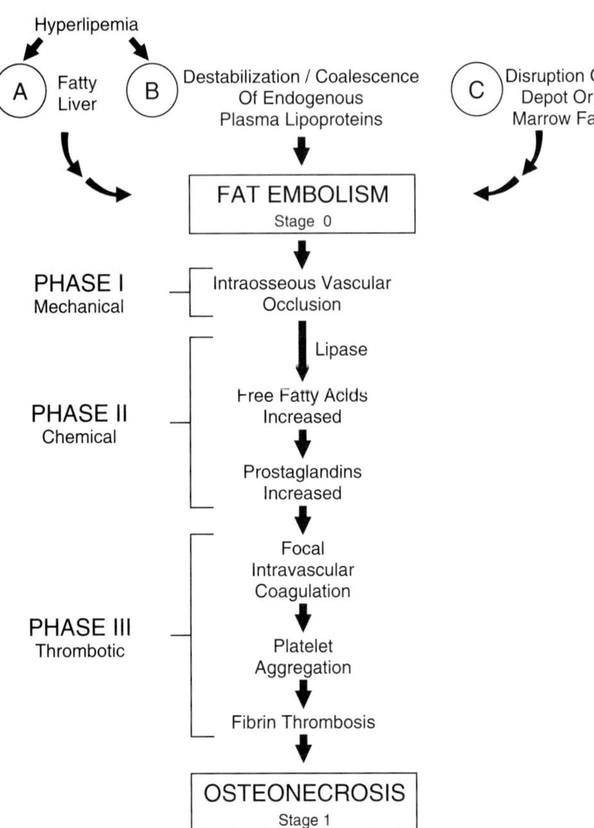

Figure 1
Schematic representation of three mechanisms potentially capable of producing intraosseous fat embolism and triggering a process leading to focal intravascular coagulation and osteonecrosis. (Reproduced with permission from Jones JP Jr: Fat embolism and osteonecrosis. *Clin Orthop* 1985;16:595–633.)

Cellular Bone Injury

Regardless of the inciting disorder, the morphologic processes of osteonecrosis are very similar. Initially and for the first few days to one week after vascular compromise has been initiated, there are no histologic changes. During the second week, the marrow contents begin to show evidence of necrosis, including death of hematopoietic cells, capillary endothelial cells, and lipocytes. The shrinking of the osteocytes produces the empty lacunae typical of necrotic bone. The death of cells within the fatty marrow releases lysosomes, and the tissue becomes acidified. Released calcium forms an insoluble soap with the free fatty acids released from dead lipocytes. Normal fatty marrow has little water; however, after it becomes necrotic, the early changes are associated with increased water. It is this change in water content that is the first abnormality that can be detected clinically. This change can be seen on a magnetic resonance imaging scan (MRI). The MRI measures the alignment of hydrogen ions and, because water is the principal source of these hydrogen ions in humans, it is quite sensitive to the water content of tissues.

Repair of Osteonecrotic Bone

The remainder of the events associated with osteonecrosis are related to replacement of the acellular bone and the time it takes for this process to occur. The initiation of repair can occur only if the surrounding viable cellular tissues receive some signal to suggest that such a process is needed. In some sites and where the area of cell death is small no signal appears to be generated to initiate this process; the bone "infarct" remains for life. If they are small enough and in an area that does not compromise the structural integrity of the bone, such lesions will be clinically silent, nonprogressive, and may be detected only as an incidental finding on an MRI or bone scan related to intramarrow fluid changes or mild peripheral reactive changes, respectively. Commonly, this occurs when necrosis of cells involves only the medullary bone with no involvement of the subchondral plate; in this situation, no symptoms and no functional abnormalities result. The necrotic tissues, especially the saponified fats, calcify and may be seen on plain radiographs forever.

If osteonecrosis involves cortical cancellous bone and a reparative response is initiated, a reactive hyperemia and vascular fibrous repair are first noted in the adjacent bony tissues. The subsequent events appear identical to those that occur with the incorporation of a bone graft and are commonly referred to as creeping substitution. Revascularization of the necrotic bone from the adjacent fibrous tissue is noted within a few weeks. Vessels grow into the medullary canal to revascularize the cancellous bone and into the haversian canals of the cortex. In the cortical bone their histologic appearance is that of "cutting cones," and is similar to what is seen at the metaphyseal end of the growth plate. At both sites, primitive mesenchymal cells accompany the vessels and differentiate into osteoblasts and osteoclasts. It is not known what stimulates the differentiation of the undifferentiated mesenchymal cells, but it is likely to be one or several bone morphogenic proteins from the necrotic bone. Other local factors, including pH, oxygen tension, and mechanical stress, also influence the differentiation of the mesenchymal cells.

In cancellous bone, the next event is the production of osteoid on the scaffolding of the necrotic trabeculae (Fig. 2). The trabeculae are thickened by the new viable bone, and, as a result, the early repair of the cancellous bone increases the density of the bone. This density, which is the result of new bone applied "over" old bone, may not reflect the strength of a similarly dense bone undergoing normal remodeling. Although calcification of necrotic marrow may account for some of the increased density seen within the osteonecrotic bone in the early stages of osteonecrosis, the majority of the changes seen on plain radiographs of osteonecrotic subchondral bone are caused by the increased size of the individual trabeculae. The appearance of the increased density requires a substantial amount of new bone formation and on plain radiographs is not obvious until between six and 12 months after the onset of necrosis.

In necrotic cortical bone, the bone in the haversian canals is reabsorbed before new bone is produced. The primitive mesenchymal cells differentiate into osteoclasts, and resorption of the necrotic haversian bone begins just after vascular invasion. Resorption continues until the majority of the haversian bone, but almost none of the interlamellar bone, has been reabsorbed. Then osteoblasts begin the process of replacing the haversian system (Fig 3). Thus, cortical bone first becomes osteoporotic and regains its original density only after it has been repaired. This resorption weakens the cortical bone, which explains the fractures observed at 18 to 24 months after the onset of necrosis. It takes that long to resorb enough bone for a pathologic fracture to occur. As the repair of the necrotic bone continues, the density, as seen on the radiograph, and the strength return to normal. This process takes at least two years.

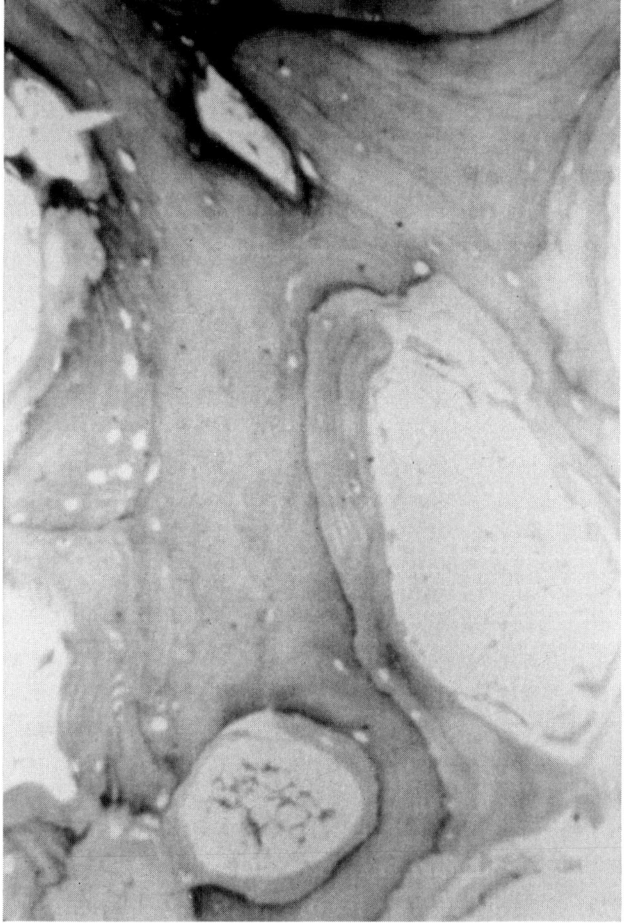

Figure 2
Photomicrograph showing the beginning of creeping substitution.

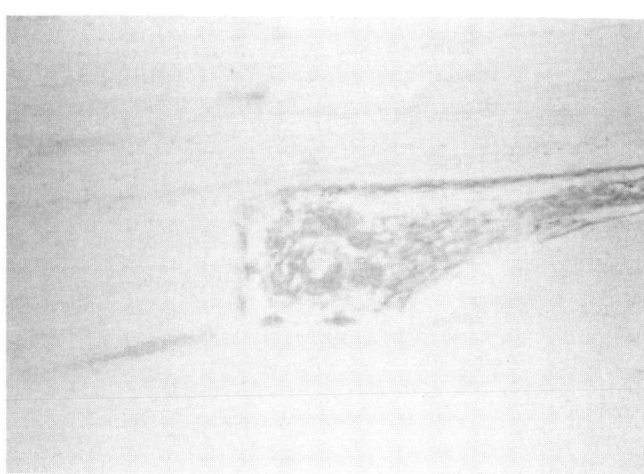

Figure 3
Photomicrograph showing a cortical cutting cone boring its way into necrotic cortex.

Structural Sequelae

Necrotic bone initially has no alteration in its mechanical properties; osteonecrosis directly affects only the cells, and structurally the bone functions normally. If, however, the osteonecrosis involves the subchondral bone, the bone eventually fractures, collapses, and leads to irregularities in the articular surface and, subsequently, to degenerative arthritis. All evidence indicates that this is a secondary mechanical phenomenon that occurs over time as a result of the absence of cells to respond to the effects of the continuation of normal daily activities. The fracture and collapse appear to be the result of multiple fatigue fractures that cannot be repaired and that are caused by repetitive loading of the bone during continued patient function. They seem to be initiated in areas of bone where: (1) the remaining avascular subchondral trabeculae oriented perpendicular to the joint surface lack the means to repair small microfractures; (2) the resorption of the subchondral bone at the periphery, where there is vascular invasion of the necrotic bone, results in osteoporotic "weakened" bone; or (3) the junction of increased bone density at the front of revascularization results in a stress riser between it and adjacent avascular bone. Prior to complete fracture and collapse, the microfractures can elicit a pain response. If functional activities are reduced, viable bone within or surrounding the osteonecrotic bone area undergoes a reduction in bone mass. The relative increased density of unresorbed necrotic bone compared to the adjacent viable osteoporotic bone permits the recognition of necrotic bone on plain radiographs. In the talus, Hawkins' sign is evidence of resorption of atrophic bone and is used to document that the bone is alive. When subchondral osteopenia is not seen, the bone is not being reabsorbed because it is necrotic.

Clinical Effects

The severity and significance of the clinical syndrome in osteonecrosis depends on the size and site of its occurrence. Involvement at the hip versus shoulder versus talus versus the foot or hand illustrates a descending order of disability, although not necessarily easier or more favorable prognoses from treatment in correcting or substituting for the osteonecrotic bone. Because treatment at different intervals in the course of the syndrome can be different and offers different prognoses, various clinical staging systems have been proposed for osteonecrosis. These have focused mainly on the femoral head and are based on the appearance of the osteonecrotic bone on the plain radiograph. These systems, which actually classify the process of repair, degree

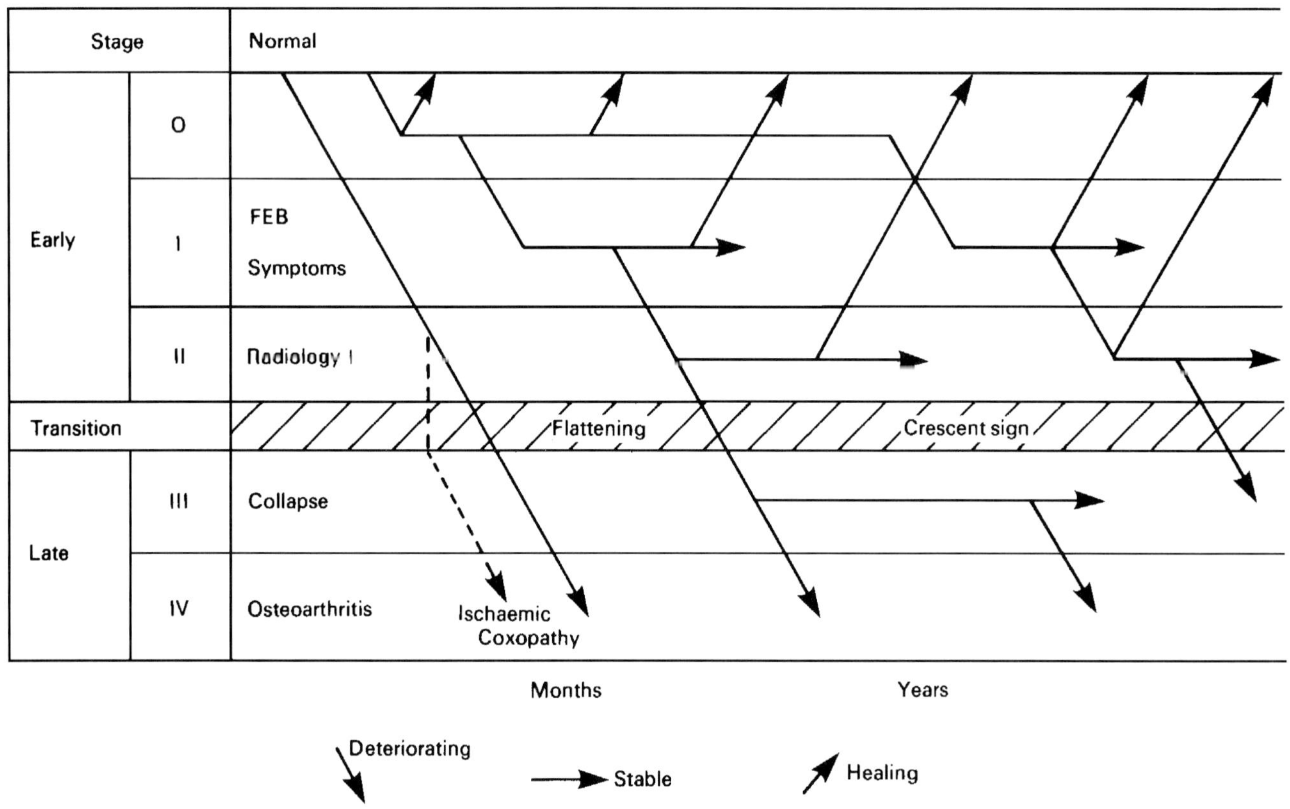

Figure 4
Diagram of the evolution of osteonecrosis. (Reproduced with permission from Ficat RP: Idiopathic bone necrosis of the femoral head. *J Bone Joint Surg* 1985;67B:3–9.)

of collapse, and degenerative changes that result from the collapse, are not a classification of osteonecrosis (Fig. 4 and Tables 1 and 2). With the introduction of MRI and the earlier recognition of osteonecrosis, new staging systems are being examined.

Table 1
Staging system for osteonecrosis

Stage	Symptoms
Stage 1	No symptoms Mottled areas of increased density on plain radiographs Histologic necrosis with areas of creeping substitution
Stage 2	No symptoms Reactive zone around infarct on plain radiographs Histologic evidence of advancing fibrovascular repair with creeping substitution
Stage 3	Onset of pain Crescent sign with no or minimal collapse on plain radiograph Subchondral fracture with intact cartilage
Stage 4	Increasing pain with activity Flattening of femoral head Collapse of the head with loose cartilage Continued creeping substitution
Stage 5	Increasing pain Flattened femoral head and early acetabular changes on plain radiographs Erosion of necrotic bone
Stage 6	Pain at rest Progressive flattening of femoral head and gross alterations of the acetabulum Little remaining necrotic bone and grossly destroyed joint

(Data taken from Marcus ND, Enneking WF, Masam RA: The silent hip in idiopathic aseptic necrosis. *J Bone Joint Surg* 1973;55A:1351–1366.)

Bone and Cartilage Grafting

The use and incorporation of a bone graft into the skeletal structure may be considered to be fundamentally the same as the process of bone repair or regeneration after osteonecrosis has occurred. A devascularized bone graft has no live cells, but has a structural scaffolding that, if needed, can be used for support. In its initial stages its mechanical structure has not changed significantly. The differences between the repair or regeneration of the osteonecrosis found in a bone graft and that commonly thought of as the clinical disease or syndrome of osteonecrosis relates to whether the bone arises from a source foreign to the host, whether a vascular network accompanies it, and the fact that, initially, no structural integrity exists between the host and the graft.

The biologic host response is significantly different between autogenic and allogeneic bone and, as in osteonecrosis, is different with either depending on whether the graft is composed of cancellous or cortical bone. Therefore, it is important to understand the biologic process of revascularization and graft incorporation not only as it relates to the type of bone needing to be regenerated but also to the source of the graft material.

Table 2
The stages of bone necrosis of the femoral head

Stage	Clinical Features	Radiographic Signs	Haemodynamics	Scintigram	Diagnosis Without Core Biopsy
Early					
0 Preclinical	0	0	+	Reduced uptake?	Impossible
I Preradiographic	+	0	++	Increased uptake	Impossible
II Before flattening of head or sequestrum formation	+	Diffuse porosis, sclerosis, or cysts	++	+	Probable
Transition		Flattening Crescent sign			
Late					
III Collapse	++	Broken contour of head Sequestrum Joint space normal	+ or normal	+	Certain
IV Osteoarthritis	+++	Flattened contour Decreased joint space Collapse of head	+	+	Arthritis

(Reproduced with permission from Ficat RP: Idiopathic bone necrosis of the femoral head. *J Bone Joint Surg* 1985;67B:3–9.)

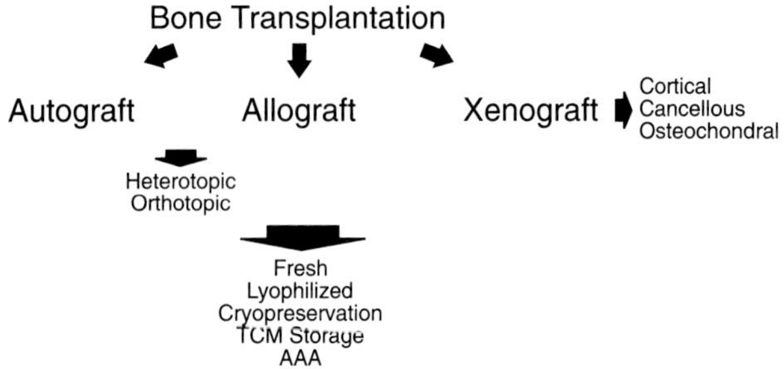

Figure 5
The nomenclature for graft materials, describing grafts by donor source, structural form, site of transplantation, and method of storage.

Figure 5 lists the current nomenclature for graft materials and describes grafts by the donor source, the structural form, the site of transplantation, and the method of storage. Tissue obtained from and implanted within the same individual is an autograft, and tissue obtained from a donor of the same species is an allograft. An orthotopic transplantation is implantation of tissue into an identical anatomic site; implantation into a distant anatomic site is called a heterotopic transplantation. Cancellous, cortical, and osteochondral grafts are currently in common clinical use as autografts or allografts.

Autogenic bone usually is used as a fresh graft. Allogeneic bone usually is stored frozen, lyophilized, or chemically sterilized; no viable cells remain. Osteochondral grafts can be used either fresh, cryopreserved, or after storage in a tissue culture environment. Each of these storage procedures significantly decreases the immunogenicity of allogeneic bone.

The incorporation of a bone graft, whether it is autogenic or allogeneic in origin, is a partnership between the transplanted tissue and the host bed into which it is placed. The graft contributions start with a passive osteoconduction, whereby the tissue acts as a trellis or scaffold for bony ingrowth of the host tissues. The graft then stimulates bone formation by the poorly understood but nonetheless real process of osteoinduction. Although a small fraction of the cells survive the transplant—more with cancellous than with cortical bone and more with rapid transplantation than with delayed, it is apparent that bone formation results from an osteoinductive recruitment of host blood vessels, which invade the graft. Figure 6 diagrams the major factors influencing bone graft incorporation. A bone graft dies after harvesting, and the success of the graft depends on the process of revascularization in its host bed. Most knowledge regarding graft incorporation comes from studies using the dog as a model.

Cancellous Grafts

For nonvascularized autogenous cancellous bone grafts, graft repair or regeneration is similar to that noted in osteonecroses of cancellous bone. The first phase is vascular ingrowth and progenitor mesenchymal cell invasion. For the dog model, this occurs during the first three weeks after implantation (Fig. 7, *top*). The second phase, which occurs in the dog model between three and 12 weeks after implantation, is a combination of osteoblastic appositional new bone formation onto the dead trabeculae of the graft and osteoclastic resorption of the graft trabeculae (Fig. 7, *middle*). The third phase, between three and six months after implantation, is that of remodeling and reorientation of the trabeculae to a mature pattern. This phase is influenced by the mechanical factors acting on the host bed. In this animal model, the process of remodeling becomes quiescent at one year after grafting (Fig. 7, *bottom*).

In a canine model, fresh cancellous bone allogeneic grafts (allografts), which do not cross major histocompatibility barriers, progress through the same sequence of incorporation steps, but twice as slowly (Fig. 8). The initial phase, which consists of hemorrhage and necrosis corresponding to the surgical placement of the graft, is identical to that for the autograft. The fibrin clot develops, and the same

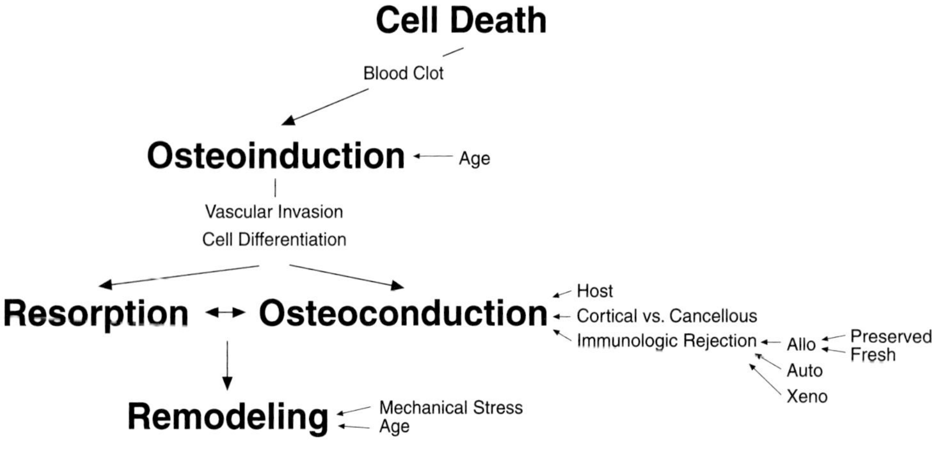

Figure 6
Major factors influencing bone graft incorporation.

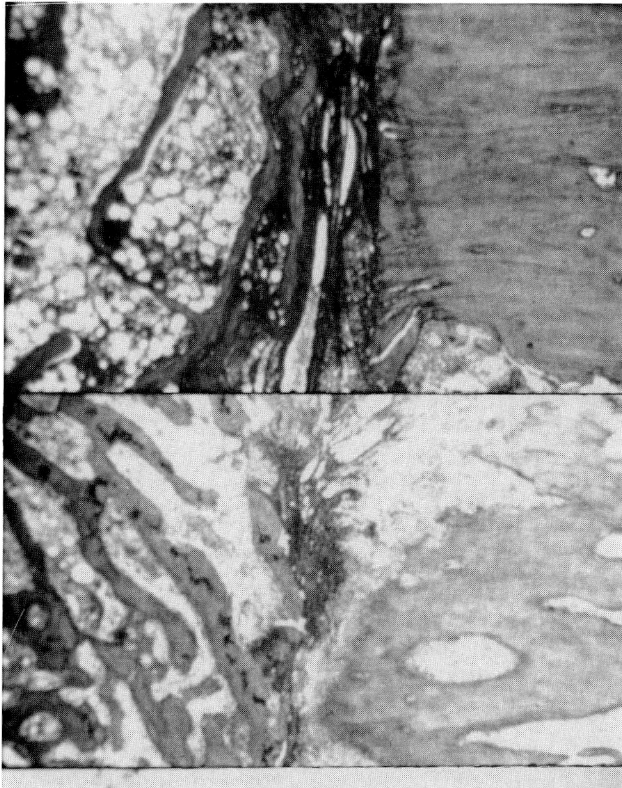

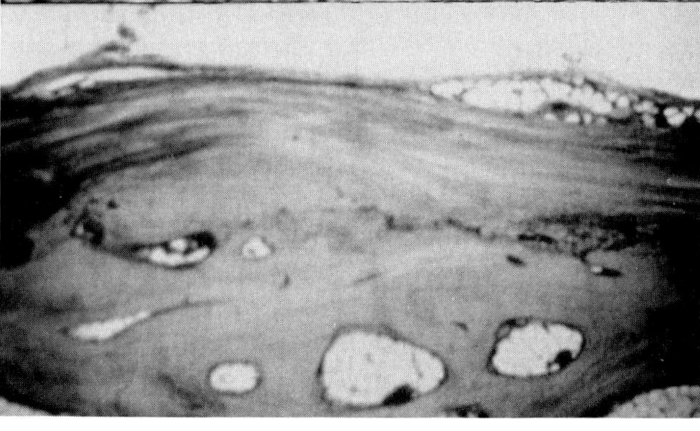

Figure 7
Composite photomicrograph showing transition from cancellous bone graft to reconstituted bone. **Top,** At one week the cancellous graft (left) is adjacent to the host cortex, and premature mesenchymal cells are accumulated at the junction. **Center,** At two weeks, new bone formation is noted in both the graft and the host. **Bottom,** By one year the autograft has been completely incorporated.

inflammatory response ensues. As in the autograft, increased vascularity in the adjacent tissues, dilation of the blood vessels, transudation, and exudation are noted but, perhaps, are greater in extent and degree.

At this point, however, the response appears to differ. The fibrin clot, clearly of great importance to the system, breaks down, and the loosely structured granulation tissue that serves as a source of cellular elements for repair becomes filled with chronic inflammatory cells rather than fibroblasts and blood vessel elements. The numbers of lymphocytes, plasma

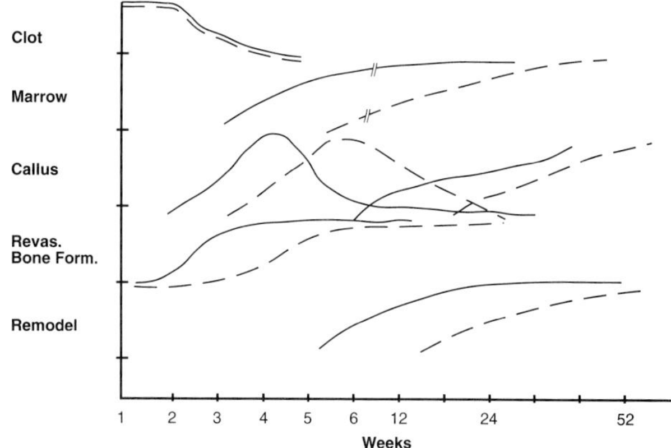

Figure 8
Time line for cancellous bone incorporation of autografts and allografts. Dashed lines are allografts.

cells, and mononuclear elements markedly increase. The major portion of the delay appears to occur in osteoclastic resorption and new bone formation. Final graft incorporation with remodeling may remain incomplete.

The use of these data in the clinical setting of patient care must be done with caution. In humans, clinical data and occasional histologic evaluation of cancellous grafts suggest that the same sequence of steps occurs, but the process takes place at approximately half the rate seen in canine studies, and large grafts may remodel even more slowly. The incorporation of allograft corticocancellous bone osteochondral segments has resulted in incomplete remodeling and incorporation of subchondral allogeneic bone as late as seven years after implantation.

Cortical Grafts

There are three major differences in incorporation of autogenous nonvascularized cortical bone in animal models as compared to that of cancellous bone grafts. First, the vascularization of cortical grafts is much slower and takes eight weeks for completion. Second, osteoclastic resorption must precede the osteoblastic new bone formation. Similar to the repair or regeneration in osteonecroses, the osteoclasts then form cutting cones within the donor bone; new bone is formed behind the cutting cones. The process is thus similarly termed creeping substitution. Third, during the process, autogenous cortical grafts generally do not demonstrate complete substitution with viable bone and, thus, are an admixture of necrotic graft bone and viable new host bone. The healing process begins at the host-graft cortical junction with bridging external enchondral bone formation from the host tissue during the first four to six weeks, followed by interstitial cortical osteoclasis and creeping substitution. The successful union between cortical graft and host bone

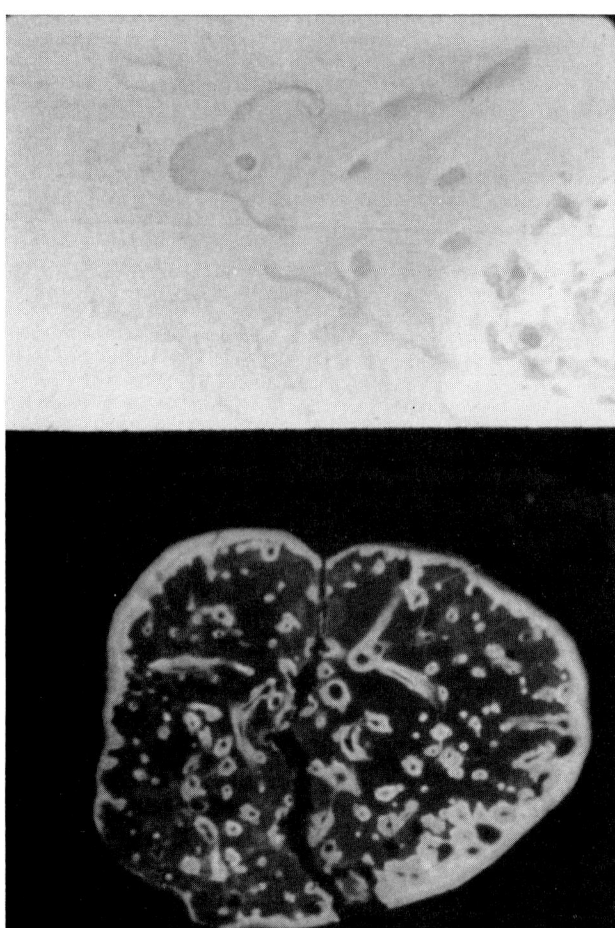

Figure 9
Photomicrograph demonstrating creeping substitution.

depends greatly upon secure and rigid osteosynthesis. Figure 9, *top,* is a photomicrograph demonstrating creeping substitution. Necrotic bone is seen on the left. New bone formation can be noted (to the right) about the haversian canal where necrotic bone has been first reabsorbed and then replaced by new bone. The bottom half of Figure 9 is a cross section of a fibular graft. Most of the cortical graft is necrotic, and numerous resorption cavities can be seen.

The function of an allograft as an osteoconductive system seems to be virtually unimpaired. With allogeneic tissues, the relationship between the transplanted tissue and the host bed into which it is placed remains functional, and the graft acts as a trellis or scaffold for bony ingrowth of the host tissues. The function of the graft as a stimulator of host bone formation by the process of osteoinduction, however, is much reduced and highly variable. Even without a significant chronic inflammatory response, which ordinarily is associated with altered immunity, the allogeneic part appears to have a very limited, or perhaps almost nonexistent, stimulatory effect on the host system.

Allograft cortical bone undergoes the same qualitative sequence of steps during graft incorporation as does autograft cortical bone. The length of time for creeping substitution is greatly prolonged in allogeneic cortical bone. The factors that stimulate host blood vessels to proliferate, invade the graft, and develop into cutting cones appear to be diminished, absent, or severely suppressed. Recruitment and differentiation of cellular elements to become both vascular invaders and the osteoblastic and osteoclastic elements essential to creeping substitution are reduced in extent and degree. Replacement of tissue by host bone is slow, and the stimulatory effect exerted on the host is virtually absent. New bone formation in either the host or the donor part is limited in degree, and repair of the host-donor junction site is also limited. Healing of a delayed or nonunion site in the host bone may respond to the mechanical aspects of the insertion of the graft, but most authorities consider that the allogeneic donor part contributes little in the form of osteoinduction. The proportion of necrotic graft bone to viable host bone is much greater in allogeneic grafts, and the active process of graft substitution may last several years.

On rare occasions, two special patterns of healing, or the lack thereof, are encountered after implantation of an allogeneic graft. Under circumstances as yet not well defined, the host soft tissues wall off the allogeneic part for an extended period of time, possibly years, and study of these tissues shows little or no vascular proliferation or attempt at invasion of the graft. Under other conditions, presumably immune directed, the graft is surrounded by inflammatory cells, is invaded rapidly by numerous blood vessels, and is destroyed. Following such a dissolution, the donor site may show no remnants of the implanted materials. Both of these responses are unusual, especially in human tissues, and, presumably, are opposite ends of the spectrum of host tissue reaction to the antigenic challenge.

Structural Properties of Cancellous Versus Cortical Grafts

The qualitative differences in graft incorporation between cancellous and cortical bone result in significant biomechanical differences. The incorporation of cancellous bone grafts with osteoblastic new bone formation onto the necrotic trabeculae of the graft tissue leads to an early increase in graft strength. Cortical bone grafts first undergo osteoclastic bone resorption, which significantly increases graft porosity. Figure 10 illustrates the quantitative temporal interrelationships between the physical integrity and the biologic processes of repair within a segmental autogenous cortical bone transplant. In the canine model, cortical grafts show the greatest compromise in mechanical strength at 12 weeks.

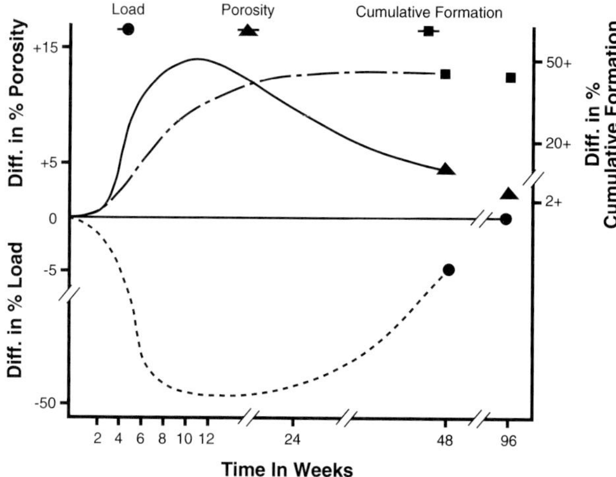

Figure 10
The quantitative temporal interrelationships between the physical integrity and the biologic processes of repair within a segmental autogeneous cortical bone transplant. (Reproduced with permission from Burchardt H: Biology of cortical bone graft incorporation, in Friedlaender GE, Mankin HJ, Sell KW (eds): *Osteochondral Allografts.* New York, Little and Brown, 1981.)

Although complete cortical graft incorporation does not occur, the biomechanical strength returns to normal between one and two years posttransplantation. In the clinical setting, histologic evaluation of nonvascularized autogenous cortical grafts in humans demonstrates that the same repair process occurs as in canine models, but takes approximately twice as long. These data suggest that human segmental cortical grafts should lose approximately half their biomechanical strength during the first six months and will persist for another six months. This process, which is related to osteoclastic graft resorption, is slowly reversed during the second year after implantation. These observations correlate with the highest incidence of mechanical graft failure between six and eight months after transplantation. The process of graft incorporation and creeping substitution is significantly prolonged with allogeneic bone grafts. These biologic factors must be considered in the clinical setting.

Osteochondral Grafting

To understand the principles necessary for the proper regeneration of a bone graft, it is interesting to look at the difference between a bone graft and a cartilage graft. The use of fresh autogeneic cartilage for transplantation is unusual in clinical orthopaedic surgery, but is more common in animal experimental protocols. There has been excellent survival for articular cartilage under these circumstances. This might be expected for a tissue not requiring a blood supply for its nutrition, but the results with epiphyseal cartilage have not been good. The question of the ultimate fate of allogeneic transplanted cartilage also has been extensively studied. Of considerable importance to such a system is the viability of the chondrocytes. In contrast to bone, there is evidence to support the concept that cartilage cells do survive in fresh grafts, remaining not only alive, but functional, for years after implantation.

If, as in composite grafts, it is necessary to freeze the graft, the use of cryoprotectants has been advocated as a method of maintaining chondrocyte viability. Recent studies have supported the original suggestion that glycerol or, more recently, dimethylsulfoxide (DMSO) can reduce the extent of cryoinjury to the chondrocytes. The best effect, however, is noted in isolated cells; when cryoprotectants are applied to intact cartilage, the results are far less salutary, and probably fewer than 50% of the cells retain their viability. The cause of the failure to translate the excellent results for chondrocyte cell suspensions to the intact tissue may have to do with the matrix, which not only limits diffusion of the cryoprotectant, but may, in fact, serve as a cold reflector. Even with successful transplantation (either as fresh graft or frozen cryoprotected graft), late degenerative changes apparently are inevitable and have been demonstrated both experimentally and clinically. It should be noted, however, that joint congruency of the graft appears to materially influence the rate at which the degeneration occurs, and grafts that are well fitted may show a long delay in appearance of degenerative changes.

Immunology of Allogeneic Bone and Cartilage

As stated, a major difference exists in the ability of an allogeneic bone graft to regenerate a viable cellular network as compared to an autograft. This is related to the immunologic response of the host to the foreign bone. Outline 1 lists the major factors in the immunologic response to allogeneic bone. The antigenicity of allograft bone is primarily the result of cell surface glycoproteins present in the heterogenous population of cells within the graft. Matrix macromolecules also have been implicated as additional

Outline 1
Immunologic response to allograft bone

- Cell HLA antigens in bone
- Greater antigenicity of fresh versus cryopreserved
- Host cell-mediated and humeral response to allografts
- Follows major histocompatibility mismatch rejection
- Major HLA mismatch improved with immunosuppression
- Vascular allografts —? successful with HLA matching

antigenic components of the graft. Most attention has been focused on the proteoglycan subunits, link protein and collagen, which are weakly antigenic in comparison to the human leukocyte cell-surface antigens. The antigenic cells in a graft include the osteogenic, chondrogenic, fibrous, vascular, and hematopoietic elements. As in other tissues, the cells of the vascular and hematopoietic system are the most immunogenic. The grouping of defined cell-surface antigens characterizes the immunogenic potential of the graft.

The recognition and immunologic response of the host to the allograft human leukocytic antigens (HLA) appears to be primarily cell mediated. This response is influenced by the HLA matching between the graft and host tissue antigens, the methods of graft preparation and storage, and the immunocompetence or pharmacologic immunosuppression of the host.

Freezing, freeze-drying (lyophilization), or chemical sterilization and antigen extraction of the bone allograft have all been shown to decrease significantly the antigenicity of the graft.

Radiographic and histologic studies of canine fibula allografts clearly demonstrate the improved rate of bone incorporation in closely matched donors as compared with strongly incompatible donors. In addition, the use of immunosuppressive agents, such as azathioprine, prednisolone, or antithymocyte sera, significantly improves the rate of incorporation of bone from antigen-incompatible donors. The data suggest the possible feasibility of vascularized allografts for closely-matched HLA donors with concurrent immunosuppressive therapy. Studies of animal species have demonstrated that antibodies may be detected in a high percentage of graft recipients. These figures are similar to the current data for humans, which have shown that about 85% of the patients who receive a massive graft show sensitization following the procedure. Class I antigens are most frequently detected but class II antigens can also be found. To date, the significance of the response of one or both of these antigens is not understood.

The major problem related to these issues, at least for humans, is the failure to find some biologic abnormalities retrospectively or, perhaps more importantly, to find predictably occurring abnormalities prospectively as a result of these host tissue antibodies. Current attempts to correlate the response of the graft with the degree or class of antibody present in the host have not been productive. Despite several animal studies that suggest that in a purer system they are likely to exert an effect, these findings have not yet been corroborated in humans.

Allogeneic bone appears to excite a host immune response characterized by the presence of humoral and cellular cytotoxic antibodies. This response apparently is dose dependent and is considerably, although not entirely predictably, ameliorated by freezing the graft. Freezing, which may derive its effect by killing the cells and disrupting their membranes, may cause the production of a blocking antibody. Freezing also has been shown to markedly inhibit collagenase activity.

The principal effect of the immune response on the allograft, particularly in the frozen state, appears to be one of inhibiting and delaying, sometimes for a very long time, the processes of vascular invasion, osteoblastic activity, and osteoclastic resorption by the host tissues. Thus, the time of onset and the rate and extent of the revascularization of the graft may vary considerably and remain unpredictable.

Articular cartilage contains numerous materials that are capable of exciting the host humoral and cellular immune response. Antibodies to the cartilage matrix and cells are readily identified following transplantation, and these are probably cytodestructive. Because the matrix of cartilage is so dense, the theoretical pore size of the tissue is minuscule. This characteristic sharply limits the egress of large antigens and, at the same time, markedly decreases the rate of ingress of antibodies or cells. These data suggest that as long as the cartilage matrix remains intact, the tissue is immunologically privileged.

Studies have shown that although both fresh and cryopreserved frozen cartilage cells survive allogeneic transplantation, they do deteriorate over time. The deteriorative process, which occurs partly on the basis of putative host immune response and partly because of the problems of joint incongruity, resembles a slowly evolving osteoarthritis. The three major complications of the allograft procedure—infection, allograft fracture, and nonunion are probably all, in part, immunologically directed and represent various forms and degrees of rejection.

Thus, it is clear that the system is still imperfect and that current knowledge remains somewhat less than complete. On the basis of clinical and experimental observations, however, it is possible to state that if a frozen osteoarticular allograft with cryoprotected cartilage is implanted into an orthotopic site and a good fit is achieved, the system has a 70% to 85% chance of success and long survival.

Biologic Response to Implants

In the strict sense, the incorporation of a synthetically made implant into the skeletal system constitutes a bone injury and requires bone repair or regeneration. Although, unlike osteonecrosis, or bone grafts, cell viability is not mandatory to maintain the structural integrity of the implant, some cell necrosis occurs in the tissue adjacent to the implant. Mechanical integrity must be achieved between the implant and bone if the bone-implant composite structure is to be functional. Thus, all features that exist in other forms of bone injury and repair exist in this situation; only the factors that play a dominant role in the success or failure of this process change.

Normal Local Tissue Response

The tissue that forms around implants results from the typical wound healing response, initiated by the surgical trauma of implantation, and from subsequent tissue remodeling. Implantation of a medical device sets into motion a sequence of cellular and biochemical processes that lead to healing by second intention, which is healing by the formation of granulation tissue within a defect, as opposed to the healing of an incision, which is healing by first intention. The first phase of healing is inflammation. This is followed by a reparative phase in which dead or damaged cells are replaced by healthy cells. The pathway that the reparative process takes depends on the regenerative capability of the cells making up the injured tissue; that is, the tissue or organ into which the implant has been placed.

Based on their capacity to regenerate, cells can be distinguished as labile, stable, or permanent. Labile cells continue to proliferate throughout life, replacing cells that are continually being destroyed. Hematopoietic tissues are examples of labile cells. Stable cells retain the capacity for proliferation, although they do not normally replicate. These cells can undergo rapid division in response to a variety of stimuli and are capable of reconstituting the tissue of origin. Stable cells include the parenchymal cells of all of the glandular organs of the body; for example, the liver, kidney, and pancreas; mesenchymal cells and their derivatives such as fibroblasts; smooth muscle cells; osteoblasts and chondroblasts; and vascular endothelial cells. Permanent cells are those that cannot reproduce themselves after birth, such as nerve cells.

Tissues composed of labile and stable cells have the capability for regeneration after surgical trauma. The injured tissue, under mechanical environments similar to those of the original tissue, is replaced by parenchymal cells of the same type, often leaving no residual trace of injury. However, tissues composed of permanent cells or of cells with limited capacity to proliferate, such as chondroblasts, are repaired to some degree by the production of fibrocollagenous scar. Despite the capability of many tissues to undergo regeneration, destruction of the supporting tissue stroma in an altered mechanical or material environment can lead to the formation of scar. The biologic response to materials, therefore, depends on the influence of the material on the inflammatory and reparative stages of wound healing. Does the material produce leachable ions or corrosion products that interfere with the resolution of surgically induced inflammation? Does the presence of the material interfere with the stroma required for the regeneration of tissue at the implant site? Does the presence of the implant material elicit an immunologic response in the host? These types of questions need to be addressed when assessing the biocompatibility of implant materials.

A number of systemic and local factors influence the inflammatory-reparative response. Systemic influences include age, nutrition, hematologic derangements, metabolic derangements, hormones, and steroids. Although there is a prevailing conventional wisdom that the elderly heal more slowly than the young, little control data and few animal experiments exist to support this notion. However, recent observations of the decreased cellularity and regenerative capability of bone and of impaired bone ingrowth with aging in dogs suggest that care must be taken in the use of implants in the elderly. Nutrition can have a profound effect on the healing of wounds. Prolonged protein starvation can inhibit collagen formation, and high protein diets can accelerate the development of tensile strength during wound healing. Local influences that affect wound healing include infection, blood supply, and the presence of a foreign body.

Osseointegration

Bonding of bone to an implant can be achieved by mechanical or chemical means. Interdigitation of bone with bone cement or with irregularities in implant topography, or bone ingrowth into porous surfaces, can yield mechanical interfaces capable of supporting shear and tensile as well as compressive forces. These types of mechanical bonding have been investigated extensively. Chemical bonding of bone to materials could result from molecular (for example, protein) adsorption/bonding to surfaces with subsequent bone cell attachment. This phenomenon is not yet as well understood as mechanical bonding.

Wound healing governs the makeup of the tissue that forms around implants. Because of its capability for regeneration, bone should be expected to appose cemented and noncemented orthopaedic prostheses and to form within the pore spaces of porous coatings. Bonding of a prosthesis to bone would enhance its stability, limiting the relative motion between the implant and bone. In addition, bonding might provide a more favorable distribution of stress to surrounding osseous tissue.

The term osseointegration has been used to describe the presence of bone on the surface of an implant with no histologically (light microscopy) demonstrable intervening nonosseous (for example, fibrous) tissue. All cemented and noncemented orthopaedic implants theoretically could become osseointegrated unless the bone regeneration process is inhibited. Initially, it was suggested that chemical bonding of bone to the implant surface was a prerequisite for osseointegration and that osseointegration occurred with commercially-pure titanium, but not with alloyed titanium or with other metals. However, observations indicate that implants fabricated from all of the orthopaedic metals, as well as polymers and ceramics, can become osseointegrated into bone. With respect to the osseointegration of bone cement, Charnley noted that in load-bearing areas, no tissue of any kind intervenes between the cement surface and the caps of changed bone on the ends of the load-bearing trabeculae. The question remains open as to whether chemical bonding of bone to any of these orthopaedic biomaterials (including commercially-pure titanium) is occurring. Mechanical tests of the attachment strength of implants to bone suggest that it is not.

The bone ingrowth into a porous-surface coating on a joint-replacement prosthesis leads to an interlocking bond that can serve to stabilize the implant. For the porous material to accommodate the cellular and extracellular elements of bone, the pore size must be greater than 100 μm. Porous coatings are produced most often by sintering techniques in which particles of the material are heat fused to form a porous structure. The increased surface area provided by porous metals and the absence of a polymethylmethacrylate (PMMA) sheath around the metallic implant provide the host tissue with significantly more contact with the metal than do cemented prostheses. This increased contact between metal and biologic tissue increases the physiologic exposure to the metal and any corrosion products released. The use of porous metals in young patients allows many years for the accumulation of metal ions and provides an extended opportunity for their effects to appear. Thus, despite considerable current interest in uncemented porous-coated total joint replacements, many issues of biologic response remain unresolved.

Chemical Bone Bonding

While there are few data that demonstrate chemical bonding of bone to the current orthopaedic biomaterials, there is evidence of bone bonding to calcium-containing bioactive glasses and to many different types of calcium phosphate. Chemical bonding is suggested by higher strength of the implant-bone interface than can be explained by a mechanical interlocking bond alone. In addition, transmission electron microscopy has been unable to detect an identifiable border between these calcium-containing implants and adjacent bone. In many recent studies the bonding of bone to hydroxyapatite has been investigated. This calcium phosphate mineral was chosen because it is closely related to the primary mineral constituent of bone; natural bone mineral is actually calcium-deficient carbonate apatite. Experiments have been performed on both hydroxyapatite-coated metallic implants and on particulate and block forms of the mineral used as bone substitute materials. Histology specimens taken from animals and retrieved from human subjects show that a shell of new bone approximately 100 μm in thickness covers most of the hydroxyapatite surface within a few weeks of implantation and remains indefinitely.

In studying the mechanism of bone bonding, researchers have found that within days of implantation, biologic apatites precipitate (from body fluid) onto the surface of the hydroxyapatite and bioactive glass implants. These biologic apatites are comparable to the carbonate apatite, which is bone mineral. Proteins probably adsorb to this biologic mineral layer, thereby facilitating bone cell attachment and the production of osteoid directly onto the implant. In this light, the bone cell responds to the biologic apatite layer that has formed on the implant and not directly to the implant itself. Data from recent studies have shown that this biologic apatite layer forms on many different calcium phosphate substances, thus explaining why bone bonding behavior has been reported for many different types of calcium phosphate materials. The clinical value of this phenomenon will depend, in part, on how well these substances can be bonded to orthopaedic implants. However, the finding that bone can become chemically bonded to certain biomaterials is a significant advance in the understanding of the implant-bone interface.

Fibrous Interface

The features of the tissue around prostheses that are not osseointegrated can vary widely. At one end of the spectrum are narrow radiolucent lines parallel to the implant surface, which are found in clinical radiographs of asymptomatic patients. These are considered to reflect stable, fibrous interfaces that might function successfully for an indefinite period. There have been, however, no systematic investigations of the mechanical properties of this fibrous tissue to validate its suitability as a supporting structure for a prosthesis. At the other end of the spectrum are interface zones around loose prostheses characterized by widening, divergent radiolucent (fibrous) seams and aggressive osteolytic lesions. Histologic examination of fibrous "capsules" around noncemented and cemented implants in bone often reveals macrophages on the biomaterial and bone cement surfaces. These cells are attracted to the prosthesis as they are to a dead space, presumably because of certain microenvironmental conditions (for example, low O_2, high lactate). In this regard it is not clear why macrophages are absent from the surface of osseointegrated implants. Perhaps stromal and osteoblast precursor cells migrate to the implant surface and begin forming new osseous tissue before macrophages have an opportunity to infiltrate. In light of the above, stable, fibrous interfaces probably should be considered metastable because they contain cellular elements (macrophages) that could be activated at some later time (by motion, particles, or metal ions) to release bone-resorbing agents that would promote loosening and cause pain.

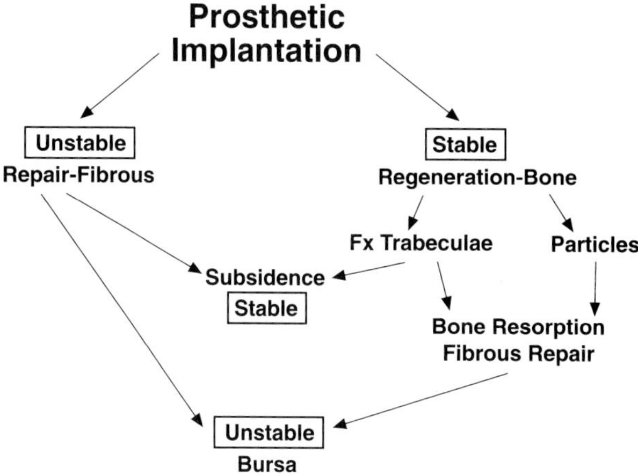

Figure 11
Paradigm for stability/instability of an implanted prosthesis.

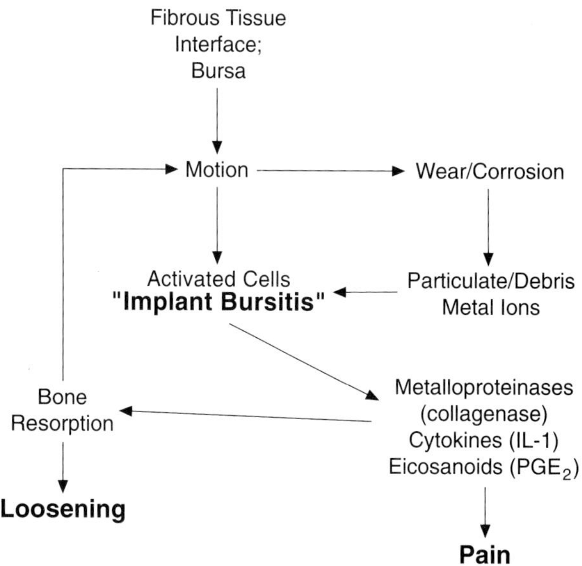

Figure 12
Paradigm for loosening of an implanted prosthesis.

Degeneration of the Interface

It is the wound-healing response that initially establishes the tissue characteristics of the implant-tissue interface. Several agents have the potential for initiating degenerative changes in the interface tissue. Others probably act as promoters to stimulate the production of inflammatory mediators that stimulate bone resorption and potentiate the process of prosthesis loosening. Of the many factors affecting the implant-bone interface, motion of the prosthetic component and particulate debris are two of the most important, because they are clearly present in most of the specimens retrieved at revision arthroplasty. However, it is difficult to determine the causal relationships between these factors and implant failure from studying only the end-stage tissue. Other histopathologic findings and laboratory study data indicate that metal ions and immune reactions might play roles in the degenerative processes leading to prosthesis loosening in certain patients. Systemic diseases and drugs used for the treatment of various disorders also could serve as factors contributing to the breakdown of the implant-bone interface. Finally, there might be individual differences in genetically determined cellular responses that could explain why prostheses fail in some patients in whom there is a low mechanical risk factor for failure.

The paradigm for loosening in Figures 11 and 12 can serve as a framework for considering the factors that influence the degeneration of the implant-bone interface and subsequent loosening. The surgical trauma of implantation initiates the wound-healing response that should be expected to result in the regeneration of osseous tissue in the surgically prepared implant site (Fig. 11). Bone will envelop a stable prosthesis, resulting in its osseointegration. Motion of a mechanically unstable implant during the initial stage of wound healing can disrupt the regenerating osseous stroma, leading to fibrous repair and encapsulation of the device. Depending on its design, subsidence of the fibrous-encapsulated prosthesis could serve to stabilize it to the extent that it might become adequately supported by bone; the interposed fibrous tissue might persist indefinitely as a stable fibrous interface.

Fibrous tissue might also replace bone around previously stable, osseointegrated devices (that is, late loosening) either because of mechanical factors, such as fracture or pressure necrosis of adjacent bone, or biologic factors, such as local bone resorption associated with particulate debris, excessive local contact stresses, and/or metal ions. These factors can act on joint synovium, infiltrate the implant-bone interface from the joint space, or cause localized lesions around the device. Fibrous tissue formation around the prosthesis (Fig. 13), regardless of the cause, is accompanied by accretion of macrophages that eventually migrate to the surface of the implant, probably attracted by the microenvironment associated with the dead space. Some macrophages on or near the implant surface fuse to form multinucleated foreign body giant cells. This giant cell formation is probably influenced by the topography of the surface and other, as yet unidentified, factors. Histologically, a layer of macrophage- and fibroblast-like cells supported by fibrous tissue is characteristic of a synovial lining (or membrane). This has led to the use of the term "pseudomembrane." Because this synovial-like lining contains a defect in tissue (implant site) and experiences friction as a result of implant micromotion, its histology is similar to that of a bursa.

Motion of the prosthesis can affect the cells around the implant in two ways. The motion can act directly to activate macrophages to produce certain

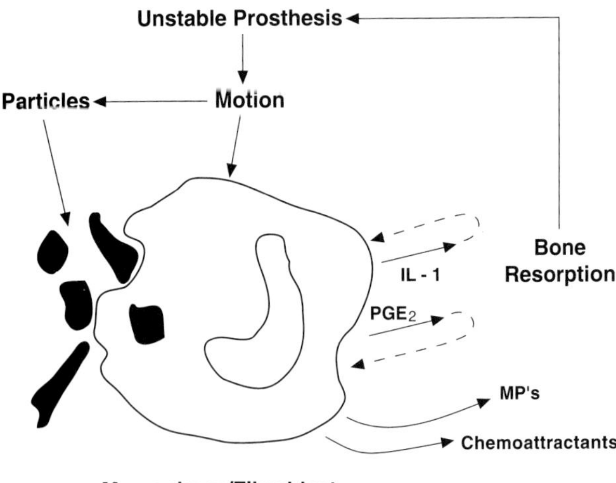

Figure 13
The response of a macrophage/fibroblast to particulate debris and motion, which can activate the cell to produce cytokines, eicosanoids, and metalloproteinases (MPs) that stimulate bone resorption. (Adapted with permission from Galante JO, Lemons J, Spector M, et al: The biological effects of implant materials. *J Orthop Res* 1991;9:760–775.)

cytokines, eicosanoids, and metalloproteinases. At the same time, this motion can create conditions that promote mechanisms of wear and corrosion. These processes can yield metallic and polymeric particulate debris and metal ions that might also activate the bursal cells to elaborate inflammatory mediators and enzymes. The inflammatory process involving the cells at the interface of the prosthesis could be referred to as "implant bursitis." Previously, this condition has been referred to as "prosthetic synovitis."

Agents such as interleukin-1, prostaglandin E_2 (PGE_2), and collagenase are known to stimulate bone resorption. Bone loss could further contribute to motion and the persistence of the inflammatory condition at the implant-tissue interface. These and other mediators of inflammation produced by the activated interfacial cells are probably responsible, at least in part, for the pain experienced by patients with loose total joint arthroplasties.

Effects of Motion

The histology of the prosthesis-tissue interface has been studied in several species. A loose fibroblast and woven bone layer forms adjacent to the implant in the early postoperative period. This layer matures into a secure interface in some cases and into a fibrous membrane in others. Studies have shown that the mechanical environment can profoundly affect the maturation of healing bone. In a fracture callus, the quality of tissue that develops between fracture fragments is a function of the relative micromotion between the fragments. The more motion there is at the interface between fragments, the softer the interposed tissue. Rigid internal fixation results in direct, primary bony union by the process of creeping substitution. Less rigid fixation produces fracture healing through an intermediary stage of cartilaginous bridging callus. Still larger interfragmentary motions result in fibrous union, and gross motion between fracture fragments prevents healing altogether, resulting in a nonunion. Similarly, micromotion has been postulated as the stimulus for the formation of a fibrous membrane at the bone-prosthesis interface. The mechanical properties of the membrane formed at the bone-cement interface differ in regions of differing stress, which suggests that the principles discussed above may be governing the formation of this membrane. In the fracture model, the initial interfacial tissue increases the rigidity of the system and is then replaced by a stiffer intermediate layer. The system thus evolves toward a solid osseous union. In the arthroplasty model this cannot happen. A fibrous membrane, being attached to only one side of the interface, decouples the bone from the prosthesis and thus increases the compliance of the system. If this decoupling is complete, a mechanical, and possibly biologic, chain of events ensues, leading to further loosening of the implanted prosthesis.

As noted earlier, motion can interfere with the wound healing response of bone regeneration by destroying the regenerating osseous stroma. Fibrous, scar-like tissue results. Another important effect of motion is the formation of a bursa within connective tissue in which shearing and tensile movement have led to disruption of tissue continuity and the formation of a void or sack lined by synovial-like cells. It is to be expected, then, that tissue around prosthetic components removed because of loosening might display features of synovial-like tissue. The presence of synovial cells, macrophages, and fibroblast-like cells is important because these cells could be activated by other agents, such as particulate debris, to produce proinflammatory molecules (Fig. 14). The process of activation of this tissue might be similar to the process that occurs in inflammatory joint synovium or bursitis.

An explanation of how prosthesis motion leads to the formation of the synovial-like tissue can be found in studies that have shown that synovial lining is simply an accretion of macrophages and fibroblasts stimulated by mechanical cavitation of connective tissue. These findings are based on experiments in which the mechanical disruption of connective tissue was produced by injection of air and/or fluid into the subcutaneous space of animals. The resulting sack was initially described as a granuloma pouch. Later studies demonstrated that the membrane lining the pouch displayed the characteristics of synovium, and referred to this tissue as facsimile synovium. Motion also can result in the prosthetic component abrading against the bone cement sheath or surrounding bone, thereby generating increased amounts of particulate debris that might contribute to activation of the macrophages and synovial-like cells at the implant-tissue interface (Fig. 13).

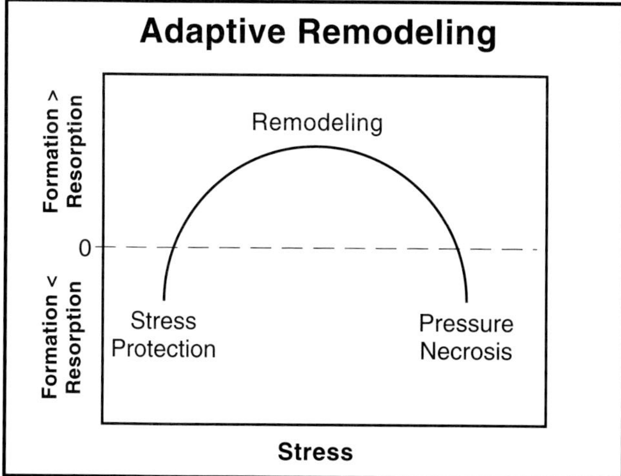

Figure 14
Adaptive remodeling as a function of mechanical environment.

Effects of Particles

Particulate debris can be generated from the wear occurring at the articulating surfaces of total joint replacement prostheses and by abrasion of the components against fragments of the bone cement sheath or against surrounding bone. This particulate debris can induce changes in the joint synovium and in the tissue around the prosthetic components. Adverse responses have been found to both metallic and polymeric particles. The biologic reactions to particles are related to the size, quantity, chemistry, topography, and shape of the particles. While it is not clear what role each of these factors plays in the biologic response, particle size appears to be particularly important. Particles small enough to be phagocytized (<10 µm) elicit more of an adverse cellular response than larger particles. This degenerative process has been referred to as small particle disease.

Particles with rough surfaces or acute angles, those that produce the greatest tissue irritation, have been found to elicit the most cellular and fibrocytic response. Motion at the interface site exacerbates this reaction. Surface charge and chemistry, as well as surface texture, influence the cellular response to particles.

Recent investigations have shown that laboratory-prepared particulate cobalt-chromium (Co-Cr) alloy particles induced rapid proliferation of macrophages and focal degeneration of synovial tissues in rats injected intra-articularly, in much the same way as seen in the articular tissues around loose total joint prostheses in human subjects. Because previous animal investigations and histopathologic studies of tissues retrieved from human subjects have suggested that titanium alloy is more biocompatible than Co-Cr alloys, it has been assumed that titanium particulate debris would be less problematic. Histology of pigmented tissue surrounding titanium implants generally has revealed considerably fewer macrophages and multinucleated foreign body giant cells than are seen around Co-Cr alloy particles and polymeric particulate debris.

However, a recent study of titanium alloy particles generated by the abrasion of femoral stems against bone cement in human subjects revealed histiocytic and lymphoplasmacytic reactions to the metallic particles. In another recent investigation, titanium particles were found to cause fibroblasts in culture to produce elevated levels of PGE_2. These findings show that the biologic response to titanium particles is not as benign as initially believed.

Many investigations evaluating the histologic response to polyethylene and PMMA particles in animals and in tissue recovered at revision surgery have revealed the histiocytic response to these polymer particles. It has been shown that this macrophage response can lead to bone resorption and, thereby, potentiate the loosening process. The ability of polymer particles to promote the destruction of the implant-bone interface and infiltrate the resulting fibrous membrane has been demonstrated in a recent animal investigation. Injection of polyethylene particles into the knee joints of rats induced resorption of bone and the formation of a membrane at the interface of a nonweightbearing plug of bone cement implanted through the knee joint into the distal part of the femur. Polyethylene particles could be found infiltrating the fibrous tissue around the acrylic plug. These data could explain how such particles are found at distal sites around femoral stems.

The effect of calcium-containing ceramic particles on synovial cells has also been investigated. Local leukocyte influx, proteinase, PGE_2, and tumor necrosis factor (TNF) levels were measured after injection of calcium-containing ceramic materials into the "air pouch model" previously described. TNF was detected in significant amounts after injection of the ceramics. These substances also provoked elevated leukocyte counts and increased levels of proteinase and PGE_2, showing that substances with surface chemistries that elicit a beneficial tissue response (for example, bone bonding) when implanted in bulk form can cause destructive cellular reactions when present in particulate form.

Recent studies have added to our knowledge of the fundamental response of cells to biomaterial chemistry and topography. In one recent investigation, macrophage-conditioned medium exposed to orthopaedic biomaterials in culture was assayed to determine its bone resorption activity. Greater bone resorption activity was present in medium conditioned with macrophages on hydrophilic and rough surfaces than on hydrophobic and smooth surfaces. When this experimental method was used, high density polyethylene (HDPE) elicited approximately 20% more bone resorption than PMMA. It has been suggested that all orthopaedic implant materials in particulate form have the capacity to elicit a cellular response. Research of this type is advancing understanding of the implant-bone interface.

Metallic Ions

Results of investigations using animal and human models have revealed elevated levels of metal ions in subjects with joint replacement prostheses and other types of implants. Knowledge of the mechanisms of metal ion release is still incomplete. Results are often variable with respect to the concentration of specific metal ions in certain tissues and fluids. The fact that metal in ionic form is often not distinguished from metal present as particles serves to confound interpretation of results. One recent investigation of 14 patients undergoing conventional cemented Co-Cr alloy hip replacement revealed postoperative rises in serum and urinary chromium levels.

However, an attempt to determine the valence of chromium as either +3 (III) or + 6 (VI) from the concentration of metal ion in blood clot was not successful. It is known that erythrocytes display a unidirectional uptake of Cr(VI) while effectively excluding Cr(III). The distinction in the valence of chromium is important because Cr(VI) is much more biologically active than Cr(III).

Unfortunately, current knowledge of the local and systemic biologic and clinical sequelae of metal ion release is not complete. The effect of metallic ions on cells in culture was explored in one recent study. Addition of cobalt ions in the form of cobalt fluoride solutions to the media of lapine (rabbit) or human synovial cells stimulated their production of neutral proteinases and collagenase. Production of PGE_2 by lapine cells was enhanced 30% to 40% by cobalt solutions that slightly depressed the production of PGE_2 by human cells. Lapine synovial cells, stimulated by $CoCl_2$, also produced a substance that provoked synthesis of collagenase, gelatinase, caseinase, and PGE_2 by monolayers of articular chondrocytes. It has been suggested that these findings may be relevant to aseptic loosening of joint prostheses in that metal ions could activate synovial cells in the joint capsule, and in the pseudomembrane at the implant-bone interface to produce agents that promote osteolysis.

Diseases and Drugs

There has been little work correlating the failure of orthopaedic prostheses with disease states and drugs used to treat various disorders. Most investigations in this area have involved the role of anti-inflammatory drugs and other agents used to prevent heterotopic ossification on the bone ingrowth into noncemented porous-coated prostheses. Generally, results of these studies have shown that these anti-inflammatory agents, as well as certain anticancer drugs, reduce the amount of bone ingrowth in the early stages of wound healing after implantation. Virtually no investigations have covered the effects of these and other agents on the remodeling and degeneration of the implant-bone interface after longer periods of implantation.

The effect of specific diseases on the formation, remodeling, and degeneration of the implant-bone interface is still unclear. In one canine investigation, estrogen deficiency was used to determine the effect that postmenopausal osteoporosis might have on bone ingrowth. The results, which were not definitive, suggested that this condition might be expected to yield greater amounts of fibrous tissue ingrowth into porous-coated prostheses. Unfortunately, there have been no studies investigating the role of selected diseases on the longer-term remodeling and degeneration of the implant-bone interface.

Adaptive Bone Remodeling

In addition to assuring a firm, strong, long-lasting implant-bone interface bond, bone repair and regeneration in response to the introduction of an implant requires changes in the structure of the bone adjacent to it. While it would be highly desirable for the implant to have the exact same material and structural properties of the bone it substitutes for or is adjacent to, this is not usually accomplished. The adjacent bone is then subjected to different stresses and strains than it is normally accustomed to and, if it does not respond properly, failure of the composite system may result.

Osteoblasts and osteoclasts are influenced by the magnitude and state of strain imposed on them by loads applied to bone (Fig. 14). Stresses or strains within a given range seem to be required to maintain a steady-state remodeling of bone, in which the rate of bone formation equals the rate of resorption. Stresses below the optimum level are often associated with stress protection leading to bone resorption. Stresses and strains exceeding upper limits can also produce resorption of bone as a result of pressure necrosis. Cyclic stresses are required to maintain osseous homeostasis; constant loads within the desired range provide insufficient stimulus to maintain bone mass. Observations of strain-related electrical potentials in bone, biopotentials, and electrical stimulation of osteogenesis combine to suggest a bioelectric phenomenon as the regulator of adaptive remodeling of bone. However, other investigations have shown that the strain imposed on the membranes of osteoblast-like cells in culture directly influences their activity, so other regulatory mechanisms are probably present in addition to electrical potentials.

Systemic Response

Immune Reactions and Genetic Determinants

Very different outcomes are not infrequent for two patients implanted with the same device by the same surgeon and matched for sex, age, weight, activity level, and other factors that might be expected to affect the performance of the prosthesis. It has been suggested that immune reactions or genetically determined responses might play a role in the failure of prostheses in some patients. Immune responses include antibody- and cell-mediated reactions and activation of the complement system. Metal ions behave as haptens, which, when complexed with serum proteins, can trigger an immune response. However, the cell types that might be expected to occur at sites of antibody- and cell-mediated reactions are not often found in tissue retrieved with revised devices. These cells include lymphocytes and plasma cells. In one recent report a lymphoplasmacytic infiltrate was found in pseudomembrane tissue containing titanium alloy particulate debris. However, this finding and the observation of occasional lymphocytic infiltrates in the pseudomembrane tissue do not provide enough information for determination of the role of immune reactions in implant loosening.

In several previous studies, it has been demonstrated that many biomaterials can activate (cleave) certain molecules (C3 and C5) in the complement system. Thus, complement activation by biomaterials could play a role in adverse reactions to certain devices. However, additional studies are required.

The delayed hypersensitivity response is one form of cell-mediated immune reaction associated with implants that has been studied. Metal allergy has been incriminated as the cause of joint prosthesis failure in certain patients. However, results obtained to date are not definitive. The incidence of metal sensitivity in the normal population is high, with up to 15% of the population sensitive to nickel and perhaps up to 25% sensitive to either nickel, cobalt, or chromium. However, the incidence of metal sensitivity reactions requiring premature removal of an orthopaedic device is very small (less than the incidence of infection). A similar situation exists with respect to sensitivity reactions to PMMA. Methylmethacrylate monomer is a strong skin sensitizer; however, failure of cemented devices has not yet been correlated with a hypersensitivity response in patients.

The fact that there is no clear etiology of the prosthesis loosening in some patients while in other individuals with multiple risk factors for failure the prosthesis functions well suggests that there may be genetic determinants for loosening. A recent investigation has shown individual differences in the in vitro cytokine and PGE_2 production by lipopolysaccharide-stimulated macrophages. HLA-DR2-positive individuals, and first degree relatives, were found to be low responders. Studies of this type suggest that in certain individuals genetic determination might play a role in the degree to which cells in the tissue around prostheses can be activated to produce proinflammatory agents that stimulate bone resorption. Additional studies of this type could be of value in identifying patients who might be high responders to prosthetic motion and particulate debris and, therefore, at high risk for prosthesis failure. Clearly there are factors not yet understood that cause one patient but not another to react.

Carcinogenicity

Chromium and nickel are known carcinogens and cobalt is a suspected carcinogen. Therefore, it is understandable that some concern might be raised about the release of these metal ions into the human body from orthopaedic prostheses. Fortunately, there have been few reports of neoplasms around orthopaedic implants. While no causal relationship has been evidenced, there is a high enough index of suspicion to warrant serious investigation of this matter through epidemiologic and other studies. The use of noncemented, porous-coated metallic stems (with large surface areas) in younger patients has added to concern about the long-term clinical consequences of metal ion release because of the significant increase in exposure.

In a recent epidemiologic investigation conducted in New Zealand, over 1,300 total joint replacement patients were followed to determine the incidence of remote site tumors. The incidences of tumors of the lymphatic and hematopoietic systems were found to be significantly greater than expected in the decade following arthroplasty. It is important to note that the incidences of cancer of the breast, colon, and rectum were significantly less than expected. The investigators acknowledged that while the association might be caused, in part, by an effect of the prosthetic implants, other mechanisms, particularly drug therapy, require consideration. Somewhat similar results were obtained from another study of the cancer incidence in 443 total hip replacement patients operated on between 1967 and 1973 and followed to the end of 1981. The risk of leukemias and lymphomas increased while the risk of breast cancer decreased. The authors concluded that the local occurrence of cancer associated with prostheses made of cobalt-chromium-molybdenum as reported in the literature as well as results of animal experiments indicate that chrome-cobalt-alloy may play some role in carcinogenesis.

Recent publications have reviewed the relationship of metallic ion release to oncogenesis, and reports of neoplasms found around orthopaedic implants have recently been reviewed. The difference in the tumor types, time to appearance, and type of prosthesis confound attempts to conclude an association of the neoplasm to the implant materials and released moieties.

Understanding of the biologic response to implanted material is in its infancy. The physiologic events, on the organ, tissue, and cellular levels, initiated by the presence of a synthetic material need further investigation. Both biologic and material factors influence the biocompatibility of implanted medical devices and both must be studied together to improve understanding of the processes involved.

Fractures and Their Fixation

Fractures of the skeletal system constitute the consummate integrated injury to bone, consisting of all aspects of potential circulatory and physical injury to the viable cellular content as well as the structural integrity of bone. Viable cells must be available; appropriate signals must be generated to have such cells produce the appropriate extracellular matrix at each phase of repair, and a sufficiently sound mechanical environment must exist, often assisted by implant devices, to assure that this can occur. Fracture injury and repair thus incorporates knowledge of all the aspects of injury and repair previously discussed in this chapter, as well as several other factors related to the uniqueness and ubiquity of this type of injury. The importance of each factor depends on the nature of the injury, its location, and the manner of its treatment.

Biomechanics of Fractures

Fractures can be classified according to the characteristics of the force that cause the fracture. A fracture may arise from forces of low magnitude that are cyclicly repeated over a long period of time or from a force having sufficient magnitude to cause failure after a single application.

The susceptibility of bone to fracture under fluctuating forces or stresses of low magnitude is related to its crystal structure and collagen orientation, which reflect the viscoelastic properties of the bone. Cortical bone is vulnerable to both tensile and compressive fluctuating stresses. Under each cycle of loading, a small amount of strain energy may be lost through microscopic cracks along the cement lines. Fatigue load under certain strain rates can cause progressive accumulation of microdamage in cortical bone. When such a process is prolonged, bone may eventually fail through fracture-crack propagation. However, bone is a living tissue and can undertake a repair process simultaneously. Periosteal callus and new bone formation near the microscopic cracks can arrest crack propagation by reducing the high stresses at the tip of the crack. This is a phenomenon commonly seen in stress fractures.

Fractures caused by a single application or injury can be classified according to the magnitude and area distribution of the force, as well as to the rate at which the force acts on the bone. When the trauma is direct, soft-tissue injury and fracture comminution are related to the loading rate; trauma energy is related to the speed of the impacting object. Fractures caused by indirect forces are produced by forces applied to bone at a distance from the fracture site itself. Fractures that are caused by strong muscle contractions across a joint with a fixed distal segment, such as those of the olecranon and patella, are but one example of this type of injury. Here, the fracture fragments are separated and distracted as a result of muscle pull rather than impacted and overridden as is seen in many fractures caused by direct trauma.

Regardless of where the force is applied, such forces may generate compressive, tensile, or shear stresses or some combination of the three in the bone. Whether each type of stress generated acts independently or with the others in various combinations, the failure patterns of long bones follow some basic rules. In general, the combination of the bone's material strength and anisometric properties, particularly its three principal planes of stress (tensile stress, compressive stress, and shear stress), dictate when, how, and along which path the fracture will occur (Fig. 15). Cortical bone, as a material, is generally weak in tension and shear, particularly along the longitudinal plane; the area where tensile stresses arise, therefore, fails first. The closer the majority of such tensile stresses are oriented to the long axes of the bone, the less force will be needed to break the bone.

Studies on dog tibias have shown that the maximum load to failure is three times higher for the production of a transverse fracture than for that of a spiral fracture. Transverse fractures are the result of pure tensile forces or bending. Failure of bone from

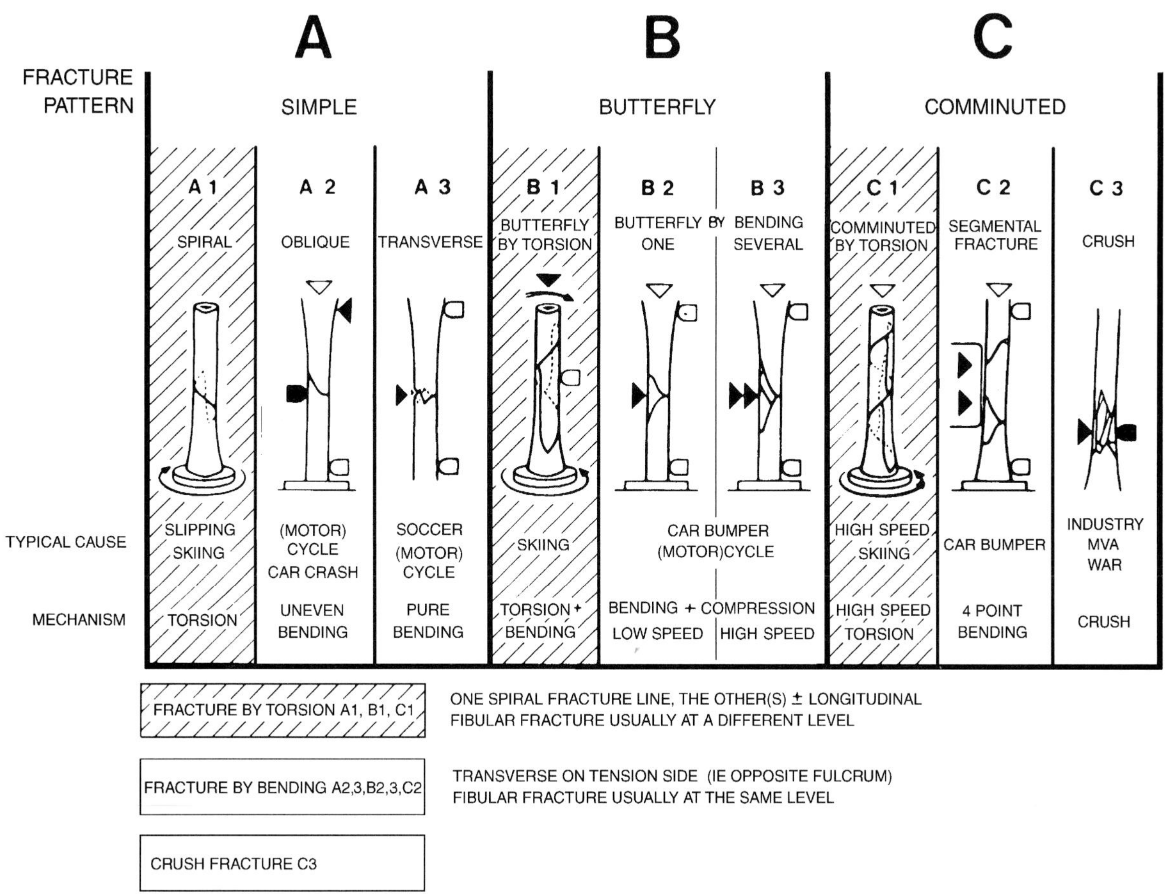

Figure 15
The nine main fracture groups; fractures are classified according to degree of comminution and etiology. (Reproduced with permission from Johner R, Wruhs O: Classification of tibial shaft fractures and correlation with results after rigid internal fixation. *Clin Orthop* 1983;178:7–25.)

a pure tensile force occurs progressively across the bone, creating a transverse fracture without comminution. The pattern of fracture arising from pure bending, similarly, is a simple transverse line as failure stresses are almost pure tensile in type. Uneven bending is more apt to produce an oblique fracture line. Occasionally, the cortex under compression breaks as a result of existing shear stress before the tension failure progresses all the way across the bone; in this situation, comminution occurs on the compression side, and may create a single butterfly fragment or multiple fragments. In contrast, spiral fractures are the result of pure torsional injuries. All spiral fractures have two different types of fracture lines: (1) an angled line turning around the circumference of the bone; and (2) a more or less longitudinal line linking the proximal and distal portions of the spiral. In experimental conditions, the average angled line of a spiral fracture is approximately 30° off the longitudinal axis, and the total angle of ascent of each spiral fracture clinically has been noted to vary from 30° to 70° and is never transverse. To a certain degree, a bending moment always exists when torsional forces are applied. Its presence is the reason for the line linking the ends of the spiral and prevents the endless propagation of the spiral fracture. Under certain circumstances it produces a butterfly fragment rather than a single linking line. In contrast, combining an axial load with torsional forces has little effect on the failure pattern of the resulting spiral fracture.

The susceptibility of a bone to fracture from a single injury is related not only to its modulus of elasticity and anisometric properties but to its energy-absorbing capacity as well. Bone undergoing rapid loading must absorb more energy than bone loaded at a slower rate. The kinetic energy of the impacting object is defined as $1/2\ MV^2$ where M is the mass and V is the velocity of the impacting object. Energy absorbed by the bone during loading is released when the bone fractures. This phenomenon helps to explain why injuries with rapid loading involving higher velocities dissipate energy and result in more significant structural changes, that is, greater fracture comminution and displacement. Thus, gunshot wounds inflicted by high-velocity bullets result in considerably more bone comminution and soft-tissue damage than gunshot wounds from low-velocity bullets. This same phenomenon is seen with the application of indirect forces as well. At low speeds, bending plus tensile stress will cause a fracture with one butterfly fragment; whereas, at high speeds the same mechanism of injury will cause several butterfly fragments. High speed torsion alone, that is, without an associated bending moment, can cause a spiral fracture with comminution. The most common etiology of segmental fractures is four-point bending, which is commonly seen when a tibia is hit by a car bumper, a high velocity injury.

How the pattern of bone injury relates to the types of forces applied to bone is not merely of concern to the bone's structural integrity, but to its cell viability as well. The importance of soft-tissue injury and cell viability has been stressed by many authors. The time to union is greatly prolonged in fractures that have more soft-tissue stripping. Experimental studies have demonstrated the retarding effect of muscle damage on bone healing. The larger load under bending failure may cause the surrounding soft tissues and periosteum to sustain more damage and, thus, may affect the fracture healing potential. Long-bone shaft fractures resulting from high-energy injuries have a higher rate of bone healing complications than fractures from low-energy injuries. In addition, open fractures have a higher incidence of nonunion than closed fractures in most large series.

Fracture Repair

Biology

At the moment of impact, the energy absorbed by the bone leads to mechanical and structural failure. Besides the actual break in continuity of the bone, there is a disruption of the blood supply to the bone at the fracture site. The biology of fracture repair is actually a tissue regenerative process rather than a healing process. That is, the injured part is ultimately replaced by bone rather than scar tissue. This regenerative process may be described as consisting of four stages: (1) inflammation, (2) soft callus, (3) hard callus, and (4) remodeling.

Stage 1 inflammation Inflammation begins immediately after a fracture is sustained and consists initially of the appearance of hematoma and fibrin clot along with platelets, polymorphonuclear neutrophils, and monocytes or macrophages at the fracture site. In addition hemorrhage and cell death are seen where blood vessels are disrupted. Figure 16 shows bone necrosis at the ends of the fracture fragments with the cellular release of lysosomal enzymes and other by-products of cell death. Fibroblasts, mesenchymal cells, and osteoprogenitor cells appear shortly thereafter. The mesenchymal and osteoprogenitor cells may arise from transformed endothelial cells in the medullary canal and/or from the periosteum and/or by osteogenic induction of cells within the surrounding muscle and soft tissue. The blood vessels of the periosteal callus are entirely new and originate from surrounding extraskeletal tissues and from the medullary canal. A tissue oxygen gradient is necessary for the maintenance of angiogenesis in these healing tissues. Angiogenesis may be con-

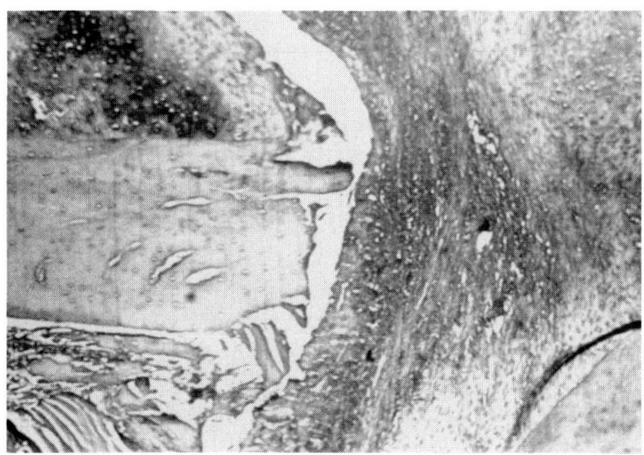

Figure 16
Photomicrograph of inflammatory stage of bone repair.

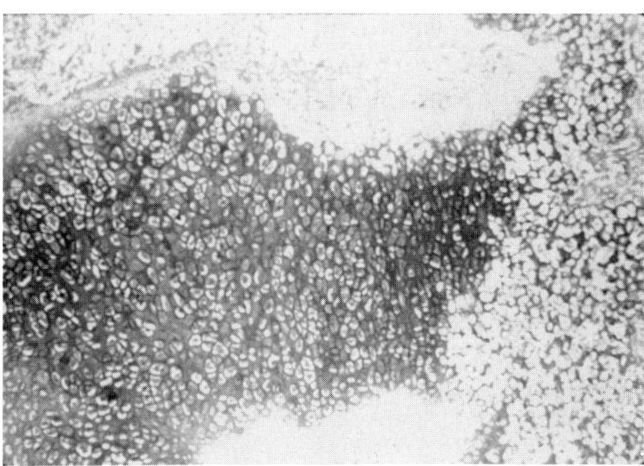

Figure 18
Photomicrograph of bone repair; soft callus stage, new cartilage formation.

trolled by macrophages, which produce angiogenic factors under hypoxic conditions.

Stage 2 soft callus The stages of soft and hard callus are rather arbitrary, because different regions within a given fracture may progress at different rates of repair. Figure 17 depicts the histology of a typical fracture and its component regions. The peripheral aspect of the external callus shows only cartilage formation, whereas that closer to the bone ends shows bone formation. Nevertheless, it is convenient to define the stage of soft callus as beginning when pain and swelling subside and lasting until the bony fragments are united by fibrous or cartilaginous tissue and are no longer freely moveable. By the end of this stage, some stability is present to prevent shortening but angulation at the fracture site can still occur. This period is marked by a great increase in vascularity at the fracture site as shown in Figure 18, a microangiograph of a dog's tibia a few days following fracture. This stage is best illustrated by the pediatric femur fracture, which has a large palpable callus, but no visible callus calcification on radiographs.

Stage 3 hard callus The repair process continues in the stage of hard callus as the callus converts from cartilaginous tissue to woven bone. The restoration of strength and stiffness seems to be related to the amount of new bone connecting the fracture fragments and less to the overall amount of uniting callus.

The typical long bone fracture exhibits both endochondral bone formation, in which new bone is formed on a cartilaginous template as in the external callus, and membranous bone formation, in which bone is formed directly from mesenchymal cells or preosteoblasts as in the periosteal callus. (With rigid internal fixation, a third type of bone formation occurs without the formation of a visible callus.

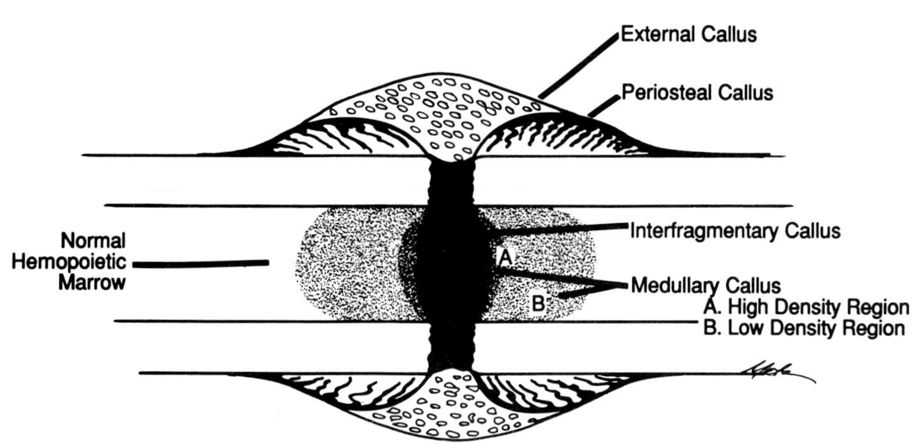

Figure 17
Histology of a typical fracture. (Reproduced with permission from Brighton CT, Hunt RM: Early histological and ultrastructural changes in medullary fracture callus. *J Bone Joint Surg* 1991;73A:832–847.)

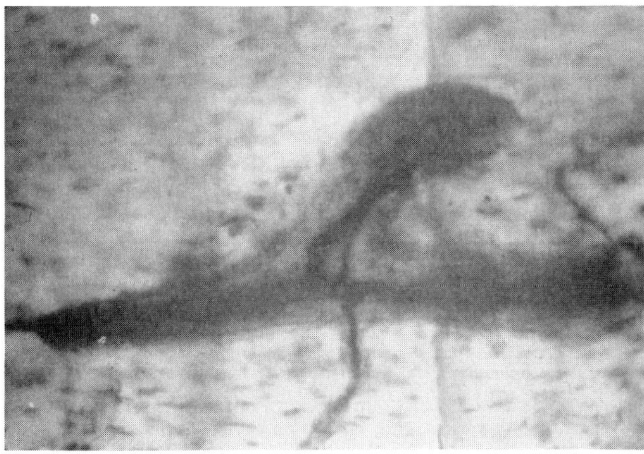

Figure 19
Photomicrograph of primary bone healing. (Reproduced with permission from Rahn BA, Gallinaro P, Baltensperger A, et al: Primary bone healing: An experimental study in the rabbit. *J Bone Joint Surg* 1971;53A:783–786.)

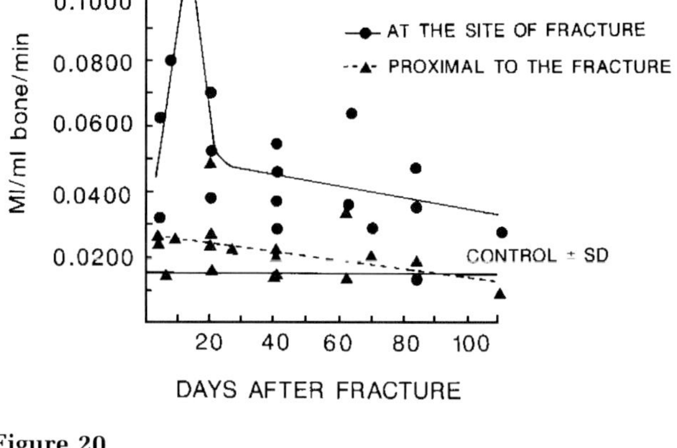

Figure 20
Blood flow rate at a fracture site as determined by a ^{125}I-labeled 4-iodoantipyrine washout technique.

Called primary bone healing, this type of bone formation results in the fracture site being bridged by direct haversian remodeling.) Figure 19 shows cutting cones extending across the fracture site and entering the other fragment to give almost a direct osteon-to-osteon hookup. Osteoclasts in the forefront of the cutting cones remove bone, while the osteoblasts trailing behind lay down new bone. It is similar in all respects to the phenomenon of creeping substitution in cortical bone described in the sections related to osteonecroses and cortical grafts.

Stage 4 bone remodeling During remodeling, the last stage of fracture repair, woven bone slowly converts to lamellar bone, and the medullary canal is reconstituted. This stage takes the longest amount of time and may not be completed for years. Angular deformities in adults will "round-off" but will not be corrected as is seen in children with open growth plates. The bone responds to its loading characteristics according to Wolff's law during this remodeling phase.

Vascular Response

The vascular response to a fracture varies with time. Initially, the blood flow rate decreases because of disruption of vessels at the fracture site. Within hours to a few days, this decrease is followed by a great increase in the blood flow rate, which peaks at two weeks. The blood flow then gradually returns to normal at around 12 weeks (Fig. 20). How the fracture is manipulated, reduced, and immobilized can have a great effect on fracture site vascularity. Internal fixation of any type obviously may disrupt vessels, especially the microvasculature. Reaming the medullary canal and inserting a tight- fitting rod significantly lowers the blood flow when compared to that of plated fractures in dogs. In the dog, blood flow is decreased in both plated and rodded tibias at 42 and 90 days postfracture, with a greater decrease in the rodded tibia. At 120 days blood flow in the rodded and plated tibias is equal. Thus, the initial decrease in blood flow following endosteal reaming is compensated, by 90 days, by development of collateral periosteal vessels.

Accompanying the above described changes in blood flow to the fracture are rather profound changes in the local tissue Po_2. Oxygen tension is very low in the fracture hematoma, low in newly formed cartilage and bone, and highest in fibrous tissue (Fig. 21). Oxygen tension in callus fiber bone remains low until the fracture is healed. Despite the great ingrowth of capillaries into the fracture callus, the increase in cell proliferation is such that the cells exist in a state of hypoxia. This hypoxic state could be favorable for bone formation, as in vitro bone growth optimally occurs in a low-oxygen environment.

Cellular Response and Biochemistry of Fracture Healing

Biochemical studies of the fracture callus have identified four steps of fracture repair: mesenchymal, chondroid, chondroid-osteoid, and osteogenic. In the mesenchymal step, fibroblasts, chondroblasts, and macrophages predominate. The first chondrocytes appear adjacent to cortical bone and originate

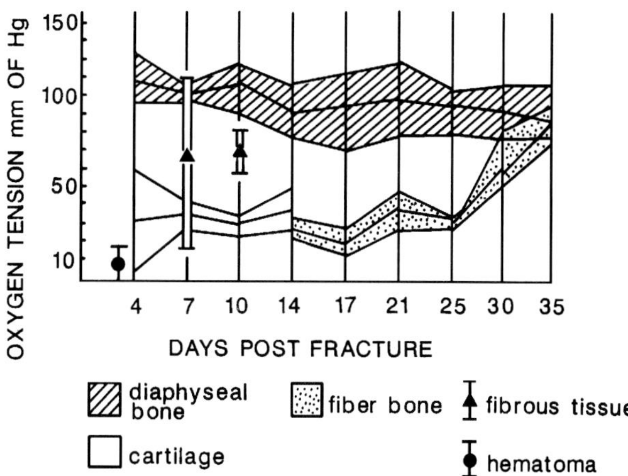

Figure 21
Changes in oxygen tension at fracture site.

by differentiation of mesenchymal cells from the cambium layer of the periosteum. Synthesis of type I collagen is increased and levels of type II are detectable. Type III collagen, expressed by fibroblasts, and type V, found in areas of fibrous tissue formation and associated with blood vessels, also are present. In the chondroid step, types II and IX collagen predominate. Type II is deposited in areas of mature cartilage production, and type IX appears to stabilize the type II collagen fibrils. In the chondroid-osteoid step, calcified bars, primary spongiosa, and types I and II collagen predominate. Type X collagen is expressed by proliferating chondrocytes as the extracellular matrix undergoes calcification. In the osteogenic step, there is a progressive shift from primary to secondary spongiosa and type I collagen predominates.

Hexosamine, hydroxyproline, and hydroxylysine reach a peak concentration in the rat fracture callus during the chondroid step, then decline during the later steps. Lipid and water contents are highest during the mesenchymal step, whereas mineral content progressively increases throughout all steps of repair (Fig. 22). During fracture callus transformation and endochondral bone formation, two main types of proteoglycans are expressed in the extracellular matrix. First, dermatan sulfate is expressed by fibroblasts in the early fracture callus and, during the second week, chondroitin 4-sulfate is expressed in large amounts by the chondrocytes. By the third week, the amount of proteoglycans and their aggregates decreases, and mineralization of the fracture callus begins.

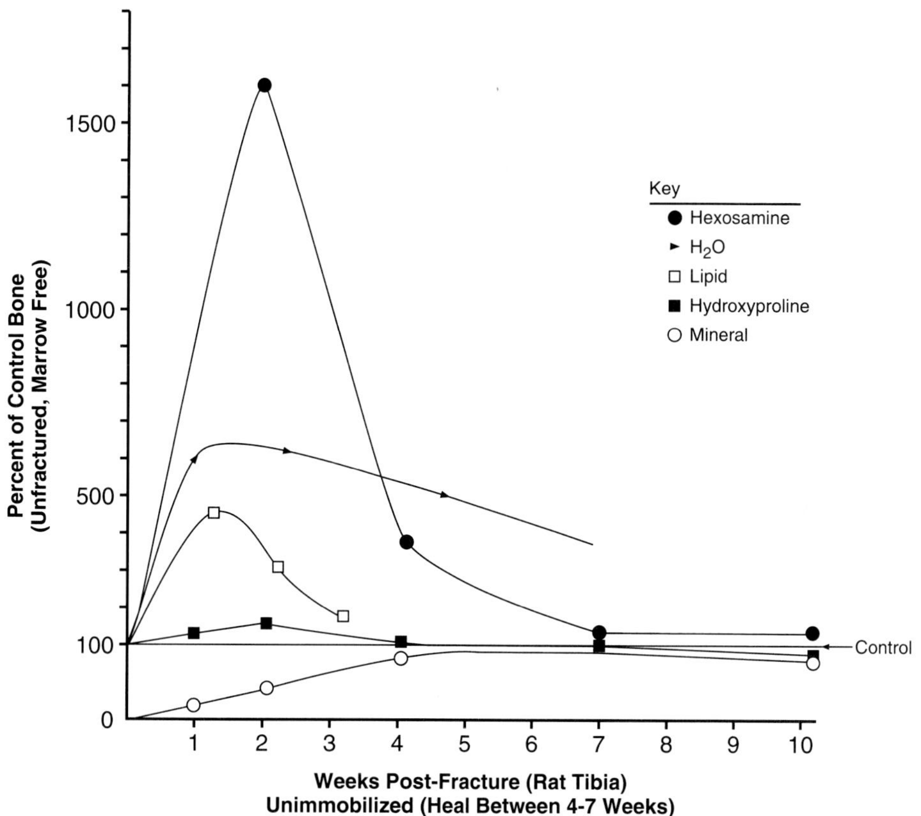

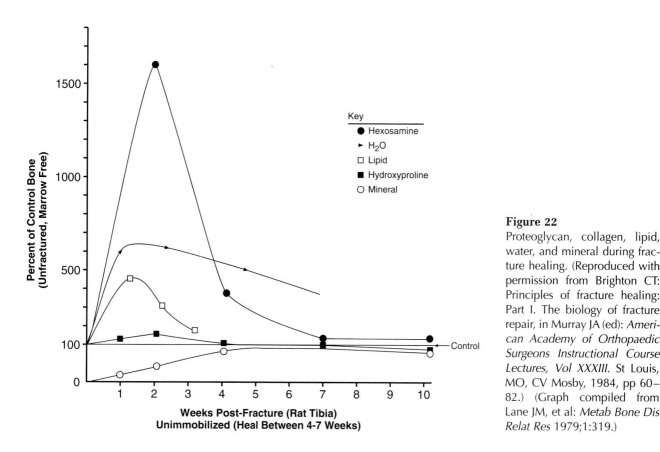

Figure 22
Proteoglycan, collagen, lipid, water, and mineral during fracture healing. (Reproduced with permission from Brighton CT: Principles of fracture healing: Part I. The biology of fracture repair, in Murray JA (ed): *American Academy of Orthopaedic Surgeons Instructional Course Lectures, Vol XXXIII.* St Louis, MO, CV Mosby, 1984, pp 60–82.) (Graph compiled from Lane JM, et al: *Metab Bone Dis Relat Res* 1979;1:319.)

Histochemical localization of calcium in the fracture callus suggests that mitochondria play an important role in matrix calcification of the cartilaginous fracture callus. These intracellular organelles may serve as calcium reservoirs in callus chondrocytes. As the cartilage matrix progressively mineralizes, chondrocyte mitochondria lose progressively more calcium. The initial site of matrix calcification in the fracture callus may be within or on matrix vesicles, collagen fibrils, or proteoglycan disaggregates or collapsed aggregates.

Bone Growth Factors

Regulation of bone volume is maintained through a continuous balance between bone formation and resorption. Two complementary regulatory mechanisms have been postulated for maintenance of bone volume: systemic control by calcium and phosphate regulating hormones and local regulation, which involves growth factors that increase cellular proliferation and biosynthetic activity. It is believed that these same factors play a significant role in the regeneration of bone after its injury resulting from a fracture.

Insulin-like growth factor II (IGF-II) is a single-chain polypeptide that consists of 67 amino acids and is cross-linked by three disulfide bridges. In serum-free cultures of bone cells from several animal species, IGF-II stimulates bone cell proliferation and cartilage matrix production in a dose-dependent manner. IGF-II also stimulates type I collagen and type I procollagen mRNA (messenger ribonucleic acid). IGF-II is produced by bone cells derived from a number of species including man. Both parathyroid hormone (PTH) and 1,25 dihydroxy vitamin D_3 (1,25 $(OH)_2$ vitamin D_3) stimulate production of IGF-II in (in vitro) cultures.

Transforming growth factor beta (TGF-β), which exists in three mammalian isoforms, is found in the fracture hematoma as early as 24 hours following fracture. TGF-β is present in platelets, mesenchymal cells, osteoblasts, and young and mature chondrocytes in the callus, and is present in hypertrophic chondrocytes adjacent to the ossification front. This factor induces the synthesis of cartilage-specific proteoglycans and type II collagen by mesenchymal cells, and stimulates collagen synthesis and proliferation by osteoblasts. Based on the high concentrations found in bone, its effect on protein synthesis by chondrocytes and osteoblasts in vitro, and its release into the fracture hematoma by platelets, TGF-β may be responsible for regulating cartilage and bone formation in the fracture callus. In vivo it is capable of initiating a repair process and callus formation when injected in the vicinity of uninjured bone.

Platelet-derived growth factor (PDGF) consists of two polypeptide chains; it stimulates replication in bone cell cultures in vitro and increases type I collagen synthesis. PDGF also stimulates bone resorption in vitro by a mechanism that involves prostaglandin synthesis. The main functions of PDGF are chemotactic; it attracts inflammatory cells to the fracture site and induces mesenchymal cell proliferation. PDGF is released from platelets and monocytes in the earliest stages of wound healing and may play a role in initiating fracture repair. Multiple subperiosteal injections of PDGF have been shown to induce subperiosteal bone formation.

Bone morphogenic protein (BMP), a low molecular weight hydrophobic glycoprotein discovered in demineralized bone matrix (DBM), can induce bone formation ectopically. BMP-3 is a bone-inductive protein also known as osteogenin. Osteogenin is extremely potent in its capacity to induce the rapid differentiation of extraskeletal mesenchymal tissue into bone. In contrast to the creeping substitution of conventional osseous transplantation, osteoinductive factors such as BMP induce tissue transformation by causing a phenotypic change of local mesenchymal cells into osteoblasts.

Collagenase, gelatinase, and stromelysin are protein-degrading enzymes that cleave components of the extracellular matrix and prepare the fracture callus for calcification. In fracture healing models, alkaline phosphatase activity increases prior to mineralization by hydroxyapatite. Interleukins (IL-1, IL-6) also regulate fracture callus matrix breakdown and stimulate the production of calcified callus.

Prostaglandins have several functions with reference to bone, and at times these functions seem contradictory. When prostaglandins are released from traumatized bone and soft tissues, they increase intracellular cyclic adenosine monophosphate (cAMP) and stimulate production of IGF, a potent bone growth factor. Several in vitro studies have shown they stimulate type I collagen synthesis. However, their effect on regulating the fracture callus in the presence of nonsteroidal anti-inflammatory agents is still unclear. Indomethacin has been reported to inhibit prostaglandin synthesis, thereby producing fracture callus weakness. Contrary to these findings, ibuprofen has been shown to have no effect on fracture healing despite being a potent prostaglandin synthesis inhibitor.

Biomechanical Properties of Fracture Callus

The structural properties of a healing fracture depend on the material properties of the uniting callus. Prior to the onset of the soft callus phase, the fracture site has little inherent stability and strength. When soft callus appears, the radiographic size of the external callus is a poor predictor of fracture strength and does not indicate, at a given healing time, the amount of chemical components in the fracture callus. In studies of fracture callus in rats, during the ossification process of external callus, there is approximately a fourfold increase in the total amount of calcium per unit volume of callus and a twofold increase in hydroxyproline (an indicator of total collagen content). The restoration of fracture strength and stiffness seems to be related more to the amount of new bone connecting the fracture fragments and less to the overall amount of uniting callus. The distinct change from a low-stiffness, rubbery quality to a hard-tissue type of resiliency occurs during a rather short period of time (Table 3). In experiments performed in rabbits, a return of stiffness in fibula fractures correlates with mature callus by 16 days. The staged differentiation and mineralization of fracture callus have a profound influence on its compressive behavior or hardness (Fig. 23) and its tensile strength, and also correlate with progressive increases in average torque and energy absorption to failure. The hardness of the fracture callus closely correlates with its calcium content. The tensile strength of the fracture site during callus formation is highly correlated with the ratio of callus/cortical bone area, and a threefold increase in the breaking strength of the callus in tensile stressing during this phase can be noted (Fig. 24).

Fracture healing, during all stages of the reparative process, is highly susceptible to mechanical factors, directly related to the amount of interfragmentary motion. In any form of fracture fixation, bone fragments under load will experience a certain amount of relative motion which, by unknown mechanisms, determines the morphologic patterns of fracture repair. The interfragmentary strain resulting from this motion is believed to govern the type of tissue that forms between the fracture fragments. Fracture healing results in a gradual decrease in interfragmentary motion. Different tissues can sustain different maximum tensile stresses before failure. Granulation tissue can tolerate 100% strain, fibrous tissue and cartilage tolerate appreciably less strain, and compact bone can resist only 2% strain. Interfragmentary strain is inversely proportional to the fracture gap size. When the fracture gap is small, even slight interfragmentary motion can increase the strain to the extent that granulation tissue may not be able to form. To circumvent this situation, small sections of bone near the fracture gap may undergo resorption; thereby making the fracture gap larger and reducing the overall strain.

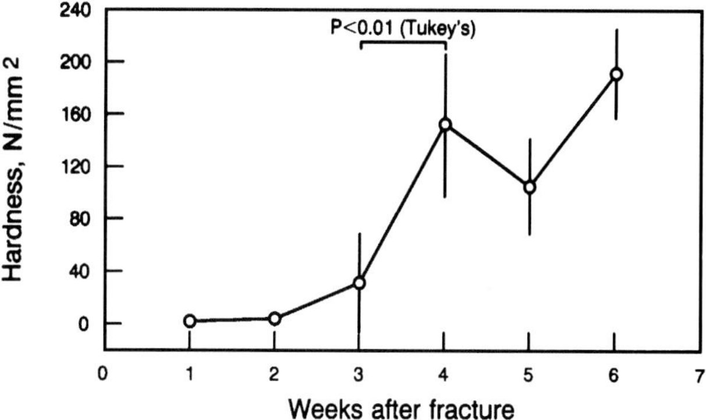

Figure 23
Compressive behavior (hardness) of fracture callus. (Adapted with permission from Aro HT, Wipperman BW, Hodgson SF, et al: Prediction of properties of fracture callus by measurement of mineral density using micro-bone densitometry. *J Bone Joint Surg* 1989;71A:1020–1030.)

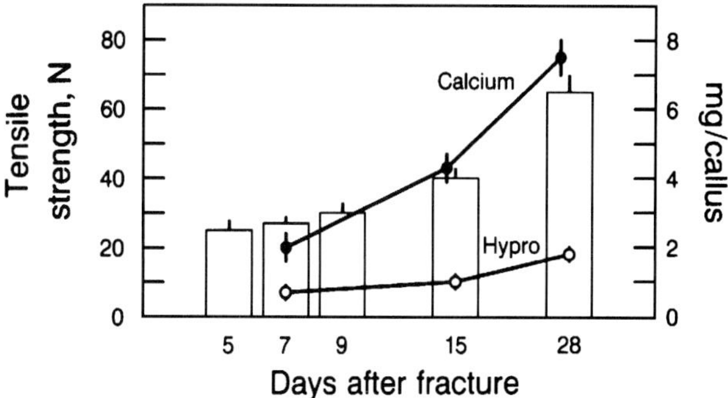

Figure 24
Breaking strength of fracture callus in tensile stressing. (Adapted with permission from Chao EYS, Aro HT: Biomechanics of fracture fixation, in Mow VC, Hayes WC (eds): *Basic Orthopaedic Biomechanics.* New York, Raven Press, 1991, pp 293–335.)

Table 3
The four biomechanical stages of fracture repair

Stage	Description
Stage 1	The bone fails through the original fracture site with a low stiffness, rubbery pattern.
Stage 2	The bone fails through the original fracture site with a high stiffness, hard tissue pattern.
Stage 3	The bone fails partially through the original fracture site and partially through the previously intact bone with a high stiffness, hard tissue pattern.
Stage 4	The site of failure is not related to the original fracture site and occurs with a high stiffness pattern.

The nature of the cellular response directly correlates with the degree of bony stability at the fracture site during repair. When mechanical stability is present and the bone ends are in intimate contact, very little cartilage will form, and a thin layer of hard callus will eventually be produced by direct haversian remodeling. When a more mechanically unstable condition exists, hard callus cannot, early on, bridge the bone ends; exuberant cartilaginous callus must first form and then, if stability is sufficient, proceed to be transformed to bone by endochondral ossification. During calcification of the soft callus, if insufficient immobilization exists in conjunction with the presence of an excessive fracture gap, a nonunion may occur because of the persistence of fibrous tissue or a failure of the fibrocartilagenous callus between the fracture fragments to transform into osteogenic callus tissue.

Biology and Biomechanics of Fracture Fixation

If a fracture is inherently stable, because of direct impaction of the bony ends or adjacent ligamentous and bony support, little additional effort is needed to maintain a minimal amount of interfragmentary motion. Cast or brace immobilization or no immobilization may be all that is needed. However for many fractures additional internal or external support is necessary. Such support alters the normal biologic process and mechanics during and after fracture repair. This section provides a review of the healing mechanisms of long bones and a discussion of the influence of stable and unstable fixation on fracture biomechanics.

Compression Plating

Rigid compression plating of an osteotomy inhibits callus formation; the bone ends unite directly by haversian remodeling. This type of healing has been referred to as contact healing in contact areas and as gap healing in noncontact areas. It is considered primary bone healing in contradistinction to the previously described secondary fracture healing, which includes callus formation and the four stages of fracture union. The haversian remodeling seen in primary fracture healing has two main functions: the revascularization of necrotic fracture ends and reconstitution of the intercortical union. The three requirements for haversian remodeling across the fracture site are the performance of an exact reduction, the production of stable fixation, and the existence of a sufficient blood supply.

When a dynamic compression plate is applied to an osteotomy in bone, the compression at the osteotomy site decays slowly over a period of time, and it is reduced by approximately 50% within two months. This same phenomenon also is seen when there is no osteotomy and a dynamic compression plate is applied to an intact bone. Therefore, this slow decay of compression is not caused by shortening of the fragments and resorption, but instead is a result of haversian remodeling under the plate and screws.

The use of a dynamic compression plate in an osteotomy model has been shown to lead to primary bone healing. When there are no gaps and the fracture fragments are rigidly held together, there is no ingrowth of mesodermal cells from the periosteum or endosteum. Active haversian remodeling is seen at approximately the fourth week via proliferation of haversian canals along the longitudinal axis of the bone. If a gap exists, which often is seen opposite the plate even if there is rigid fixation, new blood vessels and osteoblasts deposit osteoid into this gap in the first eight days. The lamellar bone that is formed in this gap is oriented 90° to the longitudinal axis. Axially oriented osteons then bridge across this perpendicularly oriented osteoid by haversian remodeling. The growth of these secondary osteons starts four weeks after fracture fixation in the dog and later in man; thus, there is always a lag period before the activation of haversian remodeling. This delay in activation has been postulated to be related to tissue damage at the fracture site.

The growth of secondary osteons from one fracture fragment to another does not occur only at sites of macroscopic gaps; it will occur in areas that seem to have intimate contact between the fracture fragments. After reduction and compression plating, incongruencies remaining at the fracture site will result in small gaps. Within weeks after fracture, these gaps are filled by direct lamellar or woven bone formation; that is, appositional bone formation. Woven bone formed within the gap acts as a spacer but does not unite the fracture ends. Secondary osteons use the gap tissue as a scaffold to grow from one fragment to another.

Although primary bone healing refers to union without callus formation and secondary bone healing to union by means of callus formation, this usage represents an oversimplification that is not always seen in vivo. The production of a small amount of callus opposite a dynamic compression plate indicates that there is sufficient interfragmentary motion opposite the plate to allow for a slight amount of callus healing. If this motion is excessive and/or long term, the plate will fail through cyclic loading. However, a small amount of motion and subsequent callus formation opposite the plate can be advantageous, leading to earlier and stronger union. Fractures also exist that heal without callus formation and, nevertheless, go through the stages previously described for secondary bone healing, which include both endochondral and intramembranous bone formation. Examples include fractures in the scaphoid and talus, which consist mostly of cartilage; the areas where blood vessels penetrate to provide the bone's vascular supply are not heavily endowed with periosteum. Additionally, neither bone is surrounded by large amounts of soft tissues or muscle.

Two theories exist to explain the remodeling under a rigidly applied plate: the vascular disturbance theory and the stress-shielding theory. These may not be mutually exclusive and may depend on the load bearing characteristics of the bone-plate construct. Additionally, although it is the crucial step for the final union, vascular ingrowth of secondary osteons results, paradoxically, in a transitory compulsory reduction of cortical bone density. The resulting porosity has been shown to be responsible for the remodeling and stress shielding seen under rigid plate fixation. This "cancellization" of cortical bone under the plate leads to thinning of the cortex and is partially responsible, along with screw holes and ununited fractures, for refractures after plate removal. This is especially true for fractures involving the forearm. The compression plate itself also affects the cortical blood supply arising from periosteal vessels.

When applying a plate for fixation the appropriate number of screws must be used to minimize stresses and achieve optimal results. A plate with less than adequate fixation and a decreased working length is at risk for failure. Recommendations are for at least four cortices on each side for the forearm and six to eight cortices for each side at the humerus. For the tibia and femur eight or more cortices on each side are preferred. Such screws traversing the medullary cavity do not significantly disturb the circulation; medullary vessels curve closely around tight screws. By one week after fracture fixation, the arterioles and capillaries of the medullary canal cross an osteotomy site, thereby effecting a medullary osseous union. At six weeks after tight plate application, vascularization of the cortex is greatly reduced.

External Fixation

While primary bone healing can be seen with plate fixation, it can also be seen with external fixation. In a study of osteotomies in canine tibias held in place with half frame external fixaters placed in the medial-lateral plane, compression was applied across the osteotomy site in one group and not in another group. Both groups showed a significantly greater amount of periosteal new bone formation in the anterior-posterior plane than in the medial-lateral plane where there was more rigidity. Primary bone healing of both the contact and gap type was seen in both groups. However, the existence of primary bone healing with external fixation does not indicate that it is the preferred method of healing. Less rigid fixation has been shown to lead to "controlled" interfragmentary motion and, therefore, to more periosteal callus and new bone formation, which may produce equally good union.

The mechanical strength of a fracture augmented by an external (or internal) fixation device must be considered to be based on a composite structure in which load sharing and motion occurs between the device and the fracture site; it is not based solely on the mechanical properties of the fixator, pins, and their connections. It has been shown that for an external fixator applied to a canine tibial fracture in which the fragment ends are not in contact, the stiffness of the composite is low and varies between 2,000 and 4,000 N/cm. In such situations, partial weightbearing of about 20 kg causes 0.5 to 1.0 mm of axial cyclic movement of fracture fragments. Thus, to avoid failure, the decision of how much weightbearing is appropriate depends not only on the frame and pin configuration but also on whether fracture reduction can yield such ideal contact. Too rigid a construct also may not be ideal. A vast improvement in healing of an osteotomy was reported when external fixation with controlled micromovement was compared to osteotomies after static rigid external fixation. More elastic fixation allows the bone to bear weight without the external fixation acting as a stress-shielding device. Making the frame more elastic by decreasing the number of pins from six to four led to an increase in the amount of periosteal callus seen in radiographs; however, there also was increased loosening of the pins as a result of the additional motion at the pin-bone junction. Thus, it is difficult to determine how rigid a frame is necessary and when a frame becomes too rigid. According to the two-column theory, if the bone is in contact, a simple anterior unilateral frame will act as a second column, and will be sufficient to allow some weightbearing and to result in union. If there is no bony contact, two columns of external fixation are necessary, initially. These would be provided by using either a stacked anterior frame or an anterior frame combined with an anteromedial frame. Others believe that a very rigid frame is necessary initially and that disassembly of the external fixation device with a sequential decrease in the stiffness is the way to achieve union (Table 4).

Many factors determine the rigidity of a frame. The pinholes should be less than 30% of the bone diameter to decrease the risk of open section frac-

Table 4
Types of axial stimulation at the fracture site under external fixation

Type	Description
Passive Dynamization	Load transmission through fracture site due to pin bending under weightbearing (rigid side-bar) Removal of additional side-bar or pins results in reduction of axial, torsional, and bending stiffness, proportionally
Active Axial Dynamization	Load transmission through fracture site under weightbearing without pin bending (telescoping side-bar) Relaxation of the axial constraint in the fixator does not affect the torsional and bending stability of the fixation
Controlled Axial Micromovement	Load transmission through fracture site using controlled force/displacement actuator (telescoping side-bar)

ture. It has been shown that a 5-mm stainless steel pin is 144% more rigid than a 4-mm pin. The difference is so large because the bending stiffness of the pin is proportional to the areal moment of inertia, which is 1/2 the radius to the fourth power. Tubular rods with an 11-mm diameter are approximately two times stiffer than solid connecting rods with an 8-mm diameter. Increasing the pin spread to 9 cm triples the resistance to anteroposterior bending, and decreasing the bone-rod distance to 2.5 cm leads to a threefold increase in resistance to transverse bending. Another way to increase stiffness of the frame is to separate half pins by greater than 45° when applying anterior and anteromedial frames together (Table 5).

Pin and pin tract complications are often difficult to avoid; however, there appear to be several distinct factors that can improve the performance of the pin-bone interface. Half pins are subjected primarily to bending loads. Some stress can be reduced by using a larger pin diameter, reducing the side-bar separation, and applying transfixation pins rather than half pins to increase the bending rigidity of the pin. As noted, weightbearing should be avoided in fractures without cortical contact. In such cases, studies have shown that locations of maximum stress are within a pin group. The site varies according to loading mode, but pin-bone failure is mainly at the entry cortex. Axial dynamization as the fracture heals restores the cortical contact in stable fractures and, therefore, decreases the bone-pin stresses. Pin insertion technique is also important. The eccentric location of pins, often seen with the use of intracortical pins, and thermal necrosis, potentially occurring when a power drill is used, may lead to loosening of the pin. Preloading in either the radial or axial direction may decrease the incidence of pin-bone loosening.

Table 5
Key factors in increasing the rigidity of external fixation

Factor	Description
1	Increased pin diameter
2	Increased pin number
3	Decreased bone-rod distance
4	Increased pin group separation
5	Half pins separated > 45°

Circular external fixation Recently circular external fixation configurations have become popular for the treatment of fractures, posttraumatic deformities, osteomyelitis, and congenital anomalies. Circular rings are connected to 1.8- or 2-mm wires that are fixed to the ring at tensions of 90 to 130 kg. The optimum orientation of the wires on the ring is 90° to each other to provide the most stability; however, because of anatomic considerations this is not always possible. Because of the circular configuration, the bending stiffness of the frame is independent of the loading direction.

When compared to the Hoffmann-Vidal frame, which has 4-mm transfixation pins applied medial to lateral and attached to half pins applied through the anterior area and is very rigid, the Ilizarov frame was half as rigid in compression. In anteroposterior bending and in torsion, the frames are comparable in rigidity. However, with lateral-medial bending, the Hoffmann-Vidal frame had a rigidity of 800 N/cm versus 80 N/cm for the Ilizarov frame. This decreased rigidity of the frame in bending resulted from bowing of the transverse wires and slippage of the bone along the smooth tensioned wires. In torsion, laxity in the system was due primarily to wire deflection.

The most critical factors in frame stability are the number, tension, and size of the cross-wires. The factors that are available to increase the stability of the circular external fixator include: (1) larger wire diameter; (2) decreased ring size; (3) use of olive wires; (4) increased number of wires; (5) crossing wires at right angles; (6) increased wire tension; (7) positioning of the center rings close to the fracture or nonunion site; and (8) closer distance between adjacent rings. However, as is the case with monoplanar and biplanar external fixation, the appropriate amount of stability and stiffness is not known. The lower rigidity of this frame, especially in compression and lateral-medial bending when compared to the Hoffmann-Vidal frame, may be advantageous in providing the appropriate amount of axial loading to the regenerate bone in order to allow it to become structurally sound.

Intramedullary Nails

In 1940, Kuntscher introduced the technique of closed intramedullary nailing of the femur, and in 1950 he added reaming of the medullary canal to improve contact between the nail and the cortical wall for more stable fixation. In the 1970s, Klemm and Schellmann added interlocking to the nail, which broadened indications for its use and allowed treatment of nonmidshaft fractures by closed nailing techniques. Closed intramedullary nailing with or without interlocking is currently the treatment of choice for fractures from the lesser trochanter to the supracondylar area of the femur. In addition, modification of the intramedullary tibial nail to allow interlocking has led to its use for fractures of the tibia that go from just below the plateau to just above the supramalleolar region.

With the addition of a loose-fitting intramedullary rod into the medullary canal, the endosteal circulation is able to regenerate rapidly and completely where space has been left between the nail and the endosteal surface. When reaming is used for placement of an intramedullary nail, the results are different.

The three major blood supplies to the long bone are the nutrient artery, the metaphyseal arteries, and the periosteal arteries (Fig. 25). The nutrient artery penetrates the cortex of the shaft and then divides into ascending and descending medullary arteries. These endosteal blood vessels are the ones that are destroyed during introduction of a reamed intramedullary nail. The metaphyseal arteries supply blood to the metaphysis and anastomose with the medullary arteries. The metaphyseal arteries, therefore, continue to feed the medullary arteries when they have been disrupted by a fracture. The periosteal arteries, which enter the cortex along heavy fascial attachments, supply blood to the outer one-third of the cortex, whereas the medullary arteries supply blood to the inner two-thirds of the cortex. However, normal periosteal blood vessels appear unable to contribute any significant blood supply to the medullary circulation after it has been disrupted. Proliferation of new extraosseous arteries arising from surrounding soft tissues is required until the medullary circulation can be reestablished.

The damage following reaming is similar to an experimental situation in which there is simultaneous ligation of the nutrient artery and interruption of the metaphyseal blood supply. Because of the anatomy of the medullary blood supply, the essential damage is caused by the first reaming, and there is necrosis of the inner 50% to 70% of the cortex. Subsequent reaming has little effect on cortical vascularity; therefore, the amount of reaming actually

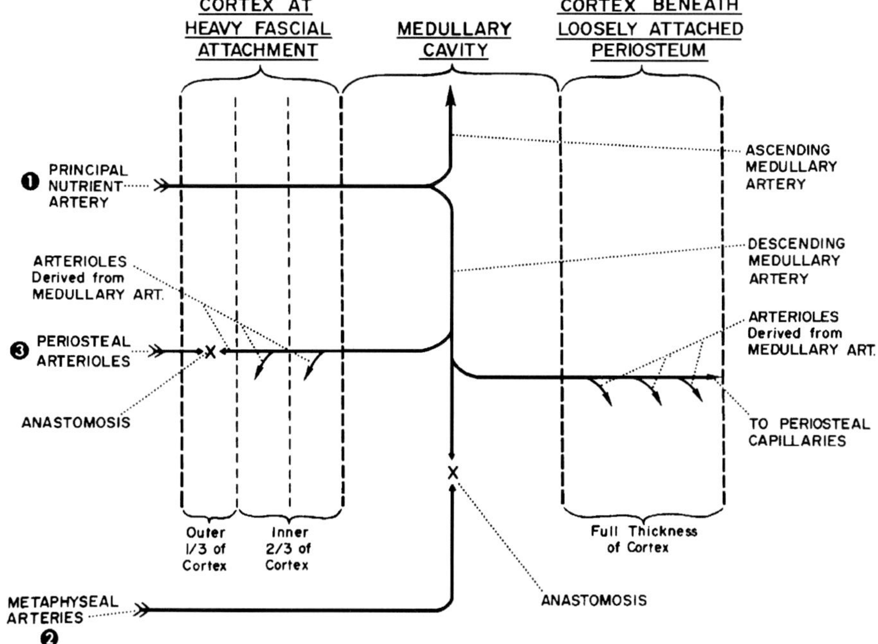

Figure 25
Diagrammatic representation of the major components of the afferent vascular system of a normal mature long bone, based on differences in the type of blood vessel observed experimentally to enter the external cortical surface at sites of heavy fascial attachment and at sites of tenuous periosteum beneath bellies of muscles. Components 1, 2, and 3 constitute the total nutrient supply to the diaphyseal cortex. Arrows indicate the direction of blood flow. (Reproduced with permission from Rhinelander FW: Circulation in bone, in Bourne G (ed): *The Biochemistry and Physiology of Bone,* ed. 2. New York, Academic Press, 1972, vol. 2.)

performed is of minor importance. After reaming and the application of a tight-fitting intramedullary nail at the four-week stage of repair, there appear to be three paths for blood supply: (1) through a regenerative endosteal membrane; (2) through the external callus at its junction with the cortex; and (3) through the substance of the cortex itself. Six weeks after medullary reaming and tight nailing, the significant regenerative blood supply to all the bony tissue appears by microangiography to be endosteal. Thus, the overall regenerative blood supply at six weeks follows the same three pathways as it did at four weeks, with a notable increase in the size of the posterior intracortical (from the nutrient artery) arteries.

Revascularization of the necrotic cortex comes from two sources. One is the regenerative medullary circulation through small arterioles in the new endosteal membrane that has been able to form within the crevices around the intramedullary nail. The other is a new extraosseous circulation supplied by large arteries derived from the surrounding soft tissues with branches traversing the full thickness of the external callus to support the osteoclastic removal of the necrotic cortex. This periosteal blood supply is not the same as the periosteal circulation of a normal long bone. These new periosteal arterioles enter the cortex where the periosteum is only loosely attached, and this new extraosseous blood supply is a transitory phenomenon helping with cortical repair. After its disruption at the endosteal surface, the principal nutrient artery turns back and produces intracortical branches that supply blood to the femoral cortex.

By 12 weeks after reaming, a thick, highly vascular endosteal membrane surrounds the entire nail tract, and large intracortical arteries appear in the posterior cortex at this time. It has been shown in dog and sheep long bones that it takes eight to 12 weeks to achieve total revascularization. In humans, this time is even longer. Based on these results, it becomes obvious that there is a higher risk of bone necrosis with intramedullary reaming of an open fracture in which the periosteal blood supply also has been stripped. This higher risk appears to be more relevant in the tibia, which does not have a large soft-tissue envelope; it is especially relevant for open tibia fractures in which reamed intramedullary nails are generally contraindicated. Data from recent experimental studies in which microsphere techniques were used following intramedullary reaming and nailing show that perfusion to the cortex at the fracture site is diminished during the early phase of fracture healing, but by 90 days, the collateral blood supply to the endosteal cortex has overcome this defect.

Fractures of the femur Intramedullary nailing has many favorable biomechanical features. Proper surgical technique is necessary so that the maximum effect can be obtained from the femoral intramedullary nail. It has been shown that an anterior starting point, medial to the greater trochanter, greatly increases hoop stresses at the fracture site and can cause comminution of the fracture when the nail is inserted. This problem can be avoided by placing the insertion site more posterior in the piriformis fossa, thus positioning the neutral axis of the nail in the center of the bone itself. Another consideration, when choosing an intramedullary nail for rodding a femur, is the location of the fracture. Unlocked nails can be used for simple transverse or short oblique fractures of the isthmus region of the shaft. These allow load sharing and, thus, may minimize the stress shielding often seen with fixation. The intramedullary nail without interlocking is based on elastic three-point fixation, and the purpose of reaming is to allow a good fit of the nail.

The treatment of fractures outside the isthmus or of comminuted fractures in which the use of conventional nails is not applicable has led to the use of interlocking intramedullary nails. With the new addition of second generation interlocking nails (reconstruction nails), the indications have expanded even more. However, fatigue fracture of interlocking nails at the more proximal of the two distal screw holes has been reported in supracondylar femur fractures in which the level of the fracture is 5 cm or less from the more proximal of the distal screw holes. In addition, several first generation intramedullary nails have been shown to break at the proximal portion where the slot meets the unslotted portion. To avoid this breakage, many of the nails come fully slotted or entirely unslotted along their length.

The stiffness of intramedullary nails varies greatly depending on the manufacturing process. Titanium has a modulus of elasticity closer to that of cortical bone than stainless steel. Posterior slotted nails have increased bending strength but less flexibility, whereas anterior slotted nails have improved flexibility. More recently, nonslotted nails have been introduced; these closed cross section nails have a marked increase in torsional stiffness as well as a small increase in bending stiffness. The other advantage to a closed cross section nail is that by eliminating the slot in the nail, the smaller diameter nails have an increased strength to allow cross fixation and cannulation. These nails were developed to make distal cross locking easier; however, because of the increased stiffness, there is a potential for added comminution during insertion of the nail. In addition, these nails must be overreamed by 1 to 2 mm, whereas the more flexible nails only need to be overreamed 1 mm. The thickness of the nail wall also has a distinct bearing on the stiffness of the intramedullary nail. Another consideration is that all nails currently have anterior bows to them; however, the radius of curvature varies depending on the nail that is used.

Two types of locked intramedullary nailing are presently in use. The first, called dynamic interlocking, is used to stabilize transverse and short oblique fractures above and below the isthmus; the screws are used to lock the smaller fracture fragment. In these cases, the isthmus is used as the second point of fixation to allow load sharing with the intramedullary nail in place. In the second type of fixation, called static interlocking, the intramedullary nail is inserted and screws are placed in both the proximal and distal parts of the nail. In static interlocking, forces from the intact bone are transmitted proximally, via the screws, through the nail that spans the fracture site to the intact cortical bone anchored distally by the transverse locking screws. This use has changed the intramedullary nail to a partial load-bearing device. Concern that static interlocking might result in a higher incidence of nonunion led to the proposal of a procedure known as dynamization. In this procedure, the patient was brought back at some time postoperatively, and the screws farthest from the fracture site were removed to allow more load sharing and to increase the stresses on the cortical bone, thereby improving healing. It recently has been shown that static intramedullary nailing does not lead to nonunion; instead it leads to union rates of 95% to 98%. Therefore, dynamization is no longer encouraged, except in those fractures that appear distracted or are going on to a delayed union or nonunion. In a recent study, the union rate with static interlock nailing was found to be 98%, and complications with dynamic nailing occurred with displacement of the fracture fragments around the rod with weightbearing. Static interlocking is now the procedure of choice for repair of most unstable femoral shaft fractures because this partial load-sharing device leads to healing and, after the reconstitution of cortical continuity, bone remodeling does take place.

Subtrochanteric fractures of the femur Subtrochanteric fractures of the femur have presented a difficult biomechanical problem. This region is an area of high stress caused by bending moments and compressive forces. Flexion and extension of the hip, even while in bed, can produce forces at the femoral head as large as 2.5 to three times body weight, and slow walking can result in hip forces of up to 4.9 times body weight. Comminution of the subtrochanteric area can further increase the stresses applied to an implant because of the greater load being borne by the implant as a result of the lack of the medial buttressing effect. In a study of simulated subtrochanteric fractures, intramedullary devices were compared with plate-bone fixation. The unlocked intramedullary nail returned 5% of the controlled femur stiffness when tested in torsion, but the torsional stiffness of the plate-bone systems was about 50% that of the intact bone. An interlocking nail system provided the highest failure loads (between 300% and 400% of body weight) under simulated weightbearing (Fig. 26). Good clinical results also have been obtained with the use of interlocking nails for the treatment of subtrochanteric fractures of the femur. With an intact lesser trochanter, first generation interlocking nails are successful; however, when the lesser trochanter is involved in the fracture, second generation nails should be used. A fracture which splits the greater trochanter may be a contraindication to intramedullary nailing. In these instances a nail-plate device may be more successful. Although the interlocking designs prevent relative rotation between the nail and the cortex, they do not change the inherent low torsional stiffness of the nail itself. This feature, in the case of intramedullary fixation, does not seem to be detrimental to fracture healing.

Fractures of the tibia Fractures of the proximal and distal ends of the tibia are best treated with plates, especially those with intra-articular extensions. However, because there is a slightly higher nonunion rate with the use of plates in midshaft tibia fractures, intramedullary nails appear to be efficacious. For stable fractures at the isthmus, unlocked intramedullary nails of the cloverleaf variety or

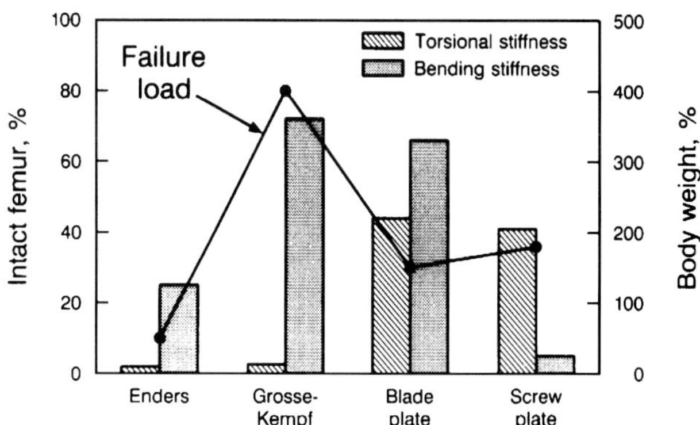

Figure 26

Comparison of intramedullary devices and plate-bone fixation of simulated subtrochanteric fractures. (Adapted with permission from Chao EYS, Aro HT: Biomechanics of fracture fixation, in Mow VC, Hayes WC (eds): *Basic Orthopaedic Biomechanics.* New York, Raven Press, 1991, pp 293–335.)

elastic nails without reaming can be used to maintain alignment and obtain healing. For the more unstable fractures, locking intramedullary nails appear to be the treatment of choice. Open tibia fractures have long been treated by external fixation, either just until the soft tissues have healed or by dynamization until union. The role of limited internal fixation in addition to external fixation is still unclear. Although bony alignment can be maintained better and there is less dead space and decreased soft-tissue injury when this technique is used, the time to union may be prolonged by not allowing for axial loading at the fracture site. The use of unreamed intramedullary nails may be indicated in some open fractures. Investigations are currently in progress to examine the type of nail, fracture configuration, and soft-tissue injury best suited for unreamed intramedullary nailing.

A large proportion of tibia fractures can be treated with casting followed by weightbearing in a brace or cast brace. Fracture bracing is based on the principles that the soft-tissue sleeve surrounding a fracture leads to union by early functional motion and weightbearing when possible. The amount of shortening is maximum at the time of injury, and further angulation is prevented by the configuration of the cast or brace. The maintenance of joint motion and a decrease in muscle atrophy are added benefits with this form of treatment. Controlled motion at the fracture site has been shown to be conducive to osteogenesis. This basic premise along with no further violation of the endosteal or periosteal blood-supply, as is seen with internal fixation, has led to very good results when there is strict adherence to the treatment principles. In a recent study of fracture bracing, the nonunion rate was only 2.5%, over 80% of patients had less than 5° of varus, 92.5% had less than 8° of varus, and 91% had a final shortening of 1 cm or less. However, there are problems with fracture bracing. Fractures with marked tibial angulation at the time of injury have a tendency to angulate further, and fractures of the tibia with an intact fibula tend to displace with the shorter tibial fragment angulating toward the fibula.

Fracture bracing also is used following the removal of an external fixator in the treatment of severe open tibia fractures. The external fixators should remain in place long enough for soft-tissue intrinsic stability to develop about the fracture site. When soft-tissue damage is extensive and associated with initial severe shortening, removal of the fixator may result in recurrence of shortening and angular deformities. Posterolateral bone grafts should be considered in these unstable open fractures to obtain union.

Comparison of Fixation Methods

Plate Fixation Versus Intramedullary Fixation

When plate fixation was compared with intramedullary rod fixation in dogs, the blood flow reached higher levels and remained elevated longer in osteotomies that were fixed with the rods than those fixed with the plates (Fig. 27). Rod-fixed osteotomies healed by periosteal callus, whereas plate-fixed osteotomies showed predominantly endosteal callus formation (Fig. 28). There were no significant differences in bone porosity between the fixation methods. The plated osteotomies displayed higher torsional stiffness values than the rod-fixed osteotomies at 90 days, but this difference was no longer apparent at 120 days.

These data show that bone heals by different mechanisms with different types of fixation. Rigid plate fixation improved the recovery of mechanical properties during the early phase of healing, although the rigidity of plate fixation inhibited periosteal callus formation. The time needed for return of normal strength and stiffness was, however, the same for both methods, indicating that the end result of the different healing patterns was the same.

Plate Fixation Versus External Fixation

Characteristics of the union of bone osteotomies achieved by means of compression plating (eight-hole prebent dynamic compression plate) were compared with those achieved by unilateral external fixation. In vitro mechanical testing showed that the plate-bone system was significantly more rigid than

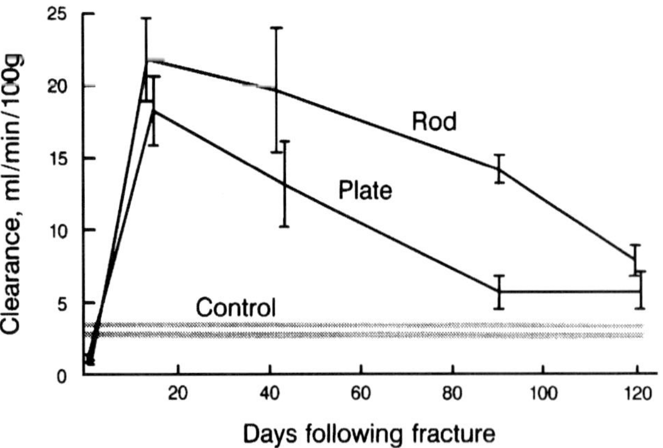

Figure 27
Fracture site clearance; mean values. (Adapted with permission from Raud JA, An KN, Chao EYS, et al: A comparison of the effect of open intramedullary nailing and compression-plate fixation on fracture site blood flow and fracture union. *J Bone Joint Surg* 1981;63A:427–442.)

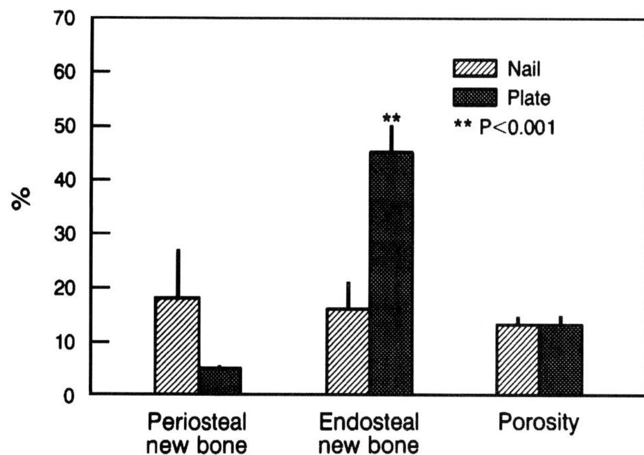

Figure 28
Callus formation in rod- and plate-fixed osteotomies. (Adapted with permission from Chao EYS, Aro HT: Biomechanics of fracture fixation, in Mow VC, Hayes WC (eds): *Basic Orthopaedic Biomechanics.* New York, Raven Press, 1991, pp 293–335.)

the external fixator-bone system in all testing modes other than lateral bending in the plane of the external fixator. The in vivo use of both methods led to osteotomy union by 120 days. However, the maximum torque and stiffness of the plated osteotomies were significantly higher than those of the osteotomies treated with external fixation.

It is again to be emphasized that the rigidity of the composite fixation system, rather than the type of device used, is an important factor in early bone healing. Data indicate that the rigidity of fixation governs not only whether the fracture will heal, but also the mechanism through which bone union will take place. Biologic and biomechanical pathways to osseous union can be changed by manipulating the rigidity of fixation during the treatment course. It has been well established that internal and external fixation devices both lead to fracture union, but do so through slightly different biologic processes, as dictated by their biomechanical characteristics. Plate fixation favors endosteal healing, while intramedullary nailing and less rigid external fixation encourage periosteal healing. Rigid external fixation prevents periosteal callus formation; thus, it relies on osteonal cortical reconstruction with minimal endosteal healing. Axially dynamized external fixation facilitates direct cortical reconstruction with periosteal new bone formation.

Fluctuating stresses induced by unstable fixation and associated fracture gap movement are important contributing factors in pin loosening. Careful pin insertion technique, an increase in pin diameter, improved pin geometry and thread design, the load-carrying capacity of the healing fracture, and the magnitude of loading under external fixation are other factors in the prevention of pin loosening and pin tract infection.

Finally, it remains unknown whether mechanical stimuli of various magnitudes and frequency will significantly improve the normal fracture healing process or whether patients with abnormal or delayed unions can be helped by such external factors. The existing data strongly support such assumptions; future studies should be encouraged to verify this exciting contention.

Factors Influencing Fracture Repair

Fracture Nonunion

A variety of local, systemic, and environmental factors may affect fracture healing. Local factors that may impede fracture healing include extensive injury sustained by the bone or the surrounding soft tissue, interruption of the local blood supply, imposition of soft tissue between fracture fragments, inadequate reduction and/or immobilization, presence of infection or malignant tissue at the fracture site, and bone death caused by avascularity, radiation, thermal or chemical burns, or infection (Outline 2). Mechanical factors may also influence healing adversely. If compression across the fracture site is too great, cell necrosis occurs. Inadequate stress between fracture fragments fails to generate an osteogenic healing response. Cyclic compression, such as that which exists with a weightbearing cast or cast brace, may have a beneficial effect on healing if introduced in the appropriate way at the appropriate time.

When bony bridging does not progress at an expected pace, the patient is said to have a delayed union or nonunion, depending on time since fracture and other factors, such as the site and severity of the injury. In delayed union (arbitrarily from three to nine months), spontaneous healing may occur, with time, for a certain percentage of patients or intervention may be required. Generally, the less severe the original insult and the more propitious

Outline 2
Factors influencing fracture healing

Systemic	Local
Age	Degree of local trauma
Hormones	Vascular injury
Functional activity	Type of bone affected
Nerve functions	Degree of bone loss
Nutrition	Degree of immobilization
	Infection
	Local pathologic conditions

the site, the more likely is a delayed union to heal with only careful management of intrinsic biomechanical factors. A fracture can be labeled as a nonunion after no progress has been carefully documented, six to eight months have elapsed since the original injury, and an informed judgment by the surgeon indicates that intervention will be required to effect healing.

At the pathologic level, a nonunion is a fracture bridged with soft tissue. It must be differentiated from a synovial pseudarthrosis in which a fluid-filled gap exists. In nonunion, healing has been interrupted at Stage II and the gap usually contains interposed cartilage, fibrous tissue, or both. Gap tissue characteristics reflect the local mechanical and nutritional factors that dominate in the first weeks of repair. Furthermore, these characteristics should dictate the type of therapeutic interaction necessary to produce bony union. Atrophic, fibrous unions are more difficult to heal and may require bone grafting, whereas hypertrophic nonunions with a predominance of fibrocartilage in the gap may just require stabilization.

The goal in treating a nonunion is to "restart" the regeneration process. Nonunions may be divided into two groups: those that have a good blood supply and are hypertrophic and those that have a poor blood supply and become atrophic. Hypertrophic nonunions require stabilization only, often without taking apart the nonunion site, in order to heal. Atrophic nonunions require both stabilization and a means to restart the repair process.

In the treatment of hypertrophic nonunions, intramedullary nailing has given the best results. With this technique union rates between 92% and 95% have been reported for noninfected nonunions of the femur and tibia.

Tho only indication for applying a bono graft to a hypertrophic nonunion would be the continued existence of a gap after correction of a deformity. Bone grafting supplies an osteoconductive surface as well as osteoinduction and, perhaps, a few live bone cells in order to stimulate the atrophic nonunion to heal. The Ilizarov technique has been used extensively for both hypertrophic and atrophic nonunions as well as infected nonunions and has been shown to be successful. However, it is a very demanding and labor intensive technique. Preliminary reports have shown that the use of ultrasound may speed up the time to union of both tibia fractures and Colles' fractures.

Electric Factors in Fracture Repair

Electric stimulation also appears to be successful in restarting the repair process in nonunions, but its use is contraindicated in synovial pseudarthrosis and nonunions with significant gaps at the fracture site. This method may also require casting, which can lead to joint immobilization and muscle atrophy. Although electric stimulation may heal a nonunion, it cannot correct associated deformities at the nonunion site. However, union rates between 70% and 90% or more have been reported with varying types of electrical stimulation and among various sites of nonunion. Other modalities under current clinical evaluation include injection of bone marrow cells or BMP into the fracture site, ultrasound stimulation, and compression-distraction using the Ilizarov technique.

Although some controversy still exists about specific clinical applications for electric fields, a body of expermental and clinical data has accumulated over the past three decades demonstrating effects on the regulation of connective tissue cells and their synthetic byproducts. There are three types of electrical stimulation: (1) direct current, (2) capacitative coupling, and (3) inductive coupling. These methods accelerate the *early phases* of fresh fracture repair by only 20% to 25%, an improvement insufficient to justify routine clinical application. However, they produce significant effects in the treatment of delayed union and nonunion. At the laboratory level, mechanisms of action for certain bioresponses to field exposure are being defined, as they are for many drugs and hormones. At the clinical level, efficacy is being examined by randomized, prospective and double blind studies for bone healing and other conditions. From such studies it has been shown that the biologic features of a fresh fracture and a chronically ununited fracture are distinctly different not only in their cellular and temporal features, but in their electric characteristics as well.

Tho oloctrical proportioo of bono and cartilago depend on the charged nature of some of the molecules that make up these materials. For example, proteoglycans in cartilage and bone become ionized in solution because of the presence of sulfate and carboxyl groups. These charges are neutralized by counterions in solution. Charges, fixed on the components of the solid phase and floating in the fluid filling the pores, give rise to continually measured electromechanical phenomena in cartilage and bone. For example, a piezoelectric effect occurs when charges in collagen are displaced by mechanical deformation. This occurs in both wet and dry bone. Streaming potential effects occur when pressures or deformations cause fluid flow, which entrains the ions. Dynamic mechanical deformation causes charge-separation by piezoelectric elements in the tissues and from streaming potentials. Streaming potentials (electrokinetic events) arise when fluids containing charged solutes are forced past sites of fixed charge in tissues, on cell membranes, or intracellularly. Both piezoelectric potentials and streaming potentials occur in wet bone. Streaming potentials dominate in cartilage because cartilage is more hydrated than bone and has a higher proteoglycan content. These two electric phenomena are both examples of stress-generated potentials. The significance of the stress-generated potentials is that they may serve as signals that modulate cellular activities, which are particularly important for fracture healing and tissue remodeling.

Another type of electric potential, a transmembrane (bioelectric) potential, is generated by cellular metabolism and depends on cell viability. Regions of greatest cellular activity (that is, growth plate or site of fracture) have the greatest negative electric potential. These endogenous electric factors seem to have their major influence during the early callus and late remodeling phases. Both stress-generated and bioelectric potentials affect cell behavior by modifying a variety of biochemical processes.

When any tissue is traumatized (for example, a fracture), injury potentials are created and steady electric fields exist locally for days after the insult. These potentials result largely from ion flux through leaky cell membranes, are basically direct current (DC) like, and decay with time. Animal studies have shown that when DC is delivered to bone by implanted electrodes, it triggers mitosis and recruitment of osteogenic cells. If current levels are appropriate (that is, 5 to 20 μA), such responses are far more brisk than those created by injury potentials. Effects of DC on subsequent phases of a fracture repair have not yet been confirmed.

Experimental studies support the presence of local stress (strain)- generated electric potentials (SGPs) in the later stages of fracture repair. These recurrent potentials appear to arise from two main sources. Evidence seems to suggest that the changes in metabolic and ionic behavior observed when cells are subjected to deforming forces may well be electrogenic in origin, both from electrokinetic and piezoelectric phenomena, depending on the rate of deformation (velocity). Although viable cells maintain transmembrane potentials, these potentials are not required for SGPs to be manifested.

Unlike injury potentials, which are comparatively steady, SGPs are time-varying; their amplitudes change in a dynamic manner and, rather than having one polarity, they are biphasic, that is, they have a positive and a negative phase. The loading velocity determines the frequency contents of these voltage waveforms (that is, potentials), as does the number of loading cycles per second (1 cycle/s = 1 Hertz). SGPs, generally, contain a broad band of frequencies that produce a voltage wave that is not sinusoidal in shape nor the same in frequency content as the loading frequency generating it. For example, if a load is applied to a bone rapidly (that is, impactively) and full deformation is reached in a few milliseconds, the leading edge of the resultant SGP will contain higher frequencies than those produced by slower loading. Frequency content has been shown to affect the type of biologic response a cell will make during exposure to an electric field and appears to confer definable levels of therapeutic specificity and efficiency. The importance of frequency content of these SGPs has become increasingly clear as experimental data from many sources indicate that specificity of various cell responses in electric fields is being governed by selective frequency/amplitude windows and thresholds. Nominal values for SGPs are in the 1 mV/cm range. In contrast, currently, it appears that streaming potentials, when produced by slowly applied deforming forces in the 0.05 to 100 Hz range, have a frequency content lying between 0.05 to 10 Hz.

When deformation is rapid (that is, impactive, as in normal, unshod heel-strike patterns), the rise time value from piezoelectric components is in the range of 5 to 20 ms. This corresponds, roughly, to a frequency content of 15 to 50 Hz in the leading edge of the voltage waveform. This frequency range has proven to be very osteogenic, both in mechanically and electrically coupled systems and to affect bone remodeling. Part of this action may stem from frequency-dependent synthesis and release of mitogens, morphogens, and growth factors observed when cells with osteogenic potential are exposed to time-varying electric fields.

Here, it is important to reemphasize the distinction between loading rate and the frequency content of that rate. The loading rate refers to the number of times a force from an external source is applied to the bone in a given period of time (for example, a gait cycle of 1 Hz). Alternatively it can be the number of pulses produced by an electromagnetic field generator as a function of time. The frequency patterns of nonsinusoidal waveforms, generally, are analyzed by a Fourier Transform, which converts events measured in the time domain (for example, milliseconds) to a frequency domain (for example, Hertz). In a nonsinusoidal voltage waveform resulting from transduction or magnetic induction, a wide range of frequencies exist (Figs. 29 and 30).

The role of endogenous electric factors in fracture repair thus seems to focus on different types of electric potentials in the first and last stages of fracture repair. Signals with different "informational" characteristics appear to be involved in each stage. Regardless of the stage both mechanical deformation

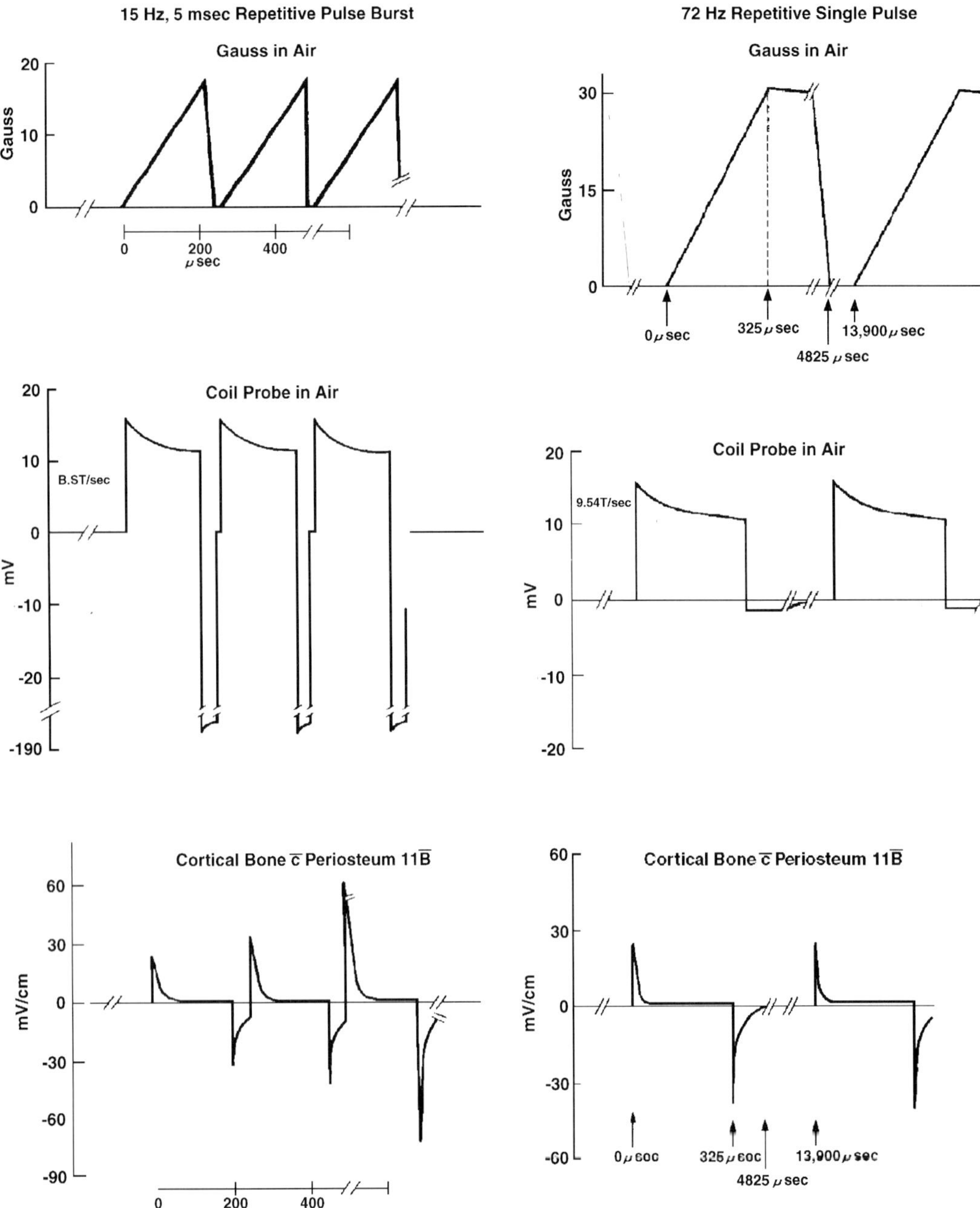

Figure 29
Diagram of the various types of pulsed electromagnetic field (PEMF) waveforms used to treat nonunions, as measured by different techniques at different levels. **Top left,** Repetitive pulse burst. A train of ≈ 20, 200-μs-wide pulses, lasting 5 ms, are repeated at 15 Hz. The magnetic (B) field is being measured (Gauss or Tesla) in air via a Hall probe. **Center left,** Same as **top left,** except the electric (E) field is being measured in air with a standardized coil probe. This field pattern is the first derivative of **top left** and is predicted by Maxwell's equations. **Bottom left,** Same as **top left,** except the voltage waveform is induced in a cortical bone sample with its long axis parallel to B (measured by Ag/AgCl electrodes, 1 cm apart on the surface of the bone). Note increasing voltage with each of the first three pulses of the burst as the result of incomplete voltage relaxation. (The B field pulse recurs in too short an interval for complete relaxation of the "negative phase.") **Top right,** Single pulse repeating at 72 Hz. Hall probe measurement of the B field in air. **Center right,** Same as **top right,** measured in air with a standardized coil probe. **Bottom right,** Same as **top right** with voltage waveforms measured as in **bottom left.** The longer interval between pulses allows complete relaxation of the "negative phase" to baseline.

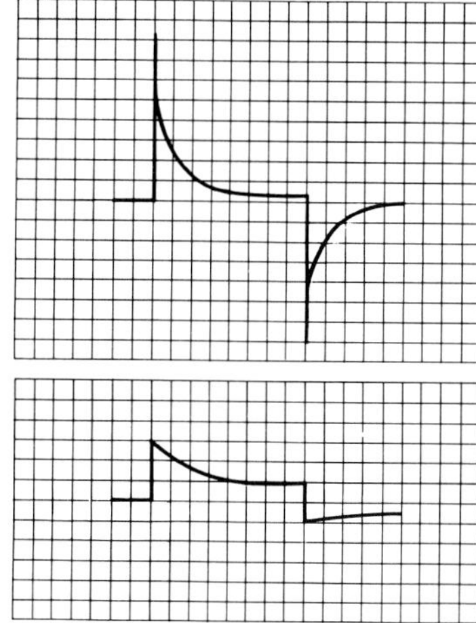

Figure 30
Diagrammatic representation of voltage waveforms recorded from rapid mechanical information of a bone specimen. **Top,** Nearly complete relaxation of voltage with a quasi-triangular waveform. **Bottom,** Less complete relaxation, with a quasi-rectangular shape. The amplitude and shape characteristics served as models for designing the parameters for inductively coupled pulsed electromagnetic fields.

and electric fields (with characteristics similar to those produced by deformation) affect cell behavior by modifying a variety of biochemical processes. These physical stimuli operate at several levels, from the cell surface to the cytoskeleton to the individual gene. Depending upon the energetic pattern, electric fields have been shown to affect cooperativity, ligand (receptor) binding, channel gating, biochemical signaling pathways (for example, cAMP, protein kinase systems, and calcium ions), intracellular calcium voltage spikes, dissociation of ions, aggregation of macromolecules (such as collagen), synthesis, secretion, migration (cytoskeletal elements), translation, transcription, and mitosis, among others. "Steady-state," DC-like injury currents drive the first stage, triggering DNA synthesis, cell division, and, perhaps, cell migration. In the remodeling stage, the frequency characteristics resulting from various types of dynamic deformation guide local reorganization, following the principles of Wolff's law.

When a nonunion exists, injury potential signals for cell activity are no longer present and SGPs generated in the bridging viscoelastic soft tissues have different voltage and frequency parameters from those resulting from impact loading of higher modulus bone. Although surgical repair will reestablish injury potentials and stage I healing, research studies have indicated that the bioelectric microenvironment of cells in the nonunion can be purposefully modified by several electric methods that can restart the healing process at stage I or II. For example, external electrical stimulation has been shown to increase the rate of the early phases of healing (stages I to III) by 20% to 30%. Furthermore, experimental and clinical evidence exists that selected pulsed electromagnetic fields (PEMFs) promote calcification of fibrocartilage, endochondral ossification, angiogenesis, and rapid revascularization of dead bone (including necrotic fragments and bone grafts).

The currently available types of electric stimulation vary in their field characteristics, but ultimately all stimulate fracture repair by altering cellular or physiologic behavior (Table 6).

DC (Direct Current) Generators

These generators are constant current devices in which the voltage is varied to overcome tissue impedance that changes as polarization products accumulate at the tissue-electrode interfaces. Since polarization (redox) products accumulating at the

Table 6
FDA-approved devices for fracture repair

Type	Source	Indications	Specifications
DC electrodes Implanted	EBI*	Nonunion Posterior Spine fusion	Constant current 5-20 μA
DC electrodes Transcutaneous	—	Nonunion 5-20 μA	Constant current
Surface Electrodes	Bio- electron	Nonunion	AC 60 kHz sine 5 V peak to peak
PEMFs	EBI* AME*	Nonunion Failed fusion Anterior spine fusion Congenital pseudarthrosis	15 Hz burst, 1.5 mV induced 15 Hz burst, 1.5 mV induced 15 Hz burst, 1.5 mV induced 72 Hz single, 1.5 mV induced
Surface Ultrasound	Interpore	Fresh fracture	1 kHz, pulsed 1.5 mHz 30 mW/cm^2

*EBI = Electro-Biology, Inc.; AME = American Medical Electronics

anode (the positive pole) may cause inflammation, this electrode is placed at a distance from the site to be treated. In practice, the generator housing becomes the anode, thereby reducing current density by increasing surface area. The cathode (negative pole) is implanted directly into the site where osteogenesis is to be stimulated. Initially, multiple cathodes were introduced, transcutaneously, into the nonunion site (a "semi-invasive" method). Present-day cathodes are helical in shape and surgically implanted in a longitudinal trough across the lesion. In general, these devices appear to be effective, mainly, because they mimic a sustained (and elevated) injury potential, triggering a faster, bulkier stage I response.

AC (Alternating Current) Generators

These surface electrodes create a sine wave. They are equipped with surface, rather than implanted electrodes and, in the past, were referred to as "capacitatively coupled" generators. Actually, current is delivered, through the skin to the fracture site, using a conductive medium such as electrocardiography paste. A sine wave, 60-kHz, 5-V peak to peak, signal is used to develop a current of 7.1 to 10.5 mA RMS (root mean square) at the skin level. Unlike DC systems, polarization at the electrodes is markedly decreased by the relatively high frequency sine waves. Generally, two electrodes are placed on opposite sides of the affected extremity (with or without casting). From limited experimental data, this frequency/amplitude pattern appears to function by affecting cAMP, collagen synthesis, and calcification during the soft and hard callus stages.

Pulsed Electromagnetic Fields (PEMF)

This inductive coupling depends on the rate of change in the magnetic field to produce changes in the electric microenvironment of the cells in the nonunion. The PEMF signal produces tissue effects in a pathway involving cAMP, the protein kinase systems, calcium-dependent intracellular mechanisms, and angiogenesis. PEMFs function mainly in the initiation of calcification of fibrocartilage in the gap; therefore, they are largely ineffective in fibrous tissue gaps until this tissue is converted to fibrocartilage by a short period of immobilization.

The process of producing electrical currents in conductors (for example, wires or tissues) by magnetic fields is called inductive coupling. If a conductor is moved through a static magnetic field, currents are induced. If the conductor is static, the field must be time-varying (changing), in order to induce current. Depending on the rate of change in the magnetic field (dB/dt); its amplitude (measured in Gauss or milliTesla); and its duration, direction, and repetition rate, a wide range of pulse shapes and frequency content characteristics can be imparted to the electromagnetic (E) field induced in a given tissue. Each tissue has unique passive electric properties (for example, dielectric constants, solid state, ferroelectric, etc.) that interact with the induced electric field to yield tissue specific pulse characteristics. The resultant E field parameters produce selective changes in cell behavior, many of which are determined by the induced frequency/amplitude pattern, the cell type, and its functional state, among other factors.

Initial PEMF waveforms (Fig 29) were developed to be similar in shape and amplitudes to SGP waveforms resulting from impactive loading of bone (that is, rise times faster than 20 ms) (Fig. 30). As a result, the E fields induced in tissues by PEMFs have biologically active amplitudes ranging from 1 mV/cm, are asymmetric, and have a broad band of frequencies. These frequencies range from ~DC to 10 MHz. Recent experimental data suggests a frequency band between 15 to 100 Hz has a specific effect on osteogenesis and remodeling. The higher amplitude frequencies in PEMFs fall mainly below 4.5 kHz. The primary cellular and subcellular mechanisms by which PEMFs exert a beneficial effect on nonunion healing are known, including signaling pathways involving cAMP, the protein kinase systems, and Ca^{2+}-dependent intracellular mechanisms. As a result, collagen and proteoglycan synthesis can be modified, calcium flux and binding altered, and angiogenesis speeded, each of which has been identified in tissue culture and animal models. Their main impact, therefore, is focused in stage III, where they initiate calcification of fibrocartilage in the gap. This sets the stage for endochondral ossification and vascular penetration. Here, it should be noted that present day PEMF characteristics are largely ineffective for inducing calcification of fibrous tissue. When this element is predominant in the gap, healing occurs only after the tissue has been converted to fibrocartilage by a short period of effective immobilization.

Summary

Each fracture fixation method, either internal or external, has advantages and disadvantages. No single method or device can be so universal as to be applicable for all fracture types and locations. The best treatment modality and fixation device must be selected according to the fracture morphology and the clinical condition of the patient. A thorough knowledge of the device's biomechanical function and expected biologic response will optimize its effectiveness.

Bone fracture union can follow any one of many combinations of pathways to the final stage. Many clinical factors such as the patient's expectations, compliance with treatment, degree of tolerance, the physician's experience, and other socioeconomic considerations are likely to play important roles in the selection of fixation methods.

Compression plate fixation has potential drawbacks, such as stress shielding, bone osteopenia, and refracture after plate removal; however, its advantages in many special circumstances appear to outweigh these considerations. Redesign of plate geometry or material composition to minimize axial stiffness appears to be ineffective. Intramedullary nailing is intended to promote axial compression of the bone ends at the fracture site. Many of the potential benefits of external fixation, such as dynamization and the change of fixation stiffness, are not yet fully appreciated. The incidence of pin tract infection and fracture nonunion has been reduced through clinical experience and basic science research results. However, the successful use of external fixators, even those of the simpler monoplanar configuration, requires learning and mastering the surgical techniques and understanding the principles of postoperative care.

The ability to balance between the biomechanical properties and the biologic behavior of different fracture fixation methods is the prerequisite to selecting the optimal treatment for each patient and fracture. Furthermore, recognizing the proper cell mediator and the physical means to stimulate cellular elements may provide a means of modulating bone fracture healing, regardless of the fixation technique used.

Medical Imaging

As medical imaging is indispensable to our assessment of the diagnoses of bone injury and to the quality of bone repair and regeneration, an understanding of the underlying principles involved in its many techniques is necessary to best interpret its results. The final section of this chapter will briefly review these principles. It is not intended to provide the reader with a comprehensive understanding of the many methods of imaging available but merely an introduction. For greater details the reader is referred to the chapter references and to the many other available publications on this subject.

Radiography

A radiographic examination is a basic and fundamental component of most orthopaedic examinations. Radiographs are produced by directing accelerated electrons through atoms. As the accelerated electrons hit electrons in the atom, they either bounce an orbiting electron to a higher orbit (excitation) or bounce it completely out of its atom (ionization). The excited or ionized atom will return spontaneously to its original (ground) state. As it does, radiation is given off in the form of a photon. In an X-ray unit, accelerated electrons are directed from a cathode toward the anode through a tungsten target. The tungsten target's atoms are excited or ionized and emit photons, which are called X rays. These X rays are then directed toward the tissue to be examined. Gamma rays are produced in a similar manner, except that in this case, photons come from the nucleus of the atom.

The photons, as X rays, interact with tissues through which they pass by one of five mechanisms: coherent scattering, photoelectric effect, Compton scattering, pair production, and photodisintegration. In clinical diagnostic radiology, photoelectric effect and Compton scattering account for the majority of interactions between the X rays and tissues being irradiated. The extent of the change depends on the density of the atoms of the tissue being irradiated. As the X rays pass through tissue, the extent to which they are altered is directly related to the atomic density of the tissue. By measuring the X rays as they exit the tissue, the atomic density is obtained. This measurement is made when the X ray exposes an X-ray sensitive film contained in an X-ray plate.

The X-ray film is usually a double emulsion film sandwiched between a pair of intensifying screens. The screens convert the X rays to a light photon distribution, which exposes the photographic emulsion. The screens also are used to magnify the sensitivity of the system and reduce the amount of irradiation necessary to produce clinically useful images. The properties of the radiographic film can change by varying the thickness and type of screen material or the thickness and grain size of the silver halide crystals in the emulsion. The quality of the image depends on the type of film and the amount of irradiation. When radiographing anatomic parts with minimal associated soft tissue (such as in hands, feet, forearms), fine detail is obtained by using less-sensitive film and high-energy irradiation. When significant soft tissue is associated with the part to be radiographed, especially the gonads, more sensitive X-ray film should be used; therefore, less irradiation will be needed. In this case, however, some detail is lost.

The adverse biologic effects of radiation vary depending on the tissues radiated and the dose. Protection from the adverse effects of radiation is important for the medical team and patient. The patient is protected by limiting the surface area exposed, the number of radiographs taken, and frequency of the radiographs. The medical team is protected by shields, usually made of lead, and the distance from the X-ray source and beam. The radiation effect is reduced by the square of the distance, thus moving from two feet to four feet reduces the effect of the radiation by a factor of four. Lead shields at least 1/32 in thick (0.79 mm) should be used by individuals immediately adjacent to the irradiation. These shields should be checked frequently for cracks. Because the shields do not cover eyes, the medical team must remember that if they can see the X ray source, their eyes receive radiation.

Computed Tomography

Computed tomography (CT) was introduced into clinical medicine in the early 1970s. This diagnostic tool provided the first three-dimensional (3-D) perspective of anatomy by creating a computerized reconstruction from a series of standard radiographic images. The scanner employs multiple X-ray units, circumferentially placed around the anatomic part to be examined. Each unit takes a radiograph of a thin slice of the anatomy. The units are then moved slightly (1, 3, or 5 mm, depending on the thickness of the "slices" desired), and another set of radiographs are taken. This process is repeated until the entire area of the anatomic site has been studied.The data from these multiple radiographs are entered into a computer and the information is used to reconstruct an image of the axial view of the patient. The images are obtained from multiple radiographs in only one plane, but it is possible to reconstruct a coronal and sagittal image from these data. Unfortunately, to obtain anatomically detailed images, the patient is exposed to more radiation than is preferred.

The information obtained from the CT scanner's computer is a measurement of the degree to which photons alter as they pass through the object that is imaged. Thus, as is the case with conventional radiographs, the information is a measurement of an object's density to radiographs. The unit of density on a CT scan is a Hounsfield unit (H) named after Dr. Godfrey Hounsfield, one of the two investigators to receive the Nobel Prize for developing the CT scanner. Zero Hounsfield units is the density of water. Normal muscle has a density of approximately 65 H; cortical bone, 1,500 H; and fat, -70 H. The computer can adjust the appearance of an image at a particular number of Hounsfield units in order to highlight tissues as desired. This is done by setting the upper and lower limits of Hounsfield units (windows) for each image. Tissues more dense than the value set as the upper limit appear white and tissues less dense than the value set as the lower limit appear black. The tissues with densities between the upper and lower limits appear as shades of gray. Thus, for example, the window level could be adjusted higher (up to 500) to enhance bony detail, or lower (down to -500) to enhance detail in the lung fields. In addition, the computer can measure the density of the tissues irrespective of the settings.

The resolution of a CT image can be improved if more radiographic slices or projections are obtained. The term "pixel" is often used to indicate the number of projections taken. Pixel refers to "picture element," and an infinite number of pixels could lead to the production of an image with ideal resolution. In practice, however, a finite number of pixels are used and this places a limit on resolution quality. Contrast materials can also be used to enhance the visualization of certain anatomic structures. Blood vessels, kidneys, ureters, bladder, bowel, spinal canal, or sinus tracts usually can be visualized better if a contrast agent is used. The ability of the computer to measure density permits an accurate determination of the vascularity of tissues if a density measurement is made before and during intravenous contrast infusion. However, intravenous contrast is insufficient to reveal the arterial supply of tissues because of the lack of sensitivity of CT scans for this application.

Magnetic Resonance Imaging

Magnetic resonance imaging (MRI) was introduced in the 1980s and has become extremely important in the evaluation of a variety of musculoskeletal conditions ranging from neoplasia and spinal lesions to torn menisci and degenerated rotator cuffs. The theory of MRI is based on the behavior of atoms to an external magnetic field and the fact that the simplest atom, hydrogen, accounts for more than two thirds of the atomic makeup of the human body. By measuring the movement of hydrogen atoms as they are subjected to altering magnetic forces, specific information about the concentration of these atoms can be assessed. With computer-aided mathematical analysis it is possible to reconstruct a picture of the tissues showing their various components.

The technique of MRI is based on the fact that atoms carry a small charge and behave as if they are polarized. When subjected to an external magnetic field, they align themselves either parallel or exactly opposite to the direction of that field (antiparallel). In fact, the atoms are actually thought to jump back and forth from parallel to antiparallel. When in equilibrium, or in the resting state, there will always be slightly more atoms parallel than antiparallel to the field. When external magnetic energy is introduced into the system, however, the atoms will be excited to a higher energy level, thus altering their alignment. When the external energy source is removed, the atoms return to equilibrium (low energy state), with slightly more atoms parallel than antiparallel to the field. The energy released with this movement back to the lower energy state is measured as the MR signal.

The MR signal depends on the density of the protons in the atom, the radiofrequency impulses that are sent through the atom, and the length of time between the end of the pulse and the recording of the emitted energy. The frequency of the pulses is called the time to repetition (TR). The time between stopping the pulse and taking a measurement is called the time to echo (TE). By altering these times, subtle differences in the makeup of the atoms can be recorded. Different types of MR images are made by adjusting the TR and TE settings. The most common types are called T1-weighted and T2-weighted images.

T1 relaxation, longitudinal, or the spin-lattice relaxation time measures the behavior of the atomic nucleus to the external magnetic fields, essentially independent of the other atomic nuclei. The time recorded is the time it takes for 63% of the nuclei to return to equilibrium. T2 relaxation, transverse, or the spin-spin relaxation time measures the behavior of the atomic nucleus as it is influenced by the external magnetic field and the adjacent nuclei. As the adjacent nuclei change their alignment, the magnetic field experienced by each atom is altered and this relationship is measured by the T2 relaxation time. The time recorded is the time it takes for 37% of the atoms to return to equilibrium.

A T1-weighted image is obtained by recording the MR signals with a short TR (about 200 ms) and a short TE (about 15 ms). A T2-weighted image is obtained by recording the measurements with a long TR (about 2,000 ms) and a long TE (about 85 ms). Another common imaging method used is called a proton density and it is obtained by recording with a long TR and a short TE.

T1-weighted images are most useful for demonstrating anatomic structures because they have a high signal-to-noise ratio. Tissues with a high signal intensity (a short T1)—fat, lipid-containing tissues, and proteinaceous fluid—will be white on a T1-weighted image. Tissues with a low signal intensity (a long T1)—normal body fluid (CSF, urine), calcium, tendons, and ligaments—will be black on a T1-weighted image. Other tissues have an intermediate length signal intensity and will be gray on the T1-weighted image (Table 7).

T2-weighted images are most useful in contrasting normal tissues with abnormal tissues. Tissues with a high-intensity signal (a long T2)—neoplasms,

Table 7
Physical properties of magnetic resonance imaging

Tissue	T1-Weighted Image*	T2-Weighted Image+
Cortical bone	Black	Black
Ligaments	Black	Black
Fibrocartilage	Black	Black
Hyaline cartilage	Gray	Gray
Bone marrow (fatty-appendicular)	Bright	Gray
Bone marrow (hematopoietic-axial)	Bright	Gray
Normal fluid	Dark	Bright
Abnormal fluid (pus)	Gray	Bright
Muscle	Gray	Gray
Intervertebral disk (central)	Gray	Bright
Intervertebral disk (peripheral)	Dark	Gray

* Time to Echo (TE), short < 1,000; time to repetition (TR), short < 80.
\+ TE, long > 1,000; TR, long > 80.

inflammation, and fluid—will be white on the T2-weighted images. Tissues with a low intensity signal (a short T2)—calcium, ligaments, and tendons—will be black on the T2-weighted images (Fig. 31).

In addition to image contrast, the signal-to-noise ratio (SNR) and spatial resolution are the most critical parameters determining image quality. SNR depends on voxel size and the number of samples collected. The term "voxel" refers to "volume element" and voxel size is determined by slice thickness (d), number of samples in the phase (Np), frequency (Nf) encoding directions, and the field of view (D) as follows: voxel volume = d × Dy/Np × Dx/Nf = (d × Dy × Dx)/Np × Nf. Increasing voxel size results in a proportional increase in SNR.

The maximum achievable SNR is determined, to a significant extent, by the strength of the external magnetic field. (This is one reason why facilities that use a stronger magnet [that is, more Tesla] may provide better images.) The amplitude of the magnetic resonance signal is proportional to the difference in spin population in the nuclear energy fields. Intrinsic SNR is a critical performance criterion of MRI systems. For visualizing small structures it is critical that the images be obtained at high spatial resolution (from small imaging voxels) without excessive SNR deterioration.

Methods to shorten the actual time required to obtain the images are being developed. One method is called gradient echo. By introducing the radiofrequency impulse at less than 90° from the primary magnetic field, the time required for the return of atomic alignment after the impulse has stopped is

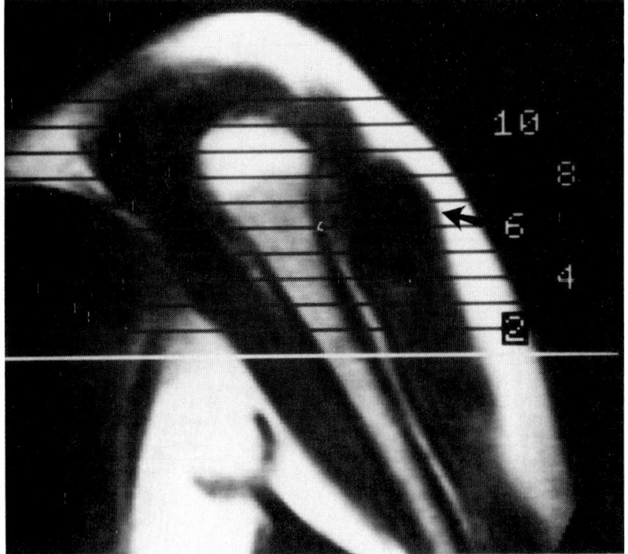

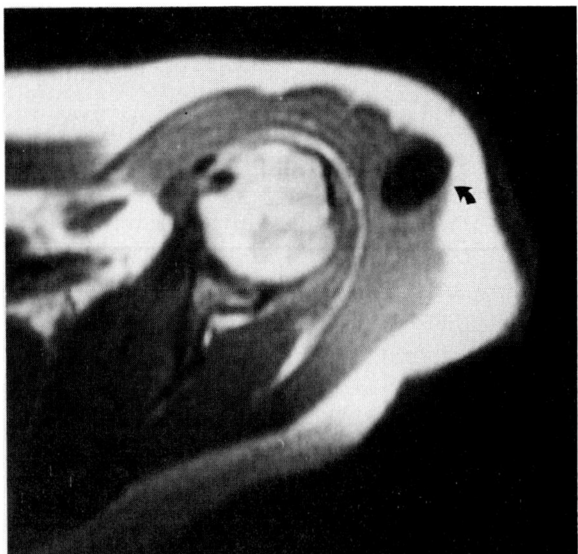

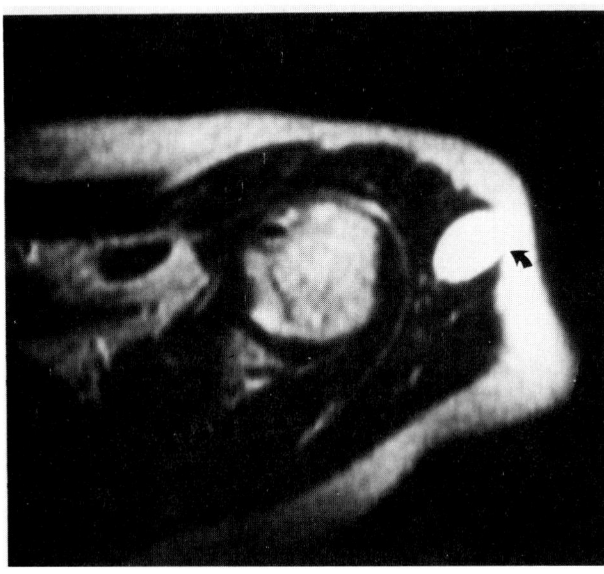

Figure 31
Scout (**top left**) and cross-sectional T1-weighted (**top right**) and T2-weighted (**bottom**) images of a benign myxoma in the deltoid region of the arm of a 42-year-old woman. Because this tumor is mostly composed of fluid, it is dark in T1 and bright in T2.

shortened. It therefore takes less time to do the entire examination. However, the images are not of the same quality as those obtained with the more conventional method. At this time, gradient echo is most often used for analysis of the spine and its associated structures.

In certain instances, an MRI can be enhanced by the injection of an intravenous contrast agent, such as gadolinium (Gd). Gadolinium, a rare earth metal with an atomic number of 64 and an atomic weight of 157.2, is a paramagnetic agent that is unique for its high magnetic movement. Because it is toxic in its free form, it is injected as a chelated complex with diethylenetriamine pentaacetic acid, thus rendering it safe for human use. Upon injection, the meglumine salt is dissociated and gadopentetate is excreted by the kidney. More than 80% is excreted by six hours without any measurable effect on kidney function. It does not cross the blood-brain barrier and, therefore, does not accumulate in normal brain tissue. Its effect is to decrease the T1 and T2 relaxation times of tissues, thus changing the signal so that tissues with gadolinium can be distinguished from tissues without gadolinium. There are no known contraindications to its use.

Selected Bibliography

Osteonecrosis

Boettcher WG, Bonfiglio M, Hamilton HH, et al: Non-traumatic necrosis of the femoral head: I. Relation of altered hemostasis to etiology. *J Bone Joint Surg* 1970;52A:312–321.

Catto M: Pathology of aseptic bone necrosis, in Davidson JK (ed): *Aseptic Necrosis of Bone.* Amsterdam, Excerpta Medica, 1976, pp 3–100.

Chryssanthou CP: Dysbaric osteonecrosis: Etiological and pathogenetic concepts. *Clin Orthop* 1978;130:94–106.

Cruess RL: Osteonecrosis of bone: Current concepts as to etiology and pathogenesis. *Clin Orthop* 1986;208:30–39.

Fisher DE: The role of fat embolism in the etiology of corticosteroid-induced avascular necrosis: Clinical and experimental results. *Clin Orthop* 1978;130:68–80.

Glimcher MJ, Kenzora JE: The biology of osteonecrosis of the human femoral head and its clinical implications: I. Tissue biology. *Clin Orthop* 1979;138:284–309.

Glimcher MJ, Kenzora JE: The biology of osteonecrosis of the human femoral head and its clinical implications: II. The pathological changes in the femoral head as an organ and in the hip joint. *Clin Orthop* 1979;139:283–312.

Glimcher MJ, Kenzora JE: The biology of osteonecrosis of the human femoral head and its clinical implications: III. Discussion of the etiology and genesis of the pathological sequelae; comments on treatment. *Clin Orthop* 1979;140:273–312.

Hawkins LG: Fractures of the neck of the talus. *J Bone Joint Surg* 1970;52A:991–1002.

Hungerford DS, Lennox DW: The importance of increased intraosseous pressure in the development of osteonecrosis of the femoral head: Implications for treatment. *Orthop Clin North Am* 1985;16:635–654.

Jones JP Jr: Fat embolism and osteonecrosis. *Orthop Clin North Am* 1985;16:595–633.

Bone and Cartilage Grafting

Berrey BH Jr, Lord CF, Gebhardt MC, et al: Fractures of allografts: Frequency, treatment, and end-results. *J Bone Joint Surg* 1990;72A:825–833.

Bos GD, Goldberg VM, Gordon NH, et al: The long term fate of fresh and frozen orthotopic bone allografts in genetically defined rats. *Clin Orthop* 1985;197:245–254.

Burchardt H: Biology of cortical bone graft incorporation, in Friedlaender GE, Mankin HJ, Sell KW (eds): *Osteochondral Allografts: Biology, Banking, and Clinical Applications.* Boston, Little, Brown, 1983, pp 51–57.

Burwell RG: The fate of bone grafts, in Apley GA (ed): *Recent Advances in Orthopaedics.* London, Churchill, 1969, pp 115–207.

Campbell CJ: Homotransplantation of a half or whole joint. *Clin Orthop* 1972;87:146–155.

Czitrom AA, Langer F, McKee N, et al: Bone and cartilage allotransplantation: A review of 14 years of research and clinical studies. *Clin Orthop* 1986;208:141–145.

Doppelt SH, Tomford WW, Lucas AD, et al: Operational and financial aspects of a hospital bone bank. *J Bone Joint Surg* 1981;63A:1472–1481.

Friedlaender GE, Mankin HJ, Sell KW (eds): *Osteochondral Allografts: Biology, Banking, and Clinical Applications.* Boston, Little, Brown, 1983.

Gebhardt MC, Roth YF, Mankin HJ: Osteoarticular allografts for reconstruction in the proximal part of the humerus after excision of a musculoskeletal tumor. *J Bone Joint Surg* 1990;72A:334–345.

Gross AE, McDermott AG, Lavoie MV, et al: The use of allograft bone in revision hip arthroplasty. *Hip* 1987;47–58.

Langer F, Czitrom A, Pritzker KP, et al: The immunogenicity of fresh and frozen allogeneic bone. *J Bone Joint Surg* 1975;57A:216–220.

Langer F, Gross AE: Immunogenicity of allograft articular cartilage. *J Bone Joint Surg* 1974;56A:297–304.

Mankin HJ, Doppelt SH, Sullivan TR, et al: Osteoarticular and intercalary allograft transplantation in the management of malignant tumors of bone. *Cancer* 1982;50:613–630.

Mankin HJ, Doppelt SH, Tomford WW: Clinical experience with allograft implantation: The first ten years. *Clin Orthop* 1983;174:69–86.

Parrish FF: Allograft replacement of all or part of the end of a long bone following excision of a tumor. *J Bone Joint Surg* 1973;55A:1–22.

Tomford WW, Duff GP, Mankin HJ: Experimental freeze-preservation of chondrocytes. *Clin Orthop* 1985;197:11–14.

Biologic Response to Implants

Black J: *Biological Performance of Materials,* ed 2. New York, Marcel Dekker, 1992.

Cohen J: Assay of foreign-body reaction. *J Bone Joint Surg* 1959;41A:152–166.

Davies JE (ed): *The Bone-Biomaterial Interface.* Toronto, University of Toronto Press, 1991.

DiCarlo EF, Bullough PG: The biologic responses to orthopedic implants and their wear debris. *Clin Mater* 1992;9:235–260.

Galante JO, Lemons J, Spector M, et al: The biological effects of implant materials. *J Orthop Res* 1991;9:760–775.

Spector M, Cease C, Xia T-L: The local tissue response to biomaterials. *CRC Crit Rev Biocompat* 1989;5:269–295.

St. John KR (ed): *Particulate Debris from Medical Implants: Mechanisms of Formation and Biological Consequences.* Philadelphia, American Society for Testing and Materials, 1992, Series: ASTM STP 11 44.

Williams DF: Biocompatibility considerations in the use of orthopaedic implant alloys, in Williams DF (ed): *Current Perspectives on Implantable Devices.* London, JAI Press, 1989.

Fracture Healing

Brighton CT: Principles of fracture healing: Part I: The biology of fracture repair, in Murray JA (ed): *American Academy of Orthopaedic Surgeons Instructional Course Lectures XXXIII.* St. Louis, MO, CV Mosby, 1984, pp 60–82.

McKibbin B: The biology of fracture healing in long bones. *J Bone Joint Surg* 1978;60B:150–162.

Biochemistry of Fracture Healing

Joyce ME, Terek RM, Jingushi S, et al: Role of transforming growth factor-Beta in fracture repair. *Ann NY Acad Sci* 1990:593:107–123.

Khouri RK, Koudsi B, Reddi H: Tissue transformation into bone in vivo: A potential practical application. *JAMA* 1991;266:1953–1955.

Mohan S, Baylink DJ: Bone growth factors. *Clin Orthop* 1991;263:30–48.

Pau WT, Einhorn TA: The biochemistry of fracture healing. *Curr Orthop* 1992;6:207–213.

Fracture Fixation

Brumback RJ, Uwagie-Ero S, Lakatos RP, et al: Intramedullary nailing of femoral shaft fractures: Part II. Fracture-healing with static interlocking fixation. *J Bone Joint Surg* 1988;70A:1453–1462.

Bucholz RW, Ross SE, Lawrence KL: Fatigue fracture of the interlocking nail in the treatment of fractures of the distal part of the femoral shaft. *J Bone Joint Surg* 1987;69A:1391–1399.

Johnson KD, Tencer AF, Sherman MC: Biomechanical factors affecting fracture stability and femoral bursting in closed intramedullary nailing of femoral shaft fractures, with illustrative case presentations. *J Orthop Trauma* 1987;1:1–11.

Kessler SB, Hallfeldt KK, Perren SM, et al: The effects of reaming and intramedullary nailing on fracture healing. *Clin Orthop* 1986;212:18–25.

Perren SM, Cordey J, Rahn BA, et al: Early temporary porosis of bone induced by internal fixation implants: A reaction to necrosis, not to stress protection. *Clin Orthop* 1988;232:139–151.

Rhinelander FW: Effects of medullary nailing on the normal blood supply of diaphyseal cortex, in *American Academy of Orthopaedic Surgeons Instructional Course Lectures, XXII.* St. Louis, MO, CV Mosby, 1973, pp 161–187.

Sarmiento A: Functional fracture bracing: An update, in Griffin PP (ed): *Instructional Course Lectures, Volume XXXVI.* Park Ridge, IL, American Academy of Orthopaedic Surgeons, 1987, pp 371–376.

Winquist RA, Hansen ST Jr, Clawson DK: Closed intramedullary nailing of femoral fractures: A report of five hundred and twenty cases. *J Bone Joint Surg* 1984;66A:529–539.

External Fixation

Hart MB, Wu JJ, Chao EY, et al: External skeletal fixation of canine tibial osteotomies: Compression compared with no compression. *J Bone Joint Surg* 1985;67A:598–605.

Kummer FJ: Biomechanics of the Ilizarov external fixator. *Bull Hosp Jt Dis Orthop Inst* 1989;49(2):140–147.

Lewallen DG, Chao EY, Kasman RA, et al: Comparison of the effects of compression plates and external fixators on early bone healing. *J Bone Joint Surg* 1984;66A:1084–91.

Weber BG: On the biomechanics of external fixation, in Weber BG, Margerl F (eds): *The External Fixator: AO/ASIF-Threaded Rod System Spine-Fixator.* Springer-Verlag, Berlin, 1985, pp 27–53.

Wu JJ, Shyr HS, Chao EY, et al: Comparison of osteotomy healing under external fixation devices with different stiffness characteristics. *J Bone Joint Surg* 1984;66A(8):1258–1264.

Electric Factors in Fracture Repair

Bassett CA: The development and application of pulsed electromagnetic fields (PEMFs) for ununited fractures and arthrodeses. *Orthop Clin North Am* 1984;15:61–87.

Bassett CAL: Fundamental and practical aspects of therapeutic uses of pulsed electromagnetic fields (PEMFs). *Crit Rev Biomed Eng* 1989:17:451–529.

Brighton CT: The semi-invasive method of treating nonunion with direct current. *Orthop Clin North Am* 1984;15:33–45.

Kempf I, Grosse A, Rigaut P: The treatment of noninfected pseudarthrosis of the femur and tibia with locked intramedullary nailing. *Clin Orthop* 1986;212:142–154.

Weber BG, Brunner C: The treatment of nonunions without electrical stimulation. *Clin Orthop* 1981;161:24–32.

Medical Imaging

Bassett LW, Gold RH, Seeger LL (eds): Magnetic resonance imaging of the musculoskeletal system. Section I: Symposium. *Clin Orthop* 1989;244:2–130.

Berquest TH: Magnetic resonance imaging of musculoskeletal neoplasms. *Clin Orthop* 1989;244:101–118.

Broders AC: The grading of carcinoma. *Minn Med* 1925;8:726–730.

Coulam CM, Erickson JJ, Rollo FD, et al (eds): *The Physical Basis of Medical Imaging.* New York, Appleton-Century-Crofts, 1981.

Fischer SP, Fox JM, Del Pizzo W, et al: Accuracy of diagnoses from magnetic resonance imaging of the knee:

A multi-center analysis of one thousand and fourteen patients. *J Bone Joint Surg* 1991;73A:2–10.

Holder LE: Clinical radionuclide bone imaging. *Radiology* 1990;176:607–614.

Iannotti JP, Zlatkin MB, Esterhai JL, et al: Magnetic resonance imaging of the shoulder: Sensitivity, specificity, and predictive value. *J Bone Joint Surg* 1991;73A:17–29.

Negendank WG, Crowley MG, Ryan JR, et al: Bone and soft-tissue lesions: Diagnosis with combined H-1 MR imaging and P-31 MR spectroscopy. *Radiology* 1989;173:181–188.

Palmer EL, Scott JA, Strauss HW (eds): *Practical Nuclear Medicine.* Philadelphia, WB Saunders, 1992.

Raunest J, Oberle K, Loehnert J, et al: The clinical value of magnetic resonance imaging in the evaluation of meniscal disorders. *J Bone Joint Surg* 1991;73A:11–16.

Saini S, Modic MT, Hamm B, et al: Advances in contrast-enhanced MR imaging. *AJR* 1991;156:235–254.

Seeger LL: Physical principles of magnetic resonance imaging. *Clin Orthop* 1989;244:7–16.

Selzer PM: Understanding NMR imaging with the aid of a simple mechanical model. *Resident and Staff Phys* 1985;31(6):30–43.

Stoller DW, Genant HK, Helms CA, et al (eds): *Magnetic Resonance Imaging in Orthopaedics and Rheumatology.* Philadelphia, JB Lippincott, 1989.

Watt I: Magnetic resonance imaging in orthopaedics. *J Bone Joint Surg* 1991;73B:539–550.

Chapter 8
Peripheral Nerve Physiology, Anatomy, and Pathology

Sue C. Bodine, PhD
Richard L. Lieber, PhD

Chapter Outline

Neurons and Signal Generation

The human brain is a complex biologic structure composed of approximately 10^{11} nerve cells (neurons). Although neurons may be classified into as many as 10,000 different types, they share many common features, including the unique ability to communicate precisely, rapidly, and over long distances with one another and with target tissues, such as muscles.

Nerve Cells—General Description

A typical neuron has four morphologically defined regions (Fig. 1, *left*): the cell body, dendrites, axon, and presynaptic terminal. The cell body contains the nucleus and the organelles for making RNA (ribonucleic acids) and proteins and is the metabolic center of the neuron although it typically contains less than 10% of the neuron's total volume. The remaining neuron volume consists of the dendrites and the axon. The dendrites are thin processes that branch off the cell body and serve as the main apparatus for receiving synaptic input from other nerve cells.

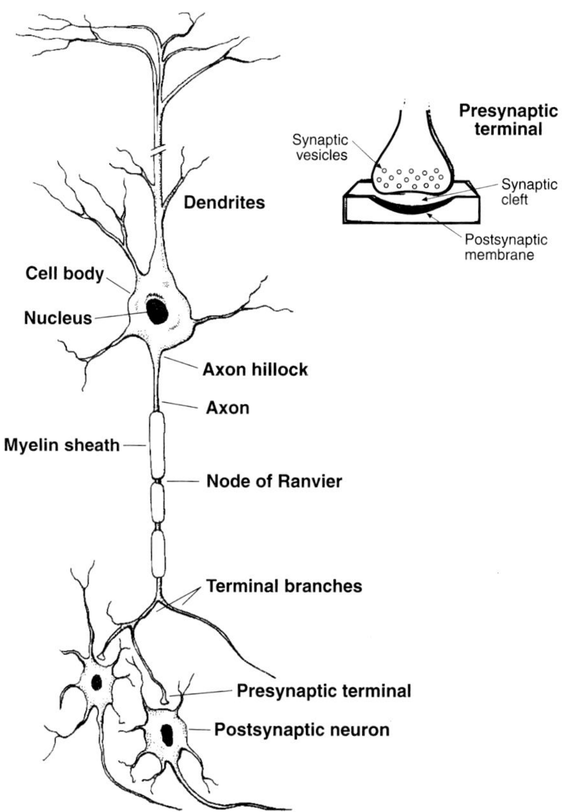

Figure 1
Left, Main features of a typical vertebrate neuron. **Top right,** Presynaptic terminal-postsynaptic receptor.

A cell body gives rise to only one axon, which is the main conducting unit of the neuron and is capable of accurately conveying information over long distances by propagating electrical signals known as action potentials. The axon arises from a specialized region of the cell body, the axon hillock, from which the all-or-none action potential is initiated once a critical threshold has been reached. The axon and its terminal branches require proteins to maintain their structural integrity, to support action potential propagation, and to effect the release of neurotransmitters; however, the axon hillock and axon cannot make proteins. To meet the requirements of the neuron, proteins are synthesized in the cell body, assembled into macromolecules, and transported down the axon via axoplasmic transport. The part of the axon nearest its target organ or termination site is divided into fine branches that have specialized endings called presynaptic terminals, which are responsible for transmitting information from the neuron to the dendrites or cell body of another neuron (Fig. 1, *left*) or a postsynaptic receptor such as the neuromuscular junction (Fig. 1, *right*).

Glial Cells and Myelin Formation

Nerve cell bodies and axons are surrounded by glial cells, which are divided into microglia and macroglia. Microglia arise from macrophages and are phagocytes that are mobilized after injury, infection, or disease. The three primary types of macroglia are oligodendrocytes, Schwann cells, and astrocytes (Fig. 2).

Oligodendrocytes and Schwann cells insulate the axons by forming a myelin sheath. Myelin is composed of 70% lipid and 30% protein, with a high concentration of cholesterol and phospholipid. Myelinated axons conduct electrical impulses at faster speeds and at higher frequencies with less energy consumption than nonmyelinated axons. Oligodendrocytes and Schwann cells form the sheath by wrapping their membranous processes concentrically around the axon in a tight spiral. Oligodendrocytes occur only in the central nervous system (CNS), and a single cell can myelinate several different axons (on average 15). Schwann cells occur in the peripheral nervous system, and each cell myelinates a region of one axon.

A single peripheral axon can be myelinated by as many as 500 Schwann cells. The genes in Schwann cells that code for myelin are turned on by the presence of an axon. Schwann cells line up along the axon at intervals of 0.1 to 1.0 mm. These intervals eventually will become nodes of Ranvier, which are specialized zones for action potential initiation. The external cell membrane of the Schwann cell surrounds the axon and forms a double membrane structure that then elongates and

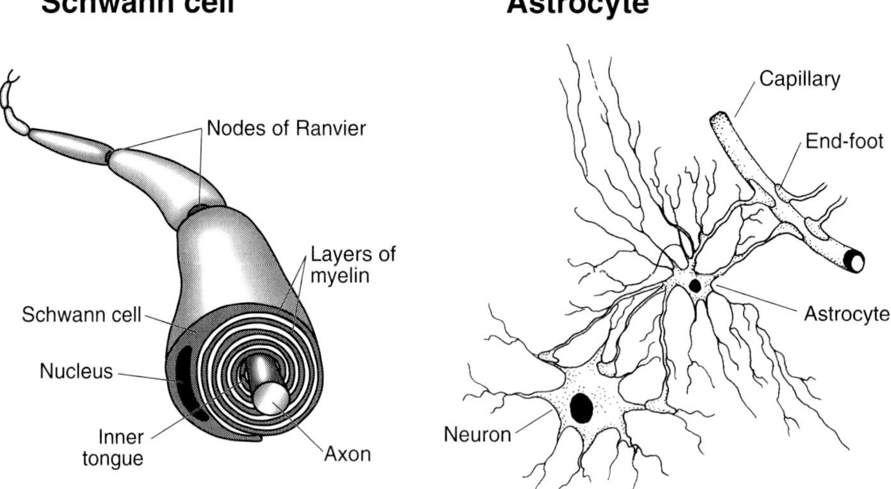

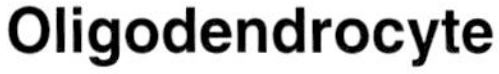

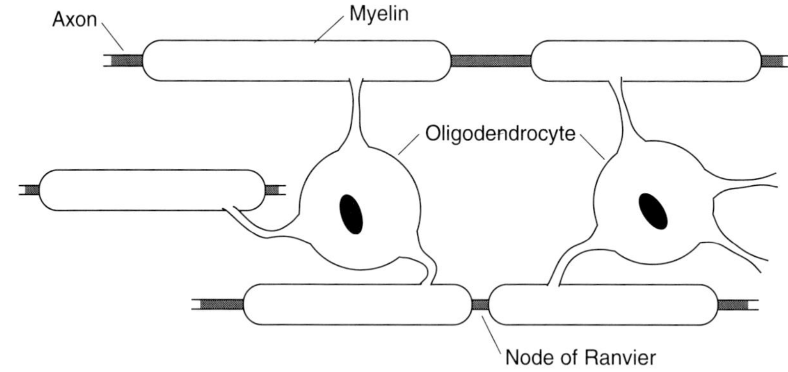

Figure 2
The principle types of glial cells. **Top left,** Schwann cells line up along the length of peripheral nervous system axons at regular intervals, each forming a segment of myelin sheath about 1 mm long. **Top right,** Astrocytes are star shaped and have end feet that contact both capillaries and neurons. **Bottom,** In white matter, oligodendrocytes participate in myelination of axons; a single oligodendrocyte can form myelin around several different axons. In gray matter, they surround the cell bodies of neurons.

spirals around the axon in concentric layers. Loss of the myelin sheath, called demyelination, can disrupt the conduction of action potentials along axons.

Astrocytes, the most common glial cells, are found only in the CNS and are thought to serve many functions. They serve as supporting structures, providing firmness and structure to the brain. Some astrocytes have processes that contact blood capillaries and neurons, thus leading to the speculation that they serve a nutritive function (Fig. 2, *top right*). Some fulfill a scavenger role, removing neuronal debris after injury. Astrocytes also have been shown to take up excess K^+ in the extracellular space and remove neurotransmitters from the synaptic cleft after synaptic transmission. Astrocytes also turn on the expression of myelin in oligodendrocytes.

Axoplasmic Transport

The neuron is a polarized cell; its cell body and presynaptic terminals often are separated by considerable distances. The proteins required to maintain the structural integrity of the axon, to support action potential propagation, and to enable neurotransmitter release at the presynaptic terminals are produced only in the cell body. Therefore, special intracellular transport systems have been developed to bring molecules synthesized in the cell body to the axon and nerve terminals and to return degradation products from the axon and terminals to the cell body for molecular reprocessing. The importance of these transport systems is demonstrated by the fact that severance of the axon from the cell body results in degeneration of the distal axon segment. Constituents move within the axon in three ways: slow and fast anterograde transport and fast retrograde transport.

Data from isotope labeling experiments reveal that motor and sensory nerves have similar transport rates. The transport rate is sensitive to temperature, slowing down with decreasing temperature and stopping at a temperature of 11°C.

Recent evidence suggests that the mechanisms for slow and fast anterograde transport are the same. Axoplasmic transport has been shown to depend on adenosine triphosphate (ATP) derived primarily from oxidative metabolism. Axon transport is blocked within ten to 30 minutes after a nerve is made anoxic by switching to a nitrogen atmosphere. The rate of transport recovers when the nerve is reoxygenated after 1.5 hours of anoxia. If, however, a nerve is kept anoxic for two to five hours, transport recovers very slowly after reoxygenation, although action potential transmission recovers immediately. After two hours of tourniquet-induced ischemia, full recovery of axoplasmic transport in the feline sciatic nerve was found to take over 24 hours. Axoplasmic transport also depends on intraneural calcium concentrations. Normally, the level of free Ca^{2+} in the nerve is maintained at 0.1 µM, with the total amount of Ca^{2+} present in the nerve being 0.4 mM. Most of the calcium is sequestered in the mitochondria and smooth endoplasmic reticulum and bound to the calcium-binding protein, calmodulin. In addition to ATP and calcium, axoplasmic transport depends on microtubules. Chemicals that cause the microtubules to disassemble block axon transport.

The model hypothesized for fast and slow transport requires ATP, Ca^{2+}-Mg^{2+} adenosine triphosphatase (ATPase), microtubules, carrier proteins, and a mechanism to control free calcium concentrations in the axoplasm (Fig. 3). An organelle or protein binds to a carrier protein that binds to the microtubule, which has side arms or associated proteins that use ATP via a Ca^{2+}-Mg^{2+} ATPase to cycle and move the carrier along the microtubule. Different carrier proteins are thought to be used in anterograde and retrograde transport. The protein kinesin has been isolated and shown to be important in anterograde transport. The microtubule-associated proteins may also control the direction of transport.

The transport filament model has been used to describe both slow and fast transport. Slow-transported proteins are loosely attached to the carrier and are dropped off early, that is, closer to the cell body; whereas, fast-transported proteins remain bound to the carrier all the way to the terminal. Differences in drop-off rates produce what are measured experimentally as slow, intermediate, and fast transport rates.

Fast axon transport also occurs from nerve terminals to the cell body, that is, in the retrograde direction. Retrograde transport is important in the returning of materials, such as empty neurotransmitter vesicles, from the terminals to the cell body either for degradation or for restoration and reuse (Fig. 4). The materials are packaged in large membrane-bound organelles that are part of the lysosomal system. The rate of retrograde transport is approximately one half to two thirds that of fast anterograde transport.

In addition to its important scavenger function, the movement of molecules from the terminals to the cell body can also be clinically important. For example, nerve growth factors released from the target organ are picked up by the growing axon and transported to the cell body, thereby influencing the direction of growth of regenerating axons after injury and nourishing the neuron. In addition, chromatolysis is initiated in the cell body when the axon is disrupted. This response may be induced by some injury signal that is given off by the target organ,

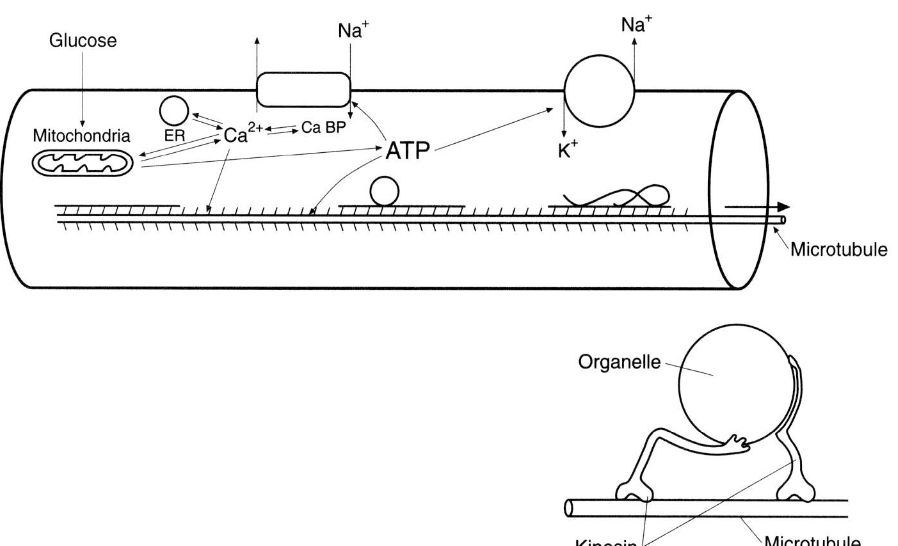

Figure 3
Model for axonal transport. CBP = calcium binding protein; ER = endoplasmic reticulum.

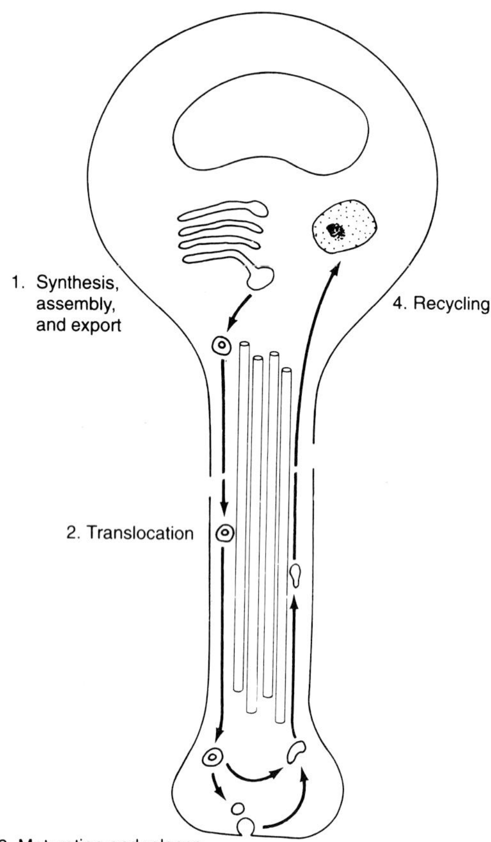

Figure 4
Synaptic vesicles and other membranous organelles involved in synaptic transmission at the nerve terminal are returned to the cell body for recycling after they are used at the synapse. 1. Proteins and lipids are synthesized and incorporated into membranes within the endoplasmic reticulum and Golgi apparatus in the neuron's cell body. 2. Organelles are then assembled from these components and exported from the cell body into the axon, where they are rapidly moved toward terminals by fast axonal transport. 3. Synaptic vesicles and their precursors reach the neuron's terminals, where they participate in the release of transmitter substances by exocytosis. At random, a small proportion of the membrane becomes degraded, and this material is returned to the cell body by fast retrograde axonal transport. 4. The degraded membrane is partly recycled, its residue is progressively accumulated in large, end-stage lysosomes that are characteristic of neuronal cell bodies. (Reproduced with permission from Kandel ER, Schwartz JH, Jessel TM: *Principles of Neural Science,* ed 3. Norwalk, CT, Appleton & Lange, 1991, p 57.)

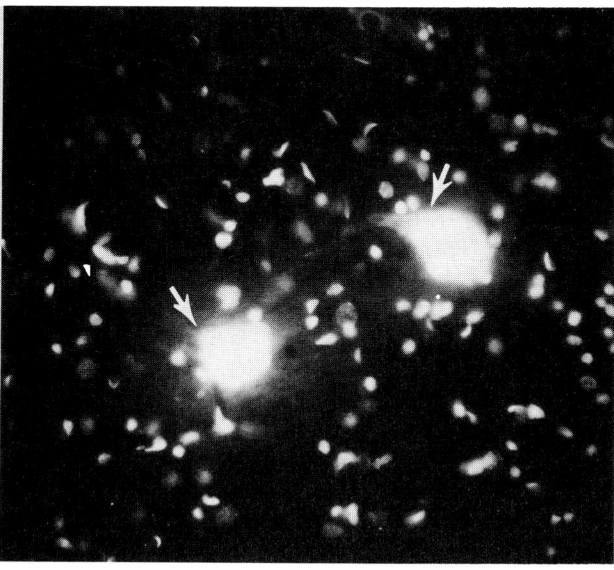

Figure 5
Labeled soleus motoneuron cell bodies in the ventral horn of the rat spinal cord. Motoneurons were labeled by injecting a fluorescent dye (fast blue) in the soleus muscles. The dye is taken up at the neuromuscular junction and transported to the cell body via retrograde axonal transport.

picked up by the damaged axon, and transported to the cell body. Retrograde transport can also have adverse effects. For example, several viruses, including herpes simplex, rabies, polio, and tetanus toxin are transported from nerve terminals to the cell body via retrograde transport.

Investigators have used the retrograde transport mechanism to trace axonal projections and label cell bodies. Horseradish peroxidase and various fluorescent dyes injected into a target organ or directly into the nerve are transported retrogradely to the cell body, allowing the investigator to trace the axonal projection or identify the location of the cell bodies in the spinal cord or spinal ganglion (Fig. 5).

Reductions in axonal transport have been observed in diseases such as diabetes and amyotrophic lateral sclerosis, and recent evidence suggests that abnormal rapid axonal transport may be involved in other peripheral neuropathies. It has not been determined, however, whether the abnormalities in axonal transport caused the associated nerve damage or whether they merely reflect structural damage to the axon from other causes. Secondary failure of axonal transport could determine the course of the neuropathy by inducing axonal atrophy, impaired nerve conduction, degeneration of nerve terminals, failure of synaptic transmission, and loss of trophic interactions.

Resting Membrane Potential and the Action Potential

The flow of information within and between neurons is conveyed by electrical and chemical signals. Nerve cells are able to process information because of the special properties of the neuronal cell membrane. Like other cell membranes, the neuronal cell membrane is composed of a lipid bilayer into which various membrane proteins are incorporated. The lipids within the membrane are hydrophobic; that is, they are immiscible with water. In contrast, the ions in the extracellular and intracellular space are hydrophilic; that is, they attract water. Ions are able to pass through the membrane by way of ion channels composed of proteins that are present in the membrane. These protein channels control the flux of ions across the membrane.

The Resting Membrane Potential

In all neurons there is an electrical potential difference between the two sides of the cell membrane, which can be measured by inserting an electrode into the cell and measuring the potential difference between the intracellular electrode and a reference electrode in the extracellular fluid (Fig. 6). By convention the reference electrode is set at 0 volts. In neurons at a resting state there is a negative potential within the cell; that is the inside of the cell is negative compared to the external environment. The potential difference of a neuron at rest is called the resting potential and usually lies between -50 and -80 mV.

The resting potential results from an unequal distribution of monovalent ions on either side of the cell membrane. The four most abundant ions on either side of the membrane are Na^+, K^+, Cl^-, and organic anions (often referred to as A^-). Early experiments that described the electrical excitability of nerve cells were performed on the giant squid axon, which is a single axon with a very large (1 mm) diameter that enables the placement of macro electrodes inside it. The distribution of ions inside and outside the membrane of the giant squid axon is given in Table 1. Na^+ and Cl^- are concentrated on the outside of the cell, and K^+ and A^- are concentrated inside the cell.

A lipid bilayer is negligibly permeable to charged ions; however, in biologic membranes, ion channels or pores in the lipid bilayer increase the permeability of the membrane to ions. Ion channels can have selective permeabilities based on the size, charge, or hydration of the specific ion. In 1902, it was hypothesized that the resting membrane potential was based on the selective permeability of the membrane to potassium. In the 1940s this theory was shown to be acceptable by comparing the actual resting potential measured using intracellular electrodes with that predicted by the Nernst equation, assuming selective permeability to potassium.

The Nernst equation is used to calculate the membrane potential at which the net flux of a specific ion across the membrane is zero. An ion's flux across the membrane depends on its concentration and electrical gradients. If the distribution of ions across a membrane equals those listed in Table 1 and the membrane is permeable only to K^+, the K^+ will diffuse down their concentration gradient from inside to outside the cell. As K^+ move from inside to outside, an excess of positive ions accumulates on the outside of the membrane, creating a potential difference across the membrane. This potential difference tends to repel the positively charged ions, moving them from outside to inside the cell. The potential difference at which the flow of K^+ from outside to inside the cell equals the flow from inside to outside is called the equilibrium potential and can be calculated using the Nernst equation:

$$E = \frac{RT}{FZ} ln \frac{[A]_i}{[A]_o}$$

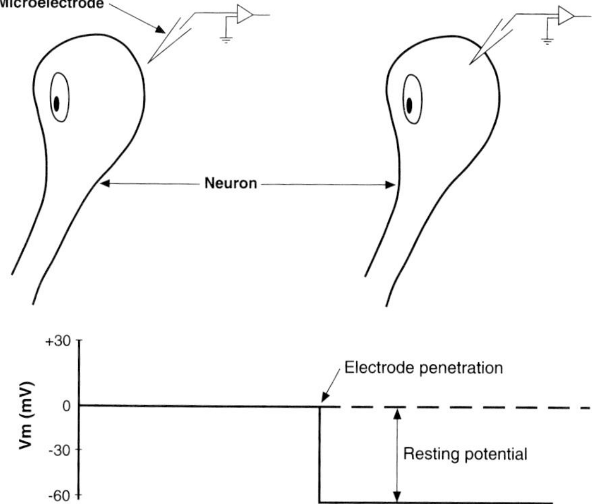

Figure 6
Measurement of the potential across a cell membrane. When a microelectrode connected to an electronic amplifier is placed outside the cell in the extracellular fluid, a potential of zero is measured. When the microelectrode is inserted through the cell membrane into the neuron, a negative potential difference is measured.

Table 1
Distribution of major ions in giant squid axon

Ion	Cytoplasm mM	Extracellular mM	Nernst Potential* mV
K^+	400	20	−75
Na^+	50	440	+55
Cl^-	52	560	-60
Organic Anion⁻	385	---	---

*The membrane potential at which there is no net flux of an ion across the cell membrane.

where E is the membrane potential, R is the universal gas constant (8.303), T is the temperature in absolute degrees Kelvin (0°C = 273°K), F is the Faraday constant, Z is the ion valence, [A]o represents the concentration of ion A outside the membrane, and [A]i represents the concentration of ion A inside the membrane.

At 25°C, RT/FZ is 26 mV and the equilibrium potential of K^+ equals -75 mV. If a neuron was permeable only to K^+, the resting membrane potential would equal the equilibrium potential for K^+. The resting membrane potential of the giant squid axon is -68 mV; therefore, the membrane must be permeable to more than one ion. Measurements of the resting membrane potential with intracellular electrodes and radioactive tracers have shown that nerve cells at rest are permeable to Na^+, Cl^-, and K^+.

Given that the equilibrium potentials of Na^+ and K^+ are -55mV and -75mV, respectively, the inside of the neuron would accumulate Na^+ and lose K^+ at a resting membrane potential of -68mV. If this process actually occurred, the concentration gradients and the electrical potential would go to 0 and the neuron would die. The neuron maintains its concentration gradients and resting membrane potential by the use of the sodium-potassium pump.

The sodium-potassium pump is an integral membrane protein that uses energy, in the form of ATP, to pump three Na^+ out of the neuron for every two K^+ it brings into the neuron (Fig. 7). When the neuron is at rest, the active fluxes (driven by the pump) and the passive fluxes (driven by diffusion) are balanced so that the net flux of Na^+ and K^+ is zero. The resting membrane potential is actually a steady-state potential, because energy must be used to maintain the ionic gradients across the membrane.

Passive Membrane Properties

Neurons process and transmit information using electrical signals produced by temporary changes in the current flow into and out of the neuron. Electrical signals come in two forms: graded potentials and action potentials.

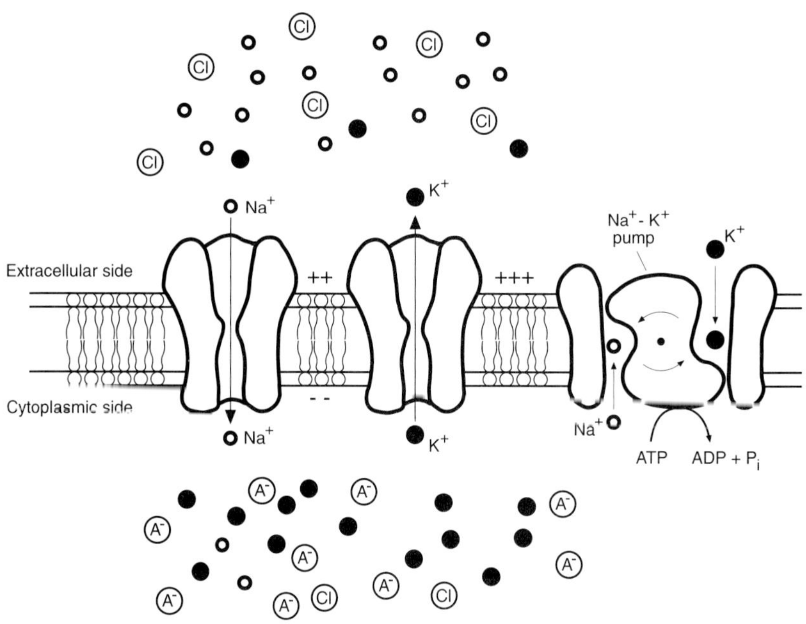

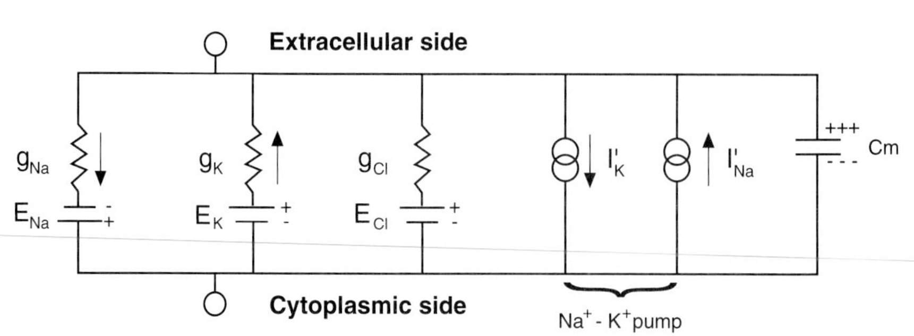

Figure 7
Permeabilities and driving forces of Na^+, K^+, and Cl^-. **Top,** When the cell is at rest, the passive fluxes of Na^+ and K^+ into and out of the cell are balanced by the energy-dependent sodium-potassium pump. **Bottom,** The electrical equivalent circuit of a neuron at rest includes the most abundant types of ion channels in parallel. Under steady state conditions, the currents resulting from passive diffusion of Na and K are balanced by active Na and K fluxes (I'_{Na} and I'_K) driven by the sodium-potassium pump.

A graded potential is a hyperpolarizing or depolarizing local change in a neuron's membrane potential (Fig. 8). In graded potentials, the amplitude of the voltage change is variable and directly related to the intensity of the external signal. Graded potentials can be one of three types: (1) Receptor (or generator) potentials are created in specialized sensory cells called receptors; for example, mechanoreceptors and pain receptors. (2) Pacemaker potentials are not found in mammalian nerve cells, but are found in the heart and smooth muscle. These are spontaneous changes in a cell's own membrane potential caused by intrinsic properties of the cell rather than by external stimuli. (3) Synaptic potentials are changes evoked at a synapse as a result of ionic currents through the membrane of the postsynaptic cell.

The conductance of graded potentials depends on the passive properties of the cell membrane: the membrane resistance R_m, internal resistance R_i, and capacitance C_m of the resting membrane. Because cell membranes act as barriers to certain ions, they are able to store charge and can be considered to be capacitors. However, cell membranes are not perfect capacitors because some ions can pass through, and they often are called leaky capacitors because pores make their resistance finite. (Refer to the glossary for definitions of basic electrical terms.)

When current I is injected into a neuron the voltage V does not rise instantaneously, but rises at an exponential rate. The amplitude of the steady-state voltage is proportional to the intensity of the stimulus because at steady state, V = IR. The change in voltage is not instantaneous because the membrane has both resistance and capacitance. Although current flows instantaneously through a resistor, it takes time to charge or discharge a capacitor. Once the capacitor has reached a steady state, current can flow through the membrane's resistance. The amount of time it takes to reach 66% of the peak voltage is defined as the time constant t, and is determined by the membrane's resistance and capacitance: t = RC. The time constant increases with the time to reach the steady state voltage (Fig. 9). The time constant can control the rate at which a neuron fires or the speed at which an action potential is propagated down the axon.

As a graded potential travels down the axon it decreases in amplitude (Fig. 10). Within an axon there are two types of resistance: the internal resistance R_i, which runs longitudinally down the axon, and the transverse resistance R_m, which is equivalent to the membrane resistance (Fig. 10). When current is injected, the amount of current will be greatest at the point of injection, and the current will go down the path of least resistance. Each time current flows across the membrane, less current flows from the point of injection and the amplitude of the voltage decreases because of the decrease in current. The distance at which voltage has decreased to 37% of its maximum is defined as lambda λ or the length constant. The length constant is dependent on both R_i and R_m: $\lambda = R_m/R_i$. If the membrane resistance is high, the length constant will be high, more current will flow down the axon, and the potential will decay at a slower rate. If the internal resistance is greater than the membrane resistance, the length constant will be low and current will flow out of the cell, causing the graded potential to decay rapidly.

The Action Potential

The action potential transmits coded messages rapidly and over long distances to other neurons or effector organs such as muscle. Graded potentials are good only for communication over short distances

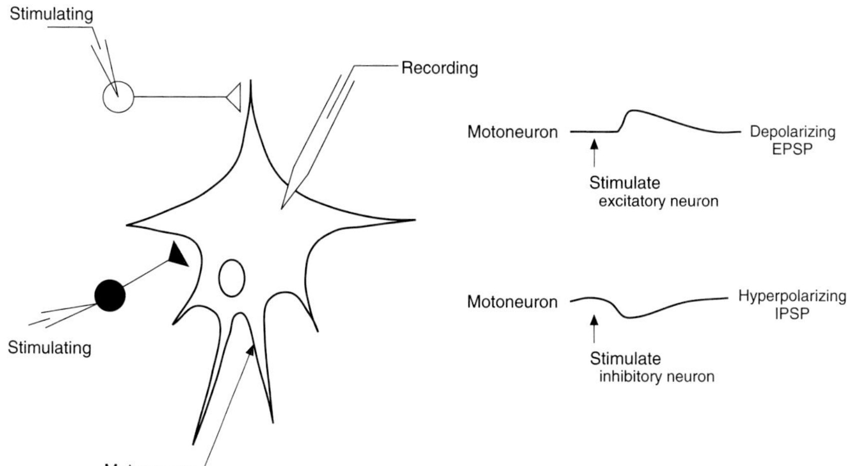

Figure 8
Graded potentials. Stimulation of an excitatory neuron that synapses onto a motoneuron produces a depolarizing synaptic potential in the cell body (excitatory postsynaptic potential, EPSP). Stimulation of an inhibitory neuron that synapses onto a motoneuron produces a hyperpolarizing synaptic potential in the cell (inhibitory postsynaptic potential, IPSP).

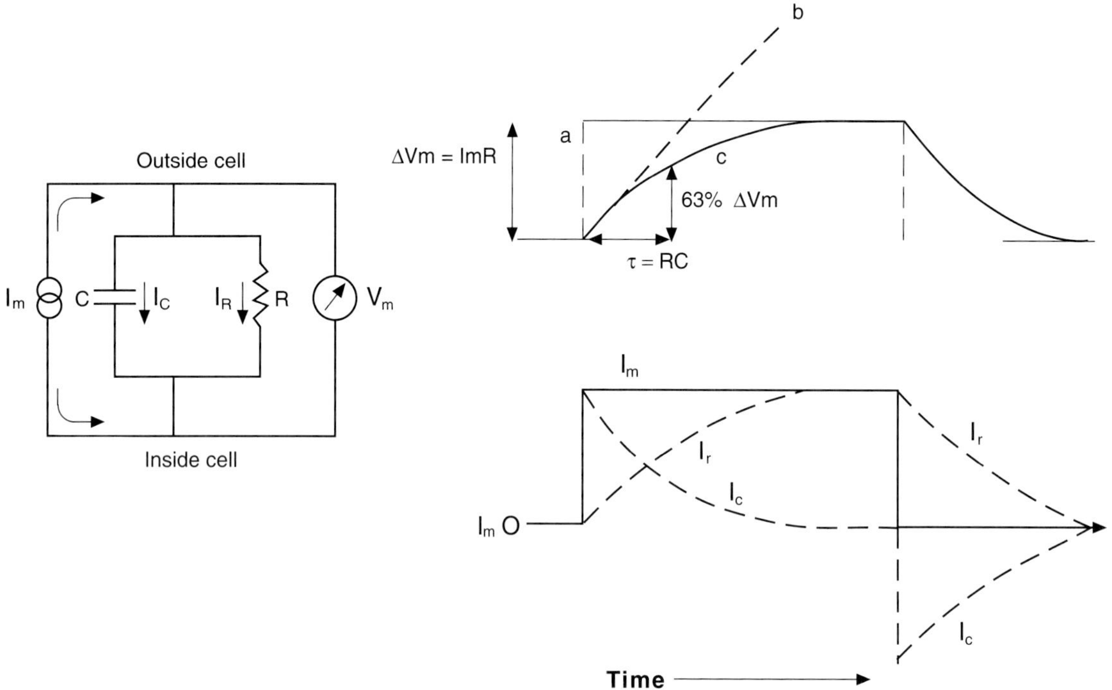

Figure 9
Membrane time constant. **Left,** Current-voltage relationship for a cell membrane consisting of resistive as well as capacitive elements. **Top right,** Time course of the change of membrane potential in response to a step of current. Line c shows the actual response of the membrane potential (ΔVm) to a rectangular current pulse; line a shows the response of a membrane containing only resistive elements; and line b the response of a membrane containing only capacitive elements. The membrane potential approaches a maximum exponentially with a time constant equal to the membrane resistance times capacitance. **Bottom right,** The time courses of the total membrane current (I_m), the ionic current (I_i), and the capacitive current (I_c).

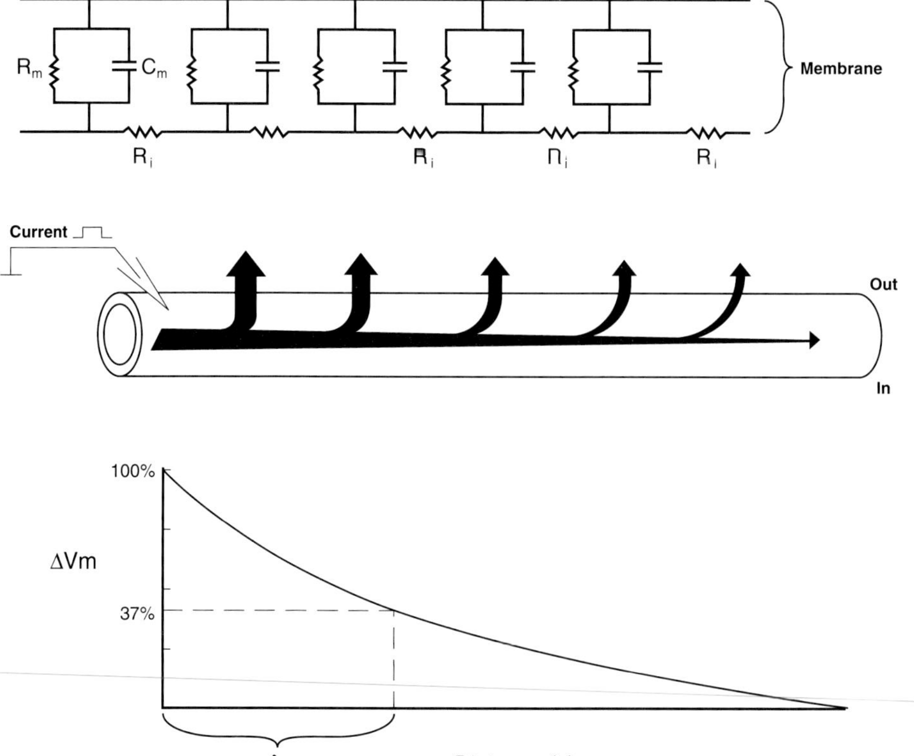

Figure 10
Length constant and passive current flow. **Top,** Equivalent circuit of a hypothetical nerve fiber consisting of membrane resistance (R_m) and internal resistance (R_i). **Center,** Current injected into a neuronal process by a microelectrode follows the path of least resistance. Current loss results when current flows out of the membrane through R_m instead of down the axon through R_i. **Bottom,** The change in membrane potential (ΔVm) decays exponentially with distance along the length of the axon or dendrite.

within a neuron because they decay over time and distance. An action potential can be described as a brief (~ 1 ms) explosive change in the membrane potential from its normal resting potential to a very positive value. Action potentials are self-regenerating potentials that occur spontaneously when the membrane is depolarized beyond a critical membrane potential called threshold (Fig. 11, *left*). The peak amplitude of the action potential is fixed and independent of the stimulus intensity above threshold. Cells that can produce action potentials are referred to as excitable cells.

Stimuli that are less than threshold create graded potentials. Graded potentials are proportional to the intensity of the stimulus, and different potentials can summate. An action potential is initiated when the graded potentials depolarize the membrane to the threshold potential. At the threshold potential, the neuron membrane resistance begins to change, and the membrane no longer obeys Ohm's law V = 1R. The membrane resistance is determined by the number of open channels. At rest the number of open channels remains constant; however, depolarization causes Na^+ membrane ion channels to actively open, allowing Na^+ to flow across the membrane into the cell.

The rising phase of the action potential results from an increase in the permeability (or conductance g) of the membrane to Na^+. The Na^+ conductance increases as a result of structural changes in gated ion channels selective to Na^+. Gated ion channels open or close as a result of structural changes that occur in response to various stimuli. The three major signals that can gate ion channels are voltage (voltage-gated channels), chemical transmitters (transmitter-gated channels), and pressure or stretch (mechanically-gated channels) (Fig. 12). Nongated channels are always open and are responsible for the resting membrane potential. The Na^+ channels responsible for the action potential are voltage-gated. Membrane depolarization causes a conformational change that opens the channels, allowing Na^+ to diffuse into the cell according to its electrochemical gradient (Fig. 13).

Action potentials are propagated down the axon by a combination of passive current flow and active membrane changes. For example, once the membrane along any point of the axon has been depolarized beyond threshold, an action potential is generated in that region in response to the opening of voltage-gated Na^+ channels. This local depolarization then spreads passively along the axon, causing the adjacent region of the membrane to reach threshold for generating an action potential (Fig. 14). The depolarization is spread by passive current flow that results from the potential difference between the active and the inactive regions of the axon membrane. Once the depolarization of the inactive region of the membrane approaches threshold, the voltage-gated Na^+ channels in this region open, Na^+ rushes into the axoplasm, and an action potential is initiated. The actively generated depolarization then spreads by passive, local circuit flow to the next region of the membrane, and the cycle is repeated.

The rate at which the action potential is conducted along the axon depends on the passive membrane properties: the capacitance C_m and the inter-

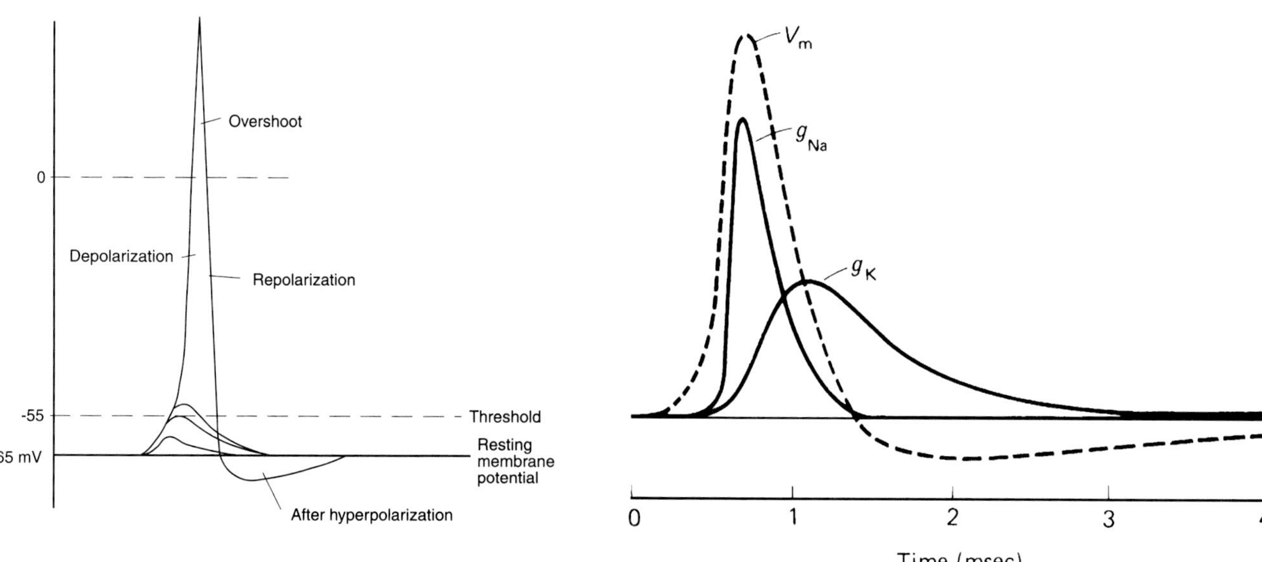

Figure 11
Left, Action potentials are generated when the membrane potential reaches a critical threshold voltage. The depolarization phase is due to the active opening of Na channels and repolarization to the active opening of K channels. **Right,** The shape of the action potential can be calculated from the changes in g_{Na} and g_K that result from the opening and closing of voltage-gated Na and K channels. (Adapted with permission from Hodgkin AL: *The Conduction of a Nervous Impulse.* Springfield, IL, Thomas, 1964.)

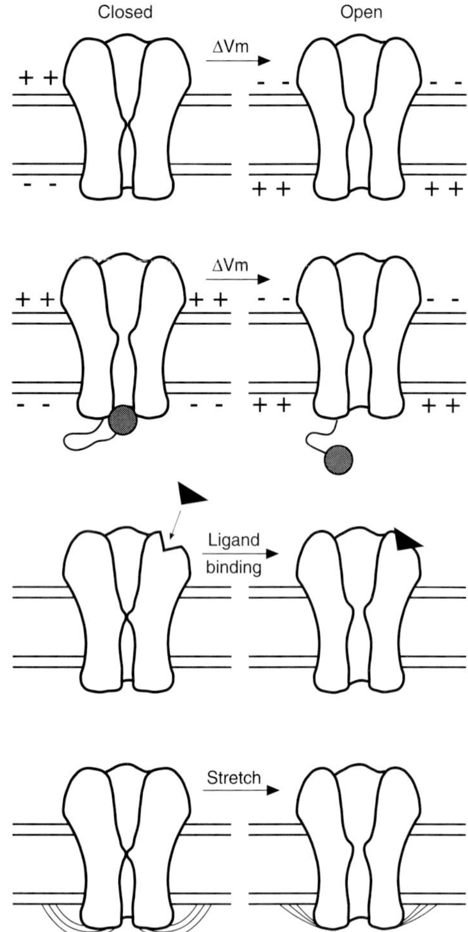

Figure 12
Channel gating is controlled by several types of stimuli. Changes in voltage can regulate a channel by causing a blocking particle to swing into or out of the channel mouth (often referred to as ball and chain model). Binding of a ligand to a receptor located on the channel or stretch or pressure can activate the channel by causing conformational changes in the channel. (Adapted with permission from Kandel ER, Schwartz JH, Jessell TM: *Principles of Neural Science,* ed 3. Norwalk, CT, Appleton & Lange, 1991, pp 75–76.)

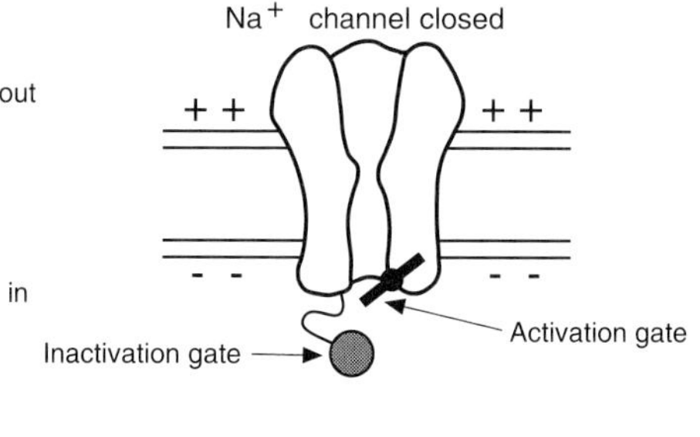

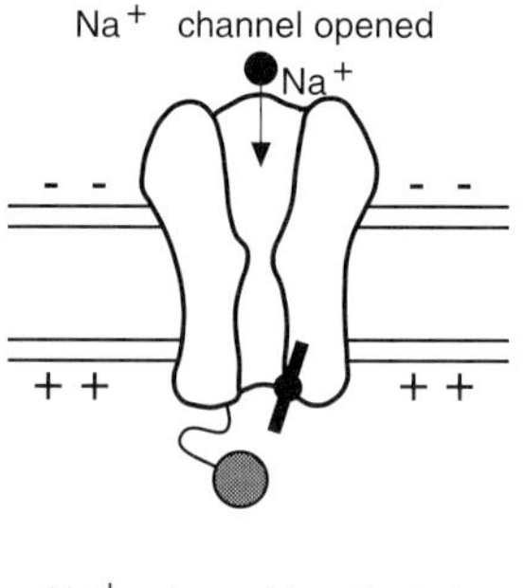

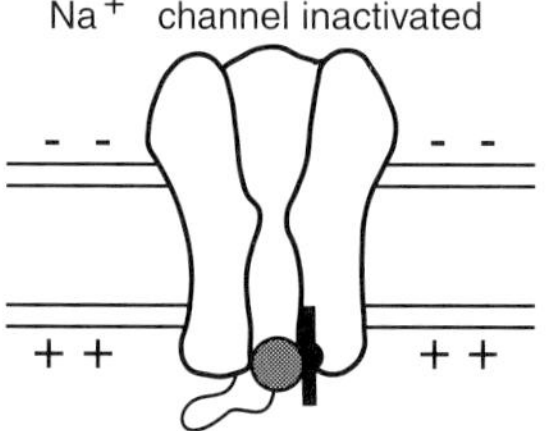

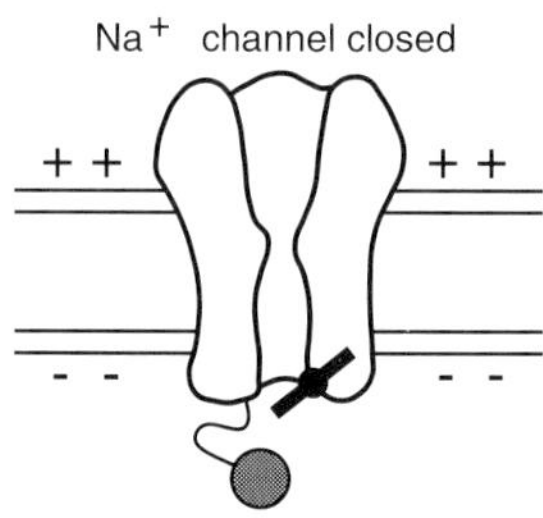

Figure 13
Response of gated Na channel during action potential. **Top,** When the cell is in the resting state, the Na activation gate is closed and the inactivation gate is open. **Top center,** Depolarization of the cell causes the Na activation gates to open and Na enters the cell. **Bottom center,** As the depolarization is maintained, channels that have opened begin to close because the inactivation gates close. **Bottom,** After the membrane is repolarized, the channel returns to its resting state. (Adapted with permission from Kandel ER, Schwartz JH, Jessell TM: *Principles of Neural Science,* ed 3. Norwalk, CT, Appleton & Lange, 1991, p 14.)

nal resistance of the axoplasm R_i. As described, an action potential generated in one segment of the axon supplies the current to depolarize the adjacent segments. According to Ohm's law, the larger the internal resistance, the less the current flow ($I = V/R$) and, thus, the longer it takes to change the charge on the membrane of the adjacent segment. Additionally, the higher the capacitance, the larger the time constant, and the longer it takes to charge the membrane and to depolarize the membrane. The rate of passive current flow varies inversely with the product R_iC_m. If this product is reduced, the rate of passive current spread and the rate of action potential conduction, that is, conduction velocity, will both increase.

One way to increase the conduction velocity is to increase the diameter of the axon. Because the internal resistance R_i decreases in proportion to the square of the axon diameter and the capacitance C_m

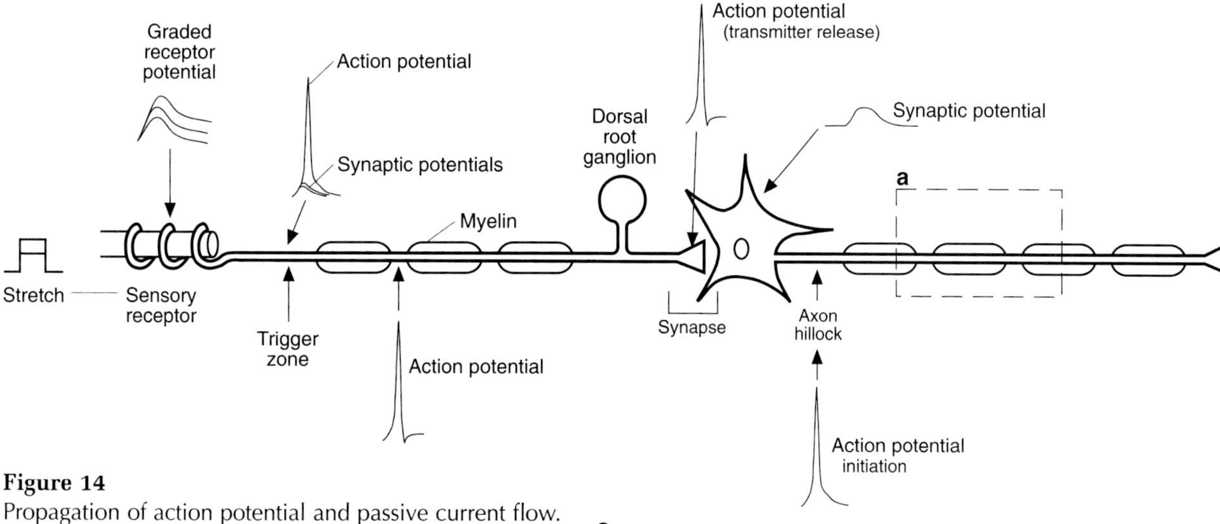

Figure 14
Propagation of action potential and passive current flow. Graded stretching of a muscle produces graded potentials in the terminal fibers of the sensory neuron. This potential spreads passively to the trigger zone and, if the potential is large enough, it will trigger an action potential, which is actively propagated without change along the axon to the terminal region. At the terminal of the afferent fiber, the action potential triggers the release of transmitter that diffuses across the synaptic cleft and interacts with the membrane of the motoneuron to initiate a synaptic potential in the motoneuron. The synaptic potential passively spreads to the axon hillock where an action potential is initiated if the membrane potential is above threshold. Action potential propagation results from the spread of local passive depolarizing currents between the nodes of Ranvier. At the nodes, voltage-gated channels open, producing an action potential.

increases in direct proportion to the diameter, the net effect of increasing the diameter is a decrease in R_iC_m. Because of the need for a large number of axons, this adaptation has not taken place in vertebrates. In vertebrates, conduction velocity is increased by increasing the membrane resistance R_m.

Vertebrate axons are wrapped in myelin, which effectively acts as an insulator, increasing the membrane resistance and decreasing the membrane capacitance. The resulting increase in the length constant and decrease in the time constant increases the rate of passive current flow. Although myelin interferes with action potential initiation, there are specialized regions of the axon that are not wrapped in myelin, the nodes of Ranvier, at which there is a high concentration of voltage-gated Na^+ channels. Action potentials are evoked at the nodes, and local currents flow quickly, largely unattenuated down the myelinated region of the axon (the internode) from one node to the next, where a new action potential is evoked; that is, action potential production jumps via saltatory propagation from node to node. This means of increasing the conduction velocity is very effective.

Several diseases of the nervous system cause demyelination; for example, multiple sclerosis and Guillain-Barré syndrome. Demyelinated regions of the axon have a higher capacitance and a lower membrane resistance; therefore, when an action potential is propagated down a myelinated axon and reaches a demyelinated region its conduction will be slowed or may be stopped completely. A decrease or loss of conduction could have devastating effects on behavior.

External Activation of Axons

To drive an axon to threshold, the current must pass through the membrane. Of the total stimulating current, only a small fraction flows across the membrane of any one axon. The current passes through the membrane, flows along the axoplasmic core, and exits through the membrane in a distant region. Larger diameter axons have a lower current threshold and their axoplasm is less resistant to current flow. Because of this, more current enters the larger axons, where it depolarizes the membrane and brings it to threshold. Once threshold is reached, the action potential is initiated and self-propagated. A gradual increase in stimulus strength will excite the larger axons first and then, at relatively large current strengths, the smaller axons.

Sensory and Motor Systems

Classification of Nerve Fibers

The CNS consists of the brain and the spinal cord. All remaining nervous tissue is referred to as the peripheral nervous system (PNS). Peripheral nerves are bundles of axons that are enclosed in sheaths of connective tissue that maintain the continuity of, nourish, and protect the individual axons.

An axon is composed of a core of axoplasm enclosed in an axolemmal membrane. The axoplasm contains subcellular structures including microtubules, neurofibrils, mitochondria, vesicles of the smooth endoplasmic reticulum, and, occasionally, dense bodies and glycogen particles. Every axon in a peripheral nerve is surrounded by a myelin sheath that is formed by Schwann cells. A nerve fiber is defined as the axon and the Schwann cell sheath surrounding it.

The outer sheath of the nerve fiber varies in structure depending on whether or not the axon is myelinated. One myelinated axon is associated with only one Schwann cell at any one level. The Schwann cell wraps spirally around the axon and produces a sheath of alternating layers of lipid and protein that are compressed together, giving the myelin sheath a characteristic laminated structure (Fig. 15, *top*). In general, an axon becomes myelinated once it reaches a diameter of 1 to 2 μm. The thickness of the myelin sheath increases with the size of the axon. The diameter of peripheral axons, excluding the myelin sheath, varies from 0.5 to 10 μm. In unmyelinated fibers, one Schwann cell surrounds many axons (Fig. 15, *bottom*). Physiologically, the primary difference between myelinated and unmyelinated fibers is the conduction velocity.

Nerve fibers can be classified into different types based on their diameter and conduction velocity or their function. Nerve fibers that transmit information from sensory receptors to the CNS are referred to as afferent. Afferent fibers from the viscera are termed visceral afferents and those from receptors in muscles, skin, and sensory organs of the head are called somatic afferents. Transmission of information from the CNS to the periphery occurs via efferent nerve fibers. Efferent fibers that innervate skeletal muscle fibers are called motor efferents. The remaining efferent nerve fibers are classified as autonomic efferents. Peripheral nerves that innervate the skin, skeletal muscles, and the joints are referred to as somatic nerves, and nerves leading to

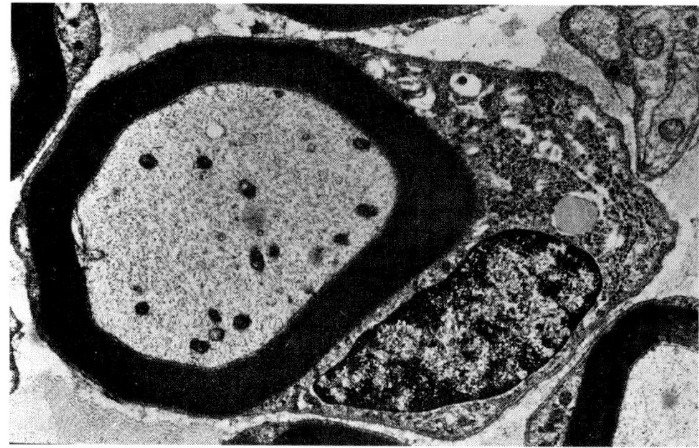

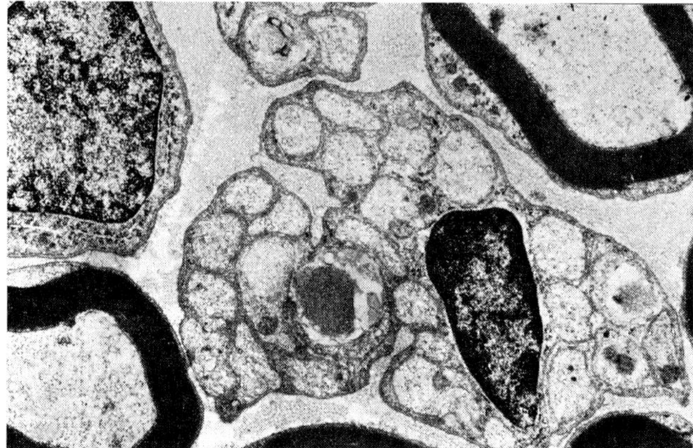

Figure 15
Photomicrograph showing myelinated (**top**) and unmyelinated (**bottom**) axons.

the viscera are called splanchnic or autonomic nerves. This chapter will focus on somatic nerves.

Two sets of nomenclature have been used to classify axons based on the diameter of the axon and the conduction velocity. The Erlanger/Gasser classification uses an alphabetical scheme and is typically used to classify afferents in cutaneous nerves. The Lloyd/Hunt classification uses Roman numerals and is typically used to classify afferents in motor nerves. The axon diameters and conduction velocities for the different types of nerve fibers are given in Table 2. The distribution of afferents in motor and cutaneous nerves is illustrated in Figure 16. Cutaneous nerves have only three peaks because the group I (Aα) afferents are absent. Group I afferents are typically primary muscle spindle afferents and afferents from muscle tendon organs. Virtually all mechanoreceptors are Aβ and Aα fibers, whereas thermoreceptors and nociceptors belong to the Aγ and C fiber groups.

A compound nerve action potential is produced by electrically stimulating a peripheral nerve at an intensity that activates all motor and sensory fibers;

Table 2:
Classification of nerve fibers

Group	Function (Examples)	Average Fiber Diameter (μm)	Average CV (ms)
	Erlanger/Gasser Classification		
Aα	Primary muscle-spindle afferents, motor axons to muscle	15	100
Aβ	Cutaneous touch and pressure afferents	8	50
Aγ	Motor axons to muscle spindle	5	20
Aδ	Cutaneous temperature and pain afferents	3	15
B	Sympathetic preganglionic	3	7
C	Cutaneous pain afferents, sympathetic postganglionic	0.5	1
	Lloyd/Hunt Classification		
I	Primary muscle-spindle afferents and afferents from tendon organs	13	75
II	Mechanoreceptors	9	55
III	Deep pressure sensors in muscle	3	11
IV	Unmyelinated pain afferents	0.5	1

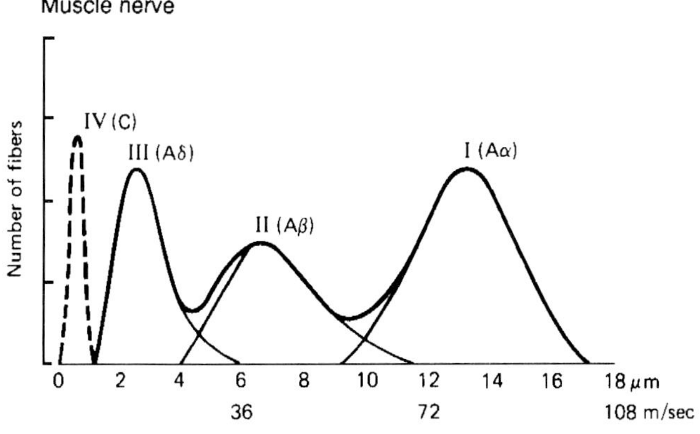

Figure 16
The distribution of different types of afferent fibers in muscle and cutaneous tissue. Axonal diameters are given in micrometers and conduction velocities are given in meters per second. (Adapted with permission from Boyd IA, Davey MR: *Composition of Peripheral Nerves.* Edinburgh, Churchill Livingstone, 1968.)

thus, it is the summation of action potentials from all activated nerve fibers. In general, the compound nerve action potential has two major deflections corresponding to the Aα (large myelinated) and Aγ (small myelinated) fibers (Fig. 17). Action potentials of unmyelinated fibers (Group C or IV) are conducted slowly and produce a small late peak that typically cannot be recorded in vivo.

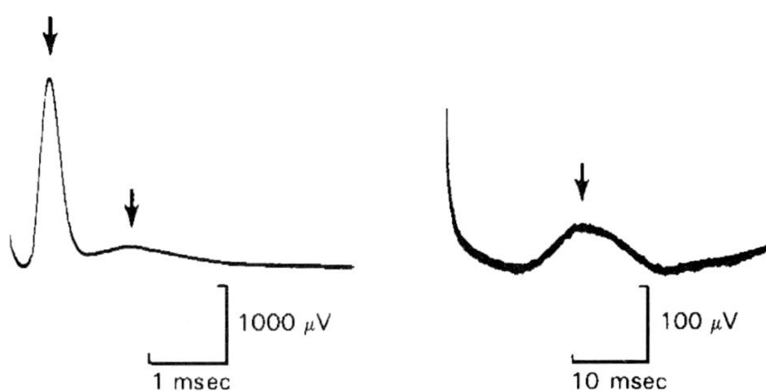

Figure 17
The compound action potential has three distinct peaks corresponding to Aα, Aδ, and C fibers. The compound action potential shown here was recorded in vitro because potentials from C fibers cannot be recorded in vivo. The nerve, from an 11-year-old boy whose leg had been amputated above the knee, was placed in a specialized recording chamber. The recording on the left shows peaks produced by Aα (left arrow) and Aδ (right arrow) fibers. The trace on the right is a high-gain, slow time scale recording of a C-fiber peak. (Reproduced with permission from Kimura J: *Electrodiagnosis in Diseases of Nerve and Muscle: Principles and Practice,* ed 2. Philadelphia, FA Davis, 1989.)

Sensory Systems

Sensory systems receive information from the environment and within the body through receptors located at the periphery of the body and transmit this information to the CNS. This information is used for three primary functions: sensation, control of movement, and maintaining arousal. Although sensation is a conscious experience, much of the sensory information used to control movement is not perceived. In addition, much of the sensory information received from within the body and used to regulate such functions as temperature, blood pressure, heart rate, respiratory rate, and reflex movement never reaches consciousness.

Sensory systems extract four attributes from a stimulus: modality or quality, intensity, duration, and location. The major modalities are described in Table 3. All sensory systems are organized in a similar manner. External stimuli are sensed by specialized neural structures called sensory receptors. Each receptor is sensitive to a specific form of physical energy: mechanical, thermal, chemical, or electromagnetic (Table 3). The external stimulus or energy is transformed into electrochemical energy through the process of sensory transduction. Sensory information is then transmitted to the CNS by action potentials. The attributes of the stimulus are neurally encoded by the action potentials. In the somatic systems, the sensory receptor is a neuron that carries out both sensory transduction and neural encoding of the action potentials.

Sensory information is transmitted to the brain via two pathways: the dorsal column-medial lemniscal tract and the anterolateral tract. The receptor neuron, which is referred to as the first order neuron or the primary afferent, projects to the spinal cord or the brainstem, where it synapses with second-order neurons. The neurons in subcortical regions are referred to as lower-order neurons. The information from lower-order neurons is passed through relay nuclei to higher-order neurons in the cerebral cortex. In the sensory system, the thalamus is an essential relay point. Sensory information is sent from the thalamus to specific sensory regions of the cortex where it is perceived.

The somatic sensory system is distinct because the receptors for somatic sensation are distributed throughout the body rather than confined to a specialized organ such as the eye and because it processes many different types of stimuli. The somatic sensory system conveys three distinct modalities: (1) mechanical, elicited by mechanical stimulation of the body surface (touch) and elicited by mechanical displacements of the muscles and joints (proprioception); (2) pain, elicited by noxious (tissue damaging) stimuli; and (3) thermal sensation, elicited by cool and warm stimuli. Within each modality there are submodalities; for example, superficial and deep touch (pressure).

Each somatosensory modality is mediated by a separate class of receptors (Table 4). However, regardless of the receptor type, all somatosensory information from the body is transmitted to the spinal cord or the brainstem by dorsal root ganglion neurons. The dorsal root ganglion neuron performs two functions: sensory transduction and transmission of encoded stimulus information. The morphology of the dorsal root ganglion neuron is illustrated in Figure 18. Dorsal root ganglion neurons are not all alike and can be distinguished by (1) the morphology of the terminal, (2) sensitivity to a stimulus, (3) the diameter of the axon and cell body, and (4) the presence or absence of a myelin sheath. The terminal of the dorsal root ganglion neuron is the only region that is sensitive to stimulus energy and is either a bare nerve ending or an end organ consisting of a nonneuronal capsule surrounding the axon terminal. Nociceptors and thermoreceptors are bare nerve endings. Mechanoreceptors are generally specialized end organs. The sensory information is transmitted to the spinal cord or brainstem

Table 3
Sensory systems

Modality	Stimulus	Receptor Type	Receptors
Vision	Light	Photoreceptors	Rods, cones
Hearing	Sound	Mechanoreceptors	Hair cells (cochlear)
Balance	Head motion	Mechanoreceptors	Hair cells (semicircular canal)
Somatic	Mechanical	Mechanoreceptors	Dorsal root ganglion cells
	Thermal	Thermoreceptors	
	Noxious	Nociceptors, chemoreceptors	
Taste	Chemical	Chemoreceptors	Taste buds
Smell	Chemical	Chemoreceptors	Olfactory sensory neurons

(Reproduced wth permission from Kandel ER, Schwartz JH, Jessel TM (eds): *Principles of Neural Science,* ed 3. Norwalk, CT, Appleton & Lange, 1991, p 334.)

Table 4
Receptor types

Receptor type	Fiber type	Quality
Nociceptors		
Mechanical	Aδ	Sharp, pricking pain
Thermal and mechanothermal	Aγ	Sharp, pricking pain
Thermal and mechanothermal	C	Slow, burning pain
Polymodal	C	Slow, burning pain
Cutaneous and subcutaneous mechanoreceptors		
Meissner's corpuscle	Aβ	Touch
Pacinian corpuscle	Aβ	Flutter
Ruffini corpuscle	Aβ	Vibration
Merkel's receptor	Aβ	Steady skin indentation
Hair-guard, hair-tylotrich	Aβ	Steady skin indentation
Hair-down	Aβ	Flutter
Muscle and skeletal mechanoreceptors		
Muscle spindle primary	Aα	Limb proprioception
Muscle spindle secondary	Aβ	Limb proprioception
Golgi tendon organ	Aα	Limb proprioception
Joint capsule mechanoreceptor	Aβ	Limb proprioception

(Reproduced wth permission from Kandel ER, Schwartz JH, Jessel TM (eds): *Principles of Neural Science*, ed 3. Norwalk, CT, Appleton & Lange, 1991, p 342.)

by the primary afferent fiber. The cell body is located in the dorsal root ganglia in the peripheral nervous system and gives rise to two processes: the peripheral and central branches of the primary afferent. Sensory information concerned with touch and limb proprioception is carried by the medial lemniscal tract and information concerned with pain and temperature by the anterolateral tract.

Motor Systems

The motor system is hierarchically organized and consists of four major divisions: (1) the spinal cord, (2) the brainstem and reticular formation, (3) the motor cortex, and (4) the premotor cortical areas that include the basal ganglia and cerebellum. Each division contains separate neural circuits that are linked to each of the other divisions. The spinal

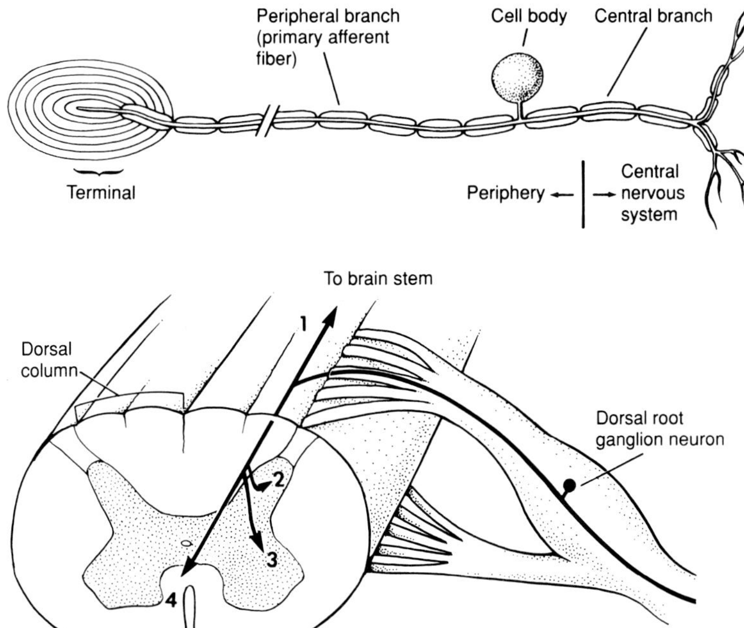

Figure 18
Top, Morphology of dorsal root ganglion cells. The cell body lies in a ganglion in the dorsal root of a spinal nerve. The axon has two branches, one projecting to the periphery and one to the central nervous system. **Bottom,** Projections of the central branch. The dorsal root ganglion cells that mediate pressure, touch, and proprioception have several central branches. The principle branch ascends in the dorsal column to the brain stem (1). The other branches terminate locally in the dorsal and ventral horns of the spinal cord (2,3), or descend a few segments and terminate in the spinal cord (4). Branches 2, 3, and 4 participate in local spinal reflexes. (Adapted with permission from Kandel ER, Schwartz JH, Jessell TM: *Principles of Neural Science,* ed 3. Norwalk, CT, Appleton & Lange, 1991, pp 287–342.)

cord contains the neural circuitry responsible for segmental and proprioceptive reflexes as well as the circuitry responsible for the reciprocal activation of flexor and extensor muscles during locomotion. Spinal cord neurons process information from the peripheral system, from each other, and from descending pathways in the spinal cord to mediate reflexes and control motor output. In addition, they send ascending projections to higher centers. The descending pathways originate from upper motoneurons in the cerebral cortex and brainstem. These pathways often are divided into pyramidal and extrapyramidal tracts. The pyramidal or corticospinal tract originates from neurons in the motor cortex, premotor cortex, and parietal lobe. The extrapyramidal tracts arise from cells in the red nucleus, reticular formation, and vestibular nucleus of the brainstem and give rise to the rubrospinal, reticulospinal, and vestibulospinal tracts, respectively.

Spinal Cord Anatomy

In the adult human, the spinal cord extends from the foramen magnum to the lower border of the first lumbar vertebra. Axons enter and exit the spinal cord via the spinal nerves, each of which consists of a ventral or efferent root and a dorsal or afferent root (Fig. 19, *top left*). The ventral roots carry output to the striated muscles from the myelinated nerve fibers of the α and γ motoneurons in the gray matter of the ventral horn. The dorsal roots carry sensory input from myelinated and unmyelinated nerve fibers that originate from somatic sensory receptors. The cell bodies of the afferent fibers are located in the dorsal root ganglia.

The spinal cord is divided into white and gray matter. The white matter is divided into columns of ascending and descending fiber tracts that contain myelinated and unmyelinated nerve axons. The gray matter, which consists of longitudinally arranged neuronal cell bodies, dendrites, glial cells, and myelinated and unmyelinated axons, is divided into the dorsal horn, intermediate zone, and ventral horn. There are three types of neurons present in the spinal gray matter: (1) neurons that send axonal projections out of the CNS via the ventral roots (α and γ motoneurons), (2) neurons that have axonal projections that remain in the spinal cord (interneurons), and (3) neurons that send ascending axonal projections to supraspinal centers (tract cells). The spinal gray matter is histologically divided by cell characteristics into nine different regions or lamina (Fig. 19, *bottom left*). Each lamina contains a specific type of neuron and receives axonal projections from specific sensory axons and descending pathways.

Lower Motoneurons

Movement is generated by the activation of striated skeletal muscles. Skeletal muscles are innervated by lower motoneurons located in the ventral gray matter of the spinal cord. The motoneurons innervating a specific muscle are arranged in columns that extend through several spinal segments. The α motoneurons are relatively large cells that have body areas ranging from 30 to 70 μm^2 and motor axons that innervate the extrafusal muscle fibers in striated muscles. Within the ventral horn, the motoneurons are located in nonoverlapping areas: axial muscles are innervated by medially located motoneurons (lamina VIII), and limb muscles are innervated by more laterally located motoneurons (lamina IX). The most medial of the lateral group of motoneurons tend to innervate the proximal muscles (muscles of the shoulder and hip), while the more lateral motoneurons in lamina IX tend to innervate the distal muscles (the muscles of the extremities and digits). The motoneurons innervating the extensor muscles tend to be located ventral to those innervating flexor muscles. The γ motoneurons are smaller than α motoneurons and innervate intrafusal fibers of the muscle spindles.

The basic functional unit of a muscle is the motor unit, which consists of an α motoneuron, its motor axon, and all the muscle fibers it innervates. The motor unit has been called the final common pathway because all information, both direct and indirect, must be processed by the α motoneuron for muscle contraction to occur. The α motoneuron receives input from three major sources: (1) the sensory system, (2) the pyramidal pathways, and (3) the extrapyramidal pathways. Although the motoneuron receives direct inputs from these systems, activity in neural circuits is coordinated primarily by interneurons. The interneurons function as a link between the peripheral nervous system, the descending pathways from the cortex and brainstem, and local spinal neurons and motoneurons.

Motor Unit Types

The function of a muscle is a reflection of the physiologic, morphologic, and biochemical characteristics of its motor units. Characterization of the physiologic properties of the muscle unit (the fibers innervated by one motoneuron) has revealed a number of interrelationships that have been the basis of the classification of units into types. Motor units most often are separated into four major types based on the physiologic properties of the muscle unit: slow, fatigue resistant (type S); fast fatigue resistant (type FR); fast fatigue intermediate (type FI); and fast fatigable (type FF). The physiologic properties

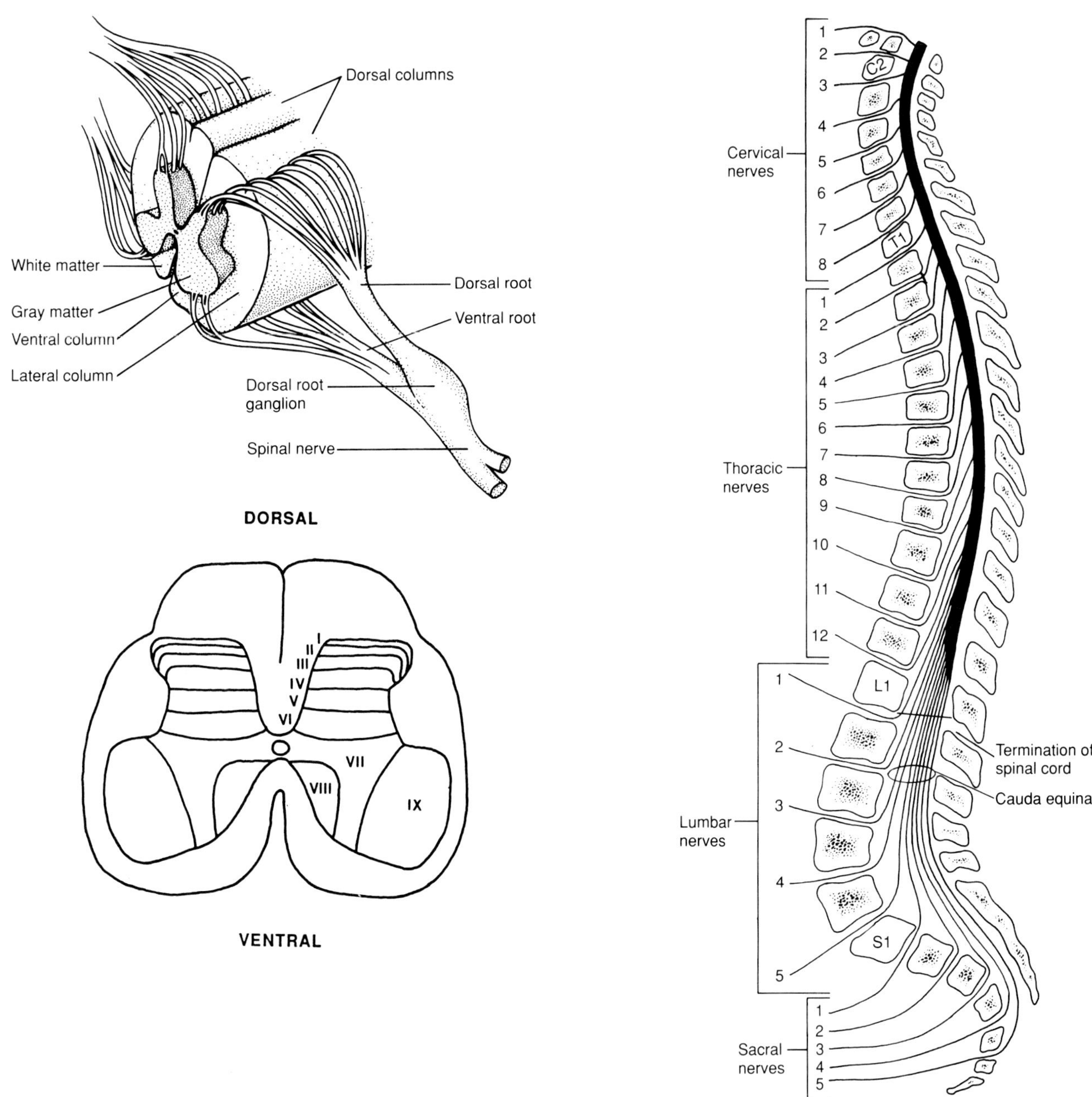

Figure 19
Spinal cord anatomy. **Top left,** Each spinal nerve has a dorsal and ventral root. The dorsal (sensory) root comprises the central branches of the dorsal root ganglion cells; the ventral (motor) root comprises the motor axons emerging from motoneurons in the ventral horn. **Bottom left,** Location of Rexed's lamina within the dorsal and ventral horns of the spinal cord. **Right,** The individual spinal nerves are related to the four levels of the spinal cord. The adult spinal cord terminates at the border of L-1. The dorsal and ventral roots of the lumbar and sacral nerves within the vertebral column are collectively termed the cauda equina. (Top left and right reproduced with permission from Kandel ER, Schwartz JH, Jessell TM: *Principles of Neural Science,* ed 3. Norwalk, CT, Appleton & Lange, 1991, pp 285–286.)

most often used to classify units are (1) contraction time, (2) the presence or absence of sag in an unfused tetanus, (3) maximum tension, and (4) the fatigue properties. The relative differences between each type are shown in Table 5. In general, type S units produce the lowest tensions, have the slowest contraction times, and are the most fatigue resistant. In contrast, units producing the largest force tend to be the fastest contracting and the most fatigable.

The fatigue resistance of a motor unit is related, in part, to the metabolic properties of the muscle fibers within the unit. The presence of three muscle fiber types has been established based on qualitative histochemical staining with succinate dehydrogenase, an oxidative marker enzyme; α-glycerophosphate dehydrogenase, a glycolytic marker enzyme; and myosin ATPase, an enzyme that is related to the rate at which ATP can be hydrolyzed. Using these histochemical stains, fibers have been classified as fast glycolytic, fast oxidative glycolytic, and slow oxidative. Glycogen depletion of physiologically classified motor units shows that type FF units are composed of fast glycolytic fibers, type FR units are composed of fast oxidative glycolytic fibers, and S units are composed of slow oxidative fibers (Table 5). The classification scheme based on the myosin ATPase staining characteristics at different pHs is also shown in Table 5. The relationship between succinate dehydrogenase activity, maximum tension, and fatigue index is shown in Figure 20. In general, there is a direct relationship between succinate dehydrogenase activity and fatigue resistance.

The fibers of the different motor unit types vary in size; fast glycolytic fibers are the largest and slow oxidative fibers are the smallest. However, the fibers of any given type range in size, and the size of the same type of fiber may be quite different in a homogeneous (all one type) and a heterogeneous (mixed types) muscle. For example, slow oxidative fibers in a heterogeneous muscle, such as the medial gastrocnemius, are significantly smaller than those in the soleus. Although fibers within a motor unit had been assumed to be identical in size, recent evidence has shown that there can be a three- to eightfold range in cross-sectional area of these fibers.

In a given muscle, the force capabilities of the component motor units differ widely. The observed range in force may be attributed to variations in (1) the number of fibers innervated by the motoneurons (the innervation ratio); (2) the size of the muscle

Table 5
General characteristics of motor unit types

Parameter	Motor Unit Types*		
	FF	FR	S
Muscle unit physiology**			
Contraction time	Fastest	Slightly slower	Slowest
Sag	Present	Present	Absent
Maximum tension	Largest	Smaller	Smallest
Fatigue index	< 0.25	< 0.75 - 1.0	0.7 - 1.0
Muscle Unit Anatomy +			
Innervation ratio	2.9	2.1	1.0
Fiber cross-sectional area	1.3	0.98	1.0
Specific tension	1.4	1.2	1.0
Muscle unit metabolism			
Fiber type++	FG	FOG	SO
Myosin heavy chain	IIB	IIA	I
Glycogen	High	High	Low
Hexokinase	Low	Intermediate	High
Glycolytic enzymes	High	High	Low
Oxidative enzymes	Low	High	High
Cyctochrome c	Low	High	High
Capillary supply	Sparse	Rich	Very rich
Motoneuron			
Cell body size	Largest	Slightly smaller	Smallest
Conduction velocity	Fastest	Slightly slower	Slowest
After-hyperpolarization duration	Shortest	Slightly shorter	Longest
Input resistance	Lowest	Slightly higher	Highest

* FF = fast fatigable; FR = fast fatigue resistant; S = fatigue resistant.
** Data relative to the FF unit.
+ Data relative to the slow unit.
++ FG = fast glycolytic; FOG = fast oxidative glycolytic; SO = slow oxidative.

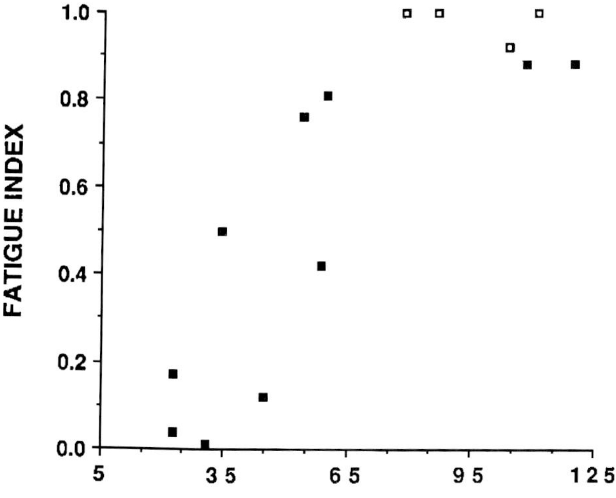

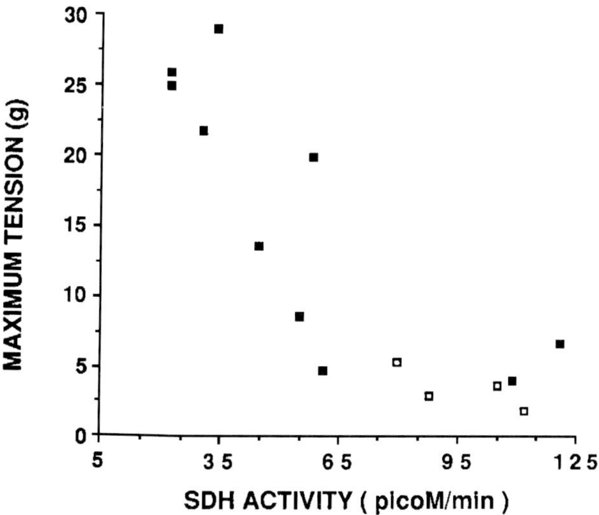

Figure 20
Relationships between succinate dehydrogenase (SDH) activity and fatigue index for 14 motor units isolated from cat tibialis anterior muscle. Fast units are represented as filled squares and slow units as empty squares. (Data taken from Martin TP, Bodine-Fowler S, Roy RR, et al: Metabolic and fiber size properties of cat tibialis anterior motor units. *Am J Physiol* 1988;255:C43–50.)

fibers belonging to the motor unit; and/or (3) the specific force output per unit area of active muscle (the specific tension). The difference in force potential between slow and fast units had been assumed to be related to differences in the specific tension of slow and fast fibers. However, recent studies have shown that the difference in tension between motor units is primarily a function of the innervation ratio. Although the specific tension of slow units is lower than that of fast units, the difference accounts for only a small part of the observed differences in maximum tension (~2%) (Table 5). The relationship between innervation ratio and maximum tension is shown in Figure 21, *left*. After the nerve to a muscle has been cut (denervation) and allowed to grow back (Fig. 21, *right*), the motor units often produce larger tensions than normal; however, there is still a direct relationship between tension and innervation ratio. Further, when a portion of the motor axons innervating a muscle have been lost (as in certain motoneuron diseases, with partial nerve injuries, and in spinal root injuries), the remaining motor axons will sprout and innervate the denervated muscle fibers. Consequently, the tension of the remaining units will increase.

The distribution of muscle fibers belonging to a motor unit has been examined using electromyographic and glycogen depletion techniques. The fibers belonging to a motor unit are not distributed across the entire cross section of a muscle but, in general, are localized to a specific region of the muscle (Fig. 22). The relative size of the motor unit territory, calculated as a percentage of the whole muscle cross section, ranges from 8% to 22% in the cat tibialis anterior muscle and 41% to 76% in the cat soleus muscle. As many as 20 to 30 units may overlap within a given region of the muscle. A motor unit's fibers are distributed such that few fibers belonging to the same unit are adjacent (Fig. 23, *top*). For example, in an average tibialis anterior unit, 71% of the motor unit fibers are not adjacent to another fiber from the same unit, 21% of the motor unit fibers occur in groups of two, and only 7% occur in groups of three. After reinnervation, there is often an increase in the number of adjacencies between motor unit fibers (Fig. 23, *bottom*).

The α motoneurons are among the largest neurons in the mammalian CNS. A single motoneuron can innervate only a few muscle fibers in muscles such as those that control eye movements or fine movements of the hand or it can innervate hundreds to thousands of fibers in muscles of the lower extremity. When a motoneuron is activated, it stimulates all of the muscle fibers that it innervates. Just as muscle unit types differ in their physiologic properties, motoneurons innervating each of the muscle unit types differ in their electrophysiologic and morphologic properties. The total cell membrane area of motoneurons is correlated with the type of muscle unit innervated in the following sequence: type FF > type FR > type S. Moreover, the diameter and conduction velocity of a motor axon are directly correlated with the size of the parent cell body, although the correlation is not precise. Consequently, the motor axons innervating the type S units are generally the slowest conducting and the smallest in diameter.

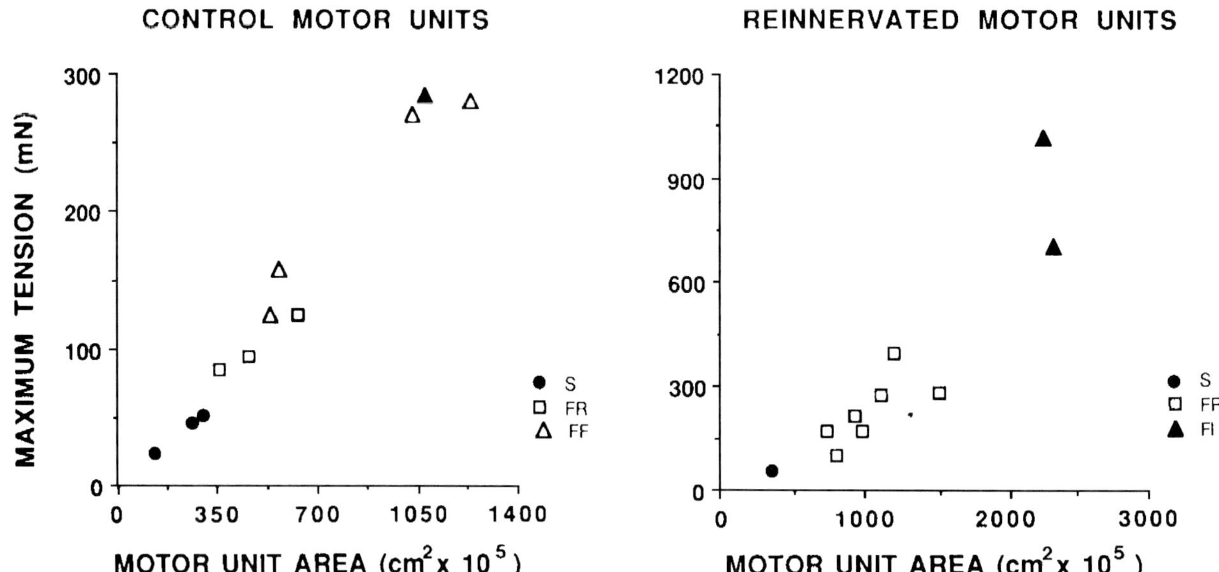

Figure 21
Relationship between motor unit maximum tension and innervation ratio for motor units isolated from control cat tibialis anterior and cat tibialis anterior six months after denervation and self-reinnervation. Units were classified into types based on the contractile properties of the muscle unit. (Data taken from Bodine SC, Roy RR, Eldred E, et al: Maximal force as a function of anatomical features of motor units in the cat tibialis anterior. *J Neurophysiol* 1987;57:1730–1745 and Unguez GA, et al: Evidence of incomplete neural control of motor unit properties in adult cat tibialis anterior after self reinnervation. *J Physiol,* in press).

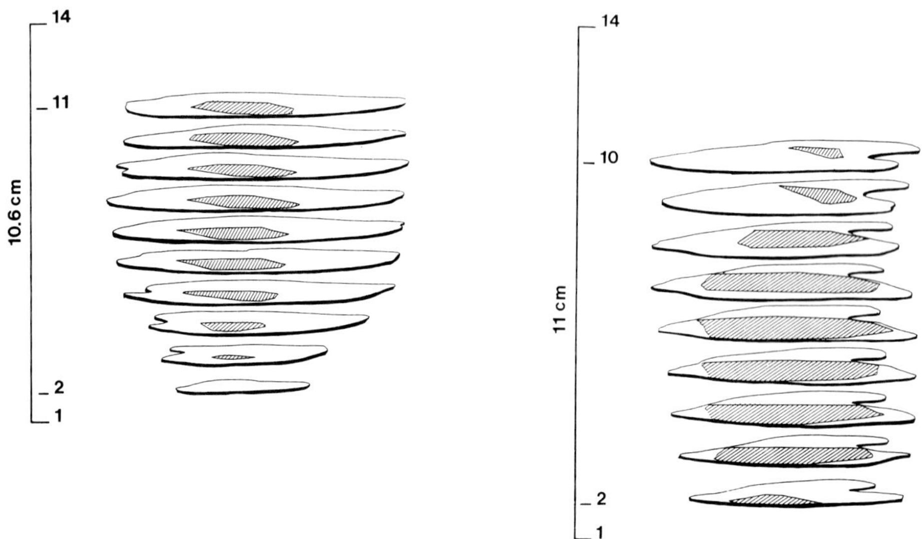

Figure 22
Distribution of motor unit fibers throughout the length of the cat tibialis anterior. The size in centimeters of the block from which each cross-section was taken is indicated. The stippled area represents the location and relative size of the territory over which the motor unit fibers were distributed. Although the motor unit territory may be distributed throughout most of the muscle, the individual muscle fibers often do not extend the length of the muscle. (Reproduced with permission from Bodine-Fowler SC, Unguez GA, Roy RR, et al: Innervation patterns in the cat tibialis anterior six months after self-reinnervation. *Muscle Nerve* 1993;16:379–391.)

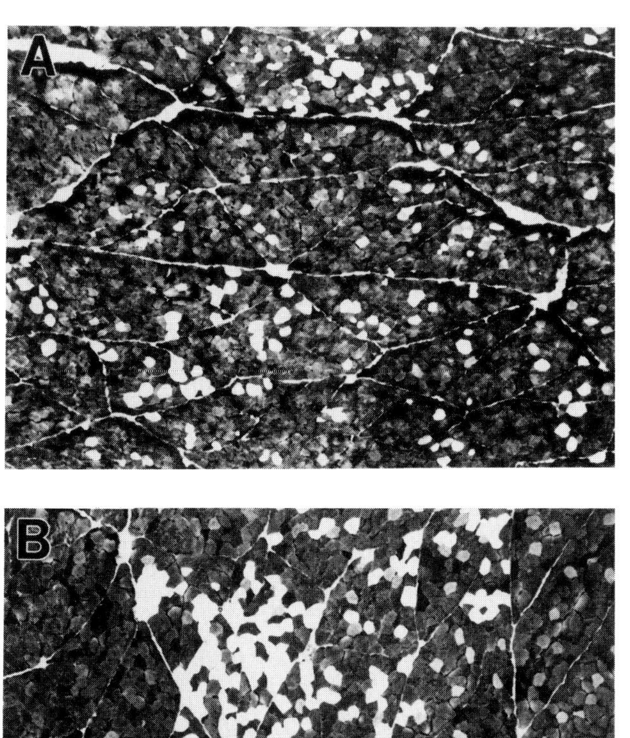

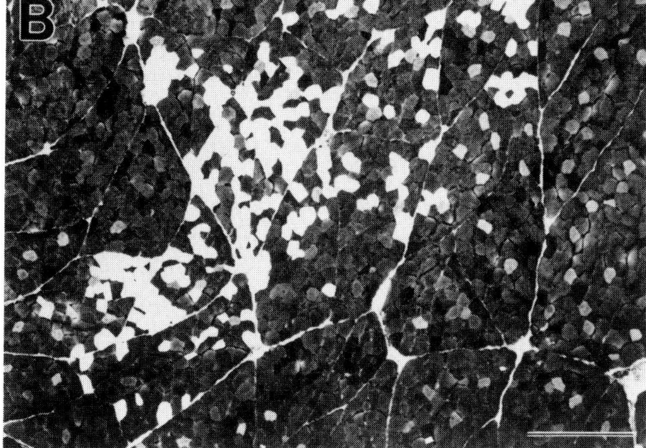

Figure 23
Cross sections from two cat tibialis anterior muscles six months after denervation (A) and self-reinnervation (B). In each muscle, a single motor unit was isolated and repetitively stimulated to deplete the muscle fibers of glycogen. Muscle cross sections were stained for glycogen using the periodic acid-Schiff reaction; the unstained fibers were identified as belonging to the stimulated motor unit. Calibration bar = 500 μm. (Reproduced with permission from Bodine-Fowler SC, Unguez GA, Roy RR, et al: Innervation patterns in the cat tibialis anterior six months after self-reinnervation. *Muscle Nerve* 1993;16:379–391.)

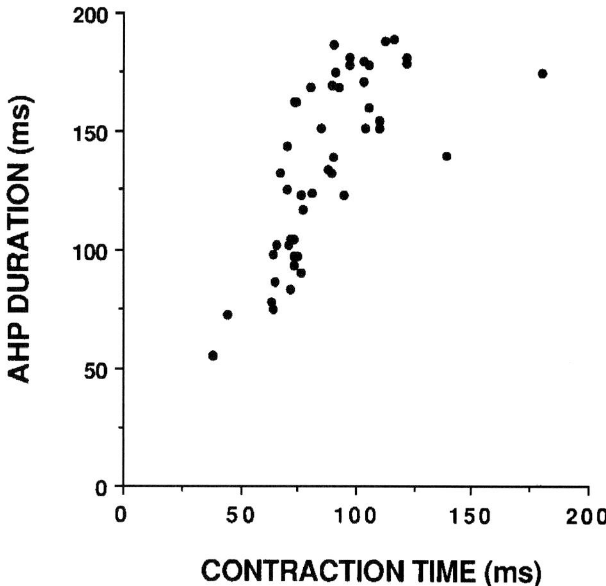

Figure 24
Relationship between motoneuron after hyperpolarization (AHP) duration and muscle unit contraction time from motor units recorded from the cat soleus muscle.

There is an inverse correlation between the measured sizes of motoneurons and their input resistance. Input resistance is a complex function of membrane area, membrane resistance, and the time and length constants of the neuron. Because slow motoneurons generally have a higher input resistance than fast motoneurons, injecting the same amount of current into each type will cause a greater change in the membrane potential of the slow motoneuron because of Ohm's law V = IR. The susceptibility of motoneuron types to discharge action potential during intracellular current injection also differs; slow motoneurons generally require less current to be excited than fast motoneurons. Lastly, slow and fast motoneurons differ in the length of their after-hyperpolarization (AHP) duration, which is important in determining the maximum frequency at which a motoneuron can fire. Slow motoneurons have a longer AHP than fast motoneurons and fire at a lower maximum frequency. The AHP duration of the motoneuron is directly correlated to the contraction time of the muscle unit (Fig. 24). The relative differences between motoneurons as related to motor unit type are summarized in Table 5. In general, the intrinsic properties of the motoneurons vary such that there is a gradient of increasing excitability: S > FR > FF.

Nerve-Muscle Interaction

As noted above, the morphologic, physiologic, and metabolic properties of the motoneuron and muscle are remarkably matched. During development, motoneurons find their appropriate muscles with remarkable accuracy. Once the axons reach their peripheral target they must synapse with individual muscle fibers. Initially, a single axon contacts many more fibers than it will maintain in the adult. For example, in the rat at birth, each muscle fiber is innervated by four to five different motoneurons. Subsequently, after a period of synapse elimination, the number of muscle fibers innervated by each motoneuron is reduced until each muscle fiber is innervated by only one motoneuron. The elimination of excess motoneuron contacts could be a random process; however, a process based solely on random elimination of synapses would likely result in some fibers becoming denervated. Synapse elimination appears to be influenced by at least two processes: (1) competition between different axons for the same fiber and (2) an inherent tendency for motoneurons to retract synapses. The specific factor(s) the axons are competing for and what determines which axons will survive are unknown.

The degree to which a motoneuron selectively innervates muscle fibers of the same type is also unknown. One general belief is that during development, a motoneuron innervates an undifferentiated population of fibers. In this situation, all the muscle fibers innervated by the same motoneuron would obtain identical physiologic and metabolic properties as a result of the specific activity pattern imposed on the fibers by the motoneuron. This mechanism implies that the motoneuron, and more specifically, the activity pattern, regulates all the properties of the muscle fibers. Recent evidence, however, indicates that muscle fibers have some degree of self-determination during development. This mechanism implies that muscle fibers differentiate into subtypes before and even without innervation.

It is not known whether motoneurons are differentiated into subtypes at the time of innervation. There is some evidence that motoneurons in 3- to 12-day-old neonatal rats have longer after-hyperpolarization durations and slower firing frequencies than adult rat motoneurons. These data suggest that neonatal motoneurons are all slow and differentiate later in development. It is possible, however, that motoneurons are predisposed to be fast or slow at the time they innervate the limb musculature. If both the motoneurons and the muscle fibers have differentiated at the time of innervation, the motoneuron could (1) selectively innervate fibers of a specific type or (2) randomly innervate muscle fibers of different types. If innervation is selective, the motor unit should be composed of a relatively homogeneous population of muscle fibers. It has been reported that motor units in the soleus of neonatal rats are composed of predominantly one fiber type. These results suggest that a motoneuron selectively innervates fast or slow muscle fibers. However, motor units in the lumbrical muscles of the neonatal rat have been reported to be heterogenous; that is, composed of a random proportion of muscle fibers of each type. Whatever is the case, the end result of development is that motor units are highly organized with regard to their anatomic, metabolic, and physiologic properties.

Recruitment Order

The majority of evidence indicates that the motor units within a specific muscle are recruited in an orderly manner. The size principle indicates that the size of the motoneuron dictates its excitability, which determines the degree of use of the motor unit, and its usage, in turn, specifies or influences the type of muscle fiber required. Data from human subjects as well as from experimental animals indicate that recruitment during slow development of force in both voluntary and reflex muscle contractions begins with the slowest contracting, lowest force units. As the demand for tension increases, the faster fatigue resistant, intermediate force units are recruited. The last units to be recruited, usually during maximal contractions, are the fastest, most fatigable, largest force units. An example of orderly recruitment in the human first interosseous muscle is shown in Figure 25.

Studies using experimental animals have shown that motor units within a muscle are recruited according to increasing maximum tension and increasing conduction velocity (Table 6). In general, the data suggest that units are recruited during normal movements in the following order: S-FR-FF (Fig. 26). Some investigators have suggested that the recruitment order can be reversed in some situations such that the fast large force units are selectively recruited before the slow low force units. Preferential activation of normally high threshold units (the FF units) has been reported during very rapid isotonic movements in humans and is implied by observations of rapid alternating isotonic movements in animals. It also has been suggested that a motoneuron may have different thresholds for firing, depending on the specific task being performed; however, this has been found primarily for motor units in multifunctional muscles. During most movements, however, motor units are recruited in an orderly manner according to the size principle. Thus, it appears that the physiologic and metabolic properties of a unit are matched such that the units recruited most often and required to maintain tension for the longest periods of time have the highest resistance to fatigue.

Spinal Cord Reflexes

Spinal cord reflexes involve the final common pathway and are an integral part of the neural circuitry believed in some way to be involved in the maintenance of posture and the production of movement. A reflex is a stereotyped response to a specific sensory stimulus. A reflex pathway consists of the receptor (the sensory organ), the effector (the motoneuron), and the interconnecting neural elements (the interneurons). A reflex that involves only one

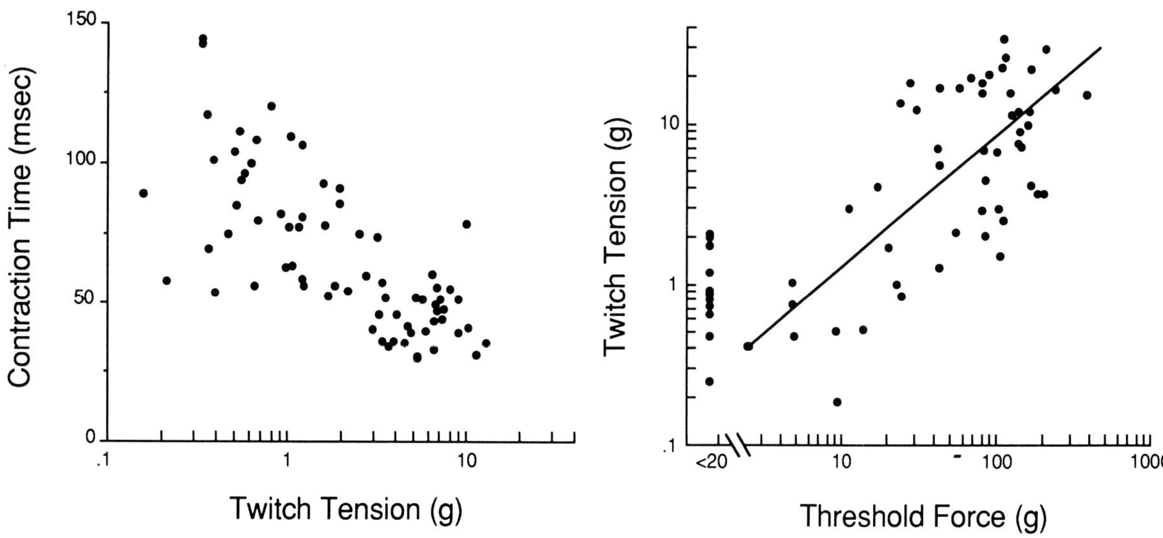

Figure 25
Left, Human motor unit twitch contraction time as a function of twitch tension recorded by spike-triggered averaging. Note that as contractile tension increases, contraction time decreases. This suggests that the motor units with larger tension have faster contractile speed, as predicted by the size principle. **Right,** Human motor unit twitch tension as a function of threshold voltage. As threshold increases, larger units are recruited, as predicted by the size principle. (Reproduced with permission from Lieber RL: *Skeletal Muscle Structure and Function.* Baltimore, MD, Williams & Wilkins, 1992, p 99.)

synapse between the receptor and the effector is a monosynaptic reflex; a reflex that involves one or more interneurons between the receptor and the effector is a polysynaptic reflex. In general, most reflexes are polysynaptic. Spinal reflex pathways can be modulated by supraspinal pathways either directly, through a mechanism known as presynaptic inhibition, or indirectly, through interneurons.

The following spinal reflexes will be reviewed in this chapter: (1) the stretch reflex, (2) the clasp-knife response, (3) autogenic inhibition, and (4) the flexion withdrawal reflex (Table 7).

The Stretch Reflex

The stretch reflex is a monosynaptic reflex initiated by an afferent discharge from the muscle spindles, which excites the α motoneurons innervating both the muscle from which the afferent discharge originated and synergistic muscles to produce a brisk, transient muscle contraction. The stretch reflex can be produced in both flexor and extensor muscles, but is generally strongest in muscles that function as physiologic extensors, that is, those muscles that oppose gravity. In humans, they are the flexors of the upper extremity and the extensors of the lower extremity.

Muscle spindles are specialized receptors distributed throughout the belly of the muscle and arranged in parallel to the extrafusal muscle fibers in striated muscles. Each spindle consists of an encapsulated group of specialized muscle fibers called intrafusal fibers (Fig. 27). The intrafusal fibers are of two types, nuclear bag fibers and nuclear chain fibers, which differ both morphologically and physiologically. The nuclear bag fibers are larger than the nuclear chain fibers, are fast-contracting, and have

Table 6
Relationship of recruitment threshold to axonal conduction velocity (CV) and maximum tension (Po) of the muscle unit

Type of Units in Pair	Number of Pairs	Number of Pairs with Lower Threshold Unit Having:			
		Slower CV	Faster CV	Smaller Po	Larger Po
Fast, Fast	20	9	10	20	0
Slow, Slow	9	8	1	9	0
Slow, Fast	13	13	0	13	0

(Data from Zajac FE, Faden JS: Relationship among recruitment order, axonal conduction velocity, and muscle-unit properties of type-identified motor units in cat plantaris muscle. *J Neurophysiol* 1985;53:1303-1322.)

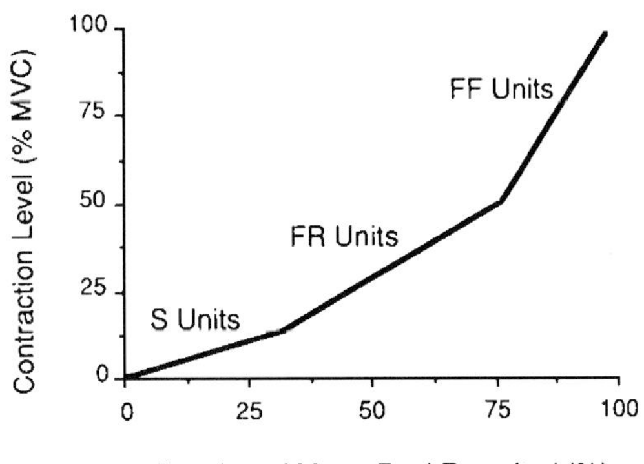

Figure 26
Schematic demonstration of predicted orderly recruitment of motor units during voluntary activity as a function of contractile force. At lower forces S units are recruited, while as force increases FR and FF units are recruited. (Reproduced with permission from Lieber RL: *Skeletal Muscle Structure and Function.* Baltimore, MD, Williams & Wilkins, 1992, p 99. Original adapted from Edgerton VR, Roy RR, Bodine SC, et al: The matching of neuronal and muscular physiology, in Borer KT, Edington DW, White TP (eds): *Frontiers of Exercise Biology.* Champaign, IL, Human Kinetics Publishers, 1983.)

clustered nuclei. The nuclear chain fibers are slow-contracting and have nuclei that are arranged in a single row.

Each intrafusal fiber within the spindle is innervated by a γ motoneuron (Fig. 27). Upon activation of the γ motoneurons, the ends or poles of the intrafusal fiber contract, causing the noncontractile equatorial region to stretch. When a muscle is shortened, the intrafusal fibers become slack or unloaded and are unable to monitor length changes. The γ-motoneuron activation provides a means of controlling the length of the intrafusal fibers and the ability of the muscle spindle to detect changes in muscle length. The γ motoneurons are generally coactivated with α motoneurons.

Two types of afferent endings, primary and secondary, are found in muscle spindles. All intrafusal fibers in the spindle have a primary ending located in the center or equatorial region of the fiber, which gives rise to a large diameter, fast-conducting afferent fiber called a type Ia fiber (Fig. 27, *right*). The primary endings are most sensitive to a sudden change in the length of the muscle and are responsible for the phasic component of the stretch reflex. The secondary endings are located primarily on the nuclear chain fibers and give rise to small diameter and slow-conducting afferent fibers called type II fibers (Fig. 27, *right*). The secondary endings are most sensitive to a steady change in muscle length and are responsible for the tonic component of the stretch reflex.

The phasic stretch reflex is elicited by muscle stretch sufficient to excite the primary afferent (Ia) fibers. Clinically, the stretch reflex is most commonly elicited by tapping on a tendon to produce stretch of the extrafusal muscle fibers, which is detected by the muscle spindle and transmitted to the central nervous system via the Ia afferent fibers.

The Ia afferent fibers project through the dorsal roots and make the following connections in the spinal cord (Fig. 28): (1) a monosynaptic, excitatory connection with α motoneurons that innervate the muscle from which the fiber originated (homonymous motoneurons); (2) a monosynaptic, excitatory connection with α motoneurons that innervate synergistic muscles (heteronymous motoneurons); and (3) a monosynaptic connection to an inhibitory interneuron referred to as the Ia inhibitory interneuron. The Ia inhibitory interneuron, in turn, connects directly to the α motoneurons that are antagonistic to the muscle from which the Ia afferent fiber originated, providing an inhibitory potential to those motoneurons. Consequently, when a muscle is stretched, the motoneurons innervating the stretched muscle and its synergists are excited, while the motoneurons innervating the antagonist muscles are inhibited. This pattern of simultaneous inhibition of antagonists and excitation of the homonymous and synergistic motoneurons is referred to as reciprocal inhibition.

The type II afferents from the secondary endings have similar connections to the type Ia affer-

Table 7
Summary of spinal reflexes

Segmental Reflex	Receptor Organ	Afferent Fiber
Phasic stretch reflex	Muscle spindle (primary endings)	Type Ia (large myelinated)
Tonic stretch reflex	Muscle spindle (secondary endings)	Type II (intermediate myelinated)
Clasp-knife response	Muscle spindle (secondary endings)	Type II (intermediate myelinated)
Flexion withdrawal reflex	Nociceptors (free nerve endings), touch and pressure receptors	Flexor-reflex afferents: small unmyelinated cutaneous afferents (A-delta, C and muscle afferents, group III)
Autogenic inhibition	Golgi tendon organ	Type Ib (large myelinated)

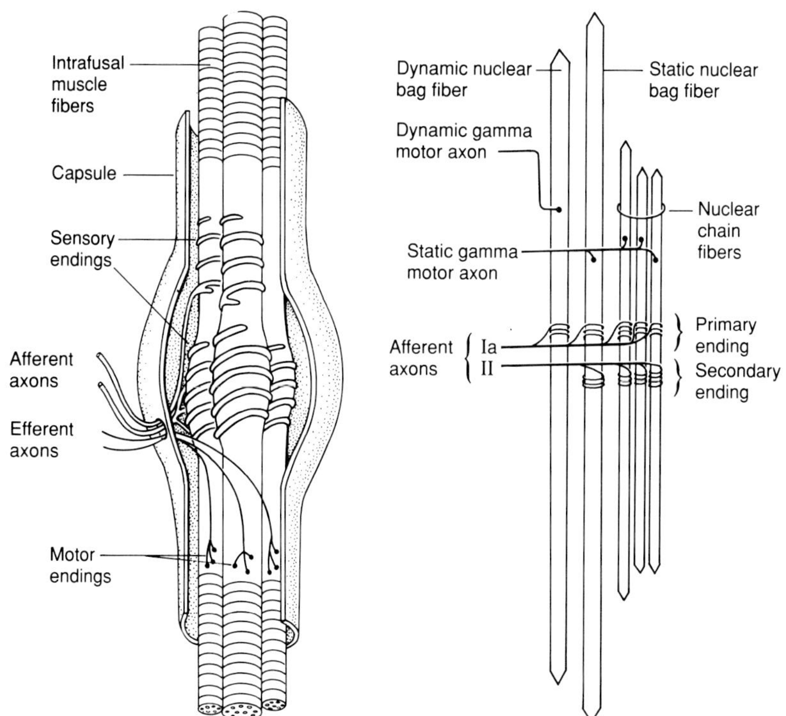

Figure 27
Left, The main components of the muscle spindle are intrafusal fibers, sensory endings, and motor axons. The intrafusal fibers are specialized muscle fibers; their central regions are not contractile. The sensory endings spiral around the central regions of the intrafusal fibers and are responsive to stretch. (Original adapted from Hullinger M: The mammalian muscle spindle and its central control. *Rev Physiol Biochem Pharmacol* 1984;101:1–110.) **Right,** The muscle spindle contains three types of intrafusal fibers: dynamic nuclear bag, static nuclear bag, and nuclear chain fibers. A single group Ia afferent fiber innervates all three types of intrafusal fibers, forming a primary ending. A group II afferent fiber innervates chain and static bag fibers, forming a secondary ending. (Original adapted from Boyd LA: The isolated mammalian muscle spindle. *Trends Neurosci* 1980;3:258–265. Reproduced with permission from Kandel ER, Schwartz JH, Jessell TM: *Principles of Neural Science,* ed 3. Norwalk, CT, Appleton & Lange, 1991, p 566.)

ents. In addition, the type II afferent fibers make widespread polysynaptic connections in the spinal cord and are thought to play a role in the flexion reflex. Because they produce a length-dependent inhibition of the stretch reflex, the type II afferent fibers are also thought to participate in the clasp-knife response. This response is characterized by an initial resistance (increase in muscle tone) at the beginning of the stretch, followed by a sudden loss of resistance (decrease in muscle tone) once the muscle has been stretched past a certain point.

Autogenic Inhibition (or Inverse Myotaxic Reflex)

Golgi tendon organs are encapsulated sensory organs located primarily near the myotendinous junction in muscle (Fig. 29). Each Golgi tendon organ is in series with approximately 15 to 20 extrafusal muscle fibers and is innervated by a Ib afferent fiber. When a muscle contracts, the Ib afferent fiber is compressed and activated. The Golgi tendon organ is most sensitive to active muscle contraction and measures muscle tension.

Activation of Ib afferent fibers results in inhibition of the muscles from which they originated and of synergistic muscles, and excitation of antagonistic muscles. Because this response is opposite to the stretch reflex, it often is referred to as the inverse myotaxic reflex. This response also is referred to as autogenic inhibition. The Ib afferent fibers make a disynaptic, inhibitory connection to the motoneurons from the homonymous and synergistic muscles, and a disynaptic, excitatory connection to the motoneurons of the antagonistic muscles (Fig. 30). The central connections of the Ib afferent fibers have three main features: (1) all connections to motoneurons are through interneurons; (2) connections to flexor muscles are weak, but connections to extensor muscles are strong; and (3) they are more widespread than those of the Ia afferent fibers.

Renshaw Cell

Another important inhibitory spinal interneuron is the Renshaw cell. Alpha motoneurons give off a collateral that makes a direct, excitatory connection to the Renshaw cell, which projects back to the same motoneuron and to synergistic motoneurons (Fig. 31). The Renshaw cell projection to α motoneurons is inhibitory. This process is called recurrent inhibition, and it regulates the activation of a particular motor pool.

The Renshaw cell also projects to the Ia inhibitory interneuron (Fig. 31). This pathway results in releasing inhibition (or disinhibition) of the antagonist motoneurons by inhibiting of the Ia inhibitory interneuron. The Renshaw cell-Ia inhibitory interneuron pathway may function to limit the duration and magnitude of the Ia afferent mediated reflex response.

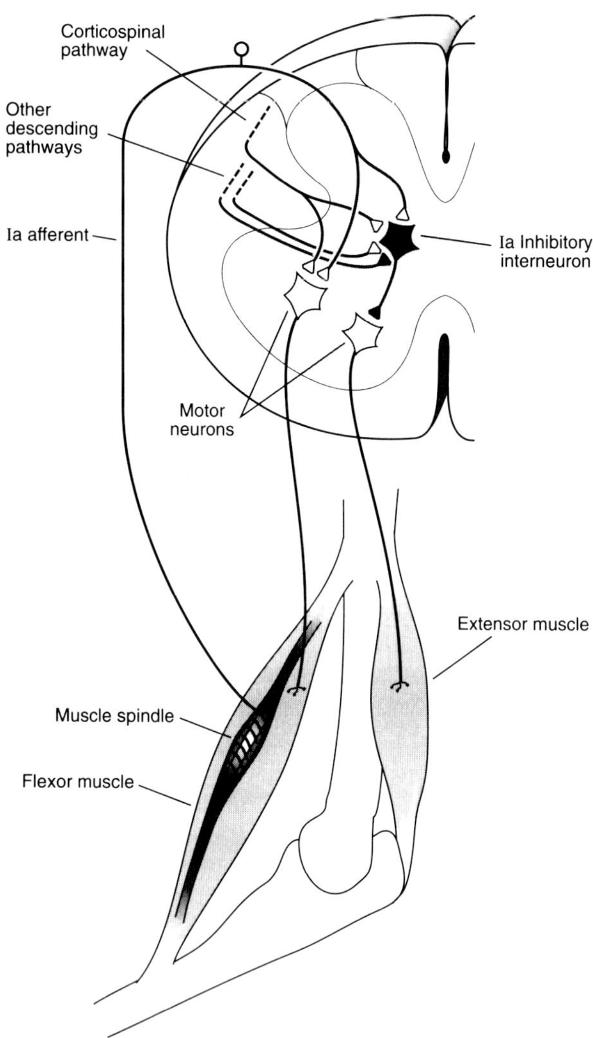

Figure 28
The Ia inhibitory interneuron allows higher centers to coordinate opposing muscles at a joint through a single command. This inhibitory interneuron mediates reciprocal innervation in stretch reflex circuits. In addition, it receives inputs from corticospinal descending axons, so that a descending signal to activate one set of muscles automatically leads to relaxation of the antagonists. Other descending pathways make excitatory and inhibitory connections to this interneuron. When the balance of inputs is shifted to greater inhibition, reciprocal inhibition will be decreased, and cocontraction of opposing muscles will occur. (Only a few of the many inputs to the Ia interneuron and motor neurons are shown in this highly simplified diagram.) (Adapted with permission from Kandel ER, Schwartz JH, Jessell TM: *Principles of Neural Science,* ed 3. Norwalk, CT, Appleton & Lange, 1991, p 584.)

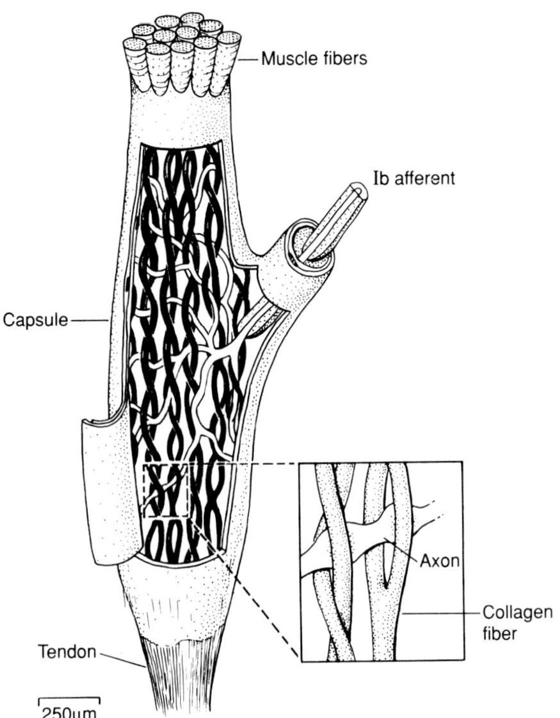

Figure 29
Golgi tendon organs are specialized structures found at the junctions between muscle and tendon. Collagen fibers in the tendon organ attach to the muscle fibers. A single Ib afferent axon enters the capsule and branches into many unmyelinated endings that wrap around and between the collagen fibers. When the tendon organ is stretched (usually because of contraction of the muscle), the afferent axon is compressed by the collagen fibers (see inset at lower right) and increases its rate of firing. (Adapted with permission from Schmidt RF: Motor systems, in Schmidt RF, Thews G (eds): *Human Physiology.* Berlin, Springer-Verlag, 1983, pp 81–110. Inset adapted with permission from Swett JE, Schoultz TW: Mechanical transduction in the Golgi tendon organ: A hypothesis. *Arch Ital Biol* 1975;113:374–382.)

Flexion Reflexes

The flexion reflex, also referred to as the withdrawal reflex, the cutaneous reflex, and the nociceptive reflex, is a polysynaptic reflex mediated by myelinated group II and unmyelinated group IV afferents. Generally, these afferents carry information from nociceptors, touch and pressure receptors, joint receptors, and muscle receptors. These afferents, which produce flexion responses, are collectively called flexor reflex afferents.

The general response to activation of flexor reflex afferents is excitation of the flexor motoneurons and inhibition of the extensor motoneurons on the ipsilateral side, and inhibition of the flexor motoneurons and excitation of the extensor motoneurons on the contralateral side. Contralateral excitation of the extensor motoneurons (also known as the crossed-extension reflex) stabilizes the body as the ipsilateral limb is flexed. The basic circuitry for the flexion reflex is diagrammed in Figure 32.

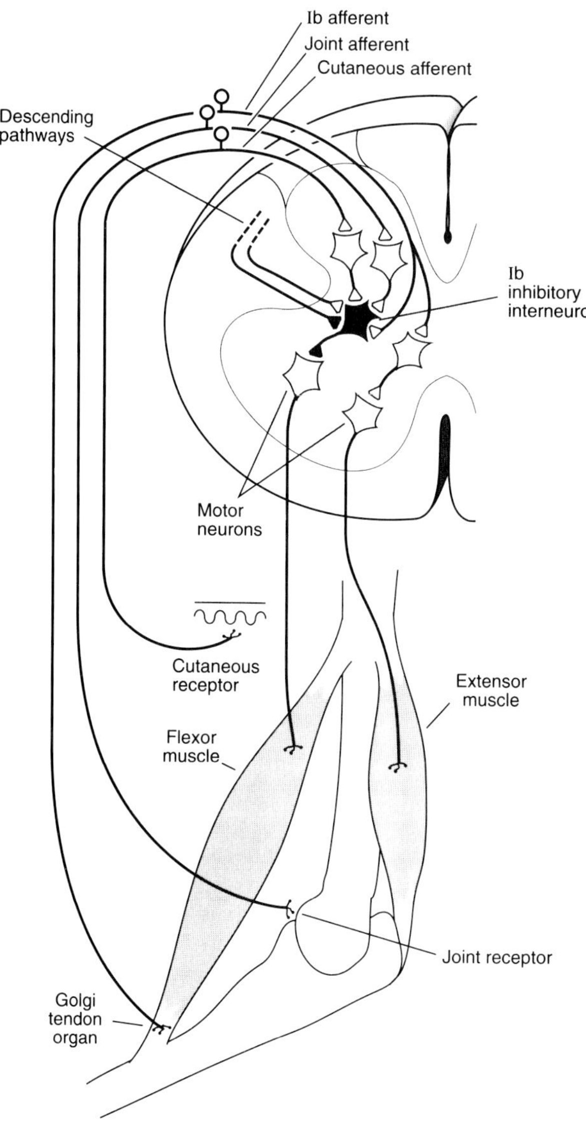

Figure 30
Ib afferent fibers from Golgi tendon organs provide a negative feedback system for regulating muscle tension. Ib afferents inhibit homonymous and synergist motor neurons (not shown) through the Ib inhibitory interneuron. They also excite antagonist motor neurons through an excitatory interneuron. Thus, the reflex effect of stimulating tendon organs is opposite to that of stimulating muscle spindles. The Ib inhibitory interneurons receive convergent input from joint and cutaneous receptors and from descending pathways, and thus mediate control of movements in which integration of different sensory modalities is important, as in touch. (Adapted with permission from Kandel ER, Schwartz JH, Jessell TM: *Principles of Neural Science,* ed 3. Norwalk, CT, Appleton & Lange, 1991, p 586.)

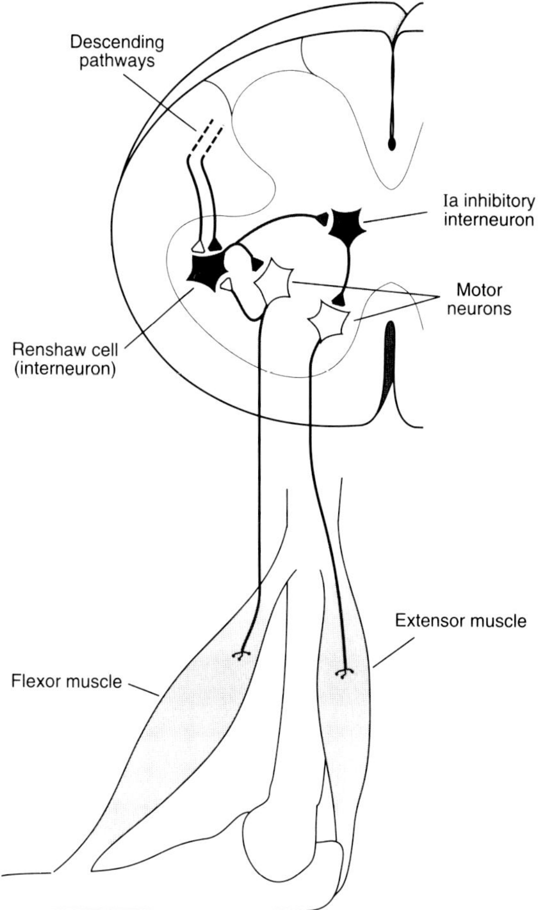

Figure 31
Renshaw cells produce recurrent inhibition of motor neurons. These spinal interneurons are excited by collaterals from motor neurons and then inhibit the same motor neurons. This negative feedback system regulates motor neuron excitability and stabilizes firing rates. Renshaw cells also send collaterals to synergist motor neurons (not shown) and to Ia inhibitory interneurons. Thus, descending inputs that modulate the excitability of the Renshaw cell adjust the excitability of all the motor neurons around a joint. (Adapted with permission from Kandel ER, Schwartz JH, Jessell TM: *Principles of Neural Science,* ed 3. Norwalk, CT, Appleton & Lange, 1991, p 585.)

Upper Motoneuron Syndrome and Spasticity

Disruption of motor pathways due to stroke, brain trauma, or spinal cord injury leads to a variety of motor dysfunctions. The term upper motoneuron syndrome is commonly used to describe patients who have abnormal motor functions as the result of lesions to descending pathways at the level of the cortex, internal capsule, brainstem, or spinal cord. Patients who have upper motoneuron syndrome suffer from both negative symptoms or performance deficits and positive symptoms or abnormal behaviors (Tables 8 and 9). Negative symptoms include weakness and/or paresis, loss of dexterity (especially fine motor control of the fingers), and fatigability. Positive symptoms include abnormal posture,

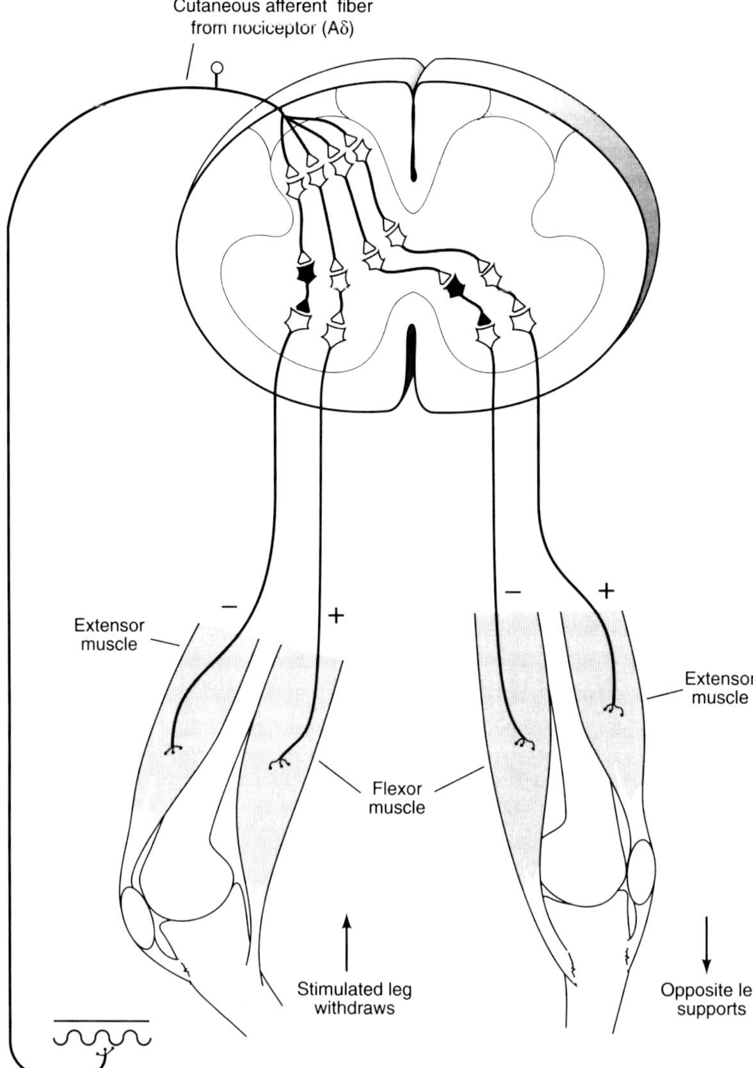

Figure 32
The flexion withdrawal reflex produces flexion of the stimulated limb and extension of the opposite limb. Stimulation of cutaneous afferents, such as an A δ fiber from a nociceptor, produces excitation of ipsilateral flexor muscles and inhibition of ipsilateral extensor muscles, while producing the opposite response in the contralateral limb (the crossed extensor reflex). The cutaneous input is distributed over many spinal segments, so that the full reflex involves contraction of muscles at all joints of both limbs. The pathways are schematically illustrated here for one spinal segment only.

Table 8
Findings in upper and lower motoneuron lesions

Findings	Upper Motoneuron Lesion	Lower Motoneuron Lesion
Strength	Decreased	Decreased
Tone	Increased	Decreased
Deep tendon reflexes	Increased	Decreased
Superficial tendon reflexes	Decreased	Decreased
Babinski's sign	Present	Absent
Clonus	Present	Absent
Fasciculations	Absent	Present
Atrophy	Absent	Present

exaggeration of proprioceptive reflexes producing spasticity, and exaggeration of cutaneous reflexes producing flexion withdrawal spasms, extensor spasms and the Babinski response. These positive symptoms can be caused by the increased excitability of a specific part of the neural circuit or by the release of one part of the neural circuit from the inhibitory control of another.

Spasticity, a common component of the upper motoneuron syndrome, is the result of changes in spinal proprioceptive reflexes; its severity and its time course depend largely on the location of the lesion(s) and the CNS pathways involved. For the clinician, the term spasticity often is used to describe such phenomena as (1) increased tendon reflexes; (2) increased resistance to passive movement of the limb; (3) flexor spasms associated with

Table 9
Positive and negative symptoms observed in upper motoneuron lesions at various levels

	Level of Damage		
Damaged pathway	Spinal	Brainstem/Caudal to the Red Nucleus	Brainstem/Rostral to the Red Nucleus
Pyramidal tract (corticospinal tract)	Weakness, loss of abdominal reflex, and Babinski's sign	Weakness, loss of abdominal reflex, Babinski's sign, hyporeflexia, and hypotonia	Weakness, loss of abdominal reflex, Babinski's sign, seizure, apraxia, hyporeflexia, and hypotonia
Extrapyramidal tract (rubrospinal, reticulospinal, and vestibulospinal tracts)	Hyperreflexia, clonus spasticity, and clasp-knife reflex	Hyperreflexia, clonus spasticity, clasp-knife reflex, and decerebrate posture	Hyperreflexia, clonus, spasticity, clasp-knife reflex, apraxia, decoricate posture

paraplegia; (4) motor dysfunctions, including decreased strength, speed, and range of voluntary movement; and (5) dystonia and rigidity. Spasticity also has been defined as a motor disorder characterized by a velocity-dependent increase in tonic stretch reflexes (muscle tone) with exaggerated tendon jerks, resulting from hyperexcitability of the stretch reflex. Because excitability of the stretch reflex is controlled by many different spinal cord circuits, a change in any one component of those circuits could modify the stretch reflex.

Diagnosis of movement disorders requires an understanding of the organization of neural networks and pathways that mediate movement as well as an understanding of the integration of the motor system with the sensory system. Because of the intermingling of fibers from the cerebral cortex and brainstem, damage is rarely restricted to a single descending pathway. Selective damage of the corticospinal tract at the level of the medullary pyramids or cerebral peduncles produces only minor movement deficits. In general, the only permanent functional defect is the loss of independent control of the fingers of the affected arm. However, damage to the extrapyramidal fibers or brainstem pathways is generally associated with the appearance of spasticity.

Spasticity is the result of changes in segmental spinal circuits, in particular, the stretch reflex arc. An enhanced reflex response to muscle stretch (hyperreflexia) could occur as the result of an increase in the excitability of the α motoneuron and/or an increase in the amount of excitatory input elicited by muscle stretch. A motoneuron is hyperexcitable if it takes less than normal amounts of excitatory input to recruit the motoneuron or alter its discharge frequency, or if the same amount of input generates a greater response. A motoneuron would be at a state of increased excitability if it were constantly depolarized, that is, if the membrane potential were closer to the threshold for action potential generation. A depolarized state could result from a change in the balance of excitatory and inhibitory input to the motoneuron. Lesions to upper motoneurons may result in a reduction in the amount of inhibitory input to the motoneuron that could be caused by a reduction in the input from inhibitory interneurons such as the Renshaw cell, the Ia interneuron, or the Ib interneuron. A motoneuron could also exhibit increased excitability if its intrinsic electrical properties were altered such that a given synaptic current generated a larger than normal voltage change in the neuron.

Another possible explanation for the hyperreflexia is that the imposed stretch on the muscle generates greater than normal excitatory input to the motoneuron. An increased synaptic current could result from the same stretch if the Ia afferent fiber showed an enhanced response to stretch, that is, greater rate of firing, because of increased fusimotor bias or if the excitatory interneurons within the neural circuit were more responsive to muscle afferent input. The second alternative could occur due to (1) collateral sprouting, leading to an increase in the number of excitatory synapses; (2) denervation supersensitivity; or (3) a reduction in presynaptic inhibition of the muscle afferent, resulting in greater transmission of the excitatory signal.

Of the mechanisms mentioned above, there is no evidence in support of increased fusimotor activity leading to excessive muscle spindle activity, decreased group II inhibition, or decreased recurrent inhibition. There is evidence, however, in support of decreased presynaptic inhibition of Ia afferent fibers, decreased inhibition of antagonists through reciprocal inhibition, and increased motoneuronal excitability. Experimental evidence suggests that motoneuron hyperexcitability is not caused by a significant change in the intrinsic properties of the motoneuron. Therefore, the changes must occur as the result of alterations in the amount of excitatory and/or inhibitory input to the cell.

In summary, patients with upper motoneuron lesions demonstrate varying degrees of spastic hypertonia, in addition to paresis and loss of dexterity, flexor spasm, clasp-knife response, and cocontraction of agonist and antagonist muscles. Changes in reflex responses can, in part, be related to a loss of inhibitory control of segmental reflex circuits by supraspinal pathways. In addition, local biochemical and/or morphologic changes at the spinal cord level may occur. These local changes could include collateral sprouting of intact dorsal root afferents, shortening of motoneuron dendrites, and/or denervation supersensitivity.

Peripheral Nerve Development, Structure, and Biomechanics

Nerve Trunk Development

The mature nervous system is composed of up to 10,000 different cell types, more than any other tissue in the body. The many classes of neurons in the brain are not randomly mixed, but are highly organized into a three-dimensional (3-D) pattern that evolves during development. The functional properties of the nervous system depend on this intricate network of neuronal connections, the development of which begins with the extension of the axon through a complex and mutable environment to reach one of many possible targets. The accuracy with which axons select pathways and synapse with the correct target organ is important not only during development, but also during regeneration after nerve fiber injury in the central and peripheral nervous systems.

Development of the nervous system begins after the formation of the three germ layers: the ectoderm, mesoderm, and endoderm. The endoderm gives rise to the gut and many of the major organs associated with the gut; the mesoderm forms muscle, skeleton, connective tissue, and the cardiovascular and urogenital systems; and the ectoderm forms the skin and the nervous system. During the neurulation stage of development in the embryo, the ectoderm further divides to form the neural tube, the neural crest, and the epidermis. During this time, mesodermal structures are also formed; the somites form adjacent to the neural tube and provide the first segmentation in the embryo. Each somite is composed of two major tissues; the dermamyotome will form the dermis and back muscle, and the sclerotome will form the vertebrae. The neural tube eventually forms the spinal cord and the brain (that is, the CNS), and the PNS originates from a distinct group of neural crest cells. The motoneurons are derived from neuroblasts in the wall of the neural tube, and the afferent neurons are derived from the cells in the neural crest.

Individual axons exit the spinal cord at discrete levels via the spinal nerves; each nerve root consists of a ventral or efferent root and a dorsal or afferent root. In humans there are 31 pairs of spinal nerves: eight cervical, 12 thoracic, five lumbar, five sacral, and one coccygeal. In a given species, the spinal nerves grow into the limb bud in a highly stereotyped way, collecting first into plexuses from which major branches emerge. From the major branches, axons diverge at highly reproducible anatomic locations to form nerves to individual muscles. In humans, three major plexuses—the cervical (C-1 to C-4), brachial (C-5 to T-1), and lumbosacral (T-12 to S-4)—provide innervation to the muscles of the upper and lower extremities. Each muscle is innervated by many motoneurons. These motoneurons are located in a specific and spatially discrete position in the lateral column of the ventral horn of the spinal cord. The motor pool, that is, the motoneurons innervating a specific muscle, forms a longitudinal column extending two to four spinal segments. Although the axons that innervate a specific muscle exit the cord through different spinal nerves, they converge to form a single nerve.

During development, motoneurons are able to find their appropriate targets with remarkable accuracy. The pathway taken by a nerve to a specific muscle is discrete, with few projection errors occurring during the developmental process. This precise patterning of the neuronal connections emerges, in part, from the interactions between the growing tips of the axons, the growth cones, and their cellular environment.

Spatial Distribution of Axons

The location of the motoneurons innervating individual muscles can be determined through use of retrogradely transported tracers, such as horseradish peroxidase. In general, the position of the individual motor pools within the spinal cord is related to the position of their target in the limb. More proximal muscles in the limb are innervated by more rostral motoneurons in the spinal cord. Analysis of the projection pattern of axons going to a particular muscle shows that, at the spinal nerve level, axons from many motor pools are intermingled. Axons to individual muscles begin to sort out into spatially discrete groups within and beyond the plexus (Figure 33). To determine whether axons follow specific cues or are passively channeled

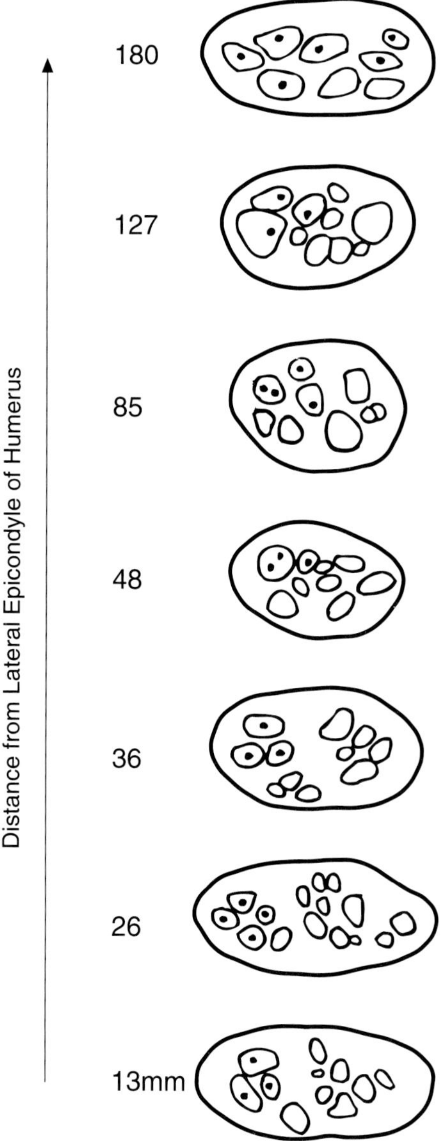

Figure 33
Selected transverse sections from a serially-sectioned radial nerve illustrating the fascicular redistribution of the different branch fiber systems brought about by fascicular plexuses. The levels are in millimeters above the lateral humeral epicondyle. The distribution of the superficial radial nerve fibers is indicated by the filled circles. (Adapted with permission from Sunderland S: *Nerve Injuries and Their Repair: A Critical Appraisal.* New York, NY, Churchill Livingstone, 1991, p 36.)

down certain paths, investigators have rotated the spinal cord in chicken embryos so that the motoneurons projecting to a specific muscle would exit the cord in a different position.

As mentioned previously, there is a topographic relationship between the location of the motor pool in the spinal cord and the location of the muscle it innervates in the limb. In the vertebrate hind limb, each muscle is derived from myoblasts that originate from somites located directly adjacent to the region of the cord in which motoneurons that will subsequently innervate that muscle originate. Consequently, motoneurons arising from a specific segment were proposed to show a specific affinity for myogenic cells from the adjacent somites. However, muscles derived from somites from foreign levels were found to be innervated with normal specificity. Further research has shown that muscles do not receive their identity from particular somites, but are patterned from the connective tissue component of the limb. These data suggest that somites are not prelabeled with guidance cues prior to axon outgrowth; however, other tissues, such as the somatopleural mesoderm from which the connective tissue is derived or ectoderm or neural crest cells, may provide such guidance cues.

When axons are forced into a foreign limb region, the nerve pattern that forms is appropriate for the limb region in question. For example, if axons from the anterior lumbar plexus are forced into the posterior sacral plexus, a normal sciatic nerve pattern will emerge even though these axons originally belonged to the femoral nerve. In addition, limbs that are made muscleless by irradiating the somites form the appropriate plexuses and nerve branches. Thus, it appears that the gross anatomic pattern of plexuses and nerve branches in the limb is determined by the surrounding connective tissue matrix. The extracellular matrix material in the limb appears to provide paths that promote growth and barriers that inhibit growth of the axonal growth cones. Some of the molecules that may promote or inhibit axon growth are discussed in the following section.

Extracellular Matrix Proteins and Axon Guidance

General cell adhesion molecules are expressed on the neural epithelial cells and mesenchymal cells through which the first axons extend, and they appear to provide permissive substrates that promote axon extension. N-cadherin and neural cell adhesion molecule (NCAM), respectively, are integral membrane glycoproteins that are the most abundant Ca^{2+}-dependent and Ca^{2+}-independent adhesion molecules present on vertebrate nerve cells. Both molecules promote cell adhesion via the binding of the same molecular species (homophilic binding) on opposing surfaces of interacting cells. Both N-cadherin and NCAM are expressed on the neural ectoderm and the axons of differentiated neurons.

Laminin, fibronectin, collagen, and tenacin are glycoproteins found in the extracellular matrix. In vitro, laminin has been shown to be the most effective in promoting neurite growth. It is not as widely expressed as N-cadherin or NCAM and, therefore, may play a more specific role in promoting directional outgrowth. Laminin promotes extension by interacting with axonal glycoproteins that are members of the integrin family of receptors. The integrins are transmembrane proteins containing two noncovalently linked subunits. Several distinct α and β subunits have been discovered, and the types of subunits expressed determine the binding specificities of the integrin receptor. Antibodies against integrins inhibit the extension of central and peripheral axons on laminin or other extracellular matrix substrates.

Molecules that promote adhesion are important for axon extension; however, they may not provide directional cues to the growing axons. Axon guidance probably is derived from contact-mediated inhibitory interactions between the growth cone and surrounding inhibitory molecules that restrict growth across a particular surface and that cause the fasciculation of "like" axons (Fig. 34). Evidence for the existence of cell surface molecules that inhibit axon extension has come from the in vitro analysis of the interaction between neurons and oligodendrocytes. Developing axons will not extend on oligodendrocyte substrates. Mature oligodendrocytes express two surface proteins that appear to mediate the inhibitory response because antibodies against these proteins neutralize the inhibitory properties of the oligodendrocytes. The presence of inhibitory proteins on oligodendrocytes is believed to be partially responsible for the inability of CNS axons to regenerate after injury in the adult. Contact-mediated inhibitory mechanisms may contribute to the selection of axonal pathways. For example, the segmentation of spinal nerves appears to be determined by inhibitory/adhesive molecules in the adjacent somites. Before axons reach the plexus region they must travel through the scelerotome of the somites. It has been shown that axons selectively project through the anterior somites and actively grow away from the posterior somites.

The segmental patterning of motor nerves may result from a combination of contract-mediated inhibition and selective adhesion between developing neurons. Glycoproteins, such as L1, G4, neurofascin, and contactin, which tend to be restricted to axonal surfaces, may play a role in the guidance of axons by causing the fasciculation of like axons. As later developing axons grow down the pathways traveled by the first growing axons, they may be attracted to axons with similar surface proteins. This type of mechanism may be important for the fasciculation of axons innervating a particular muscle.

Growth cones also may be oriented by diffusible chemotrophic molecules that are secreted by re-

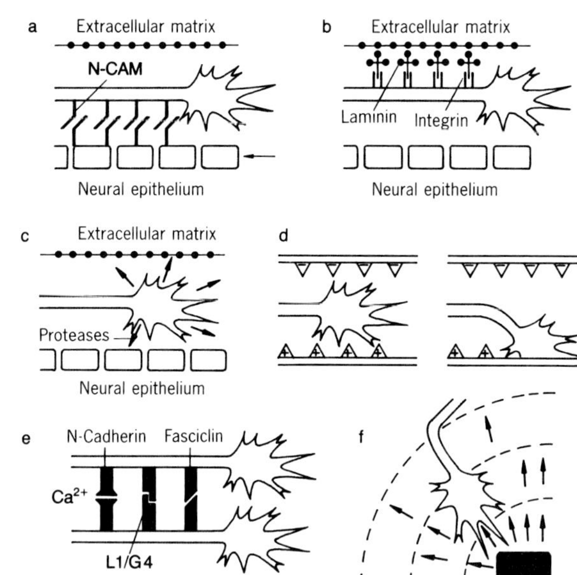

Figure 34
Mechanisms of neuronal navigation. Outgrowing neurites are guided by interactions with their surroundings. (a) Adhesion between neurons and neural epithelium by homophilic interactions between cell adhesion molecules. (b) Interactions between glycoproteins of the extracellular matrix and receptor molecules on the axon surface. (c) Progression of growth cone by release of proteases. (d) Selective attraction or repulsion between growth cones and cell- or substrate-bound molecules. (e) Fasciculation of nerve fibers induced by glycoproteins on different growth cones or neurites. (f) Chemotactic response of a growth cone to diffusible substances (after Dodd and Jessel). (Reproduced with permission from Reichert H: *Introduction to Neurobiology.* Stuttgart, Georg Thieme Verlag, 1992, p 197.)

stricted populations of intermediate or final cellular targets (Fig. 34). Experiments have shown that in the absence of a muscle target the outgrowth of the axons is random, whereas, in the presence of denervated muscle, the outgrowth of the motor axons is directed toward the muscle. Additional experiments suggested that the motor axons were responding to a diffusible substrate being released from the denervated muscle. Extracts of denervated muscle have been shown to increase neuron survival and promote neurite extension of cells in culture. Consequently, diffusible factors that could influence axonal outgrowth may be released from muscle after denervation; however, the distance over which these factors work is unknown. Additional chemotrophic molecules may be released from the distal stump of the damaged nerve.

Several experiments have shown that substances released from the distal stump of a damaged nerve can promote and direct the outgrowth of regenerating axons. The precise contribution of chemoattractants in vivo, however, remains to be determined. The demonstration of directed growth does not exclude the possibility that other factors, in addition to chemoattractants, are influencing the growth. A complete understanding of directional growth and the role of chemoattractants will require the isolation and biochemical characterization of specific chemoattractants.

Anatomy of the Peripheral Nerve

A peripheral nerve is a complex structure made up of individual nerve fibers, blood vessels, and supporting connective tissue. Individual nerve fibers collect into fascicles, which are surrounded by a connective layer called the perineurium. Within the fascicles, the individual nerve fibers are separated by a connective tissue framework called the endoneurium. Nerve fascicles are embedded in a connective tissue matrix called the epineurium, which provides a supporting and protective framework for the fascicles (Fig. 35).

Fascicular Organization

Individual fascicles are often grouped together into "fascicular bundles" separated by the deep, inner, or interfascicular epineurium. Nerves composed of one fascicle are referred to as monofascicular (Fig. 36). Nerves composed of many fascicles are categorized by the number and size of the fascicles: type 1 has few large fascicles; type 2 has many small fascicles that are approximately the same size; and type 3 has large and small fascicles combined together (Fig. 36). The general organization of fascicles in a nerve is summarized as follows: (1) Fascicles repeatedly divide and unite to form fascicular plexuses and, therefore, are not arranged as parallel uninterrupted strands along the entire length of a nerve. (2) No fascicle runs an unaltered course along the length of a nerve; however, at a given level, some fascicles may not participate in plexus formation. (3) The precise form of a plexus varies from nerve to nerve, level to level, side to side, and individual to individual. (4) The size and number of fascicles are inversely related at any given level. (5) The diameters of most fascicles range from 40 mm to 2 mm. (6) Fascicles are smaller and more numerous where a nerve crosses a joint, presumably to allow for nerve deformation without damage. (7) For a given fascicular area, nerve tensile strength increases with the number of fascicles. (8) The fascicular structure of a nerve changes rapidly and often along its length; the greatest length of a major nerve with an unchanged fascicular pattern is about 15 to 20 mm (Fig. 37).

Fascicular anatomy is relevant to the consequences of partial injury, the pathology and classification of nerve injuries, and surgical nerve repair. A nerve with many small fascicles as opposed to a few fascicles of various sizes may sustain only partial injury after mechanical trauma because of the greater amount of epineurium (Fig. 38). In addition,

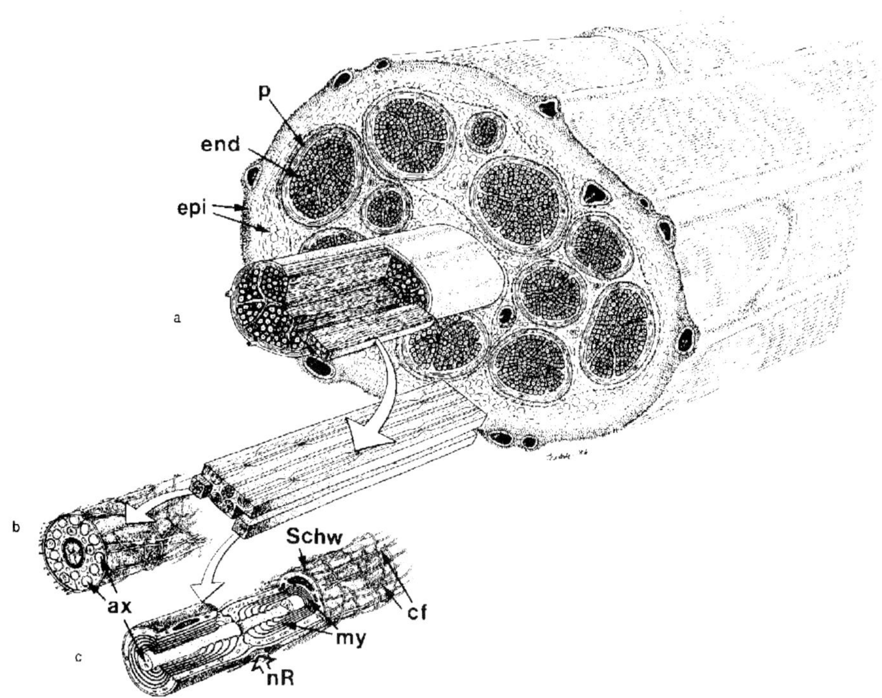

Figure 35
Microanatomy of a peripheral nerve trunk and its components. (a) Fascicles surrounded by a multilaminated perineurium (p) are embedded in a loose connective tissue, the epineurium (epi). The outer layers of the epineurium are condensed into a sheath. (b) and (c) illustrate the appearance of unmyelinated and myelinated fibers respectively. Schw = Schwann cell; my = myelin sheath; ax = axon; nR = node of Ranvier; cf = collagen fibrils. (Reproduced with permission from Lundborg G: *Nerve Injury and Repair.* New York, Churchill Livingstone, 1988, p 33.)

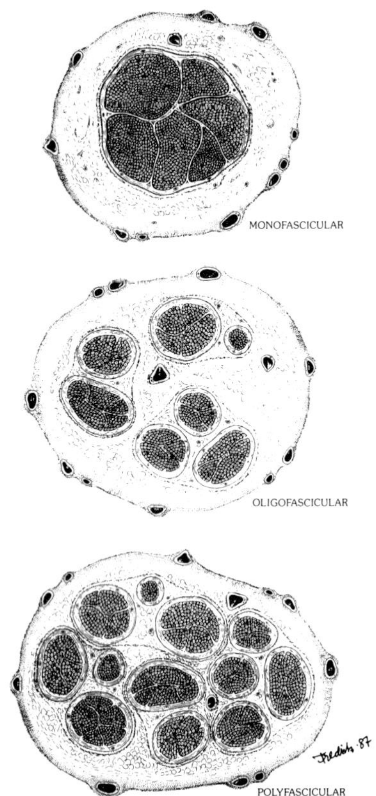

Figure 36
Basic patterns of interneural structure. **Top,** Monofascicular; **Center,** oligofascicular; **Bottom,** polyfascicular. (Reproduced with permission from Lundborg G: *Nerve Injury and Repair.* New York, Churchill Livingstone, 1988, p 198.)

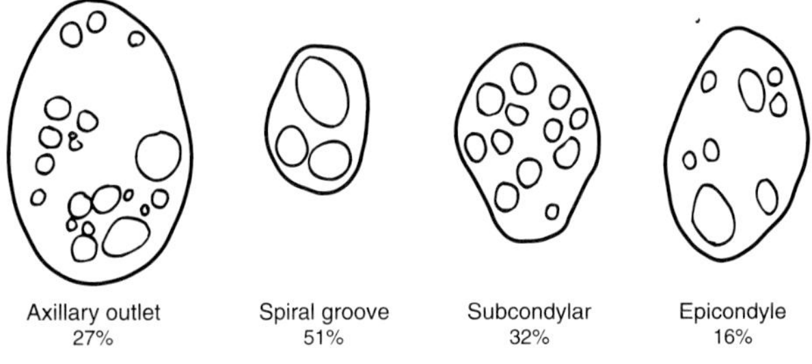

Figure 37
Variations in the size, number, and arrangement of fasciculi in a specimen of the radial nerve between the axilla and the elbow. The figures given are the percentage of cross-sectional area of the nerve devoted to fasciculi. (Adapted with permission from Sunderland S: *Nerve Injuries and Their Repair: A Critical Appraisal.* New York, Churchill Livingstone, 1991, p 33.)

nerve ends must be properly aligned during repair to maximize the potential for correct reinnervation.

Peripheral Nerve Connective Tissue

Endoneurium The endoneurium is a loose collagenous matrix that surrounds the individual nerve fibers within the fascicle. The matrix has large extracellular spaces and contains fibroblasts, mast cells, and a capillary network. Collagen fibrils predominate within the endoneurium and are closely packed around each nerve fiber to form a supporting framework. The collagen fibrils in the endoneurium of spinal nerves are fewer and finer than those in the endoneurium of peripheral nerves. The endoneurium forms a thin bilaminar sheath around each nerve fiber. This bilaminar sheath forms the wall of the "endoneurial tube," which contains the axon, the Schwann cell layer, and the myelin when it is present.

Perineurium The perineurium is a thin, dense connective tissue sheath that surrounds each fascicle. The sheath is composed of three identifiable layers. The internal layer is composed of a single layer of flattened mesothelial cells that form a smooth inner surface with tight junctions at cell boundaries. The outer layer merges with the epineurium. At this junction, the perineurial cells are replaced by fibroblasts, and the collagen fibers become thicker and their arrangement is less orderly. The middle layer is composed of flattened perineurial cells arranged in a series of three to 15 concentric lamellae. The lamellae are separated by spaces containing longitudinally oriented capillaries, collagen fibrils, and, occasionally, elastin fibers that are aligned longitudinally and obliquely. The perineurial cells in the middle layer have a basement membrane and tight junctions, and they function as a bidirectional diffusion barrier. The perineurium varies in thickness from 1.3 to 100 µm; there is a linear relationship between its thickness and the diameter of the fascicle. The tensile strength of the perineurium is high; the perineurium resists and maintains an interfascicular pressure that can be experimentally raised to 750 mm Hg before it ruptures. The perineurial diffusion barrier protects the fibers in the endoneurial space by preventing the penetration of the epineurial edema caused by ischemia. Spinal nerves do not have perineurial or epineurial tissue, which increases their vulnerability to stretch and compression injuries and to injury resulting from infections and exposure to chemicals.

Epineurium The epineurium is a loose meshwork of collagen and elastin fibers that provides a supporting and protective framework for the fascicles. Collagen fibers in the epineurium are thicker than those in the endoneurium and perineurium. The amount of epineurium varies from nerve to nerve and level to level and is generally thicker where the nerve crosses a joint. The epineurium is thought to protect the nerve from compressive forces. The epineurium contains a well-developed vascular plexus with numerous longitudinal main vascular channels feeding the endoneurial plexus.

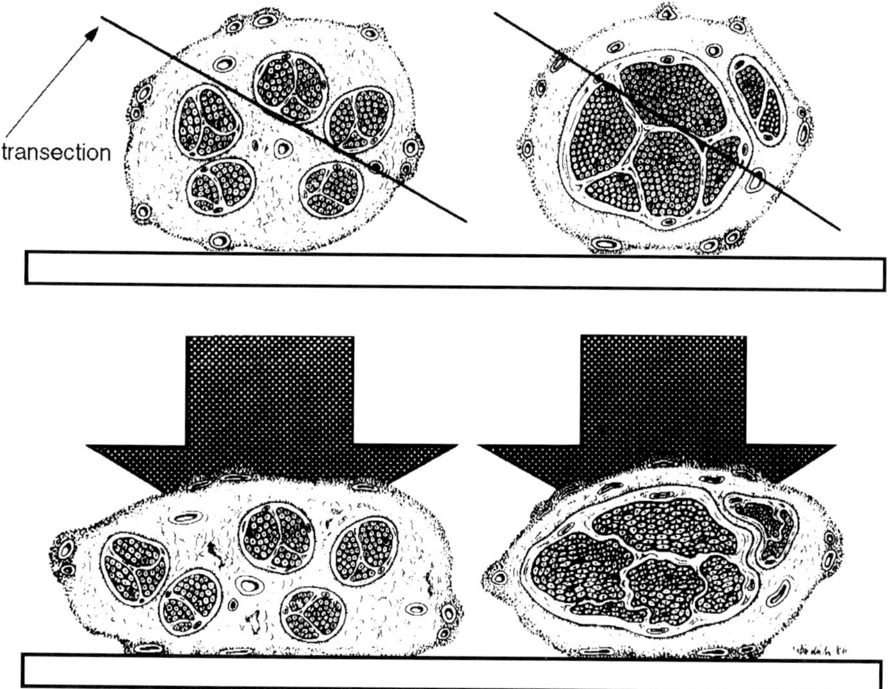

Figure 38
Protective effects of the epineurium when a nerve is subjected to mechanical trauma. Several small fascicles embedded in a large amount of epineurium (**left**) are less vulnerable to transection injuries and compression than large fascicles in a small amount of epineurium (**right**). (Adapted with permission from Lundborg G: *Nerve Injury and Repair.* New York, Churchill Livingstone, 1988, p 65.)

The Blood Supply

The nerve fiber requires a continuous energy source to maintain impulse conduction and axonal transport. Consequently, peripheral nerves are supplied by a well-developed intraneural microvascular system consisting of separate but interconnecting microvascular networks within the epineurium, perineurium, and endoneurium. The microvascular system of human nerves has been studied extensively. The vascular systems, both intrinsic and extrinsic, are characterized by longitudinally oriented vessels that communicate with each other via a great number of anastomoses. The intrinsic vascular system consists of the vascular plexa in the epineurium, perineurium, and endoneurium (Fig. 39). The extrinsic vascular system is made up of segmental regional vessels that approach the nerve trunk at various levels along its course; these vessels run in the loose connective tissue meshwork that surrounds the nerve trunk.

In the epineurium, large arterial and venular vessels, which run longitudinally along the nerve in close apposition to the fascicles, supply both the superficial and deep layers. The epineurial vessels anastomose with the perineurial vascular plexus, which consists of individual vessels located at various depths between the lamellae of the perineurium. The perineurial vessels travel longitudinally between the perineurial lamellae layers for a long distance before they pierce through the inner layer into the endoneurial space in a characteristic oblique manner. The perineurial vascular plexus and the endoneurial vascular plexus represent an anatomically well-defined vascular unit that can be isolated and spared when fascicles are teased apart. The individual fascicles, which often run together as a fascicular group, have a common vascular unit, which also can be defined and spared during surgery.

The endoneurial microvascular network consists of capillaries, arterioles, and venules; their vascular bed appears to form a continuous anastomotic network throughout the length of the fascicles. Their capillaries are unusually large, with the smallest capillaries having diameters of 6 to 10 μm compared to muscle capillaries with diameters of 3 to 6 μm. These capillaries have structural and functional characteristics similar to those of capillaries in the CNS. Consequently, the blood-nerve barrier is similar to the blood-brain barrier, being impermeable to a large range of macromolecules, especially proteins. The blood-nerve barrier and the diffusion barrier of the perineurium are essential for maintaining the appropriate endoneurial environment. The diffusion barriers can be damaged by metabolic and infectious diseases, intoxication, and irradiation, which can bring about changes in the ionic equilibrium, osmotic pressure, and endoneurial fluid pressure.

Response to Trauma

The PNS, like most other highly vascularized systems, responds to trauma with an inflammatory response. The epineurial vessels, which lack a

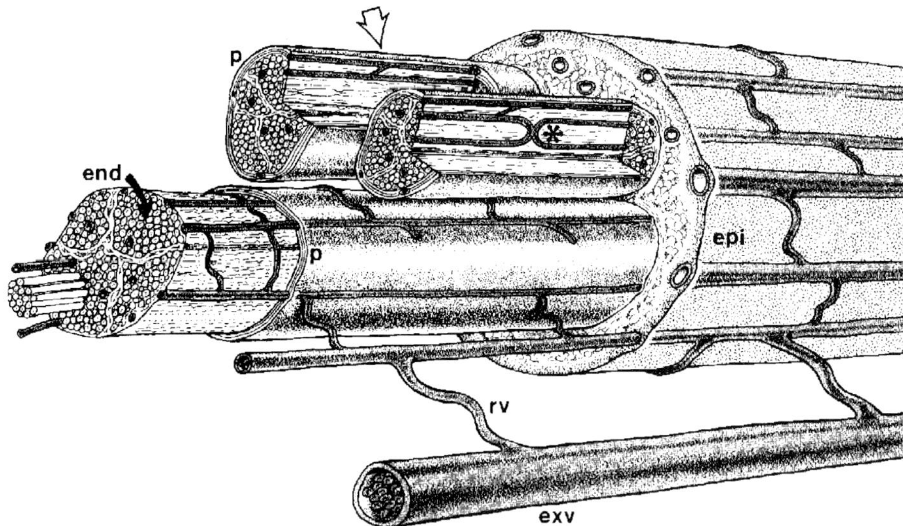

Figure 39
Interneural vascularization. Vessels are abundant in all layers of the nerve, forming a pattern of longitudinally oriented vessels. Extrinsic vessels (exv) are, via regional feeding vessels (rv), supporting vascular plexa in superficial and deep layers of the epineurium (epi), perineurium (p), and endoneurium (end). Note the oblique course of vessels penetrating the perineurium (arrows) and the intrafascicular 'double loop formations' (*). (Reproduced with permission from Lundborg G: *Nerve Injury and Repair.* New York, Churchill Livingstone, 1988, p 43.)

blood-nerve barrier, respond to even slight trauma by increasing their permeability, leading to epineurial edema. The perineurial diffusion barrier prevents the edema from reaching the endoneurial space. However, severe trauma, such as crush or transection lesions, can induce increased vascular permeability of the endoneurial capillaries. This increased vascular permeability probably is caused by direct trauma to the blood vessels, but may also be caused by the liberation of endogenous chemicals that increase permeability. It has been suggested that mast cells, located in both the epineurium and endoneurium, release histamine and serotonin, thereby increasing vascular permeability.

Crush and transection injuries damage the barriers in the endoneurial and perineurial vessels. Compression injuries and ischemia may, under some circumstances, induce vascular changes in the endoneurial vessels without affecting the perineurial vessels. Under these conditions, edema would occur in the endoneurial space and would not be drained because of the functioning perineurial diffusion barrier. Normally, there is a positive pressure inside the fascicles, the endoneurial fluid pressure. However, edema-caused increases in the endoneurial fluid pressure could affect blood flow and the exchange of nutrient and waste products. Changes in the ionic content of the endoneurial fluid or a decrease in oxygen delivery and energy production may affect the nerve fiber conduction of action potentials and axonal transport. Chronic nerve compression or irritation may cause chronic intraneural edema, which could profoundly affect nerve function.

Nerve Biomechanics

Peripheral nerves, like any other structure that involves a connective tissue matrix surrounding other structures, have biomechanical properties characteristic of soft tissues. For example, a nerve can be stretched and the load supported by the nerve measured. If such experiments are performed under controlled conditions, it can be demonstrated that nerves have a typical stress-strain relationship (see the chapter on biomechanics), with a compliant toe region observed at low strain and increasing stiffness at higher strains. This type of relationship has been thoroughly defined for other tissues, such as bone, tendon, ligament, and muscle.

A review of the literature reveals a wide variety of values for ultimate strain (that is, the strain at which a nerve fails), ranging from 20% to 60%. Table 10 gives some of the values that have been reported. Unfortunately, many of the ultimate strain values were historically derived by attaching a nerve to a stretching machine and deforming it until it failed. The distance between the clamps at the time of failure was used to calculate strain based on the original length (see the chapter on tendon,

Table 10
Comparison of Ultimate Elongation and Stress

Reference	Nerve	Ultimate Elongation (%)	Ultimate Stress
Beel and associates	Mouse sciatic control	43	3.2×10^{-7} dynes/cm^2
	Crush, day 2	63	2.6×10^{-7} dynes/cm^2
	Crush, day 6	55	3.0×10^{-7} dynes/cm^2
	Crush, day 12	51	4.2×10^{-7} dynes/cm^2
	Crush, day 24	40	3.8×10^{-7} dynes/cm^2
Clark and associates	Rat sciatic	17	3.4 N
Denny-Brown and Doherty	Cat peroneal	43-316	NA
Haftek	Rabbit tibial	69.3	NA
Okamoto	Human median	18.4	1.32 kg/mm^2
	Human femoral	18.5	1.30 kg/mm^2
	Human sciatic	18.5	1.28 kg/mm^2
	Pig sciatic	18.8	1.25 kg/mm^2
	Pig median	18.6	1.35 kg/mm^2
	Dog sciatic	18.1	0.83 kg/mm^2
	Dog median	18.3	0.95 kg/mm^2
	Cat sciatic	19.2	0.95 kg/mm^2
	Cat median	19.0	1.12 kg/mm^2
	Rabbit sciatic	22.0	0.67 kg/mm^2
	Rabbit median	22.2	0.94 kg/mm^2
	Mouse sciatic	19.4	0.64 kg/mm^2
Rydevik and associates	Rabbit tibial	38.5	11.7 MPa
Sunderland and Bradley	Human median	19	1.7 kg/mm^2
	Human ulnar	18	1.6 kg/mm^2
	Human tibial	23	1.1 kg/mm^2
	Human peroneal	20	1.3 kg/mm^2
Yoshimura and associates	Rabbit tibial	31.8	NA

ligament, and meniscus). The problem with this approach is that it is difficult to securely fasten nerves to clamps and, as the tissue is deformed, slippage around the clamp occurs. As a result, the distance between the clamps overestimates the actual strain in the nerve material, and many of these ultimate strain values were probably artificially inflated. Several recent biomechanical studies of peripheral nerve, however, have been performed under conditions in which surface strain has been measured directly. In a study of the rabbit tibial nerve in which the nerve was slowly deformed from its "slack" length (defined as zero strain) to failure, ultimate strain was 38% ± 2% and the in situ strain of the material was recorded to be 11% ± 1.5%. In a study of the rat sciatic nerve, zero strain was defined at that point where the load rose above the noise level and continued to rise. In this study, mean ultimate strain was 16% ± 4.3%, and the mean in situ strain was 1.9% ± 0.58% (Fig. 40). These data indicate that the nerve is under some degree of tension in the resting tissue and suggest that under normal physiologic conditions the nerve functions in the very compliant toe region of the stress-strain curve, where it probably produces low tension. This relationship may be dramatically altered, however, in those cases where nerves are repaired and the retracted stumps of the nerve are brought together under tension. In human nerves, gaps of 3 to 5 cm are often overcome to reappose the proximal and distal nerve stumps. Additionally, although nerves may not rupture until strains approaching 20%, the nerve undergoes ischemic damage at strains approaching 15%.

The speed at which the nerve regains its structural strength is important because limbs are often immobilized for periods of three to six weeks following nerve repair in order to protect the repair site. In an experimental study on rat sciatic nerve, end-to-end epineurial repair was performed immediately following a transection injury. The nerve regained 66% of its strength almost immediately after repair (within seven days) and maintained a relatively constant level of ultimate stress and ultimate strain throughout the testing period, which extended up to 84 days. These data challenge the dogma that extended limb immobilization is required after peripheral nerve repair. However, because the study was performed in rats, which have a higher tissue turnover than primates or humans, it is not clear to what extent these results transfer to the clinical situation. It does appear, however, that

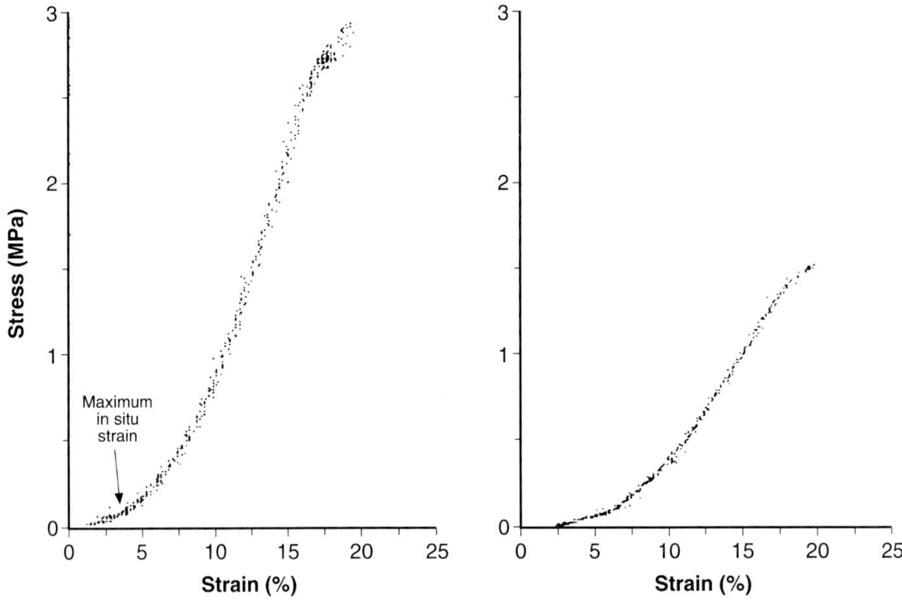

Figure 40
Stress-strain curves showing in situ strain in rat sciatic nerve. Control (**left**) and seven days after repair (**right**).

nerves repair themselves much faster than ligaments and tendons. More studies are required, which define the tensile properties of repaired nerve.

Like many other biologic tissues, nerves demonstrate time-dependent biomechanical properties (viscoelasticity). The familiar tests used to quantify viscoelasticity are the creep test and the stress relaxation test (Fig. 41). In the creep test, a load is rapidly applied to a nerve, and the nerve slowly elongates or "creeps" to a new length. The length of time required for the creep to occur is a measure of the viscoelasticity of the nerve itself. Similarly, a deformation can be applied to a nerve, immediately raising the load on the nerve. When the deformation is held constant, that load slowly decays; this phenomenon is known as stress relaxation, which is another measurement of nerve viscoelasticity. The parameters related to these properties are time constants. These properties have been derived for rabbit tibial nerves and show that nerves are not highly viscoelastic compared to tendon and ligaments. These data indicate that rapid movement of limbs, which results in rapid elongations of nerves, would probably not have a major impact on the stress experienced by the nerve and, therefore, would probably not contribute in a significant way to nerve injury.

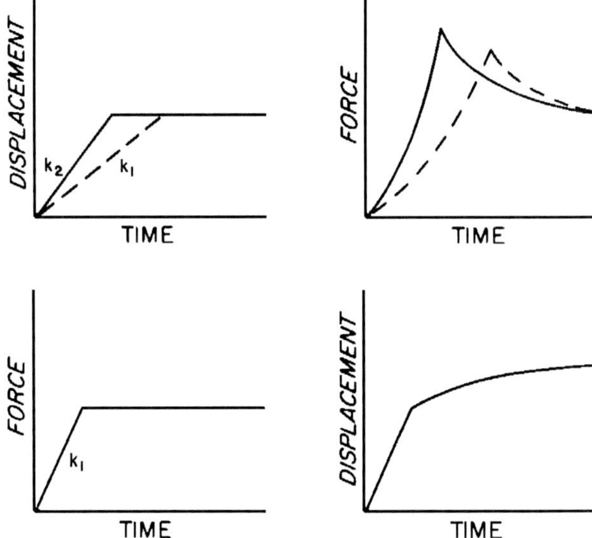

Figure 41
Curves for force relaxation (**top**) and creep (**bottom**) tests. Input loading curves are on the left, and typical output curves are on the right. (Reproduced with permission from Butler DL, Noyes FR, Grood ES: Measurement of the biomechanical properties of ligaments, in Bahnuik G, Burstein A (eds): *Handbook of Engineering and Biology*. West Palm Beach, FL, CRC Press, Inc, 1978.)

Electrodiagnosis of Peripheral Nerves

Nerve conduction studies and electromyography can be used to evaluate the function of motor and sensory nerves and skeletal muscle, and have become invaluable tools for the diagnosis of neuropathies and myopathies. The objectives of electrical diagnosis are: (1) Differentiation of weakness due to lower motoneuron versus upper motoneuron dysfunction and ventral horn motoneuron lesions versus more peripheral lesions; (2) identification of the involved muscles to determine the level of the injury and degree of dysfunction; and (3) demonstration of (a) muscle denervation to differentiate between a complete lesion and a reversible nerve conduction block, (b) reinnervation as proof of regeneration, (c) aberrant reinnervation following a peripheral nerve lesion, (d) diffuse or localized disturbances of nerve conduction in peripheral nerves, and (e) disturbances of neurotransmission at the motor end plate.

Nerve Conduction Studies

Nerve conduction studies can be used to determine the presence and severity of any peripheral nerve dysfunction, its localization (that is, cell body, spinal roots, plexus, or peripheral nerve), its distribution (focal, multifocal, or diffuse), and the pathophysiology (for example, axonal degeneration versus axonal demyelination). It should be pointed out that nerve conduction studies evaluate only the large myelinated nerve fiber function. Nerve fiber function is routinely evaluated in the following nerves: the ulnar, medial, radial, and tibial nerves (motor and sensory fibers); the sciatic, femoral, and peroneal nerves (motor fibers only); and the musculocutaneous, superficial peroneal, sural, and saphenous nerves (sensory fibers only).

Stimulation and Recording Procedures

Electrical activity can be recorded extracellularly from muscle or nerve using surface electrodes. Surface electrodes come in a variety of shapes and sizes. Commonly used types are small silver disc electrodes that are applied to the skin or ring electrodes that fit around the fingers. Stimulating electrodes come in pairs that usually are placed 2 to 3 cm apart. Several terms used to describe the electrodes are listed in the glossary and are illustrated in Figure 42.

The stimulus artifact, which is the deflection from the baseline resulting from direct conduction of the stimulus, is often used for latency measurements as a marker of the onset of a sweep. It often is so large that it masks the onset of the response being measured. This phenomenon is related to excessive cutaneous spread of the stimulating current to the recording electrodes and is particularly noticeable during sensory stimulation in which the higher amplification of the signal is often needed.

The standard stimulus is a 0.1- to 0.2-ms square wave pulse at a slow repetitive stimulation rate of 1 to 2 per second. The intensity is gradually increased to get the maximal response and then increased 20% to 30%. This is referred to as supramaximal stimulation and is used to ensure activation of all the nerve fibers. The action potentials that are recorded have either a biphasic or triphasic configuration (Fig. 43). According to the convention of clinical electrophysiology, an upward deflection reflects a relative negativity of the active electrode (G1) with respect to the reference electrode (G2); that is, depolarization, and a downward deflection reflects a relative positivity of the active electrode.

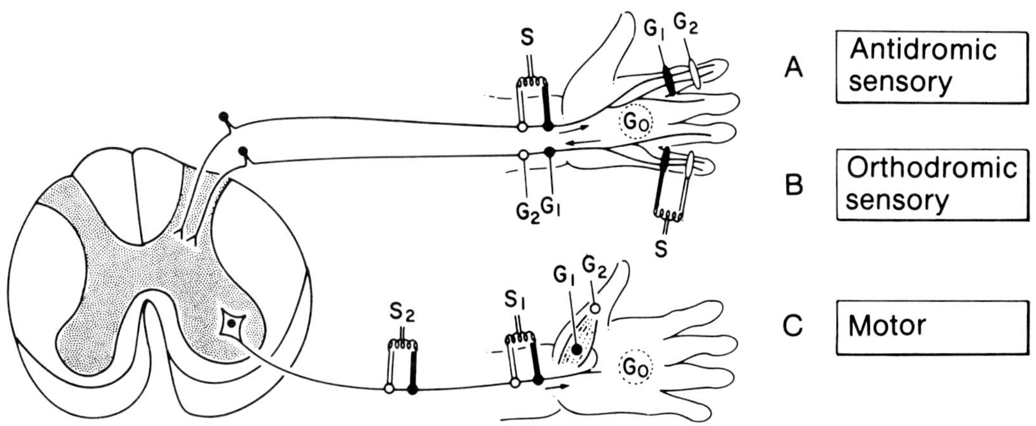

Figure 42
Diagrammatic illustration of electrode placement for nerve conduction studies. Antidromic sensory study (A); orthodromic sensory study (B); and motor nerve conduction study (C). G_1 = active recording electrode; G_2 = reference recording electrode; G_o = ground electrode; S = stimulating electrode; S_1 = distal stimulation site; S_2 = proximal stimulation site. Cathode is black; anode is white. (Reproduced with permission from Sethi RK, Thompson LL: *The Electromyographer's Handbook,* ed 2. Boston, Little Brown and Company, 1989, p 4.)

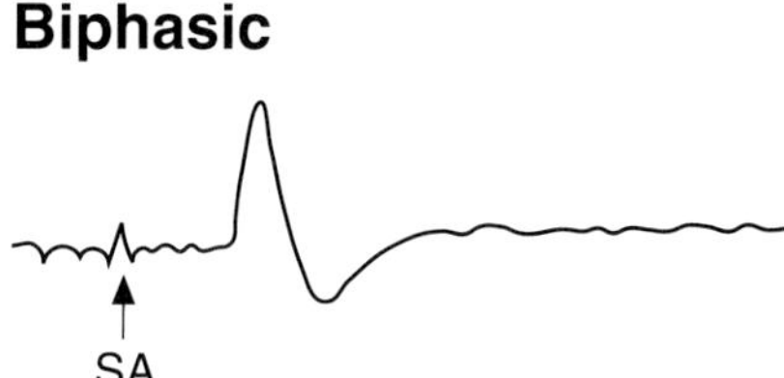

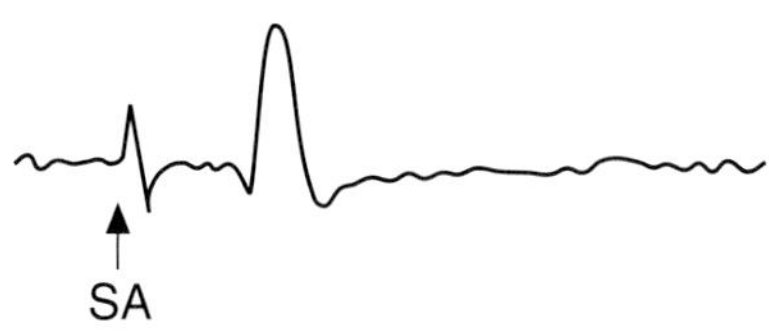

Figure 43
Biphasic (**top**) and triphasic (**bottom**) wave forms. SA = stimulus artifact.

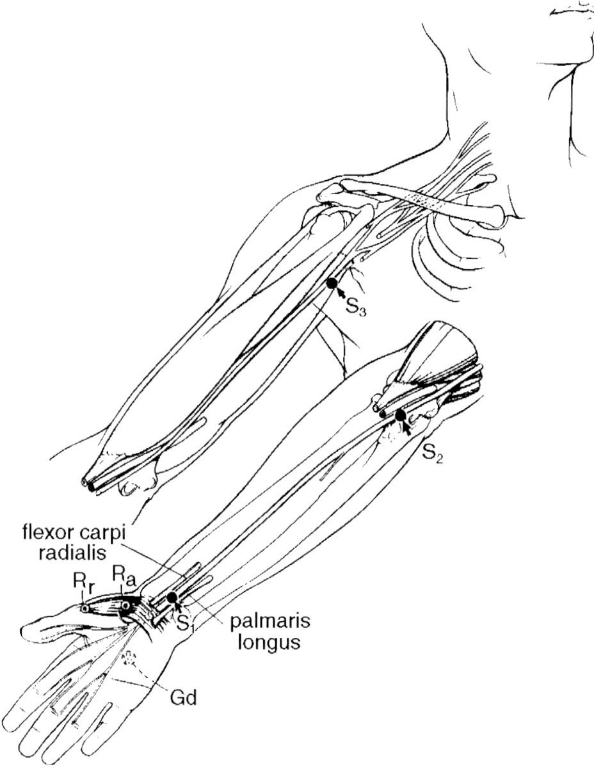

Figure 44
Motor conduction set up for median nerve (motor). (Reproduced with permission from Liveson JA, Ma DM: *Laboratory Reference for Clinical Neurophysiology.* Philadelphia, FA Davis Co., 1992, p 84.)

Motor Nerve Conduction

To study motor conduction, the nerve is supramaximally stimulated where it is most superficial at two or more points along its course (Fig. 44). The motor response is recorded from a distal muscle that is innervated by the nerve (Fig. 42). In the recording of muscle potentials, the active electrode is placed over or close to the end plate region in the muscle, and the reference electrode is placed over the tendon. The evoked motor response is a sum of the action potentials of the individual muscle fibers and is called a compound muscle action potential (CMAP). It also is referred to as the M-wave. If the recording electrode is directly over the end plate region, the evoked response will be a biphasic potential with an initial large upward (negative) deflection followed by a smaller downward (positive) deflection (Fig. 43). If the initial deflection is downward or positive (Fig. 43), this suggests that (1) the recording electrode is not over the end plate region, (2) the active and reference electrodes have been transposed, (3) stimulation of neighboring nerves has occurred because of incorrect placement of stimulating electrodes or by spread of stimulus as a result of its high intensity, or (4) there is an anomalous innervation. The CMAP is described by its latency, amplitude, area, and duration, which are measured as shown in Figure 45.

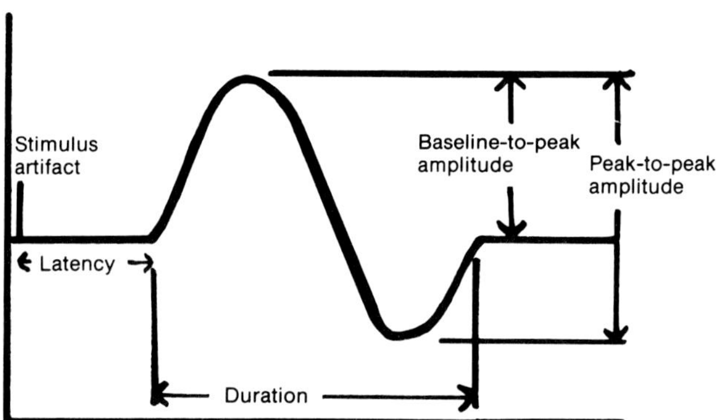

Figure 45
Measured parameters of a compound motor action potential (CMAP). (Reproduced with permission from Sethi RK, Thompson LL: *The Electromyographer's Handbook,* ed 2. Boston, Little Brown and Company, 1989, p 10.)

Latency and conduction velocity The latency is the time in milliseconds from the application of the stimulation to the initial deflection from the baseline. The onset latency is a measure of the fastest-conducting motor fibers and includes the time required to travel from the site of stimulation to the nerve terminal (nerve conduction time), the time required for the stimulus to activate the postsynaptic terminal on the muscle fibers (neuromuscular transmission time), and the time required for the action potential to propagate along the muscle membrane to the recording electrode. To measure the nerve conduction time, the CMAP is recorded after stimulation from at least two sites along the nerve. Because the neuromuscular transmission time and muscle fiber propagation time will be the same, the latency difference between the two represents the time required for the nerve impulse to travel from one stimulation site to the other (Fig. 44). The conduction velocity is calculated using the following equation: CV (m/s) = *distance (mm) between proximal and distal stimulating sites*

proximal latency (ms) - distal latency (ms)

Normative values for individual nerves in children and adults can be found in several textbooks. Table 11 lists some normative data for a few nerves at different ages.

In myelinated axons, conduction velocity is influenced by myelin thickness, internode distance, age, and temperature. Nerve conduction velocities at birth are about 50% of adult values, increasing to about 75% by 12 months and 100% by 4 to 5 years. The relative increase in speed is due to myelination and increase in size of axons, which is usually complete by age 5. Temperature has a considerable effect on conduction velocity. As surface temperature decreases below 34°C, there is a progressive increase in latency and a decrease in conduction velocity.

Conduction velocity measurements vary between the upper and lower extremities and between proximal and distal segments of the same nerve. Upper extremity conduction velocities are generally 10% to 15% faster than those of the lower extremity. The lower limit of conduction velocity is around 50 m/s in the upper extremity and around 45 m/s in the lower extremity. Conduction velocity in the proximal segments is generally 5% to 10% faster than in the distal segments. This variation may be related to lower temperatures and smaller nerve fibers distally. In general, there is an error of about 5% to 10% in the measurement of conduction velocity caused by observer errors in measuring distance and latency.

Amplitude and duration The amplitude of the CMAP is measured from the baseline to the negative peak or between negative and positive peaks and is expressed in millivolts (Fig. 45). With supramaximal stimulation, the area under the negative peak is directly proportional to the number of muscle fibers depolarized. Both amplitude and area provide an estimate of the amount of functioning axons and muscle, although area is a better measurement than amplitude. The duration of the CMAP is a reflection of the range of conduction velocities and the synchrony of contraction of the muscle fibers. The duration is measured as the time, in milliseconds, from the onset to the end of the initial negative phase. If the axonal conduction velocities vary widely, the muscle fibers will be activated at different times, and the duration of the negative phase will be long. Dispersion of the CMAP, which occurs when some axons conduct slowly; for example, in acute demyelinating diseases, is shown on the recording as an increase in the duration and number of turns (spikes without baseline crossings) or phases (spikes with baseline crossings).

Sensory Nerve Conduction

Sensory potentials are unaffected by lesions proximal to the dorsal root ganglion even though there is sensory loss. Consequently, sensory potentials are useful in localizing a lesion either proximal (root or spinal cord) or distal (plexus or nerve) to the dorsal root ganglia. Sensory nerve action potentials (or compound nerve action potentials) are much smaller in amplitude than compound motor action potentials and are often obscured by other electrical activity and artifacts. Consequently, techniques that use digital averaging of multiple potentials and high amplification are often required.

Sensory axons are evaluated by (1) stimulating and recording from a cutaneous nerve, (2) recording from a cutaneous nerve while stimulating a mixed nerve, (3) recording from a mixed nerve while stimulating a cutaneous nerve, or (4) recording from the spinal column while a cutaneous or mixed nerve is stimulated. The recording electrodes are placed 3 to 4 cm apart, with the active recording electrode (G1) placed 10 to 15 cm from the cathode of the stimulating electrode (Fig. 46). Larger distances tend to increase dispersion and decrease the amplitude. Potentials recorded by an electrode that is placed closer to the spinal cord than the stimulating electrode are said to be orthodromic potentials (in the

Table 11
Mean motor nerve conduction velocities at different ages

Average Age	Ulnar Nerve m/sec	Median Nerve m/sec	Peroneal Nerve m/sec	Tibial Nerve m/sec
5 weeks	34.5	33.1	37.2	34.2
1 year	46.1	41.8	44.1	38.3
4 years	52.4	49.4	44.2	43.1
6 years	56.1	54.9	52.2	48.4

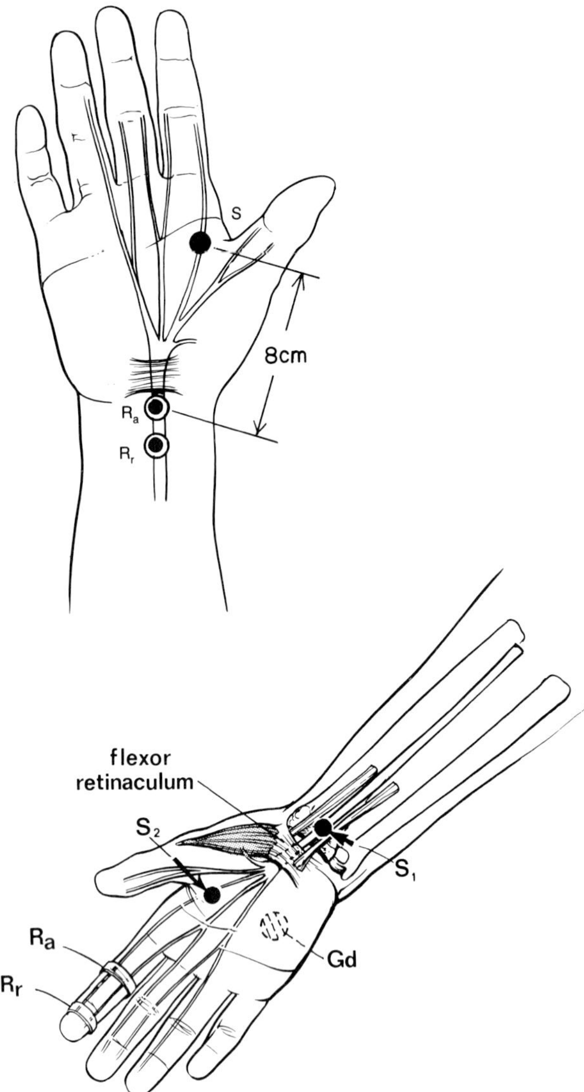

Figure 46
Carpal tunnel studies. **Top,** Orthodromic palmar stimulation. **Bottom,** Antidromic palmar stimulation. S = stimulating electrode; R_a = active recording electrode; R_f = reference recording electrode; Gd = ground. (Reproduced with permission from Liveson JA, Ma DM: *Laboratory Reference for Clinical Neurophysiology.* Philadelphia, FA Davis Co., 1992, pp 116, 120.)

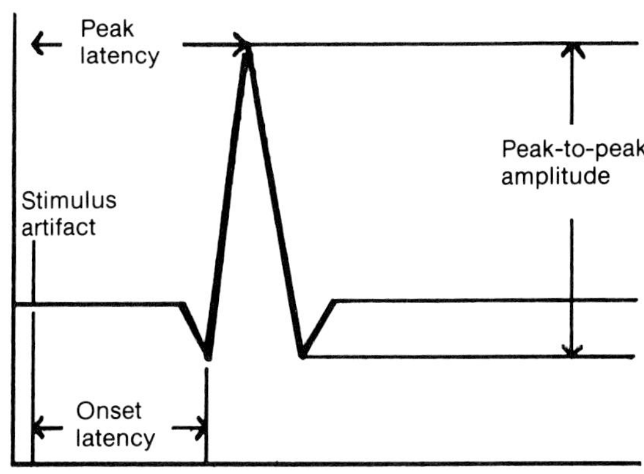

Figure 47
Measured parameters of a sensory nerve action potential (SNAP). (Reproduced with permission from Sethi RK, Thompson LL: *The Electromyographer's Handbook,* ed 2. Boston, Little Brown and Company, 1989, p 16.)

direction of the physiologic conduction), while those recorded by an electrode that is distal to the stimulating electrode are antidromic (in the direction opposite the physiologic conduction). The speed of conduction is the same in both directions; however, the amplitude is generally larger with antidromic recording because the recording electrode is closer to the nerve (Fig. 46).

An orthodromically recorded compound nerve action potential typically is a triphasic wave with an initial small downward (positive) deflection (Fig. 47). Antidromic recordings typically have a biphasic wave with an initial large upward (negative) deflection. The sensory latency is measured from the stimulus onset to the onset of the negative peak or to the top of the initial positive peak (Fig. 47). This latency measurement represents the conduction in the fastest sensory fibers. Latencies to the peak of the negative phase (peak latency) are often used because they are more easily defined, especially in noisy recordings. The conduction velocity (m/s) is calculated by dividing the conduction distance (in mm) by the sensory latency (in ms).

The amplitude of the response is measured from the positive to negative peak and is an estimate of the total number of fibers activated, although it is heavily influenced by the distance between the recording electrode and the nerve. The area under the peak is often difficult to measure because of the difficulty in defining the measurement points.

The F-Wave

The F-wave is a long-latency motor response to antidromic activation of α motoneurons in the spinal cord. The F-wave is evoked by supramaximal stimulation of peripheral nerves and can be recorded in almost all skeletal muscles. Supramaximal stimulation of a nerve results in an impulse that travels orthodromically toward the muscle and antidromically toward the spinal cord (Fig. 48). The short latency orthodromic response is called the M-wave and the late response occurring after the M-wave is called the F-wave. The latency of the F-wave includes the time required for the evoked potential to travel antidromically to the ventral horn of the spinal cord, the delay time to activate the α motoneurons (~1 ms), and the time required for the signal to travel orthodromically from the spinal cord to the muscle. With more proximal stimulation, the latency of the M-wave increases and the latency of the F-wave decreases (Fig. 48). The F-wave is small in comparison to the M-wave because not all of the motor axons activated in the M-wave are activated in the F-wave. The F-waves usually vary considerably in amplitude, latency, and shape with repeated stimulation because different groups of motoneurons are activated with each stimulus (Fig. 49). In general, the motor unit potentials activated in the F-waves represent the highest threshold, largest amplitude motor units. The shortest latency in a series of recorded F-waves is a measure of the fastest conducting fibers. The percentage of stimuli that elicits an F-wave is termed F-persistence and is normally 90% to 100%. Inconsistency of F-waves may be an early sign of a neuropathy.

To record the F-wave, two sets of recording electrodes are placed over the end plate region of the muscle and over the tendon. The M- and F-waves must be recorded from different electrodes because a higher gain and different time base are required to record the F-wave. Usually ten or more F-waves are recorded, and the shortest latency is measured. Other parameters of the F-wave that are measured are minimum-maximum latency differences, F-wave amplitude, F-wave persistence, and duration of the F-wave complex.

The F-wave is often measured to supplement routine nerve conduction studies because the F-wave permits evaluation of the proximal segments of peripheral nerves. F-waves are valuable in evaluating disorders involving the nerve roots, plexuses, and the proximal segments of peripheral nerves. Determination of F-wave latencies is particularly valuable in evaluating patients with demyelinating polyradiculoneuropathies.

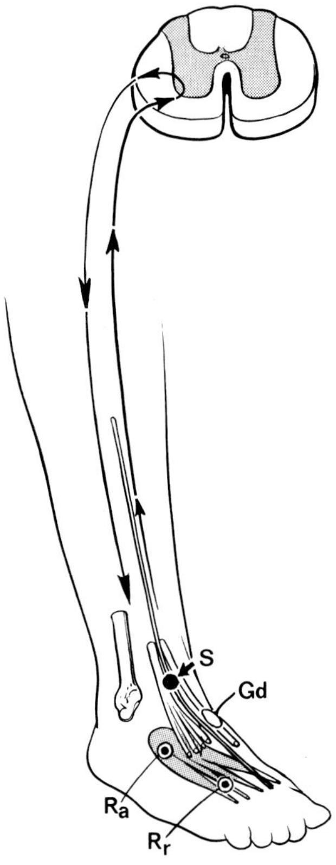

Figure 48
F-wave test. (Reproduced with permission from Liveson JA, Ma DM: *Laboratory Reference for Clinical Neurophysiology.* Philadelphia, FA Davis Co., 1992, p 250.)

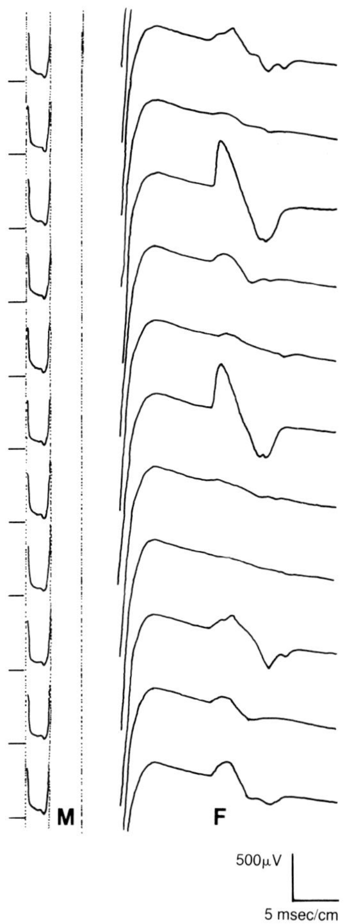

Figure 49
F waves. Median nerve stimulation at wrist with surface recording from abductor pollicis brevis. Calibration: 500 μV, 5 ms/cm. M = direct response, F = F waves. Note intermittent and varying configuration of F waves. (Reproduced with permission from Liveson JA, Ma DM: *Laboratory Reference for Clinical Neurophysiology.* Philadelphia, FA Davis Co., 1992, p 253.)

The H-reflex

The H-reflex is an electrically evoked spinal monosynaptic reflex involving the Ia afferent fibers from the muscle spindles and motor axons. A submaximal stimulus activates the Ia afferents (large myelinated fibers with the lowest threshold for activation) in a mixed nerve, which in turn evokes a monosynaptic reflex contraction in the corresponding muscle. The motoneurons activated in the H-reflex are the lowest threshold, slow-conducting motoneurons. In contrast, the axons activated by the peripheral stimulation and recorded in the M-wave are the large, fast-conducting motor axons. The amplitude of the H-reflex is indirectly related to the amplitude of the M-wave (Fig. 50) and is maximal near the threshold for the M-wave. With increasing stimulation intensity, motor fibers in the nerve are activated, with the resulting antidromic motor impulse colliding with the reflex impulse and obliterating it.

The H-reflex has several characteristics that differ significantly from the M-wave: (1) The stimulus threshold is lower than that required to elicit an M-wave; (2) the latency and waveform tend to be constant at a fixed stimulus intensity because the same motoneurons are activated each time; (3) the amplitude often exceeds that of the M-wave at low stimulus intensity, and the mean amplitude can be 50% to 100% of the M-wave; and (4) after the first year of life, the H-reflex is consistently found only in the calf muscles and flexor carpi radialis.

The H-reflex from the soleus is primarily mediated by the S-1 spinal root and is the analog of the ankle reflex. A unilateral abnormality is useful in differentiating an S-1 from an L-5 radiculopathy. The H-reflex in the quadriceps is used to study the L-3, L-4 spinal roots. Bilateral H-reflex abnormalities are a sensitive indicator of a peripheral polyneuropathy, but must be differentiated from bilateral S-1 radiculopathies. H-reflex abnormalities occur early in the course of demyelinating neuropathies.

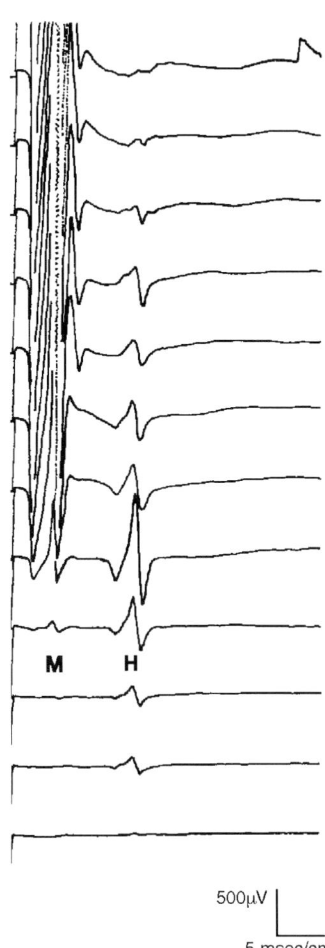

Figure 50
H-reflex. Popliteal stimulation of tibial nerve; surface recording from soleus. Calibration: 500 μV, 10 ms/cm. M = direct response, H = H-reflex. Increasing stimulus strength progressing from lowest to highest sweep. Note appearance of H reflex at low stimulus intensity, and its subsequent inverse relationship to the M wave with increasing stimulus intensity. (Reproduced with permission from Liveson JA, Ma DM: *Laboratory Reference for Clinical Neurophysiology.* Philadelphia, FA Davis Co., 1992, p 240.)

Electromyography

Electromyography refers to the methods used to study the electrical activity of individual muscle fibers and motor units. Electromyographic (EMG) examination often is used in conjunction with nerve conduction studies and permits determination of the origin of the lesion, that is, neural, muscular, or junctional. If the lesion is of neural origin, EMG studies can help localize the level of the lesion to the motoneuron, spinal root, nerve plexus, or peripheral nerve. EMG studies also can assist in determining the prognosis of a peripheral nerve lesion.

The electrical activity of a muscle is studied by inserting a recording electrode directly into the muscle. In screening patients for EMG studies attention should be paid to bleeding tendencies and unusual susceptibility to recurrent systemic infections. In addition, repeated EMG studies should not be done before muscle biopsies because the repeated insertion and movement of the electrodes will induce local muscle damage and inflammation that could interfere with the interpretation of subsequent muscle biopsies and histologic evaluation.

EMG Electrodes

Two types of electrodes are commonly used for EMG studies: the concentric needle electrode and the monopolar needle electrode (Fig. 51). The con-

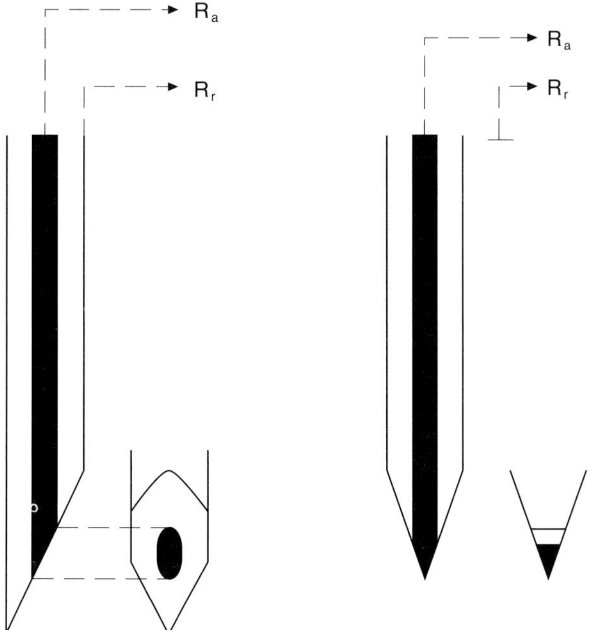

Figure 51
Concentric (**left**) and monopolar (**right**) needles. R_a = active electrode; R_r = reference electrode.

centric needle consists of an outer stainless steel cannula through which runs a single wire that is insulated except at the tip. The inner wire serves as the recording electrode, the outer cannula serves as the reference electrode, and the patient is grounded by a separate surface electrode. The potential difference between the outer cannula and inner wire is recorded. Monopolar electrodes consist of a solid steel needle, usually stainless steel, that is insulated except at the tip. The potential difference is measured between the tip of the needle and a reference electrode that is either a conductive plate attached to the skin or a needle inserted subcutaneously. The concentric needle records from a smaller area in the muscle than the monopolar needle and has an asymmetric pick-up area as opposed to the circular pick-up area of the monopolar needle. The electrode records motor unit action potentials with biphasic or triphasic waveforms.

A typical EMG recording session generally proceeds as follows. A needle is inserted into a muscle while the muscle is relaxed so that the presence and extent of any insertion activity can be noted. Then, the muscle is explored systematically with the electrode for the presence of spontaneous activity. The patient is then asked to contract the muscle voluntarily to submaximal force levels, and the parameters of individual motor units are studied at several different sites within the muscle. The parameters that are measured are the shape and dimensions of the potentials, the initial firing frequency, the rate at which a unit must fire before additional units are recruited, and, finally, the number of units recruited.

Insertional Activity

When a needle is inserted into a muscle or moved within a muscle, there is a single burst of activity that usually lasts 300 to 500 ms. The activity is related to movement of the electrode and is thought to result from mechanical stimulation or injury of the muscle fibers. Insertional activity that lasts longer than 300 to 500 ms may be an early sign of denervation and is found in polymyositis, the myotonic disorders, and some of the other myopathies. In contrast, a reduction of insertion activity is found after prolonged denervation when muscle fibers have been replaced by connective tissue and with fibrosis.

EMG Activity in Resting Muscle

In healthy muscles, EMG activity usually cannot be measured at rest, except at the end plate region where two types of end plate activity can be identified. Table 12 lists the characteristics of end plate activity that can be recorded in normal muscle. End plate noise represents nonpropagated end plate depolarization (miniature end plate potentials) caused by random release of transmitter from the motor nerve terminals. End plate spikes are nonpropagated single muscle fiber discharges caused by excitation in the intramuscular nerves.

Spontaneous activity recorded from relaxed muscles that is not from the end plate and continues after the insertional activity has ceased is abnormal. The basic types of spontaneous activity that can be recorded include fibrillation potentials, positive sharp waves, fasciculation potentials, myokymic discharges, and complex repetitive discharges.

Fibrillations are action potentials that arise spontaneously from single muscle fibers. These po-

Table 12
Normal spontaneous activity

Parameter	End Plate Noise	End Plate Spikes
Amplitude	10-15 μV	100-200 μV
Duration	1-2 ms	3-5 ms
Frequency	20-40 Hz	5-50 Hz
Firing interval	Irregular	Irregular
Sound	Hissing	Crackling
Waveform	Monophasic (negative)	Biphasic (initial negative)

(Reproduced with permission from Sethi RK, Thompson LL: *The Electromyographer's Handbook,* ed 2. Boston, Little, Brown, 1989, p 128.)

tentials usually occur rhythmically and are thought to be due to oscillations of the resting membrane potential in denervated fibers. They are typically biphasic or triphasic waveforms that are distinguished from end plate potentials by their initial positive phase and the high-pitched repetitive click that can be heard when the recordings are listened to over the loudspeaker. Other waveform characteristics are listed in Table 13.

Positive sharp waves often are found in association with fibrillation potentials, but tend to precede them in appearance after a nerve lesion. Positive sharp waves arise from single fibers that have been injured. Their waveform consists of an initial positive phase followed by a slow negative phase that is much lower in amplitude and much longer (~10 ms) in duration.

Fibrillation potentials and positive sharp waves are found in denervated muscle, but may not appear for three to five weeks after the nerve lesion. They are most often seen in neurogenic lesions affecting the motoneurons, spinal roots, plexus, or peripheral nerves. They remain until the muscle fibers become reinnervated or the fibers become fibrotic. Fibrillation potentials alone are not diagnostic of denervation, because they occur in primary muscle diseases such as polymyositis and muscular dystrophy. Because these potentials can be found in healthy muscles, pathologic significance should not be attributed to their appearance unless they are detected in at least three different sites within the muscle.

Fasciculation potentials are caused by the spontaneous discharges of a group of muscle fibers representing a whole or part of a motor unit, and usually produce a visible twitching in the muscle. Fasciculation potentials most commonly occur in diseases of the anterior horn cells. Grouped fasciculation potentials result from the discharge of multiple units and commonly occur in amyotrophic lateral sclerosis, progressive spinal muscular atrophy, or other degenerative diseases of the anterior horn cells such as poliomyelitis and syringomyelia. These discharges are referred to as myokymic discharges. During these discharges, multiple units fire repetitively, usually two to 10 spikes at a frequency of 30 to 40 Hz, recurring at regular intervals of 0.1 to 10 seconds. Myokymic bursts are thought to be generated ectopically in demyelinating motor nerve fibers.

EMG Activity During Voluntary Movements

Individual motor unit potentials can be measured during submaximal voluntary contractions using EMG electrodes. The motor unit action potential (MUAP) represents the summated electrical activity of the muscle fibers innervated by a single motoneuron that are within the recording range of the electrode. MUAPs are generally triphasic waveforms (Fig. 52) that are characterized by their shape, amplitude, and duration. With careful electrode placement and a patient who is able to control a minimal effort, a single MUAP can be recorded.

For quantitative measurements, two to three motor units that can be clearly identified are recorded from each site. Several sites can be examined from a single needle insertion by advancing or withdrawing the needle in small steps and changing the direction of the needle. Typically, amplitude, duration, and shape of the waveform are measured for 20 or more MUAPs in a single patient during mild voluntary contractions. These values are compared with data from the same muscle in age-matched normal subjects examined in the same laboratory under similar recording conditions. The general characteristics of MUAPs in normal subjects are listed in Outline 1.

The rise time is measured from the initial positive to the subsequent negative peak (Fig. 52) and is a measure of the distance between the EMG electrode and the muscle fibers generating the major spike potentials. It should be less than 500 ms for

Table 13
Spontaneous activity with denervation

Parameter	Fibrillations	Positive Sharp Waves
Amplitude (peak to peak)	20-300 μV (<1 mV)	20-300 μV(<1 mV)
Duration	1-5 ms	10-30 ms (<100 ms)
Frequency	1-50 Hz	1-50 Hz
Firing interval	Usually regular	Usually regular
Sound	Crisp clicks	Dull popping
Waveform	Biphasic and triphasic (initial positive, then sharp negative)	Biphasic (initial sharp positive, then long negative wave)

(Reproduced with permission from Sethi RK, Thompson LL: *The Electromyographer's Handbook,* ed 2. Boston, Little, Brown, 1989, p 129.)

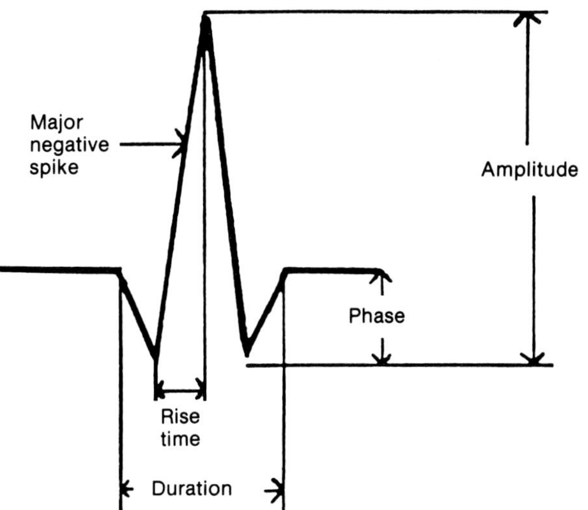

Figure 52
Measured parameters of a motor unit action potential (MUAP). (Reproduced with permission from Sethi RK, Thompson LL: *The Electromyographer's Handbook,* ed 2. Boston, Little Brown and Company, 1989, p 136.)

Outline 1
Characteristics of motor unit action potentials in normal subjects

Amplitude:	Variable (up to 3 mV)
Duration:	Variable (< 15 ms)
Frequency:	Depends on degree of effort (up to 50 per second)
Shape:	Biphasic or triphasic, 5% to 12% polyphasic (more than four phases)
Firing pattern:	Semirhythmic
Sound:	Sharp and crisp

the MUAP to be acceptable for measurements. The amplitude of the major spike is determined primarily by those muscle fibers that are within a 1-mm radius of the recording electrode. In general, the higher the amplitude, the closer together are the muscle fibers belonging to the unit. Hence, the amplitude assists in determining the muscle fiber density within a motor unit. The duration measured from the initial deflection from the baseline to final return to the baseline reflects the activity of most of the muscle fibers in the motor unit and is a good indicator of motor unit territory. The shape of the waveform also is used for diagnostic purposes. An increase in the percentage of polyphasic potentials suggests desynchronized discharge or drop-off of individual fibers within a motor unit. The changes in the motor unit potential in myopathic and neuropathic disorders will be discussed at the end of this section.

Another way to measure changes in the structural and functional properties of motor units is the assessment of recruitment patterns during submaximal and maximal voluntary contractions. According to the size principle, small tension units are recruited before large tension units. As the demand for tension increases, the units that already are recruited increase their rate of firing, and additional units are recruited. The recruitment frequency is defined as the firing frequency of a unit at the time an additional unit is recruited. In normal subjects, the recruitment ratio (the average firing frequency divided by the number of active units) should not exceed five. An increase in the ratio suggests a loss of motor units.

The interference pattern is the electrical activity recorded from a muscle during full effort. With maximal contractions, a complete or full interference pattern is recorded, implying that individual units cannot be recognized. The average amplitude of the cumulative response is an estimate of the number of firing units. In disorders that reduce the number of excitable motor units, the recruitment of additional units as force demand increases is limited; therefore, the surviving units must fire at an inappropriately high rate to compensate for the loss in number of units. In paralysis resulting from upper motoneuron lesions, the firing frequency during maximal contractions is generally lower than expected. In myopathies, the motor units are smaller in size than normal; consequently, a greater number of units are recruited to produce a given submaximal force. In advanced myogenic disorders, recruitment patterns are similar to those observed in neurogenic disorders because of the loss of entire motor units.

Single-Fiber EMG

In conventional EMG, a concentric or monopolar electrode is used to study the temporal and spatial relationship of action potentials from a restricted number of muscle fibers within a motor unit. Several other techniques recently have been developed to examine the activity of individual muscle fibers and motor end plates, the territory of a motor unit, and the cumulative activity of the whole motor unit. These techniques include single-fiber, scanning, and macro EMG.

Single-fiber EMG can be used to assess both the density of motor unit fibers and neuromuscular transmission. The electrode consists of a 0.5-mm steel cannula with one to 14 platinum wires, each

25 μm in diameter, exposed in a side port a few millimeters behind the tip (Fig. 53). The small size of the electrode surface allows selective recording of one muscle fiber. Under certain conditions, the activity from two fibers belonging to the same unit can be recorded and neuromuscular transmission can be studied (Fig. 53). The time interval between the two action potentials varies between consecutive discharges. This variability, called jitter, results primarily from the variability in transmission time in the two motor end plates being recorded. Jitter is expressed as the mean consecutive difference (MCD). The MCD is the mean value of the differences between interpotential intervals of consecutive discharges and is calculated as

$$MCD = [D1 - D2] + [D2 - D3] + ...+ [D (n - 1) \quad Dn] / n - 1$$

where D = individual interpotential intervals and n = the number of discharges.

At least 50 discharges for each fiber pair and a minimum of 20 pairs should be analyzed when the abnormalities are minimal. Normal values for jitter range from 20 to 50 μs, but occasionally can be as low as 5 μs. Increased jitter is observed in myasthenia gravis and following reinnervation.

Single-fiber EMG can also provide information regarding the local distribution or density of motor unit fibers that are within a 300-μm uptake radius of the recording electrode. The electrode is placed close to one active fiber, and the number of synchronously firing fibers is counted. To be counted, an action potential must have an amplitude exceeding 200 μV and a rise time less than 300 μs. The fiber density of a unit is calculated by taking measurements at 20 different sites within the motor-unit territory. In the extensor digitorum communis in young adults, the density is normally less than 1.5. After reinnervation, the density of motor unit fibers usually increases (Fig. 54).

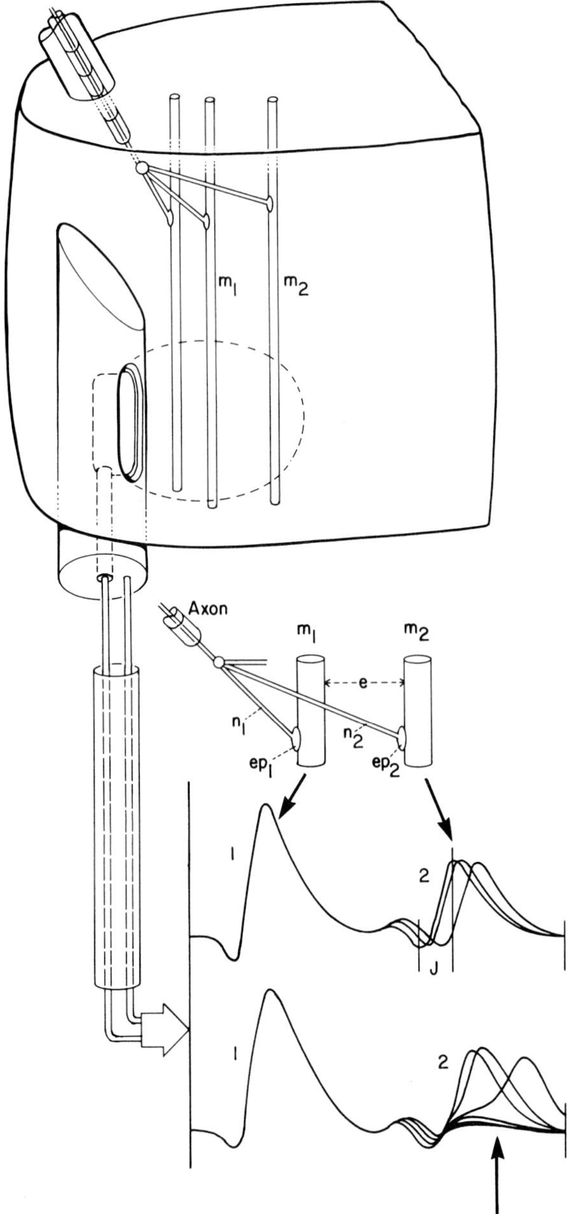

Figure 53
Single-fiber electromyography. Paired single-fiber action potentials are studied by using one to trigger a sweep. This permits the variation between the pair (J = "jitter") to be measured (upper record), and "blocking" to be demonstrated (arrow, bottom record). (Reproduced with permission from Liveson JA, Ma DM: *Laboratory Reference for Clinical Neurophysiology*. Philadelphia, FA Davis Co., 1992, p 373.)

Evaluation of Neuromuscular Disorders

Nerve lesions can affect either the axon or the myelin and can predominate in motor or sensory axons. Localized peripheral nerve lesions are characterized by three basic types of abnormalities: (1) reduced amplitude with normal or slightly increased latency; (2) increased latency with relatively normal amplitude; and (3) absent responses. Table 14 summarizes some of the patterns observed.

Axonal Neuropathies

Axonal neuropathies involve axonal degeneration and are characterized by reduced sensory and motor amplitudes with only mild slowing of the conduction velocities and latencies. The reduction in conduction velocity is generally less than 40% of the normal mean. Diabetes and alcohol abuse are the most common causes of axonal neuropathies. Most neuropathies affect motor and sensory fibers, but selective involvement of sensory fibers can occur with lesions affecting only the dorsal root ganglia.

Demyelinating Neuropathies

Demyelinating neuropathies are characterized by slowing of conduction velocities and latencies,

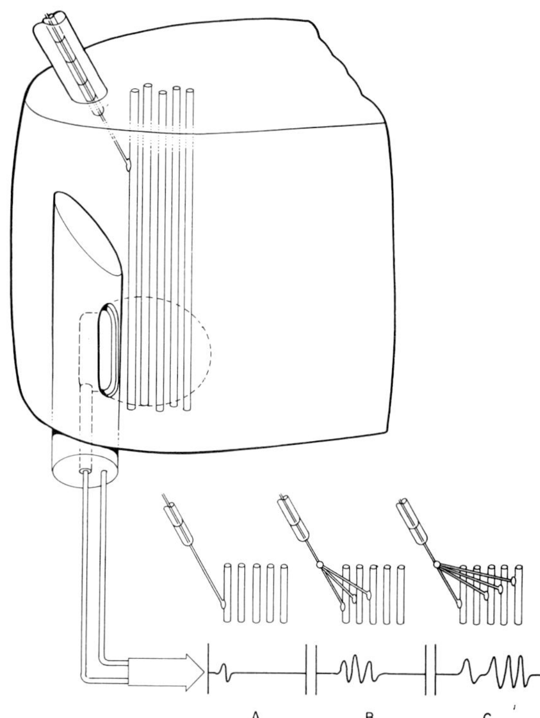

Figure 54
Fiber density studies. With the use of a single-fiber electromyography needle, multiple readings are taken of the number of single-fiber action potentials subtended by the field of the needle. These reflect the number of muscle fibers triggered by a single axon. Increasing reinnervation is represented in the figure from left (A) to right (C). (Reproduced with permission from Liveson JA, Ma DM: *Laboratory Reference for Clinical Neurophysiology.* Philadelphia, FA Davis Co., 1992, p 378.)

Table 14
Patterns of Abnormality in Nerve Conduction Studies of Peripheral Neuromuscular Disorders

	Motor Nerve Studies				Sensory Nerve Studies		
	Action Potential*				Action Potential		
Disorder	Amplitude	Duration	Conduction Velocity	F-Wave Latency	Amplitude	Duration	Conduction Velocity
Axonal neuropathy	↓	Normal	>70%	Mild ↑	↓↓	Normal	>70%
Demyelinating neuropathy	↓ proximal	↑ proximal	<50%	↑	↓	↑proximal	<50%
Mononeuropathy	↓	↑	↓	↑	↓↓	↑	↓
Regenerated nerve	↓	↑	↓	↑	↓	↓	↓
Motor neuron disease	↓↓	Normal	>70%	Mild ↑	Normal	Normal	Normal
Neuromuscular transmission defect	(↓)	Normal	Normal	Normal	Normal	Normal	Normal
Myopathy	(↓)	Normal	Normal	Normal	Normal	Normal	Normal

*↑, increase; ↓, decrease; ↓↓, greater decrease; (↓), occasional decrease.

including those of late responses such as F-waves. The slowing of conduction velocity is often greater than 40% of the normal mean. Values $<$ 40 m/s in the upper extremity and $<$ 30 m/s in the lower extremity are suggestive of demyelinating neuropathy. Slow conduction and dispersion can also be observed in immature regenerating axons.

Myopathies

Myopathies are characterized by motor unit potentials that have small amplitudes and short duration and are polyphasic (Table 15). These changes are related to a loss of muscle fibers within the motor units. There is rapid recruitment of motor units with a complete interference pattern of reduced amplitude on weak effort. Fibrillations and positive sharp waves can be seen in inflammatory myopathies, muscular dystrophies, and some toxic myopathies.

The electrophysiologic approach to the diagnosis of specific clinical disorders will be outlined next. These descriptions are taken from *The Electromyographer's Handbook.*

Table 15
Typical motor unit action potential characteristics

	Myopathy	Normal	Neuropathy
Duration	< 5 ms	5-16 ms	> 16 ms
Amplitude (mean)	< 200 μV	200-400 μV	> 400 μV
Waveform	Polyphasic	Triphasic	Polyphasic

(Reproduced with permission from Sethi RK, Thompson LL: *The Electromyographer's Handbook*, ed 2. Boston, Little, Brown, 1989, p 142.)

Motoneuron Diseases

EMG examination is the most useful test for evaluation of the motoneuron diseases. To diagnose diffuse degenerative diseases of α motoneurons, widespread and progressive neurogenic changes must be demonstrated, which could not result from a focal structural spinal cord lesion. The following criteria can be used as guidelines.

The EMG shows abnormal spontaneous activity with fibrillations, positive sharp waves, and fasciculations. The motor unit potentials are reduced in number and increased in amplitude and duration, and there is an increased incidence of polyphasic potentials. These changes should be demonstrated in at least three extremities based on study of two or three muscles in each limb innervated by different nerves and roots.

In addition, motor conduction, including F-wave and H-reflex latencies, is either normal or shows mild slowing, and reduction of conduction velocity is less than 40% of the normal mean. Finally, sensory nerve conduction studies are normal.

Radiculopathy

The relative inaccessibility of roots and plexuses make radiculopathies difficult to diagnose. EMG examination is generally used rather than nerve conduction studies. Objective abnormalities on EMG may be absent if only the sensory roots are involved or if the lesion is purely demyelinating. Positive EMG examinations have a 70% to 95% correlation with myelograms. Clinical and EMG abnormalities caused by single-root lesions are generally partial because of multisegmental innervation. The following criteria can be used as guidelines.

The EMG diagnosis must demonstrate that denervation activity or chronic motor unit recruitment changes are restricted to a single root. The abnormalities should be documented in at least two or more limb muscles innervated by the same root but different peripheral nerves and absent in muscles not innervated by that root. Fibrillation potentials take two to five weeks to develop, whereas reinnervation changes take at least six to eight weeks after the onset of symptoms. Neurogenic changes start in the more proximal muscles and progress to the distal muscles. Reduced recruitment with increased firing frequency may be seen even before other EMG findings have developed.

Paraspinal muscle involvement is corroborative evidence of a proximal lesion, but its absence does not exclude a radiculopathy. Segmental sensory stimulation of appropriate cutaneous nerves is normal in spite of any sensory loss, because the peripheral sensory axons remain intact with preganglionic lesions. F-wave latencies are usually normal because the short involved segment is diluted by a long, normally conducting distal segment, but the H-reflex is often abnormal in S-1 root lesions.

Entrapment Neuropathies

Mononeuropathies resulting from mechanical compression are referred to as entrapment neuropathies. The pathophysiology is focal demyelination, with secondary axonal degeneration as severity of compression increases. The three most common entrapment neuropathies are (1) median nerve at the wrist, (2) ulnar nerve at the elbow, and (3) common peroneal nerve at the fibular head. A combination of a nerve entrapment and a radiculopathy (for example, carpal tunnel and a C-6 or C-7 radiculopathy) is not uncommon and is sometimes referred to as the double crush syndrome. Entrapments are characterized by the following electrophysiologic findings.

Focal slowing of conduction and/or conduction block is seen across the suspected site of the entrapment (Fig. 55). Sensory conduction studies across the entrapment are generally more sensitive than motor studies. Reduced motor and sensory amplitudes to stimulation distal to the entrapment indicate the severity of compression because they are a reflection of the amount of axonal degeneration. Moreover, with axonal degeneration, EMG evidence is seen of denervation and/or reinnervation restricted to the muscles innervated by the entrapped nerve distal to the site of entrapment.

Traumatic Neuropathies

Nerve conduction studies can assist in distinguishing between the three major types of nerve injuries: neurapraxia, axonotmesis, and neurotmesis. Table 16 lists the sequence of posttraumatic findings on electrophysiologic testing.

With neurapraxia there is immediate conduction block across the site of injury with normal conduction distally. With severe trauma, there is focal demyelination without disruption of the axons, and slowing of the conduction velocity can be demonstrated across the lesion.

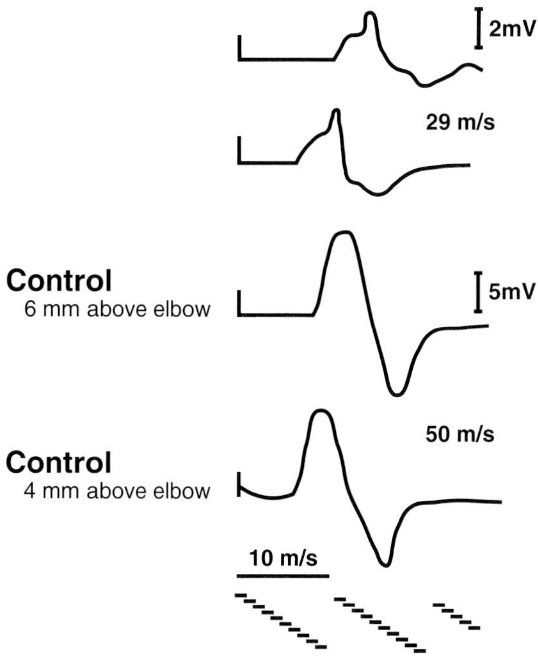

Figure 55
Ulnar entrapment neuropathy with stimulation 6 cm above (**top**) and 4 cm below (**top center**) the ulnar sulcus. Normal ulnar nerve conduction with same stimulation site is shown below for comparison. (Adapted with permission from Sethi RK, Thompson LL: *The Electromyographer's Handbook,* ed 2. Boston, Little Brown and Company, 1989, p 165.)

Table 16
Sequence of events after traumatic nerve injury

Electrophysiological Abnormality	Timing of Onset
Conduction block across injury site	Immediate
Reduced amplitudes on distal stimulation	> 7 days
Denervation changes on EMG	2-5 weeks
Reinnervation on EMG (partial lesion)	> 6-8 weeks

(Reproduced with permission from Sethi RK, Thompson LL: *The Electromyographer's Handbook*, ed 2. Boston, Little, Brown, 1989, p 166.)

With axonotmesis, there is interruption of the axons, resulting in immediate conduction failure across the site of injury. Axonal degeneration occurs distally; however, conduction velocity is preserved distal to the injury site for up to seven days. There is a decline in amplitude of evoked responses on distal stimulation during the first week, progressing to complete failure of neuromuscular transmission. Denervation activity with fibrillation and positive sharp waves appears in the affected muscle in two to five weeks, depending on the distance from the injury site.

With neurotmesis, there is interruption of the entire nerve trunk. The electrophysiologic findings are identical to those seen with axonotmesis, but regeneration does not occur as expected and, therefore, surgical repair of the nerve is required.

Traumatic Nerve Injury

Localized nerve injuries fall into two main categories: (1) those causing a temporary block of nerve conduction at the site of injury without loss of axon continuity, and (2) those in which axons are severed or damaged to a degree that causes axonal degeneration below the site of injury and for a variable distance above the injury. The reaction to the second category of injury proceeds in two phases. In the first phase, the axon and the myelin sheath disintegrate along the entire distance distal to the site of injury and for some distance proximal to the site of injury. These changes, referred to as Wallerian degeneration, result in the separation of the neuron cell body from the target organ; that is, denervation. Depending on both the injury's location along the axon and its severity, the cell body may respond by regeneration of the injured axon or by its own degeneration, that is, cell death. In most instances, the cell body's reaction is one of axonal elongation and restoration of axon continuity with the peripheral target organ. The details of axonal degeneration and regeneration will be discussed in a later section. The degree to which functional recovery occurs depends on several variables, including whether or not the endoneurial tubes have been transected or damaged.

Classification of Nerve Injuries

Prior to World War II, nerve injuries were categorized according to general terms such as contusion, concussion, stretch, compression, laceration, and division. In 1943, three classifications were introduced based on the pathology of the nerve fiber and nerve trunk: neurapraxia, axonotmesis, and neurotmesis. In 1951, a classification scheme was introduced, which included the three types listed above, but added two additional categories. This classification scheme describes five degrees of nerve injury increasing in severity from loss of conduction through loss of continuity of the entire nerve trunk (Fig. 56). This classification scheme is based on the histopathology of the nerve rather than the cause of the injury. Each of these injuries can be caused by a variety of agents; for example, mechanical, thermal, chemical, and ischemic. The site of injury may be localized to a short segment of the nerve or it may extend over a considerable length. A description of the degrees in this scheme follows.

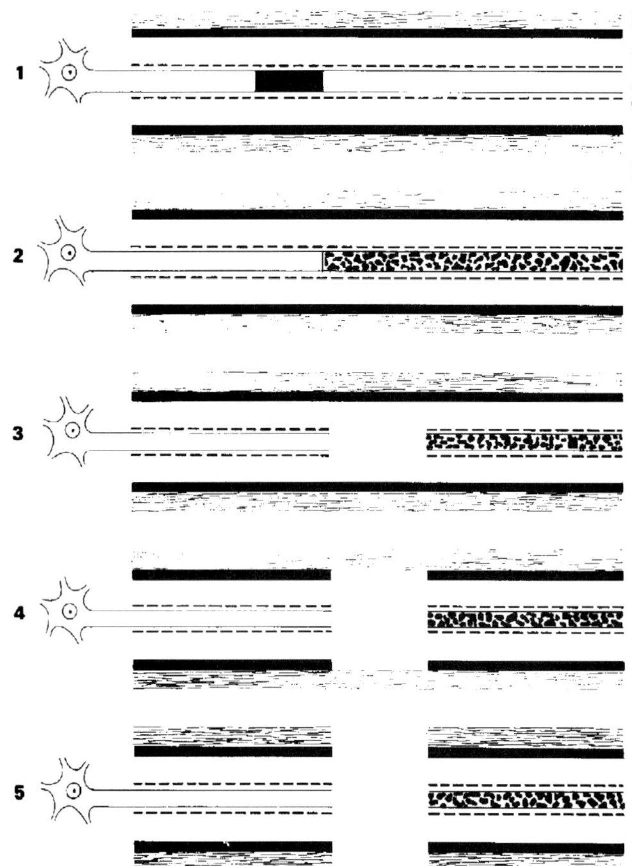

Figure 56
Diagram illustrating the five degrees of nerve injury. 1. Conduction block. 2. The lesion confined to the axon within an intact endoneurial sheath and resulting in Wallerian degeneration. 3. Loss of nerve fiber continuity (axon and endoneurial sheath) inside an intact perineurium. 4. Loss of fascicular continuity with nerve trunk continuity depending solely on epineurial tissue. 5. Loss of continuity of the entire nerve trunk. (Adapted with permission from Sunderland S: *Nerve Injuries and Their Repair: A Critical Appraisal.* New York, Churchill Livingstone, 1991, p 222.)

First Degree Injury

The first degree injury corresponds to neurapraxia and is characterized by an interruption of conduction at the site of injury. The severity of the injury, as measured by the duration of the conduction loss, is influenced by the magnitude of the deforming force, the rate of application of the force, the time over which it acts, and the manner in which it is applied. Conduction blocks are classified as either brief, mild, or severe and have the following characteristics in common: (1) the lesion is localized, (2) the continuity of the axon is preserved, (3) there is no Wallerian degeneration, and (4) all changes are reversible providing the offending agent is removed. As a general rule, motor fibers are more susceptible to injury than sensory fibers, and large myelinated fibers are more susceptible than fine or nonmyelinated fibers. Motor and sensory nerve fibers generally fail sequentially in the following order: motor, proprioceptor, touch, temperature, and pain. Recovery occurs sequentially in the reverse order.

The principle causes of conduction block are mild compression and ischemia. The mechanisms responsible for the cessation of conduction across a localized segment of nerve are not fully understood. This cessation probably is related to pathologic changes resulting from mechanical trauma and/or impaired blood supply, which could alter the ionic composition, nutrient supply, energy metabolism, and/or axonal transport and could produce segmental demyelination.

In first degree injury, there is conduction above and below the lesion, but not across the lesion. There is complete or partial loss of motor function depending on the number of motor nerves affected. However, there are no fibrillation or denervation changes in the affected muscles. In a severe first degree injury, in addition to loss of motor function, there may be loss of all forms of sensation in those areas innervated by the injured nerves. Frequently, however, the only sensory defect that can be detected is loss of proprioception. There is complete functional recovery after first degree injuries because axonal continuity is preserved and the changes responsible for the conduction loss are fully reversible. Full restoration of function may take as long as three to four months after the injury. A residual motor deficit indicates a loss of axons and suggests a more severe injury.

Second Degree Injury

The second degree injury corresponds to axonotmesis. These injuries involve severe damage or severance of the axon, leading to Wallerian degeneration. The continuity of the endoneurial sheath and the basal lamina of the Schwann cell layer is maintained. Consequently, the axon regenerates within its original endoneurial tube and is guided back to its original target, thereby ensuring complete and functional restoration of motor and sensory functions.

A second degree injury results in complete loss of motor and sensory functions. The distal segment can be electrically activated immediately after the lesion; however, conduction distal to the lesion is lost within 24 to 72 hours after the injury. Fibrillation and other electromyographic signs of denervation are evident in the muscles, and the denervated muscles begin to atrophy. The interval between injury and the onset of recovery is influenced by the severity and the level of the injury because regenerating axons must elongate over a greater distance after proximal as opposed to distal lesions.

The next three classifications correspond to divisions of the neurotmesis classification of nerve injury. The injuries progress from damage to the axon and endoneurial tube, to damage to the perineurium and fascicular organization, to complete severance of the epineurium.

Third Degree Injury

The third degree injury involves degeneration of the axons and loss of endoneurial tube continuity. The internal structure of the fascicle is disorganized; however, the arrangement of the individual fascicles is preserved, that is, the perineurium remains intact. Intrafascicular damage may include hemorrhage, edema, and ischemia. Intrafascicular fibrosis may occur, which can seriously impede axon regeneration and elongation across the injury site. If the axons are injured at proximal levels (close to the spinal roots), loss of axons may be caused by degeneration of the cell bodies within the spinal cord.

A third degree injury results in complete loss of motor and sensory functions in the region served by the nerve. The onset of recovery is delayed for longer periods than in second degree injuries because of the more severe retrograde disturbances to the cell body and the additional time taken by the regenerating axons to traverse the disorganized and possibly fibrotic internal structures of the fascicles. In addition, the muscles remain in a denervated state for a longer period of time and, consequently, additional time may be required for functional recovery when the muscles are reinnervated.

The outcome of third degree injuries varies depending on the loss of axons, the extent and severity of intrafascicular fibrosis, and the extent of incomplete and incorrect reinnervation of the denervated muscles. Because of the loss of continuity of the endoneurial tube, axons may be misdirected and reinnervate inappropriate targets. The degree to which inappropriate reinnervation occurs depends on the nerve fiber composition of the affected fascicles. If the nerve fibers within the fascicles innervate the same or functionally similar targets, then the functional outcome will be minimally affected. However, if the fascicles are composed of nerve fibers from functionally unrelated targets and, in particular, if motor and sensory fibers are intermingled, the reinnervation is often misdirected and incorrect leading to poor functional recovery. In general, the more proximal the injury the worse the prognosis for functional recovery because the nerve fibers from distal targets are intermingled and more widely distributed over the fascicles.

Fourth Degree Injuries

In the fourth degree injury, the continuity of the nerve trunk is preserved; however, the fascicles are ruptured or so disorganized that they can no longer be demarcated from the epineurium. Wallerian degeneration follows the usual pattern. The retrograde neuronal effects are more severe than in third degree injuries and, consequently, there is a higher incidence of neuronal cell-body degeneration and axon loss. In addition, axon regeneration and elongation are complicated by extensive intraneural scarring and complete disruption of the fascicular structure. Thus, the number of axons which make it back to their original targets is greatly reduced.

A fourth degree injury results in complete loss of motor and sensory functions in the region served by the nerve. There may be spontaneous regeneration; however, it rarely proceeds in a useful manner. Generally, this type of injury requires excision of the damaged segment and surgical repair of the nerve.

Fifth Degree Injury

A fifth degree injury is one in which there is loss of continuity of the nerve trunk. Generally, the nerve ends remain separated, and varying amounts of scar tissue may form between the cut ends. Often, a neuroma forms on the proximal stump. Wallerian degeneration occurs in the distal stump. Although some axons may regenerate and elongate along the distal stump, the chances for restoring function are minimal because the number of axons that regenerate across the lesion are few in number and the reinnervation is usually incorrect. These types of injuries require surgical nerve repair.

Causes of Nerve Injuries

Nerve injuries can be caused by a variety of agents. A nerve can be damaged by physical trauma in the form of compression, stretch, or friction. Compression is defined as a force applied to the nerve that results in an alteration in the cross-sectional dimensions of the nerve. Stretch or traction is a deforming force applied along the long axis of the nerve, resulting in increases in its length. Friction is applied to a nerve when it rubs across a rough surface or structure. Compression and stretch injuries can be open or closed and can be first through fifth degree injuries. Friction-based injuries are closed injuries; the most common are entrapment nerve lesions.

Nerve injuries can also be caused by ischemia; that is, a reduction in blood supply to the nerve resulting from constriction or obstruction of a blood vessel. Ischemia often is a component of nerve injuries resulting from physical trauma. A nerve can be damaged by therapeutic agents that are inadvertently injected into the nerve or purposely injected into the nerve with the intention of decreasing abnormal activity in the nerve fibers, for example, phenol and lidocaine. Other miscellaneous causes of nerve injury include dislocations, closed and open fractures, high velocity and other missile wounding, childbearing, and compression injuries caused during anesthesia, coma, drug narcosis, and the undisturbed sleep of the fatigued and wasted individual.

Compression Nerve Injury

Nerve compression injuries fall into two major categories: (1) acute injuries of immediate onset and (2) chronic injuries of delayed and gradual onset. The deforming force can be from either an external or internal source. The primary underlying cause of the impaired nerve function in acute and chronic compression lesions is related to a combination of mechanical and ischemic factors.

Categories of Compression Injuries

The extent and severity of the compression lesions are determined by the magnitude and rate of application of the force, the duration over which the force is applied, and the manner in which it is applied. The magnitude of the force can be mild, intermediate, or severe. Mild compression produces first and second degree injuries, intermediate forces produce third degree injuries, and severe forces can cause damage resulting in fourth and even fifth degree injuries. Nerves can tolerate greater magnitudes of force when the deforming force is applied gradually and slowly increases over long periods of time (months and years versus milliseconds and seconds). The manner in which the force is applied (Fig. 57) will also influence the severity of the lesion. The force may be localized to a point on the surface of the nerve, leading to a penetrating or puncture injury; it may slice obliquely or transversely across the nerve; or it may be applied to a length of the nerve and crush or lacerate that segment.

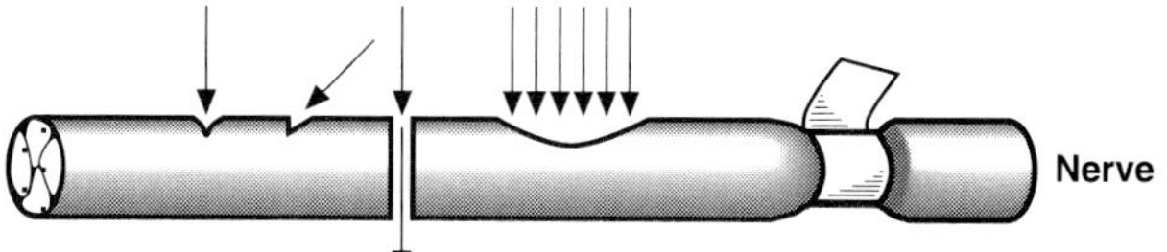

Figure 57
Manner in which compressive force can be applied to nerve. (Adapted with permission from Sunderland S: *Nerve Injuries and Their Repair: A Critical Appraisal.* New York, Churchill Livingstone, 1991, p 131.)

Features That Increase the Vulnerability to Compression Injury

Not all nerve fibers respond the same way to compression. Nerve fibers that are collected into a single or a few large closely packed fascicles with little epineurium are more susceptible to injury than nerve fibers collected into several small fascicles embedded in a large amount of epineurium. This phenomenon is thought to be related to the manner in which the compressive forces are dispersed through the epineurium (Fig. 38). Spinal nerve roots are more vulnerable to compression injury than peripheral nerves because they lack epineurial and perineurial tissues. Within a fascicle, the damage to a nerve fiber may be related to its position, with fibers situated near the surface of the fascicle suffering more than fibers situated more centrally, and size, with large fibers more susceptible than small fibers.

A nerve is at particular risk in areas at which (1) it is in direct contact with an unyielding surface against which it can be compressed, for example, the ulnar nerve behind the medial humeral epicondyle, the radial nerve in the musculospiral groove of the humerus, and the common peroneal nerve near the head of the fibula; (2) it passes through, or is contained within, a compartment with unyielding walls, for example, the median nerve in the carpal tunnel and the lumbar plexus in the psoas compartment; or (3) it is intimately related to a structure that would stretch or compress the nerve if enlarged, for example, aneurysmal swelling of a vessel in contact with the nerve.

Biologic Effects of Pressure

The effects of compression on intraneural tissues are illustrated in Figure 58. In severe acute injuries, the mechanical deformation of the nerve

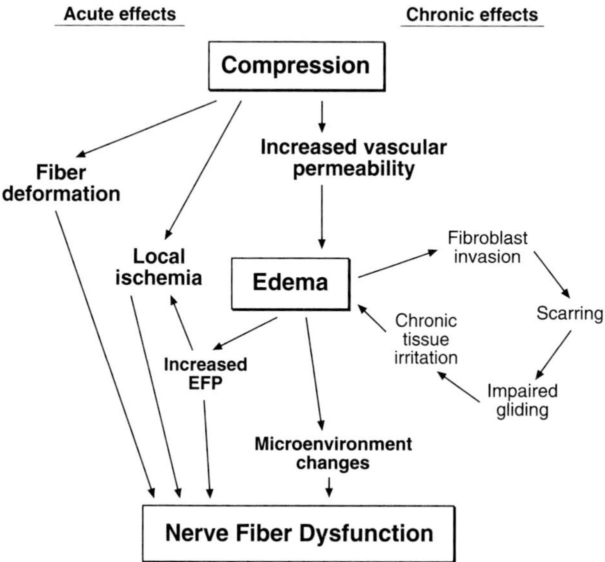

Figure 58
Effects of compression on intraneural tissues. (Adapted with permission from Lundborg G: *Nerve Injury and Repair.* New York, Churchill Livingstone, 1988, p 64.)

fibers is primarily responsible for the pathologic changes in the nerve. In chronic compression, ischemia becomes a significant factor in the genesis of the injury. Delayed secondary effects include edema, hemorrhage, neural fibrosis, and the formation of adhesions that impair the gliding of the nerve.

The mildest compression injury is the prolonged conduction block or first degree injury. In these injuries, the block is rapidly reversible when the deforming force is released, suggesting that it is associated with impaired oxygenation caused by partial or total occlusion of intraneural vessels. Extended periods of vascular occlusion may result in edema, which will extend the period required for recovery. Under higher compressive forces, there is not only vascular obstruction, but also mechanical deformation of nerve fibers and blood vessels. Examples of this type of injury include unrelieved pressure on the radial nerve and tourniquet compression. In these instances, long-lasting conduction block may result from local intraneural edema and segmental demyelination. Severe compressive forces may lead to further damage to the various connective tissues, resulting in third and fourth degree injuries.

Recent studies have addressed the question of critical pressure levels for peripheral nerve viability in humans. Patients who have carpal tunnel syndrome have intracarpal canal tissue pressures of 32 mm Hg as compared to an average pressure of 2.5 mm Hg in control subjects. Based on these data, a human model was developed to study the effects of induced intracarpal pressures of various levels on sensory and motor function of the median nerve. At a tissue pressure of 30 mm Hg in the carpal tunnel, mild neurophysiologic changes and symptoms were found, including paresthesia and a slight increase in latencies. Complete blockage of motor and sensory conduction was found at tissue fluid pressures of 50 to 60 mm Hg. The sensory action potential decreased rapidly and disappeared after 25 to 50 minutes, and the motor potential disappeared 10 to 30 minutes after the disappearance of the sensory potential.

There is experimental and clinical evidence that tourniquet ischemia can cause compression lesions and nerve dysfunction. Cuff pressures sufficient to occlude blood flow in the upper arm result in a block of nerve conduction within 15 to 45 minutes. At a cuff pressure of 150 mm Hg, sensory loss and paralysis develop at the same rate as when a pressure of 300 mm Hg is used, suggesting that ischemia rather than mechanical pressure is the underlying cause of the conduction block. Complications have been reported, which vary from slight disturbances in sensibility to total paralysis involving the median, ulnar, and radial nerves in the forearm and hand. In most cases, complete recovery occurred within three to six months. The majority of cases involved faulty pressure gauges, with the actual applied pressures varying from 350 to 1,200 mm Hg. There are also reports of nerve injuries following the use of a tourniquet to the lower extremity. In a study of 48 arthrotomy patients where the cuff pressure was between 350 and 450 mm Hg, more than 50% had EMG changes postsurgery. In those surgeries that exceeded one hour, 85% of the patients had abnormal EMGs postsurgery. To minimize the effects of tourniquet ischemia on muscle and nerve, it is recommended that the pressure in the cuff used for upper extremity surgery be no more than 50 to 100 mm Hg above the systolic pressure. For lower extremity surgery, twice the systolic pressure is recommended. Tourniquets should not be applied for more than two hours.

External compression of a nerve causes obstruction of intraneural blood vessels, jeopardizing the microcirculation in the nerve. Ischemia induced by compression may cause anoxic and mechanical damage to endothelial cells of the intraneural microvessels, resulting in increased permeability to water, various ions, and proteins. Consequently, ischemia may lead to intraneural edema when the blood flow is restored. The extent of the edema is influenced by the magnitude and duration of the compression. In the rabbit tibial nerve, compression at 50 mm Hg for two hours induced edema that was restricted to the epineurium. Increasing the pressure to 200 mm Hg caused endoneurial edema at the edge of the nerve segment, but not in the center. When the duration was increased to four and six hours at a pressure of 200 mm Hg, endoneurial edema was observed in the center as well as the edges of the compressed segment.

Endoneurial fluid pressure can be measured following ischemia/compression. A threefold increase of pressure was observed after compression at 30 or 80 mm Hg for eight hours. The endoneurial fluid pressure was still elevated to the same level 24 hours after the compression was removed. The increase in pressure was associated with a marked endoneurial edema, with separation of nerve fibers and nerve fiber injury of varying degrees beneath the perineurium. Demyelination of superficial fibers within the fascicles could be seen at pressures of only 30 mm Hg. At higher pressures (80 mm Hg), axonal damage was observed.

The results show that compression causes increases in endoneurial fluid pressures, which parallel the occurence of endoneurial edema. If sustained, such pressure increases have been shown to cause nerve fiber damage, changes in the electrolyte composition of the endoneurial fluid, and impairment of endoneurial capillary blood flow. Compression may also influence nerve function by impairing axonal transport directly through production of a mechanical block or secondarily through induction of anoxia, because both slow and fast transport depend on ATP derived from oxidative metabolism. Several studies have shown that both slow and fast transport are impaired in a graded manner with compression. These results indicate that pressures comparable to those found in patients with carpal tunnel syndrome may interfere with both the slow and fast axonal transport systems. Impairment of axonal transport systems is thought to be partially responsible for the double crush syndrome.

Compression could also induce nerve injury via direct mechanical trauma to the nerve. Extreme tourniquet pressures (1000 mm Hg) have been shown to cause nerve injury to single fibers by displacement of the nodes of Ranvier. The damage was found to be restricted to large, myelinated fibers under the edge of the cuff. In summary, the majority of the data suggest that in chronic compression nerve lesions, the primary pathology is based on vascular complications. However, the contribution of direct physical deformation cannot be disregarded.

Double Crush Syndrome

Patients who have symptoms of a nerve entrapment at one level commonly also have symptoms that indicate compression of the same nerve at another level of the same extremity. Of 115 patients with either carpal tunnel syndrome or ulnar neuropathy, 70% also showed evidence of cervicothoracic root lesions. The term double crush syndrome was introduced to describe this phenomenon. From the clinical observations, it was postulated that a partial lesion at one level of nerve makes the nerve more susceptible to compression at another site. These ideas are not universally accepted, but have raised interesting questions that are being studied.

One of the postulated mechanisms is that proximal compression of a nerve fiber leads to impairments in slow and fast transport. The disruption of axonal transport systems decreases the delivery of cytoskeletal components, such as tubulin and actin and other membrane proteins, to the distal axons. This decrease impairs the quality of the axoplasm as well as the axonal membrane in the distal segment, making the distal nerve more vulnerable to physical trauma, such as compression. The reverse situation may also occur, that is, a distal impingement of a peripheral nerve may contribute to the development of an entrapment neuropathy at more proximal levels. A typical example is ulnar nerve entrapment at the wrist level caused by a local blow to the wrist, which later changes in nature, resulting in symptoms that indicate ulnar nerve compression at the elbow level. Additional explanations for the occurrence of multiple compressive injuries in a nerve include: (1) endoneurial edema proximally affecting neural circulation distally; (2) intrinsic susceptibility of the nerve to compression as a result of diabetes or other peripheral neuropathies; (3) mechanical effects of loss of nerve elasticity; and (4) connective tissue abnormalities.

Nerve Stretch Injuries

Categories and Causes of Stretch Injuries

Nerve injuries caused by traction or stretch fall into two major categories: (1) the acute injury caused by an abrupt application of force of considerable magnitude and (2) the chronic injury in which the nerve is slowly stretched over an extended period of time. Stretch-induced nerve injuries can range from first to fifth degree, the extent and severity of the damage are determined by the magnitude of the force and the rate of deformation. The deforming forces can be arbitrarily assigned one of three magnitudes: mild, intermediate, or violent. In general, mild stretch produces first and second degree injuries, intermediate stretch produces structural damage leading to third degree injuries, and violent stretch causes widespread trauma and tearing resulting in fourth degree injuries or complete loss of continuity. When a nerve is slowly stretched over months or years, it can be stretched well beyond its normal limits and deformed to a remarkable degree without showing symptoms of loss of function. However, if this same nerve is rapidly stretched over milliseconds or seconds, conduction and structural failure can be instantaneous. For example, human nerves stretched at an elongation rate of 7.5 cm/min have an elastic limit at approximately 20% elongation. However, with rapid stretch the elastic limit may be as low as 2% to 4% elongation.

Stretch injuries have a variety of causes. A stretch injury can be caused by the severe displacement of two parts of the body that have a nerve passing between them. For example, stretch injuries of the brachial plexus occur when the arm and shoulder girdle are forcibly displaced in relation to the trunk. Stretch injuries can also occur with joint dislocation or fractures. The passage of a high velocity missile through the limb can create a range of forces within the limb that can stretch the nerves, creating injuries ranging from first degree conduction blocks to gross lacerations and loss of continuity. Stretch on the nerve ends brought together during end-to-end nerve repair may produce stretch lesions at other levels along the nerve. Premature and forcible postoperative extension of a joint immobilized in flexion to permit tension free nerve repair may induce stretch lesions along the nerve or cause rupture at the repair site. Nerve fibers may also experience stretch and compression forces leading to injuries at a point where the nerve is in direct contact with a slowly enlarging aneurysm, cyst, ganglion, or tumor.

Features That Increase the Vulnerability to Stretch Injury

Certain anatomic features increase the susceptibility of a nerve to stretch injuries. Nerve fibers in a nerve with one or a few large fascicles with minimal epineurial tissues are more susceptible to stretch injuries than nerve fibers in a nerve with many small fascicles embedded in a lot of epineurial tissue. A nerve that crosses the extensor aspect of a joint is under tension during full flexion and vulnerable to injury. Examples of this include the ulnar nerve at the elbow and the sciatic nerve at the hip joint. A nerve in close proximity to a joint is predisposed to stretch injury when the joint is dislocated. Nerves at risk include the axillary nerve with dislocation of the shoulder, the median and ulnar nerves at the elbow, and the common peroneal nerve at the knee joint.

Nerve Elasticity

Information regarding the sequence of events that occurs with nerve stretch is important in understanding the nature and prognosis of the lesion (Fig. 59). When first stretched, a nerve elongates rapidly and easily as the slack in the nerve trunk and its fascicles is taken up and the undulations are eliminated. Although the epineurium assists in maintaining the undulations in the nerve trunk, the component primarily responsible for the tensile strength and elasticity of the nerve is the perineurium. As stretching continues, the nerve fibers become taut and are stretched with the perineurium. As the

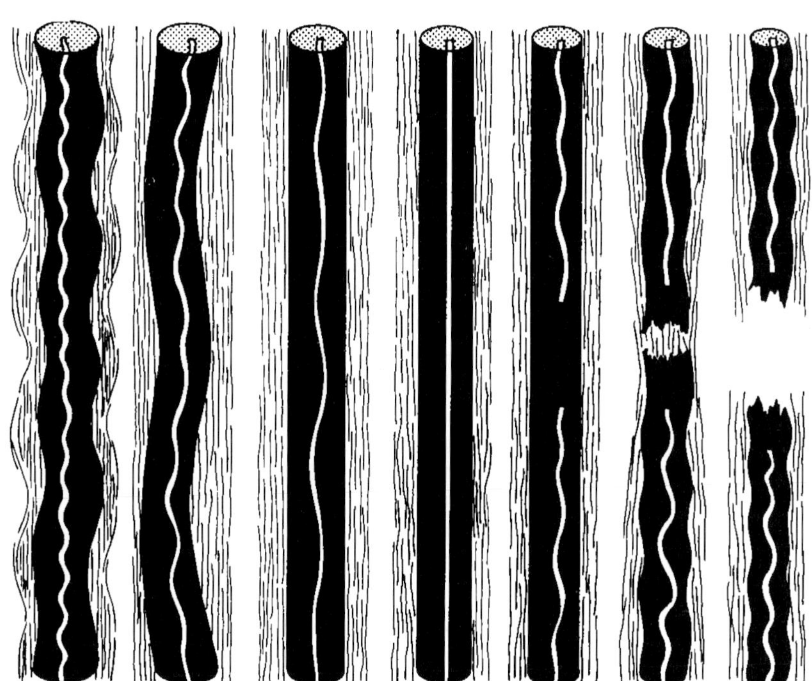

Figure 59
Diagram illustrating the changes occurring in a nerve as it is gradually stretched to mechanical failure. For simplification only one fasciculus and one nerve fiber are shown. (Reproduced with permission from Sunderland S: *Nerve Injuries and Their Repair: A Critical Appraisal.* New York, Churchill Livingstone, 1991, p 148.)

fascicles are stretched, their cross-sectional area is reduced, raising the intrafascicular pressure and leading to compression deformation and ischemia. As elongation approaches the elastic limit, nerve fibers begin to rupture inside the fascicles (second degree injury). With increasing stretch, the endoneurial tubes rupture within the fascicles (third degree injury), and then the perineurium tears (fourth degree injury). Further stretching results in tearing of the epineurium and loss of continuity (fifth degree injury). The rupture of nerve fibers and fascicles can occur over a considerable length of the nerve. These injuries are associated with extensive intrafascicular damage and fibrosis, which can impede regeneration.

A contrasting sequence of events in which the epineurium is the first tissue to rupture has been presented based on experimental data. According to this theory, damage to the nerve caused by stretching up to the elastic limit corresponds to neurapraxia or axonotmesis. At the limit of elasticity, the epineurium ruptures but the fascicles remain intact and continue to elongate. Further elongation ruptures the perineurium. Ultimately, the nerve fibers rupture, resulting in a loss of continuity.

Neural Degeneration

Trauma to peripheral nerve trunks results in various degrees of nerve fiber injury as described in the previous section. The most serious injury is the complete severance of the nerve trunk. Healing of nerve injuries is unique in that it consists of a process of cellular repair as opposed to tissue repair. In order to reestablish function, the neuron cell body must send out new axonal processes, which find the appropriate target organ and establish synaptic connection. Although the number of neurons does not increase, the repair occurs in an environment of intense cellular proliferation (fibroblasts, endothelial cells, Schwann cells, etc.). The initial response to nerve injury is axonal degeneration followed by regeneration (Fig. 60). This section will review changes that occur immediately after the injury, and the discussion will concentrate on changes that occur after the complete severance of a nerve trunk.

Zone of Injury

When a nerve trunk is severed, the two ends retract, and a gap is left between the proximal and distal nerve stumps. Within the first 24 hours after the injury, capillary permeability increases and reaches a peak between days 7 and 14. The increase in capillary permeability is thought to be mediated by serotonin and histamine, which are released from the mast cells during degranulation of the axoplasm. A swelling composed of a disorganized edematous matrix of Schwann cells, fibroblasts, capillaries, macrophages, and collagen fibers soon develops at the end of each nerve stump. Eventually, the growing tips of the proximal axons will enter this swelling and must navigate through this matrix to the distal stump. Many of the axons will be arrested, forming whorls, spirals, and other abnormal endings; others will be deflected back to the proximal stump; and some will find the way to the distal stump. With the passage of time, the zone between the two stumps is converted into scar tissue. During secondary surgical repair of an injury that has severed the two ends, this traumatized zone of injury is resected and the two stumps are reapposed with sutures or a nerve graft.

Wallerian Degeneration

When a nerve fiber is disconnected from its cell body, a series of metabolic and structural events occur in the segment distal to the lesion. The process of Wallerian degeneration involves changes in the axon, myelin sheaths, Schwann cells, and endoneurial collagen.

Axonal Degeneration

The first stage of Wallerian degeneration involves granular disintegration of axoplasmic microtubules and neurofilaments as a result of proteolysis. This process is initiated within hours of the injury. Neural conductance within the distal segment is completely lost within 48 to 96 hours after the injury. All traces of the axon debris are usually lost within two weeks of the injury. The disintegration of the axoplasm appears to be triggered by a large increase in axoplasmic calcium and mediated by calcium-sensitive proteases. In normal nerves, intra-axonal calcium concentration is very low (~0.3 μM). Transection of the nerve fiber results in a rise in the intra-axonal calcium throughout the distal stump. Chelation of calcium in the extracellular fluid delays the time of granular disintegration, suggesting that the entry of extracellular calcium is involved in initiating the axoplasmic degradation.

The breakdown of myelin follows the disintegration of the axoplasm by only hours. Within 36 to 48 hours of the injury, myelin breakdown is well advanced, and within three days myelin fragments are collecting into ovoids. The myelin debris is removed by the phagocytic action of macrophages and Schwann cells, occurring over a one week to three month period. In the final stages of Wallerian degeneration, the interior of the nerve fiber is occupied by an amorphous mass of axon and myelin debris. Axon degeneration begins at the site of injury and progresses distally to the peripheral target organ.

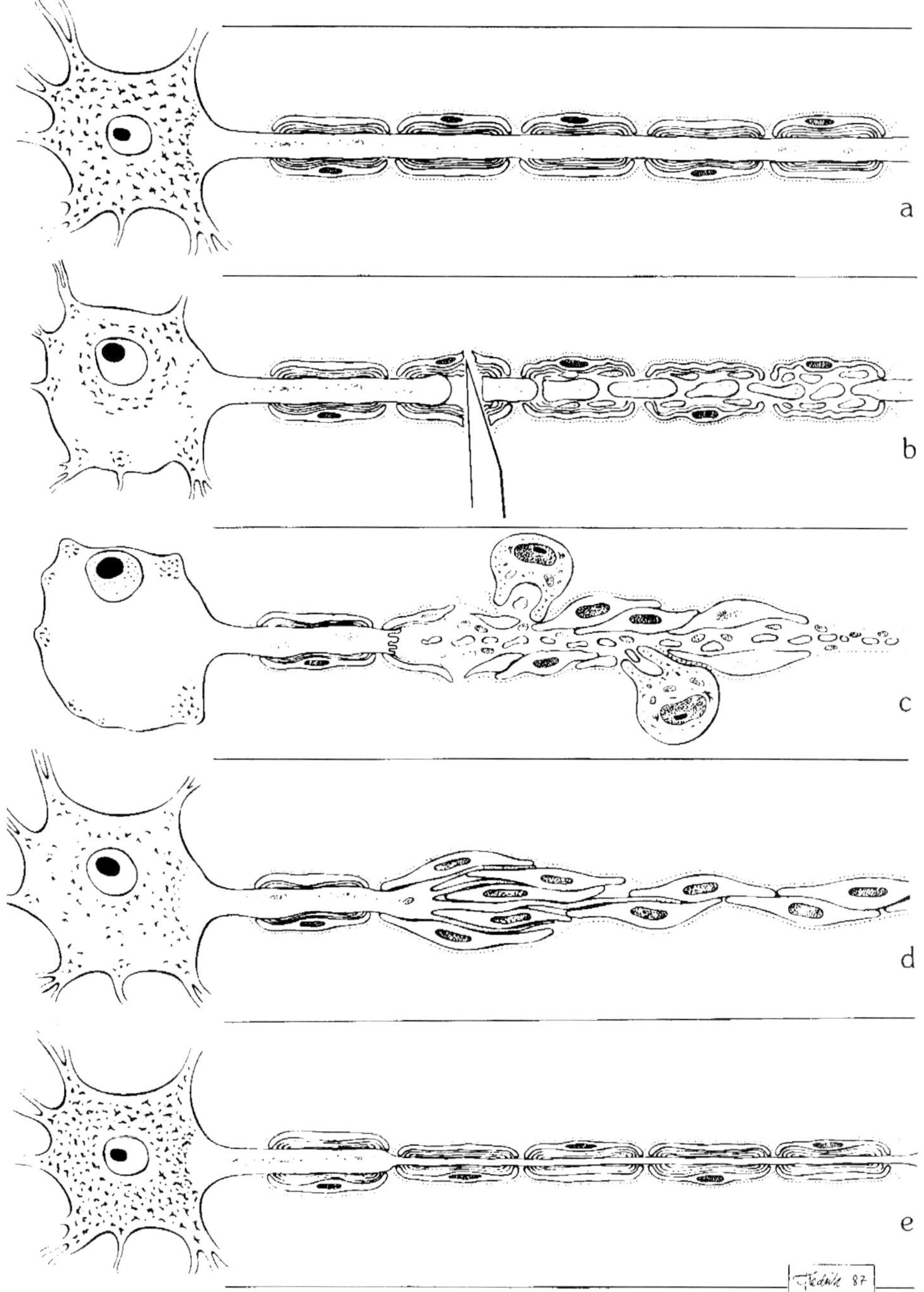

Figure 60
Degeneration and regeneration of myelinated fiber. (a) Normal appearance. (b) Transection of the fiber results in distal fragmentation of axon and myelin. In the proximal segment degeneration occurs at least to the nearest node of Ranvier. (c) In the distal segment Schwann cells proliferate. Macrophages and Schwann cells phagocytose debris material. (d) The Schwann cells in the distal segment have lined up in bands of Büngner. Sprouting occurs from the cut axonal stump. Advancing sprouts are embedded in Schwann cell cytoplasm. (e) "Axonal" connection with periphery, maturation of nerve fiber. Sprouts that do not link up with the periphery may atrophy and disappear. The cell body response during these phases includes swelling, migration of the nucleus to the periphery, and condensation of basophilic material (chromatolysis). (Reproduced with permission from Lundborg G: *Nerve Injury and Repair.* New York, Churchill Livingstone, 1988, p 151).

Schwann Cell Response

The Schwann cells of normal intact myelinated fibers do not divide. Within 24 hours of nerve transection, Schwann cells throughout the distal segment undergo a series of mitoses. Schwann cell proliferation continues for at least two periods, with the peak of mitosis occurring around day 3 after the injury. A second wave of Schwann cell proliferation occurs during the regenerative stage. The stimulus for Schwann cell proliferation is unknown; however, the onset of Schwann cell mitogenesis is synchronous with that of other endoneurial cells, including fibroblasts, endothelial cells, and mast cells. The newly divided Schwann cells maintain cytoplasmic processes that interdigitate and line up in rows beneath the original basal lamina of the nerve fiber. These tubes are referred to as the bands of Bungner. The Schwann cell basal lamina produces fibronectin and laminin, which have been shown to promote the growth of neurites in culture. The proliferating Schwann cells also synthesize nerve growth factor and nerve growth factor receptors. In the absence of axonal growth down the endoneurial tubes or bands of Bungner, the tubes atrophy.

Macrophage Response

After nerve injury (day 1 to 3), there is an accumulation of macrophages around the degenerating fibers. The early macrophages express Ia, the major histocompatibility class II antigen, and are not phagocytic. Once the cells pass through the basal lamina of the degenerating fiber, they lose their Ia expression and become phagocytic. Throughout their cycle, macrophages in Wallerian degeneration express interleukin 1, a cytokine that influences the behavior of the Schwann cells. In particular, macrophage-derived interleukin 1 is required to stimulate Schwann cells to produce nerve growth factor.

Nerve Cell Body Response

When an axon is severed, the nerve cell body goes through structural and functional changes reflecting an alteration in metabolic priority from the production of neurotransmitters needed for synaptic transmission to the production of proteins needed for axonal repair and growth. The degree of the response varies with the severity of the injury, the level of the injury, the type and size of the neuron, whether functional connections are restored, and also age and species. The closer the injury is to the cell body (or the greater the loss of axoplasm), the more severe the reaction. In general, the reaction occurs more rapidly and to a greater degree in sensory than in motor neurons. Within the sensory neuron population, the cell body reaction is more severe in nonmyelinated than myelinated axons.

The response of the cell body can be divided into several phases: a reactive or chromatolytic phase, a recovery phase, and a degenerative phase. The reactive phase includes an increase in cell body volume, displacement of the nucleus to the periphery, and the disappearance of basophilic material from the cytoplasm. This phase is followed by the complete or incomplete recovery of the cell or its degradation. The synthesis of neurotransmitters and neurofilament proteins is decreased, and the synthesis of cytoskeletal proteins such as tubulin and actin is increased. In addition, there is an increase in the synthesis of several growth-associated proteins (GAPs) that promote axonal growth and extension. One specific growth-associated protein that is enhanced is GAP-43.

Proximal Segment Response

With transection of the nerve, axonal degeneration occurs over one or several internodal segments in the proximal stump, leaving the endoneurial tubes of the last centimeter or so of the proximal stump occupied only by Schwann cells. The fate of the axons above the injury depends on whether the cell body survives and regenerates a new axon or degenerates. If the cell body degenerates, the entire proximal length of the axon undergoes Wallerian degeneration. If the cell body survives, the proximal nerve fibers undergo a reduction in axon diameter and myelin thickness that proceeds distally from the cell body. As regeneration proceeds and the axons make functional contact, axon diameter increases but remains smaller than normal. This permanent reduction in axon diameter and myelin thickness is accompanied with a slowing of the conduction velocity.

Within the first few days after transection, proximal myelinated axons produce a great number of collateral and terminal sprouts that advance distally and are confined to the endoneurial tubes until they reach the injury site. The behavior of the axons at this point depends on the degree of the injury. Collateral sprouts arise from the nodes of Ranvier at the level where the axons are still intact, whereas terminal sprouts arise from the tips of the remaining axons (Figure 61). The growing sprouts from a single axon form an anatomic unit called the regenerating unit. The regenerating units consist of clusters of nonmyelinated axons originating from the same myelinated axon and surrounded by a single Schwann cell and its basal lamina. Occasionally, regenerating units are found, which contain several Schwann cells surrounded by a single basal lamina. With time, the average number of sprouts per group diminishes. The reduction in the number of sprouts occurs because some axons fail to make functional contact with a peripheral target.

Axonal Regeneration

Axon Elongation Across the Zone of Injury

Regenerating axons from the proximal stump must cross a critical zone to reach the distal stump. The final success of regeneration depends largely on what happens at this level. When a nerve trunk has been severed, the nerve ends are left separated by a gap or are reunited surgically. In either case, the tissue that develops between the ends is essentially the same, except that the tissue between separated nerve ends is more extensive and usually is denser and more disorganized than is the tissue between surgically reunited nerve ends.

The zone between the stumps is similar to other wound-healing environments. It is characterized by exudation, cell proliferation, and collagen synthesis. Initially, the gap is filled with an exudate containing blood corpuscles and macrophages, and then a fibrin clot is formed. Subsequently, there is an ingrowth of capillaries and fibroblasts from the nerve stumps as well as from surrounding tissues.

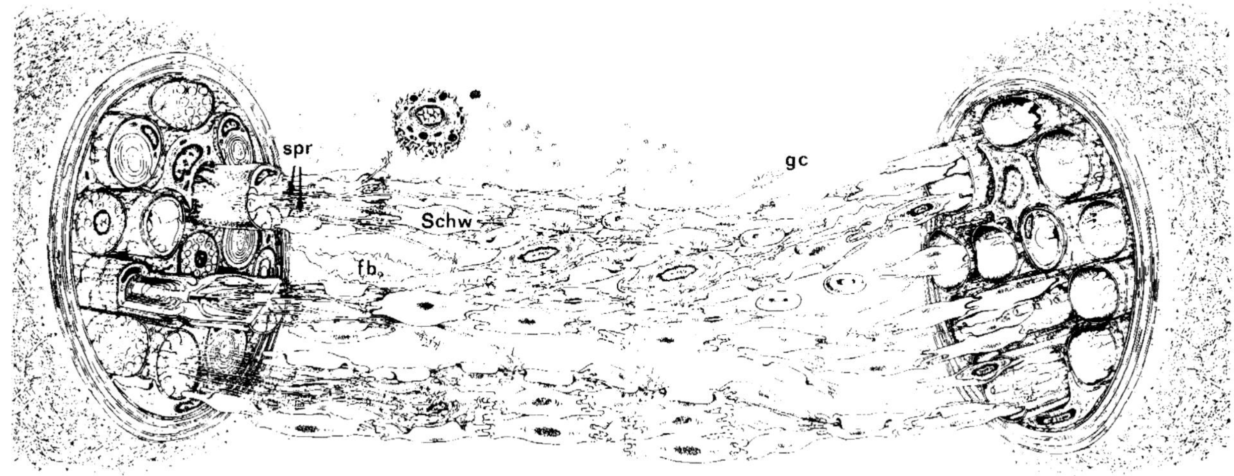

Figure 61
Local cellular response to nerve transection. Schw = Schwann cells; spr = sprouts; fb = fibroblasts; gc = growth cone. (Reproduced with permission from Lundborg G: *Nerve Injury and Repair.* New York, Churchill Livingstone, 1988, pp 152–153.)

Schwann cells migrate into the gap from the proximal and distal stumps, forming columns and groups. The tissue that forms between the stumps is generally not as suitable for growth as that in the endoneurial tubes of the distal segment. In general, the tissue is obstructive to axonal growth and results in delays and misdirection of axonal growth. The direction taken by each growing axon tip is influenced by the structural organization of the medium through which it regenerates. Resistance is minimal where collagen fibrils are organized in parallel. The direction of axonal growth may also be influenced by chemotropic molecules released into the microenvironment of the growing axons. This topic will be discussed in greater detail in the next section.

The overall effect of scar tissue in the zone between the nerve stumps is to: (1) obstruct the advance of some regenerating axons, thereby reducing the number of axons that reinnervate denervated end organs; (2) delay the advance of regenerating axons; (3) retard the development of those axons that have regenerated by delaying and limiting their maturation; and (4) misdirect axons into functionally unrelated endoneurial tubes.

Axon Elongation in the Distal Segment

Regenerating axons that make it across the zone of injury enter endoneurial tubes in the distal segment. Generally, an excess number of sprouts invade the distal segment, resulting in endoneurial tubes occupied by multiple axons (usually from the same parent neuron). The original basal lamina eventually disintegrates, releasing new fibers into the fascicle. With time, however, the number of axons in the distal segment decreases as axons that do not make functional connections with the periphery atrophy and disappear. The excess sprouts in the distal segment suggest that axon counting is not a reliable method for assessing regeneration. In fact, an excess number of axons in the distal segment may be a response to obstacles in the zone of injury and, therefore, is an indication of poor regeneration.

The signal for myelination comes from the regenerating axon. The regenerating axons of an originally myelinated neuron instruct the enveloping Schwann cells of the distal segment to form myelin, while unmyelinated fibers remain unmyelinated even when regenerating into a distal segment originally containing myelinated fibers. The maturation of an axon depends on its innervating the appropriate peripheral target.

The rate of regeneration varies depending on the type and location of the injury. In general, axonal elongation is slower after a complete nerve lesion than after a crush injury. Regeneration rates in nerves from experimental animals range from 2.0 to 3.5 mm/day after transection and repair, and 3.0 to 4.4 mm/day after crush. Regeneration of human peripheral nerves has been reported to be nonlinear, with a gradually decreasing regeneration rate in more distal regions of the limb (Table 17). For example, regeneration rates are faster in the axilla than in the wrist. In humans, an average outgrowth of 1 to 2 mm/day is generally quoted.

Factors Influencing Axonal Regeneration

Neuronal growth consists of several processes including neuron survival, neurite formation, axonal elongation, synaptogenesis, and synthesis of

Table 17
Axonal regeneration rate

Location of Injury	Rate (mm/day)
Rates of uncomplicated axon regeneration	
Root of limb	6.0
Elbow	4-5.0
Wrist	1-2.0
Hand	1-1.5
Lower limb	1-2.0
Ankle	1.0
Rates of axon regeneration after nerve suture	
Lower forearm	2.0
Wrist and hand	1.0
Upper leg	2.0
Lower leg	1.5
Ankle	1.0

neurotransmitters and other related enzymes. The number of neurons that survive, the rate of axonal elongation, and the direction of axonal outgrowth may be influenced by several local and systemic factors, the majority of which are incompletely known. This section will review some factors that may enhance axonal regeneration.

Regeneration Across A Gap: Use of Nerve Guide Tubes

Neurotmesis is an interruption of nerve continuity that leads to Wallerian degeneration and disruption of the endoneurial tubes. Clinically, the preferred technique for the repair of this type of injury is the direct coaptation of the proximal and distal nerve stumps using epineurial sutures. In many cases, however, direct coaptation of the severed ends of a nerve is not possible, and a gap must be bridged. Tubes composed of biologic and synthetic materials, such as arteries, muscle, veins, millipore, collagen, silicone, and various other materials, have been used to provide a guiding structure and an optimal environment for the advancing sprouts. Studies have recently been carried out with the purpose of understanding the cellular and biochemical events occurring during regeneration and to determine if nerve guide tubes provide a better means of bridging a nerve deficit than do nerve grafts.

Experimental data have demonstrated that, in rats and primates, axonal regeneration can occur across gaps of 5 to 15 mm, which have been bridged with either synthetic or biodegradable tubes. The quality of the regeneration usually is assessed by measuring the rate of elongation, the number of sprouts, and/or the maturity of the regenerating axons. These data suggest that contact guidance is extremely important during the early stages of axonal elongation. Axons forced to elongate into an empty chamber will do so only when fluid is injected into the chamber or when the chamber fills with fluid from the external environment. Axonal elongation is enhanced, however, if the fluid in the chamber forms a linear fibrin matrix or the chamber is prefilled with a matrix that supports longitudinal growth of axons. The rate of elongation and the number of axons that regenerate are increased if the tube is filled with laminin and/or other extracellular matrix proteins. Extracellular matrix proteins, such as collagen, laminin, and fibronectin, have been shown to promote the growth of axons in culture. These molecules may play an important role in cell-cell recognition and cell adhesion, which are important processes in axonal outgrowth and guidance. Schwann cells may also play a crucial role in axonal regeneration in that they may provide a source of neuronotropic factor(s).

Neuronotropic Factors

Neuronotropic factors are macromolecular proteins derived from various sources that promote the survival and growth of specific neuronal populations. These factors are present in the target of innervation (muscle or sensory receptor) or in the distal structure to be innervated (distal nerve segment). In the early 1950s a factor was isolated from mouse tumor cells that stimulated the growth of sensory and sympathetic neurons in culture. This factor, called nerve growth factor, was later found to be synthesized in tissues innervated by sensory and sympathetic neurons. Nerve growth factor recently has been found to be synthesized in Schwann cells distal to the site of axonotmesis in rat sciatic nerve and is presumed to have survival and directional effects on the regenerating proximal axons.

Other factors that may promote regeneration after nerve injury are ciliary neuronotropic factor, acidic and basic fibroblast growth factor (aFGF and bFGF), and insulin-like growth factor (IGF). An additional factor, motor nerve growth factor, has been isolated from normal, denervated, and embryonic muscle. These factors may function to enhance regeneration by increasing the survival of neurons or the rate of regeneration, and they may also provide directional cues to regenerating axons. Additional research is needed to determine the exact function of these factors in regeneration.

Axon Promoting Factors

Axon promoting factors are molecules that specifically promote the growth of axons without necessarily influencing neuronal survival. These factors may be: (1) surface-bound to cellular or extracellular structures in the substrate; (2) humeral; or (3) confined to the medium or microenvironment. Surface-bound glycoproteins have been shown to play a significant role in axon extension in vitro and in vivo. One such protein is laminin, which is a major component of the basal lamina of Schwann cells and endothelial cells. The addition of a laminin-collagen gel to a nerve guide tube increases the rate of axonal regeneration across a gap. Another component of the basal lamina that has been shown to promote axon extension is fibronectin. The neuronal response to fibronectin is weaker than that to laminin, and fibronectin does not exert a directional cue as does laminin. Axon promoting factors appear to influence axon outgrowth independently of their ability to affect growth cone adhesion.

Other membrane glycoproteins that influence cell adhesion are nerve cell adhesion molecule and N-cadherin. These molecules are present on axons during development and after injury; antibodies to these molecules reduce the outgrowth of peripheral axons in vitro.

Other Factors

Several other agents have been shown to promote nerve regeneration. Exogenous application of gangliosides, which are a major structural component of the neuronal plasma membrane, has been reported to stimulate axonal sprouting in vivo, to stimulate sprouting at the neuromuscular junction, and to promote axon extension in vitro. Hormones also have been reported to enhance the rate of regeneration. Testosterone has been shown to stimulate regeneration of transected hypoglossal and facial nerves and crushed sciatic nerves. Administration of thyroid hormone (T3) has been reported to increase protein synthesis in the nerve cell body, increase the rate of axonal outgrowth, and improve maturation of regenerating axons. However, it also has been reported that experimentally induced hyperthyroidism does not enhance peripheral nerve regeneration. It has been hypothesized that the protease inhibitor, leupeptin, may enhance regeneration because of its ability to inhibit Wallerian degeneration in the distal segment and reduce the amount of atrophy in denervated skeletal muscles. Administration of leupeptin after transection of the rat sciatic nerve or primate median nerve has been reported to lead to an increase in the number of regenerating axons. Table 18 lists some of the factors thought to play a role in axon elongation and survival. Clearly, axonal growth is influenced by numerous factors. The discovery of factors that can increase the rate of regeneration, the number of surviving axons, and the specificity of reinnervation should lead to better functional recovery after nerve injury.

Table 18
Factors reported to enhance nerve regeneration

Factor	Proposed Mechanism
Nerve growth factor (NGF)	NTF
Ciliary neuronotropic factor (CNTF)	NTF
Motor nerve growth factor (MNGF)	NTF
Fibronectin	NPF
Laminin	NPF
Neural cell adhesion molecule (NCAM)	NPF
N-cadherin	
Hormones	IPS
Estrogen	
Testosterone	
Thyroid hormone	
Insulin	
Acidic fibroblast growth factor (aFGF)	NTF
Basic fibroblast growth factor (bFGF)	NTF
Insulin-like growth factor (IGF)	NTF
Forskolin	IPS
Leupeptin	ITD
Gangliosides	?

NTF: promotes neuron survival; NPF: promotes axonal extension; IPS: Increased protein synthesis; ITD: inhibits traumatic degeneration.

Functional Recovery After Nerve Injury

The outcome of peripheral nerve injuries is quite variable. Variables hypothesized to have an important role in determining the outcome of nerve repair include: (1) the age of the patient; (2) the type of nerve injured; (3) the distance the regenerating axons must grow to reach the target organ; (4) the length of the injury zone; (5) the timing of the nerve repair; (6) the status of the target organ at the time it is reinnervated; and (7) the technical excellence of the surgeon.

Functional recovery is generally complete after a crush injury because the basement membrane and endoneurium are left intact, and the damaged axons can regenerate within their original endoneurial tubes and reinnervate their original target organ. After a complete lesion to the nerve, however, functional recovery of movement is often quite poor. The loss of functional recovery probably is related to the failure of axons to regenerate and the misdirection of regenerating axons, which leads to inappropriate innervation of denervated muscles. Inappropriate innervation is thought to result in a loss in the ability to accurately recruit individual muscles and motor units within a muscle, resulting in the loss of motor control.

Specificity of Reinnervation

Although regeneration of axons across a lesion is a prerequisite for recovery, it is generally believed that their misdirection is primarily responsible for the lack of functional recovery. Specificity of reinnervation can occur at many levels. Specificity at the tissue level is characterized by growth of an axon toward the severed nerve segment as opposed to tendon, muscle, or visceral organs. Once inside the nerve, the axon must move in the appropriate direction at those intersections where the nerve branches, that is, toward a sensory or motor branch or toward one of two major motor branches, such as the peroneal or tibial branch of the sciatic nerve. The axon must then be attracted toward the target organ it is to innervate. Motor nerves may innervate different muscles and sensory nerves may attach to various types of sensory receptors. The final attachment(s) must be made within the target organ. For example, once a motor axon has innervated a muscle, the number and type (that is, fast versus slow) of fibers to be innervated must be determined.

During development, motoneurons find their appropriate targets with remarkable accuracy. This precise patterning of neuronal connections emerges, in part, from the interactions between the growth cones and their cellular environment. The question is, can damaged axons in the adult reach the correct target with the same specificity as developing axons? If not, what can be done to increase the probability of correct reinnervation after injury? Some of the mechanisms thought to be responsible for the generation of specific connections are shown in Figure 62.

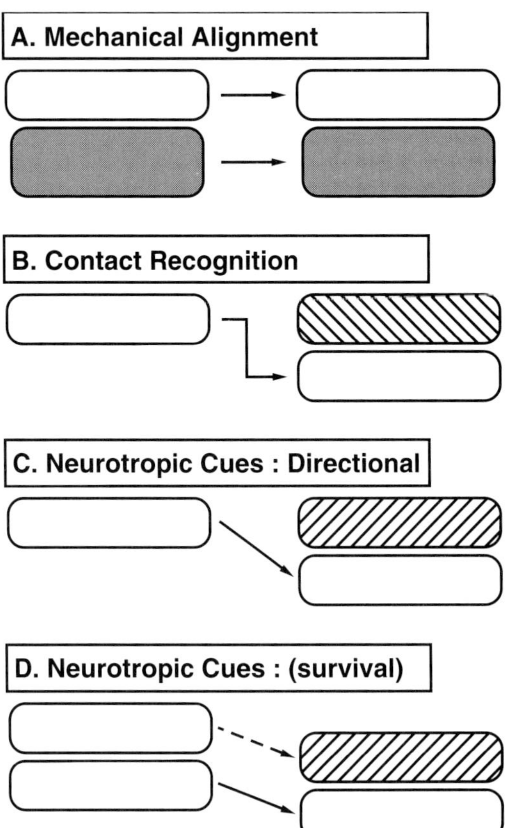

Figure 62
Guidance mechanisms.

Traditionally, the surgeon has attempted to improve specificity by operative alignment of the proximal and distal nerve stumps. The mechanical approach forces axons to take a certain path. If the axon is allowed to explore its environment, humeral mechanisms may also be available to guide it to the appropriate target. Contact recognition permits an axon to select the appropriate path based on the molecular composition of the environment. Axons would selectively propagate down distal tubes that had the appropriate molecular signature. Neurotropism refers to diffusion of factors from distal targets guiding axons to the appropriate target. Neurotrophism refers to a mechanism in which axons randomly grow to a target, and only those entering a correct pathway or innervating the correct target receive a trophic or nutritive factor that allows the axon to continue to develop and become myelinated. Axons that receive no trophic support would degenerate.

Selectivity of reinnervation has been reported to occur after the transection of motor axons in the neonatal rat, whereas, reinnervation in adult rats appeared to be random. It has been suggested that during development there are target-derived cues that serve to guide the motor axons to their correct targets. Target-specific regeneration, however, has been considered impossible in the mammalian adult peripheral nervous system. A high degree of nonselectivity has been shown to occur in rats after section and resuture of the sciatic nerve, as well as in humans after severance and surgical repair of the ulnar nerve branch at the wrist.

Recent evidence suggests that injured axons in mature animals may be capable of detecting and following specific neurotropic cues. A neurotropic factor is a substance that provides directional cues. Studies have shown that a regenerating sprout will preferentially grow towards a tube that contains nerve as opposed to tendon or muscle. Additional evidence of target-specificity has been provided by experiments that demonstrated that motor axons in the proximal portion of a Y-shaped silicone tube preferentially reinnervated the distal branch that contained the motor stump rather than the sensory stump. Moreover, the distance between the proximal and distal stumps was found to be important. Motor axons in the proximal stump of a cut nerve would selectively grow into a distal tube containing a motor stump as opposed to a sensory stump if the cut ends were separated by 5 mm; however, selective innervation was not apparent if the distance between the stumps was only 2 mm.

Several investigators also have shown that selectivity of axon growth occurs at the level of the nerve trunk. Using a Y-shaped Silastic tube, they demonstrated that the proximal stump of the tibial and peroneal branches of the sciatic nerve of the rat and cat preferentially innervated that portion of the tube containing the appropriate distal stump, that is, proximal tibial to distal tibial and proximal peroneal to distal peroneal. These studies raise the possibility that target-specific reinnervation can occur in the adult, given the appropriate conditions.

Muscle Recovery After Denervation

Partial recovery of hindlimb muscles is thought to be a major factor that limits the recovery of motor function after long-term denervation. An inability of the muscle to recover its tension-producing capabilities after reinnervation may be related to (1) a loss of muscle fibers, (2) a loss of motor units, or (3) a loss in the ability to increase muscle fiber size and reverse the atrophy that occurs after denervation. Long-term denervation has been shown to result in both a loss of muscle fibers and increased connective tissue proliferation within the muscle. The ability of a muscle to recover from denervation is thought to be related, in part, to the number of motor axons that reinnervate the muscle. A decrease in the number of axons that reinnervate a muscle may result in fibers remaining denervated and, subsequently, a loss of muscle fibers. However, a reduction in motor axons may not necessarily lead to denervated muscle fibers. The motor axons that reinnervate the muscle may have the capacity to sprout and maintain synaptic connections with more fibers than they would in a normal muscle. This should lead to an increase in the number of large motor units. An increase in motor unit size, that is, mean motor unit tension, has been observed after injury to the sciatic nerve and in muscles that have been partially denervated. A change in the distribution of motor unit tensions may influence the manner in which units are recruited, which, in turn, may cause a deficit in motor control.

The reason for a lack of muscle recovery may also reside in the muscle itself. If the muscle tissue cannot reverse the atrophy that occurs after denervation, the fibers will remain smaller than normal, and tension will not be fully recovered. The inability to recover muscle mass may reside in the satellite cells and their ability to proliferate and increase fiber size. Growth factors such as fibroblast growth factor (FGF), insulin-like growth factor (IGF), and transforming growth factor-β have been suggested to have a role in myogenesis and satellite cell proliferation and differentiation. FGF and IGF have both been shown to stimulate satellite cell proliferation. Moreover, the expression of IGF has recently been shown to be increased in muscles during regeneration after ischemic injury. Further studies are needed to determine the exact role of growth factors during muscle degeneration and regeneration.

Surgical Nerve Repair

Nerves had been distinguished as different from tendons as long ago as the 3rd century BC by Herophilus, who also traced nerves to the spinal cord and separated them into motor and sensory components. The repair of severed nerves, however, was not looked upon with favor until well into the 19th century. The overriding belief from the Middle Ages through the 19th century was that although the ends of transected nerve could join and form a scar, the nerve permanently lost the ability to produce movement. Real progress began in 1795 when Cruikshank showed that anatomic continuity of a severed nerve could be restored by healing, and that the function of the reunited nerve had been restored.

A dramatic change in attitudes toward repairing severed nerves occurred in the second half of the 19th century, with the improvement of the compound microscope and the introduction of improved stains and staining techniques. These permitted study of the fine structure of nerves and their response to injury. The advances that occurred during the 19th century depended primarily on two sets of investigations: the histologic investigations that revealed the fine structure of nerve fibers and experiments that demonstrated that following transection of a nerve, the nerve fibers left attached to the parent cell body survived, whereas those fibers separated from it underwent degenerative changes that came to be known as Wallerian degeneration. From these observations it was concluded that recovery of function required restoration of axonal continuity with the periphery.

Prior to World War II, nerves were still regarded as cord-like structures and were treated the same as other tissues during surgery. The period following World War II marked the beginning of many breakthroughs in trauma surgery and peripheral nerve repair. The effective control of wound infection by antibiotics was a major advance. In addition, a better understanding of the internal structure of nerves and the physiology of the nervous system, along with improved surgical techniques and surgical instruments, made nerve repair potentially more successful.

The period of technical achievement can be attributed to several factors including: (1) clinicians' recognition of the significance of basic science data; (2) the realization that nerve repair involved far more than the simple restoration of nerve trunk continuity; (3) the recognition that nerve repair had become a highly specialized undertaking, demanding a detailed knowledge of the internal anatomy of nerves and regenerative processes and calling for great technical skill and experience, meticulous observance of atraumatic techniques, and the use of operative methods, instruments, and suture materials specially designed for this type of work; (4) the application of microsurgical techniques to the repair of nerves; and (5) the emergence of hand surgery as a recognized specialty.

The objectives of surgical repair of a damaged nerve are to maximize (1) the number of axons that regenerate across the lesion site and (2) the accuracy with which these axons reinnervate denervated peripheral targets. The surgeon can influence the result by the way the damaged tissue is handled and by the method used to reapproximate the severed ends.

The four basic steps of nerve repair are: (1) preparation of the stumps, often involving resection or interfascicular dissection with separation of individual fascicles or groups of fascicles; (2) approximation, with special reference to the length of the gap between the stumps as well as the amount of tension present; (3) coaptation of the nerve stumps; and (4) maintenance of coaptation, involving the use of, for example, stitches, glue, or a natural fibrin clot. Coaptation describes the apposition of corresponding nerve ends with special attention to bringing the cross-section of the fascicles into optimal contact. A direct coaptation (neurorrhaphy) can oppose stump to stump, fascicle to fascicle, or fascicle group to fascicle group in the corresponding ends. An indirect coaptation can be performed by interposing a nerve graft. Other factors that may influence the results are the timing of the surgery and the postoperative rehabilitation. These topics have been addressed extensively in several textbooks.

Selected Bibliography

Neurons and Signal Generation

Goldman DE: Potential, impedance and rectification in membranes. *J Gen Physiol* 1943;27:37–60.

Hirokawa N, Pfister KK, Yorifuji H, et al: Submolecular domains of bovine brain kinesin identified by electron microscopy and monoclonal antibody decoration. *Cell* 1989;56:867–878.

Hodgkin AL: Change and design in electrophysiology: An informal account of certain experiments on nerve carried out between 1934 and 1952. *J Physiol (Lond)* 1976;263:1–21.

Hodgkin AL, Huxley AF: A quantitative description of membrane current and its application to conduction and excitation in nerve. *J Physiol (Lond)* 1952:117; 500–544.

Hodgkin AL, Katz B: The effect of sodium ions on the electrical activity of the giant axon of the squid. *J Physiol (Lond)* 1949:108:37–77.

Kandel ER, Schwartz JH, Jessell TM (eds): *Principles of Neural Science,* ed 3. New York, Elsevier Science Publishing, 1991.

Nicholls JG, Martin AR, Wallace BG (eds): *From Neuron To Brain: A Cellular and Molecular Approach to the Function of the Nervous System,* ed 3. Sunderland, MA, Sinauer Associates, 1992.

Ochs S: Fast transport of materials in mammalian nerve fibers. *Science* 1972;176:252–260.

Ochs S, Brimijoin WS: Axonal transport, in Dyck PJ, Thomas PK, Griffin JW, et al (eds): *Peripheral Neuropathy,* ed 3. Philadelphia, WB Saunders, 1993, pp 331–360.

Rall W: Core conductor theory and cable properties of neurons, in Kandel ER (ed): *Handbook of Physiology, Section 1: The Nervous System.* Bethesda, MD, American Physiological Society, 1977, pp 39–97.

Reichert H: *Introduction to Neurobiology.* New York, Oxford University Press, 1992.

Sensory and Motor Systems

Bodine SC, Garfinkel A, Roy RR, et al: Spatial distribution of motor unit fibers in the cat soleus and tibialis anterior muscles: Local interactions. *J Neurosci* 1988;8:2142–2152.

Bodine SC, Roy RR, Eldred E, et al: Maximal force as a function of anatomical features of motor units in the cat tibialis anterior. *J Neurophysiol* 1987;57:1739–1745.

Brandstater ME, Lambert EH: Motor unit anatomy, in Desmedt JE (ed): *New Developments in Electromyography and Clinical Neurophysiology.* Basel, S. Karger, 1973, vol 1, pp 14–22.

Brown AG (ed): *Organization in the Spinal Cord: The Anatomy and Physiology of Identified Neurones.* Berlin, Springer-Verlag, 1981.

Burke D: Spasticity as an adaptation to pyrimidal tract injury. *Adv Neurol* 1988;47:401–423.

Burke RE: Motor units: Anatomy, physiology and functional organization, in Brooks VB (ed): *Handbook of Physiology, Section I, The Nervous System.* Bethesda, MD, American Physiological Society, 1981, pp 345–422.

Daube JR, Reagan TJ, Sandok BA, et al (eds): *Medical Neurosciences: An Approach to Anatomy, Pathology, and Physiology by Systems and Levels.* Boston, Little, Brown, 1986.

Delwaide PJ, Young RR (eds): *Clinical Neurophysiology in Spasticity: Contribution to Assessment and Pathophysiology.* Amsterdam, Elsevier, 1985.

Edstrom L, Kugelberg E: Histochemical composition, distribution of fibres and fatiguability of single motor units: Anterior tibial muscle of the rat. *J Neurol Neurosurg Psychiatry* 1968;31:424–433.

Guyton AC: *Basic Neuroscience: Anatomy and Physiology,* ed 2. Philadelphia, WB Saunders, 1992.

Henneman E, Mendell LM: Functional organization of motoneuron pool and its inputs, in Brooks VB (ed): *Handbook of Physiology: Section 1, The Nervous System.* Bethesda, MD, American Physiological Society, 1981, pp 423–507.

Jansen JK, Fladby T: The perinatal reorganization of the innervation of skeletal muscle in mammals. *Prog Neurobiol* 1990;34:39–90.

Katz RT, Rymer WZ: Spastic hypertonia: Mechanisms and measurement. *Arch Phys Med Rehabil* 1989;70:144–155.

Kugelberg E: Properties of rat hind-limb motor units, in Desmedt JE (ed): *New Developments in Electromyography and Clinical Neurophysiology.* Basel, S. Karger, 1973, vol 1, pp 2–13.

Lance JW: The control of muscle tone, reflexes, and movement: Robert Wartenberg lecture. *Neurology* 1980;30:1303–1313.

Matthews PBC: Muscle spindles: Their messages and their fusimotor supply, in Brooks VB (ed): *Handbook of Physiology, Section 1, The Nervous System.* Bethesda, MD, American Physiological Society, 1981, pp 189–228.

Nickel VL, Botte MJ: *Orthopaedic Rehabilitation,* ed 2. New York, Churchill Livingstone, 1992.

Park TS, Phillips LH II, Peacock WJ (eds): *Neurosurgery: State of the Art Reviews: Management of Spasticity in Cerebral Palsy and Spinal Cord Injury.* Philadelphia, Hanley and Belfus, 1989, vol 4.

Purves D, Lichtman JW: *Principles of Neural Development.* Sunderland, MA, Sinauer Associates, 1985.

Romanes GJ: The motor cell columns of the lumbo-sacral spinal cord of the cat. *J Comp Neurol* 1951;94:313–363.

Schmidt RF (ed): *Fundamentals of Neurophysiology,* ed 2. New York, Springer-Verlag, 1978. Translated by Bederman-Thorson, MA.

Van Essen DC: Neuromuscular synapse elimination: Structural, functional, and mechanistic aspects, in Spitzer NC (ed): *Neuronal Development.* New York, Plenum, 1982, pp 333–376.

Wernig A (ed): *Plasticity of Motoneuronal Connections.* Amsterdam, Elsevier, 1991.

Peripheral Nerve Development, Structure, and Biomechanics

Beel JA, Groswald DE, Luttges MW: Alterations in the mechanical properties of peripheral nerve following crush injury. *J Biomech* 1984;17:185–193.

Clark WL, Trumble TE, Swiontkowski MF, et al: Nerve tension and blood flow in a rat model of immediate and delayed repairs. *J Hand Surg* 1992;17A:677–687.

Denny-Brown D, Doherty MM: Effects of transient stretching of peripheral nerve. *Arch Neurol Psychiatry* 1945;54:116–129.

Dodd J, Jessell TM: Axon guidance and the patterning of neuronal projections in vertebrates. *Science* 1988;242:692–699.

Hall ZW: *An Introduction to Molecular Neurobiology.* Sunderland, MA, Sinauer Associates, 1992.

Haftek J: Stretch injury of peripheral nerve: Acute effects of stretching on rabbit nerve. *J Bone Joint Surg* 1970;52B:354–365.

Lance-Jones C: Motoneuron axon guidance: Development of specific projections to two muscles in the embryonic chick limb. *Brain Behav Evol* 1988;31:209–217.

Landmesser LT: The generation of neuromuscular specificity. *Annu Rev Neurosci* 1980;3:279–302.

Landmesser L: The development of specific motor pathways in the chick embryo. *Trends Neurosci* 1984;7:336–339.

Lundborg G: The intrinsic vascularization of human peripheral nerves: Structural and functional aspects. *J Hand Surg* 1979;4:34–41.

Lundborg G: *Nerve Injury and Repair.* Edinburgh, Churchill Livingstone, 1988.

Okamoto T: Study on strength of peripheral nerve tissue of human beings and various animals. *J Kyoto Pref Med Univ* 1955;58:1007–1029.

Rydevik BL, Kwan MK, Myers RR, et al: An in vitro mechanical and histological study of acute stretching on rabbit tibial nerve. *J Orthop Res* 1990;8:694–701.

Sanes JR: Extracellular matrix molecules that influence neural development. *Annu Rev Neurosci* 1989;12:491–516.

Sanes JR, Schachner M, Covault J: Expression of several adhesive macromolecules (N-CAM, L1, J1, NILE, uvomorulin, laminin, fibronectin, and a heparan sulfate proteoglycan) in embryonic, adult, and denervated adult skeletal muscle. *J Cell Biol* 1986;102:420–431.

Sunderland S: *Nerve Injuries and Their Repair: A Critical Appraisal.* Edinburgh, Churchill Livingstone, 1991.

Sunderland S, Bradley KC: Stress-strain phenomena in human peripheral nerve trunks. *Brain* 1961;84:102–119.

Yoshimura M, Amaya S, Tyujo M, et al: Experimental studies on the traction injury of peripheral nerves. *Neuro-Orthop* 1989;7:1–7.

Electrodiagnosis of the Peripheral Nerve

Aminoff MJ (ed): *Electrodiagnosis in Clinical Neurology,* ed 3. New York, Churchill Livingstone, 1992.

Kimura J: *Electrodiagnosis in Diseases of Nerve and Muscle: Principles and Practice.* Philadelphia, FA Davis, 1983.

Kugelberg E, Edstrom L, Abbruzzese M: Mapping of motor units in experimentally reinnervated rat muscle: Interpretation of histochemical and atrophic fibre patterns in neurogenic lesions. *J Neurol Neurosurg Psychiatry* 1970;33:319–329.

Liveson JA: *Peripheral Neurology: Case Studies in Electrodiagnosis,* ed 2. Philadelphia, FA Davis, 1991.

Liveson JA, Ma DM: *Laboratory Reference for Clinical Neurophysiology.* Philadelphia, FA Davis, 1992.

Luff AR, Hatcher DD, Torkko K: Enlarged motor units resulting from partial denervation of cat hindlimb muscles. *J Neurophysiol* 1988;59:1377–1394.

Mumenthaler M, Schliack H (eds): *Peripheral Nerve Lesions: Diagnosis and Therapy.* New York, Thieme Medical Publishers, 1991.

Peyronnard J-M, Charron L: Muscle reorganization after partial denervation and reinnervation. *Muscle Nerve* 1980;3:509–518.

Sethi RK, Thompson LL: *The Electromyographer's Handbook,* ed 2. Boston, Little, Brown, 1989.

Stalberg E: Single-fiber electromyography and some other electrophysiologic techniques for the study of the motor unit, in Dyck PJ, Thomas PK, Griffin JW, et al (eds): *Peripheral Neuropathy,* ed 3. Philadelphia, WB Saunders, 1993, pp 645–657.

Traumatic Nerve Injury

Dahlin LB, McLean WG: Effects of graded experimental compression on slow and fast axonal transport in rabbit vagus nerve. *J Neurol Sci* 1986;72:19–30.

Flatt AE: Tourniquet time in hand surgery. *Arch Surg* 1972;104:190–192.

Gasser HS, Erlanger J: The role of fiber size in the establishment of a nerve block by pressure or cocaine. *Am J Physiol* 1929;88:581–591.

Gelberman RH, Hergenroeder PT, Hargens AR, et al: The carpal tunnel syndrome: A study of carpal canal pressures. *J Bone Joint Surg* 1981;63A:380–383.

Gelberman RH, Szabo RM, Williamson RV, et al: Tissue pressure threshold for peripheral nerve viability. *Clin Orthop* 1983;178:285–291.

Haftek J: Stretch injury of peripheral nerve: Acute effects of stretching on rabbit nerve. *J Bone Joint Surg* 1970;52B:354–365.

Klenerman L: The tourniquet in operations on the knee: A review. *J R Soc Med* 1982;75:31–32.

Lundborg G, Gelberman RH, Minteer-Convery M, et al: Median nerve compression in the carpal tunnel: Functional response to experimentally induced controlled pressure. *J Hand Surg* 1982;7A:252–259.

Lundborg G, Myers R, Powell H: Nerve compression injury and increased endoneurial fluid pressure: A "miniature compartment syndrome". *J Neurol Neurosurg Psychiatry* 1983;46:1119–1124.

Myers RR, Powell HC: Endoneurial fluid pressure in peripheral neuropathies, in Hargens AR (ed): *Tissue Fluid Pressure and Composition.* Baltimore, Williams & Wilkins, 1981, pp 193–207.

Ochoa J, Fowler TJ, Gilliatt RW: Anatomical changes in peripheral nerves compressed by a pneumatic tourniquet. *J Anat* 1972;113:433–455.

Rorabeck CH: Tourniquet-induced nerve ischemia: An experimental investigation. *J Trauma* 1980;20:280–286.

Rydevik B, Lundborg G, Bagge U: Effects of graded compression on intraneural blood flow: An in vivo study on rabbit tibial nerve. *J Hand Surg* 1981;6A:3–12.

Seddon HJ: Three types of nerve injury. *Brain* 1943;66:237–288.

Seddon HJ: *Surgical Disorders of the Peripheral Nerves,* ed 2. Edinburgh, Churchill Livingstone, 1975.

Sunderland S: A classification of peripheral nerve injuries producing loss of function. *Brain* 1951;74:491–516.

Sunderland S: *Nerves and Nerve Injuries,* ed 2. Edinburgh, Churchill Livingstone, 1978.

Neural Degeneration, Axonal Regeneration, and Functional Recovery After Nerve Injury

Anzil AP, Wernig A: Muscle fibre loss and reinnervation after long-term denervation. *J Neurocytol* 1989;18:833–845.

Archibald SJ, Krarup C, Shefner J, et al: A collagen-based nerve guide conduit for peripheral nerve repair: An electrophysiological study of nerve regeneration in rodents and nonhuman primates. *J Comp Neurol* 1991;306:685–696.

Bain JR, Mackinnon SE, Hunter DA: Functional evaluation of complete sciatic, peroneal, and posterior tibial nerve lesions in the rat. *Plast Reconstr Surg* 1989;83:129–138.

Brushart TM: Preferential reinnervation of motor nerves by regenerating motor axons. *J Neurosci* 1988;8:1026–1031.

Brushart TM, Mesulam MM: Alteration in connections between muscle and anterior horn motoneurons after peripheral nerve repair. *Science* 1980;208:603–605.

Brushart TM, Seiler WA IV: Selective reinnervation of distal motor stumps by peripheral motor axons. *Exp Neurol* 1987;97:289–300.

Brushart TM, Tarlov EC, Mesulam MM: Specificity of muscle reinnervation after epineurial and individual fascicular suture of the rat sciatic nerve. *J Hand Surg* 1983;8A:248–253.

Cabaud HE, Rodkey WG, McCarroll HR Jr: Peripheral nerve injuries: Studies in higher nonhuman primates. *J Hand Surg* 1980;5A:201–206.

Cabaud HE, Rodkey WG, McCarroll HR Jr, et al: Epineurial and perineurial fascicular nerve repairs: A critical comparison. *J Hand Surg* 1975;1A:131–137.

Danielsen N, Pettmann B, Vahlsing HL, et al: Fibroblast growth factor effects on peripheral nerve regeneration in a silicone chamber model. *J Neurosci Res* 1988;20:320–330.

Daniloff JK, Levi G, Grumet M, et al: Altered expression of neuronal cell adhesion molecules induced by nerve injury and repair. *J Cell Biol* 1986;103:929–945.

Dellon AL, Mackinnon SE: Selection of the appropriate parameter to measure neural regeneration. *Ann Plast Surg* 1989;23:197–202.

Evans PJ, Bain JR, Mackinnon SE, et al: Selective reinnervation: A comparison of recovery following microsuture and conduit nerve repair. *Brain Res* 1991;559:315–321.

Fawcett JW, Keynes RJ: Peripheral nerve regeneration. *Annu Rev Neurosci* 1990;13:43–60.

Fields RD, Ellisman MH: Axons regenerated through silicone tube splices: I. Conduction properties. *Exp Neurol* 1986;92:48–60.

Fields RD, Ellisman MH: Axons regenerated though silicone tube splices: II. Functional morphology. *Exp Neurol* 1986;92:61–74.

Fields RD, LeBeau JM, Longo FM, et al: Nerve regeneration through artificial tubular implants. *Prog Neurobiol* 1989;33:87–134.

Hardman VJ, Brown MC: Accuracy of reinnervation of rat internal intercostal muscles by their own segmental nerves. *J Neurosci 1987;7:1031–1036.*

Harsh C, Archibald SJ, Madison RD: Double-labeling of saphenous nerve neuron pools: A model for determining the accuracy of axon regeneration at the single neuron level. *J Neurosci Methods* 1991;39:123–130.

Hollowell JP, Villadiego A, Rich KM: Sciatic nerve regeneration across gaps within silicone chambers: Long-term effects of NGF and consideration of axonal branching. *Exp Neurol* 1990;110:45–51.

Irintchev A, Draguhn A, Wernig A: Reinnervation and recovery of mouse soleus muscle after long-term denervation. *Neuroscience* 1990;39:231–243.

Keynes RJ: Schwann cells during neural development and regeneration: Leaders or followers? *Trends Neurosci* 1987;10:137–139.

Knoops B, Hurtado H, van den Bosch de Aguilar P: Rat sciatic nerve regeneration within an acrylic semipermeable tube and comparison with a silicone impermeable material. *J Neuropathol Exp Neurol* 1990;49:438–448.

Kuffler DP: Regeneration of muscle axons in the frog is directed by diffusible factors from denervated muscle and nerve tubes. *J Comp Neurol* 1989;281:416–425.

Kuno M: Target dependence of motoneuronal survival: The current status. *Neurosci Res* 1990;9:155–172.

Laskowski MB, Sanes JR: Topographic mapping of motor pools onto skeletal muscles. *J Neurosci* 1987;7:252–260.

Laskowski MB, Sanes JR: Topographically selective reinnervation of adult mammalian skeletal muscles. *J Neurosci* 1988;8:3094–3099.

Le Beau JM, Ellisman MH, Powell HC: Ultrastructural and morphometric analysis of long-term peripheral nerve regeneration through silicone tubes. *J Neurocytol* 1988;17:161–172.

Lieberman AR: The axon reaction: A review of the principle features of perikaryal responses to axon injury. *Int Rev Neurobiol* 1971;14:49–124.

Longo FM, Hayman EG, Davis GE, et al: Neurite-promoting factors and extracellular matrix components accumulating in vivo within nerve regeneration chambers. *Brain Res* 1984;309:105–117.

Lundborg G, Dahlin LB, Danielsen N, et al: Tissue specificity in nerve regeneration. *Scand J Plast Reconstr Surg* 1986;20:279–283.

Mackinnon SE, Dellon AL, Lundborg G, et al: A study of neurotrophism in a primate model. *J Hand Surg* 1986;11A:888–894.

Madison RD, Da Silva CF, Dikkes P: Entubulation repair with protein additives increases the maximum nerve gap distance successfully bridged with tubular prostheses. *Brain Res* 1988;447:325–334.

Manthorpe M, Engvall E, Ruoslathi E, et al: Laminin promotes neuritic regeneration from cultured peripheral and central neurons. *J Cell Biol* 1983;97:1882–1890.

Nurcombe V, Hill MA, Eagleson KL, et al: Motor neuron survival and neuritic extension from spinal cord explants induced by factors released from denervated muscle. *Brain Res* 1984;291:19–28.

Politis MJ: Specificity in mammalian peripheral nerve regeneration at the level of the nerve trunk. *Brain Res* 1985;328:271–276.

Politis MJ, Ederle K, Spencer PS: Tropism in nerve regeneration in vivo: Attraction of regenerating axon by diffusible factors derived from cells in distal nerve stumps of transected peripheral nerves. *Brain Res* 1982;253:1–12.

Rosario CM, Fry KR, Madison R: Rabbit retinal ganglion cells survive optic transection and entubulation repair with type I collagen nerve guide tubes. *Restor Neurol Neurosci* 1989;1:31.

Seckel BR: Enhancement of peripheral nerve regeneration. *Muscle Nerve* 1990;13:785–800.

Seckel BR, Chiu TH, Nyilas E, et al: Nerve regeneration through synthetic biodegradable nerve guides: Regulation by the target organ. *Plast Reconstr Surg* 1984;74:173–181.

Seckel BR, Ryan SE, Gagne RG, et al: Target-specific nerve regeneration through a nerve guide in the rat. *Plast Reconstr Surg* 1986;78:793–800.

Sumner AJ: Aberrant reinnervation. *Muscle Nerve* 1990;13:801–803.

Tessier-Lavigne M, Placzek M: Target attraction: Are developing axons guided by chemotropism? *Trends Neurosci* 1991;14:303–310.

Thomas CK, Stein RB, Gordan T, et al: Patterns of reinnervation and motor unit recruitment in human hand muscles after complete ulnar and median nerve section and resuture. *J Neurol Neurosurg Psychiatry* 1987;50:259–268.

Wasserschaff M: Coordination of reinnervated muscle and reorganization of spinal cord motoneurons after nerve transection in mice. *Brain Res* 1990;515:241–246.

Williams LR: Exogenous fibrin matrix precursors stimulate the temporal progress of nerve regeneration within a silicone chamber. *Neurochem Res* 1987;12:851–860.

Williams LR, Danielsen N, Muller H, et al: Exogenous matrix precursors promote functional nerve regeneration across a 15-mm gap within a silicon chamber in the rat. *J Comp Neurol* 1987;264:284–290.

Woolley AL, Hollowell JP, Rich KM: Fibronectin-laminin combination enhances perpheral nerve regeneration across long gaps. *Otolaryngol Head Neck Surg* 1990;103:509–518.

Yamada S, Buffinger N, DiMario J, et al: Fibroblast growth factor is stored in fiber extracellular matrix and plays a role in regulating muscle hypertrophy. *Med Sci Sports Exerc* 1989;21(5 Suppl):S173–S180.

Surgical Nerve Repair

Brunelli G, Monini L, Brunell F: Problems in nerve lesions surgery. *Microsurg* 1985;6:187–198.

Cabaud HE, Rodkey WG, McCarroll HR Jr, et al: Epineurial and perineurial fascicular nerve repairs: A critical comparison. *J Hand Surg* 1976;1A:131–137.

Gelberman RH (ed): *Operative Nerve Repair and Reconstruction.* Philadelphia, JB Lippincott, 1991.

Mackinnon SE, Dellon AL: *Surgery of the Peripheral Nerve.* New York, Thieme Medical Publishers, 1988.

Millesi H: Nerve grafting. *Clin Plast Surg* 1984;11:105–113.

Millesi H: The nerve gap: Theory and clinical practice. *Hand Clin* 1986;2:651–663.

Millesi H: Brachial plexus injuries: Nerve grafting. *Clin Orthop* 1988;237:36–42.

Millesi H: Progress in peripheral nerve reconstruction. *World J Surg* 1990;14:733–747.

Moberg E: Nerve repair in hand surgery: An analysis. *Surg Clin North Am* 1968;48:985–991.

Nicholson OR, Seddon HJ: Nerve repair in civil practice: Results of treatment of median and ulnar nerve lesions. *Br Med J* 1957;2:1065–1071.

Orgel MG, Terzis JK: Epineurial vs. perineurial repair: An ultrastructural and electrophysiological study of nerve regeneration. *Plast Reconstr Surg* 1977;60:80–91.

Omer GE Jr: The evaluation of clinical results following peripheral nerve suture, in Omer GE Jr, Spinner M (eds): *Management of Peripheral Nerve Problems.* Philadelphia, Saunders, 1988, pp 431–442.

Suematsu N: Tubulation for peripheral nerve gap: Its history and possibility. *Microsurgery* 1989;10:71–74.

Sunderland S: The intraneural topography of the radial, median and ulnar nerves. *Brain* 1945;68:243–299.

Sunderland S: Funicular suture and funicular exclusion in the repair of severed nerves. *Br J Surg* 1953;40:580–587.

Terzis JK, Smith KL: *The Peripheral Nerve: Structure, Function and Reconstruction.* New York, Raven Press, 1990.

Yahr MD, Beebe GW: Recovery of motor function: Peripheral nerve regeneration: A follow-up study of 3,656, world War II injuries, in Woodhall B, Beebe GW (eds): *VA Medical Monograph.* Washington, DC, U.S. Government Printing Office, 1959.

Chapter 9
Biomechanics

Van C. Mow, PhD
Evan L. Flatow, MD
Robert J. Foster, ScD

Chapter Outline

Chapter Outline

Behavior of Simple Structures
- Size and Shape of Geometric Forms
- Areas and Centroids
- Uniaxial Tension and Compression of Bars
- Torsion of Circular Shafts
- Bending of Beams
- Combined Compression and Bending
- Stress Concentration
- Finite Element Analysis

Biotribology of Diarthrodial Joints
- Introduction
- Synovial Fluid
- Newtonian and Non-Newtonian Fluids
- Anatomic Forms of Diarthrodial Joints
- Motion and Forces on Diarthrodial Joints
- Friction
- Wear
- Diarthrodial Joint Lubrication
- Interstitial Fluid Flow and Diarthrodial Joint Lubrication
- Summary of Joint Lubrication

Clinical Applications
- Prosthetic Design Considerations: Shoulder

Conclusions

Selected Bibliography

Introduction

The musculoskeletal system, although complex, obeys the basic laws of mechanics. Biomechanics is the branch of science that deals with the effects of energy and forces on biologic systems. The study of biomechanics involves the application of Newton's laws of mechanics to models of biologic objects in order to describe their behavior and their functions. Orthopaedic biomechanics has focused on the effects, motions and deformation, of forces and moments acting on tissues such as bone, cartilage, growth plate, ligament, meniscus, synovial fluid, and tendon. The study of biomechanics has been important in the development and design of many of the joint replacement and fracture fixation devices commonly used in orthopaedic surgery today. Kinematics describes motions within the musculoskeletal system, such as those of diarthrodial joints (hip, knee, shoulder, etc.), as well as locomotion and gait. Biotribology is the study of friction, lubrication, and wear resulting from the interaction of apposed articular surfaces in relative motion.

In addition to describing normal structure and function, clinical orthopaedic biomechanics seeks to examine specific pathologic conditions through the study of joint instability, gait pathologies, and fracture healing. Furthermore, surgical procedures designed to restore normal mechanics may be critically evaluated, using techniques such as force analysis of tendon transfer, kinematic studies of ligament repair, and finite element analysis of joint replacements.

This chapter provides a review of some fundamental principles of mechanics and demonstrates the use of these principles in some specific orthopaedic biomechanics problems. It includes definitions of forces and moments and examples of their calculation in specific cases (knee, hip, shoulder, spine, etc.), as well as definitions of stresses and strains and examples of how these provide the intrinsic material properties of biologic materials. Furthermore, this chapter covers the friction, lubrication, and wear mechanisms existing in diarthrodial joints. Finally, some basic concepts of biomaterials and prosthesis design will be surveyed.

Skeletal Forces

Vectors and Forces

There are many types of physical quantities. Temperature, mass, volume, density, etc., are scalar physical quantities. Only one number is needed to quantify the magnitude of a scalar quantity. For example, temperature is quantified in degrees Celsius, mass in kilograms, volume in meters^3, and density in kilograms/meter^3. Vectors are quantities that have direction and magnitude. Velocity, acceleration, force, and moment are all vectors. A vector is portrayed by an arrow; its direction is indicated by the direction of the arrow, and its magnitude is represented by the length of the arrow. For example, the velocity of a car going from east to west at 80 km/hr is defined by a vector; its direction is east to west and its magnitude is the speed 80 km/hr. Although body weight commonly is thought of as a magnitude; for example 150 lb; it also has direction, which is down. Thus, the weight of a limb or body segment must always be portrayed by a vector in the direction of gravity (down), with its length defined relative to the weight of the limb applied at its center of gravity. The importance of direction is illustrated in Figure 1. When the arm is at the side of the body, the weight of the forearm will tend to

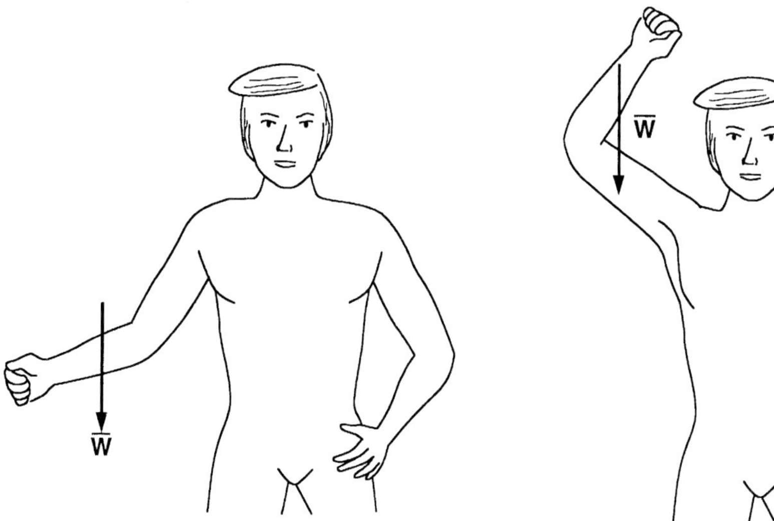

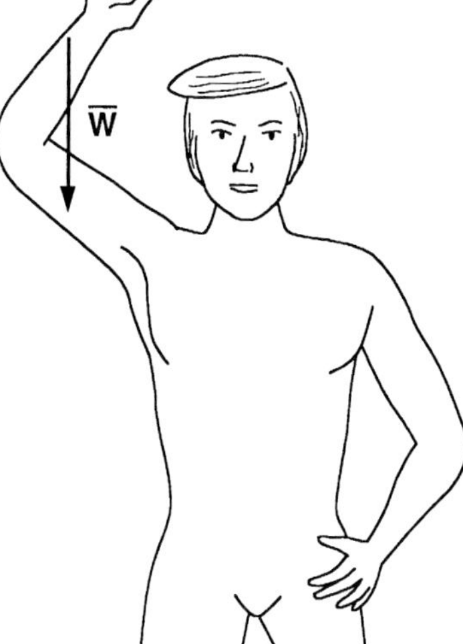

Figure 1
A force is a vector. The importance of direction is illustrated here.

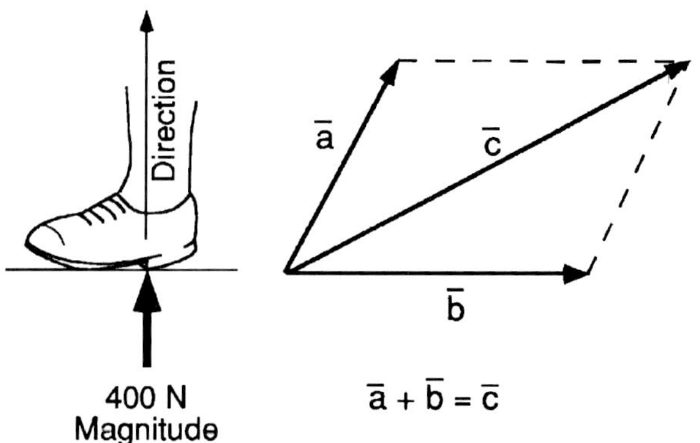

Figure 2
Left, An example of the reaction force exerted on the foot by the floor. **Right,** Two vector quantities are added according to the parallelogram law of vector addition; a and b are the sides of the parallelogram and c is the diagonal, which is known as the resultant vector.

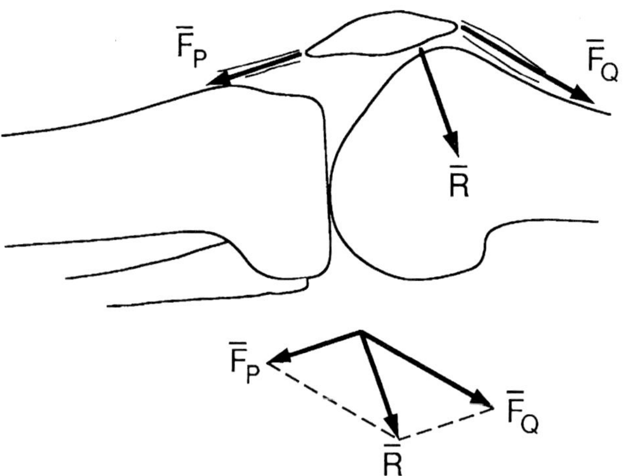

Figure 3
The force of the quadriceps $\mathbf{F}_Q$ added to the force of the patellar tendon $\mathbf{F}_P$ in accordance with the parallelogram law, produces the resultant force **R,** which tends to compress the patella against the femur.

extend the elbow; when the arm is elevated overhead, this weight will act to flex the elbow.

A force, in its most elementary definition, is a "push" or a "pull." For example, when the foot contacts the floor during standing, a force exists between the foot and the floor. The foot pushes on the floor and the floor pushes back, because according to Newton's 3rd law, for every force (action) there is an equal and opposite force (reaction). Figure 2, *left,* illustrates an example of a force exerted on the foot. The unit most commonly used for force is the newton (N).

Two vector quantities, such as forces, may be added according to the parallelogram law of vector addition. This is done by using the two vectors as two sides of a parallelogram and then drawing a new arrow along the diagonal (Fig. 2, *right*). A vector is usually denoted by a boldface letter or a letter with an arrow, →, or bar, -, over it. Figure 3 shows that the force of the quadriceps $\mathbf{F}_Q$, pulling the patella proximally, added to the force of the patellar tendon $\mathbf{F}_P$, pulling it distally, results in a force **R,** which tends to compress the patella against the femur.

A bit of reflection will show that the parallelogram law also means that any vector may be broken down into component forces along any specified mutually perpendicular coordinate axes. The original vector **F** is the sum of its components along these axes:

$$\mathbf{F} = \mathbf{F}_x + \mathbf{F}_y + \mathbf{F}_z,$$

as shown in Figure 4. The magnitudes of $\mathbf{F}_x$, $\mathbf{F}_y$, $\mathbf{F}_z$ are denoted by $|\mathbf{F}_x|$, $|\mathbf{F}_y|$, $|\mathbf{F}_z|$, or F_x, F_y, F_z, and they are known as the components of the vector **F** with respect to the xyz coordinate system.

The magnitude of the force **F**, denoted by $|\mathbf{F}|$, is given by the Pythagorean theorem:

$$|\mathbf{F}|^2 = |\mathbf{F}_x|^2 + |\mathbf{F}_y|^2 + |\mathbf{F}_z|^2.$$

Figure 5 illustrates how the force of the deltoid $\mathbf{F}_D$, acting on the humerus may be broken down into a compressive force $\mathbf{F}_C$ acting perpendicularly ("normal") to the glenoid joint surface and a "shear" force $\mathbf{F}_S$ acting parallel (tangential) to the surface. This deltoid force also creates a moment (or rotation), which is defined next.

Moments

A force applied to an object may both push or pull and twist that object. That action of a force applied to an object, which tends to rotate the object about an axis is called a moment. The force applied to the wrench handle in Figure 6 will generate a moment about the axis OO′ of the bolt. The magnitude of the moment about the axis OO′, M_o, caused by this force is equal to the magnitude of the force F multiplied by the perpendicular distance d from the axis OO′ of the bolt to the line of action A-A of the force; $M_o = F \times d = F \times l\sin\theta$. Clearly, M_o is also equal to $F\sin\theta \times l$, that is, to the component of F perpendicular to the wrench multiplied by the length of the wrench l. The distance d is often referred to as the moment arm. The units used for a moment are N·m. In the example shown in Figure 6, there is a 200 N force applied on the handle at a perpendicular distance of 25 cm from the bolt. The moment applied to the bolt is therefore 200 N × 25 cm or 50 N·m. The magnitude of a moment is a torque. Using

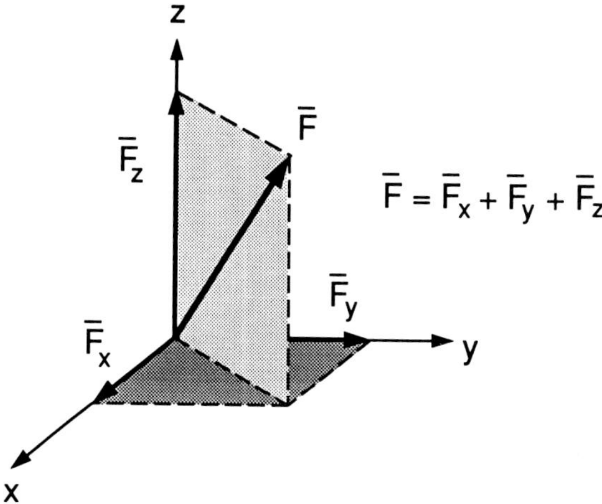

Figure 4
The parallelogram law of vector addition permits any vector to be resolved into its component vectors along any set of mutually orthogonal coordinate axes. This resolution is expressed by the equation $\mathbf{F} = \mathbf{F}_x + \mathbf{F}_y + \mathbf{F}_z$.

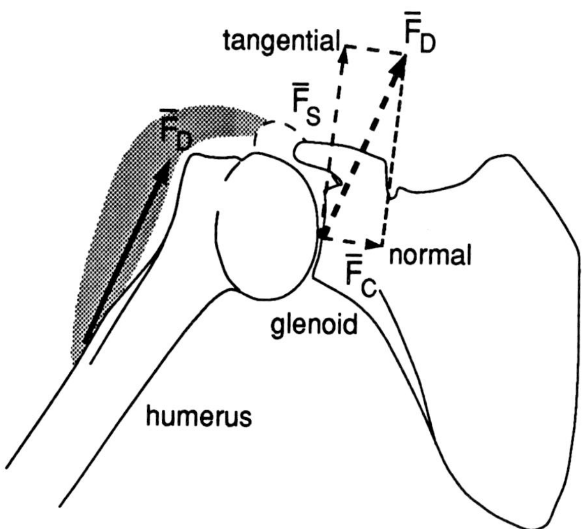

Figure 5
The force of the deltoid muscle $\mathbf{F}_D$ acting on the humerus may be resolved into a compressive force $\mathbf{F}_C$, acting perpendicularly or normal to the glenoid joint surface, and a shear force $\mathbf{F}_S$, acting parallel or tangential to the surface. $\mathbf{F}_D$ also creates a moment, which is not shown.

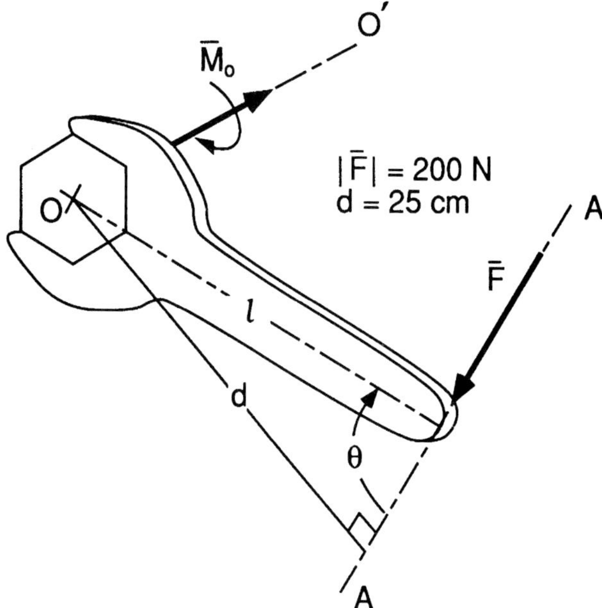

Figure 6
The magnitude of the moment about 00′, perpendicular to the face of the wrench, caused by the force **F**, parallel to the face of the wrench, is equal to the magnitude of the force multiplied by the perpendicular distance d from the axis 00′ to the line of action A-A of the force; $M_o = F \times d = F \times l\sin\theta$. The direction of the moment is given by the right hand rule.

the right hand rule, the direction of the moment is given by the thumb of the right hand when the fingers of the right hand are taken to be along the direction of rotation caused by the force. Note that a moment corresponds to a specific axis about which it turns. It does not matter whether any rotation ever occurs. Thus, it is possible to choose the most convenient axis for the problem at hand, and, indeed, any force will exert a moment around any point not located along its line of action.

When a moment is created by two equal, noncolinear, parallel but oppositely directed forces **F** and **-F**, the moment created is called a couple. The simplest examples are the thumb and index fingers twisting off a bottle cap, or two hands turning a steering wheel. Figure 7, *top*, shows such a pair of forces in the xy plane. Obviously, the resultant force is zero. The magnitude of the couple is **F**d, where d is the perpendicular distance between the two forces. Although the torque created by a single force is dependent on the location of the reference point O (Fig. 6), the torque of the couple is not. Thus, a couple is a free pure moment vector with no resultant force, and may be applied anywhere in the plane determined by the two vectors **F** and **-F.** The couple is a very important concept, because the effects of any force may be made equivalent to a couple and a force. This is shown in Figure 7, *bottom*, by a force **F** applied at a point A. The line of action of **F** is closest to O at A′; the distance d is the moment arm of **F** relative to point O. A pair of imaginary forces **F** and **-F** is added at the origin O. The original problem has

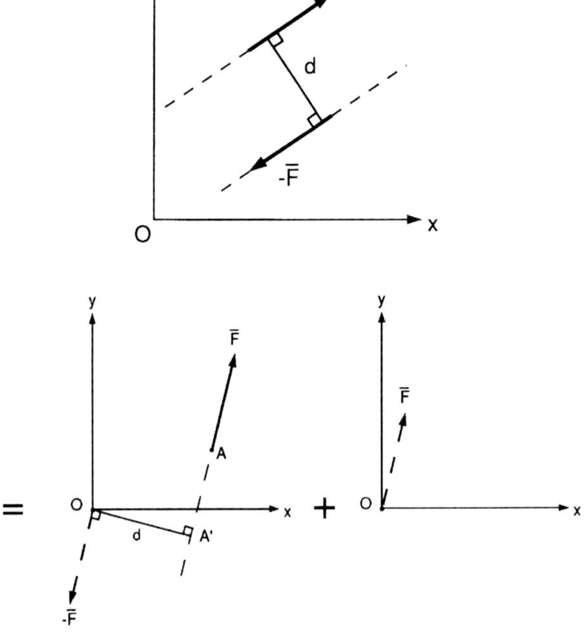

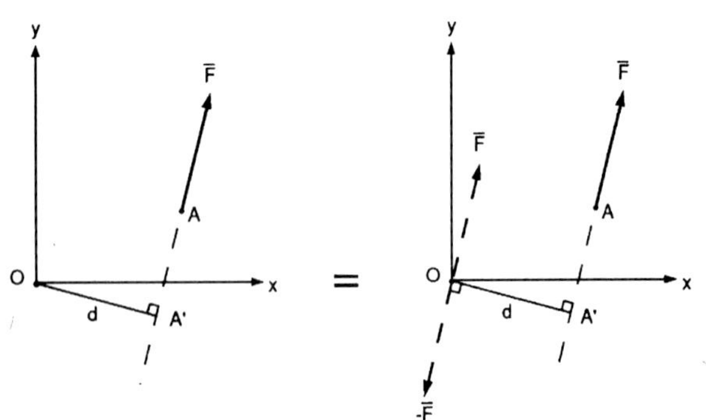

Figure 7
Top, A couple is created by two equal, noncolinear, parallel but oppositely directed forces **F** and **-F.** The magnitude of the couple is Fd, where d is the perpendicular distance between the two forces. The resultant force of a couple is zero. **Bottom,** A single force **F** applied at a point A acting along A-A′, whose perpendicular distance to 0 is d, is equipollent to a force acting at 0 and a couple of magnitude F_d.

not changed because these opposite forces cancel each other. The pair of forces composed of **-F** at O and the original force **F** at A is a couple. Its magnitude is **F**d, and it is a free pure moment acting in the xy plane. The remaining force is the force **F** acting at O. Thus the force **F** acting at A is equipollent to a force **F** acting at O and a couple. This important result is very useful in understanding the effects of muscle action around a joint.

Dynamics

An unopposed force acting on an object will accelerate the object, that is, it will change the velocity of the object. This is known as a nonequilibrium (dynamic) condition. It is important to note that, because velocity is a vector, a change of velocity could mean a change of direction or of speed (magnitude) or of both. For example, a ball on the end of a string being twirled around at a constant speed moves in a circular path. Because its direction is constantly changing, there is an acceleration. In this case the tension (force) in the string produces a centripetal (toward the center) acceleration. If the string breaks, the ball will fly off in a straight line.

An acceleration produced by a force occurring along a straight line is called a linear acceleration. An acceleration produced by a torque occurs about an axis of rotation, and is called an angular acceleration.

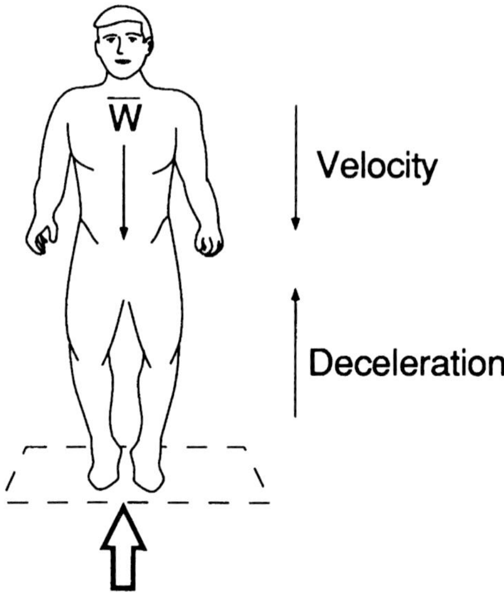

Figure 8
The reaction force provided by the floor pushing up on the feet of a person landing from a jump decelerates his/her downward motion.

Figure 8 shows an example of linear deceleration. Here, the force of the floor is pushing up on the feet of a person who has just landed from a jump. This force is acting to decelerate, and eventually stop, the person's downward motion and, therefore, would be much greater than if the person were standing, when the force from the floor was balancing only body weight. The increase in force is proportional to the deceleration, which is, on average, equal to the change in speed divided by the time interval during which the change occurs. Thus, factors that lengthen this time interval, such as soft, compressible running-shoe heels or bending the knees, will diminish the decelerating force, that is, soften the impact.

Figure 9 shows an example of angular acceleration. The knee extensor force $\mathbf{F}_e$ generates a moment about the center of rotation O in the knee. The magnitude of the moment is given by $M_o = F_e \times d$. It provides an angular acceleration to the lower leg in rotation about the center of rotation of the knee O. The greater the magnitude of the force $\mathbf{F}_e$, the greater the impact will be at the instant the foot strikes the football. The moment $\mathbf{M}_o$ can be changed in only two ways: (1) change d (for example, total knee replacement or tibial tubercle elevation); or (2) change the magnitude of $\mathbf{F}_e$. The first option is surgical; the second option is exercise or physical therapy.

The knee extensor force $\mathbf{F}_e$ is equivalent to a force $\mathbf{F}_e$ acting at the center of the knee O, causing compression of the tibial plateau and femoral condyle surfaces, and a pure moment (couple) $M_o = F_e \times d$, rotating the lower leg about O. Thus, contrary to popular notions, during a "free" swing of the upper or lower extremity, compressive forces may be generated at the articulating surfaces when the muscles are active; the faster the swing, the larger the compressive force.

Most musculoskeletal movements are caused in this way. Limbs are rotated about joints as a result of the moments produced by the skeletal flexor and extensor muscles. Thus, it is apparent that the musculoskeletal system is essentially a collection of lever systems (shoulder, hip, knee, ankle, etc.) linked together. The facts that the lever arms of muscles and tendons are generally very small and the moment arms of the extremities themselves are generally large result in a mechanical disadvantage that requires generation of large muscle forces to create moments large enough for movement.

Statics

Biomechanical Modeling Concepts

Biomechanics and, indeed, mechanics provide a means to study a problem through its representation by a physical model. Assumptions about the isolated unit must be made to construct the model. These assumptions deal with the geometry of the unit (size and shape) and the nature of the material(s) of which the unit is composed. Furthermore, assumptions must also be made about the nature of forces and moments acting on the surface of the object. These forces and moments move and deform the object. Clearly, the accuracy and acceptability of predictions based on the model depend on how well the model is constructed, especially on how closely it represents the actual unit with respect to the specific types of questions being pursued in the study. For example, modeling the action of a muscle on a bone as a single resultant force applied to the muscle's point of insertion may be reasonable if the aim of the study is to understand the muscle's moment about an adjacent joint, or to help predict the effect of a tendon transfer on gait. However, this

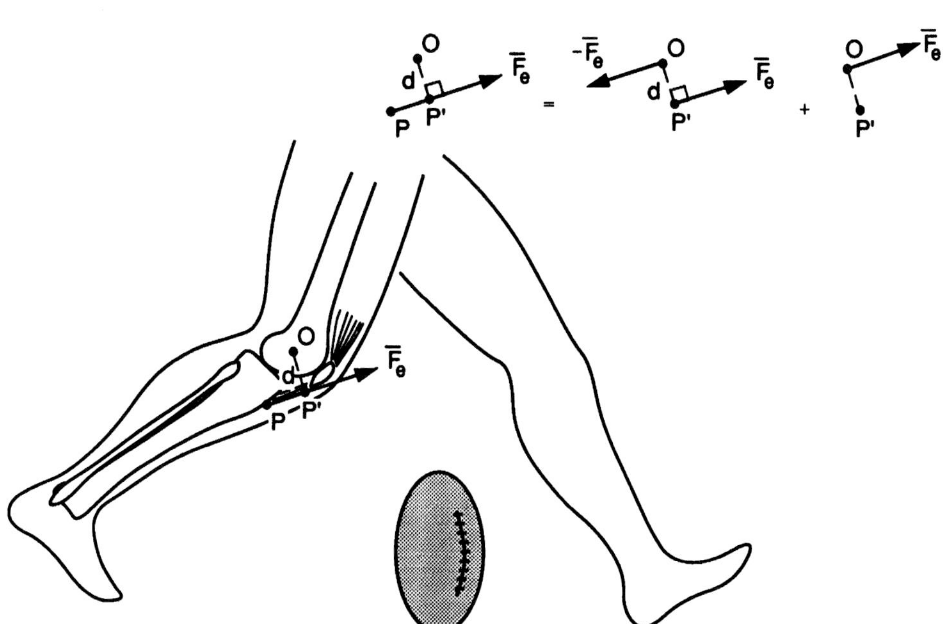

Figure 9
The knee extensor force $\mathbf{F}_e$ generates a moment about the center of rotation O in the knee. The magnitude of the moment is given by $M_o = F_e \times d$. Note that from the concept of the equipollent force systems, the knee extensor force $\mathbf{F}_e$ is equivalent to a force $\mathbf{F}_e$ acting at the center of the knee 0, compressing the tibial plateau and femoral condyle surfaces together, and a pure moment $M_o = F_e \times d$, rotating the lower leg about 0.

model would be totally inadequate in a study aimed at understanding modes of tendon failure in tension, in which the precise geometry of the tendon and its insertion, the pattern of stress and strain within the tendon under load, and the material properties of the tendon are crucial to the problem.

A rigid body is an idealization of a real object; it assumes that the body is absolutely rigid so that it does not stretch, compress, or otherwise deform no matter how large are the forces and moments acting on it. This assumption, for example, usually is made in gait analysis models. Here, the model for the musculoskeletal system assumes bones to be absolutely rigid rods (stick figures) and joints to be rigid frictionless hinges. The important elements of rigid body mechanics are: (1) the magnitude and direction of forces and moments acting on the object; (2) the total mass of, and its distribution within, the object; and (3) the size and geometric form of the object.

Equilibrium

When the sum of all forces acting on an object is zero and the sum of all moments acting on an object also is zero, there will be no linear or angular acceleration; the object is said to be in equilibrium, at rest, or at constant velocity.

Large forces may be involved within a system at equilibrium, although the sum of all forces is zero when added together. For example, two evenly matched men playing tug-of-war will be at equilibrium so long as they pull equally hard on each end of the rope. Static analysis examines systems in equilibrium in this fashion. Although biologic systems are rarely in complete equilibrium, static analysis often is helpful in estimating skeletal forces.

Figure 10 illustrates the concept of both force and moment equilibrium. In this example two children, one weighing 600 N and the other weighing 300 N, are sitting on the seesaw. At equilibrium, the amount of force applied at the hinge support of the seesaw must equal the sum of the weight of the two children. Thus, the reaction force **R** at the hinge may be calculated by summing all the forces acting on the seesaw: – 300 N (down) – 600N (down) + **R** (up) = 0. Hence, the reaction force **R** at the hinge is a vector of magnitude 900 N pointing up.

For an object to be in equilibrium, the sum of all the moments must also equal zero. In this example, because the seesaw is not rotating, the net moment about the hinge supports must equal zero. Thus, for the sum of the moments about the hinge O to balance, the 300-N child must be sitting at a distance of 2 m to the right of the hinge to cancel the moment of the 600-N child sitting 1 m to the left of the hinge. The moment 300 N × 2 m clockwise must be equal to the moment 600 N × 1 m counterclockwise. The reaction force of 900 N at the hinge does not cause a moment about the hinge, because the moment arm of this force is zero. For many applications, a hinge is used because it cannot transmit a moment.

Thus static equilibrium analysis examines a system at rest in which all the forces are balanced, allowing unknown forces, which must exist to balance the known forces, to be determined.

Problem:

When an object is in static equilibrium, any point may be used to calculate the moment, and the sum of all these moments will still be zero. Demonstrate this principle by calculating the moments caused by the two children and the reaction force about A.

Free-Body Diagrams

The forces acting on any limb or body part may be identified by isolating that body part as a free

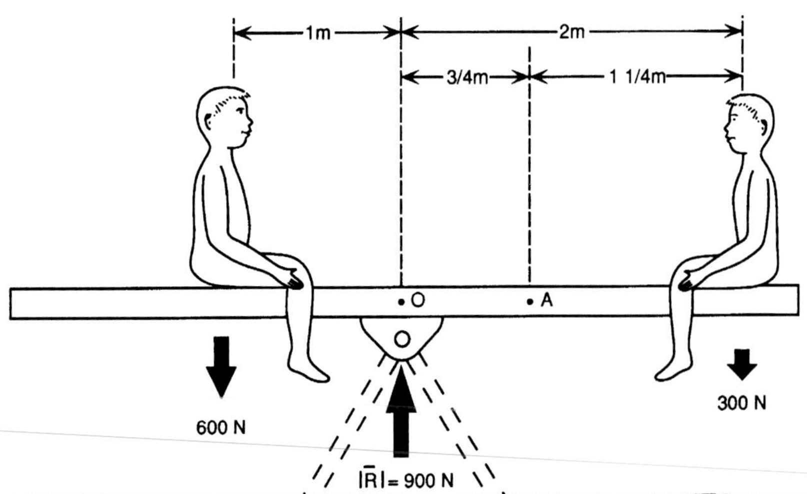

Figure 10
Force and moment balance must occur for motion equilibrium to exist. The reaction force at the hinge (900 N) may be determined by setting the sum of all vertical forces to zero. The sum of the moments must also equal zero so that the seesaw does not rotate.

body. For a portion of the body to be at equilibrium, the sum of all forces must be zero, and the sum of all moments must be zero. Because both forces and moments are vectors, they must sum to zero in each of three perpendicular directions. Thus, in three dimensions, there are a total of six equations of equilibrium, and a maximum of six unknowns may be solved.

Statically determinate problems are ones in which the number of unknown forces and moments is equal to the number of available equations. These equations may then be solved to determine the unknown forces. In statically indeterminate problems, the number of unknowns exceeds the number of equations available. Thus, there are not enough equations to solve for the unknowns, and if a solution for the unknowns is available, it will not be unique. To illustrate this point, consider the seesaw problem shown in Figure 10. Is it possible to determine the weights of two persons by seating them at known distances from the hinge at one side when the weight of the third person at the other side of the hinge is known, and that person's seating position relative to the hinge is specified so that the seesaw is balanced horizontally? The seesaw is similar to the old fashioned, lever-arm balance scale used to determine weights. However, in this seesaw problem, there are three unknowns: the vertical reaction force at the hinge and the weights of the two persons, and there are only two equations: the vertical component of force and the moment about an axis perpendicular to the plane of the seesaw (the axis may be taken to be the hinge). Clearly, in this problem, no unique solution can be found, because an infinite variation of weights for the two individuals may be chosen to balance this seesaw. Unfortunately, in nearly every problem encountered in orthopaedic biomechanics, which involves the determination of muscle and joint forces, the situation is statically indeterminate because of the large number of muscles spanning the joint. This problem may be remedied by drastically simplifying the model, sometimes even in an unrealistic manner, so that an estimate of the important muscle or joint force may be obtained. Once again, of course, the reliability and accuracy of any model calculations depend on how realistic that model is in replicating the actual anatomic and physiologic circumstances.

A method frequently used in modeling is to assume that a muscle force exists only in tension; that is, to assume that muscles cannot exert compressive forces. Another commonly used method is to assume that the joint-reaction force only can be compressive, that is, tension force at the joint will cause the joint surfaces to lose contact. If the line of action of the muscle force is defined by assuming that it always acts along the center of the cross-sectional area of the muscle mass, the magnitude of the muscle force is the only remaining unknown. Another common simplifying assumption is to model a joint as a hinge (for example, the ankle), eliminating two of three possible axes of rotation and ignoring translations.

In this method of solving for the forces and moments around a joint at equilibrium, only the external forces and moments acting on the free body are considered. Internal forces within the free body cancel out. However, if care is taken in choosing the part to be modeled as a free body, it is possible to expose an internal force.

Forces on the Hip Joint

The free-body method of solution will be illustrated by calculating the abductor and joint-reaction forces at the hip. Figure 11, *left,* illustrates the case of a person standing on the right leg. In this free-body diagram, the body and the left leg have a weight of 5 W/6, where W is the total weight of the person. This weight must be supported and balanced by the force acting on the right acetabulum, joint-reaction force $\mathbf{F}_j$, and by the action of the abductor muscles, $\mathbf{F}_{AB}$. The moment equilibrium equation can be applied to determine the abductor force acting about the hip joint. The weight, 5 W/6, which tends to rotate the upper body about the center of the femoral head O, is counteracted by the pull of the abductor muscles on the pelvis. The hip joint is assumed to be frictionless so no reaction moment exists. Thus, for the body to be in equilibrium, the unknown counterclockwise moment (+) created by the abductor muscles must be balanced by the known clockwise moment (-) created by the gravitational forces of 5 W/6. In this model, the point of application and direction of the abductor force $\mathbf{F}_{AB}$ are assumed to be known from anatomic data; thus only the magnitude of $\mathbf{F}_{AB}$ is unknown. Taking the moments about the center of the femoral head O, with b the distance from O to the line of action of the 5 W/6 weight and a the distance from O to the abductor muscle force $\mathbf{F}_{AB}$, the magnitudes of the two moments are $-(5\ W/6) \times (b)$ and $(F_{AB}) \times (a)$, respectively. For equilibrium, the sum of these two moments must equal zero. Thus, given a body weight W and a measured distance of a = 5 cm and b = 15 cm, the magnitude of the abductor muscle force F_{AB} will be 2.5 W (Fig. 11, *left*). The reaction force at the joint $\mathbf{F}_j$ does not create a moment about the joint center (center of rotation), similarly to the reaction force at the hinge in the seesaw.

The hip-joint-reaction force $\mathbf{F}_j$ can be calculated by applying the force equilibrium condition that the sum of all forces acting on the pelvis must equal zero. This calculation is made by using a force triangle, based on the parallelogram law of vector addition

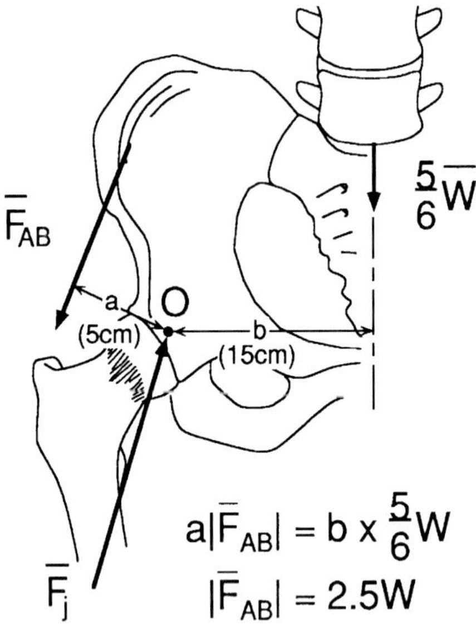

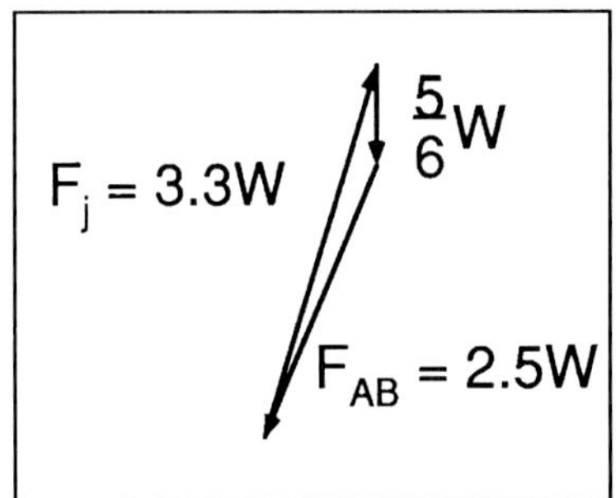

Figure 11
Left, A free-body diagram of the hip of a man standing on his right leg; the body and the left leg weighs 5 W/6, where W is the total weight of the person. The magnitude of the abductor muscle force F_{AB}, the direction of which is assumed known, may be determined by setting the sum of the moments about O equal to zero. **Right,** A force triangle may be constructed to determine the joint-reaction force $\mathbf{F}_j$.

(Fig. 11, *right*). When only three forces are acting on a body in equilibrium, these forces must form a closed force triangle, because the two forces 5 W/6 and $\mathbf{F}_{AB}$ must add, by the parallelogram law, to equal the third unknown force $\mathbf{F}_j$. Therefore, by simple geometric construction with the two known sides of the triangle, the gravitational force on the body, 5 W/6, and the abductor muscle force, 2.5 W, drawn to scale, the third side of the triangle also can be drawn to scale. The length of this third side is the magnitude of $\mathbf{F}_j$ and the direction of the arrow is the direction of the force $\mathbf{F}_j$. In this simple example, the magnitude of the joint-reaction force F_j is calculated to be 3.3 W. Both the muscle force and the joint-reaction force are considerably greater than the weight of the body and leg they are supporting because of the lever action of muscle forces around the hip joint.

Problem:

During osteoarthritis of the hip, where the near frictionless cartilage has been totally worn away, frictional force of significant magnitude exists between the femoral head bone and the acetabular bone. This frictional force exerts a resisting moment so that the perfectly frictionless ball and socket joint is not a good modeling assumption. To account for this, suppose in a model for the osteoarthritic hip that friction between the two articulating surfaces can exert a resisting torque of 25 N·m. In this model, calculate the abductor reaction force required to maintain this osteoarthritic hip in equilibrium in the above example.

Forces on the Spine

The free-body diagram (model) shown in Figure 12 can be used to show how the musculoskeletal lever system can magnify the compressive force acting on the spine during an ordinary daily activity such as holding a weight W_1 with an outstretched hand. Calculation of the compressive force F_N in the spine begins with consideration of the moment equilibrium condition about the center of a vertebral body O. The moment that the weight W_1 creates about O is clockwise and is equal to $-(W_1) \times (b)$. Similarly, the moment of the upper body weight is $-(W) \times (c)$. The extensor muscle force $\mathbf{F}_e$ creates a counterclockwise moment about O given by $+ (F_e) \times (a)$. For equilibrium, these three moments must balance; therefore, $F_e = (W_1b + Wc)/a$. For an upper body weight W = 500 N (2/3 of a body weight of 750 N), a held weight of W_1 = 100 N, and the distances a = 5 cm, b = 50 cm, and c = 8 cm, the magnitude of the extensor muscle force F_e required to hold this weight is calculated to be (1,000 + 800)N. Note that the 100-N weight held at 50 cm produces a 1,000-N force in F_e while the 500-N upper body weight produces only 800 N in F_e.

For the portion of the upper body to be at equilibrium, the sum of the vertical components of all forces must add to zero: $F_N\cos\theta - F_e\cos\theta - W - W_1 + F_t\sin\theta = 0$. The sum of the horizontal components of all forces must also add to zero: $F_N\sin\theta - F_e\sin\theta - F_t\cos\theta = 0$. If $\theta = 60°$, then the two equations can be solved to give $F_t = (W + W_1)\sin60° = 520$ N and $F_N = F_e + (W + W_1)\cos60° = 2{,}100$ N. Hence the component of the compressive force acting perpendicularly to the face of the vertebral body $\mathbf{F}_N$ is many times the weight supported. The major contribution to the compressive force on the vertebral body derives from the extensor muscle force (1,800 N), and the major component of that force (1,000 N) results from holding the relatively small force (100 N) at 50 cm in the outstretched hand. If the distance b is reduced by holding the weight W_1 closer to the

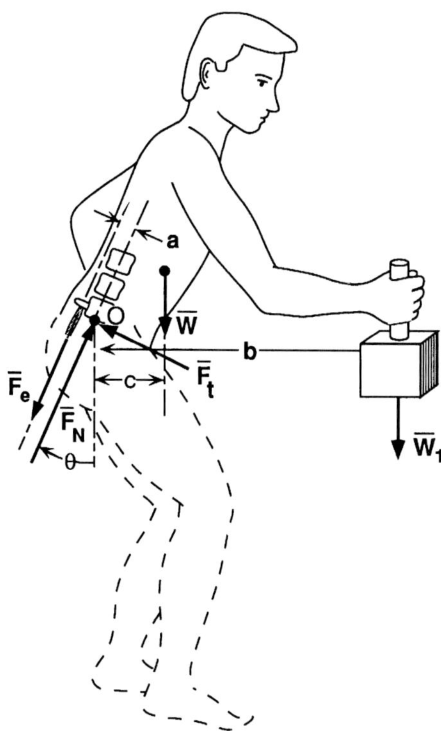

Figure 12
A free-body diagram of the spine. The normal compressive force F_N acting on the spine is 2,100 N even during an ordinary daily activity such as holding a 100-N weight by an outstretched hand (at 50 cm).

body, the magnitude of the normal compressive force F_N acting on the vertebral body will be reduced dramatically. The contribution of body weight to the compressive force is usually much less than that of a weight held by an outstretched hand. This finding illustrates the large forces that may be generated in the spine from simple activities, causing fracture in some patients, especially those with osteoporosis.

Problem:

Assuming everything else remains the same as in the example discussed above, describe how the compressive force on the lumbar intervertebral discs will vary going from L-1 to L-5.

Forces on the Shoulder

Figure 13 shows how the muscle and joint-reaction forces acting about the shoulder can be calculated when a weight is held at arm's length. In this problem, the free-body diagram consists of the extended arm with three forces acting on it: the weight **W** being held; the deltoid muscle force $\mathbf{F_D}$; and the joint-reaction force $\mathbf{F_J}$ between the humeral head and the glenoid fossae. In this example, the weight of the arm (30 N) is neglected while determining only the extra deltoid muscle force and the glenohumeral joint force resulting from the held weight W (100 N). In this free-body diagram, four modeling assumptions for the unknown forces have been made: (1) a two-dimensional (2-D) plane model is chosen; (2) the location of the deltoid force

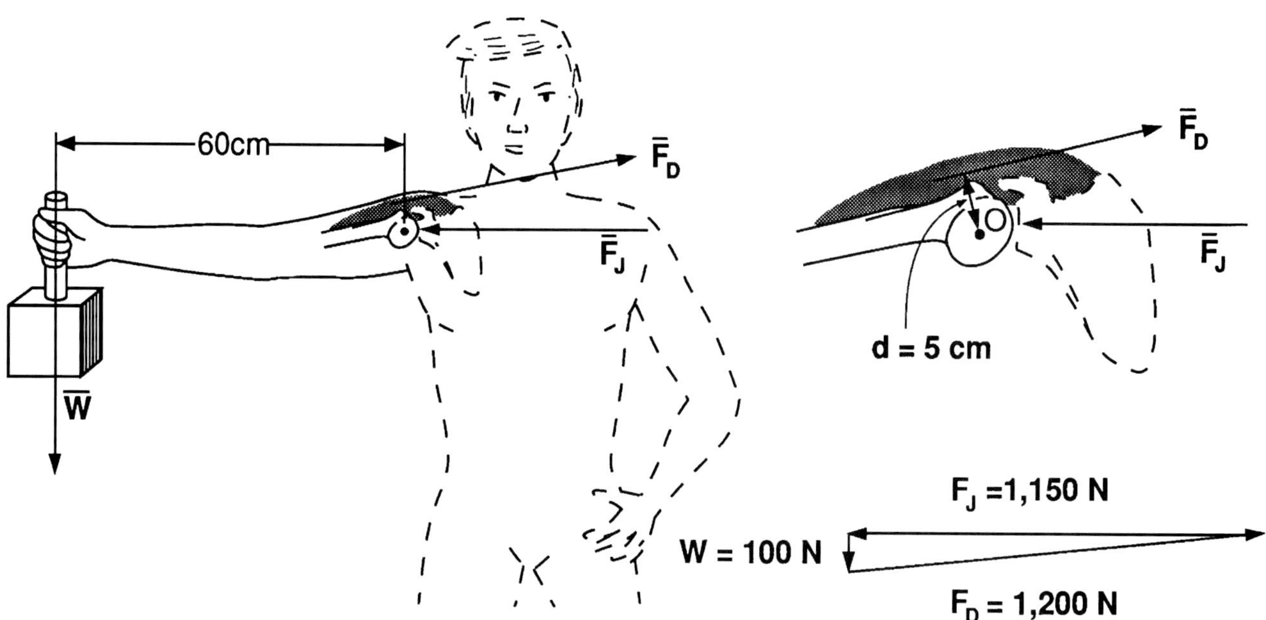

Figure 13
A man holds a weight W at a distance of 60 cm from the center of rotation of the humeral head. After determining the magnitude of the deltoid muscle force F_D (its direction is given) by summing the moments about O, F_J may be found from the force triangle.

is at the centroid of the muscle (d = 5 cm from the center of the humeral head) and is given from anatomic data; (3) the deltoid force is tensile; and (4) the glenohumeral joint force is compressive. The held weight W is 100 N in the direction of gravity (down), and is located 60 cm from the center of the humeral head O. When the arm is in equilibrium, these three forces and their moments must sum to zero. Again, by taking the moments about O, the clockwise moment of the deltoid muscle force is -(F_D) × d and must balance the counterclockwise moment of the weight + (W) × 60; thus, F_D = 1,200 N. This equals about 1.5 times the average body weight of an adult; this is a result of lever action.

The joint-reaction force $\mathbf{F_J}$ can be found by using the force triangle concept shown in the lower right-hand side of the figure. By drawing the sides of the triangle proportional to the length of the forces, the joint-reaction force is found to be 1,150 N in the direction shown.

Problem:

Find the total joint-reaction force $\mathbf{F_J}$ and the total deltoid muscle force $\mathbf{F_D}$ if the weight of the arm (30 N), located at the centroid of the arm 30 cm from O, is also included in the above problem.

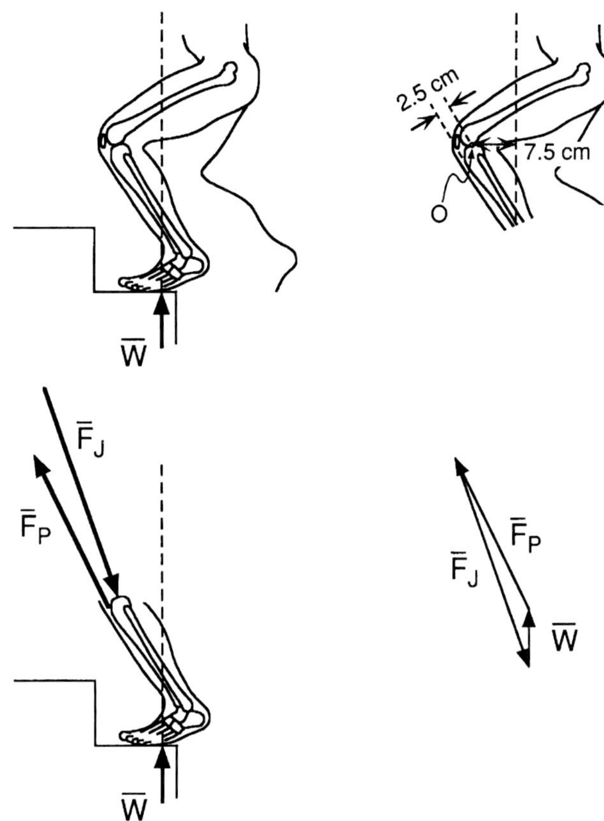

Figure 14
Top left, If during slow stair-climbing the inertial force on the leg may be neglected, then the ground-reaction force on the foot is **W,** the weight of the person. **Top right,** The knee is flexed so that the ground-reaction force passes 7.5 cm posterior to the center O of the knee joint. The patellar tendon force F_p acts 2.5 cm from O. **Bottom left,** The three major forces acting on the lower leg are the ground-reaction force **W,** the patellar tendon force $\mathbf{F_P}$, and the compressive force on the tibial plateau of the knee joint $\mathbf{F_J}$. **Bottom right,** Force triangle to determine the joint-reaction force $\mathbf{F_J}$ acting on the lower leg.

Forces on the Knee Joint

If a person is slowly climbing steps, the inertial force (that is, force due to acceleration) on the leg may be neglected. Thus, the leg may be considered to be in static equilibrium (Fig. 14, *top left*). The floor is pushing up on the foot with a force equal to body weight; otherwise the body would be falling. This ground-reaction force passes 7.5 cm posterior to the center O of the knee joint, creating a counterclockwise flexion moment about the knee (Fig. 14, *top right*). For the lower leg to be in equilibrium, three major forces must be acting: the ground-reaction force **W**; the tension on the patellar tendon $\mathbf{F_P}$; and the compressive force on the tibial plateau of the knee joint $\mathbf{F_J}$, (Fig. 14, *bottom left*). Here $\mathbf{F_P}$ is assumed to be acting at 2.5 cm from the center O of the knee (Fig. 14, *top right*). To satisfy moment equilibrium about the center of the knee joint O, the flexion moment (counterclockwise) caused by the ground-reaction force + (W) × (7.5) must equal the extension moment (clockwise) caused by the patellar tendon force - (F_P) × (2.5). Thus, the magnitude of the patellar tendon force F_P is 3 W, showing the lever action again. By using the force triangle, the joint-reaction force F_J is determined to be 3.5 W (Fig. 14, *bottom right*). Thus, large forces can be created at the knee even during very slow stair-climbing and other ordinary activities.

Problem:

Specifically identify the modeling assumptions used to arrive at the free-body diagram for the lower leg of the illustrative example discussed above.

Problem:

If during a sudden application of stepping, the reaction force at the foot is 2 W, find $\mathbf{F_P}$ and $\mathbf{F_J}$ in this problem.

Forces on the Ankle

When a person does a bilateral toe raise, large forces may also be generated on the ankle. One-half of the body weight (W/2) is supported by each foot. As illustrated in Figure 15, the ankle dorsiflexion moment (counterclockwise) created by the ground

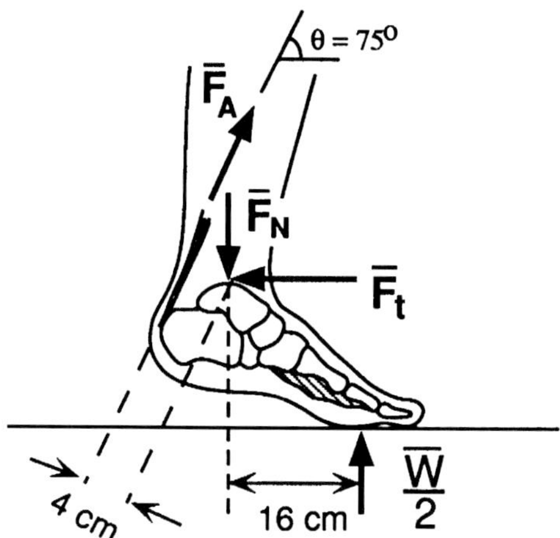

Figure 15
Free-body diagram of the ankle during dorsiflexion. The major forces acting on the foot are the Achilles tendon force $\mathbf{F}_A$, the tangential $\mathbf{F}_t$ and the normal $\mathbf{F}_N$ components of the joint-reaction force, and the floor-foot reaction force **W**/2.

reaction is + (0.5W) × 16 and is balanced by the plantarflexion moment (clockwise) created by the tension of the Achilles tendon, equal to - (F_A) × (4). The moment arms for both of these forces were obtained from radiographic measurement. For equilibrium, these two moments are equal; thus the force F_A in the Achilles tendon must be 2 W. If θ = 75°, then $F_t = F_A\cos 75° = 0.52$ W and $F_N = F_A\sin 75° + (W/2) = 2.43$ W. Therefore, the joint-reaction force is $(F_N^2 + F_t^2)^{1/2} = 2.49$ W.

In all the examples discussed, the large forces at the joint surface $\mathbf{F}_J$ result from the lever action of the muscle forces required to balance the relatively low applied loads. If the applied loads are high, then the joint-reaction loads will be proportionally higher. For high-performance athletes, such as a baseball pitcher accelerating a baseball up to 150 km/hr during a pitch, or soccer players kicking the ball at 80 km/hr, very high muscle forces are required to accelerate the limb and ball. These forces will produce a correspondingly higher joint-reaction force.

Kinematics

Kinematics is the study of the relationships between positions, velocities, and accelerations of rigid bodies, without concern for how the motions are caused (that is, without concern for forces and moments acting on the body). In other words, kinematics describes the geometry of motion.

Position Vectors

The position of an object at any time is always defined relative to a reference frame. In this chapter, the reference frame is assumed to be the x-y plane with origin O. The position of an object such as the femur (Fig. 16), which is assumed to be a rigid body in this discussion, may be defined by two points P and Q (in three dimensions (3-D) three points would have to be specified to fully define an object's

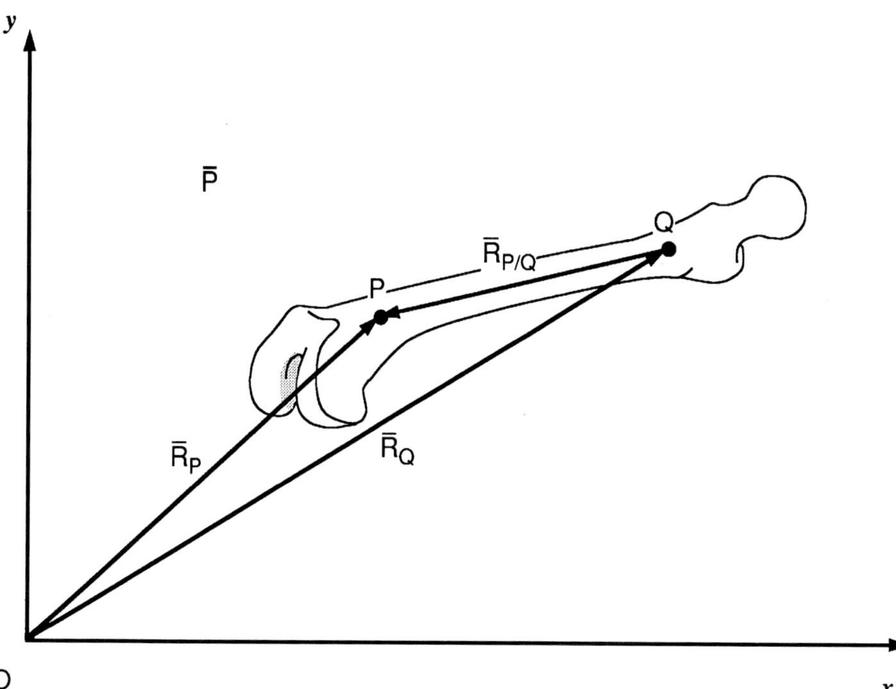

Figure 16
The position of the rigid body (femur) is defined by the two points P and Q located in the x-y plane by the two vectors $\mathbf{R}_P$ and $\mathbf{R}_Q$. The vector locating the point P relative to Q, $\mathbf{R}_{P/Q}$, is given by the parallelogram law of vector addition: $\mathbf{R}_{P/Q} = \mathbf{R}_P - \mathbf{R}_Q$.

position). These points are located in the x-y plane by two vectors $\mathbf{R}_P$ and $\mathbf{R}_Q$. The vector locating the point P relative to Q, $\mathbf{R}_{P/Q}$, is given by the parallelogram law of vector addition:

$$\mathbf{R}_Q + \mathbf{R}_{P/Q} = \mathbf{R}_P \text{ or } \mathbf{R}_{P/Q} = \mathbf{R}_P - \mathbf{R}_Q.$$

Because P and Q are arbitrarily chosen on the femur, the definition of a rigid body is given by:

$$|\mathbf{R}_{P/Q}| = \text{constant}.$$

This means that the distance between any pair of points on the femur remains constant. If it were to change, then internal deformation would be taking place, and the body would no longer be rigid.

In 3-D space, six coordinates are required to locate and orient the rigid body. These six coordinates may be defined as: (1) the three coordinates of a point such as Q; and (2) the three orientation angles of the body relative to an x,y,z reference frame. This corresponds to the intuitive notion that a rigid body may be translated in three perpendicular directions, and rotated about three axes. In Figure 17, the center of the humeral head is placed at the origin O defined by the three coordinates (0,0,0) in the x,y,z reference frame. The position of the humerus relative to the origin can be defined by the three angles θ,ϕ,ψ. The humerus may be translated anteroposterior (x-direction), superior-inferior (z-direction), or toward or away from the glenoid (joint compression or distraction; y-direction). Possible rotations of the humerus are abduction/adduction θ in a vertical plane, for example, the scapular plane; flexion/extension ϕ relative to the scapular plane, or axial rotation ψ around the longitudinal axis of the humerus. These six possible motions corresponding to the six coordinates are described as the six degrees of freedom of a rigid body. If a fixed fulcrum were implanted (for example, a constrained shoulder replacement), then translation would no longer be possible, and only three degrees of freedom, corresponding to rotation, would remain.

Velocity Vectors: Translation and Rotation

Velocity is defined as the change of position with respect to time. Because the position of any point P is defined by a vector, velocity is also a vector, having both magnitude (speed) and direction. Velocity is measured in units of meters/second (m/s).

Translation occurs when all points on a body are moving in the same direction. If two points on the rigid body are moving in two different directions, then the body will be both translating and rotating. The rotation of an object is described by an angular velocity vector, usually denoted by ω. In general, the motion of any rigid body can be described in terms of a combination of a translation plus a rotation. The velocity of a point P on any rigid body is given by the velocity of any point Q, $\mathbf{V}_Q$, plus the relative velocity of point P with respect

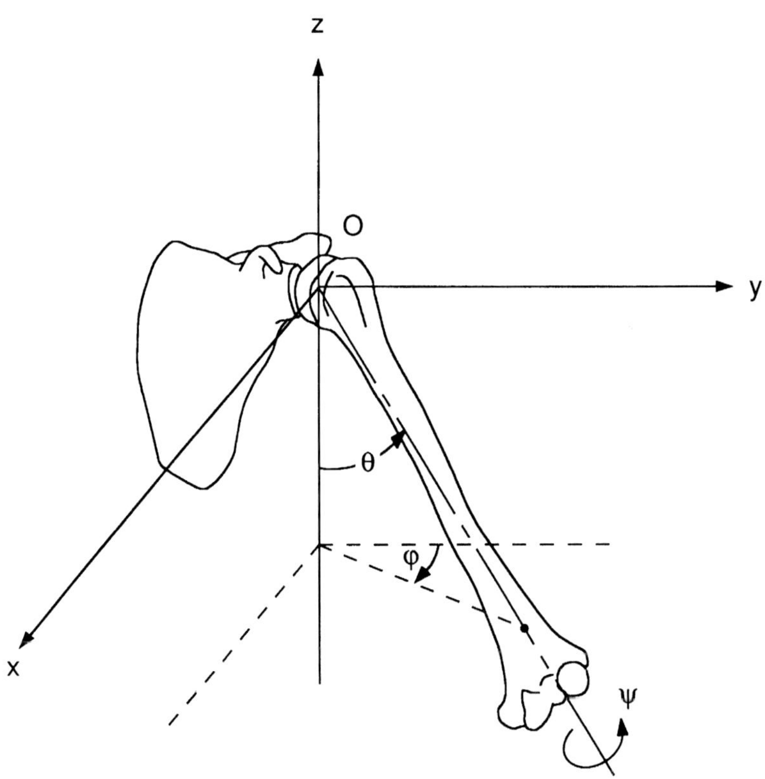

Figure 17
Illustration of the six degrees of freedom of a rigid body: the position of one point of the rigid body must be specified (for example, the three coordinates locating the humeral head); and the three angular orientations θ,ϕ,ψ are relative to a set of xyz coordinate axes.

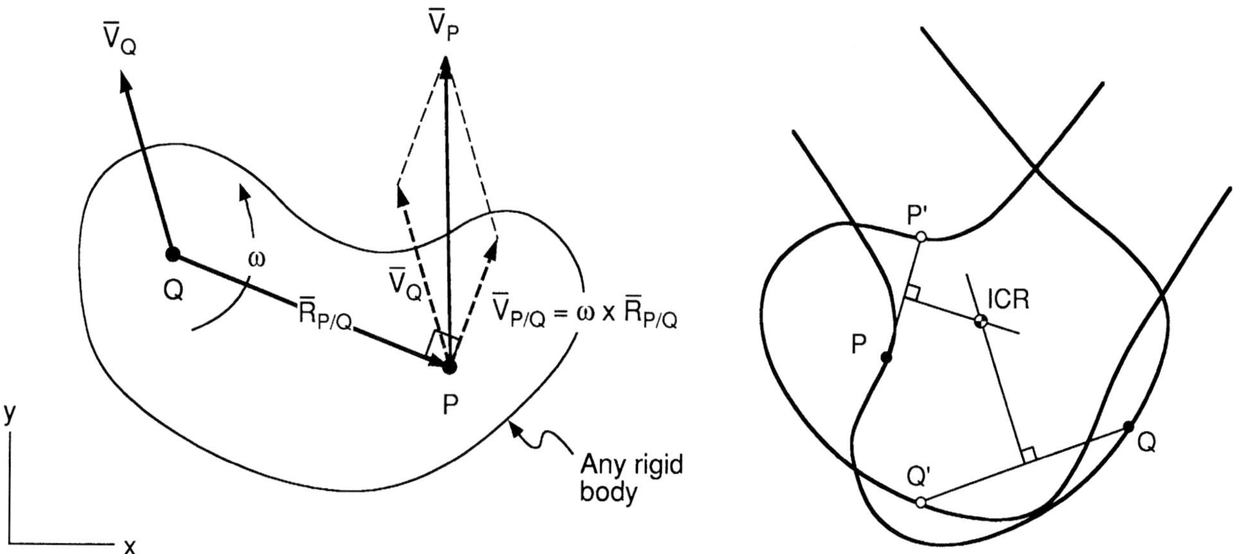

Figure 18
Left, For rigid bodies, the velocity of point P, $\mathbf{V}_P$, is equal to the sum of the velocity of point Q, $\mathbf{V}_Q$, plus a relative velocity $\mathbf{V}_{P/Q}$ of point P with respect to Q ($\omega \times \mathbf{R}_{P/Q}$): $\mathbf{V}_P = \mathbf{V}_Q + \mathbf{V}_{P/Q} = \mathbf{V}_Q + \omega \times \mathbf{R}_{P/Q}$. **Right,** The ICR (instant center of rotation) may be found by drawing: (1) lines connecting two nearby successive positions P-P′ and Q-Q′ of two arbitrary points P and Q on the body; and (2) lines perpendicular to two lines P-P′ and Q-Q′ at their midpoints. The intersection of these two perpendicular bisectors locates the ICR. The reason why this construction works is that all points must rotate about the ICR.

to Q, $\mathbf{V}_{P/Q}$ (Fig. 18, *left*). For rigid bodies, this relative velocity $\mathbf{V}_{P/Q}$ is equal to the product ω x $\mathbf{R}_{P/Q}$. This simple result means, for example, that if the motion of the center of a ball is known, as well as the way the ball is turning about the center, then the motion and position of the ball have been described fully.

Instant Center of Rotation

When a 2-D body is rotating without translation, for example, a rotating stationary bicycle gear, any marked point P on the body may be observed to move in a circle about a fixed point called the axis of rotation or center of rotation. When a rigid body is both rotating and translating, for example the motion of the femur during gait, its motion at any instant of time can be described as rotation around a moving center of rotation (Fig. 18, *right*). The location of this point at any instant, termed the instant center of rotation (ICR), is determined by finding the point (ICR) which, at that instant, is not translating. Then by definition, at that instant, all points on the rigid body are rotating about the ICR. For practical purposes the ICR is determined by noting the paths traveled by two points, P and Q, on the object in a very short period of time to P′ and Q′. The paths PP′ and QQ′ will be perpendicular to lines connecting them to the ICR because they approximate, over short periods, tangents to the circles describing the rotation of the body around the ICR at that instant. Perpendicular bisectors to these two paths (Fig. 18, *right*) will intersect at the (approximate) center of rotation.

Problem:

Suppose two roentgenograms of a patient's knee were taken at two slightly different flexion angles, say 30° and 35°. Describe how to find the ICR of the knee of this patient.

Screw Axis

In 3-D, instead of describing a body's motion with respect to an ICR, the concept of a screw (or helical) axis is used. Any rigid body's motion may be described, at any instant, as a combination of rotation about an axis and translation along (parallel to) that same axis. This axis does not have to be within the body. In fact, as the rotational component of the motion becomes smaller, the axis comes to be farther and farther away, approaching infinity for pure translation. At the other extreme, a ball-and-socket joint such as the hip will have more rotation than translation, and its screw axis will pass close to the geometric center of the femoral head. The screw axis description is often used for its elegance and an intuitive conceptualization of 3-D motion, but motions may be described in other ways. For example, because a rigid body's position may be specified by the location of one point and the orientation of the body around it, any motion may be described as the translation of any given point (from its original to its final location) plus a rotation of the body around an axis passing through that point.

Relative Motion at the Articulating Surfaces of Diarthrodial Joints

Although in principle two objects may move relative to one another in any combination of rotation and translation, diarthrodial joint surfaces are constrained in their relative motion, by their surface geometry, the ligamentous restraints, and the action of muscles spanning the joint. In general, joint surface separation (or gapping) and impaction are small compared to overall joint motion.

When surfaces remain in contact in this fashion, they may move relative to each other in either sliding or rolling contact. In rolling contact (Fig. 19, *top left*), the contacting points on the two surfaces have zero relative velocity, namely, no slip. In such a case, the rolling contact by an automobile tire would leave a clear impression of its treads. Because the point P on the wheel, which contacts the ground at any instant, is not moving, it is, by definition, the instant center of rotation for the wheel during rolling (Fig. 19, *top right*), and the arrows define the actual velocities of points on the wheel. Rolling and sliding contact occur together (Fig. 19, *bottom left*) when the relative velocity at the contact point is not zero. The instant center will then lie between the geometric center and the contact point. Under these conditions, in the example of a tire, a skid mark would be left on the ground. In spinning motion (Fig. 19, *bottom right*), the center of rotation will be the axis of the vehicle. This is the case if there is a total loss of traction between a tire and the ground, and the wheel is in pure rotation, with no forward translational motion of the vehicle. This situation often occurs with the tire spinning on icy pavement.

All diarthrodial joint motion consists of both rolling and sliding motion. In the hip and shoulder, sliding motion predominates over rolling motion. In the knee, both rolling and sliding articulation occur simultaneously. These simple concepts affect the design of total joint prostheses. For example, some total knee replacements have been designed for implantation while preserving the posterior cruciate ligament, which appears to help maintain the normal kinematics of rolling and sliding in the knee. Other knee prostheses substitute for ligament control of kinematics by alterations in articular surface contour.

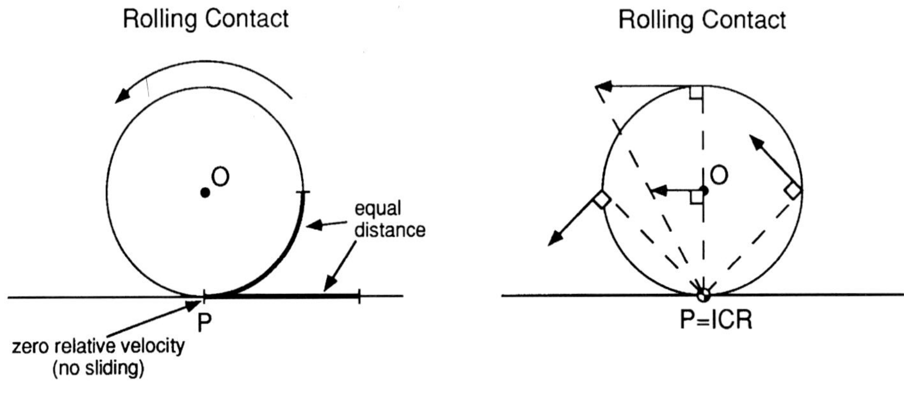

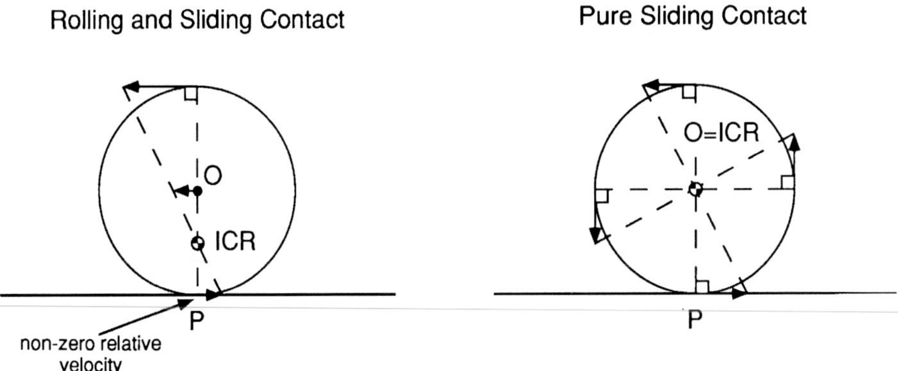

Figure 19
Top left, Rolling contact occurs when the circumferential distance of the rolling object equals the distance traced along the plane. This can only occur when there is no sliding, that is, the relative velocity at the point of contact P is zero. **Top right,** For rolling contact, the point P of the wheel has zero velocity because it is in contact with the ground. Therefore, P is the ICR of the wheel. This diagram shows the actual velocity of points along the wheel as it rolls along the ground. **Bottom left,** Sliding contact occurs when the relative velocity at the contact point is not zero. **Bottom right,** Pure sliding occurs when the wheel rotates about a stationary axis O. In this case, the car would have no forward motion.

Mechanical Properties of Materials

Although modeling skeletal members as rigid bodies can be very useful in many orthopaedic applications, for example, gait analysis, the deformation experienced by the object is of major concern in many problems. Deformation must be considered to understand how a bone may be fractured, how the anterior cruciate ligament may be torn or avulsed, or how the prosthetic femoral stem may be fatigued and fail. In these problems, the rigid body model is no longer appropriate. Understanding these problems requires analysis of the stresses and strains produced inside the body when forces and moments are applied onto the surface of the body.

Forces and moments (excluding electromagnetic effects) can be applied only to the external surface of a body, and stresses and strains inside the body can only be calculated, they can never be measured. However, strains on the surface may be measured experimentally. This distinction between the loading conditions on a body (forces and moments applied to a body) and the state of stress within a body is very important. For example, a frictionless joint surface can be loaded only in compression, but this loading will still produce shear and tensile stresses, as well as compressive stress inside the compressed articular cartilage.

All musculoskeletal tissues, for example, bone, cartilage, intervertebral disk, ligament, meniscus, and tendon, are deformable to some degree. Some are more deformable than others; cartilage is more deformable than bone. The degree of deformability depends on the intrinsic properties of the material of the object (for example, bone versus intervertebral disk) as well as its size and shape. When the deformational response of a material object depends on its size and shape, as well as its intrinsic properties, this response is called a structural property. For example, a 1.0-cm diameter rod would be structurally four times stiffer than a 0.5-cm diameter rod even if both were made of the same material, because the structural stiffness of each rod depends on its cross-sectional area $A = \pi r^2$.

Deformational properties of an object that do not depend on its size and shape are called intrinsic material properties. Load-deformation tests often are used to describe the structural response of a material object. For example, the structural response of the femur-prosthesis composite structure (Fig. 20, *left*), could be measured by loading the entire structure in a testing machine and measuring its bending behavior. To determine the intrinsic material properties of bone or steel, the effect of geometry must be eliminated. This may be done by making geometrically precise specimens for testing (Fig. 20, *right*), by dividing the load (force) by the object's cross-sectional area to determine stress, F/A, and by dividing the elongation by the original length to determine strain, $\Delta l/l_o$. For metals, the strain is usually very small and is measured in microstrain units. The stress-strain behavior of the object describes its intrinsic material response, and all physical quantities obtained from the stress-strain response are intrinsic material properties. In biomechanics, unfortunately, it is often difficult to obtain geometrically well defined specimens from which stress-strain tests may be performed.

Directional Properties

Isotropy

Isotropy is the property of a material such that its intrinsic material properties do not depend upon the direction of loading. In general, the internal structure of such materials is very small and randomly dispersed. Metals, glasses, and plastics are isotropic materials. For isotropic elastic materials, there are only two material constants: Young's modulus

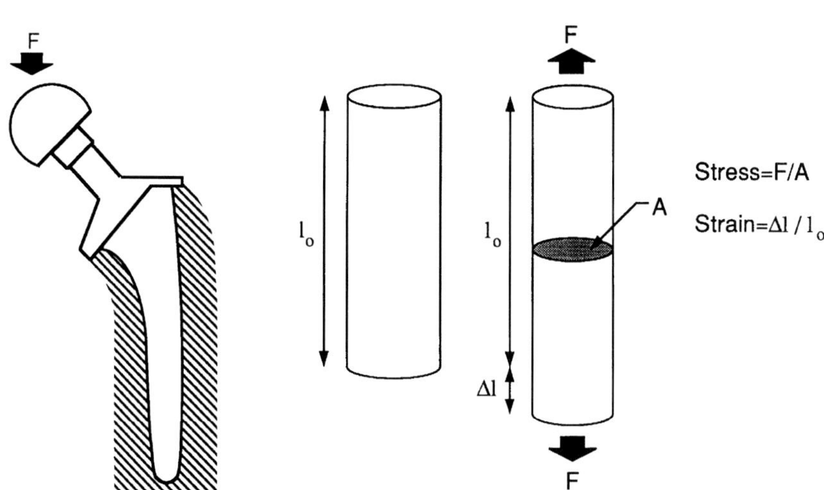

Figure 20
Left, A femur-prosthesis composite structure is loaded for its structural response. The deformation of the structure depends on its geometry (size and shape) as well as the materials it is made of. **Right,** To determine the intrinsic material properties, the stress-strain behavior of the material must be measured. Stress is defined as force/area F/A, and strain is defined as change of length/ original length $\Delta l/l_o$.

E and Poisson's ratio υ. Once these two constants have been determined for an isotropic material, its elastic properties have been fully characterized.

Often, in the literature, other moduli are presented: shear modulus G, bulk compressive modulus k, aggregate modulus H_A, modulus of rigidity G or μ, Lamé coefficients λ,μ. All these moduli are related to each other; once any two are known, the others may be calculated using very simple formulas. Investigators use different forms for these two isotropic coefficients because, in a particular experiment, a specific modulus may be the easiest to use and the most meaningful in terms of physical interpretation.

Anisotropy

Anisotropy is the property of a material such that its intrinsic material properties depend upon the direction of loading. In general, the internal structures of such materials are large and observable, similar in size to the specimens, and arranged in an orderly manner. Wood, fiber-reinforced composite materials, and practically all materials of interest in the musculoskeletal system, such as articular cartilage, cancellous and cortical bone, intervertebral disk, ligament, meniscus, and tendon, are anisotropic. For such materials, more than two material constants are required, although the "apparent" Young's modulus E and Poisson's ratio υ still are used commonly to describe their stress-strain behavior. For example, the meniscus is highly anisotropic. Table 1 provides the tensile modulus of bovine meniscus for specimens taken parallel to the predominant collagen fiber direction and radial to the collagen fiber direction. Bone, ligament, and tendon are often considered to be transversely isotropic. Five constants are required to determine the elastic properties of this type of material. Articular cartilage and meniscus are considered to be orthotropic, and nine constants are required to determine their elastic properties. Besides the isotropic coefficients, very little is known of the other coefficients for these materials.

Strain

Figure 21, *left,* shows how a rectangular block of material (solid lines) will deform when stretched by a force $\mathbf{F}_x$ in the x-direction. This deformation will be an elongation Δl in the x-direction and a contraction - Δd in the y-direction. The original lengths of the sides are l_o and d_o. The lineal strain in the x-direction is defined by

$$\epsilon_{xx} = \Delta l / l_o.$$

The contraction in the y-direction is also a lineal strain, but it is caused by the force applied in the x-direction. In a similar manner, it is possible to define ϵ_{yy} and ϵ_{zz} caused by forces applied in the y- and z-directions, respectively. The Poisson's ratio, if only $\mathbf{F}_x$ is applied, is defined as the ratio:

$$\upsilon = -(\Delta d/d_o)/(\Delta l/l_o).$$

Because Δd and Δl are always in opposite directions, one being (+) and one being (-), the Poisson's ratio is always positive. The Poisson's ratio, which is an important intrinsic property of deformable materials, may be thought of as a measure of how much a material thins when it is stretched (as with a piece of taffy being pulled) and how much it bulges when compressed (as with a piece of clay or intervertebral disk being squeezed). Obviously, the Poisson's ratio may be defined in the y- and z-directions also. These three Poisson's ratios may or may not be equal depending on the microscopic structure of the material. Poisson's ratio is a measure of a material's compressibility. For isotropic materials, a Poisson's ratio of 0 indicates a highly compressible material, such as cork, a cylinder of which does not bulge sideways when compressed. A ratio of 0.5 indicates an incompressible material, such as natural rubber, a cylinder of which will bulge just enough to maintain a constant volume.

Table 1
Material properties of cartilage and meniscus

	Tensile Modulus (MPa)		
	Bovine (| |)*	**Human (| | Normal)**	**Human (| | Fibrillated)**
Cartilage			
Surface zone	42.2	10.1	8.5
Middle zone	13.0	5.9	8.4
Deep zone	2.6	4.5	4.0
Meniscus			
	198 (c)	93–160 (M)	
	4.6 (r)	159–294 (L)	

* | | = parallel specimen; c = circumferential direction parallel to the collagen fibrillar network; r = radial direction perpendicular to the collagen fibrillar network; M = medial meniscus in the circumferential direction; and L = lateral meniscus in the circumferential direction

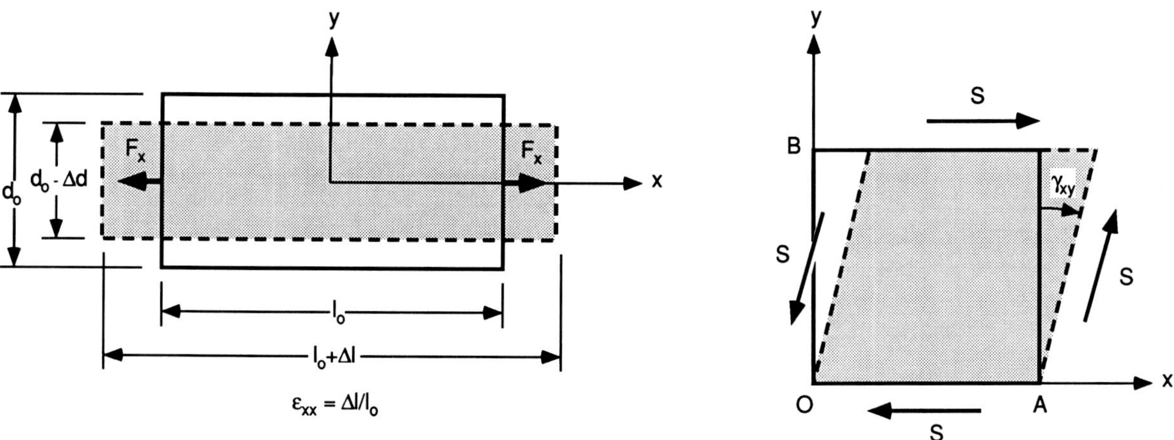

Figure 21
Left, A rectangular block of material (solid lines) will deform when stretched by a force $\mathbf{F}_x$ in the x-direction. This deformation will be an elongation Δl in the x-direction. The lineal strain in the x-direction is defined by $\epsilon_{xx} = \Delta l/l_o$. $\mathbf{F}_x$ causes a contraction $-\Delta d$ in the y-direction. **Right,** A square block of material (solid lines) will deform when sheared by two pairs of forces **S** as shown. The deformation will be a change of angle between the lines OA and OB, denoted by γ_{xy}.

Figure 21, *right,* shows how a square block of material (solid lines) will deform when sheared by two pairs of forces **S** in the x- and y-directions as shown. (For both force and moment equilibrium, the magnitude of forces in the x- and y-directions must be equal.) The deformation caused by these forces will be a change of the angle between the lines OA and OB, which were originally perpendicular. This change of angle is called the shear strain and is denoted by γ_{xy}. Obviously, if the square block of material is taken in the y-z plane or in the x-z plane, and sheared in a similar manner, then shear strains γ_{yz} and γ_{xz} will be created, respectively. For most hard materials, the shear strain is small.

In summary, the complete description of deformation in an object is given by the three lineal strain components, ϵ_{xx}, ϵ_{yy}, ϵ_{zz}, and the three shear strain components, γ_{xy}, γ_{yz}, γ_{xz}. These *six* components define the strain *tensor,* which is a mathematical construct that fully specifies the strain state at each point within deforming objects (for example, bone). The details of how tensors are manipulated are beyond the scope of this book, but it is important to understand that these six components completely define the state of strain. However, to actually analyze the strain, a coordinate system must be chosen. This is an extremely important concept. For example, in Figure 22, *top,* a strip is being loaded in uniaxial tension. The corners of a small block of material oriented parallel to the loading direction will all remain right angles, and no shear strain will be observed in this x-y orientation. If, on the other hand, the block is oriented at 45°, the angles at the corners will change, and shear strain will be observed. How is it that a test in uniaxial tension can cause shear? The force acting on each face of the block oriented at 45° in Figure 23, *top,* can be resolved into two components; one parallel and one perpendicular (Fig. 23, *bottom left*). The parallel components are shear stresses that will distort the square block of material. This simple example shows that the stress state is a sum of the normal stresses and shear stresses (Fig. 23, *bottom right*). This notion is very counter-intuitive at first, and much confusion will occur if the loading condition

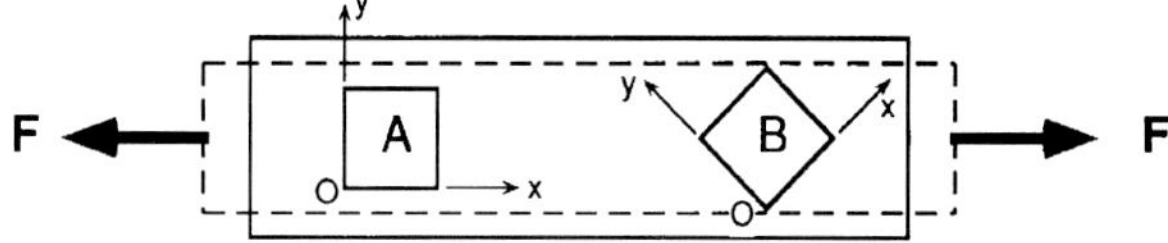

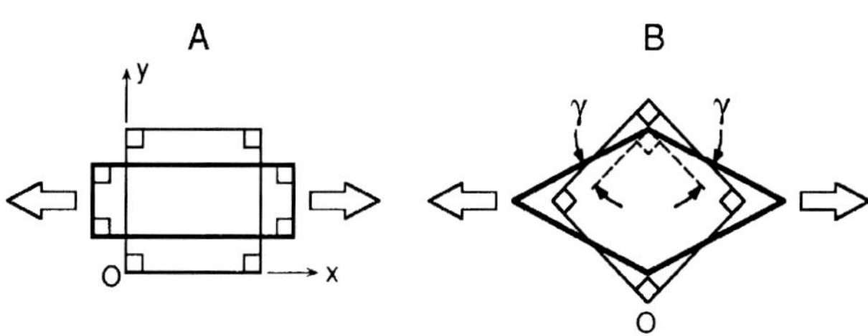

Figure 22
A strip loaded in uniaxial tension. No shear strain will be observed for block A but shear strain will be observed for block B.

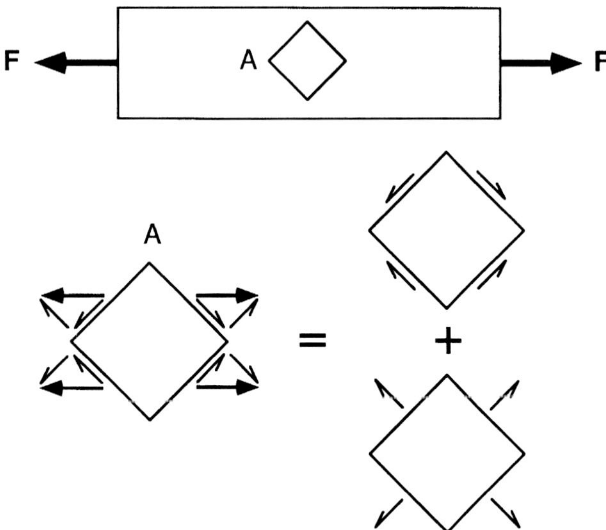

Figure 23
A strip loaded in uniaxial tension (**top**); the stresses acting on block A (**bottom left**) are equivalent to the normal stresses plus the shear stresses (**bottom right**).

(tensile force **F**) is not carefully distinguished from the states of stress and of strain within the material. These stresses are complex and depend on the coordinate system chosen. As with strain, there are six components of stress; three normal stress components and three shear stress components. These components define the stress tensor.

Normal Stress and Shear Stress

Determination of forces acting on the femur in rigid body models has been discussed. Figure 24 shows how these externally applied forces on the femur (Fig. 24, *top left*) will produce internal forces within the bone. Figure 24, *top center,* shows a thin section of the femur and a cube of the diaphyseal bone within the thin section. Only those forces acting on the top and bottom faces of this cube are shown in Figure 24, *top right.* The top and bottom faces of this cube are subjected to two types of forces: F_y, which is perpendicular (normal force), and S, which is parallel (shear force), to these faces (Fig. 24, *bottom*). The normal stress σ_{yy} is defined by F_y/A. This stress can be either compressive or tensile in nature. For the shear force **S** acting on this y-plane, there are two components: $\mathbf{S}_x$ and $\mathbf{S}_z$. Thus, the components of the shear stress acting on the y-planes (top and bottom planes of the cube) are defined by

$$\tau_{xy} = S_x/A \text{ and } \tau_{zy} = S_z/A.$$

Similarly, it is possible to define σ_{xx}, τ_{yx}, τ_{zx} acting on the x-planes (left and right planes), and σ_{zz}, τ_{xz}, τ_{yz} acting on the z-planes (front and back planes). Because the moments must balance,

$$\tau_{xy} = \tau_{yx}, \tau_{zx} = \tau_{xz}, \text{ and } \tau_{yz} = \tau_{zy}.$$

Thus, the six components of stress are the three normal stresses σ_{xx}, σ_{yy}, and σ_{zz} and the three shear stresses τ_{xy}, τ_{yz}, and τ_{xz} corresponding to the six components of strain.

Stress Analysis

These definitions can be used to analyze the state of stress in the simplest of all possible problems. Figure 25, *top left,* shows a rectangular bar being stretched by a single tensile force **F**. By the definition of stress, to determine the state of stress at point P inside the bar (Fig. 25, *top right*), the plane (the coordinate system) on which the stress will be defined must be identified. On the plane defined by $\theta = 0°$, the normal stress $\sigma_o = F/A_o$, and the shear stress $\tau_o = 0$. If the plane is at an angle $\theta \neq 0°$ from the horizontal (Fig. 25, *bottom*), the force **F** has two components with respect to this plane: a normal component given by $F\cos\theta$ and a shear component $F\sin\theta$. However, the area on which these normal and shear forces are acting is also different from the $\theta = 0°$ case. This area A_θ, by simple trigonometry, is equal to $A_o/\cos\theta$ (Fig. 25, *bottom*). Thus, the normal stress σ_θ acting on the θ-plane is given by $\sigma_\theta = (F\cos^2\theta)/A_o$ and the shear stress by $\tau_\theta = (F\sin 2\theta)/2A_o$. The normal stress σ_θ goes from a maximum of F/A_o on the $\theta = 0°$ plane (Fig. 25, *top right*) to zero on the $\theta = 90°$ plane. The shear stress τ_θ goes from zero on the $\theta = 0°$ plane to a maximum of $F/2A_o$ on the $\theta = 45°$ plane; beyond the 45° plane the shear stress decreases to zero at $\theta = 90°$. This analysis is also valid if **F** is taken to be compressive.

This stress analysis of the simplest possible problem indicates that, even for uniaxial tensile loading, shear stresses exist inside the object. Thus, material weak in shear will fail along the $\theta = 45°$ plane when subject to tension or compression. Concrete is such a material. When a concrete bar is overloaded in compression, its failure surface is oriented at 45° from the line of loading. Materials weak in tension, such as cast iron, will fail in a plane perpendicular to the line of loading. Once again, the distinction between loading condition and stress inside the object is crucial.

Figure 26, *left,* shows a square block of material being sheared by the forces **S** acting on each side of the element. Again, obviously, this system of forces is in equilibrium. A free-body diagram of the section of the square created by passing a plane through P along BPD shows that there must be a force **F** given by $\sqrt{2S^2}$ (Fig. 26, *center*). This is from the Pythagorean theorem for right triangles. Using the definition A =

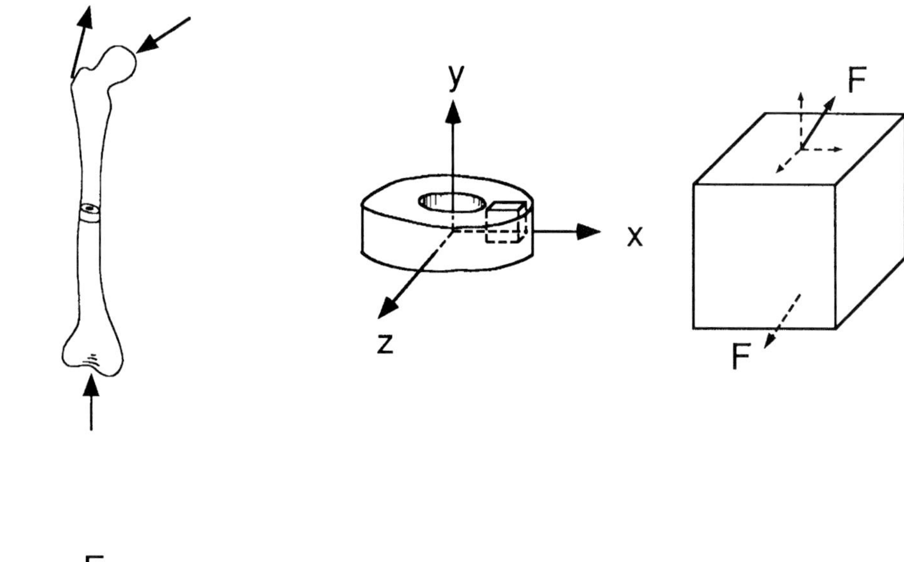

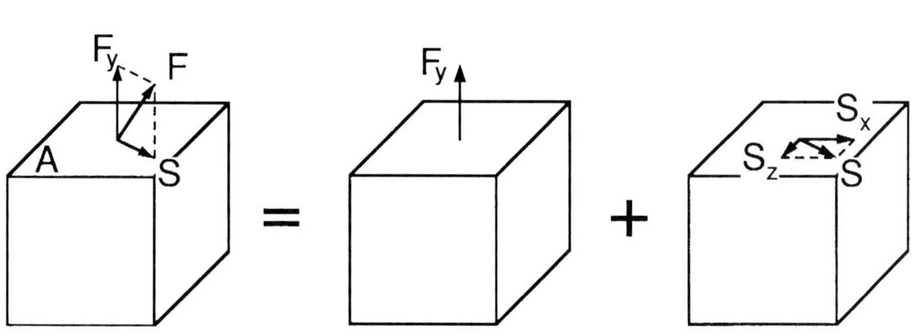

Figure 24
Top left, Externally applied forces on a femur will cause internal stresses to be developed. **Top right,** A thin section of the femur, and a cube of diaphyseal bone. Forces are shown acting on the top and bottom faces of a cube (y-plane). Similar forces also act on the left and right (x-plane), and front and back faces (z-plane) of the cube and have been omitted for clarity. **Bottom,** Resolution of the force acting on the top face of the cube into a normal component F_y and a shear component S. The normal stress σ_{yy} is defined by F_y/A. The shear force S acting on this y-plane has two components: S_x and S_z. The components of the shear stress acting on the y-planes are defined by $\tau_{xy} = S_x/A$ and $\tau_{zy} = S_z/A$.

$A_o/\cos\theta$ (Fig. 25, *bottom*), at 45° the tensile stress acting on the BPD plane is S/A_o. On this plane no shear stress exists, and this is the maximum tensile stress acting inside the square block under the pure shear condition. Similarly, it can be shown that the maximum compressive stress acts on the APC plane (Fig. 26, *right*). Thus, if a material such as bone, which is weak in tension, is sheared, it will fail along the 45° plane BPD. This is the basis for the often observed spiral fracture of the tibia from skiing injuries in which the tibia is torqued by the ski during a fall. The failure surface forms a spiral whose tangent is very close to 45° from the long axis of the tibia.

The results of these stress analyses are valid regardless of the nature of the material, for example, steel, titanium, bone, cartilage, etc. The results of these two stress analysis problems indicate that it is important to know the intrinsic properties of materials. Knowledge is required of materials' intrinsic stiffness in tension, compression, and shear; their respective strengths; and for materials used in prostheses, their fatigue life.

Elastic Properties of Metals and Biologic Tissues

A linear elastic material has three fundamental stress-strain characteristics: (1) stress and strain are directly proportional to each other; (2) the strain is totally recovered when the stress is removed; and (3) the material is insensitive to the rate of loading. For a linear elastic material (Fig. 27, *bottom left*), the straight line OP shows the stress σ to be proportional to the strain ϵ (Hooke's law), that is,

$$F/A = E(\Delta l/l_o),$$

where F, A, Δl, and l_o are all measured quantities on precisely prepared specimens (Fig. 27, *top*). Young's modulus E, an important property of the material, is expressed in units of MPa or GPa. For elastic materials, if in an experiment the maximum load is below point P, Δl will vanish if the load is released.

The proportional limit P is the point beyond which stress is no longer proportional to the strain. The elastic limit (not shown) is the point beyond which further deformation is no longer purely elastic. These two limits are generally regarded to be the same. If the specimen is stretched beyond P, a small but permanent plastic deformation is created, that is, if the load F is released (shown by the down arrow), a small residual or permanent deformation remains (Fig. 27, *bottom left*). This permanent deformation is caused by damage to the internal micro-

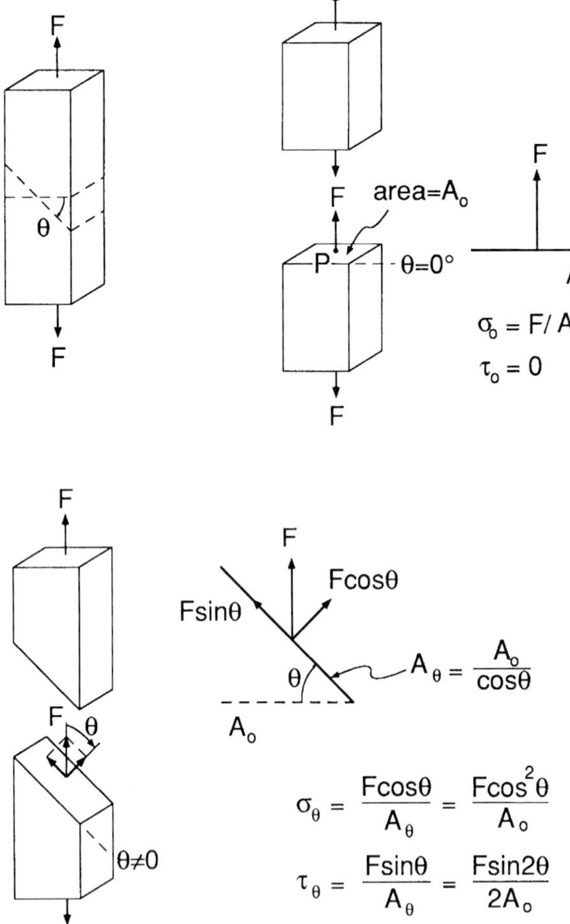

Figure 25
Top left, A rectangular bar being stretched by a single tensile force **F. Top right,** The normal stress F/A_o acting at point P on a plane defined by $\theta = 0°$. No shear stress exists on this plane. **Bottom,** On an inclined plane ($\theta \neq 0°$) the force F has two components with respect to this plane: a normal component, Fcosθ, and a shear component, Fsinθ. The area A_θ on this inclined plane is $A_o/\cos\theta$. Thus, the normal stress σ_θ acting on the θ-plane is equal to $F\cos^2\theta/A_o$ and the shear stress τ_θ is equal to $(F\sin 2\theta)/2A_o$.

structure of the specimen. The yield strength Y is the point at which a large plastic flow occurs, such that strain increases with little or no increase in stress. The ultimate tensile strength U (failure stress) is the point at which the specimen fails. The maximum stress that a material attains is known as its strength; this usually coincides with U. The strain at which failure occurs is known as the failure strain ϵ_f. Tables 1 to 3 provide some material constants for some common orthopaedic materials.

Toughness

Figure 27, *bottom,* shows the typical stress-strain behavior of solid materials such as steel, titanium, or bone and collagenous tissues. The energy a structure absorbs as it is deformed by an applied force is equal to the work done by that force. This energy is calculated as the magnitude of the force times the deformation produced and is equal to the area under the load-deformation curve. The energy required to bring the structure to failure can thus be calculated. This concept is useful because many injuries may impart a specific energy to the body. For example, a fall from a height may turn the potential energy of the body weight at the original height into the energy of deformation of the lumbar spine or hip, causing fracture. To eliminate the effects of size, this energy is divided by the volume of the material being deformed. Because volume equals area × length:

energy/volume = [force × deformation]/[area × length]
= [force/area] × [deformation/length]
= stress × strain
= area under the stress-strain curve

The amount of energy/volume a material can absorb before failure defines the intrinsic toughness of the material. For example, a brittle material often will fail at point P of the stress-strain curve. Such materials as ceramics and cast iron are brittle materials that are easily fractured. Although they are very stiff, these materials are not tough because they cannot absorb much energy. Ductile or annealed steel will fail only after significant amounts of stretching. These materials are intrinsically stiff and tough. Plastics and rubber are relatively soft (not stiff), but will stretch a great amount before failure. Thus, these materials are intrinsically soft and tough. This is the reason why rubber or similar substances are used for bumpers or tires. Collagenous tissues are soft and not particularly tough (Fig. 27, *bottom right*); thus, these tissues fail easily.

Fatigue

Thus far material behavior has been discussed without considering the number of times the loading cycle is repeated. If subjected to large numbers of such cycles, most materials will fail at a stress lower than their ultimate tensile stress U, which is the stress at failure from only one cycle. The number of loading cycles required to cause failure is determined by performing a cyclic stress-strain experiment on the material. For such an experiment, the number of loading cycles required to cause specimen failure is plotted against the maximum stress level attained during the cyclic test. This is known as a σ-n curve (Fig. 28). As the magnitude of the stress decreases from the ultimate stress σ_{ult} (for one cycle), the number of cycles required to induce failure increases until a stress is reached for which failure will not occur, no matter how often the cycle is repeated. This is known as the endurance limit σ_E.

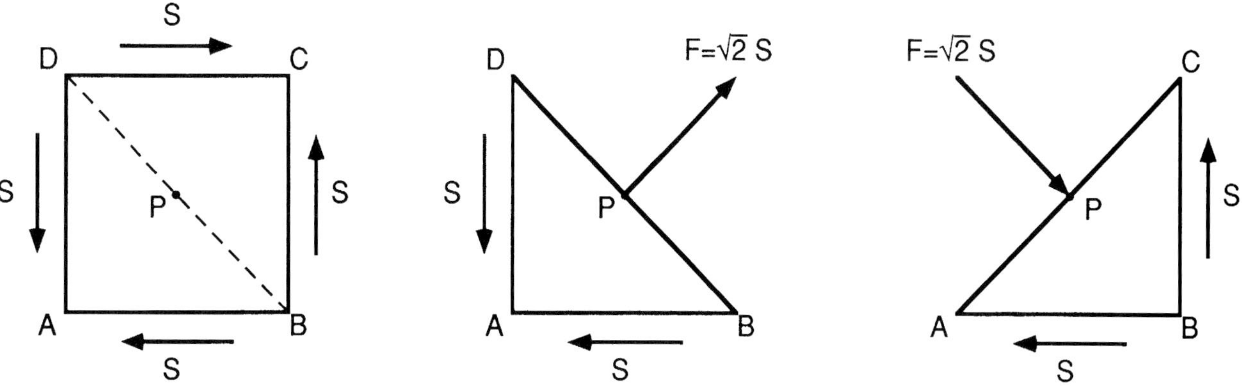

Figure 26
Left, A square block of material being sheared by the forces **S** acting on each side of the element. **Center,** A free-body diagram of a section of the square created by passing a plane through P along BPD. The force **F,** acting on the plane BPD, is equal to $\sqrt{2S^2}$. This is the maximum tensile stress created during pure shear and it always acts on a plane inclined at 45° with respect to the directions of shear. **Right,** A free-body diagram of the section APC. This is the plane of maximum compressive stress created during pure shear. Its magnitude is the same as that for maximum tension.

Viscoelasticity

Linear elasticity is an idealized model for real material stress-strain behavior. It is the basis for practically all structural analysis of buildings, bridges, airplanes, etc. Modern orthopaedic prostheses are usually developed using finite element analysis with an elastic model for the bone, the prosthesis, and polymethylmethacrylate (PMMA).

As a reminder, linear elasticity has three fundamental stress-strain assumptions: (1) stress and strain are directly proportional to each other; (2) the strain is reversible when the stress is removed; and (3) the material is insensitive to the rate of loading. The proportionality relationship between stress and strain is given by $\sigma = E\epsilon$. The definitions of σ and ϵ are used to obtain the relationship

$$F/A = E(\Delta l/l_o), \text{ or } F = k\Delta l$$

where $k = AE/l_o$ is the structural stiffness of the material (in N/m), depending on the geometry of the object, A, l_o. This relationship between F and Δl is often written as $F = kx$ and the structure is designated by a spring (Fig. 29, *top left*). Thus, for this linear, elastic spring, the F-x diagram (load-deformation) is a straight line, the slope of which defines the stiffness (Fig. 29, *top right*). According to the elastic modeling assumptions stated, this straight line behavior does not change with time, nor does it depend on the rate of loading. In other words, as long as the deformation x (stretch) is maintained on the spring, a constant force is required to maintain the elongation, and vice versa.

This type of behavior often fails to occur, particularly in soft collagenous tissues. Articular cartilage, intervertebral disk, ligament, tendon, and even bone exhibit pronounced viscoelastic behavior, in which there is time-dependence. A syringe with a thin needle exhibits time-dependent behavior, because the faster the plunger is compressed the greater is the resistance generated.

These viscoelastic behaviors are the manifestations of the internal friction within the material, which may arise from many sources. To describe the viscoelastic behavior of materials, this friction is usually modeled by a linear viscous dashpot (Fig. 29, *bottom left*) analogous to the linear elastic spring element already described. For the linear viscous dashpot, the relationship is

$$F = \eta\, \dot{x},$$

where force F is the applied force, $\dot{x}$ is the rate of deformation (speed) or flow, and η is the "structural" viscosity of the dashpot. Figure 29, *bottom right,* shows the linear load-rate of deformation response of this dashpot. Implicit in this linear viscous dashpot model are the following: (1) if flow velocity is zero, no force exists (even if the element has been deformed); (2) if a force exists, flow will always occur; (3) the force response increases with the speed of deformation. These response characteristics are those of a viscous fluid, and are fundamentally different from the response characteristics of a solid. Thus, any material model that includes a dashpot will have some of these basic flow characteristics.

For such materials, a constant force will produce creep, that is, the deformation will increase with time as long as the force is maintained on the material (like the motion of a bicycle pump plunger), until equilibrium is reached. Conversely, for viscoelastic materials a constantly held deforma-

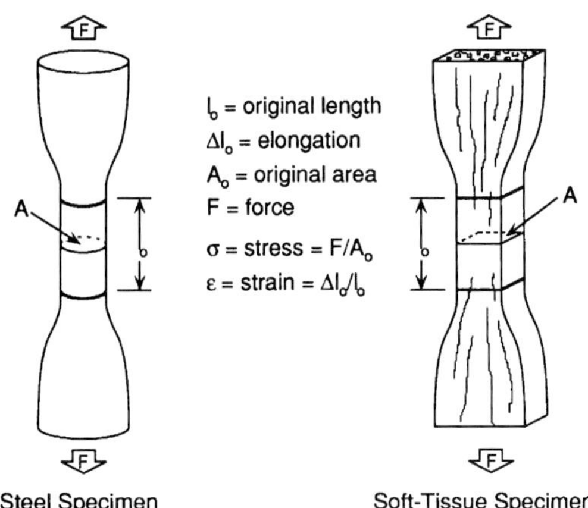

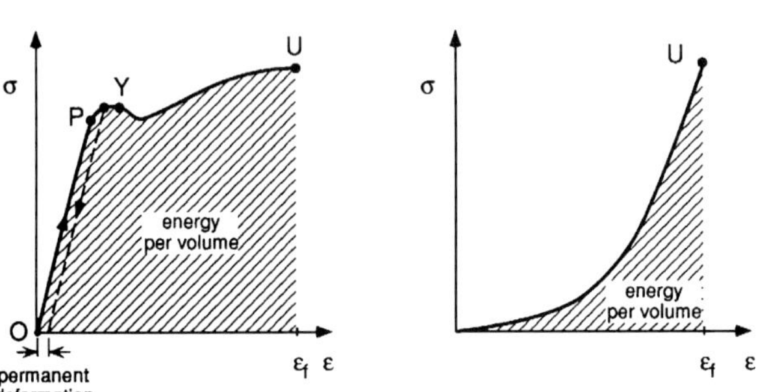

Figure 27
Top, Two typical well prepared specimens for stress-strain testing. The circular cylindrical specimen is usually used for hard solid materials. The thin dumbbell strip is usually used for fibrous collagenous tissues. Dumbbell-shaped specimens are used to avoid gripping effects, and the middle section of the dumbbell is used for strain measurement. **Bottom left,** Typical stress-strain curve of a ductile metal or cortical bone: P is the proportional limit; Y is the yield strength; and U is the ultimate tensile strength. **Bottom right,** Typical stress-strain curve of collagenous tissues; U is the ultimate tensile strength.

Table 2
Material properties of commonly encountered prosthesis materials

Material	Tensile Modulus E (GPa)	Ultimate Tensile Strength U (MPa)	Yield Strength Y (MPa)
Aluminum alloy	7.0	300	275
Alloy steel	20.6	600	540
Titanium	110.0	650	550
PMMA	2.07	30	

Table 3
Material properties of bone

	Tensile Modulus E	Shear Modulus G	Ultimate Tensile Strength U
Cortical bone	17 GPa	3.3 GPa	130 MPa
Trabecular bone	100 MPa	(N.A.)	50 MPa

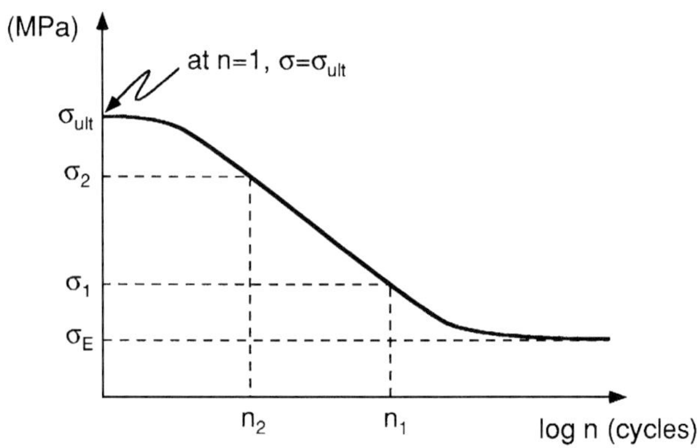

Figure 28
The number of loading cycles n required to fail the specimen plotted against the maximum stress level σ attained during the cyclic test. This is known as a σ-n curve. The endurance limit σ_E is the stress below which cyclic fatigue of the material will not occur.

tion will cause stress relaxation to occur, that is, the force required to maintain the deformation will diminish with time until equilibrium is reached. For example, when a rubber ball is stepped on in a muddy field, the ball initially is elastically compressed by the force applied by the foot. Gradually, however, the ball sinks into the mud, and less and less force need be applied to keep the foot at a constant position. Figure 30 shows compressive creep and recovery and ramp loading and stress-relaxation behavior typical of hydrated soft collagenous tissues such as articular cartilage, intervertebral disk, and meniscus. All viscoelastic materials are sensitive to strain rate. Structures made of these viscoelastic materials (all diarthrodial joints and each spinal motion segment) will also exhibit creep and stress-relaxation behavior.

Viscoelastic materials are modeled by linking the elastic springs and viscous dashpots in series or parallel, or some other combination. Figure 31 illustrates three commonly used viscoelastic models: the

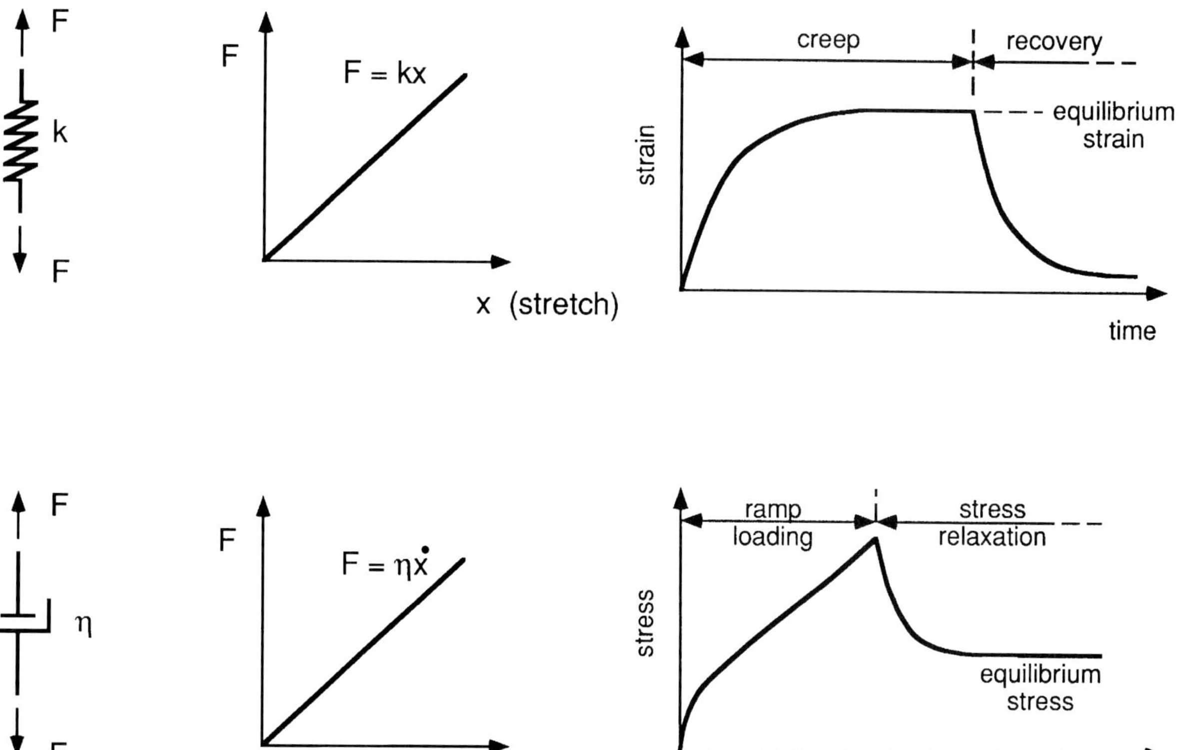

Figure 29
A linear elastic spring element (**top left**) and its linear load-deformation (stretch) response (**top right**). A linear viscous dashpot element (**bottom left**) and its linear load-rate of deformation (speed) response (**bottom right**).

Figure 30
Typical compressive creep and recovery (**top**), and ramp loading and stress-relaxation behaviors (**bottom**) of hydrated soft collagenous tissues such as articular cartilage, intervertebral disk, and meniscus.

Maxwell viscoelastic fluid where the spring and dashpot are linked in series *(left)*; the Kelvin-Voigt solid where the spring and dashpot are linked in parallel *(center)*; and the standard three element solid *(right)*.

When loaded, the Maxwell fluid will respond instantaneously (spring) and flow indefinitely (dashpot) by virtue of the serial arrangement. However, when loaded, the Kelvin-Voigt solid, by virtue of the parallel spring-dashpot arrangement, cannot respond instantaneously because this would require an infinite force on the dashpot, and it will not flow indefinitely because a force balance between the stretched spring and the load must exist at equilibrium. The creep and stress-relaxation of these idealized materials may be determined using engineering analysis. Figure 32 shows the creep and stress-relaxation response of three linear viscoelastic models. By comparing these responses with real

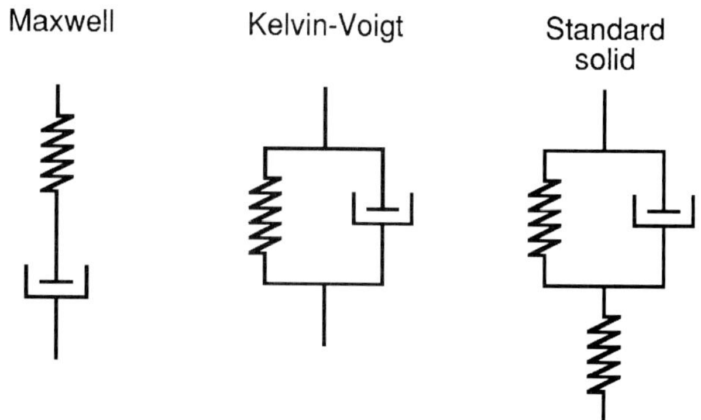

Figure 31
Left, A Maxwell viscoelastic fluid with a spring and dashpot linked in series. **Center,** A Kelvin-Voigt viscoelastic solid with a spring and dashpot linked in parallel. **Right,** A standard three-element viscoelastic solid.

creep and stress-relaxation responses, it is easy to see which is the most realistic model to use. Indeed, in principle, the number of springs and dashpots

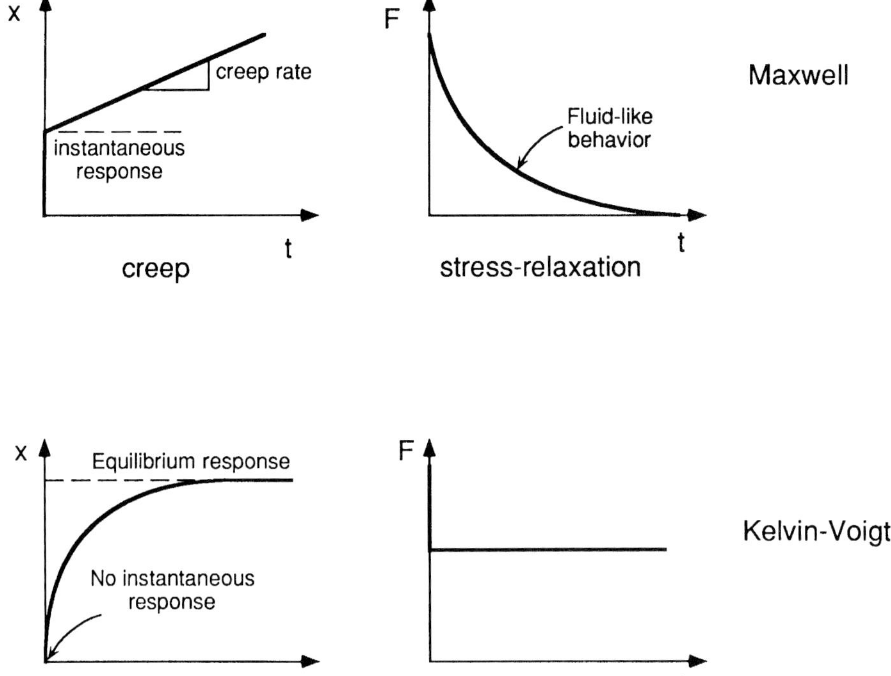

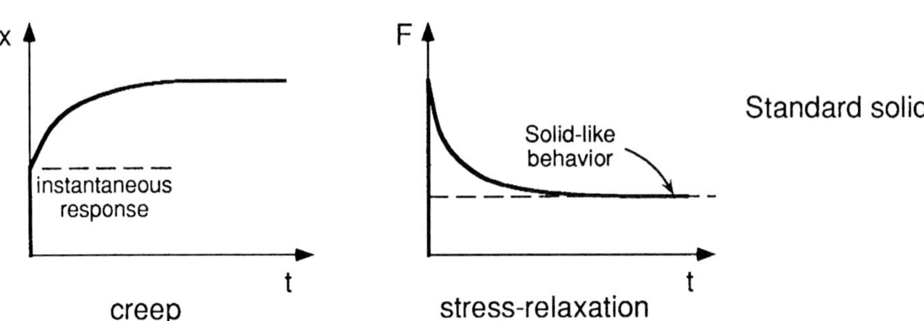

Figure 32
Top, The creep and stress-relaxation response of a Maxwell viscoelastic fluid. **Center,** The creep and stress-relaxation response of a Kelvin-Voigt viscoelastic solid. **Bottom,** The creep and stress-relaxation response of a standard three-element viscoelastic solid.

can always be increased in series or parallel ad infinitum to model the behavior of any real viscoelastic material. However, this usually is not done because of the complexity of the calculations involved.

Tensile Stress-Strain Behavior of Articular Cartilage and Meniscus

Because the composition of biologic materials often is complex (for example, collagen and proteoglycans of the extracellular matrices and water) and their structures are observable (for example, trabecular bone, ligament, and tendons) their intrinsic properties are more complex. These properties often depend on the orientation of the specimen relative to, for example, the predominant directions of the collagen fibrous ultrastructure (anisotropic) and the location (inhomogeneous) from which the specimen is obtained. As examples, the swelling properties of the annulus fibrosus are not the same as those of the nucleus pulposus, and the tensile properties of the articular cartilage surface are very different from those of the deeper regions. In addition, in many hydrated soft materials (for example, articular cartilage, meniscus, and intervertebral disks), the movement of the interstitial fluid during deformation exerts the major force in governing their viscoelastic behaviors. The tensile properties of two important orthopaedic materials will be presented in this section.

The anisotropic properties of these collagenous tissues are closely related to their composition and fibrillar structure. At the articular surface, collagen is arranged in a specific pattern, which depends on the joint. This may be illustrated by puncturing the surface with a round awl. The holes produced are not round, but rather oblong in shape, much like a split formed in lumber when punctured by a large nail. Figure 33 shows a split-line pattern on the surface of a human femoral condyle. This pattern is believed to reflect the predominant collagen fibril arrangement along the surface of the joint. Each joint surface, for example, femoral head, glenoid, humeral head, patella, etc., has specific characteristic split-line patterns. Each feature mentioned here has an influence on the properties of articular cartilage, and, thus, on its function in the joint. (See the chapter on articular cartilage for more details.)

Figure 34 is a schematic depiction of the collagen fibrillar structure of the meniscus. The articulating surfaces of meniscus are composed of fine collagen fibrils organized in a random fashion. These surface layers are approximately 300 µm thick. In the deeper regions, very large collagen fiber bundles, visible to the naked eye, are found coursing around the circumferential direction. Occasionally small radial fibers are seen randomly distributed around the circumference. These radial fibers are believed to function as ties that hold the large circumferential fiber bundles together. Figure 27, *bottom right,* illustrates a typical exponential tensile stress-strain curve for collagenous tissues such as articular cartilage and meniscus. The exponential shape means that the tangent to the stress-strain curve increases with increasing strain. Remember, for linearly elastic materials the slope, that is, the Young's modulus, is a constant. The explanation for

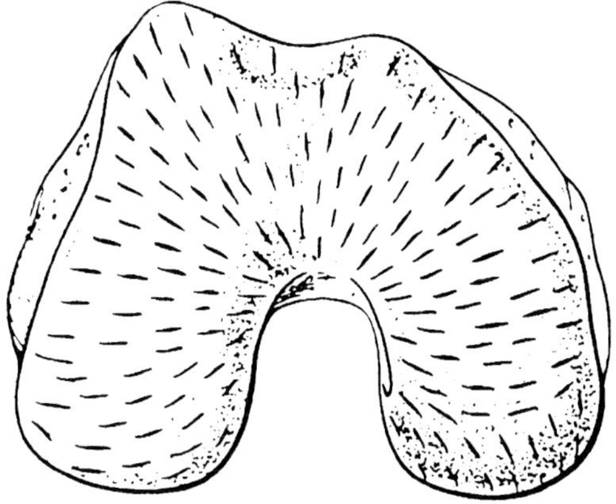

Figure 33
The split-line pattern on the surface of a human femoral condyle. This pattern is believed to reflect the predominant collagen fibril arrangement along the surface of the joint. (Reproduced with permission from Norden M, Frankel VH, Forseen K: *Basic Biomechanics of the Musculoskeletal System.* Philadelphia, Lea & Febiger, 1989, p 323.)

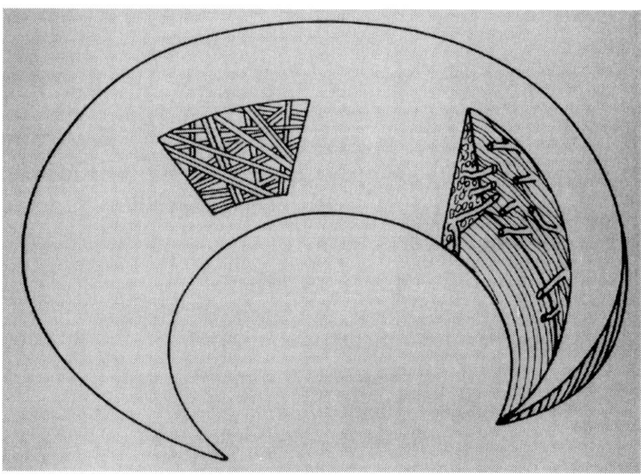

Figure 34
Schematic depiction of the collagen fibrillar structure of the meniscus. The articulating surfaces are composed of fine collagen fibrils and organized in a random fashion. In the deeper regions, very large collagen fiber bundles are found coursing around the circumferential direction. Small radial fibers are seen randomly distributed around the circumference serving to tie the large circumferential fiber bundles together. (Reproduced with permission from Fithian DC, Kelley MA, Mow VC: Material properties and structure function relationships in the meniscus. *Clin Orthop* 1990;252:19–31.)

this increasing stiffness with strain may be found in the collagen ultrastructure. In these tissues, collagen is never laid down straight nor organized in a linear fashion. There is always slack or "crimp." Thus, as strain increases during a tensile test, more and more collagen fibers are straightened, and thus "recruited" to bear load. Usually, before the ultimate stress U is attained, there is a linear region in the stress-strain curve. It is believed that in this region all the available collagen fibers in the specimen are straight and have been recruited to bear load. Indeed, under the microscope, researchers have shown that the crimp pattern may be removed by stretching the collagenous tissue. (See the chapter on tendon, ligament, and meniscus for more details). This "recruitment model" for the tensile stress-strain behavior of collagenous tissues is also an idealization. The behavior of most tissues does not follow this neat pattern. Other organic matter such as proteoglycan and physical interactions between collagen and proteoglycan often play important roles in influencing the properties of tissues such as cartilage and meniscus. Swelling, which is an aspect of this, will be discussed below.

The anisotropic and inhomogeneous tensile properties of articular cartilage and meniscus are shown in Figure 35. For cartilage specimens taken parallel to the split-line pattern (Fig. 35, *top left*) the surface zone is much stiffer than the middle and

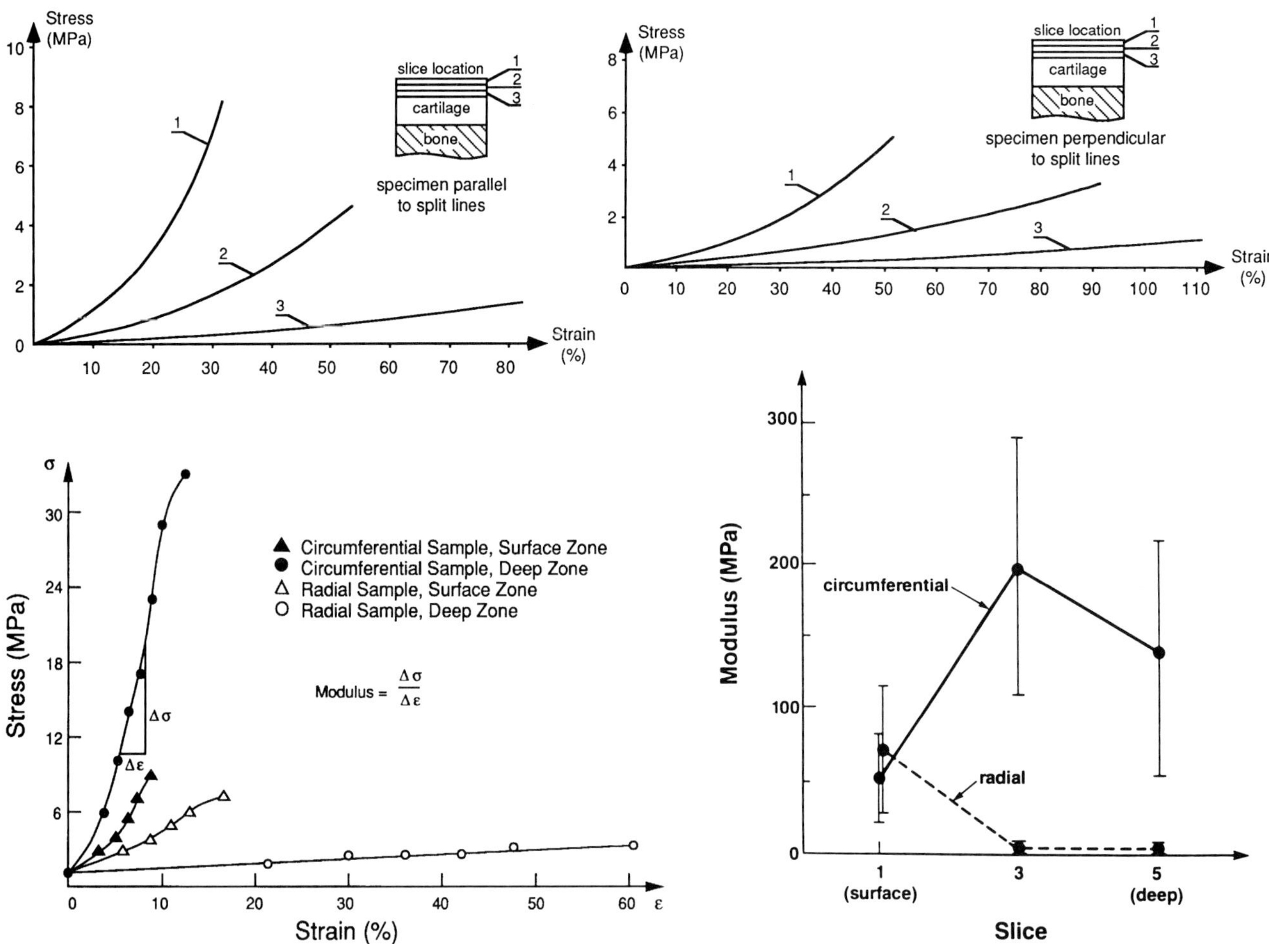

Figure 35
The anisotropic and inhomogeneous tensile properties of articular cartilage; specimens parallel to the split-line pattern (**top left**) and specimens perpendicular to the split-line pattern (**top right**). The surface zones are stiffer than the deep zones. **Bottom left,** Tensile stress-strain behavior of meniscal specimens taken in the circumferential and radial directions. In the deep zone, circumferential specimens are much stiffer than radial specimens. **Bottom right,** The anisotropic (circumferential versus radial) and inhomogeneous (surface versus deep) tensile properties of meniscal tissue. (Bottom left and right reproduced with permission from Proctor CS, Schmidt MB, Whipple RR, et al: Material properties of the normal medial bovine meniscus. *J Orthop Res* 1989;7:771–782.)

deep zone tissue. This situation is consistent with the layering morphology of the collagen network inhomogeneity. The tensile stiffness of specimens taken perpendicular to the split-line pattern is much less than that of specimens taken parallel to the split-line (Fig. 35, *top left* and *top right*). Again, this is consistent with overall understanding of the cartilage collagen network organization. Also, all these stress-strain curves do not strictly follow the idealized exponential recruitment model. Figure 35, *bottom left,* shows the tensile stress-strain behavior of meniscal specimens taken in the circumferential and radial directions. In the deep zone, circumferential specimens are much stiffer than the radial specimens. No statistically significant differences for the surface zone have been reported between these two directions. Figure 35, *bottom right,* shows the dramatic anisotropic (circumferential versus radial) and inhomogeneous (surface versus deep) characteristics of meniscal tissue. These two tissues clearly illustrate the profound effect collagen structure has on their material properties.

Swelling Behavior of Articular Cartilage

An example of collagen-proteoglycan interaction may be seen from studies on the swelling properties of articular cartilage. In general, proteoglycan tends to produce swelling while collagen tends to limit swelling. Changes in proteoglycan content or damage to the collagen network will cause an increase in the tissue's water content. This is a very important area of investigation because in the earliest stages of osteoarthritis, articular cartilage swells because of a weakened collagen network.

Figure 36 shows the nature of cartilage swelling, which also is anisotropic and inhomogeneous. Figure 36, *left,* shows that increased NaCl concentration in solution around a cartilage specimen will produce greater contraction, and the relationship between NaCl concentration and contraction is linear. The slope of this linear relationship is known as the coefficient of chemical contraction. Because there is less collagen and more proteoglycan in the deeper zones than in the surface zone, contraction increases with depth: deep > middle > surface. Figure 36, *right,* shows that the contraction coefficient is anisotropic. Swelling is greatest in the thickness direction where there is a significant amount of crimping of the collagen fibers and least in the direction parallel to the split-lines (length direction) where the collagen fibers are likely to be straight.

Flow-independent and Biphasic Flow-dependent Viscoelastic Material Properties

There are two basic mechanisms responsible for the viscoelastic behavior of tissues: (1) internal friction due to sliding of one microstructural element past another (for example, collagen fibrils rubbing against collagen fibrils); and (2) viscous drag of interstitial fluid as it flows through the porous-permeable solid matrix (analogous to the resistance encountered when water is forced through coffee grounds in an espresso machine). Internal friction caused by interlamellar sliding within osteons has been reported as being responsible for the long-term creep behavior of bone. For ligaments and tendons under tensile loads, the major cause of internal friction arises from the "uncrimping" of the collagen fiber bundles as they slide through the thick viscous proteoglycan gel.

Viscous drag of interstitial fluid flow becomes the dominant cause of the viscoelastic response of articular cartilage, intervertebral disk, and meniscus, where the dominant mode of loading is compression. To account for this, these tissues have been modeled as biphasic materials. The solid phase is linearly elastic and porous (70% to 85% porosity). The fluid phase (mostly water) is incompressible. The solid matrix compresses elastically, thereby forcing out fluid, like water being squeezed out of a sponge. The frictional drag of this fluid is greater, the faster it is being forced (time-dependent). Obviously, if the cartilage is compressed very slowly the frictional drag will be negligible, and the cartilage will behave nearly elastically. Furthermore, the smaller the pores (lower permeability), the harder it is to force fluid through them; thus, the greater the drag. Because the pores are part of the solid matrix, compressive strain of the matrix makes the pores smaller, increasing the viscous drag. Thus the vis-

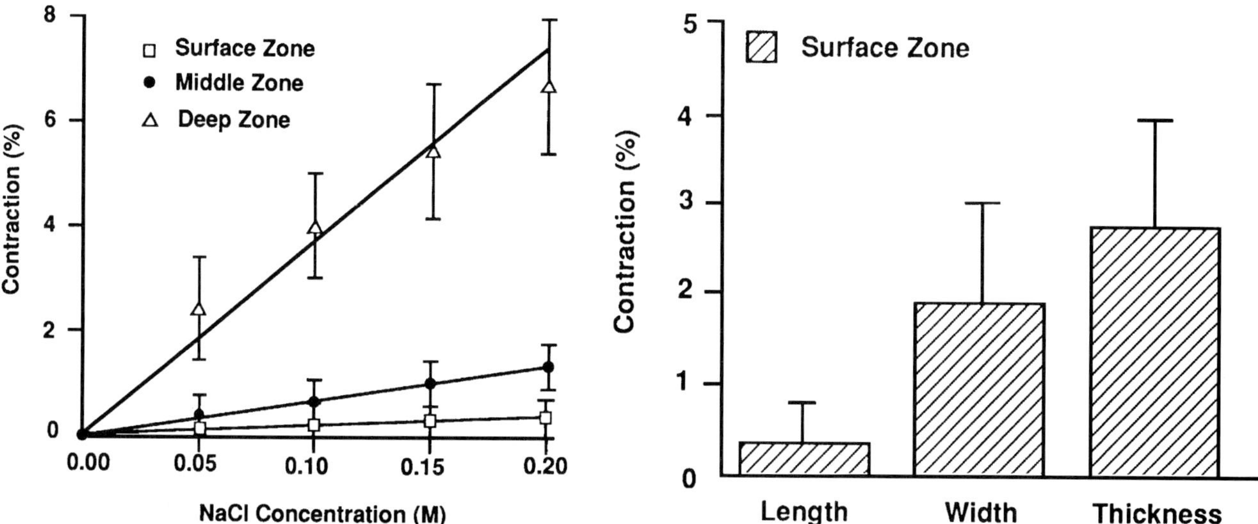

Figure 36
Left, The inhomogeneous swelling properties of articular cartilage. With increased NaCl concentration, the cartilage specimen will contract. This swelling behavior increases with depth from the surface. **Right,** The anisotropic swelling property of cartilage. The contraction coefficient is greatest in the thickness direction and least in the direction parallel to the split-lines (length). (Reproduced with permission from Myers ER, Lai WM, Mow VC: A continuum theory and an experiment for the ion-induced swelling behavior. *J Biomech Eng* 1984;106:151–158.)

cous behavior is both time- and strain-dependent. Finally, at equilibrium, when the fluid ceases to flow, all of the load is borne by the solid matrix at the same position on the stress-strain curve that it would have reached if it had been elastically compressed. (For details, see the chapter on articular cartilage.)

Behavior of Simple Structures

Size and Shape of Geometric Forms

If an object is rectangular, its size may be described by the length of its sides, a,b,c. To characterize a sphere, it is necessary only to specify the radius r. How then is the size of a femur quantitatively defined? If shaft fracture from a bending load is of concern, shaft diameter and length are important. If joint-reaction force is of concern, the trochanter-head distance (abductor moment arm) is crucial. If femoral neck fracture is of concern, the size of the femur from the femoral head to the distal medial condyle is less important than the length of the femoral neck. In general, it is important to remember that different geometric parameters are important in determining the structural response to different loading conditions. For an object of given shape and size, different orientations of the load with respect to the object will produce different responses. For example, it is far easier to bend a flat ruler perpendicular to its flat surface than along its edge. Thus, how tissue functions as a *structure* depends not only on its intrinsic material properties but also on its size and shape. This section covers the important geometric properties of objects, which influence the structural behavior of material objects.

Areas and Centroids

Recall that in describing the behavior of a bar of a material in tension, the two important geometric quantities are A (cross-sectional area) and l_o (the length along the direction of applied load). In many other problems, the "geometric center" of an area or a volume must be known. The geometric center is known as the centroid. For areas such as a circle or a rectangle, at least two lines of symmetry are obvious. Intuitively, the geometric center of these areas may be thought of as the intersection of these lines of symmetry. For volumes such as spheres and cubes, the geometric center may be thought of as the intersection of three planes of symmetry. How then is it possible to find the centroid of a more complex shaped object (triangle, trapezoid, etc) or an arbitrarily shaped object (femur, patella, etc) that does not have lines or planes of symmetry? This is done by defining the first moment of an area or volume.

Consider a very small bit of area $\triangle A$ (for example, $\triangle A = 0.005\ mm^2$) located at a point x and y (3 cm and 4 cm) in the x-y plane. The first x-moment of this bit of area $\triangle A$ is defined to be x times $\triangle A$ (that is, $30\ mm \times 0.005\ mm^2 = 0.15\ mm^3$), and the first y-moment to be y times $\triangle A$ (that is, $40\ mm \times 0.005\ mm^2 = 0.2\ mm^3$). Note that for areas, the first x- and y-moments are also known as the first moments about the y and x axes, respectively. Now, any arbitrarily shaped area with a total area A ($500\ mm^2$) may be subdivided into tiny bits. In this example, the $500\ mm^2$ area could be divided into 100,000 equal bits of $\triangle A$, and each $\triangle A$ in the x-y plane would have a contribution to the first x- and y-moments of area. The shape of the area comes into play in computation of the contribution of each $\triangle A$ to the first moment. The contribution of each $\triangle A$ would depend on where it is located relative to a set of reference axes x and y; the farther away from the axes, the greater would be the contribution to the first moment of area. The first x-moment of the area A is calculated by simply adding the contributions (that is, $x\triangle A$) of all the $\triangle A$s. The first y-moment may be similarly calculated. The x coordinate of the centroid (denoted by x_c) of any arbitrary area is defined by dividing the first x-moment of the area A by the total area A; y_c is similarly defined. If the object is a 3-D volume, then there are first x-, y-, and z-moments of volume with respect to the yz, xz, and xy planes, respectively.

Example:

If the x-axis lies along the center line of a straight intermedullary rod with uniform circular cross section, and y and z axes are perpendicular to the rod and at the end of the rod, then the rod would have zero as the first y- and z-moments and a large first x-moment. In this case, the x axis is known as the centroidal axis.

It is important to remember that the first moment of area (or volume) is a measure of how far the centroid of the area (or center of the volume) is with respect to a coordinate system used to describe the area (or volume).

Physically, if the area A is a thin homogeneous steel plate weighing W (for example, 10 N), it is held in the x-y plane, and the z axis is the direction of gravity (down), then the first moments of area of the plate are proportional to the components of the moment vector exerted by the weight of the plate about the x and y axes; the proportionality constant being the specific weight of the steel plate (N/mm^2). The centroid of the plate located at x_c, y_c is then defined as the point at which the weight W may be considered to be located. In other words, the moment components $M_x = y_cW$ and $M_y = x_cW$ are proportional to the first moments of area of the steel plate.

Problem:

Explain why it is possible to balance this plate with one finger located at the centroid.

For each bit of the steel plate $\triangle A$, gravity exerts a bit of force $\triangle W$. The total weight W is the sum of all the $\triangle W$s because all these gravitational forces are parallel. This simple example illustrates the general principle that any arbitrary distribution of parallel forces $\triangle W$s all acting in one direction may be represented by an equipollent single force W acting at the centroid. This is a very fundamental result and it is commonly used in musculoskeletal biomechanics. Almost always, researchers will use the centroid of the physiologic cross-sectional area (commonly denoted as PCSA) of a muscle as the point through which the resultant muscle force acts. In ligament and tendon biomechanics studies, the resultant force also always is assumed to act through the centroid. The implication of this assumption is that the investigator has assumed that all the collagen fiber bundles in ligaments and tendons are parallel, are stretched by the same amount, and have the same material properties, so that the force per unit area is the same everywhere.

Problem:

In light of what you know about the structure of the human anterior cruciate ligament (ACL) in the knee, provide arguments for and against the assumption that the force carried by the ACL must pass through the centroid of the cross section.

For other loading states, different aspects of the geometry come into play. For example, in the case of bending of the long stem of a hip prosthesis, an entirely different aspect of structural geometry must be considered. To resist bending, the second moment of area or moment of inertia plays the dominant role. To define the second moment of area, consider again an area A in the x-y plane, in which A is subdivided into many tiny bits of $\triangle A$s, and x and y specify the location of $\triangle A$ in the x-y plane. The second moment of area of A with respect to the x-axis (second y-moment) is the sum of the product of y^2 and $\triangle A$ over all subdivided areas; this is always denoted by the symbol I_{xx}. Similarly I_{yy} is the sum of the product of x^2 and $\triangle A$ over all the subdivided areas.

While the second moments of area I_{xx} or I_{yy} are important in resisting bending, the polar moment of inertia, usually denoted by I_p or I_{zz}, is fundamental in resisting torsion. The polar moment of inertia is also a second moment of area, but is given by the sum of the products $(x^2 + y^2)\triangle A = r^2\triangle A$ over all subdivided areas. More simply, the polar moment of inertia is given by the formula

$$I_p = I_{xx} + I_{yy}.$$

Figure 37 provides the location of the centroid, x_c,y_c, of three common simple areas and the second moment of area about a set of x and y axes and the centroidal axes x_c and y_c.

Problem:

For the rectangular area shown in Figure 37, describe how you would determine the second moment of area I_{xx} from $I_{x_cx_c}$ and knowledge of the position of the centroid C.

The concept of the second moments of area naturally arises when bending of beams and torsion of shafts are considered (for details, see sections below). In bending, the resistance to a bending moment is inversely proportional to the second moment of the cross-sectional area, say I_{yy}, and in torsion the resistance to a torque is inversely proportional to the polar moment of the cross-sectional area I_p.

To explain why a meter stick of length x = 1,000 mm, thickness y = 2 mm and width z = 30 mm will appear very flexible in the thickness direction and very stiff in the width direction, consider a small area $\triangle A = 0.02$ mm^2 in the cross section (y-z plane) of the meter stick. If, for example, in the thickness direction, the centroid of this $\triangle A$ is located at 0.25 mm below the surface (that is, y = 0.75 mm), then its second moment of area about the z axis I_{zz} will be $y^2\triangle A = (0.75\text{ mm})^2 0.02\text{ mm}^2 = 0.01125\text{ mm}^4$. Now, if in the width direction z, the centroid of this $\triangle A$ is also located at 0.25 mm below the surface (that is, z = 14.75 mm), then its second moment of area about the y axis I_{yy} will be $z^2\triangle A = (14.75\text{ mm})^2 0.02\text{ mm}^2 = 4.351\text{ mm}^4$. Thus, the same $\triangle A$ (0.02 mm^2) located at the same relative position will contribute 386.8 times more to the resistance of bending in the width direction when compared to that in the thickness direction.

There are three other second moments of area, I_{xy}, I_{yz}, I_{xz}. These are given by the sum of the products of $xy\triangle A$, $yz\triangle A$ and $xz\triangle A$, respectively, and are known as the products of inertia of the area A. They are a measure of the symmetry of an area with respect to the set of coordinates x,y,z used to describe that area. If x is an axis of symmetry for the area A, for every $\triangle A$ above the axis x there is an identical $\triangle A$ below x, that is, the locations of the two $\triangle A$s above and below the x-axis are identical. For example, in Figure 37, x_c is an axis of symmetry for the rectangle and the circle, but not for the triangle. If x is an axis of symmetry of A, then at each value of x, for each $xy\triangle A$ there is a $-xy\triangle A$, and when $xy\triangle A$ and $-xy\triangle A$ are summed they must

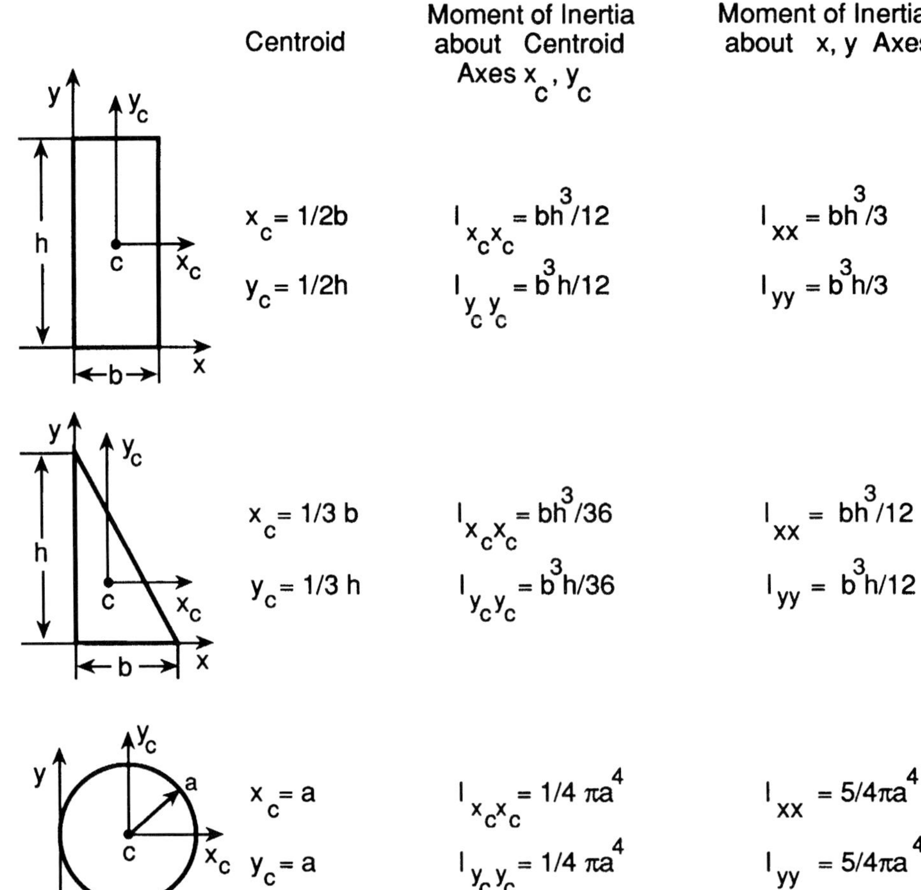

Centroid
Moment of Inertia about Centroid Axes x_c, y_c
Moment of Inertia about x, y Axes
$x_c = 1/2b$
$y_c = 1/2h$
$I_{x_cx_c} = bh^3/12$
$I_{y_cy_c} = b^3h/12$
$I_{xx} = bh^3/3$
$I_{yy} = b^3h/3$
$x_c = 1/3\ b$
$y_c = 1/3\ h$
$I_{x_cx_c} = bh^3/36$
$I_{y_cy_c} = b^3h/36$
$I_{xx} = bh^3/12$
$I_{yy} = b^3h/12$
$x_c = a$
$y_c = a$
$I_{x_cx_c} = 1/4\ \pi a^4$
$I_{y_cy_c} = 1/4\ \pi a^4$
$I_{xx} = 5/4\pi a^4$
$I_{yy} = 5/4\pi a^4$
y
y_c
h
c
x_c
x
b
a

Figure 37
The centroid, and second moment of area (or moment of inertia) about the centroid axes x_c,y_c and the x,y axes of some common areas.

cancel each other. Thus, I_{xy} must be zero. A similar argument must hold if the y axis is an axis of symmetry. That is, if either x or y is an axis of symmetry, $I_{xy} = 0$. In general, even if there are no axes of symmetry, there exist at least three directions for which all three products of inertia, I_{xy}, I_{yz}, I_{xz}, will be zero.

For 3-D objects, there are six components of the second moment of area, I_{xx}, I_{yy}, I_{zz}, I_{xy}, I_{xz}, I_{yz}, that have the same mathematical properties as the stress tensor and the strain tensor, thus the identical tensorial analysis may be used to describe the second moments of area, otherwise known as the moment of inertia tensor.

Problem:

In Figure 37, x_c,y_c are axes of symmetry for the rectangle, therefore $I_{x_cy_c} = 0$. For another set of coordinate axes x′,y′ chosen to be rotated at an arbitrary angle θ with respect to the x_c,y_c axes, but sharing the same origin, is the product of inertia $I_{x'y'}$ with respect to x′,y′ also zero? Yes or no, and explain why.

Uniaxial Tension and Compression of Bars

Structures are materials fashioned into specific sizes and shapes to serve a specific function. Thus, structures have dimensions and shapes. The simplest load-carrying structural element is a straight bar of cross-sectional area A and length l_o that is loaded in a uniaxial manner, for example, the gauge section of a test specimen (Fig. 27). When a bar is loaded in uniaxial tension (or compression), the elongation Δl will be inversely proportional to the cross-sectional area A and stiffness of the material (Young's modulus E), and directly proportional to the load F and length l_o. Thus, Δl is given by the simple relation $\Delta l = Fl_o/AE$. Clearly, this gives Hooke's law $\epsilon = \sigma/E$ where $\epsilon = \Delta l/l_o$ and $\sigma = F/A$, as discussed in an earlier section. Again, for the bar, the structural stiffness is $k = AE/l_o$ and the intrinsic material modulus is E. The bar, as an example of a simple structure, clearly demonstrates the difference between structural response, which depends on the geometry of the structure, and material response, which depends only on the intrinsic properties of the material. For many linearly elastic materials, or even for materials that are not linearly elastic, the uniaxial test is universally used to determine the stiffness k or Young's modulus of the material.

Problem:

The stress-strain behavior of soft biologic tissues such as the cruciate ligaments of the knee, glenohumeral ligaments, etc, usually looks like that shown in Figure 27, *bottom right.* Describe how to determine the stiffness of such materials, using the simple linear relationship $\sigma = E\epsilon$.

Torsion of Circular Shafts

A cylinder loaded in torsion is a common model used to help understand problems such as a tibia being twisted in a skiing accident, or a femoral intramedullary nail resisting torsion. Figure 38, *top left,* shows a circular shaft of radius a and length l_o subject to twisting couple M_t on either end; thus, both force and moment equilibrium conditions are satisfied. In this figure, x is the coordinate along the axis of the shaft through the center of the circular cross-sectional area, and y,z are axes perpendicular to the shaft. Under this torque, any line along the shaft AB will be twisted. This twist follows a helical path from the left face to the right face, assuming the left face is fixed. From theory of elasticity, the total angle of twist θ between the right face and the left face is given by $\theta = (M_t l_o / GI_p)$, where I_p is the polar moment of inertia (Fig. 38, *top right*), and G is the linear elastic shear modulus. For a given applied torque, the angle of twist θ (the structural response) will depend directly on the length of the rod (the longer the rod the larger the angle) and inversely on its polar moment of inertia. Many geometric properties will affect the polar moment; for example, adding slots on the surface of an intramedullary nail will greatly reduce it. For a cylindrical rod, the polar moment will vary as the fourth power of the radius, so a rod or bone that is twice as thick has 16 times the torsional rigidity.

To determine the shear modulus G of the material of the shaft, look at the twist angle $\triangle\theta$ between two nearby surfaces, separated by $\triangle l$ (Fig. 38, *bottom left*). Thus, in an experiment, if the twist angle $\triangle\theta$ and the geometry of the circular-cylindrical specimen, I_p, are prescribed, and the torque M_t response is measured, it is possible to calculate $G = (M_t \triangle l)/(\triangle\theta I_p)$. The shear modulus determined in this manner satisfies the shear component of Hooke's law $\tau_{xy} = G\gamma_{xy}$ in the same way the Young's modulus satisfies the lineal component of Hooke's law $\sigma_{xx} = E\epsilon_{xx}$. For isotropic materials there are only two independent elastic coefficients E,G; all other material coefficients may be derived from these two coefficients. For example, the Poisson's ratio may be calculated from the simple relationship $\upsilon = (E-2G)/2G$. Figure 38, *bottom right,* shows how a square area is deformed when sheared. In the torsional configuration, the shear stresses τ_{xy} shown are acting on each face of a rectangular element; this is known as the pure shear state. A word of caution: There are no other easy test configurations for which a state of pure shear may be achieved. Often, for expediency,

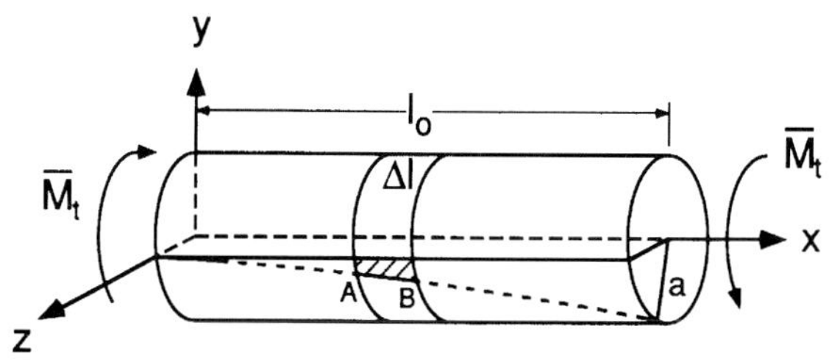

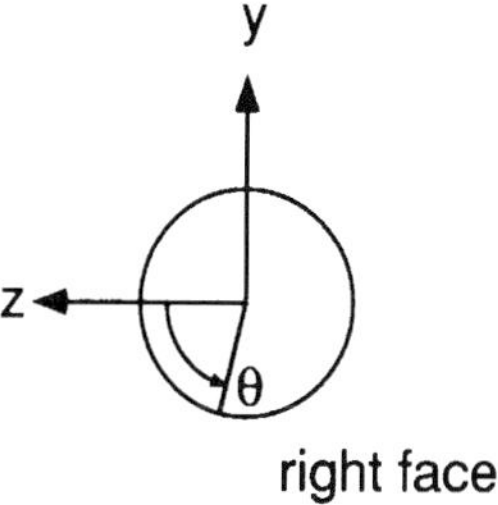

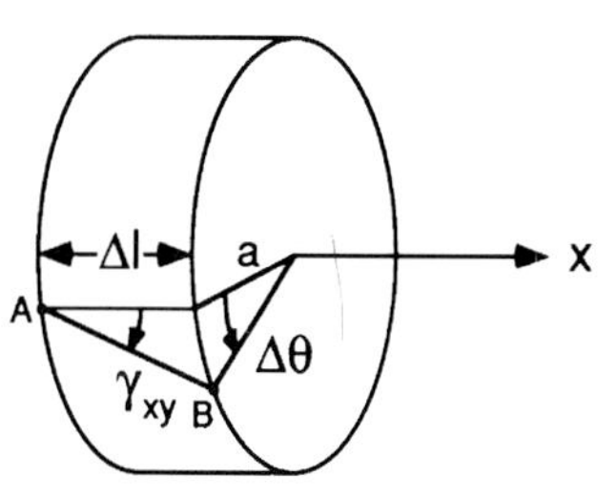

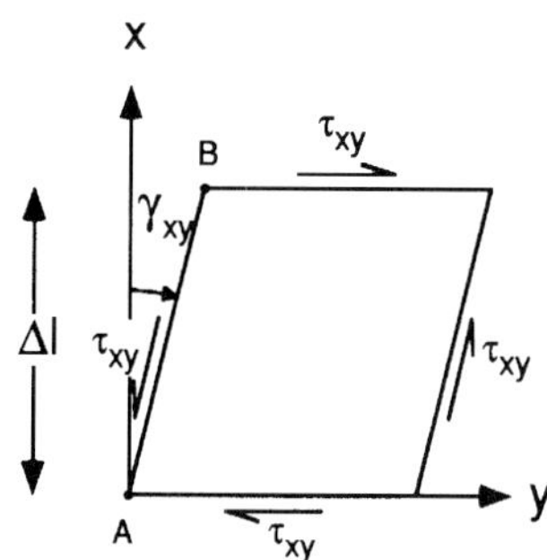

Figure 38
Top left, A circular shaft subject to twisting by a couple $\mathbf{M}_t$ at either end. **Top right,** The angle of twist θ between the right and left faces is given by $\theta = M_t l_o / GI_p$. **Bottom left,** The shear modulus G may be determined from the twist angle $\triangle\theta$ between two nearby surfaces separated by $\triangle l$: $G = (M_t \triangle l)/(\triangle\theta I_p)$. **Bottom right,** In the pure shear state, the shear stresses τ_{xy} act on each face.

experimenters use a simple shear test, where the stresses τ_{xy} are applied to the top and bottom surfaces. Such a test clearly is not in rotational equilibrium; thus, other stresses (normal stresses) must be added at the top and bottom face to balance the torque. Because of this addition, results from simple shear tests are difficult to interpret.

Inside the circular cylindrical shaft, the magnitude of the shear stress τ increases linearly with the distance r from the center; this relationship is given by $\tau = M_t r/I_p$. This shear stress increases with the applied torque M_t and decreases inversely with I_p. If this shear stress were plotted along an arbitrary circle of radius r in the shaft, the shear τ would be tangent to that circle, (Fig. 39, *left*), and its magnitude would increase in the manner shown in Figure 39, *right*. The maximum shear stress would occur at the circumference of the cross-section.

For stress analysis, look at the specific case of a hollow circular shaft (tibia) with inner radius a and outer radius b (Fig. 40, *top left*). As indicated in the preceding discussion, the square denoted by ABCD in the section Δl will be sheared as shown. The magnitude of the shear stress τ varies from a to b as shown in Figure 40, *top right*. For the hollow tube, the polar moment of inertia I_p must be equal to I_p(outer cylinder) minus I_p(inner cylinder).

Problem:

The average inner and outer diameters of the humerus for males are 2.45 cm and 0.97 cm, respectively, and for females they are 2.07 cm and 0.87 cm, respectively. For an applied torque of 5 N·m, calculate the maximum shear stress acting inside the humeral shaft. If the shear moduli of males and females are the same (800 MPa), and the length of the humeral shafts are 30 cm and 28 cm, respectively, calculate the angle of twist between the humeral head and the epicondylar axis of the elbow.

Figure 40, *bottom left*, illustrates that plane BC in the deformed square ABCD is the plane on which the tensile stress inside the shaft is a maximum given by $\sigma_{max} = M_t b/I_p$. This maximum always occurs at the surface, and the plane is always orientated at 45° from the horizon. Figure 40, *bottom right*, shows the orientation of a failure surface along the cylinder under pure shear for materials weak in tension. This forms a 45° spiral along the surface of the shaft. Clinically, this failure surface resembles that seen in a spiral fracture of the tibia in ski injuries resulting from torsion, because cortical bone is weak in tension.

Bending of Beams

A straight beam of cross-sectional area A and length l_o is subject to pure bending $\mathbf{M}_b$ on either end (Fig. 41, *top*). Again, x is the coordinate along the axis of the beam through the centroid C of the cross section; y and z are perpendicular to the beam axis as shown. For pure bending, any cross-sectional plane such as AA′ perpendicular to the centroidal axis remains a plane after bending (Fig. 41, *bottom left*). Because of this, the normal stress σ_{xx} acting on the planes AA′ or BB′ must vary linearly from the plane containing the centroidal axis (known as the neutral plane) (Fig. 41, *bottom right*). The stress is compressive from O to A′ and O to B′, and it is tensile from O to A and O to B. Maximum tension occurs along AB, and maximum compression occurs along A′B′. The normal stress along line OO is zero. Line OO is also known as the neutral axis. For a straight beam, the neutral axis and the centroidal axis are coincident. These axes are not coincident for curved beams. This difference is the origin of the often discussed tension-band concept in the orthopaedics literature.

As in torsion, the state of stress within the beam may also be calculated. In the bending configuration

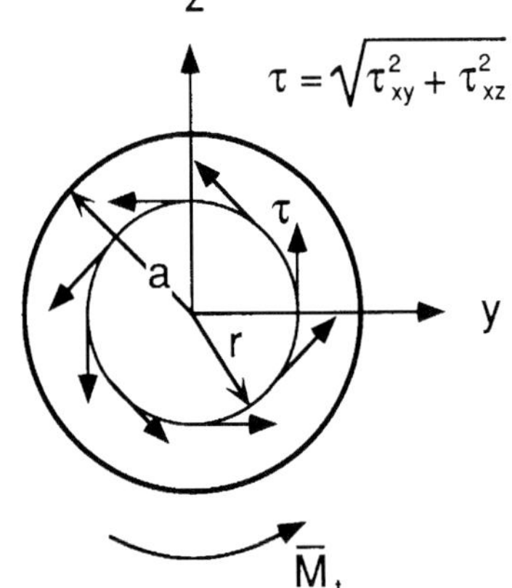

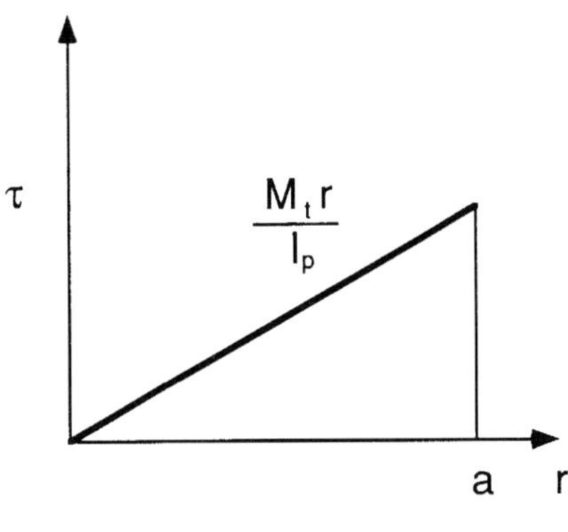

Figure 39
Shear stress along an arbitrary circle in a shaft subject to torsion (**left**). The magnitude of the shear stress varies from 0 to $M_t a/I_p$ (**right**).

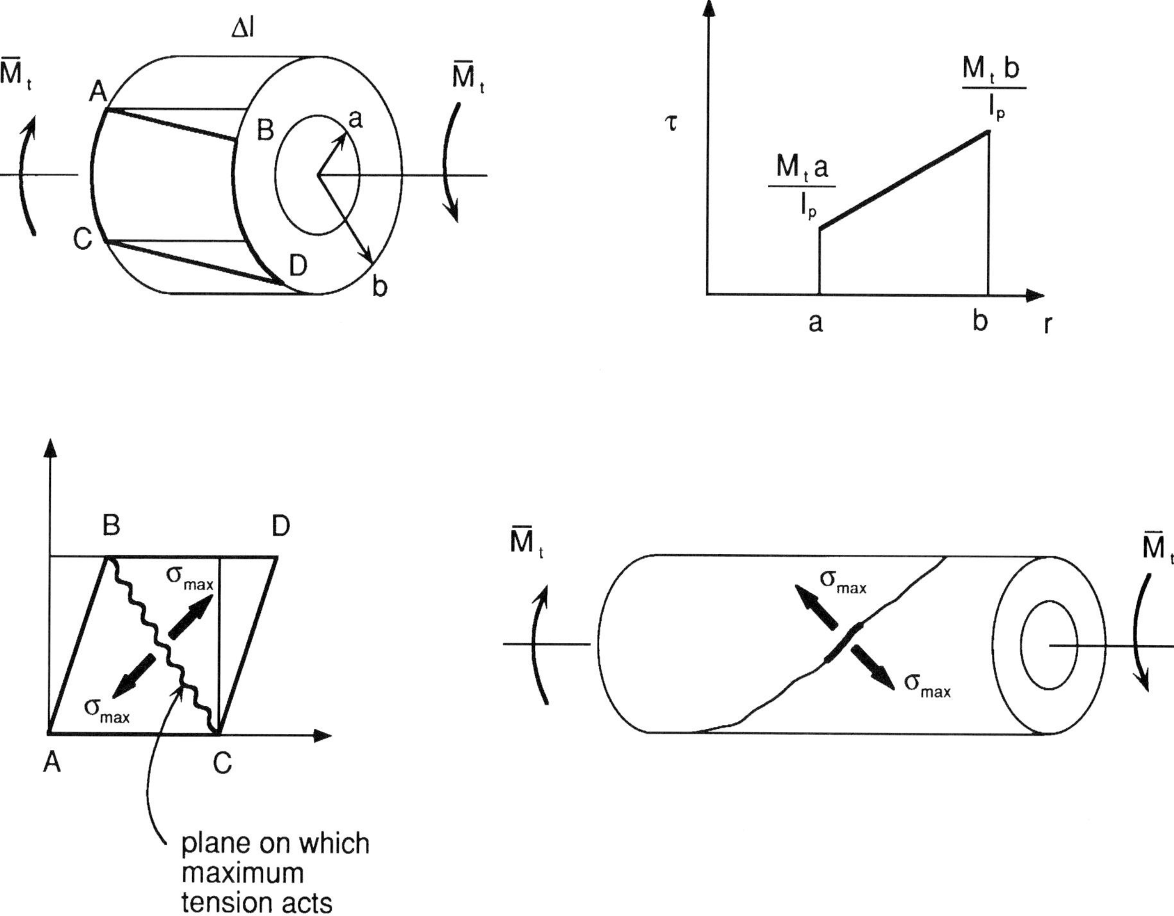

Figure 40
Top left, Stress analysis of a hollow circular shaft with inner radius a and outer radius b. The square denoted by ABCD in the section Δl is sheared as shown. **Top right,** The magnitude of the shear stress τ varies from a to b. **Bottom left,** The plane BC in the square ABCD is the plane on which the tensile stress inside the shaft is a maximum. This plane is oriented at 45° from the horizontal. **Bottom right,** The orientation of a tensile failure surface along the cylinder under pure shear for materials weak in tension.

(Fig. 41), the normal stress σ_{xx} acting on any plane (for example, AA′) is given as $\sigma_{xx} = M_b z/I_{yy}$, which is known as the simple flexure formula in bending. Maximum compression occurs at $z = -h/2$ $(-M_b h/2I_{yy})$ and maximum tension occurs at $z = h/2$ $(M_b h/2I_{yy})$. Hooke's law $\sigma_{xx} = E\epsilon_{xx}$ may be used to calculate the lineal strain ϵ_{xx} from the flexure formula, and the change of length Δl may be calculated from the relationship $\epsilon_{xx} = \Delta l/l_o$.

The three formulas (bar, torsion, and bending) are very important, and they are the most frequently used formulas in structure mechanics. However, biologic structures such as bone are usually more complex geometrically; they are hetereogeneous and anisotropic, and they are subjected to more complex forms of loading, which involve combinations of these pure forms. Thus, caution is always advised in interpreting data based on the three simple structure formulas.

Problem:

For femoral cortical bone, the tensile strength is 60 MPa. If the femoral shaft is modeled as a straight, hollow, circular cylinder that is 42-cm long with inner and outer radii of 1.5 cm and 2.0 cm, respectively, and if a bending moment of 20 N·m is applied, calculate the maximum tensile stress. Will the femoral shaft fail?

Large tensile, compressive, and shear stresses exist inside the beam as a result of pure bending. From stress analysis, the plane of maximum shear stress occurs at 45° from the horizontal direction (Fig. 42). If, for example, a long bone such as the

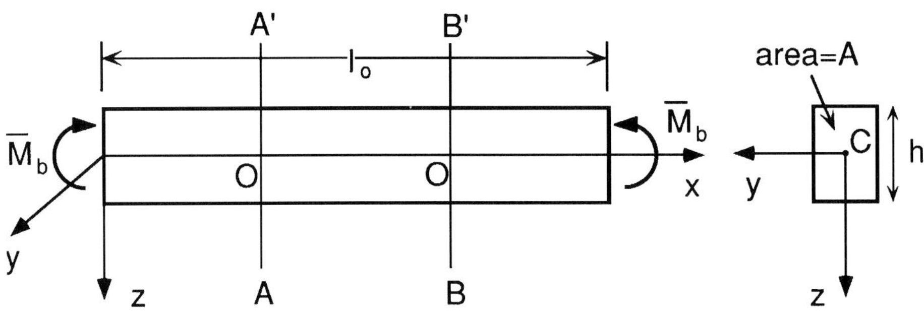

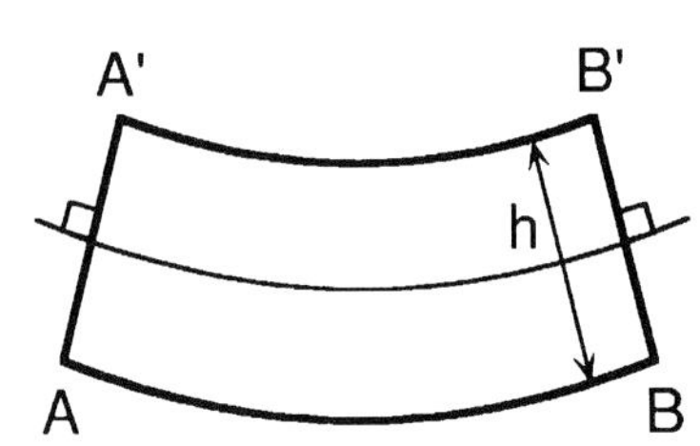

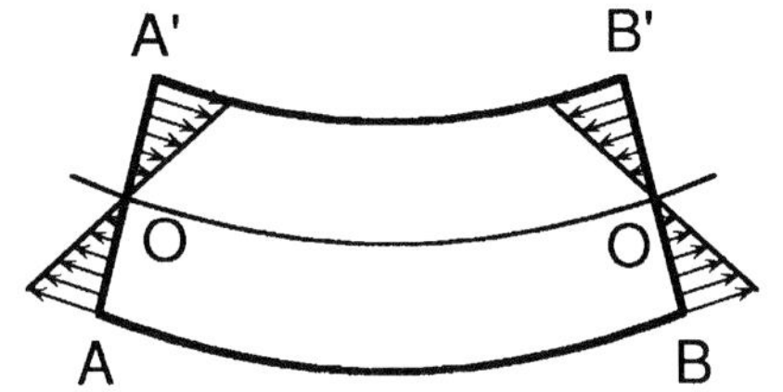

Figure 41
Top, A straight beam of cross-sectional area A, length l_o, and centroid C subject to pure bending $\mathbf{M}_b$ on either end. **Bottom left,** Any straight plane such as AA′ perpendicular to the centroidal axis remains a plane after bending. **Bottom right,** The normal stress on the plane AA′ or BB′ varies linearly from the plane containing the centroidal axis O-O.

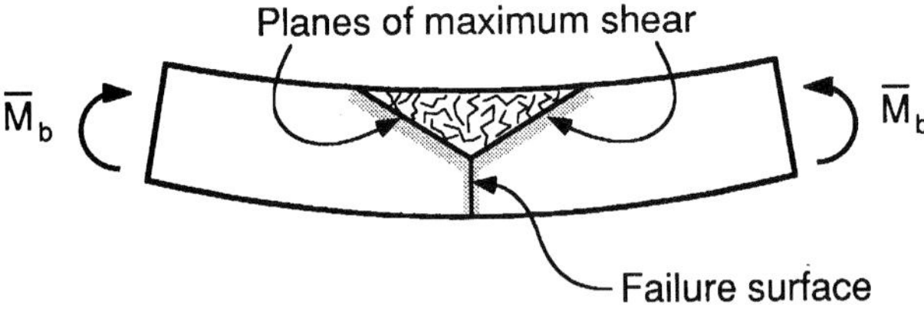

Figure 42
If a long bone subject to bending begins to crack at the side under tension, failure could be induced in the shear mode along the planes of maximum shear stress (45° from the horizontal direction) creating a butterfly fragment.

tibia is subject to large bending moments and begins to fail at the tension side, it also could induce failure in the shear mode as the tensile crack propagates into the bone. These two failure modes are responsible for the often observed butterfly fragment in bone fractures.

Problem:

In finding the stress in the beam, the intrinsic material properties *do not* enter into consideration, for example, the stress in the beam would be the same if the meter stick were made of steel or wood. Does that mean any material may be used to construct a bridge, for example?

Combined Compression and Bending

So far, the behavior has been considered of only simple structures subjected to pure tension or compression, pure shear (or torsion), or pure bending. In this section, the case of combined compression and bending will be considered as an illustration of how more complex loading conditions may be described. This model often has been applied to describe the state of stress within the femoral neck and fractures (Fig. 43).

The stress distribution in the femoral neck resulting from loading of the femoral head by the acetabulum can be described as follows. The resultant force produced by the acetabulum occurs at an angle to the transverse plane through the femoral neck. This situation cannot be analyzed by considering any one of the pure forms of loading alone. However, the state of stress may be determined by considering the components of the resultant force acting parallel to and perpendicular to this transverse plane (Fig. 43, *top left*). The x axis is taken perpendicular to this plane and through the centroid of the cross-sectional area, and the y axis is taken parallel to this plane. The z axis is taken perpendicular to the x-y plane through the centroid of the cross-sectional area. Assume that $\mathbf{F}_R$ has no component in the z direction for this example. The resultant force may then be resolved into its x and y components F_x and F_y.

To see how these force components contribute multiple effects, first isolate the femoral neck, cut by the imaginary plane of interest as a free body (Fig. 43, *top right*). If forces in the y direction are summed, a force $\mathbf{F}'_y$, which is equal and opposite to $\mathbf{F}_y$, must act at O to balance the force $\mathbf{F}_y$. When forces are summed in the x direction, a force $\mathbf{F}'_x$, equal and opposite to $\mathbf{F}_x$, must act at O. This force

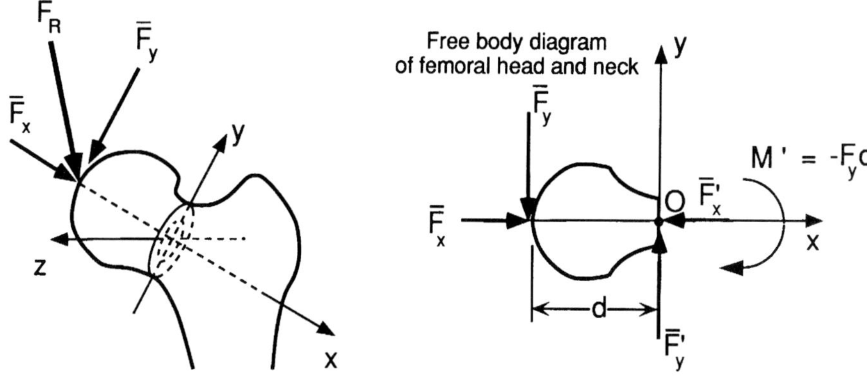

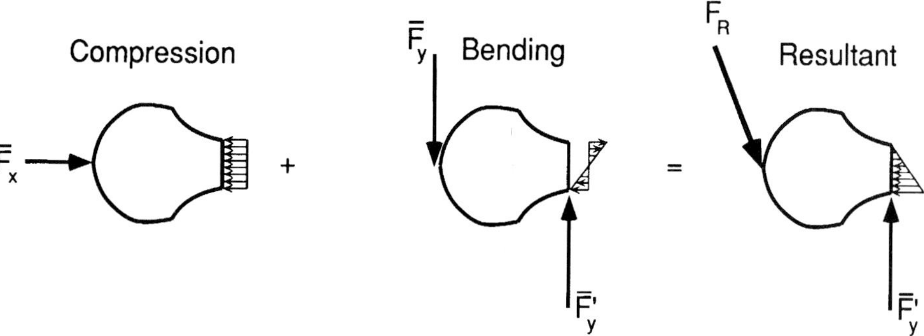

Figure 43
Top left, The force $\mathbf{F}_R$ acting on the femoral head may be resolved into components $\mathbf{F}_x$ and $\mathbf{F}_y$. **Top right,** Free-body diagram of the femoral head. The effects of $\mathbf{F}_x$ and $\mathbf{F}_y$ are balanced at the right side by the moment M′ and the forces $\mathbf{F}_y'$ and $\mathbf{F}_x'$. **Bottom,** The resultant effect of the compressive and bending loads on the femoral head.

results in a normal (compressive) stress $\sigma_{xx} = -F_x/A$, where A is the cross-sectional area of the cut surface (bar formula). Now summing moments about O, the force $\mathbf{F}_y$ produces a counterclockwise moment M equal to + (F_y) x (d), which must be balanced by a clockwise moment M′ on the right side of the section equal to - (F_y) x (d). The effect of these moments may be approximated by the pure bending case discussed above. It results in a stress σ_{xx}' on the cut surface equal to My/I_{zz}. The resultant stress across the cross-sectional area must then be the sum of σ_{xx}, produced by compression, and σ_{xx}', produced by bending, and is therefore equal to $(-F_x/A) + (My/I_{zz})$ (Fig. 43, *bottom*). There is also a shear component acting through the femoral neck as a result of F_y' at the section. This force produces a shear stress $\tau_{xy} = -F_y'/A$. As the resultant force $\mathbf{F}_R$ acting on the femoral head approaches the direction perpendicular to the axis of the femoral neck, large bending moments and shear forces will be developed, resulting in tensile stresses at the superior aspect of the femoral neck and a large shear stress across the neck.

Problem:

If the force $\mathbf{F}_R$ applied to the femoral head is 1,500 N at an angle of 45°, d = 4 cm, and the outer and inner diameters of the femoral neck cortex are assumed to be 3 cm and 2.5 cm, respectively, what is the maximum value of σ_{xx} on the cut surface? If the tensile strength of the cortical bone there is 100 MPa, will the femoral neck break?

Stress Concentration

These analyses compute average stresses over uniform geometries and loading conditions. In fact, structural imperfections, sudden changes in cross-sectional area, discontinuities, cracks, drill-holes, and other irregularities may concentrate stress locally, resulting in failure if the local material's ultimate strength is exceeded. The stress-concentration factor K_c is defined as the ratio of the maximum stress at the site of the discontinuity to the average stress in the region. This may be determined empirically, with a photoelastic method, or estimated by other techniques. Tables of stress-concentration factors for defects of known geometry are available. A more complete discussion of the stress-concentrating effects of cracks in cortical bone may be found in the chapter on bone.

Finite Element Analysis

The discussions provided above are only for structures such as the bar, beam, and shaft under simple loading conditions such as uniaxial tension or compression, pure bending, and pure shear. For more complicated geometric forms and loading conditions, and for more complex materials, the state of stress inside the material becomes very complex. Thus, when the idealized assumptions are not met, the simple analyses cannot be used to assess the state of stress inside the body, or they must be used with great caution. For example, to treat the stress analysis problem of an actual femur with a femoral head prosthesis in place, the following must be known: (1) the actual loading conditions on the bone and the prosthesis; (2) the actual geometric form of the femur-prosthesis configuration; (3) the material properties of bone (inhomogeneous and anisotropic) and the prosthesis; and (4) the interface conditions between the bone and the prosthesis. Obviously, none of the required information is known precisely. First, better estimates of joint loadings may be obtained by increasing the sophistication of the statically indeterminate problems to solve for muscle and joint forces. Second, better geometric data may be obtained from mechanical sectioning or radiographic imaging procedures. Third, more tests may be made on the material properties of the femur. Finally, better educated guesses may be made on the mechanical interactions occurring at the prosthesis-bone interface. Suppose all this information is now available. Has the bone-prosthesis interface problem been solved? The answer is no. A detailed stress analysis must be performed of the bone-prosthesis problem by calculating the stresses and strains inside the bone, the PMMA, and the prosthesis. But the geometric form and other complexities prevent simple solutions from being obtained. This is where finite element analysis is used.

To solve a problem with complex geometric form and material property distributions, the finite element approach is to break the problem up into smaller "finite elements" with simple geometric form. Usually triangular or quadrilateral elements are used. A computer program is written to balance the forces and moments acting on each element, and match these forces and moments with those of its neighboring elements. For large structures with a large number of elements, the computer must solve thousands of algebraic equations to make sure all the forces are balanced in the interior of the body and at the surface where the forces are applied. Usually, in finite element analysis of linear elastic material structures, the principle of minimum energy is invoked, that is, the energy of deformation caused by the external loading is a minimum at equilibrium. While the finite element procedure is conceptually simple, the technical details for actual implementation of the computer programs are very complex. For most finite element analyses of bone and prostheses, linear elasticity is assumed as the model for their stress-strain behavior.

Biotribology of Diarthrodial Joints

Introduction

Diarthrodial joints have some common features. First, they are all enclosed by a strong fibrous capsule lined with the metabolically active synovium (Fig. 44, *left*). Second, the load-supporting bony ends of these joints are lined with a thin layer of articular cartilage (see the chapter on articular cartilage for more details). These two linings form the joint cavity, which contains the synovial fluid (Fig. 44, *right*). The synovial fluid, articular cartilage, and supporting bone form the smooth, nearly frictionless bearing system of the body. For the human knee, the intra-articular fibrocartilaginous meniscus is also important for load bearing.

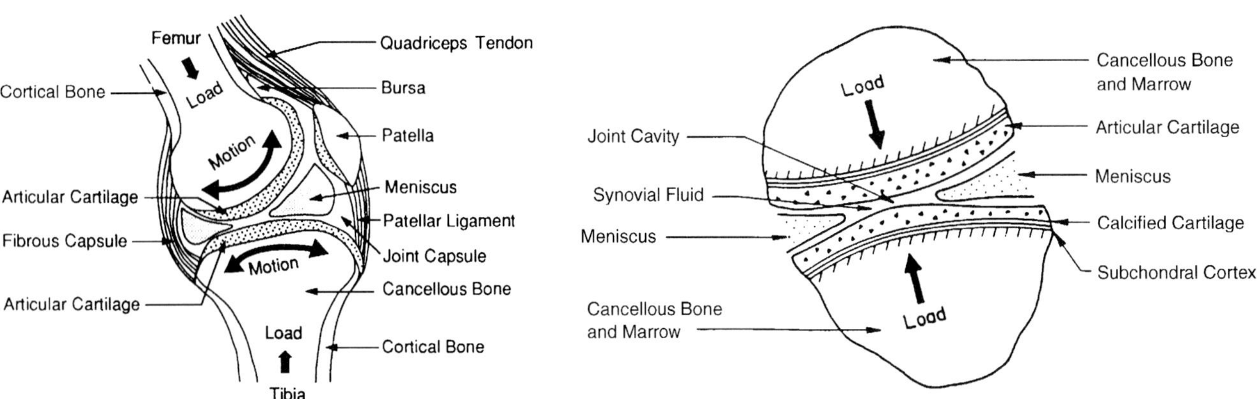

Figure 44
Schematic of a diarthrodial joint showing the strong fibrous capsule, articular cartilage (**left**), synovial fluid, and joint cavity (**right**).

Although diarthrodial joints are subjected to an enormous range of loading conditions, the cartilage surfaces undergo little wear and tear under normal circumstances. For example, the human hip joint sustains a variety of loading conditions. Under relatively high speed motion, for example, during the swing phase of walking or running, low loads are sustained. However, during stance phase, especially at heel-strike, forces five to ten times body weight across the hip and knee joints may be generated. Human diarthrodial joints must be capable of functioning effectively under these very high loads and stresses, and at generally very low operating speeds for seven or eight decades. This demands an efficient lubrication process to minimize friction and to prevent wear of cartilage in the joint. Breakdown in cartilage by either biochemical or biomechanical means may lead to arthritis.

Tribology is defined as the science that deals with the friction, lubrication, and wear of interacting surfaces in relative motion. Biotribology, the branch of tribology that focuses on the understanding of the friction, lubrication, and wear phenomena found in diarthrodial joints, has been an intense area of investigation for over 50 years. Precise and meticulous measurements have been made on the frictional properties of joints and wear properties of cartilage. The biphasic nature of articular cartilage is important in these functional characteristics of diarthrodial joints.

Synovial Fluid

Synovial fluid is a clear, or sometimes slightly yellowish, highly viscous liquid secreted into the joint cavity by the synovium. Minute amounts of this fluid are contained in various human and animal joints. Approximately 1 to 5 ml of fluid is contained in a healthy human knee joint. Synovial fluid is a dialysate of blood plasma, without clotting factors, erythrocytes, or hemoglobin, but containing hyaluronate, an extended glycosaminoglycan and a lubricating glycoprotein (LGP) that aids in friction reduction. A typical long-chain hyaluronate molecule has a molecular weight of one to two million daltons.

Newtonian and Non-Newtonian Fluids

Synovial fluid exhibits non-Newtonian flow properties, which include a shear thinning viscosity effect and viscoelastic effects. Newtonian viscosity of a fluid is defined by an equation very similar to the dashpot equation $F = \eta\dot{x}$ except it is now written for shear stress τ and shear-rate $\dot{\gamma}$: $\tau = \mu\dot{\gamma}$. This equation is entirely analogous to Hooke's law for linearly elastic solids, that is, a Newtonian fluid is a linearly viscous fluid. The viscosity μ is an intrinsic property of the fluid, whereas η is the structural viscosity or the damping coefficient of the dashpot, and they both represent resistance to flow. A Newtonian fluid has no shear stiffness. For Newtonian fluids such as air and water, the viscosity coefficient μ is a constant at a given temperature. For non-Newtonian fluids, the viscosity coefficient μ is not a constant; instead, it depends on the shear-rate $\dot{\gamma}$. Newtonian fluids are also purely dissipative materials (analogous to the dashpot). They cannot store energy, that is, there is no elastic spring element in the fluid. If the fluid contains a macromolecule in solution that is capable of forming networks, the energy of deformation may be stored by deforming the network. Such fluids are also known as viscoelastic fluids, and they may be modeled, for example, by the Maxwell model.

Figure 45 shows the shear-rate dependent viscosity η and shear stiffness (or modulus) G of synovial fluid. These characteristics demonstrate that synovial fluid is a non-Newtonian fluid. In this figure, the viscosity of synovial fluid from normal knee joints decreases from 1,000 to 0.01 poise as the shear rate increases from 0.01 to 1,000 s^{-1}. Normal synovial fluid also has significant shear stiffness (1 to 10 Pa), which remains relatively constant. The shear-rate dependent viscosity derives from the alignment of the long-chain hyaluronate molecules as the synovial fluid is sheared in the viscometer, and the shear stiffness derives from the entanglement of these long chain molecules forming elastic networks (springs) in the synovial fluid. The "stringiness" of synovial fluid is caused by the hyaluronate network in solution.

Synovial fluids from rheumatoid patients usually contain enzymatically degraded hyaluronate molecules. The viscosity of rheumatoid synovial fluid does not have these non-Newtonian flow properties; thus, researchers believe that rheumatoid

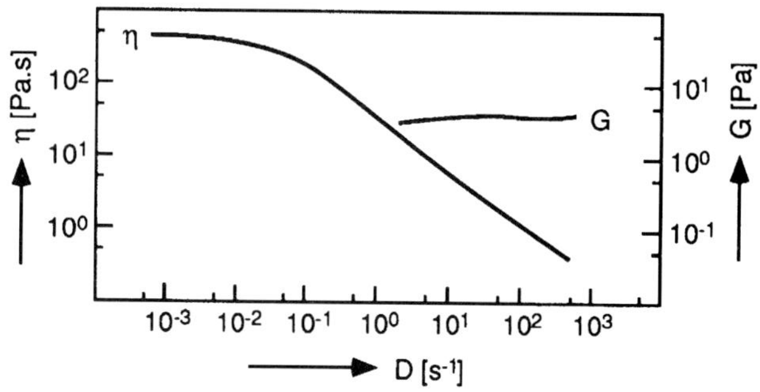

Figure 45
The shear-rate dependent viscosity η and the shear modulus G of normal synovial fluid: D = shear rate.

synovial fluid is less effective as the lubricant in diarthrodial joints. Hyaluronates of synovial fluids from osteoarthritic joints (without inflammation) are not degraded. They maintain their non-Newtonian fluid properties.

Synovial fluid not only aids in lubrication, but also provides the necessary nutrients for cartilage. Furthermore, synovial fluid acts as a medium for osmosis between the joint and the blood supply, and as protection for cartilage against enzyme activity.

Anatomic Forms of Diarthrodial Joints

A major consideration in determining the frictional characteristics between two surfaces sliding over each other is the topography of the given surfaces. Changes in the anatomic form affect the way in which loads are transmitted across joints, altering the mode of lubrication in that joint and, thus, the physiologic state of cartilage.

Microscopically, articular surfaces are relatively rough compared to machined bearing surfaces (Table 4). In fact, the natural surfaces are much rougher than joint replacement prostheses. The mean of the surface roughness R_a for articular cartilage ranges from 1 to 6 µm, while the metal femoral head of a typical artificial hip has a value of approximately 0.025 µm, that is, the metal femoral head is much smoother. Topographic features on the joint surfaces are commonly described as follows: (1) primary anatomic contours; (2) secondary roughness less than 0.5 mm in diameter and less than 50 µm deep; (3) tertiary hollows on the order of 20 to 45 µm deep; and, (4) quaternary ridges 1 to 4 µm in diameter and 0.1 to 0.3 µm deep.

Scanning electron micrographs of arthritic cartilage usually depict a large degree of surface irregularity. Normal articular surface texture is shown in Figure 46, *top left,* which depicts a tightly woven texture with fine pores. Degenerative tissues often exhibit tears (Fig. 46, *top right*) and peeling (Fig. 46, *bottom*) on their surfaces. These surface irregularities have profound effects on the lubrication mechanism involved, and thus greatly affect the friction and the rate of degradation of the articular cartilage.

Table 4
Typical values of mean surface roughness (R_a) for various surfaces

Components	R_a (µm)
Plain bearings	
bearing (bush or pad)	0.25 to 1.2
journal or runner	0.12 to 0.5
Rolling bearings	
tracks	0.2 to 0.3
rolling element	0.05 to 0.12
Gears	0.25 to 1.0
Articular cartilage	1.0 to 6.0
Endoprostheses	
metal (eg, femoral head)	0.025
plastic (eg, acetabulum)	0.25 to 2.5

On the macroscopic level, the types of surface interactions occurring between different joints in the body vary greatly. For example, the hip joint is a deep congruent ball and socket joint; this differs greatly from the femoral condyles of the knee joint, which are bicondylar in nature, or from the saddle shape of the carpometacarpal joint of the thumb. Furthermore, these anatomic forms can vary with age and disease. The degree of matching between the various bones and articulating cartilage surfaces comprising a joint is a major factor affecting the distribution of stresses in the cartilage and subchondral bone.

Motion and Forces on Diarthrodial Joints

In vivo experimental measurements on the relative motions between articulating surfaces of a joint, which correspond to daily activities, are limited. Most quantitative information is obtained from gait studies that do not provide the detailed information required for lubrication studies. However, simple calculations show that translational speeds between two articulating surfaces can range from approximately 0.06 m/s between the femoral head surface and the acetabulum surface during normal walking, to approximately 0.6 m/s between the humeral head surface and the glenoid surface of the shoulder when a baseball pitcher throws a fastball.

The loads transmitted across a joint may be carried by the opposing joint surfaces by means of cartilage to cartilage contact, through a fluid-film layer, or a mixture of both. As in joint motion, the load on the joint surface is dependent on the type of activity, that is, the loading sites change drastically as the articulating surfaces move relative to each other. During a normal walking cycle, the human hip, knee, and ankle joints can be subjected to loads on the order of six times body weight, with these peak loads occurring just after heel-strike and just before toe-off. The average load on the joint is approximately three to five times body weight, which lasts as long as 60% of the walking cycle. During the swing phase of walking, only light loads are carried. During this phase, the articular surfaces move rapidly over each other. In addition, extremely high forces occur across the joints in the leg during jumping.

Friction

Basic Concepts

Friction is defined as the resistance to motion between two bodies in contact. The first type of friction, called surface friction, comes either from

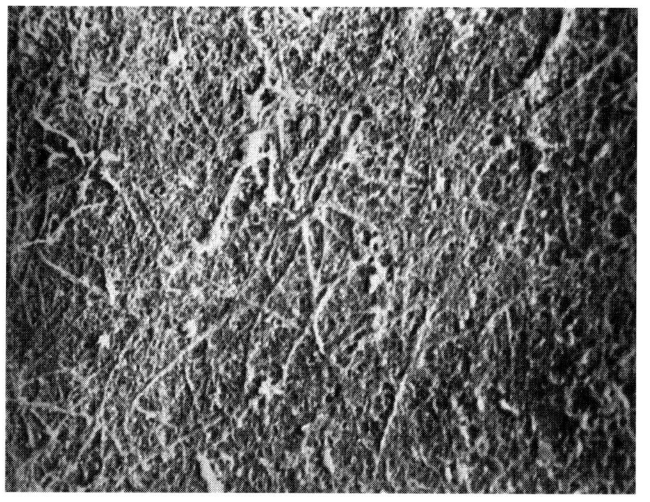

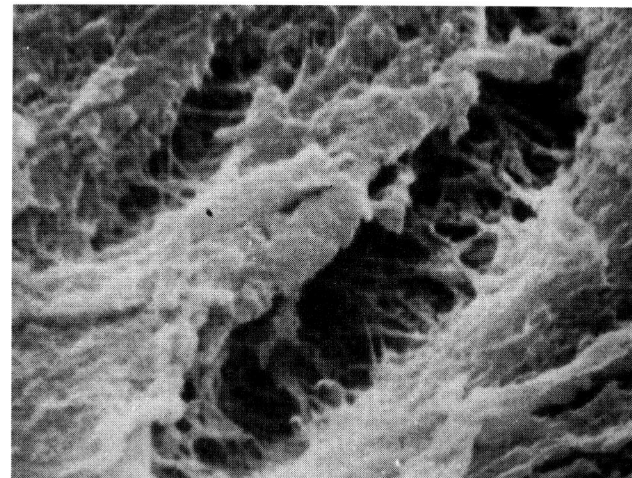

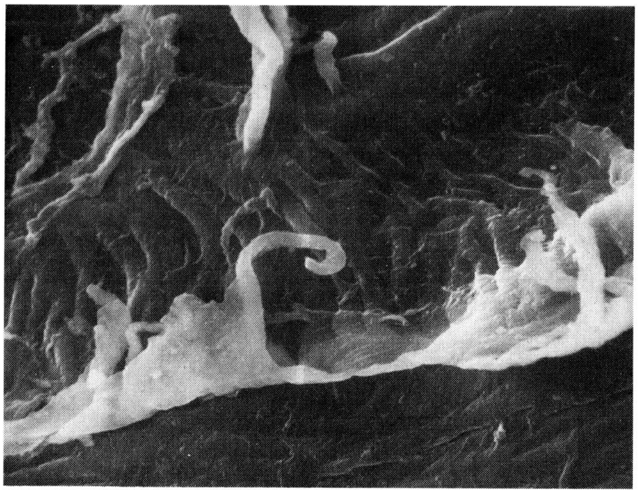

Figure 46
Normal articular surface texture depicting a tightly woven texture with fine pores (**top left**). Degenerative tissue exhibiting tears (**top right**) and peeling (**bottom**) on their surfaces.

adhesion of one surface to another caused by roughness on the two surfaces or from the viscosity of the sheared lubricant film between the two surfaces. In the case of "dry friction," that is, surface friction without a lubricant, three laws have been defined by Amonton (1699) and Coulomb (1785): (1) Frictional force F is directly proportional to the applied load W; (2) F is independent of the apparent area of contact; and (3) the kinetic F is independent of the sliding speed V. These laws help to define a coefficient of friction μ_f by the simple well-known equation $F = \mu_f W$.

The second type of friction, called bulk friction, occurs from the mechanisms for dissipation of internal energy within the material (viscoelasticity) or within the lubricant (viscosity). For cartilage, an internal friction is produced by the viscous drag caused when interstitial fluid flows through the porous-permeable solid matrix. Ploughing friction is a specific form of internal friction and occurs, for example, in diarthrodial joints when a load moves across a joint surface causing interstitial fluid flow.

Measurements of Coefficients of Friction

For friction between articular surfaces, μ_f has remarkably low values in comparison to other engineering materials (Tables 5 and 6). This friction coefficient μ_f for articular surfaces of joints has been measured in two ways. First, specially designed "arthrotripsometers" or pendulum devices have

Table 5
Coefficients of friction for typical materials

Material Combination	Coefficient of Friction
Gold on gold	2.8
Aluminum on aluminum	1.9
Silver on silver	1.5
Steel on steel	0.6–0.8
Brass on steel	0.35
Glass on glass	0.9
Wood on wood	0.25–0.5
Nylon on nylon	0.2
Graphite on steel	0.1
Ice on ice at 0°C	0.1

Table 6
Coefficients of friction for articular cartilage in synovial joints

Joint Tested	Coefficient of Friction
Human knee	0.005–0.02
Porcine shoulder	0.020–0.35
Canine ankle	0.005–0.01
Human hip	0.010–0.04
Bovine shoulder	0.002–0.03

been used on intact joints. The second method involves sliding excised pieces of cartilage over another surface. The pendulum type experimental configuration uses a diarthrodial joint, usually the hip, as the fulcrum of a simple pendulum where one of the joint surfaces rocks freely over the other (Fig. 47, *left*). When the pendulum is set into motion, the frictional dissipation between the sliding surfaces and the dissipation within the bearing materials would eventually bring the motion to a stop (Fig. 47, *center*). The parameter α denotes the damping coefficient. This method provides a way to calculate the coefficient of friction. From these studies, the coefficient of friction of diarthrodial joints has been calculated to range from 0.003 to 0.06. However, this method includes the combination of both ploughing friction and surface friction. The second type of experimental configuration involves the sliding of small pieces of cartilage over another surface (Fig. 47, *right*). The advantage of this technique is that the effects of surface friction can be measured directly, as compared with measuring the combination of surface and ploughing friction as was done using the pendulum technique. Because the entire surface of a flat specimen is loaded (hypothetically), no ploughing can occur. The coefficient of friction μ_f from this experiment ranged from 0.003 (Fig. 48). This interfacial friction has the following characteristics: (1) μ_f increased with time after application of the load; (2) μ_f increased with magnitude of the load; (3) μ_f was lower when synovial fluid was used as the lubricant than with buffer saline; and (4) μ_f was very sensitive to small vertical oscillations of the annular plug of cartilage and actually decreased in magnitude under such motions. This last observation is due to efflux of interstitial fluid caused by the applied dynamic compressive load. The exudate from cartilage creates a fluid film gap that has the effect of converting the lubrication mechanism from boundary to fluid-film (see discussion below).

Role of Synovial Fluid

Many experiments have been performed in an attempt to assess the role of synovial fluid or its components in joint lubrication. This role has been difficult to quantify because it differs under varying circumstances and with different material properties of cartilage and synovial fluid. In general, synovial fluid affects joint lubrication in the following manner: (1) It reduces the cartilage-cartilage interface frictional coefficient significantly at light loads (Fig. 48); (2) it reduces the cartilage-glass interface frictional coefficient from 0.02 to 0.01; (3) it reduces the cartilage-synovium friction from 0.4 to 0.2; and (4)

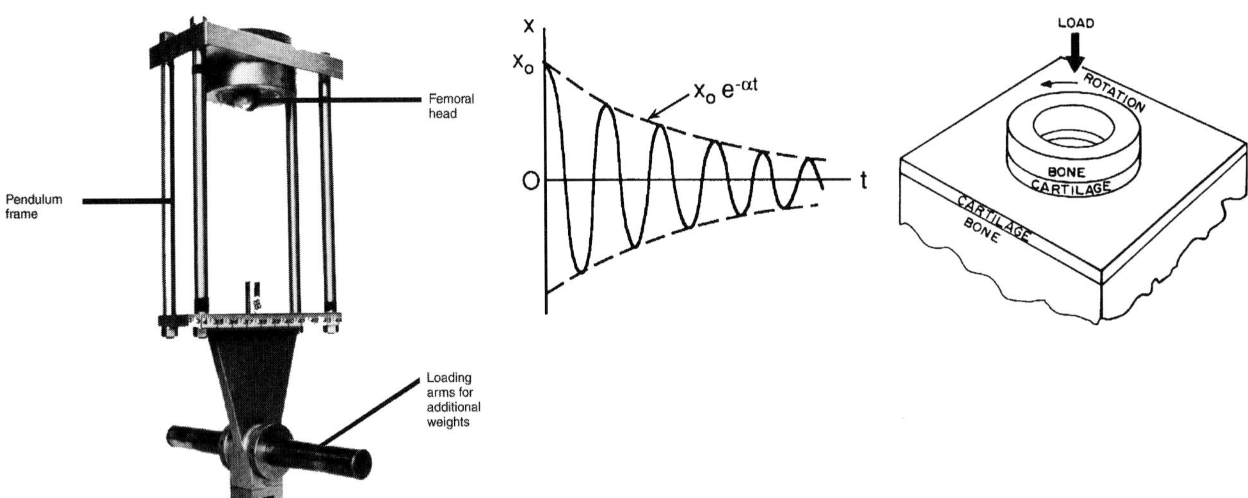

Figure 47
Left, The pendulum type experimental configuration in which one of the joint surfaces (femoral head) rocks freely over the other (acetabulum, not shown). **Center,** When the pendulum is set into motion, the frictional dissipation eventually brings the motion to a stop. The coefficient of friction may be calculated from the damping coefficient α. **Right,** An experimental configuration in which small pieces of cartilage slide over another surface. This configuration is effective in preventing ploughing friction.

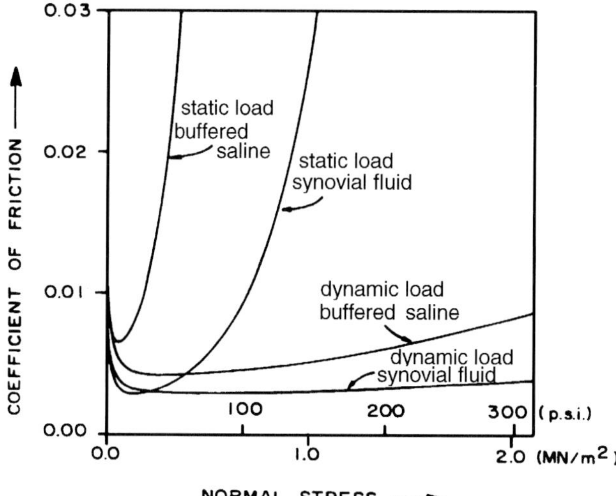

Figure 48
The coefficient of friction μ_f determined from sliding small pieces of cartilage over another surface under various lubrication and loading conditions.

at high loads, no additional benefit is seen with synovial fluid.

In summary, very low friction appears to exist within diarthrodial joints regardless of the presence of synovial fluid. Dynamically applied loads, as is almost always the case physiologically, and oscillations or sliding tend to lower the coefficient of friction, and static loads act to increase frictional resistance.

Wear

Wear of bearings is a progressive loss of bearing substance from the material as a result of chemical or mechanical action. Chemical wear is usually a result of corrosion (see the chapter on biomaterials). The two conventional types of mechanical wear are fatigue wear and interfacial wear. Fatigue wear is independent of the lubrication phenomena occurring at the surfaces of the bearing. It occurs because of the cyclic stresses and strains generated within the cartilage as a result of the application of repetitive loads caused by joint motion. A typical human joint has been estimated to experience one million cycles of loading in a year. These large cyclical stresses and strains may cause fatigue failure within the bulk material and may grow by an accumulation of microscopic damage within the material (Fig. 46, *top right* and *bottom*). These internal failures within diseased tissues have been observed in the forms of collagen fiber buckling and loosening of the normally tight collagen network. Eventually, the internal failures can extend to the material surface, causing cracks and fissures. If the rate of damage exceeds that by which the cartilage cells may regenerate the tissue, an accumulation of fatigue microdamage will occur, which may lead to bulk tissue failure. Thus, in vivo wear is a balance of mechanical attrition and biologic synthesis.

Interfacial wear occurs as a result of solid-solid contact at the surface of bearing materials. There are two basic types of interfacial wear. Adhesive wear, the most common, occurs when a junction is formed between the two opposing surfaces as they come into contact. If this junction is stronger than the cohesive strength of the individual bearing material surface, fragments of the weaker material may be torn off and adhere to the stronger material. Abrasive wear occurs when a soft material comes into contact with a significantly harder material. Under these circumstances, the microasperities of the harder material surface may cut into the softer counterpart causing abrasive wear. This harder material may be either the opposing bearing surface or loose particles between the bearing surfaces. When loose particles between the surfaces cause abrasive wear, the process is termed three-body wear. This type of wear occurs frequently in orthopaedics, for example, when PMMA cement particles are trapped in the joint space between an endoprosthesis and cartilage.

Wear is measured either as the mass of material removed from interacting surfaces per unit time, or as the volume lost. At present, wear measurement is mostly an empiric science. Therefore, it is difficult to predict either wear rates or their dependency on other physical parameters. Little or no quantitative information exists on wear mechanisms or wear rates for biologic materials. For hydrated tissues such as cartilage, it is very difficult to quantify either loss of mass or of volume as a result of the phenomenon of swelling. The only available data on cartilage wear were obtained from rubbing cartilage against stainless steel plates. Figure 49 shows the measured wear and wear rates for cartilage using collagen and hexosamine as markers at two compression levels.

In general, different types of wear produce different wear rates. Fatigue wear depends on the frequency and magnitude of the applied loads and on the intrinsic material properties of the bulk material. Interfacial wear depends on the roughness of the bearing surfaces, the true size of the contact area of the two surfaces, and the magnitude of the applied load. Some general rules on wear are: (1) wear rates increase with increasing applied normal load; (2) wear rates increase with increasing sliding contact area between the two opposing bearing surfaces; and, (3) the wear rate of the softer bearing surface is higher than that of the harder bearing surface.

The function of typical engineering bearings often is impaired if even a relatively small amount of

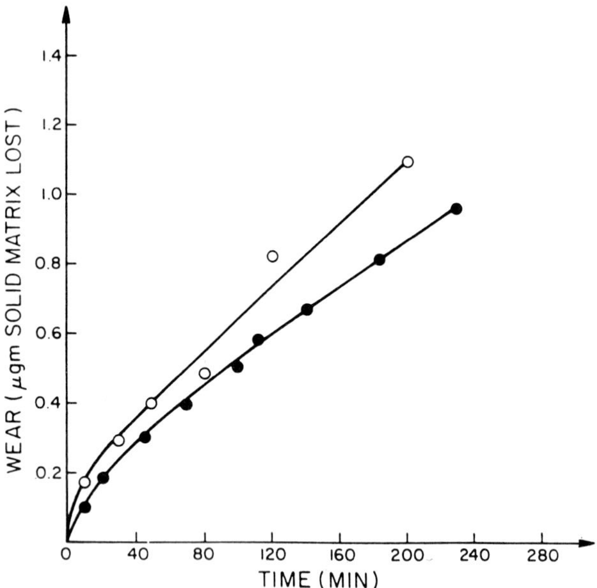

Figure 49
The measured wear and *wear rates* for cartilage at two compression levels: open circle, 4.62 MPa; closed circle, 1.66 MPa.

the bearing volume is lost. Minute changes of bearing surface geometry can greatly affect the hydrodynamics of the thin lubricant film, usually no more than 25 μm thick, in the worn bearing. Despite its topographic roughness, an extremely low wear rate is seen for articular cartilage.

Repetitive joint motion and loading could cause cartilage fatigue damage and wear. Usually, normal chondrocyte activity and turnover are sufficient to maintain tissue homeostasis. Cartilage damage may be accelerated by blunt impact loading. As normal cartilage is compressed, redistribution of fluid within the tissue occurs, causing stress relaxation. Because fluid redistribution in the tissue is not possible during high speed impact loading, high pressures are built up within the tissue and high tensile stresses are built up near the articular surface. Experiments have shown that a single impact on the patellofemoral joint can cause cartilage damage at the surface and shear fracture at the tidemark. Early accelerated biologic remodeling of patellar cartilage after impact in the region of the tidemark also has been observed. This impact-induced mechanical damage, followed by biologic remodeling, causes tidemark advancement and thinning of cartilage. The number of tidemarks has been found to increase with age. In general, cartilage thins dramatically during aging. Thus, these studies indicate that in vivo wear of articular cartilage is fundamentally different from wear of machine bearings. Biologic wear really is caused by an imbalance of biologic turnover and mechanical attrition. (See the chapter on "Form and Function of Articular Cartilage" for a more detailed discussion on cartilage pathology.)

Diarthrodial Joint Lubrication

Many modes of lubrication exist to provide the minimal friction and wear characteristics of cartilage found in diarthrodial joints. Each mode of lubrication accounts for friction and wear of these joints under specific loading and motion conditions. For fluid film lubrication to exist, the minimum fluid film thickness predicted must exceed the known average surface roughness of cartilage. If the predicted fluid film gap is too thin to produce fluid film lubrication at given loading and motion conditions, then boundary lubrication must be present. Basically, there are only two lubrication mechanisms: fluid film and boundary, a fact that gives rise to two questions. How is the fluid film created? What substance provides the boundary lubrication in diarthrodial joints?

Fluid-film Lubrication

Hydrodynamic Lubrication To address the question of how the fluid films are created in joints, many models have been suggested (Fig. 50). Hydrodynamic lubrication occurs when the speed of sliding and the viscosity of the fluid are sufficient to create a thin fluid film capable of supporting the applied load (Fig. 50, *top left*). The essential assumptions of this model are: (1) the bearing surfaces are rigid and non-porous; (2) the surfaces form a wedge-shaped gap; (3) the lubrication viscosity is constant (Newtonian); (4) the relative sliding speed is high; and (5) loads are light. In general, obviously, higher speeds and viscosities promote greater load-carrying capacities. These model approximations might prevail during high-speed, nonaccelerating, rotatory motion of the femur during the swing phase of gait. However, if acceleration occurs, high compressive joint-reaction forces must exist. If the joint-reaction force exceeds the capacity of the lubricant film to support the load, the fluid film gap will close.

Elastohydrodynamic Lubrication The hydrodynamic lubrication model assumptions are really far from reality. Improvement may be gained by considering the "elastic" deformation of the cartilage. In this model, cartilage surface deformation acts to: (1) spread the joint load over a larger surface area; (2) decrease the shear-rate between the two surfaces; and, (3) by virtue of item (2), increase synovial fluid viscosity. All three effects produce gains in the capacity of the fluid film to carry load as well as decreasing stresses within the cartilage. In engineer-

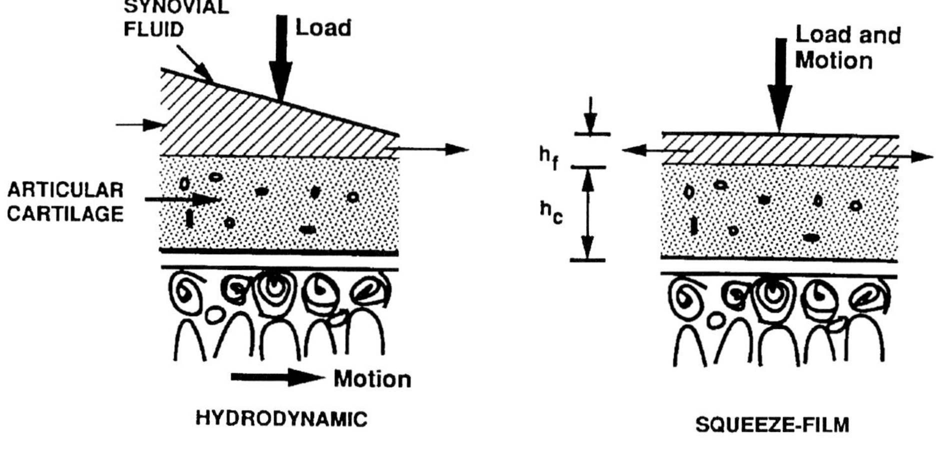

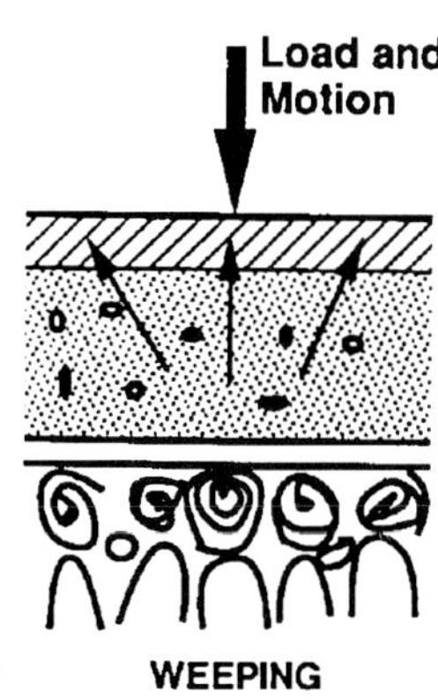

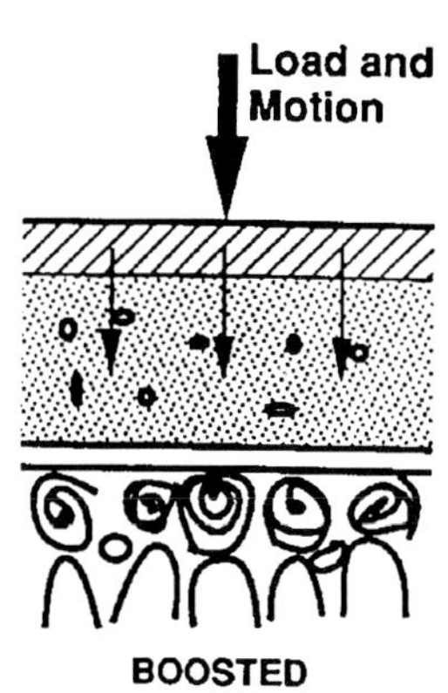

Figure 50
Models of fluid film lubrication: Hydrodynamic (**top left**), squeeze-film (**top right**), weeping (**bottom left**), and boosted (**bottom right**). (Reproduced with permission from Mow VC, Soslowsky LJ: Friction, lubrication and wear of diarthrodial joints, in Mow VC, Hayes WC (eds): *Basic Orthopaedic Biomechanics.* New York, Raven Press, 1991, pp 245–292.)

ing terminology, this lubrication mode, where both the viscous resistance of the lubricant and the elastic deformation of the bearing surfaces play a prominent role, is called elastohydrodynamic lubrication. For the hip and knee joints, film thickness has been estimated by this mechanism to range up to 2.5 μm.

Squeeze-film Lubrication In squeeze-film lubrication, two bearing surfaces simply approach each other without sliding over each other (Fig. 50, *top right*). Because a viscous lubricant cannot instantaneously be squeezed out from the gap between two surfaces that are approaching each other, a pressure is built up as a result of the viscous resistance offered by the lubricant as it is being squeezed from the gap. The pressure field in the fluid film formed in this manner is capable of supporting large loads. Because the bearing surfaces are deformable layers of articular cartilage, the large pressure generated can cause localized depressions where the lubricant film can be trapped. Typically, with rigid bearings, a 20-μm thick film of fluid can resist several MPa of pressure for many seconds before the film becomes depleted. The non-Newtonian behavior of synovial fluid prolongs the squeeze-film time.

Weeping Lubrication In many engineering applications, hydrostatic lubrication is developed by providing an externally pressurized source of liquid to supply the lubricant film. Exotic applications such as large astronomic telescopes are floated on precisely ground smooth plates separated by a thin film of pressurized gas, and ordinary hydraulic lifts in many auto garages work on this principle. If the fluid in articular cartilage somehow could be imagined to flow out of the tissue, then a similar mechanism could occur in diarthrodial joints. In this model, the fluid in cartilage is assumed to be "self-pressurized" and "wept" uniformly from the tissue into the joint space, serving as the lubricant in joints (Fig. 50, *bottom left*). According to this weeping lubrication theory, lubricant fluid film between the two articulating surfaces is generated by the compression of articular cartilage during joint function.

Boosted Lubrication Another model of lubrication for diarthrodial joints is known as boosted lubrication. In this model, as the articulating surfaces approach each other, the solvent component of synovial fluid, that is, water, passes into the articular cartilage over the entire load-support region during squeeze-film conditions, leaving behind a concentrated pool of hyaluronic acid-protein complex to lubricate the surfaces (Fig. 50, *bottom right*). During squeeze-film lubrication, as the size of the gap between articulating surfaces decreases, the resistance of sideways efflux of the lubricant will eventually become greater than the resistance of flow into the articular cartilage (Fig. 50, *top right*). Because the pores in normal articular cartilage (20 to 70 Å) are much smaller than the hyaluronate molecules (solution diameter range: (1 to 4) × 10^3 Å), the molecules cannot penetrate the cartilage surface and, thus, are left behind in the joint gap. In this manner the articulating surfaces act as filtration membranes through which only water and low molecular weight electrolytes and nutrients are capable of passing into cartilage. During this process, the hyaluronate concentration increases in the joint space, and synovial fluid viscosity is correspondingly increased; hence, the load-carrying capacity of this fluid is boosted.

Boundary Lubrication

A monolayer of glycoprotein is adsorbed on the articular surface. This monolayer functions like the pile of a carpet to provide a cushioning layer and protect the articular surface from abrasion (Fig. 51). Its thickness ranges from 10 to 1,000 Å, and it has the ability to carry weight and reduce friction. Indeed, it has an excellent lubricating capacity. The glycoprotein that makes up this monolayer is called lubricin, and its molecular weight is approximately 2.5 × 10^2 kd. It is a single polypeptide chain with many oligosaccharides distributed along its length. In the joint under heavy loading, some combination of fluid-film lubrication and boundary lubrication must coexist (Fig. 52).

Interstitial Fluid Flow and Diarthrodial Joint Lubrication

Detailed studies of cartilage flow and deformational behavior have determined how interstitial fluid flow at the articular surface may occur rapidly. Because lubrication and fluid flow within a joint depend on many conditions such as joint loading, material properties of articular cartilage and synovial fluid, and joint anatomy, theories can be developed only for specific joints and individual conditions or for very general idealized conditions. From the results of these general idealized studies, it is now clear that no global lubrication theory for synovial joints is possible. Thus, joint lubrication mechanisms should be joint specific (that is, shoulder, elbow, hip, knee, ankle, etc.), using the properties and anatomy of the joint.

From general idealized conditions in which cartilage is modeled as a biphasic medium, some broad conclusions can be made. The fluid efflux pattern at the articular surface depends on (1) the intrinsic stiffness and permeability of cartilage; (2) the porosity of the tissue, (3) the loading conditions at the articular surface; and (4) the rate of loading and the sliding speed. In general, under moderate to high loading conditions and for normal cartilage properties, as the contact area moves across the articulating surface during joint function, fluid exudation appears to begin ahead of the oncoming load and increases as the load approaches (Fig. 53). After

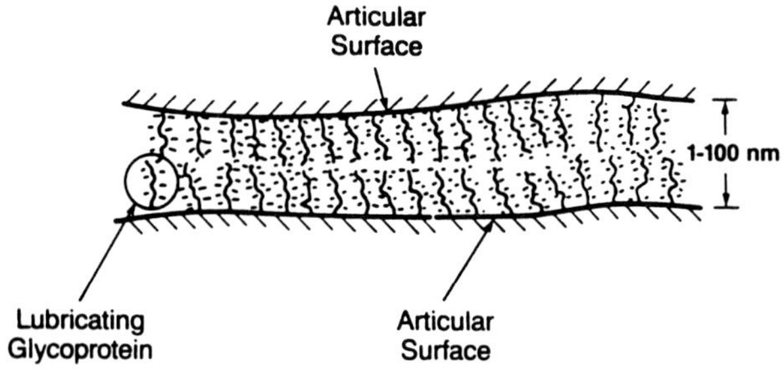

Figure 51
Boundary layer lubrication. A monolayer of glycoprotein provides a cushioning layer, protecting the articular surface from abrasion. (Reproduced with permission from Mow VC, Soslowsky LJ: Friction, lubrication and wear of diarthrodial joints, in Mow VC, Hayes WC (eds): *Basic Orthopaedic Biomechanics.* New York, Raven Press, 1991, pp 245–292.)

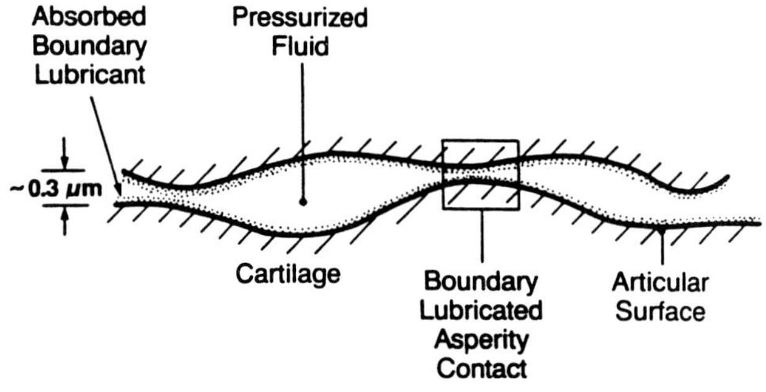

Figure 52
A combination of fluid-film lubrication and boundary lubrication. (Reproduced with permission from Mow VC, Soslowsky LJ: Friction, lubrication and wear of diarthrodial joints, in Mow VC, Hayes WC (eds): *Basic Orthopaedic Biomechanics.* New York, Raven Press, 1991, pp 245–292.)

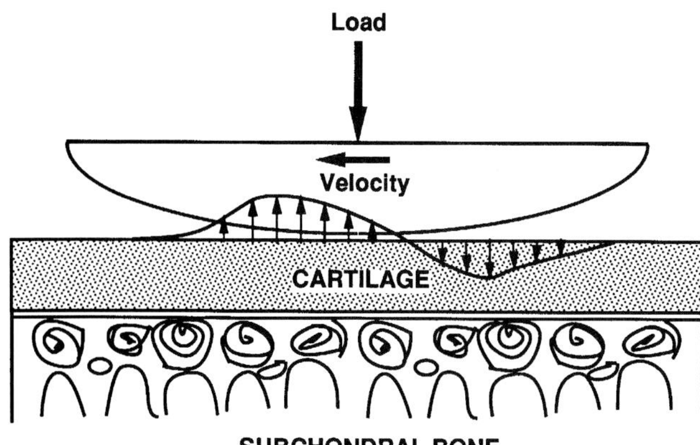

Figure 53
A biphasic model of articular cartilage showing fluid exudation ahead of and fluid imbibition behind the moving load. (Reproduced with permission from Mow VC, Soslowsky LJ: Friction, lubrication and wear of diarthrodial joints, in Mow VC, Hayes WC (eds): *Basic Orthopaedic Biomechanics.* New York, Raven Press, 1991, pp 245–292.)

the load has passed, the expelled fluid is resorbed as the porous-permeable solid matrix recovers its lost fluid. Because of the high water content, particularly near the articular surface, this provides an ideal mechanism to create a fluid lubricant film. However, as the properties of the tissue change, for example, with osteoarthritic cartilage (increased porosity and permeability, and decreased compressive stiffness) or as the loading and sliding speed increases (for example, during injury), the fluid efflux pattern will be altered. Under these conditions, no lubricant film will be created, leaving boundary lubrication as the sole protector of the bearing surface. Because the normal flow pattern is circulatory in nature, this self-generating lubricant film may not only provide superb lubrication, but also may create a mechanically generated circulation system required by the chondrocytes in the tissue.

Summary of Joint Lubrication

There are two fundamental types of lubrication, fluid-film and boundary. Fluid-film lubrication can operate in many forms such as hydrodynamic, elastohydrodynamic, or squeeze-film lubrication. The lubricant for fluid-film lubrication can come from either synovial fluid or the interstitial fluid exuded from cartilage, depending on conditions. The non-Newtonian properties of synovial fluid, specifically its shear thinning effect, act to increase the load-carrying capacity, the area over which a load is spread, and the duration of the squeeze-film time. The self-generating mechanism in which fluid is exuded over the leading-edge region of the advancing load and fluid imbibition occurs over the trailing-edge region of the passing load appears to be the prevalent mode of lubricant film creation. Boundary lubrication involves a monolayer of lubricant molecules, which is adsorbed on each bearing surface. It is active when the surface roughnesses of the opposing articular surfaces come into contact, or when the fluid film is depleted under severe loading conditions. The details of specific lubrication mechanisms depend on the specific joint in question and the particular type of loading applied. Under pathologic conditions, the lubrication mechanisms within a joint will be affected as the properties of the synovial fluid and/or the properties of the articular cartilage are altered as a result of degenerative changes.

Clinical Applications

Prosthetic Design Considerations: Shoulder

In this section, a clinical problem is discussed, using some of the basic biomechanics concepts presented. The design of a shoulder prosthesis must take into account a variety of factors peculiar to that joint. The glenohumeral joint functions in concert with the acromioclavicular, sternoclavicular, and scapulothoracic articulations during normal shoulder use. Thus, knowledge of shoulder anatomy and cartilage material properties is needed to define shoulder motion and articulation. The ligamentous stabilizers are complex, and because of the unique anatomy of the coracohumeral and glenohumeral ligaments, stress is distributed among varying regions depending on arm elevation and rotation. The muscles, especially the rotator cuff, not only are important for dynamic stability, but their precise lever arms and lines of action are vital to generating the moments required to rotate the arm. Required knowledge includes the tensile properties of the glenohumeral ligament and lines of action of forces exerted by the shoulder muscle forces. Clearly, from this description, all the biomechanical concepts discussed must be brought to bear to understand shoulder biomechanics.

Constrained total shoulder replacements have had the same difficulties with loosening and mechanical failure as constrained replacements of other joints. The ideas of fatigue and failure stress within the bone and PMMA must be appreciated here. The initial appeal of the concept was the hope that the constrained articulation would provide stability to a joint whose small socket (glenoid) could not enclose the entire ball (humeral head). This articulation also was expected to assure a fulcrum for the deltoid in cases without a functioning rotator cuff. Joint-reaction loads and contact areas within the glenohumeral articulation must be determined by biomechanical investigations.

Figure 54, *top,* shows a two-dimensional model of a total shoulder replacement, which is assumed to be frictionless; the deltoid force and the rotator cuff force have been drawn. Both forces tend to abduct the humerus and, along with the weight of the arm, can be resolved into a resultant force acting at the center of the glenoid. This resultant force produces a uniform compressive loading pattern on the cement and bone. If the rotator cuff is torn or nonfunctional, the unopposed deltoid force will tend to act superiorly and eccentrically load the humerus, thus producing a tendency to sublux the humeral component (Fig. 54, *bottom*). A rocking action would then be generated, causing the glenoid component to rotate against the restraining cement in the bone. This action has been clinically associated with glenoid component loosening.

Figure 55 shows the contact stresses on the surface of the humeral component. With the prosthetic surfaces assumed to be frictionless, only normal contact stresses may be developed. If the rotator cuff muscle force is present, the resultant force on the glenoid component may be centered to give a uniform contact stress pattern (Fig. 55, *top*). If the rotator cuff muscles are weak, a greater stress will be exerted on the "overhang" of the glenoid component (Fig. 55, *bottom*) used in some prostheses to "substitute" for the head-depressing effect of the rotator cuff. However, as shown in the figure, these forces have the same tendency to rock the glenoid as noted before. The risk of loosening rises as more constraint is added, because the moment arm will be increased.

It is often stated that the normal shoulder has a relatively flat glenoid articulating with a more curved humeral head, and, thus, that even a glenoid component of normal size adds constraint if it is manufactured to the same radius of curvature as the humeral component. However, recent precise quantitative assessments of glenohumeral articular geometry have shown that the normal humeral head and glenoid surfaces are conforming spheres within less than a mil-

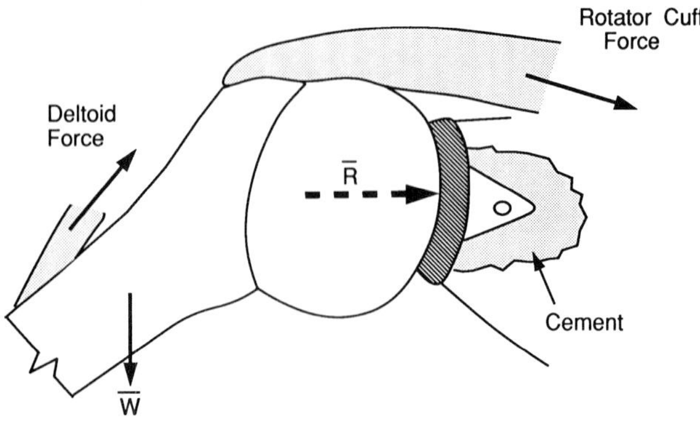

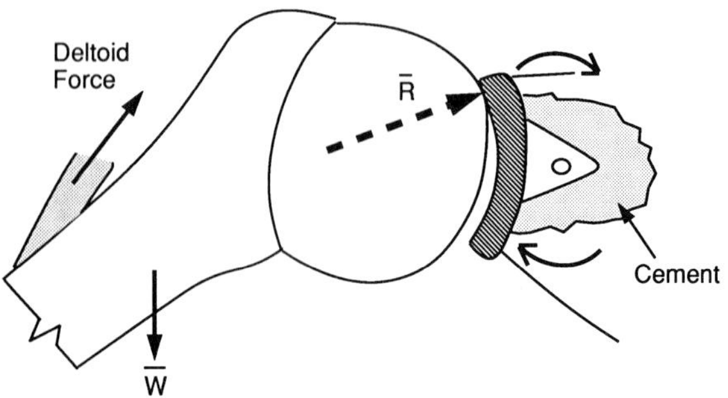

Figure 54
Model of a total shoulder replacement. **Top,** With a functional rotator cuff, the resultant force is centered toward the glenoid, resulting in a uniform compression of the cement and bone. **Bottom,** With a nonfunctional rotator cuff, the deltoid will eccentrically load the glenoid causing it to rotate against the restraining cement in the bone.

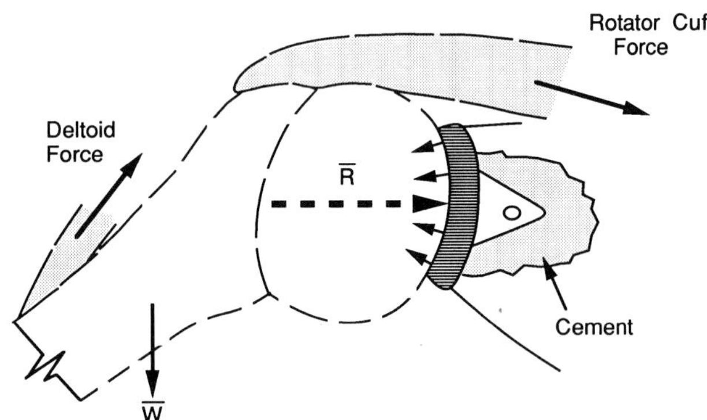

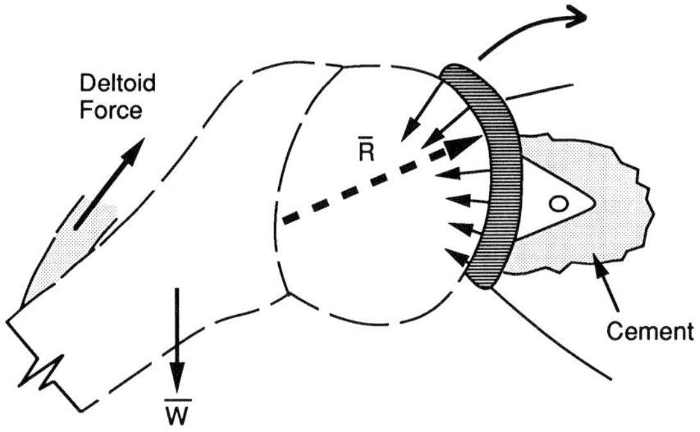

Figure 55
The contact stresses on the surface of the humeral component. **Top,** The rotator cuff resists the superiorly directed force exerted by the deltoid. **Bottom,** If the rotator cuff muscles are weak, stress will be exerted on the overhang of the glenoid component, which will tend to rock the glenoid.

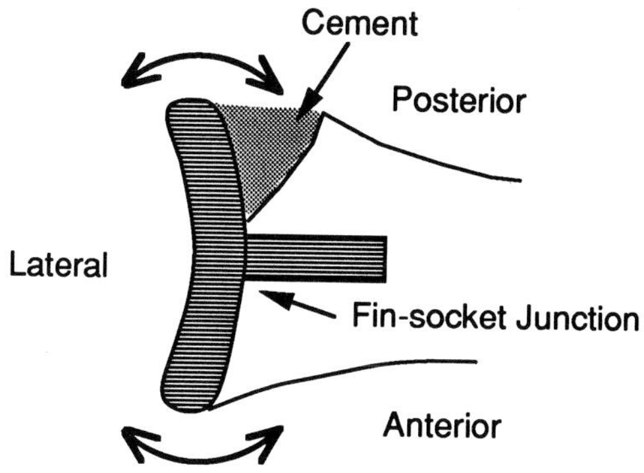

Figure 56
Area of glenoid wear built up with cement. The differences in the Young's moduli of bone and cement result in a different amount of displacement between the two sides, thus toggling and fatiguing the fin-socket junction.

limeter difference. Impressions of glenoid shallowness probably resulted from its flatter appearance on radiographs that show only the subchondral bone, because cartilage thickness is greatest peripherally on the glenoid. Thus, the need to obtain precise anatomic information in prosthesis design is obvious.

Early experience with total shoulder replacement revealed an occasional fracture of a glenoid component at the junction of the fin and the socket. This fracture may have been caused in part by the stress concentration effect of a notch at that junction, which was eliminated on subsequent designs. Also, however, early techniques often built up areas of uneven glenoid wear with cement (Fig. 56). Given the different Young's moduli of bone and cement, a uniformly distributed load on the glenoid would nevertheless result in a different displacement on the side of the cement buildup, thus toggling around and fatiguing the fin-socket junction. Therefore, the surgical technique was altered, either lowering the "high" side, bone grafting the "low" side, or altering the component version (or a combination) so that the glenoid component rests on bone evenly.

Metal backing of the glenoid component has been suggested to improve the evenness of stress transfer to bone according to finite element analysis, but clinical evidence of this is not yet available. Modular heads have been introduced to allow precise tensioning of the soft tissues and adjusting of muscle moment arms. Clearly, an understanding of the biomechanical principles presented in this chapter facilitates understanding of these considerations.

Conclusions

Although all material objects are subject to the laws of mechanics, the precise relation between form and function, so dear to the orthopaedist, may be, in practice, difficult to work out. This difficulty is due not only to the technical and mathematic complexities involved, but also to the variation in the anatomy and constitution of living tissues. Furthermore, living systems change rapidly, so that, for example, a bone undergoing stress remodeling may be difficult to subject to precise stress analysis.

Nevertheless, this chapter should enable the reader to: (1) work out forces and moments to estimate loads in clinical situations; (2) understand the assumptions that underlie biomechanical modeling; (3) understand the principles of deformation mechanics, especially the distinction between loading conditions and the states of stress and strain within the material; (4) understand the difference between a structural response and a material property; (5) feel comfortable with kinematic analysis; and (6) have a general grasp of the frictional and wear properties of diarthrodial joints.

Selected Bibliography

Elementary Engineering Textbooks

Lai WM, Rubin D, Krempl E: *Introduction to Continuum Mechanics.* New York, Pergamon Press, 1978.

Shames IH: *Engineering Mechanics: Statics,* ed 2. Englewood Cliffs, NJ, Prentice Hall, 1966.

Shames IH: *Engineering Mechanics: Dynamics,* ed 2. Englewood Cliffs, NJ, Prentice Hall, 1966.

Advanced Engineering Textbooks

Hertzberg RW: *Deformation and Fracture: Mechanics of Engineering Materials,* ed. 3. New York, John Wiley & Sons, 1989.

Johnson KL: *Contact Mechanics.* Cambridge, Cambridge University Press, 1985.

Moore DF: *Principles and Applications of Tribology.* Oxford, Pergamon Press, 1975.

Timoshenko SP, Goodier JN: *Theory of Elasticity.* New York, McGraw Hill, 1969.

Yih CS: *Fluid Mechanics: A Concise Introduction to the Theory.* New York, McGraw Hill, 1969.

General Biomechanics

Fung YC: *Biomechanics: Mechanical Properties of Living Tissues.* New York, Springer-Verlag, 1981.

Fung YC: *Biomechanics: Motion, Flow, Stress and Growth.* New York, Springer-Verlag, 1990.

Skalak R, Chien S: *Handbook of Bioengineering.* New York, McGraw Hill, 1987.

Orthopaedic Biomechanics

Mow VC, Hayes WC (eds): *Basic Orthopaedic Biomechanics.* New York, Raven Press, 1991.

Mow VC, Ratcliffe A, Woo SL-Y (eds): *Biomechanics of Diarthrodial Joints.* New York, Springer-Verlag, 1990, vols I and II.

Ozkaya N, Nordin M: *Fundamentals of Biomechanics: Equilibrium, Motion, and Deformation.* New York, Van Nostrand Reinhold, 1991.

Woo SL-Y, Buckwalter JA (eds): *Injury and Repair of the Musculoskeletal Soft Tissues.* Park Ridge, IL, American Academy of Orthopaedic Surgeons, 1988.

Articular Cartilage

Brandt KD (ed): *Cartilage Changes in Osteoarthritis.* Indianapolis, IN, University of Indiana Press, 1990.

Mow VC, Ratcliffe A (eds): *Structure and Function of Articular Cartilage.* Boca Raton, FL, CRC Press, 1993.

Bone

Cowin SC: *Bone Mechanics.* Boca Raton, FL, CRC Press, 1989.

Ligaments

Daniel DM, Akeson WH, O'Connor JJ: *Knee Ligaments: Structure, Function, Injury and Repair.* New York, Raven Press, 1990.

Chapter 10
Biomaterials

Alan S. Litsky, MD, ScD
Myron Spector, PhD

Chapter Outline

The term biomaterials generally refers to synthetic and treated natural materials that are used to replace or augment tissue and/or organ function. Implanted devices, such as total joint replacement prostheses, play a critical role in many facets of orthopaedic practice. The longevity of these implanted materials often is related directly to the clinical result. An understanding of the physical properties of materials used to fabricate orthopaedic devices is important for the judicious selection and implementation of these devices and provides a foundation for realistic expectations of clinical performance. The physical properties of materials result from their chemical composition and structure. Therefore, an understanding of the molecular structure and chemical bonding of biomaterials can provide a basis for understanding their physical properties. Knowledge of their chemistry is not sufficient to predict the functional properties of most materials; manufacturing and processing variables significantly affect their final properties. After an introduction to the fundamental concepts of materials science, this chapter will address relationships between molecular structure and properties of biomaterials. Friction, lubrication, and wear will then be discussed. A review of the various classes of synthetic biomaterials comprises the final section of the chapter.

Fundamentals of Materials Science

A force applied to an object either accelerates the object or deforms it. When the object is constrained so that it cannot move or if equal and opposite forces are applied, the object is deformed. Any material subjected to a force or a torque deforms to some degree. The assumption of rigid body motion that underlies much of mechanics is useful on a large scale but is uniformly false on a smaller scale. This section deals with the information that can be ascertained about a material by the way it deforms when subjected to various forces.

Elastic Deformation

Stress

When a force acts on an object, tending to produce a deformation in that object, an internal resistance to that deformation is produced in the material. That internal reaction to the externally applied force is called stress; it is equal to the applied force in magnitude but is opposite in direction. This stress is distributed over the cross-sectional area of the specimen and thus has the units of force per unit area:

Stress = σ = Force/Area

The SI unit for stress is the pascal, which is a one-newton force distributed over one square meter, that is, 1 Pa = $1 N/m^2$.

An applied external force can be directed at a specimen from any angle producing complex stress patterns in the material. All stresses can be resolved into three types—tension, compression, and shear. Tension is produced in a material when two forces are pulling away from each other along the same straight line. The resistance to tensile forces comes from the interatomic attractive forces that keep the material from being torn apart. The ultimate tensile strength of a material is a measure of this cohesive force. Compression results from two forces, again along the same line, pushing toward each other. The interatomic repulsive force that rises sharply at short interatomic distances resists compressive forces. Bending produces a combination of tension on the convex side of the specimen and compression on the concave side (Fig. 1). In between there is a plane where the stress is zero; this plane is called the neutral axis, and its location depends on the geometry of the specimen. Two forces directed parallel to each other, but not along the same line or in the same direction, produce shear. The ease with which one portion of a material slides over another determines the material's resistance to shear defor-

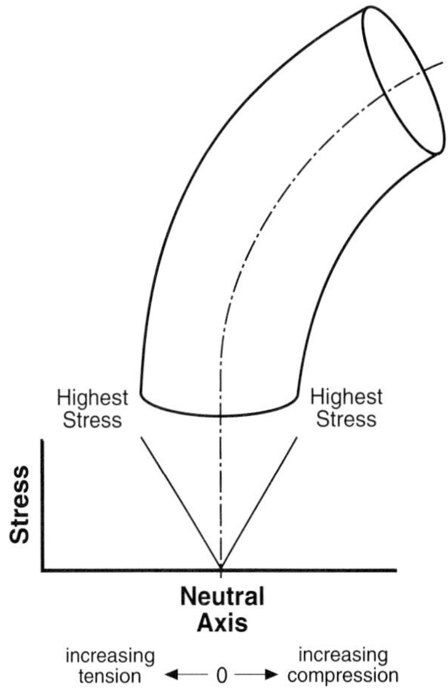

Figure 1
Bending stress in a cylinder demonstrating tensile and compressive forces. The neutral axis is the plane of zero stress. The magnitude of the stress increases with distance from the neutral axis. (Adapted with permission from Radin EL, Rose RM, Blaha JD, et al: *Practical Biomechanics for the Orthopedic Surgeon,* ed 2. New York, Churchill Livingstone, 1991.)

mation. Torsion or twisting produces shear stresses in the material. Figure 2 depicts the three basic types of stress. Most actual stress patterns are complex combinations of these three types.

Strain

Stress produces deformation. Figure 3 demonstrates the effect of various stress types; a rectangular grid is drawn on the surface of a specimen to show more clearly the deformations that occur. The measurement of deformation, normalized by the original length of the specimen, is called strain:

Strain = ϵ = Change in length/Original length
= (Deformed length - Original length)/Original length
= (DL - OL)/OL

Strain is dimensionless. It is often reported as a percent or in terms of microstrain $\mu\epsilon$. (One microstrain is a change in length of 10^{-6} for each unit of original length, 0.000001 mm/mm; 1,000 $\mu\epsilon$ is a change in length of 1 mm/m of initial length.) Peak strains in bone have been measured in the 2,000 to 3,000 $\mu\epsilon$ range.

When a material is deformed in one dimension, its other dimensions undergo smaller opposite changes. For example, when a bar is elongated by tensile forces it becomes somewhat narrower. The negative of the ratio of the transverse strain to the

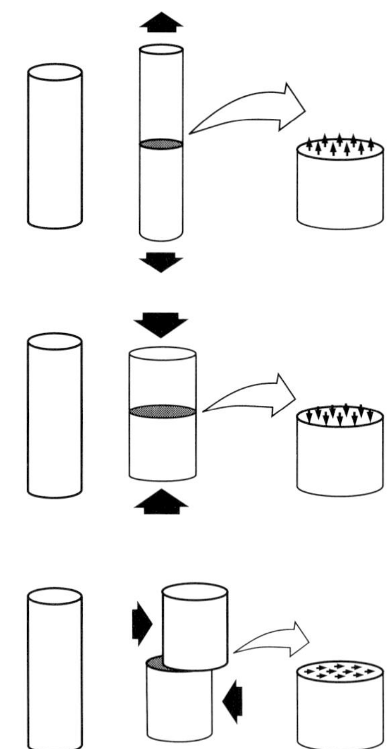

Figure 2
Tension, compression, and shear stress. The stress developed in a material opposes the externally applied load. (Adapted with permission from Nordin M, Frankel VH: *Basic Biomechanics of the Musculoskeletal System,* ed 2. Philadelphia, Lea & Febiger, 1989.)

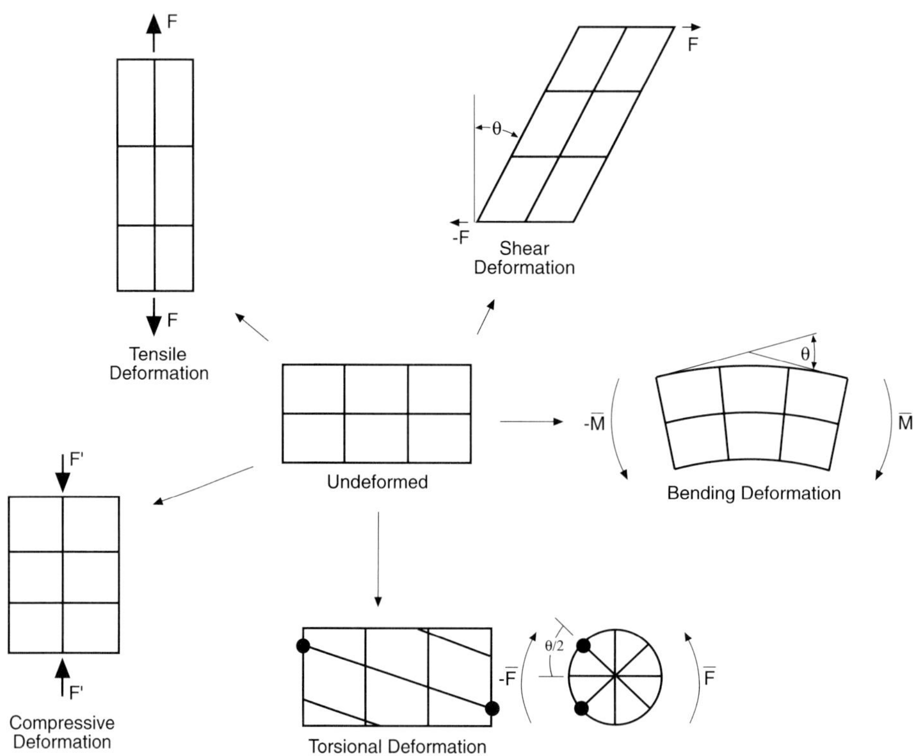

Figure 3
Deformations produced by tensile, compressive, shearing, bending, and torsional stresses. (Adapted with permission from Black J: *Orthopaedic Biomaterials in Research and Practice.* New York, Churchill Livingstone, 1988.)

longitudinal strain is called Poisson's ratio. Being a ratio of two strains, Poisson's ratio is a dimensionless quantity. Values for Poisson's ratio υ range from 0, indicating a material that is fully compressible, to 0.5 for a material that is totally incompressible. Many fluids are incompressible materials that maintain a constant volume during deformation. Most solid materials have Poisson's ratios between 0.2 and 0.5. Ratios less than zero, indicating a material that expands on deformation, are found only in foam materials specifically designed and manufactured to achieve this property.

Stress-Strain Curve

When a material is tested under controlled laboratory conditions, the force(s) applied and the deformation(s) produced can be measured, and the measurements used to produce a plot of load versus deformation. If the specimen size is known, this information can be expressed in terms of stress and strain. By convention, the stress is plotted on the ordinate and the strain on the abscissa. Figure 4 is a stress-strain plot of cortical bone. Stress-strain curves reveal much useful and important information about the material being tested because geometric factors have been removed from the load-deformation data.

Stress-strain curves are intrinsic measures of material properties, that is, they do not depend on the dimensions of the specimen. Data obtained from one set of experiments on a specimen convenient for laboratory testing can be used to design any size structural component. At low levels of stress there is a linear relationship between the applied stress and the resultant deformation. This proportionality is called the modulus of elasticity or Young's modulus. It is a measure of the stiffness of the material and is computed by dividing the stress by the strain at any point along the linear portion of the curve.

Modulus of Elasticity = E = stress/strain

The modulus has the same units as stress because strain is a dimensionless quantity. The higher the modulus of a material, the more it resists deformation when a force is applied; the higher the modulus, the stiffer the material. (It is important to distinguish between the material stiffness and the structural stiffness of a real object. The latter includes geometric factors that the former does not.) Stress-strain curves can also be drawn for materials subjected to shear stresses. The proportionality constant between shear stress and shear strain is called the shear modulus and is abbreviated by the letter G. The underlying concept is identical. The linear relationship between stress and strain is invalid at higher stress levels in some elastic materials. Figure 5 shows the stress-strain curves of three idealized elastic materials. The proportional limit is defined as the greatest stress that a material will sustain without deviating from this linearity. Point b in Figure 5 represents the proportional limit of material B.

The elastic limit is defined as the maximum stress that a material can withstand without permanent deformation or failure. It is the same as the proportional limit for many materials. Up to the elastic limit, energy put into the material stretches or bends atomic bonds but does not rearrange the atomic organization of the material. This energy can be recovered by releasing the applied load. The point at which the material fails, indicated by the X's in Figure 5, determines the ultimate strength and the ultimate strain. Material A has the highest strength of the three while material C has the greatest ultimate strain. The area under the stress-strain curve is the work necessary to produce a given

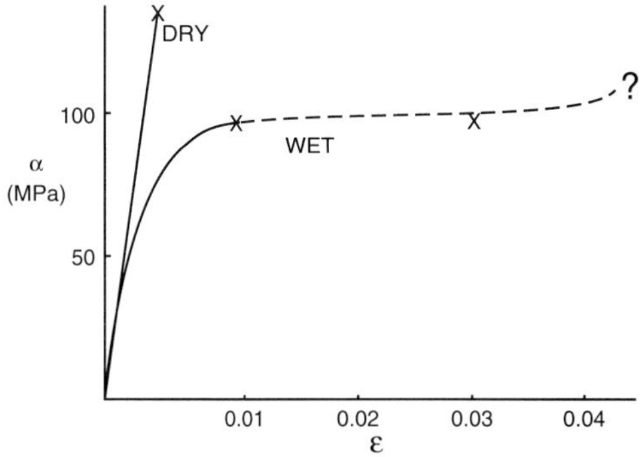

Figure 4
Stress-strain curves of cortical bone at a strain rate of 0.01 per second. (Reproduced with permission from Black J: *Orthopaedic Biomaterials in Research and Practice.* New York, Churchill Livingstone, 1988.)

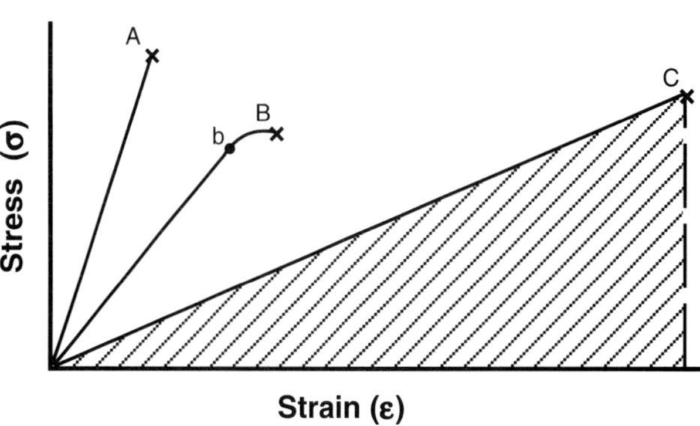

Figure 5
Stress-strain curves of three idealized elastic materials. Point b is the proportional limit; X represents the failure of each material.

deformation. Work is defined as force times distance, and is expressed in Joules.

1 Joule = J = 1 N·m

The area under the load-deformation curve is the work required to produce a given deformation. The area under the stress-strain curve is a measure of the work per unit volume required to produce a given strain. This is the strain energy density, expressed in Joules/meter^3 (1 J/m^3 = 1 N·m/m^3 = 1 N/m^2). The area under the entire stress-strain curve, up to the point of failure (the shaded area under curve C in Figure 5), is the amount of energy required to break a unit volume of the material under the given test conditions. Energy put into deforming a purely elastic material to any point before failure can be recovered by removing the stress. Resilience is the energy returned and is a measure of the energy storage capability of the material (Fig. 6).

True Versus Nominal Stress and Strain

The stress-strain curves normally extracted from load-deformation data are based on the original geometry of the specimen. With ductile materials, a localized reduction in cross-sectional area occurs before failure. This is called necking. The true stress is the applied load distributed over the instantaneous local area, and the true strain is the local strain (local change in length/original length). These values are greater than the nominal values, which are based on the original dimensions of the specimen (Fig. 7). Because of the practical difficulties in ascertaining these quantities, virtually all stress-strain curves show nominal or engineering stress and strain.

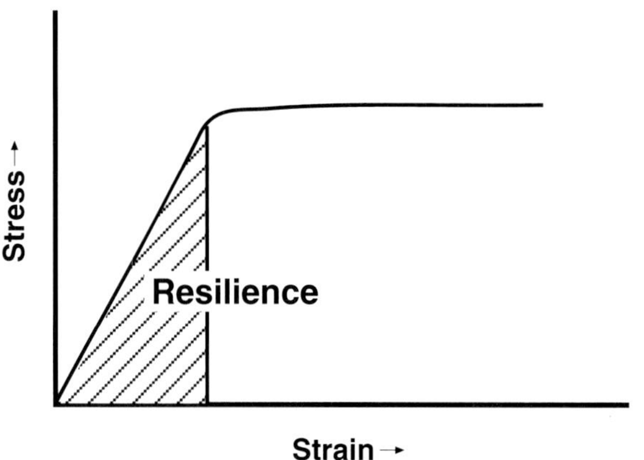

Figure 6
Resilience is the energy returned upon release of a material strained in the elastic region. (Adapted with permission from Craig RG: *Restorative Dental Materials.* St. Louis, CV Mosby, 1989.)

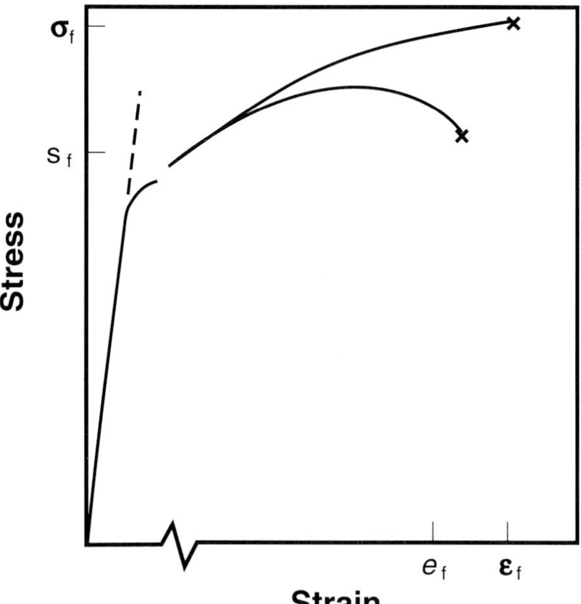

Figure 7
The true stress σ and true strain ϵ are based on the actual area at the site of failure rather than the original area of the specimen. In materials that develop a local decrease in area prior to fracture, true stress and true strain are higher than the nominal values. Therefore, the true fracture stress σ_f exceeds the nominal breaking strength s_f. Also, because the strain is localized, the true strain at the point of fracture ϵ_f exceeds the nominal strain to fracture e_f. (Adapted from Van Vlack LH: *Elements of Materials Science,* ed 6. Redding, MA, Addison Wesley, 1989.)

Permanent Deformation

Figure 8 shows a stress strain curve that extends significantly beyond the elastic limit of the material. This curve represents a material that undergoes permanent deformation when stress is applied in excess of a given value. Elastic deformation is not permanent after the stress is removed, whereas plastic deformation is a residual deformation remaining after all initial stresses have been removed.

Yield

The yield strength of a material is defined as the stress at which the material exhibits a specified deviation from the linear proportionality between stress and strain. Some materials have a clearly defined yield point, beyond which the strain continues to increase with no additional stress. For other materials, such as the one shown in Figure 8, the stress-strain curve passes the proportional limit and begins to level off without a distinct demarcation. A fixed amount of nonelastic deformation is selected so that various materials can be compared. This is often 2%, as shown in the figure. A line is drawn

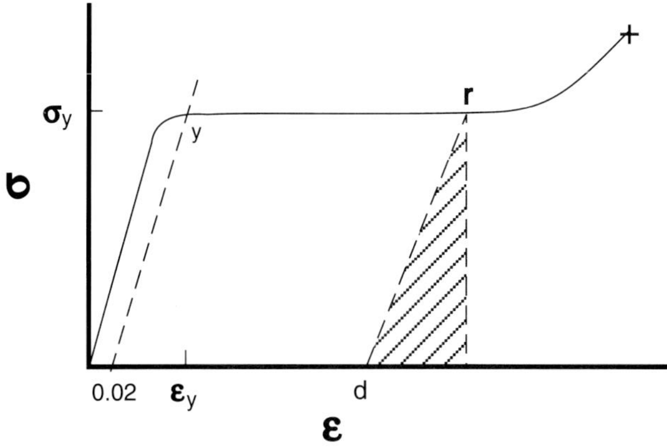

Figure 8
Stress-strain curve of an idealized elastic-plastic material. The dotted line indicates the 2% strain line; its intersection with the stress-strain curve defines the yield point. σ_y represents the yield strain, ϵ_y the yield stress. A material strained to point r will return the elastic energy and recoil to a deformed length, point d.

parallel to the initial slope of the stress-strain curve through the point on the abscissa corresponding to 2% strain. The intersection of that line with the stress-strain curve is the yield point y. The yield stress σ_y and yield strain ϵ_y are the corresponding values of stress and strain.

Ductility

Some materials fracture or fail before they undergo any permanent deformation. These materials are called brittle and have straight stress-strain curves. Ceramics typically behave in a brittle manner; bone usually fractures without permanent deformation.

Materials that reach a yield point and then undergo further deformation before fracture are termed ductile. Energy put into a material to produce this permanent or plastic deformation is not recoverable. The resilience previously discussed is not lost when a material is stressed beyond the yield point. The energy absorbed to produce elastic deformation is still recoverable (Fig. 8). The plastic deformation remains. The irrecoverable, permanent deformation represents a change in the molecular structure of the material and often indicates a change in properties. If the above material is stressed again, it may have different yield and ultimate strengths. This is what occurs when a metal is work-hardened.

Toughness

The area under both the elastic and the plastic portions of the stress-strain curve is a measure of the material's toughness, that is, the total energy required to stress the material to the point of fracture. A brittle material can be tough because it has a high modulus and high strength without any ductility. A less stiff material can absorb an equal amount of energy by undergoing a large plastic deformation before failing. Both materials in Figure 9 absorb the same amount of energy prior to failure; the areas beneath their stress-strain curves are equal, so both are equally tough.

All of the material properties previously mentioned can be determined from the stress-strain curve of a material. This makes stress-strain curves a very compact and convenient way to document a large amount of information about any material (Fig. 10).

Fatigue

Repeated loading and unloading of a material will cause it to fail, even if the loads are below the ultimate stress. Each loading cycle produces a minute amount of microdamage that accumulates with repetitive loads until the material fails. The orthopaedic relevance of this phenomenon is obvious considering the multiple loading cycles that each portion of the musculoskeletal system undergoes as a consequence of normal human activities; the average person walks between one and two million steps per year. Devices designed to bear weight must withstand their share of the applied load repeatedly for an extended period. Whereas biologic tissues have repair mechanisms for coping with the microdamage as it occurs, implant materials do not.

The fatigue life of a material is recorded on a curve of stress σ versus number of cycles, or S-N curve. The ordinate is the peak stress per cycle and the abscissa is the number of cycles to failure, usually drawn on a logarithmic scale to compress the data into a reasonable curve. Higher stresses produce failure in fewer cycles (loading to the ultimate stress produces failure in one cycle), while

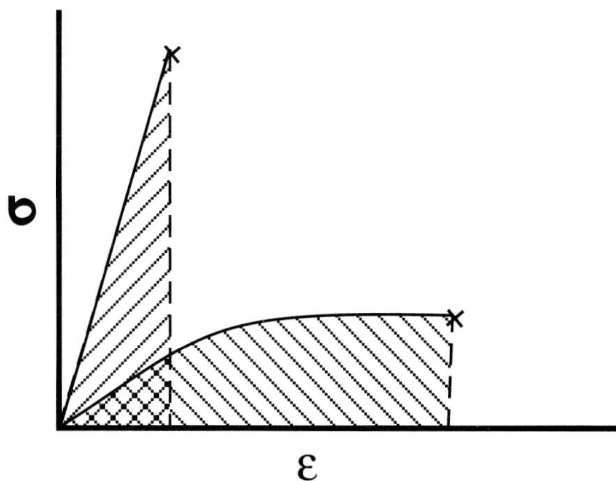

Figure 9
Toughness is the energy absorbed prior to failure, indicated by the area under the stress-strain curve. The two materials whose stress-strain curves are drawn here are equally tough even though one is stiff and brittle and the other is flexible and ductile.

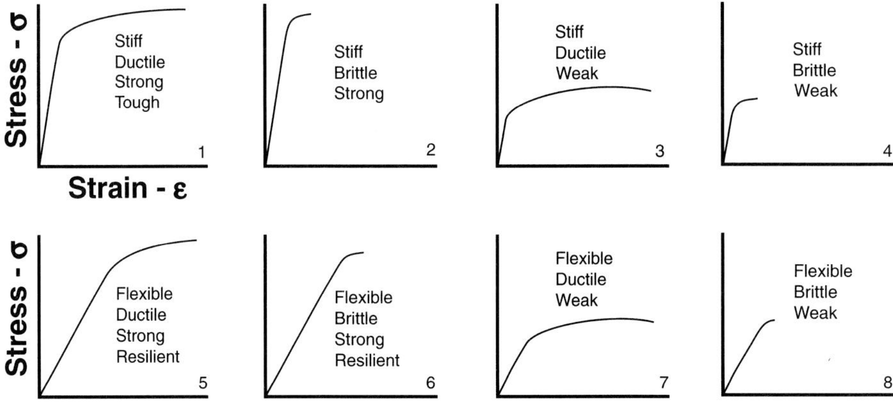

Figure 10
Stress-strain curves for idealized materials with various combinations of material properties. (Adapted with permission from Craig RG: *Restorative Dental Materials.* St. Louis, CV Mosby, 1989.)

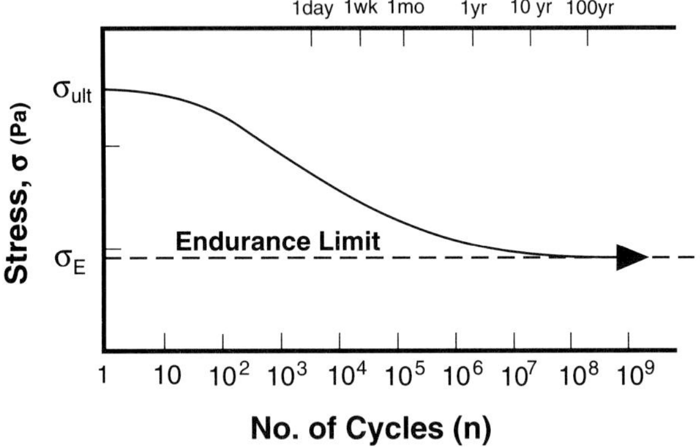

Figure 11
S-N curve. (Adapted with permission from Black J: *Orthopaedic Biomaterials in Research and Practice.* New York, Churchill Livingstone, 1988.)

lower stresses are tolerated for an extended period. Figure 11 shows a typical S-N curve. Many materials, including all the clinically used implant and fracture fixation alloys, have S-N curves that have limited values at low stress levels. This stress is called the fatigue or endurance limit. Implants designed for long-duration cyclic loading must be designed to keep the peak stress below this level. The fatigue life of some materials (for example, stainless steel) is profoundly affected by the functional environment.

There are two distinct stages to fatigue failure. The first, crack initiation, occurs at a chemical, structural, or geometric weakness. Surface scratches, nicks from surgical instruments, and sharp changes in cross section are typical sites for fatigue cracks to start. (See the chapter on biomechanics for a discussion of stress risers.) In the second stage, crack propagation, the localized crack grows with each application of the load by a process that depends on both the load and the material. The growing fracture decreases the structural area of the remaining material, thereby increasing the true stress. When this exceeds the true ultimate stress, the material fails.

The resistance to fatigue fracture of a material can be enhanced in two ways: by decreasing the population of intrinsic flaws, which nucleate cracks, or by increasing the intrinsic fracture toughness of the material, which retards the crack propagation rate. Both approaches have been applied in attempts to improve the fracture toughness of acrylic bone cement: centrifugation to reduce the population of voids that may serve as crack initiation sites, and the inclusion of fibers or soft polymer domains to enhance the fracture toughness of the cement.

Hardness

For many materials, the mechanical properties at the surface differ from those found in the bulk of the material. Hardness is the ability to resist plastic deformation at the material surface. It is measured by pressing an indenter into a surface under controlled conditions and measuring the resultant surface impression. All hardness scales are relative, with higher numbers indicating harder surfaces. An early test, the Mohs hardness scale, is based on the ability of a harder mineral to scratch the surface of a softer one. Common hardness scales are the Rockwell, Brinell, and Vickers scales. Figure 12 shows how orthopaedic materials rate on these various scales.

Hardness is an important design consideration in articulating surfaces; hard surfaces or debris tend

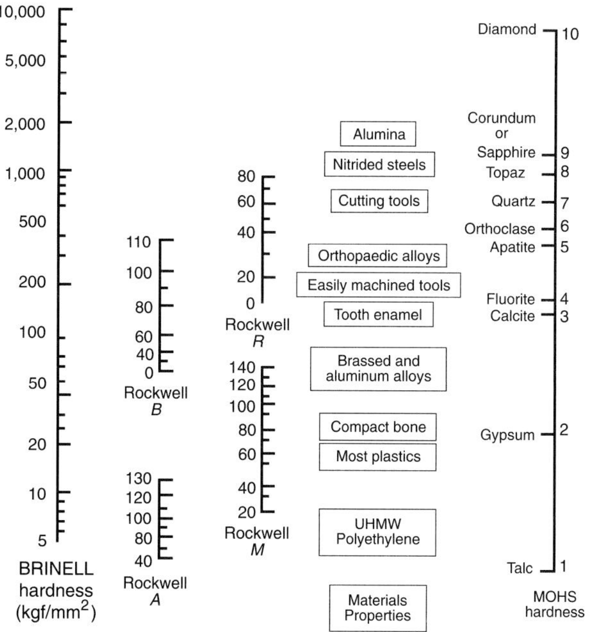

Figure 12
Comparison of orthopaedic materials using relative hardness scales. (Adapted with permission from Black J: *Orthopaedic Biomaterials in Research and Practice.* New York, Churchill Livingstone, 1988.)

to gouge softer ones, and soft materials can form transfer films on hard surfaces. Both processes contribute to the wear of articulating surfaces. Hardness is not, however, the only determinant of wear, and knowing the hardness of two materials is not sufficient to predict their wear behavior.

Surfaces can be modified to alter their properties without changing those of the bulk of the material. A surface coating can be formed or enhanced. Examples include formation of surface oxides on implant metals for increased corrosion and wear resistance and carburization of steel to produce a very hard cutting edge. Mechanical means also can be used to alter surface geometry; polishing produces smooth articulating surfaces, and grit blasting roughens and work hardens load-bearing stems. Alteration of surface layer composition by nitriding or ion implantation is currently under investigation as a means of improving wear characteristics of titanium surfaces.

Nonideal Materials

The behavior of real materials is similar to that of the ideal materials previously described, but usually is not as neat and simple. Biologic materials often have oriented structural elements that produce very different material properties when the material is tested in different directions and when different parts of the structure are tested. Each of these elements will be discussed briefly below.

Anisotropy

Ideal materials are homogeneous and behave the same regardless of orientation. A material is called isotropic when its properties in each of the three coordinate axes, the x, y, and z directions, are identical. Biologic tissues, on the other hand, are structured to achieve optimal material properties in a given orientation with the minimum weight and metabolic load. They therefore have different properties in different directions, a characteristic referred to as anisotropy.

The directional nature of tissue materials must be considered and documented when obtaining specimens for materials testing. Reproducible orientation in the testing device is important if the resultant data are to have any meaning. An anisotropic material has different tensile properties when tested in different orientations (Fig. 13), as is obviously true of ligaments and tendons. This concept should not be confused with the differences between tensile and compressive properties found in many materials, such as bone.

Heterogeneity

Biologic tissues are composed of many structural elements, each with its own function and a corresponding set of material properties. Such a material has different properties in different areas. The importance of this heterogeneity depends on the scale of the experiment; the smaller the test specimen the more of an effect the compositional heterogeneity will have.

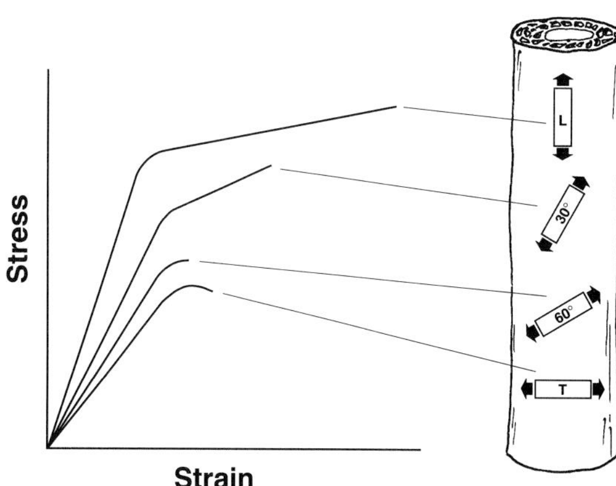

Figure 13
Anisotropic behavior of cortical bone specimens from a human femoral shaft tested in tension. (Adapted with permission from Nordin M, Frankel VH: *Basic Biomechanics of the Musculoskeletal System,* ed 2. Philadelphia, Lea & Febiger, 1989.)

Viscoelasticity

Time has not been a factor in the stress-strain relationships discussed thus far; the elastic-plastic behaviors of the materials are solely a function of stress and strain. Elastic-plastic materials respond instantly to applied loads or strains. Many materials can be treated as purely elastic-plastic. The behavior of most metals and ceramics used in orthopaedic biomaterials is not time dependent.

All biologic tissues, plastics, and most structures composed of more than one material (composites) flow to some extent under an applied load, and this flow or creep behavior is time dependent. The faster a load is applied, the less creep can occur and the stiffer the material seems. Figure 14 shows that for a single material, an increase in the rate of loading, or strain rate, increases the modulus and the ultimate strength while decreasing the ultimate strain. At low strain rates the material has no appreciable elastic deformation; instead it flows like a viscous liquid. At high strain rates, the same material can behave as a brittle, elastic solid. These materials are called viscoelastic because they exhibit both kinds of behavior. A familiar viscoelastic material is Silly Putty. When left at room temperature overnight (low strain rate), it exhibits viscous flow and slowly forms a flat puddle. If molded into a ball and thrown against a wall (high strain rate), it bounces back in an elastic manner. Each loading pattern in this example is so extreme that one behavior dominates. Under more normal conditions, viscoelastic materials exhibit both viscous and elastic behavior simultaneously. In reporting the results of materials testing of viscoelastic materials, it is essential to specify the strain rate used. Without this information, in addition to the other experimental data required in all materials testing, the results are not interpretable in any meaningful manner.

Hysteresis

The elastic recovery of a viscoelastic material stressed below its yield point does not always coincide with the deformation curve (Fig. 15). The area between the two curves represents energy that is dissipated, usually as heat, and is not recoverable. An easily observable example of this is the increase in temperature of an elastic band that is rapidly stretched and released many times. The loss of strain energy, or hysteresis, is an important factor both in materials testing (the specimen heats up and material properties are often temperature dependent) and in the physiologic behavior of exercising muscles.

Anelasticity

The dimensional recovery of strained materials when a load is released is also a viscoelastic phenomenon. Some portion of the deformation is recovered immediately, some is recoverable over a more extended period, and some is permanent. Whereas elastic-plastic materials lose no energy to irrecoverable processes below the elastic limit, viscoelastic materials dissipate energy immediately at any stress by viscous flow. The loss of energy depends on stress level, time, and temperature.

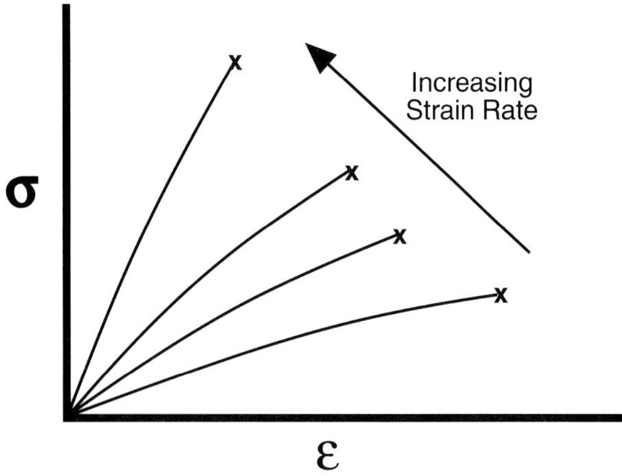

Figure 14
Stress-strain curves for a viscoelastic material showing increase in elastic modulus and ultimate strength with increasing strain rate. (Adapted with permission from Black J: *Orthopaedic Biomaterials in Research and Practice.* New York, Churchill Livingstone, 1988.)

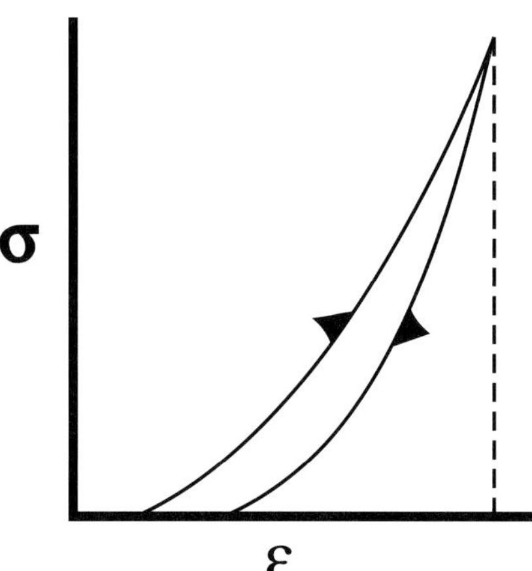

Figure 15
Hysteresis. The area between the deformation and recovery curves represents the energy that is dissipated, usually as heat. (Adapted with permission from Black J: *Orthopaedic Biomaterials in Research and Practice.* New York, Churchill Livingstone, 1988.)

Fluids

Viscosity η is the resistance of a fluid to flow and is equal to the shear stress divided by the shear rate. It characterizes the internal resistance of a fluid to shear deformation.

The viscosity of many fluids is independent of shear rate; such fluids are called newtonian. Water and plasma are newtonian. Other fluids do not behave as simply (Fig. 16). Shear thinning fluids show decreasing viscosity with increasing shear rate; the faster they are loaded the easier they flow. Ketchup, whole blood, and synovial fluid are examples of shear thinning fluids. The opposite behavior, increasing viscosity with increasing shear rate, is exhibited by dilatant fluids. No biologic fluids exhibit this behavior.

The complexities of structure and substance often make testing actual materials, and particularly biologic tissues, a major undertaking. Natural materials usually are tested after removal from their physiologic environment. Isolating the material of interest from surrounding materials in this manner inevitably affects the tissue of interest. Experimental results from tests done under nonliving conditions are used to report the condition of living tissues. This situation obviously is not ideal for any tissue. While the change should be small for most hard tissues, it is an extremely important consideration for contractile tissues such as muscle.

Material Versus Structural Properties

Material properties are normalized to eliminate geometric considerations; stress and strain are independent of area and length. However, size and shape considerations play an important role in the design of actual devices or components and must be reintroduced. Often the approximate size is dictated by the application; for example, a total hip stem can be only as large as the medullary cavity, and an appropriate material must be found that can withstand the imposed stresses when manufactured to the appropriate size. In nonuniform loadings, which encompass all real applications, geometric factors determine the location and magnitude of the maximum stresses. An analysis of the expected stresses, which must include size and shape considerations, must precede material selection.

Bending

When subject to a bending load, one side of a beam undergoes tensile loading while the other side is compressed (Fig. 17). In the simple case of a rectangular beam, the stress distribution varies continuously across the beam and changes from tension to compression at the neutral axis, a plane of zero stress through the center of a simple beam. The magnitude of the compressive or tensile stresses varies linearly with distance from the neutral axis:

$$\sigma = My/I$$

where M is the bending moment, which is equal to the applied force times the distance from the point of interest, y is the linear distance from the neutral axis, and I is the areal moment of inertia. This last value is the resistance to bending created by the shape of the beam (Fig. 18). It is independent of material factors, involving only geometry. The material from which the beam was made is not a factor in the bending stress. The deformation of a beam subjected to a bending moment is a function of both its geometry and the material of which it is made. The

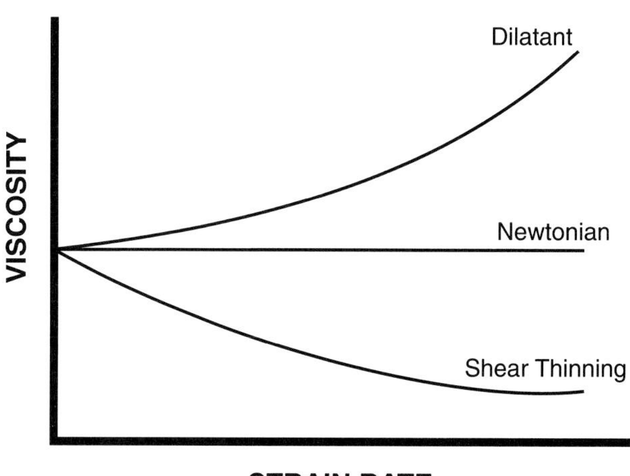

Figure 16
The viscosity of newtonian fluids is independent of shear rate; that of viscoelastic fluids varies with shear rate. Some fluids are shear thinning; others are shear thickening.

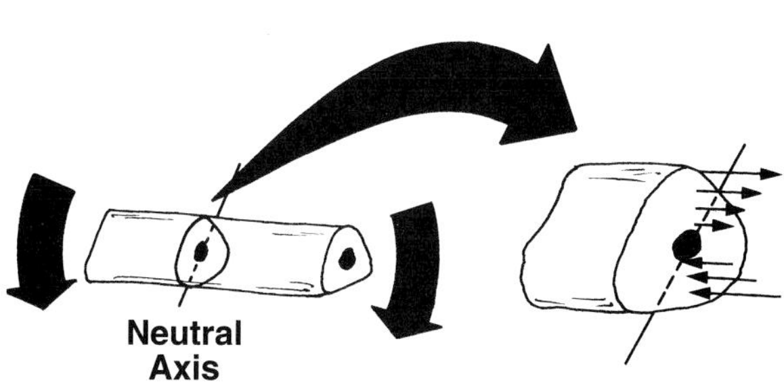

Figure 17
Cross section of bone subjected to bending showing distribution of stresses around the neutral axis. The stresses are highest at the periphery and zero at the neutral axis. The tensile and compressive stresses are unequal because the bone is asymmetric. (Adapted with permission from Nordin M, Frankel VH: *Basic Biomechanics of the Musculoskeletal System,* ed 2. Philadelphia, Lea & Febiger, 1989.)

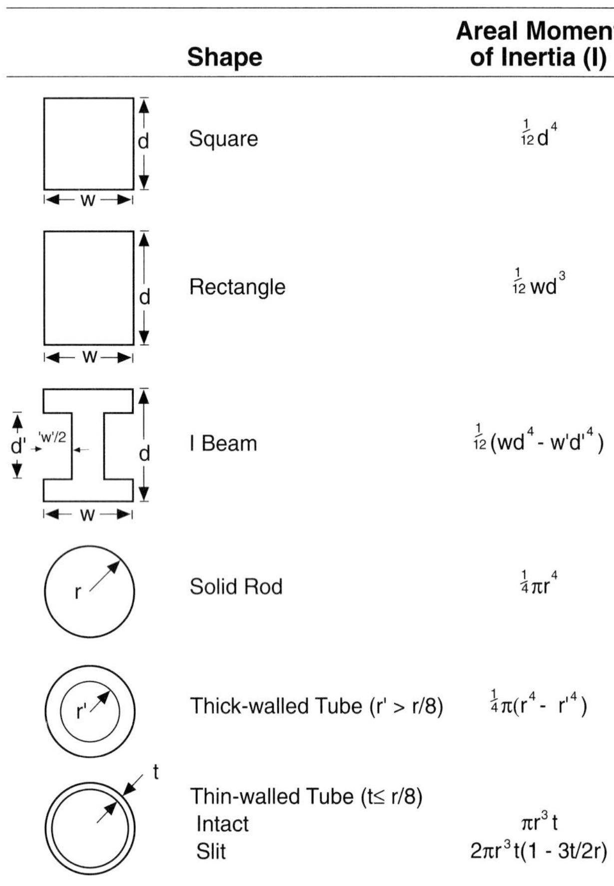

Areal Moments of Inertia

Shape	Areal Moment of Inertia (I)
Square	$\frac{1}{12}d^4$
Rectangle	$\frac{1}{12}wd^3$
I Beam	$\frac{1}{12}(wd^4 - w'd'^4)$
Solid Rod	$\frac{1}{4}\pi r^4$
Thick-walled Tube (r' > r/8)	$\frac{1}{4}\pi(r^4 - r'^4)$
Thin-walled Tube (t≤ r/8)	
Intact	$\pi r^3 t$
Slit	$2\pi r^3 t(1 - 3t/2r)$

Figure 18
Areal moments of inertia for simple shapes. (Adapted with permission from Black J: *Orthopaedic Biomaterials in Research and Practice.* New York, Churchill Livingstone, 1988.)

bending stiffness of a structure is obtained as the slope of a load-deformation curve with bending moment plotted as a function of angular deflection.

Torsion

When a specimen is twisted, similar geometric factors have to be considered. Torsion applies a shear load whose magnitude increases with the distance from the center of rotation (Fig. 19). Mass further from the center of rotation imposes a greater restriction to twisting than does an equal amount of mass more centrally located. This is reflected in the polar moment of inertia (Fig. 20). The physiologic effect of mass location is seen in the diaphyseal expansion of bone with age. Thinner or weaker cortices with a larger internal diameter can have torsional strength equal to that of thicker or stronger bone of smaller diameter. Greater strength is achieved with less mass. However, there are limits to this structural efficiency; thinner structures are more susceptible to localized deformations in regions of increased stress or of focal material weakness. Buckling and kinking are two such localized deformation processes.

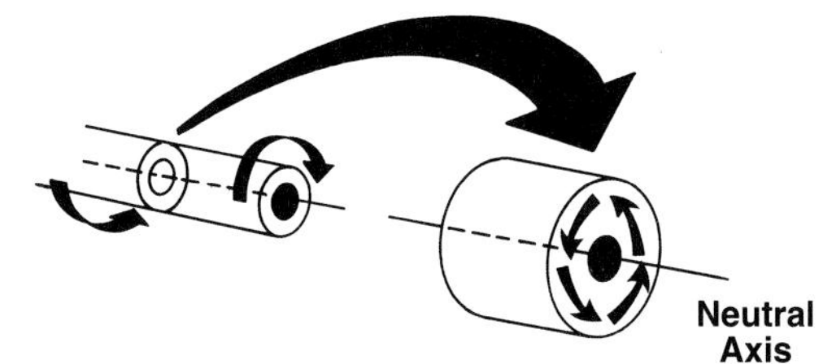

Figure 19
Cross section of cylinder loaded in torsion showing the distribution of shear stresses around the neutral axis. (Adapted with permission from Nordin M, Frankel VH: *Basic Biomechanics of the Musculoskeletal System,* ed 2. Philadelphia, Lea & Febiger, 1989.)

Polar Moments of Inertia

Shape	Polar Moment of Inertia (K)
Square	$0.141a^4$
Triangle	$(\sqrt{3}/80)a^4$
Solid Rod	$\frac{1}{2}\pi r^4$
Thick-walled Tube	$\frac{1}{2}\pi(r^4 - r'^4)$
Thin-walled Tube	$\frac{1}{2}\pi r^3 t$
Thin-walled Tube, open	$\frac{2}{3}\pi r t^3$

Figure 20
Polar moments of inertia. (Adapted with permission from Black J: *Orthopaedic Biomaterials in Research and Practice.* New York, Churchill Livingstone, 1988.)

Axial Load Sharing

Two materials placed adjacent to one another in a structural application, such as a fracture fixation plate attached to a bone, will each carry part of the applied load. The stress distribution will depend on the material properties and cross-sectional areas of the two materials and on the nature of the bonding between them. In an idealized construct with two materials of equal area under a uniformly distributed load, each will undergo the same strain (Fig. 21). The stress developed in each will depend on the modulus, and the stiffer material will support most of the load. The less stiff material will be "stress shielded." When a bone is fixed with a metallic plate having six (titanium) to 12 (cobalt-chromium, stainless steel) times its modulus, it supports only a small fraction of the applied load. The exact amount of stress shielding depends on the relative areas of the plate and the fracture surface. Because the cross section of a bone plate is usually less than that of the bone to which it is applied, the load borne by the bone after plating is still significant.

Material Properties and Mechanical Design

The structural efficiency of material placement is only one design factor involved in constructing an efficient implant device. Geometric and material considerations must be dealt with in a coordinated manner to arrive at an optimal design.

An important concept in design is that of stress concentration, the magnification of the applied stress in a local region by some discontinuity in shape or structure. A surface defect or internal structural imperfection (grain boundary, impurity, void) magnifies the overall stress at a local level. This multiplier, the stress intensity factor, depends on the shape and size of the imperfection. Gross geometric factors also increase local stresses: sharp edges, holes, changes in area, and other design features each exact a price in terms of ultimate strength. The material selected for a given application must withstand these local stresses as well as the overall nominal stress pattern. Stress concentration diminishes with distance from the imperfection. For this reason, multiple holes in a material, particularly in a brittle material like bone, should be separated by a distance greater than three times the size of the hole.

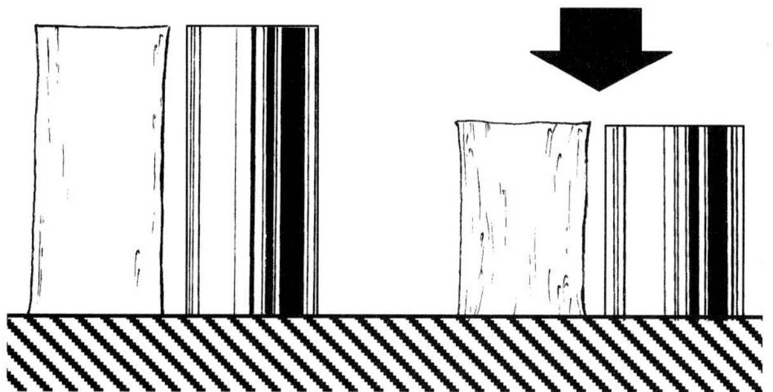

Figure 21
The strain in both materials is the same: $\epsilon_1 = \epsilon_2 = \epsilon$. The stress in each will vary directly with the modulus: $\sigma_1 = E_1\epsilon$, $\sigma_2 = E_2\epsilon$. The stiffer material will bear a larger share of the load; the less stiff material will be "stress shielded": $\sigma_1 \neq \sigma_2$.

Materials Testing

The controlled laboratory testing of materials relies on precise instrumentation to determine the true characteristics of a material. Each specimen must be precisely made to minimize structural and geometric irregularities that would taint the results. All parameters of specimen fabrication, preparation, and testing must be reported to permit independent interpretation and validation of results.

Stress-strain curves are generated from load and deformation data obtained under controlled conditions. A typical material testing system consists of a rigid frame in which a specimen can be placed between a mobile actuator and a load cell. A wide variety of instruments are used for materials testing, depending on the property being investigated. These machines can apply tensile or compressive forces, and newer versions also can be used for torsional testing. The specimen shape, specimen size (particularly as it relates to intrinsic defects), and gripping devices are key elements of the construct.

Most single cycle materials testing (quasistatic testing) is done at low strain rates to minimize dynamic factors such as inertia and impact. For biologic tissues or implanted materials, the rate of physiologic loading is a natural test parameter. Certain properties, such as impact resistance, can be determined only at high strain rates.

Cyclic loading is used for fatigue testing. A given stress or strain pattern is repeatedly applied to a test specimen at a given frequency, and the number of cycles to failure is monitored by the machine. The data obtained are used to determine the fatigue life and endurance limits of individual materials or actual devices. Fatigue testing of biologic or other viscoelastic materials is particularly sensitive to experimental variables. The strain rate sensitivity of the material properties and the heat generation resulting from anelasticity often restrict the rate at which an experiment can be run. This makes obtaining high cycle fatigue data on biologic tissues or viscoelastic implant materials very time-consuming and costly. One million cycles take 11.6 days at one cycle per second.

Molecular Structure—Chemical Bonding

The physical properties of materials, including biomaterials, depend on the nature of the chemical bonds between the atoms. A simplified scheme of the interatomic bonding in various materials is shown in Figure 22. Each of these bonding types and the material properties they produce will be explained in more detail in this section. Knowledge of the bonding patterns in a class of materials serves as a strong foundation for understanding their mechanical and physical properties.

Metals—Metallic Bonding

In metals, closely packed arrays of positively charged atomic nuclei are held together in a loosely associated "cloud" of free electrons. The essential features of the metallic bond are that it is nondirectional and the electrons are freely mobile. Nondirectional bonding results in dense atomic packing; the atoms are free to associate in any direction relative to their nearest neighbors and can fill in gaps and crevices. Metallically-bonded materials thus are able to undergo significant permanent deformation without fracture; the nondirectional bonding imparts the characteristic ductility to metals.

Metallic bonding involves outer-shell electrons that are mobile throughout the crystal. Metals can be viewed as an orderly array of ionic nuclei in a cloud of free electrons. The free electron cloud in metals allows them to be excellent conductors of both current and heat because electrical and thermal conductivity are functions of electron flow.

The nuclei in metals, held together by their shared electron cloud, pack as densely as possible, usually in one of three common patterns. Each pattern can be described as the continuous three-dimensional (3-D) repetition of a unit cell. The unit cell displays the relative atomic positions of the ionic nuclei and represents the crystal symmetry (Fig. 23). At body temperature, metallic calcium forms a face-centered cubic crystal, and cobalt and titanium assume a hexagonal close packed configuration.

The lack of a directional bonding requirement in metals allows the introduction of other elements into a metal's crystal matrix. If the atomic sizes of the two metals are close enough (atomic radii within approximately 15%) and the electronic structures are similar, two metals can form a single-phase solid solution. (A phase is a region of homogeneous structure.) Commercially pure titanium (cp-Ti) is a single-phase solid so-

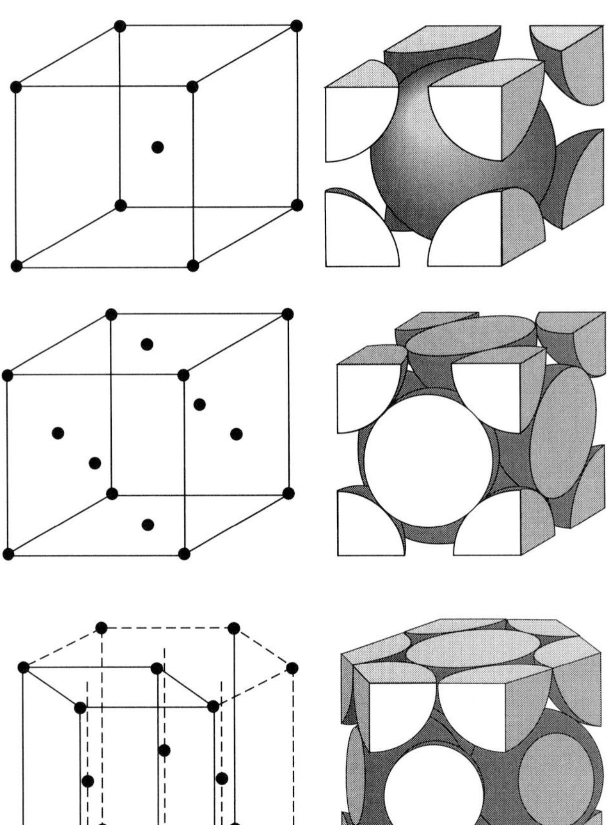

Figure 23
Unit cell structure for body-centered cubic **(top),** face-centered cubic (center), and hexagonal close packed **(bottom)** crystal structures. (Adapted with permission from Ralls KM, Courtney TH, Wulff J: *Introduction to Materials Science and Engineering.* New York, John Wiley & Sons, 1976.)

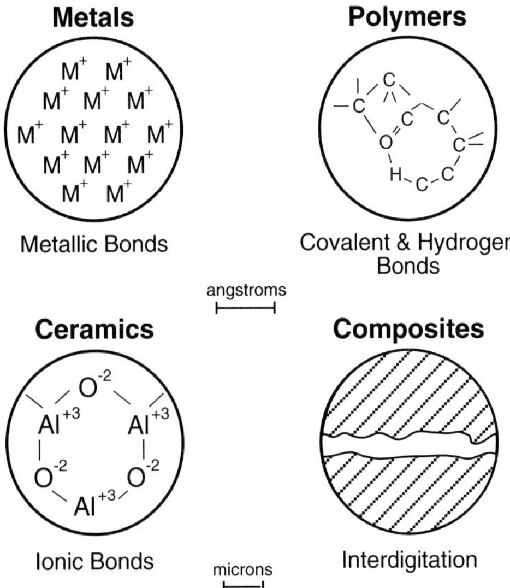

Figure 22
Schematic representation of interatomic bonding patterns.

lution of oxygen in titanium. If these requirements are not met, two-phase solid solutions are formed. Titanium-6 aluminum-4 vanadium is a two-phase solid solution; α and β phases are both present. These mixtures of multiple elements into a single metal are called alloys.

When metals are solidified from their molten state, crystals nucleate at several sites and grow until they reach other growing crystals. This results in a solid composed of irregularly shaped crystals or grains. Impurities and/or alloying elements are often concentrated at the boundaries between the growing grains. This gives the grain boundaries mechanical, chemical, and electrical properties that differ from those of the grains. As a result, grain size and grain shape are important in determining the material properties of a metal, and mechanical or thermal processes that alter grain size and shape can significantly affect the metal's subsequent behavior. This will be described in greater detail later in this chapter.

Polymers and Biologic Molecules—Covalent Bonding

Polymers consist of long chains of molecules, often carbon based, held together by covalent chemical bonds that, like ionic bonds, are strong and localized, but are also highly directional. The bonds have a fixed length and a preferred angle. Covalent bonds are formed when valence electrons are shared between two adjacent nuclei; they are held in fixed orbits. This type of bonding imparts strict limitation on certain structural elements of polymers. The localization of electrons severely restricts the electrical and thermal conductivity of covalently bonded structures. Most polymeric materials are good insulators; only specially designed polymers are conductive.

Bonding between polymer chains results from secondary forces—hydrogen bonds or van der Waals forces—that are much weaker than covalent bonds. This weak bonding allows the individual polymer chains to slide past one another when a polymeric material is stressed, and it gives rise to irrecoverable plastic deformation. Physical entanglements of the long polymer chains, the degree of crystallinity, and chemical cross-linking between chains play important roles in determining polymer properties.

The backbone of a polymer chain can be a linear arrangement of carbon atoms or a more complicated structure with branching (Fig. 24). The side groups on the backbone can have a wide variety of chemical functions that strongly influences polymer structure and properties. Additionally, these pendant groups can be arranged in regular or random patterns along the chain (Fig. 25). Both of these factors play a major role in determining chain flexibility, chain folding, crystallinity, and interchain forces. These subsequently are the determinants of chain mobility, which directly affects a polymer's physical characteristics and behavior. The flexibility of macromolecular chains permits a wide array of random conformations, analogous to those of a strand of wet spaghetti. A more ordered arrangement is sometimes more stable because of secondary forces, such as hydrogen bonds, between chains. Polymer chains may

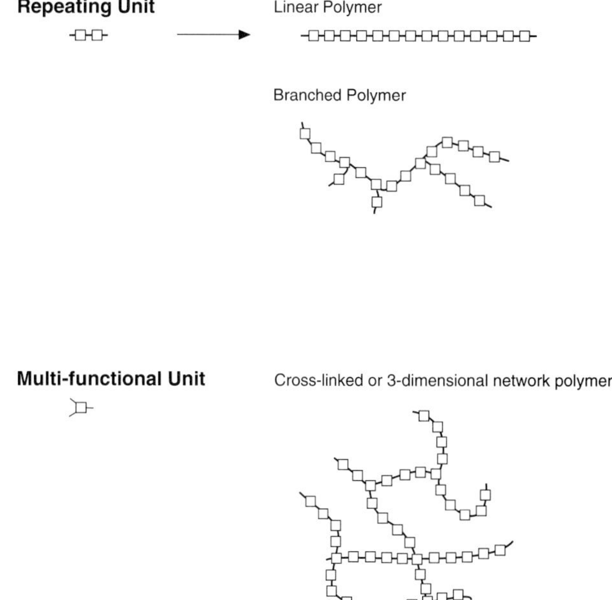

Figure 24
Linear, branched, and cross-linked polymer backbones.

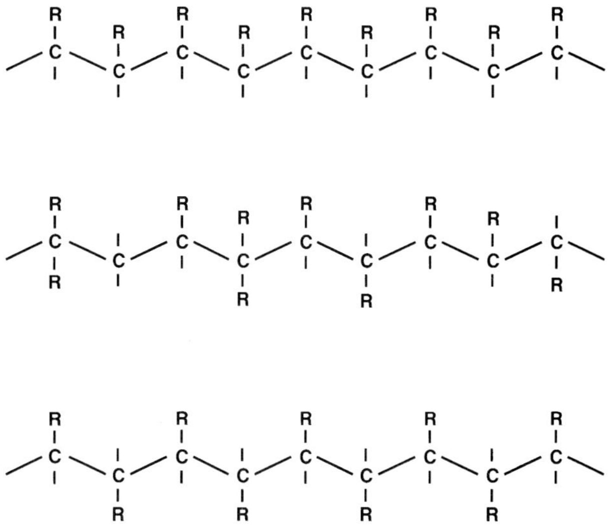

Figure 25
Stereoregularity of side groups along a polymer backbone. **Top,** Isotactic, all side groups on one side; **center,** atactic or random placement; **bottom,** syndiotactic or regularly alternating placement of side groups.

then form small crystalline domains, resulting not in the long-range order of a true crystal but rather in a semi-crystalline polymer with crystalline regions of aligned chains interspersed in a matrix of randomly oriented amorphous chains (Fig. 26). It also is possible to covalently link polymer backbone chains, thereby restricting mobility and increasing structural properties. This is known as cross-linking.

Monomer units can be mixed to form a chain with varying properties along the backbone, and polymer chains of different types can be blended together. Both processes produce copolymers. Figure 27 shows a few of the types of copolymers that can be produced; the possibilities are endless. Knowledge of the relationship between molecular structure and physical properties allows the design of polymers for specific applications. The primary determinant of polymer properties is the molecular weight of the chains. In biologic polymers, each molecule has identical length and structure. However, man-made polymerization processes give a distribution of molecular weights (Fig. 28). These distributions are characterized by the number-average ($\overline{MW}_n$) and weight-average ($\overline{MW}_w$) molecular weights. Knowing both gives a fair estimate of the shape of the distribution curve. Because high and low molecular weight polymers behave very differently, this information is important to any polymer application. An example of how the properties of materials with the same chemical composition can be affected by changes in molecular weight and crystallinity is shown for polyethylene (Fig. 29). Surgical-grade ultrahigh molecular weight polyethylene has a molecular weight in excess of one million daltons.

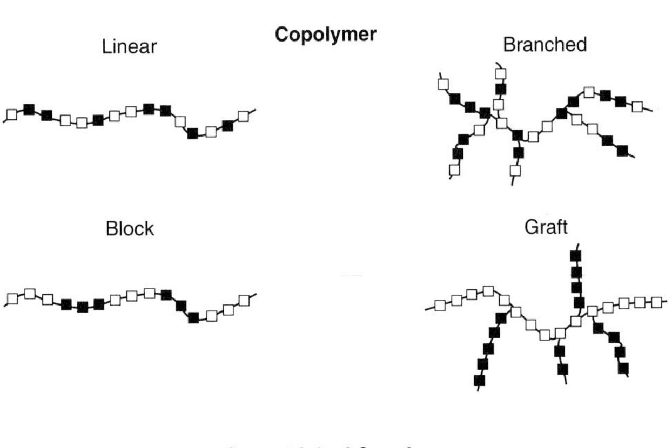

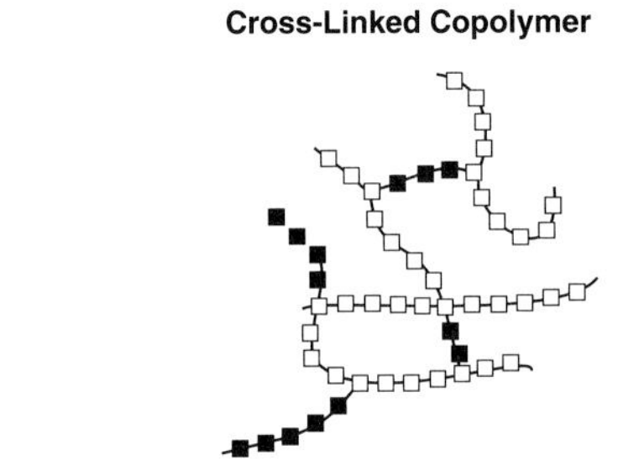

Figure 27
Copolymer arrangements.

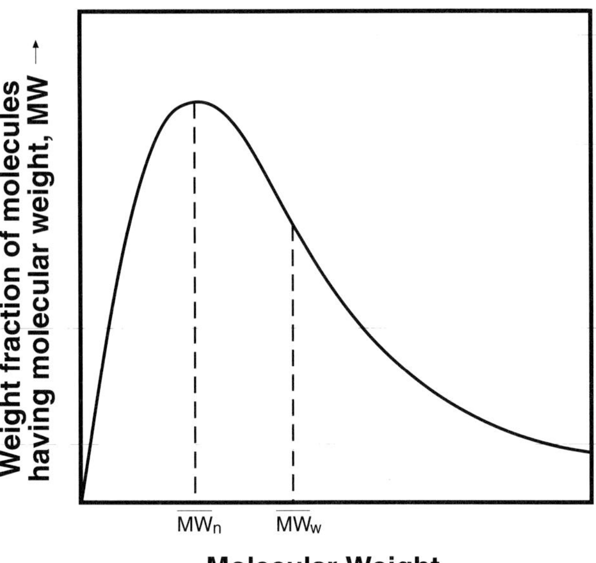

Figure 28
Typical molecular weight distribution of a polymer. (Adapted with permission from Ralls KM, Courtney TH, Wulff J: *Introduction to Materials Science and Engineering.* New York, John Wiley & Sons, 1976.)

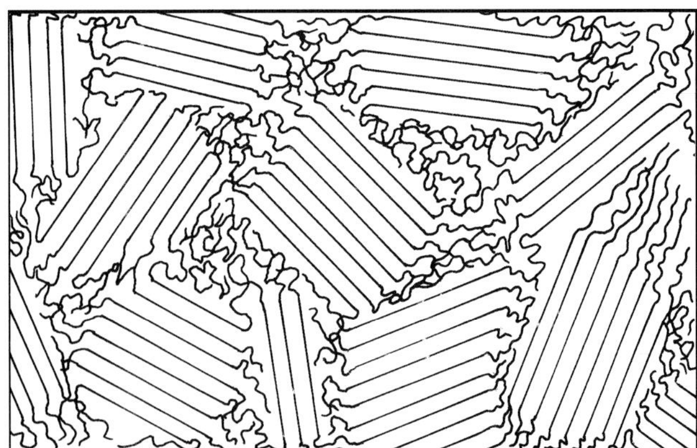

Figure 26
Model of semi-crystalline polymer including crystalline regions of aligned chains in a matrix of randomly oriented, amorphous chains. (Adapted with permission from Ralls KM, Courtney TH, Wulff J: *Introduction to Materials Science and Engineering.* New York, John Wiley & Sons, 1976.)

Ceramics—Ionic Bonding

Ceramics are typically 3-D arrays of positively charged metal ions and negatively charged nonmetal ions, often oxygen. The ionic bond between adjacent

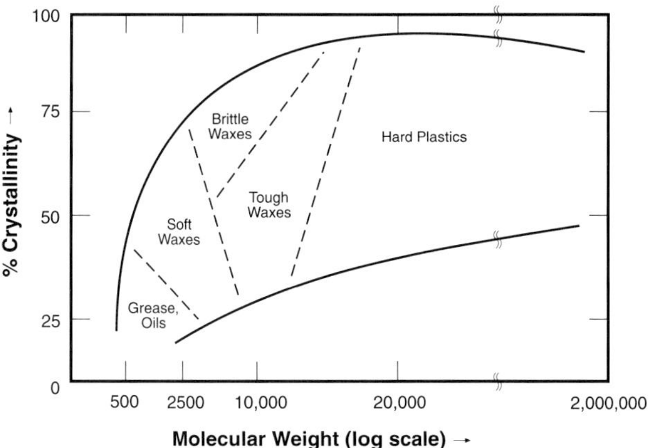

Figure 29
Variations in molecular weight and crystallinity have a profound effect on the material properties of polymers, as shown here for polyethylene.(Adapted with permission from Ralls KM, Courtney TH, Wulff J: *Introduction to Materials Science and Engineering.* New York, John Wiley & Sons, 1976.)

nuclei localizes all the available electrons in the formation of the bond. This localization of electrons makes most ceramics insulators, both electrical and thermal. Network organization ranges from highly organized, crystalline, 3-D arrays to amorphous, random arrangements in glassy materials.

Other Materials—Bonding Considerations

Composites are formed by the mechanical association of different materials, most frequently by fibers of one material in a matrix of another. The bonding force between the materials can be chemical, physical, or mechanical. Many naturally occurring biologic materials are composites, including bone, which is a composite of polymeric collagen molecules in an inorganic matrix of mineralized apatite. A great variety of properties can be achieved in bulk composites by varying the orientation of the reinforcing fibers within the matrix. The alternating orientation of collagen fibers in the layers of haversian bone is a natural example of this reinforcing strategy.

The properties of composite materials are directly related to the arrangement of the material constituents. Such arrangements can include particulate fillers in a polymer matrix (carbon black in automobile tires), fiber strands in a solid matrix (steel-reinforced concrete, fiberglass), or laminates of different materials or one material with different orientation (plywood).

Composite materials, by definition, include interfaces between the matrix and the reinforcing material or between the laminate layers. These interfaces profoundly influence the material properties of the composite. The stability of these interfaces also affects the useful lifetime of the composite in a particular application.

Processing—Its Effect on Structure

The mechanical properties of any material are closely linked to its ultrastructure. Any chemical, thermal, or physical process that alters the structure of a material will affect its physical and mechanical properties. For example, anything that changes the phase structure, grain size, or grain orientation of a metal will change its material properties. Altering the cross-linking or crystallinity of a polymer changes its behavior. Mechanical processing of ceramics is limited because of their brittle nature, but the sintering variables (time, temperature, temperature gradients, pressure) used in the manufacturing process can profoundly affect the ceramic's material properties.

The vast variety of properties that can be achieved with different metals and with different processing operations allows metals to be used for a tremendous variety of applications. Mechanically deforming a metal beyond its yield stress will produce, in addition to a macroscopic shape change, an elongation of the grains in the direction of the the stress and a thinning in other directions; grain volume remains unchanged. The increased grain boundary area results in a material of higher energy. This process, called cold working, includes hammering, forging, rolling, and drawing. Any mechanical deformation occurring below the temperature at which the grain crystals can reform results in work hardening. Cold working changes the shape of the material and results in increased yield and ultimate stresses and a higher endurance limit. The resultant material is less ductile than the initial material.

A cold-worked structure can be returned to a strain-free condition by heating it sufficiently for the grains to reform in a lower energy configuration. This process, called recrystallization, can occur below the melting point of the metal. Metals are often heat-treated or annealed in this manner to soften or relax work-hardened shapes. The time and temperature used in heat treatment determine the effectiveness of the process and the resultant material properties. Cold working and annealing can be cycled to achieve the desired combination of shape and physical properties. Heating above the recrystallization temperature adds the additional factor of grain growth. Typically, microstructures with small, uniform grains produce the strongest metals.

Casting is the pouring of molten metal into a mold to produce, upon cooling, a specific shape. Voids and other flaws are a major problem with casting. Impurities tend to migrate to the grain boundaries, resulting in areas of mechanical weakness. Forging is a process by which a blank of metal is heated and pressed into a die by the application of a large, single force. This produces a part with fewer defects than a casting. Parts formed by both of these processes can be annealed to allow stress relaxation and grain reorganization and growth. Hot isostatic pressing (HIPing) involves the consolidation under high temperature and pressure of metal powder into a fine-grained material. This is done to achieve superior strength.

Many ceramic materials are produced by a sintering process in which a fine powder of the inorganic starting material is pressed and heated into a glassy solid matrix. Figure 30 shows the influence of sintering temperature on ceramic grain size and strength. High porosity is often a problem in sintered ceramics, which can be reduced by a controlled heat treatment that is essentially a process of grain growth. Some residual porosity usually remains, which, when combined with the increase in grain size, has a detrimental effect on the material properties of the ceramic.

Another class of ceramics, produced by vitrification, consists of two-phase composites of crystalline particles in an amorphous glass matrix. These two-phase materials are sensitive to thermal shock because of variation in the thermal expansion of the two components. Controlling the nucleation and growth of the crystalline phase in vitreous ceramics can result in extremely fine-grained, nonporous ceramic materials with excellent strength. The development of this technology has enabled the production of larger and stronger ceramic parts, expanding the range of applications for which ceramics can now be used.

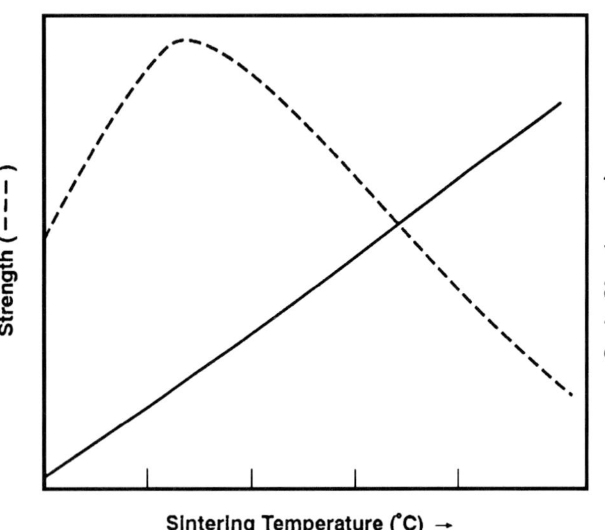

Figure 30
The effect of sintering temperature on grain size (solid line) and strength (dashed line) of a ceramic material. (Adapted with permission from Ralls KM, Courtney TH, Wulff J: *Introduction to Materials Science and Engineering.* New York, John Wiley & Sons, 1976.)

Polymers also can be amorphous, semicrystalline, or crystalline. This is largely determined by their molecular architecture as previously discussed. Crystalline regions serve as mechanical cross-links, and the strength of a given polymer increases monotonically with the degree of crystallinity. The amount of crystallinity and the size of the crystalline phase domains can be controlled by the processing temperature and the rate at which it is varied. As with metals, polymers with fine-grained crystalline domains have superior mechanical properties.

Polymer additives can be used to affect physical and material properties. These materials either dissolve into the polymer or become segregated into small domains. Such fillers can be used to serve a particular function (coloration, radiopacity, resistance to solvents, improved insulating properties) or can be used solely to add bulk and reduce the cost of the finished product.

Tribological Properties

Friction

When two materials in contact are in relative motion, the resistance to movement or frictional force (F_f in Fig. 31) that exists is proportional to the load across the interface. The ratio between the frictional force and the load R is called the coefficient of friction μ.

$$\mu = F_f/R$$

Because this ratio is always a finite value, the expenditure of some energy is required to initiate and/or maintain motion. Work must be done to overcome the frictional resistance to motion. When the relative motion begins, the initial value is called

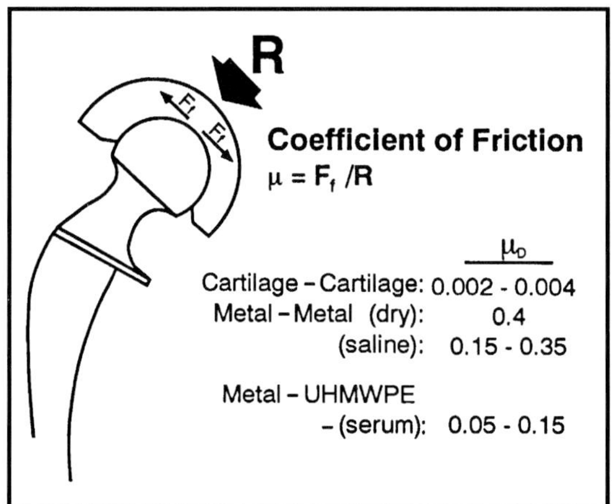

Figure 31
Coefficient of friction of natural and replacement joint surfaces.

Table 1
Frictional coefficients of natural and artificial joint materials

Material Combination	Coefficients	
	μ_S	μ_D
Rubber tire/concrete (dry)	1.0	0.7
Rubber tire/concrete (water)	0.7	0.5
Leather/wood	0.5	0.4
Steel/steel		0.5
Co-Cr/Co-Cr (saline)		0.35
UHMWPE/steel (serum)	0.35	0.07-0.12
UHMWPE/steel (synovial fluid)	0.07	0.04-0. 5
UHMWPE/Co-Cr (serum)		0.05-0.11
UHMWPE/Ti6Al4V (serum)		0.05-0.12
Al_2O_3/Al_2O_3 (saline)		0.09
UHMWPE/Al_2O_3 (saline)		0.05
Hip joint (natural)(saline)		0.005-0.01
Hip joint (natural)(synovial fluid)		0.002

(Adapted with permission from Black J: *Orthopaedic Biomaterials in Research and Practice.* New York, Churchill Livingstone, 1988.)

the static coefficient of friction μ_S. As motion continues, the value of the coefficient of friction decreases to the dynamic value μ_D. The purpose of lubrication is to reduce resistance to motion by reducing the values of the static and dynamic coefficients of friction for any pair of materials. The coefficient of friction of cartilage on cartilage is less than any yet achieved for synthetic bearing surfaces (Table 1).

Lubrication

Lubrication acts to reduce frictional resistance and to separate surfaces, thereby reducing local stress concentrations. The effectiveness of lubrication is a function of the contacting materials, their surface roughness, the separation between the materials, their relative velocity, and the lubricant. The more viscous the lubricant and the greater the separation of surfaces at a given relative velocity, the lower the value of the dynamic coefficient of friction μ_D. Several lubrication mechanisms are illustrated in Figure 32.

Hydrodynamic Lubrication

In hydrodynamic lubrication the surfaces are fully separated by the lubricant. This is the design objective in many rapidly rotating or sliding machine parts; the relative motion of the surfaces keeps the fluid film thick enough to prevent surface-to-surface contact. The viscosity of the lubricant is of primary importance. (Some industrial equipment relies on externally pressurized lubrication to force the surface apart; this is known as hydrostatic lubrication.)

Boundary Lubrication

Boundary lubrication relies on a very thin, slippery, surface-adherent layer to minimize the contact between asperities of smooth rubbing surfaces. Friction and wear rates are significantly higher than in lubrication schemes where the surfaces can be separated.

Elastohydrodynamic Lubrication

In elastohydrodynamic lubrication, the elasticity of the bearing surfaces allows adaptation of surface irregularities without producing plastic deformation. This deformation of the local surface geometry maintains a thicker lubricant film and, thus, a lower coefficient of friction. Relatively low wear rates result but subsurface fatigue becomes an important concern.

Weeping Lubrication

If at least one of the contacting surfaces is porous, the elastohydrodynamic regime can be augmented by fluid expressed from the deforming surface, forming a pressurized lubricating mechanism called weeping lubrication. This is believed to be an

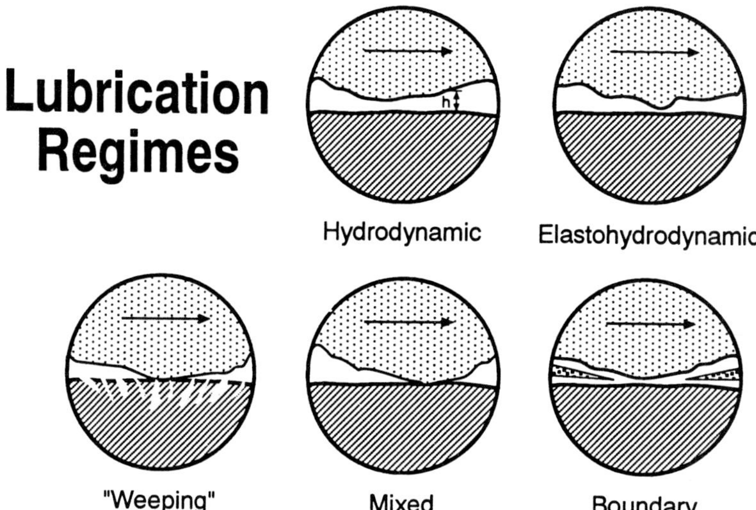

Figure 32
Types of lubrication.

important lubrication mechanism in normal articular cartilage.

Articular cartilage normally displays a combination of elastohydrodynamic, weeping, and boundary lubrication. Total joint arthroplasties rely on elastohydrodynamic and boundary lubrication.

Wear

Even in situations of low friction coefficients, surface interaction can produce local mechanical damage and loss of material. This process is called wear. The essential feature of the wearing process is the loss of material from one of the bearing surfaces (as opposed to creep, which involves a dimensional change in a material by plastic deformation without the loss of material). Wear results when two surfaces, in relative motion, temporarily join together. When they separate, the local mechanical and tribological factors dictate where the new interface is formed. Five important wear mechanisms are illustrated in Figure 33.

Adhesive Wear

When two smooth bodies slide over one another, small fragments of each surface adhere to the other surface. This happens because of the strong local forces produced by two atoms in intimate contact. When subsequent movement occurs and this contact is broken, there is a finite probability that the break will not occur at the original interface, but instead will occur through one of the two materials. A fragment of one material will have been transferred onto the other material.

Abrasive Wear

When a rough, hard material or a soft surface contaminated with hard particles slides on a relatively soft surface, it can plow through the softer material and produce needles or curls of loose debris, analogous to those produced by a cutting tool on a lathe.

Transfer Wear

In some cases, a film of the softer material may be transferred to the harder surface, changing the nature of the interface. These transfer films are usually unstable.

Fatigue Wear

Local strain gradients in the softer material may cause sufficient subsurface stress concentrations to produce fatigue failure after repetitive or cyclic loading. Such a surface demonstrates a characteristic array of surface cracks resembling a dried mudflat. This mechanism has been postulated as a cause for polyethylene delamination in total knee arthroplasties.

Third Body Wear

Trapping of wear debris within the moving interfaces or the introduction of foreign particles, such as bone, polyethylene, or polymethylmethacrylate fragments, produces local stress concentrations and results in abrasion of one or both moving surfaces. This is often classified as a specific form of abrasive wear rather than a separate wear mechanism.

Corrosive Wear

This is a combined process in which the corrosion debris at a moving interface is scraped away from the point of contact, allowing corrosion to occur more rapidly than it would in the absence of motion. Because the loss of substance is primarily a result of chemical attack rather than mechanical factors, corrosive wear is frequently considered a subset of corrosion rather than a wear mechanism. This combi-

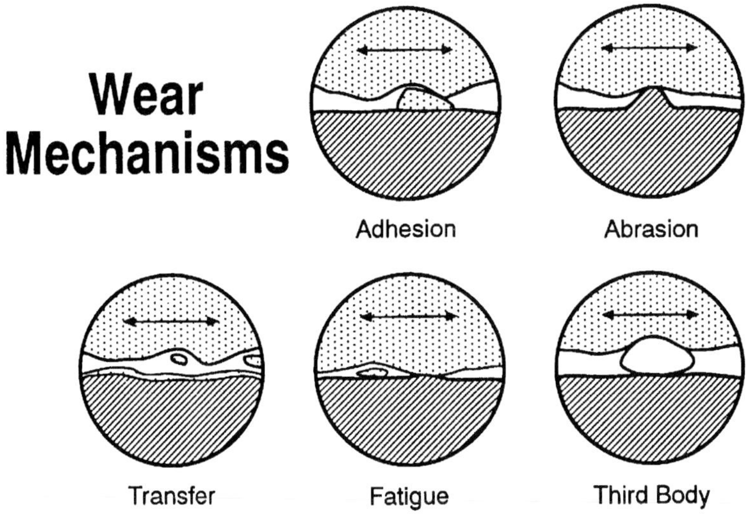

Figure 33
Wear mechanisms.

nation of corrosion accelerated by motion is also called fretting. This type of wear occurs between plates and screw heads and in the Morse taper connections of modular total joint components.

After an initial high wear rate or wearing-in period, the volume of wear debris is proportional to the force across the interface and the total distance traveled.

Volume of Debris = K × load × distance

The proportionality factor (K = Archard's constant) depends on the material, the lubricant, and the wear mechanism (Fig. 34). In general, dissimilar material pairs show the lowest rates of debris production. Ceramic-polymer combinations produce the least amount of wear of any arthroplasty system.

Wear of Total Joint Components

Measuring the wear properties of implanted materials is extremely difficult. Accurate measurement requires that the wear debris be retrieved and quantitatively analyzed. This is impossible in vivo because the synovial lining of the joint traps, and to some extent processes, this debris. The best experimental results come from joint simulators in which the debris can be retrieved and studied. Measuring the shape change of components gives the combined effects of both wear and cold flow. The latter process, called creep, involves a change of shape without the loss of material, an essential feature of wear.

Polyethylene

Attempts to measure polyethylene wear in vivo date back to the earliest series of total hip arthroplasties. Charnley, using radiographic measurements, reported a wear rate for acetabular cups of 0.15 mm per year. Far lower values were found in subsequent laboratory tests in which the true wear rates were measured. Current understanding explains the difference; a large proportion of the shape change in polyethylene is a result of creep rather than wear. Acetabular cup wear is primarily abrasive, and the most crucial factor affecting the true wear rate of polyethylene acetabular cups under weightbearing conditions is the molecular weight of the material. Cups of insufficient molecular weight show a dramatic deterioration of wear properties. In total knee geometries, where the surface contours differ significantly, local contact stresses and subsurface fatigue wear become the dominant mechanism of tibial tray degradation.

Titanium

The poor wear characteristics of titanium alloy heads on femoral components articulating against polyethylene acetabular cups have been well documented. The surface becomes burnished by a wear process believed to be predominantly adhesive. The presence of debris in the joint results in third body wear and accelerates the process. Ion implantation processes are being investigated as a means to increase the stability of the surface oxide and thus decrease the wear rate.

Wear particles from total joint arthroplasties have the potential for detrimental consequences of several types. The fragmentation of the implant vastly increases the surface area of material in contact with biologic tissues, thereby increasing the rate and volume of material exchange. This may have both local and systemic effects. Small wear particles can be phagocytized and interfere with intracellular processes. Debris also can be transported to remote sites, such as lymph nodes, spleen, and lungs, and could affect the function of these organs.

Metals

Composition and Properties

Metallic materials have certain properties that make them ideal for load-bearing applications and, therefore, frequently are used as structural elements for skeletal repair or reconstruction. These materials

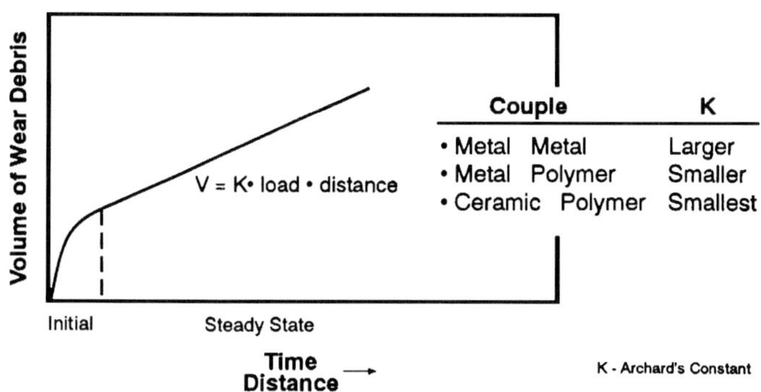

Figure 34
Proportionality of wear rate with time or distance traveled.

can achieve very high strength and are ductile (able to withstand irreversible, or plastic, deformation under load), which confers a resistance to fracture. The biocompatibility of metals is directly related to their corrosion resistance. Several families of metallic alloys are well tolerated by biologic systems.

Only rarely are metals used in their pure elemental form; their manufacturing and service properties are usually enhanced by the addition of other elements to form alloys. Three metallic alloys are used extensively in orthopaedic applications: stainless steel, cobalt-chromium alloys, and titanium and its alloys. The elemental composition of these implant metals are depicted in the pie charts in Figure 35. Standardization of alloys is regulated by the American Society for Testing and Materials (ASTM), which sets specifications of composition, manufacture, and properties. Manufacturers each have their own trade names for these standard alloys.

Stainless Steel (ASTM F-55-56)

There are at least 50 alloys and grades of alloys identified as commercial stainless steel. Only a few are used as implant biomaterials in orthopaedic surgery. Nonalloyed iron and carbon steels cannot be used because they corrode in oxygenated saline solutions. Surgical stainless steels, despite their very good general corrosion resistance, are subject to several other types of electrochemical processes, including crevice, intergranular, and stress corrosion. This not only degrades the mechanical properties of the alloy but also can lead to the release of metal ions into the surrounding tissue with undesirable biologic consequences.

The stainless steels designated as ASTM F-55-56 (grades 316 and 316L) are used extensively when the properties of stainless steel are appropriate for a clinical application. Type 316L stainless steel is an iron-based alloy with 17% to 20% chromium, 10% to 14% nickel, 2% to 4% molybdenum, and less than 0.03% carbon. Minor elements include less than 2% manganese and less than 0.75% silicon. Alloying with chromium generates a protective, self-regenerating oxide film that resists perforation, has a high degree of electrical resistance, and, thus, provides a major protection against corrosion. Nickel imparts more corrosion resistance and facilitates manufacturing. The molybdenum addition provides excellent resistance to pitting corrosion. Limited quantities of manganese and silicon are added to control manufacturing problems.

The presence of carbon in this alloy is undesirable. Under certain conditions, the carbon segregates from the major elements of the alloy, taking with it a substantial amount of chromium in the form of chromium carbide precipitates. Local depletion of chromium deprives some areas of corrosion resistance, and because the carbides form most frequently at the grain boundaries, the resultant corrosion occurs selectively at those grain boundaries. Type 316L stainless steel has a very low level of allowed carbon to minimize this problem.

The 316 stainless steels are capable of substantial yield strength, ranging from 260 to 896 MPa. The elastic modulus of stainless steel is in the range of 200 GPa and is, therefore, approximately 12 times higher than the elastic modulus of cortical bone.

All metallic materials are subject to fatigue fracture under conditions of fluctuating load, such as those experienced by implants used to fix or replace a weightbearing bone in the lower extremity. Fatigue fracture begins with small flaws within the material. Cracks can begin at defects in the structure of the material (grain boundaries, voids, inclusions) or at

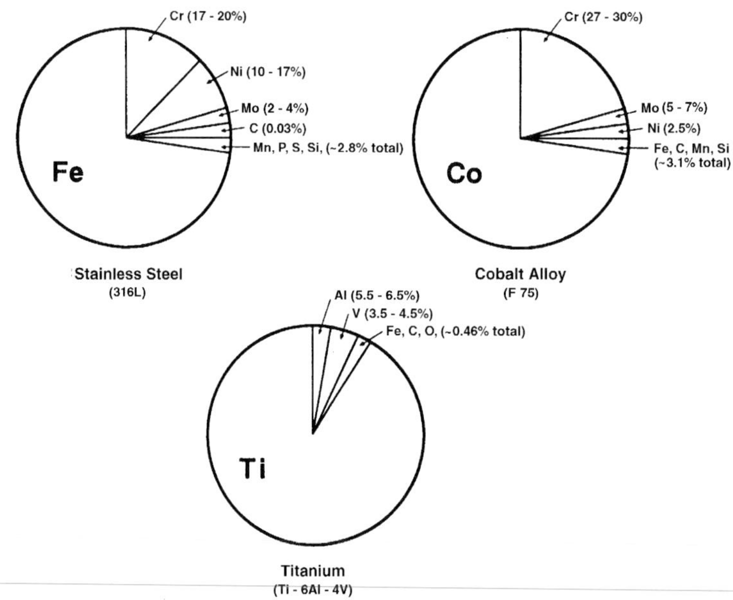

Figure 35
Composition of common orthopaedic alloys.

mechanical defects on the surface (scratches, notches, bends). To increase resistance to fatigue failure, 316L stainless steel is available in a special grade with smaller and more widely spaced inclusions. This grade, designated as AISI 316LVM and specified by ASTM F-138, is produced using a special vacuum-melting procedure that results in a cleaner metal.

All stainless steels are prone to crevice corrosion. When two parts of a stainless steel device, such as plate and screw, are fitted closely together, the fluid in the gap between them has a lower concentration of dissolved oxygen than the surrounding fluid. This phenomenon establishes an oxygen concentration cell with sufficient voltage to overcome the passive film intrinsic to the steel, thereby allowing local corrosion to proceed more rapidly. This type of corrosion is commonly seen at the junction of plates and screws removed after use as fracture fixation devices. Crevice corrosion is not expected in a monolithic device, such as a femoral stem, unless the device is placed in contact with another implant, such as the wires used to secure a detached greater trochanter.

Most metallic devices are exposed to a passivation process after forming and machining operations but before use as a finished product. This process involves immersion of the device in a strong nitric acid solution for 10 to 30 minutes. The solution dissolves imbedded iron particles from the machining operations and also generates a thin, transparent but dense oxide film on the surface of the alloy. This process is important in enhancing the corrosion resistance of the finished implant device.

As a strong, stiff, biocompatible material, 316L stainless steel is well suited for use as an orthopaedic implant material. Its slow but finite corrosion rate and concerns about the long-term effects of nickel ions suggest that this material be used primarily for devices that will be removed once their mission is completed. Therefore, the major orthopaedic application for stainless steel devices is in fracture fixation.

Cobalt-Chromium Alloys

Cobalt-chromium-molybdenum alloy (ASTM F-75) consists of 27% to 30% chromium, 5% to 7% molybdenum, and less than 0.35% carbon in a cobalt base. For many years this material was used primarily as a casting alloy, but the inevitable casting defects doomed femoral stems cast from the material. Although the mechanical properties of the cast alloy (yield strength 517 MPa) are adequate for most orthopaedic applications, they are not sufficient for high stress, high cycle loading in a femoral stem. As the casting alloy solidifies, carbides segregate into continuous bands and shrinkage leads to voids at the grain boundaries. Both of these factors lead to intrinsic weakness in cast cobalt-chromium (Co-Cr) implants.

Forging and hot isostatic pressing can improve the yield strength and fatigue life of this alloy by producing a material with fewer defects. In forging, implants are formed from a bar of the alloy produced with specific composition and properties. Hot isostatic pressing involves atomization of the liquid alloy into a fine powder followed by high-pressure consolidation into a virtually void-free component. The modulus of elasticity of Co-Cr produced in this manner is about 200 GPa (cast Co-Cr has the same modulus), but the yield strength increases 80% to almost 900 MPa. This increased strength is a direct result of the smaller grain size produced by hot isostatic pressing, 0.01 mm compared with 5 to 15 mm for cast Co-Cr. Both forging and hot isostatic pressing produce rough products that must be finished by various machining operations.

As with stainless steels, the chromium content of this alloy generates a highly resistant passive film that contributes substantially to corrosion resistance. The F-75 alloy has better corrosion resistance than F-138 stainless steel, and particularly superior resistance to crevice corrosion. The biocompatibility of this alloy has been documented by extensive long-term experience with both animal models and humans. The high strength coupled with excellent corrosion resistance and biocompatibility make cobalt-chromium an excellent material for high-stress applications such as the femoral stems of total hip prostheses.

Cobalt-chromium-tungsten-nickel alloy (ASTM F-90) is very different from the F-75 alloy. The F-90 alloy is cobalt based with 19% to 21% chromium, 14% to 16% tungsten, 9% to 11% nickel, and 0.05% to 0.15% carbon. This alloy is not suitable for use as a casting material, but it can be hot forged or cold drawn. Yield strength can be controlled by processing and can range from 690 MPa, when fully annealed, to greater than 6,000 MPa for severely cold drawn wire. In clinical practice it is used to make wire and internal fixation devices, including plates, intramedullary rods, and screws.

Commercially-pure Titanium (ASTM F-67)

Titanium and its alloys are of particular interest for biomedical applications because of their outstanding biocompatibility. In general, their corrosion resistance significantly exceeds that of the stainless steels and the Co-Cr alloys. In saline solutions of near neutral pH, the corrosion rate is extremely small, and there is no evidence of pitting, intergranular, or crevice corrosion. Data from in vivo animal models and from human clinical retrievals confirm truly superior biocompatibility.

Nonalloyed or commercially-pure titanium actually is alloyed by the level of oxygen dissolved into the metal. In large amounts, oxygen embrittles titanium and its alloys; however, in small, regulated amounts it helps control the yield strength of the materials. ASTM F-67 is a specification for oxygen concentration calling for 345 MPa yield strength for grade III and at least 485 MPa for grade IV. Other contaminating elements in commercially-pure titanium (cp-Ti) are limited to a maximum of 0.07% nitrogen, 0.15% carbon, 0.015% hydrogen, and 0.35% iron. Any excess of these elements degrades the material properties of the metal.

Commercially-pure titanium is not used extensively in orthopaedic surgery today but it does have an important application. Because it is easier to sinter than titanium-aluminum-vanadium (Ti-Al-V) alloy, it is the material of choice for the porous layer in titanium-based cementless total joint prostheses and is used to form the fiber-metal pads on arthroplasty components.

Titanium-Aluminum-Vanadium Alloy (ASTM F-136)

ASTM F-136 specifies a titanium-based alloy with 5.5% to 6.5% aluminum and 3.5% to 4.5% vanadium, which commonly is referred to as Ti6Al4V. The standard restricts impurities to a maximum of 0.25% iron, 0.05% nitrogen, 0.08% carbon, 0.0125% hydrogen, and 0.1% other, with a maximum total impurity of 0.4%. Developed by the aircraft industry for its high strength-to-weight ratio, this alloy is used for biomedical applications in a slightly weaker annealed condition because of the enhanced ductility. ASTM F-136 limits the oxygen concentration to an especially low level of 0.13%, known as the ELI (extra low interstitial) grade. Limiting the level of dissolved oxygen improves the mechanical properties of the material, particularly increasing its fatigue life. One disturbing quality of this alloy is its fatigue sensitivity to notching. Any external stress risers dramatically shorten its fatigue life. Therefore it is not a suitable material for porous coatings on cementless total joint components.

Titanium and its alloys have an elastic modulus approximately half that of the stainless steels and Co-Cr alloys. The lower stiffness of titanium-based fracture fixation plates has been reported by some to reduce the severity of stress shielding and cortical osteoporosis under these devices. It must be recalled that their modulus of 100 GPa is still roughly six times that of cortical bone (17 GPa). Controversy still exists regarding the potential advantages of titanium alloys over more rigid metals for femoral stems.

Another important feature of titanium alloys that must be considered in designing total joint prostheses is their wear characteristics. Significant wear of titanium femoral heads has been observed after articulation with ultrahigh molecular weight polyethylene (UHMWPE). This wear has been seen in wear simulators and in clinical retrievals. The problem is thought by some to relate to the mechanical stability of the passive surface film on the titanium alloys. When the alloy surface is hardened through ion implantation technologies, the wear rate of the titanium head reportedly has decreased.

Corrosion

Corrosion, the gradual degradation of materials by electrochemical attack, is a concern when a metallic material is placed in the electrolytic environment of the body. Corrosion weakens the implanted material, changes the surface of the material, and releases metal ions into the body fluids. The response of the implant to the biologic environment, both chemical and mechanical, and the biologic response to the implanted material surface and to the metal ions that are released must be investigated to fully predict the biocompatibility of a potential implant material.

Corrosion is arbitrarily defined as a reaction that produces a concentration of metal ions greater than 10^{-6} M. Materials with a stable surface that produce less than this concentration of ions are called immune. The production of a stable surface coating, often an oxide, which decreases a metal's corrosion rate, is called passivation. Some metals, such as titanium, owe their low corrosion rate to rapid, spontaneous self-passivation.

Whether corrosion, passivation, or immunity occurs in a single part of a homogeneous metallic implant depends on the pH and the oxygen tension at the implantation site. Generally, tissue conditions (pH 7.4) are such that chromium alloys with preformed oxide layers are stable. Some tissue locations and occasional transient conditions, such as the acid pH shift associated with infection, may damage the chromium oxide layer and produce corrosion. Titanium rapidly forms a stable surface oxide and is self-passivating in an oxygenated environment. A particular material may be well suited for one implant application, but inappropriate for another. Although all of them involve the same chemical reactions, there are several distinguishable types of corrosion.

Uniform Attack

Metal ions are released and either hydrogen or oxygen serves as an electron receptor (Fig. 36). A conductive, electrolytic solution (most physiologic fluids) is required for this means of corrosion. Metals that corrode uniformly under physiologic conditions are obviously not suitable for use as orthopaedic implants.

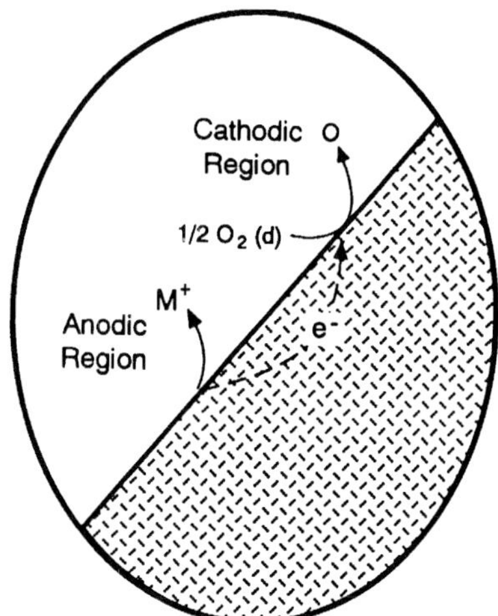

Figure 36
Uniform corrosion. (Adapted with permission from Black J: *Orthopaedic Biomaterials in Research and Practice.* New York, Churchill Livingstone, 1988.)

Galvanic Attack

When two different metals are placed in contact in an electrolytic environment, one material gives up electrons to the other (Fig. 37). This metal, the anode, is oxidized, releasing ions and electrons that flow to the cathode. The relative electron-holding capacity of different metals under standard conditions is called the electromotive force (EMF). The EMFs of various metals are tabulated in most metallurgy texts and reference books and give a quantitative assessment of corrosion resistance. The electrical potential established between two metals with different EMFs is the driving force for galvanic corrosion.

In general, metals in implant systems should not be mixed. One fortuitous exception is the galvanic compatibility of Co-Cr alloys and Ti6Al4V. This resistance to galvanic corrosion results from the rapid and spontaneous self-passivation of the titanium alloy; the interface actually consists of Co-Cr in contact with titanium dioxide (TiO_2), preventing the formation of a galvanic couple. Their galvanic compatibility allows the use of Co-Cr heads, with their superior wear properties, on titanium stems in total hip prostheses. Recent evidence suggests that this combination of materials may not completely avoid corrosion problems. Crevice and fretting corrosion has been reported at the junction between the Co-Cr femoral head and the Ti-alloy neck.

Crevice Corrosion

Intense localized corrosion frequently occurs within crevices on metal surfaces exposed to corrosive environments (Fig. 38). Corrosion in isolated areas with restricted fluid conduction is self-accelerated by the accumulation of positive metal ions and the resultant influx of negative chloride ions to maintain chemical neutrality. Metals and alloys that depend on oxide films or passive layers (for example, Co-Cr, Ti) for corrosion protection are particularly susceptible to crevice corrosion. High concentrations of chloride or hydrogen ions destroy these films and the local corrosion rate increases. Defects such as scratches and macroscopic crevices formed by the ap-

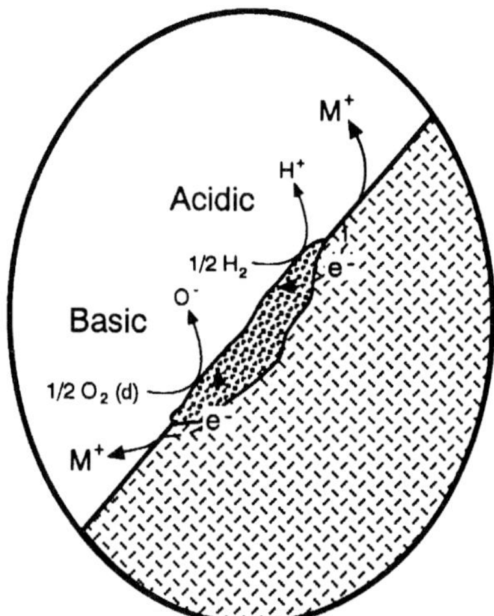

Figure 37
Galvanic corrosion. (Adapted with permission from Black J: *Orthopaedic Biomaterials in Research and Practice.* New York, Churchill Livingstone, 1988.)

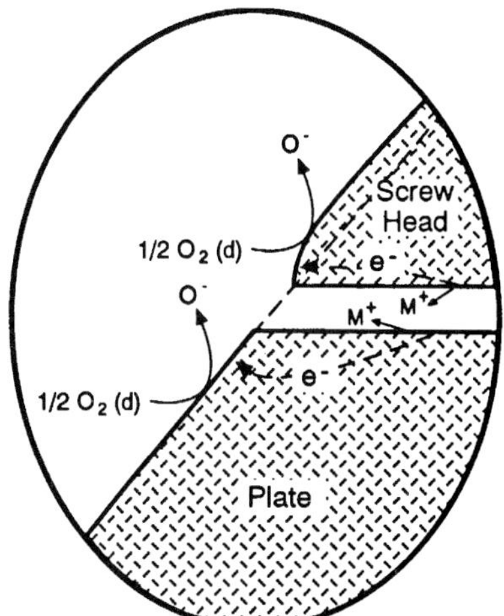

Figure 38
Crevice corrosion. (Adapted with permission from Black J: *Orthopaedic Biomaterials in Research and Practice.* New York, Churchill Livingstone, 1988.)

position of two pieces of an implant (for example, beneath screw heads) result in localized crevice corrosion of implanted metal hardware.

Pitting

This is an extremely localized corrosion mechanism that is similar to crevice corrosion. Starting at a defect in the passive surface layer, corrosion proceeds into the metal setting up the self-accelerating concentration gradients previously discussed (Fig. 39). Chromium, nickel, or molybdenum are added to stainless steels to increase the resistance to pitting corrosion.

Intergranular Attack

If impurities aggregate between grains of relatively pure alloy, a localized galvanic cell may exist between the crystals and the alloy in the grain boundaries (Fig. 40). This phenomenon focuses corrosion in these intergranular regions resulting in the formation of intergranular cracks. Depletion of chromium in the grain-boundary regions of stainless steels, often caused by the intergranular precipitation of chromium carbide, results in intergranular corrosion. This problem explains the extremely low level of carbon specified in the standard for surgical stainless steel.

Stress Corrosion

Stress-corrosion cracking refers to cracking caused by the simultaneous presence of tensile stress and a corrosive medium (Fig. 41). The metal or alloy is virtually immune over most of its surface but fine cracks progress through it. The combination of stress level and corrosive environment that leads to this phenomenon is specific to each metal or alloy. High mechanical stresses may alter the activity of a metal and rupture a protecting passive surface layer, thereby increasing the susceptibility to corrosion. If conditions are right, the material may repassivate, forming a new protecting oxide. Cyclic loading and/or the presence of organic molecules may interfere with this process. Localized corrosion can lead to stress concentration and premature failure.

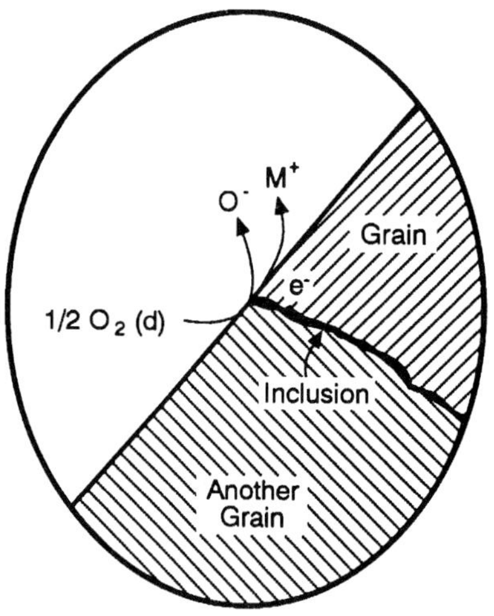

Figure 40
Intergranular corrosion. (Adapted with permission from Black J: *Orthopaedic Biomaterials in Research and Practice.* New York, Churchill Livingstone, 1988.)

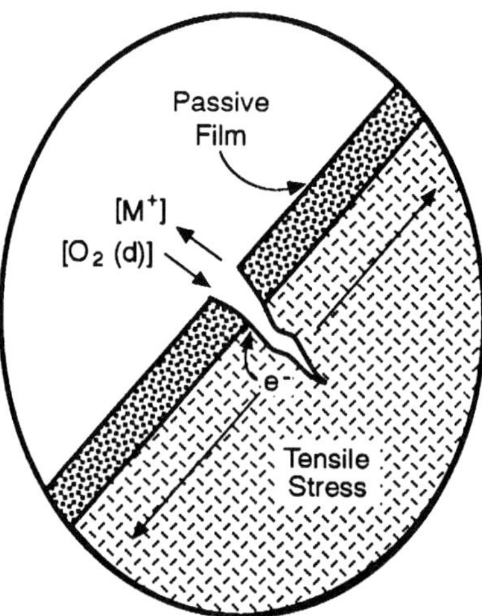

Figure 41
Stress corrosion. (Adapted with permission from Black J: *Orthopaedic Biomaterials in Research and Practice.* New York, Churchill Livingstone, 1988.)

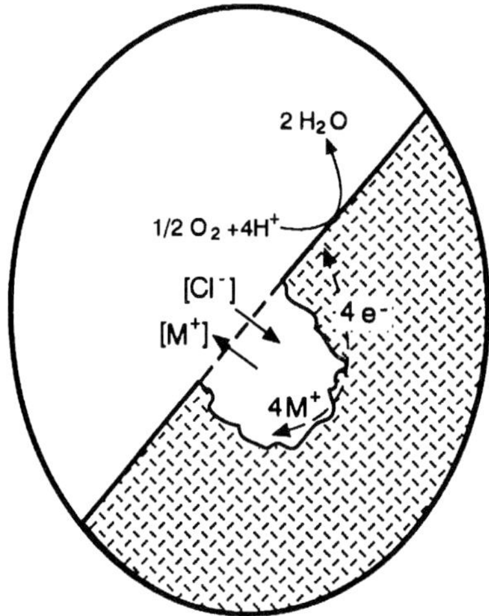

Figure 39
Pitting corrosion. (Adapted with permission from Black J: *Orthopaedic Biomaterials in Research and Practice.* New York, Churchill Livingstone, 1988.)

Fretting Corrosion

Fretting describes corrosion occurring at contact areas between materials under load subjected to vibration and slip. The relative motion necessary to produce fretting corrosion is extremely small; displacements of as little as 10^{-7} mm (1 Å) can produce fretting damage. Repeated oscillatory motion is required, such as when multicomponent implanted devices are placed in weightbearing limbs.

Metal Failure in Clinical Practice

Failure of metallic implants is uncommon in current clinical practice. High-strength alloys and improved knowledge of the functional loads applied in various situations have made static failure virtually a thing of the past. Any metal failure seen today is the result of fatigue. All metal components have a finite fatigue life unless loads are kept below the components' endurance limit. Inserting a metallic implant into a situation where the load is greater than the endurance limit begins a race between the completion of the implant's designated functional task and the fatigue failure of the device. Unless unloaded or removed, the metal will eventually fail.

Only rarely do major intrinsic material defects play a significant role in the fatigue failure of orthopaedic implants. The fabrication techniques and manufacturing practices have been developed such that quality control is excellent. Extrinsic defects, such as scratches, bends, and divots from surgical clamps, act as stress risers and can decrease the fatigue life of an implant.

In fracture fixation devices, the plate or rod is designed to share the load bearing with the fractured bone. The bone is expected to heal and to assume a larger share of the load with the passage of time. This unloads the fracture fixation device and prolongs its fatigue life. Failures do occur when the loads are excessive, such as when the fracture is comminuted and the bone is unable to assist in load bearing. Fatigue failures also occur when the period of load bearing is longer than the device was designed to endure. Fatigue life thus can be important in cases of delayed union or nonunion. Most fracture stabilization devices are overdesigned to minimize the occurrence of fatigue failures.

With endoprostheses, the problem is complicated by their function as full weightbearing devices and their longer expected functional lifetime. The rate of hip stem failure has decreased with the introduction of newer alloys and better designs. All recovered failures have been found to be fatigue fractures. Most fatigue fractures begin at the anterolateral corner of the prosthesis as a result of the longitudinal and torsional loads applied to the femoral head during normal activities.

Those fatigue failures that do occur are invariably associated with conditions that place high stress on the stem. These conditions include design variables such as sharp lateral corners and porous coatings on the lateral surface; surgical variables such as varus positioning; and patient variables such as overactivity, excessive weight, and limited range of hip motion. Fatigue failures can be identified by scanning electron microscopy of the fracture surface. A series of concentric striations originating at the point of crack initiation are characteristic of fatigue failure (Fig. 42).

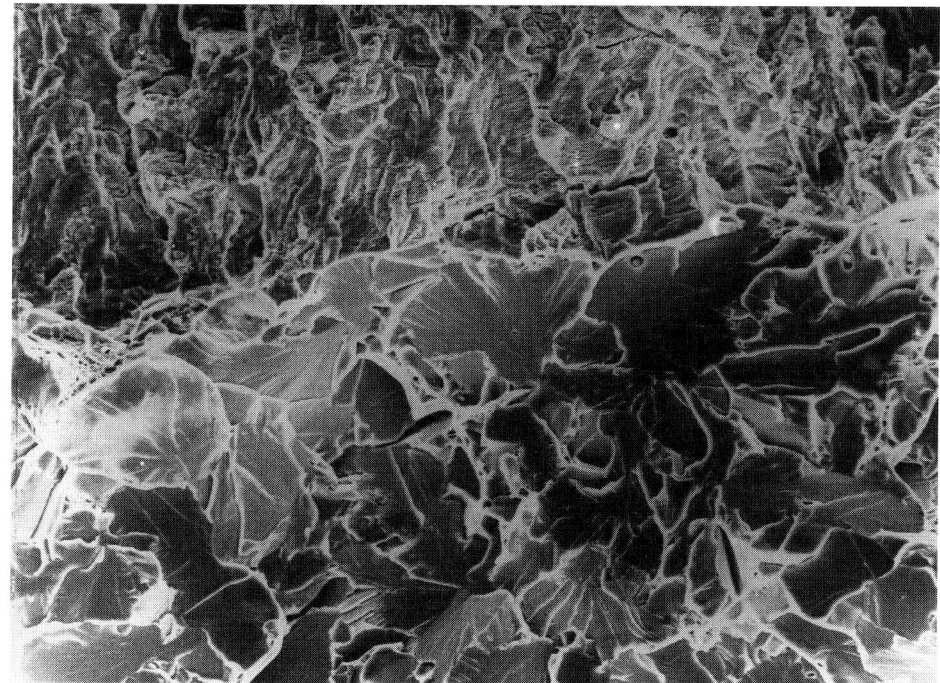

Figure 42
Fatigue fracture showing striations and abrupt junction with region of rapid failure. (Courtesy of Professor Robert M. Rose, Department of Materials Science and Engineering, Massachusetts Institute of Technology.)

Physiologic variables place the highest tensile stresses along the lateral edge, particularly the anterolateral edge, of the device. Microstructural defects in the stem often serve as the localizing point for the start of fatigue fractures. In stainless steel devices, a large surface grain or carbide precipitates often are found near the focus of the fatigue striations. A micropore resulting from shrinkage or gas expulsion is the most common nucleating defect in cast Co-Cr alloys. Inclusions are the most common microstructural defects in the newer alloys and newer processing techniques. Any defect can cause a significant decrease in the fatigue resistance of an alloy by initiating a crack that subsequently grows with each load application. In addition to controlling the surgical and patient-related variables that increase stress on the prosthesis, the choice of alloys is critical. Currently used alloys, Ti6Al4V and hot isostatically pressed Co-Cr, have outstanding yield and fatigue strength. Their use is an important improvement in total joint surgery.

Polymers

Polyethylene

The term polyethylene refers to plastics formed from the polymerization of ethylene, $CH_2{=}CH_2$. The dominant variable determining the functional properties of polyethylene is the molecular weight of the polymer chains. Clinical conditions require the use of very high molecular weight material. Low density polyethylene is used routinely in packaging and for other short-term, low-load situations. High density polyethylene (HDPE) is a linear, more crystalline material with improved physical and material properties. Both materials have molecular weights of up to 500,000. Neither has any orthopaedic biomaterial application. Ultrahigh molecular weight polyethylene is the material used for acetabular cups and tibial trays. This material is less dense and less crystalline than HDPE; however, with a molecular weight in excess of one million, it has superior mechanical properties. It is extremely tough (a 0.357 magnum bullet fired from 25 feet bounces back from a 1-inch thick slab of UHMWPE) and is exceptionally wear resistant.

Molecular weight is the most important, but not the only, variable determining the properties of polyethylene components. Molding conditions, sterilization procedures, and environmental conditions during storage also affect the material. Radiation sterilization produces free radicals that can either combine to form cross-links between the chains or oxidize, starting a cascade of environmental degradation reactions. Keeping radiation dosages low and performing the sterilization in a nitrogen atmosphere minimize the damage. Repeated doses of radiation, as would occur with resterilization, are not recommended.

The wear debris produced in both controlled laboratory tests and in hip simulators has shown wear rate to depend largely on molecular weight. There is a tenfold drop in wear rate when the molecular weight is increased from 500,000 to two million. The presence of acrylic debris in the articulation of total joint arthroplasties is postulated to increase the abrasive wear of polyethylene components. Whether or not substantial true wear is caused by loose acrylic debris has not been proved. On the other hand, it is known that substantial true wear can occur in the absence of loose third bodies.

Subsurface fatigue has proved to be a major cause of polyethylene delamination in total knee replacements in which the local contact stresses are high because of the incongruent geometries of the tibial and femoral components. Recent reports from an industrial research laboratory show that ion implantation of Co-Cr increases the surface energy and, hence, the wettability of the metal. The resultant increase in lubrication efficiency leads to a sizable decrease in polyethylene wear during in vitro testing.

Polyethylene in other forms also finds applications in orthopaedics. Produced as a closed-cell foam, polyethylene can be made into sheets of lightweight, heat-moldable splint material. Plastazote is commonly used for corrective or therapeutic splints not subjected to high loads.

Polymethylmethacrylate

Polymethylmethacrylate (PMMA) is used in a self-curing form as a grouting agent for total joint arthroplasties, as a supplement to spinal fixation, and as a filler for pathologic fractures. It can be shaped during surgery prior to polymerization and thus makes a custom implant for each use. The formulation used today is essentially unchanged from that of the cement developed for John Charnley by Dennis Smith, a dental materials scientist at the University of Manchester. Because PMMA is polymerized intraoperatively, it is imperative that the surgeon understand the processes involved and the effects of operating room conditions and practices on the properties of the cement.

Polymerization and Curing

About 70% of the mass of cured bone cement is composed of preformed polymeric beads that are the major constituents of the powder component. The rest of the bone cement mass consists of the additional matrix that forms on polymerization of the liquid monomer and an additive to make the bone cement radiopaque.

The requirements for a surgical bone cement include several that relate directly to its mixing and polymerization. Reliability is critical in cements for operative use—the handling characteristics, consistency, working time, and setting time must be predictable within narrow tolerances to permit adequate planning of the surgical procedure (Fig. 43). The working time must be adequate to allow the surgeon time to properly seat the prosthesis without hurrying; the setting time must be reasonably short to reduce the incidence of implant motion during the curing. The initial polymerization must proceed to a sufficient degree to achieve secure, immediate fixation. The amount of heat given off by the reaction must be predictable to minimize the risk of thermal necrosis to the bone. The components must be sterilizable, and the mixing must be possible with relative ease under sterile conditions. As supplied by the manufacturer, the powder contains 88% by weight (wt%) polymer, 10 wt/% radiopaque agent (either barium sulfate, $BaSO_4$, or zirconium oxide, ZrO_2), and a small amount (about 2 wt%) of an initiator (often benzoyl peroxide). The prepolymerized beads from some manufacturers consist solely of PMMA; other manufacturers include a copolymer of PMMA-polystyrene or polymethylacrylate to facilitate mixing and handling properties. The liquid component is a colorless, flammable, slightly acrid smelling solution of methylmethacrylate monomer, 97.4% by volume (vol%), with an activator (2.6 vol% N,N-dimethyl-p-toluidine), and a small amount of hydroquinone (75 ± 15 ppm). The hydroquinone serves as a free radical scavenger and stabilizes the monomer to prevent spontaneous polymerization and increase its shelf life. The powders of commercial bone cements are sterilized by gamma irradiation, the monomers by ultrafiltration.

When the powder and liquid components are mixed, the activator cleaves the initiator, forming two free radicals that begin a chain-growth polymerization of the monomer. Mixing triggers both chemical and physical events that occur at various rates. Physical processes include swelling of the prepolymerized beads in the monomer, diffusion of the liquid components into the beads toward the initiator, and evaporation of the monomer. These events combine to produce a doughy stage within three to seven minutes, depending on environmental conditions. Chemical reactions of chain initiation, growth, and termination dominate during the setting period. The polymerization reaction, once initiated, is

$$(R^\bullet) + (M) \longrightarrow (RM^\bullet)$$

self-catalyzing and exothermic. Sufficient temperature increases may occur in adjacent tissues to cause thermal necrosis. The physical escape of excess monomer through the increasingly viscous mass of polymerizing bone cement determines the amount of residual monomer in the cement mass and is another example of the interdependence of physical and chemical processes.

An important determinant of final bulk properties is the degree of interpenetration of the preformed polymer chains from the beads with the newly polymerizing chains. Incomplete penetration results in focal areas of microscopic delamination and weakness, which can precipitate microfractures, particularly when pressed into an irregular geometry, and increase the formation of acrylic debris. The relative speeds of the physical and chemical processes are, therefore, very important to achieving a good cement mass.

Environmental conditions influence both the physical and chemical processes and thus affect the properties of the bone cement. The entire setting curve and all phases of it are shortened by increased ambient temperature. Increasing the relative amount of monomer increases the amount of heat given off during polymerization, prolongs the setting time, and increases the amount of free monomer available to the tissues,

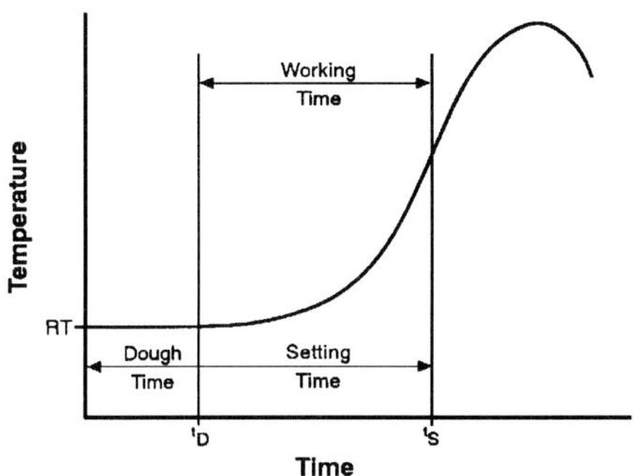

Figure 43
Curing curve of polymethylmethacrylate bone cement. (Adapted with permission from Black J: *Orthopaedic Biomaterials in Research and Practice.* New York, Churchill Livingstone, 1988.)

with potential increases in toxicity. Entire batches of premeasured cement as supplied by the manufacturer should be mixed, taking care to avoid spilling of either component because changes to the powder-liquid ratio can affect both handling and final properties.

Size, both thickness and weight, of the cement mass determines the peak exothermic temperature. Heat generation is a function of the amount of reacting monomer, and heat dissipation is a function of surface area and the temperature of surrounding structures. The balance of these two processes determines the temperature increase produced in the tissues. (The significance of exothermic insult to surrounding tissues and any role this might play in the loosening process has been extensively debated in the literature.) There is another cause for concern about the peak temperature of PMMA; if acrylics are heated too quickly or allowed to become too hot, there is an increase in porosity and a resultant decrease in mechanical strength.

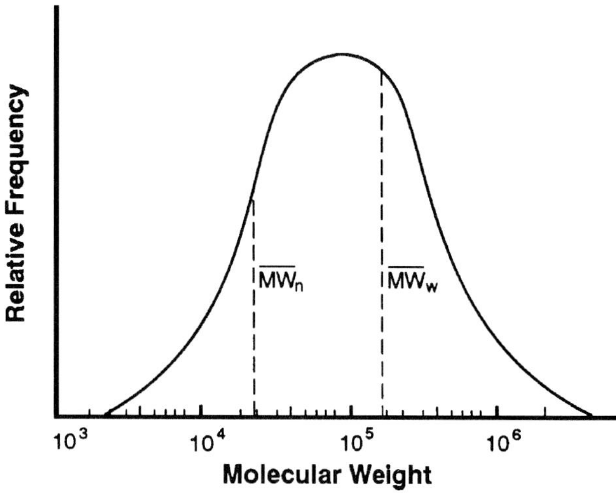

Figure 44
Molecular weight distribution of bone cement. (Reproduced with permission from Lautenschlager EP, Stupp SI, Keller JC: Structure and properties of acrylic bone cement, in Ducheyne P, Hastings GW (eds): *Functional Behavior of Orthopaedic Biomaterials.* Boca Raton, FL, CRC Press, 1984, vol 2.)

Physical Properties

The bulk mechanical properties of any polymer specimen reflect its molecular weight and its molecular weight distribution. For amorphous polymers below their glass transition temperature (T_g), such as PMMA at body temperature (T_g (PMMA) = 114°C), tensile strength, hardness, ultimate strain, and other bulk properties are molecular weight-dependent below a critical level. For PMMA, the critical molecular weight is approximately 150,000. Surface properties, such as abrasion and wear resistance, tend to be less sensitive to molecular weight. As shown in Fig. 44, the molecular weight distribution of cured surgical acrylic is broad. The number average molecular weight $\overline{MW}_n$ is about 30,000 while the weight-average molecular weight $\overline{MW}_w$ is somewhat under 200,000. Other authors have reported slightly higher values.

Industrial processes can produce void-free, transparent PMMA suitable for windows. In a clinical setting, bone cement has 3% to 11% porosity, which alters the mechanical and physical properties. Small spherical voids account for much of the porosity and are thought to result from volatilization of monomer when heat is generated during polymerization. The poor thermal conductivity of PMMA prevents the efficient dissipation of heat and, during curing, causes local hot spots that can exceed the boiling point of methylmethacrylate monomer (100.3°C). The application of external pressure can raise this boiling point and, thus, decrease the porosity of the bone cement. External pressurization also reduces the irregularly shaped pores that result from insufficient penetration of monomer into the polymer beads. Pressures of 27.6 MPa (4,000 psi), far in excess of surgically achievable pressurization, are necessary to produce acrylic cements free of porosity. Recent research has demonstrated that much of the porosity found at the implant-cement interface results from air carried down into the cement when the prosthesis is inserted.

The polymerization process itself creates voids in the final cement. During the early stages of mixing, when the monomer is dissolving and swelling the beads, the cement mass increases in volume by 3% to 5%. Later, the volume contracts by 5% to 7% as the monomer polymerizes. At this stage, however, the cement mass is partially set and cannot fully contract, so internal pores are formed. Internal pores, whether spherical or irregular, are stress risers that undermine the optimal material properties of the bone cement. Voids decrease the cross-sectional area of the cement and also serve as crack initiators. Several research groups have experimented with centrifugation and vacuum mixing to decrease the porosity of the cement mass. Each technique has proved successful in producing cement specimens with a lower level of porosity. Of particular importance, both techniques virtually eliminate large voids, which can have catastrophic effects on strength. The clinical effect of porosity reduction has been debated based on both experimental and clinical evidence. The jagged external surface of a well-interdigitated cement mantle will necessarily have many stress risers and discontinuities, so the role of internal porosity in crack initiation is questionable.

Cured bone cement has the capacity to imbibe small amounts of fluid by both absorptive and adsorptive mechanisms. An increase in weight of cement specimens has been documented. The equilibrium moisture content leads generally to a 3% reduction in ultimate compressive strength in comparison with dry specimens. When water, or biologic fluid, fills the pores of PMMA, it can act as a plasticizer and increase the amount of deformation before fracture. Water also can inhibit crack growth at defects and dissipate stresses more evenly throughout the bulk material. This effect is small; one study showed that storing Simplex-P bone cement for two years in bovine serum at 37°C had a negligible effect on mechanical properties.

Mechanical Properties

The properties of PMMA bone cement are not the same as those of commercial PMMA resins such as Plexiglass. The requirement for polymerization under ambient conditions results in a polymer of lower average molecular weight with a broader dispersion of molecular weights. Both factors have detrimental effects on the material properties (Table 2). The literature values for the properties of PMMA bone cements show wide variation, which is caused partly by the dependence of mechanical properties on polymerization conditions, preconditioning, and testing methods (including strain rate). Polymers, including acrylic bone cement, are viscoelastic and thus are stiffer and stronger at higher strain rates (Fig. 45). Direct comparison of the data is often difficult because of the variation in testing conditions, and the failure of some authors to report the details of their test conditions. PMMA bone cement is brittle at body temperature and, like many brittle plastics, has a much higher strength in compression than in tension or shear. Below their glass transition temperature, acrylic bone cements fracture in a brittle fashion. The introduction of plasticizers (barium sulfate, serum, water) increases the fatigue life by reducing the rate of crack propagation through the matrix. The addition of fibers within the cement matrix also increases the fatigue life of the cement. The endurance limit of PMMA bone cement in fatigue has been found to be higher in compression tests than in tension tests. The mechanical weakness of PMMA has been implicated in the failure of total hip and knee arthroplasties.

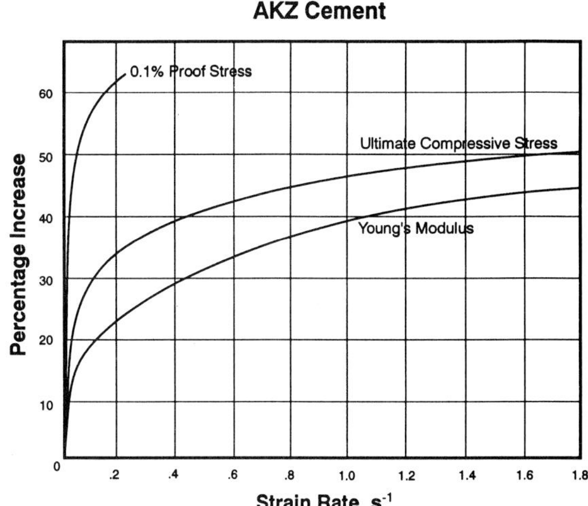

Figure 45
Effect of strain rate on the mechanical properties of bone cement. (Adapted with permission from Lee AJ, Ling RS, Vangala SS: Some clinically relevant variables affecting the mechanical behavior of bone cement. *Arch Orthop Trauma Surg* 1978;92:1–8.)

The surgical team controls a number of variables that potentially are critical in the mechanical behavior of the acrylic cement. Use of a slow beating frequency while mixing the monomer with the poly-

Table 2
Physical properties of bone cement and commercial acrylic resins

	Radiopaque Bone Cement*	Commercial Acrylic Resins**
Tensile strength (MPa)	28.9 ± 1.6	55 –76
Compressive strength (MPa)	91.7 ± 2.5	76 –131
Young's modulus (compressive loading, MPa)	2,200 ± 60	2,360–3,280
Endurance limit (ultimate tensile strength)	0.3	0.3
Density (g/ml)	1.10 –1.23	1.18
Water adsorption (%)	0.5	0.3 –0.4
Shrinkage after setting (%)	2.7–5	—

* From Haas SS, Brauer GM, Dickson G: A characterization of PMMA bone cement. *J Bone Joint Surg* 1975;57A:380–391.
** From *Modern Plastic Encyclopedia.* New York, McGraw-Hill, 1980, vol 57, p 533.
(Adapted with permission from Park JB: *Biomaterials Science and Engineering.* New York, Plenum, 1984.)

mer and limiting the mixing time to 90 seconds can maximize the ultimate compressive strength of the polymerized acrylic. Rapid beating while mixing decreases this strength by 10% and mixing for 2 ½ minutes leads to an 11% strength reduction. The viscosity of the acrylic cement increases slowly at first and then more rapidly after mixing. Early insertion of the acrylic cement, while the viscosity is low, prevents laminations that significantly weaken the polymerized cement mass. Because the acrylic mass is not controllable in the surgeon's hands during the early stages of mixing, it is necessary to handle it in an injection device. This technique also permits pressurization of the cement within the bone, which can enhance both the ultimate compressive and tensile strengths by as much as 30%, depending on the amount of pressure applied. The application of two atmospheres (29.4 psi = 0.2 MPa) for 15 seconds on insertion of the dough can increase the ultimate compressive strength by 11%.

Other operating room variables that influence the mechanical behavior of the acrylic cement are only partially controllable by the surgeon. These variables include blood and tissue inclusions, stress risers, and cement thickness. The inclusion of blood within the cement mass can have a dramatically detrimental influence on the mechanical behavior of the cement, with reductions of up to 77% in tensile strength and 69% in shear strength. Although it is rarely possible to eliminate blood totally from bony surfaces during total hip arthroplasty, the degree of blood contamination can be minimized with use of hypotensive anesthesia, epinephrine rinse, jet lavage of the bone surface, and/or the use of suction prior to insertion of the acrylic. Acrylic cement is brittle and exhibits a limited plastic deformation before failure. Exposure of polymerized cement to stress risers leads to mechanical failure at lower levels; therefore, prosthetic devices should not have sharp edges or corners. Bone cement does not immediately reach a state of equilibrium with reference to its physical properties following polymerization. When polymerized at 37°C, PMMA achieves 90% of its strength in four hours and ultimate strength in 24 hours. Plugging of the medullary canal, insertion in a low viscosity state, and pressurization of the cement mass all contribute to improved interpenetration of cement into cancellous bone. These techniques have resulted in a reduced incidence of radiolucency at the bone-cement interface.

Cement Interfaces

Acrylic bone cement is not an adhesive. The only source of mechanical integrity between bone cement and the adjacent structure is mechanical interlock. Bone-cement interface strengths are directly related to the surface area of fixation and the degree of penetration (up to a maximum of about 5 mm). The density of the cancellous bone on the biologic side of the interface is an important factor in the bone-cement interface bond strength. Shear strengths at the bone cement interface with cancellous bone have been reported in the range of 3 MPa (450 psi). In dense cortical bone, where cement penetration is poor, the interface strength suffers. Early insertion of the cement when its viscosity is lower, thorough cleaning and lavage of the osseous bed, and pressurization of the cement mass improve the mechanical integrity and strength of the bone-cement interface.

The interface between the bone cement and the prosthesis has been receiving increased attention in light of new studies showing the effect of debonding at this interface on the stresses in the rest of the system. Clinical studies of asymptomatic retrievals indicate that the cement-prosthesis interface may be a site of early failure in the loosening process. Surface finish on the metal obviously plays a key role in prosthesis-cement interface bond strength; increased surface roughness gives superior shear strength. Polished surfaces have an interfacial shear strength of 0.5 MPa; sandblasting the surface increases this value to 6.84 MPa. Precoating the metallic implant industrially with a thin layer of PMMA can achieve an interfacial shear strength of 2,340 MPa.

Toxicity

Occasional cardiovascular collapse or irreversible cardiac arrest has been associated with the surgical use of PMMA. Monomeric methylmethacrylate is metabolized to methacrylic acid, a normal intermediate in the catabolism of valine. Methylmethacrylate released during the curing of bone cement is metabolized to carbon dioxide by the tricarboxylic acid cycle. No quantitative correlation has been found between the maximum concentrations of either methylmethacrylate or methacrylic acid and the patient's reduction in arterial blood pressure. The onset of hypotension (usually 30 to 75 seconds following the insertion of acrylic cement) always precedes the appearance of methylmethacrylate or methacrylic acid in the serum.

In patients who develop cardiac collapse, fat emboli and other marrow contents are consistently identified in the pulmonary system during postmortem examinations. A transient elevation of intramedullary pressure is correlated with the insertion of bone cement into the femoral canal during total hip arthroplasty. It has been hypothesized that elevated intramedullary pressures might precipitate fat embolization, and pressures up to 120,000 Pa (900 mm Hg) have been recorded during insertion of the femoral component. Radioactive albumin placed in the femoral canal before insertion of the cement or the prosthetic component appears in the lung 10 to 120 seconds after cementing. Thus, it seems that the cardiovascular changes result from embolization of fat and marrow contents, which initiate aggregation of platelets and fibrin in the pulmonary circulation.

Modification to Bone Cement

There has been considerable interest in the use of antibiotic-impregnated PMMA to treat osteomyelitis or infected total joint replacements. If 1 g of powdered antibiotic is thoroughly mixed with the powder component of commercial bone cement formulations, the final cement has a 4% decrease in ultimate compressive strength. The elution of antibiotics from the PMMA varies with the type of cement used; the copolymer composition of the powder is believed to be the reason. Several antibiotics have been demonstrated to leach out of bone cement in bactericidal concentrations. Impregnated-PMMA cement can deliver locally high concentrations of those antibiotics that can withstand the heat of polymerization without loss of potency. Because the elution rate of antibiotics is related to surface area, the introduction of beads of polymerized antibiotic-impregnated acrylic cement on a wire produces increased surface area and provides a means of removal. Implantation of acrylic bone cement with antibiotic into the defect following debridement of an osteomyelitic cavity is as efficacious as conventional treatment with intravenous antibiotics.

The superior interpenetration of PMMA with cancellous bone when handled in a less viscous state led to the development of low viscosity PMMA. However, the mechanical behavior of low viscosity cement was inferior to that of standard formulations and the cement required reinforcement with carbon fibers. This addition decreased crack velocity in the acrylic mass by one order of magnitude and increased the tensile fracture strength by 20%. The presence of the carbon fibers, however, adversely affected the flow behavior of low viscosity cement, making it more difficult to obtain good interdigitation with cancellous bone and reducing bone-cement interface strength.

In addition to the carbon fibers added to low viscosity cement, aramid fibers have been tried in an attempt to improve the fracture toughness of PMMA. The increase in viscosity precluded adequate interdigitation with trabecular bone so the composite never made it to clinical use.

Several attempts have been made to decrease the voids in bone cements, which often are sites of failure both experimentally and clinically. The two most successful approaches are centrifugation of the mixed cement in its low viscosity state and mixing of the powder and liquid components under a partial vacuum. Both approaches, which are now common in clinical practice, have been shown to significantly reduce the overall porosity and to eliminate the large voids that seriously compromise the local strength. An alternative means of increasing the fracture toughness of bone cement is to decrease the rate of fracture propagation by including rubbery beads in the brittle PMMA matrix. Such cements are currently under investigation.

The locally high contact stresses at geometric and material discontinuities along the bone-cement interface are thought to be a stimulus for bone resorption, which is a critical step in the loosening of total joint components. More compliant, viscoelastic bone cements, designed to dissipate and distribute the loads more evenly, have been developed. Those that retain the structural integrity to support the imposed loads have yielded excellent results in preliminary animal studies.

Materials for Orthotics and Prosthetics

The use of a wide variety of new and improved materials by the prosthetic and orthotic industry has resulted in improved design and better clinical results. Durability, function, and cosmesis have improved simultaneously as prosthetic and orthotic practitioners innovatively combine the new materials with traditional metal and leather components. The array of materials currently being used to manufacture prostheses and orthoses indicates that no single material will serve all purposes, because distinctly different properties are required for varying clinical applications or even for parts of the same device.

Materials Used for Orthoses

For optimal orthotic management, the mechanical demands to be placed on an orthosis for any given treatment must be understood prior to material selection. Selection of the correct material is often the difference between success and failure; therefore, the skilled orthotist will attempt to match the characteristics of the material to the biomechanical and functional needs of the patient.

Orthoses are constructed from two main groups of materials, plastics and metals; a single device often is a combination of both. The metals most suitable for orthotic fabrication are steel and aluminum alloys; the choice depends on the application. Steel is stronger and stiffer than aluminum alloy; aluminum alloy has a lower density, making it lighter. A clinical example of this would be the upright of a lower extremity orthosis in which deformation under bending stresses is very important. The alignment of the patient's lower extremity, the patient's weight, and the patient's activity level, together with the loading pattern on the upright, are considered before selecting either a steel or an aluminum component.

The major advantage of steel in orthotics is its low cost, abundance, and relative ease of fabrication. Steel is fatigue resistant and combines high strength with high rigidity or ductility depending on the alloy used. Steel is widely used in prefabricated joints, metal uprights, metal bands and cuffs, springs, and bearings. The main disadvantage of steel is its weight.

The main benefit of aluminum in orthotics is its high strength-to-weight ratio. Thus, aluminum is used whenever light weight is a major consideration, as in upper extremity orthoses. Aluminum does, however, have a lower endurance limit under repeated dynamic loading conditions than does steel. Therefore, if loading conditions are known to be great or highly repetitive, steel is superior to aluminum.

Plastic materials play an extremely important role in the provision of orthotic care and have become increasingly popular; many would suggest their availability has revolutionized orthotic practice. Two major groups of plastics are used for orthotic design, thermoplastics and thermosets. Low temperature thermoplastics, those classified as requiring no more than 80°C to become workable, may be molded directly to the body. These materials have gained increasing popularity, particularly for upper extremity applications in which the rapid provision of an assistive or protective orthosis is desirable. Minimal equipment is required: a source of hot water, scissors, and a heat gun. Low-temperature thermoplastics typically are not effective when high stress is anticipated.

High-temperature thermoplastics usually are molded under vacuum to a plaster model that has been prepared by the orthotist. Polyethylene and polypropylene are the high-temperature thermoplastics most widely used for orthotic design. Polyethylene generally is classified as being of low, medium, or high density, and it is important when selecting this plastic to realize that varying densities will produce very different mechanical characteristics in the finished orthosis. Low density polyethylene is a good option for nonweightbearing applications, for example, a supportive wrist and hand orthosis. High density polyethylene is commonly used in a wide variety of orthotic situations but perhaps it is chosen most often as an appropriate material selection for varying spinal orthotic treatments.

Polypropylene is a thermoplastic polymer with low specific gravity and good resistance to chemicals and fatigue. Its unique flexing capability coupled with its resistance to fatigue accounts for wide acceptance, particularly for lower extremity orthotic applications. However, the plastic most often used for orthotic design is a copolymer of polypropylene and polyethylene. This copolymer, polypropylene with 5% to 25% polyethylene, has much better fatigue resistance than either constituent. Because the thickness of the plastic may be varied and the rigidity of the orthoses determined by changing trimlines, any number of designs are possible. A wide range of clinical objectives and biomechanical requirements thus can be satisfied.

The provision and design of foot orthoses is an area in which the choice of materials is of paramount importance. If the function of the orthosis is to support, leather or felt with or without a more sturdy underliner are appropriate; if the function is to reduce shear force, a viscoelastic polymer may be used. Commonly, foot orthoses are required to cushion or absorb shock; closed-cell polyethylene foams and nitrogen filled rubbers have proved successful for this use. As is the case in most areas of prosthetic and orthotic design, clinical devices typically are manufactured from more than one material as the functional requirements demand varying characteristics from each component; for example, the diabetic patient with significant tissue loss and adherent scar tissue will require both shock absorption and reduction of shear.

Materials Used for Prostheses

Many of the most significant advances in prosthesis development have been related to new materials and the improved design features that they permit. Throughout the 18th century, prostheses designers innovatively used such readily available materials as leather, steel, tin, and wood to construct limbs. Today a much wider selection of materials is available, and amputees are being given lightweight functional limbs constructed from such materials as thermoplastics, improved acrylic resins, titanium, graphite, and carbon composites. The choice between an exoskeletal and an endoskeletal prosthesis should be made after reviewing the patient's lifestyle. The exoskeletal design provides strength via the hard laminated surface of the prosthesis; the endoskeletal system provides strength through a central pylon, which commonly is constructed of aluminum alloy or a graphite composite to give the patient a very strong, lightweight prosthesis. Cost and durability are advantages of the exoskeletal design. However, with the endoskeletal system it is possible to interchange modular components, to use soft cosmetic coverings, and to conveniently make alignment changes.

Modern prostheses usually are made of a combination of materials and consist of varying modules and components. Only the socket of the prosthesis is custom fabricated; the other components (feet, knees, ankles, wrists, elbows, etc.) are premanufactured in an array of sizes and varying levels of sophistication. Components, and thus the materials used for prosthetic design, are selected by the prosthetist to match the biomechanical and functional needs of each patient.

Prosthetic sockets can be manufactured from either thermoplastic materials or fiber-reinforced thermosetting plastics. The use of thermoplastics for this important part of the prostheses is gaining wide acceptance as both patient and prosthetist come to appreciate the advantages. Manufacturing time is reduced, and the overall process is simpler and cleaner. Patients have reacted positively to the greater flexibility and reduced weight of thermoplastic sockets.

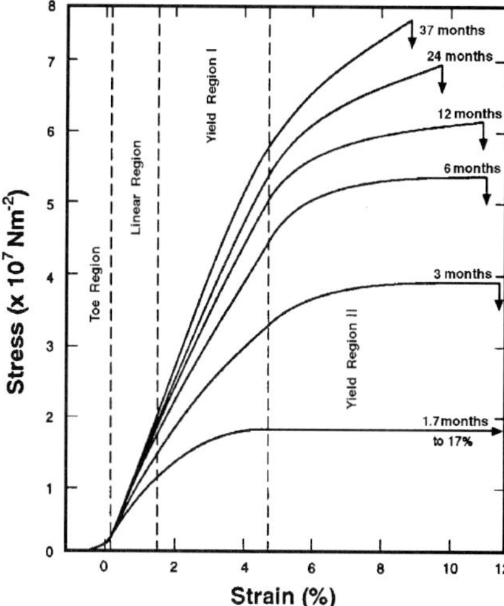

Figure 46
Load-deformation curve of rat tail tendon showing the various mechanical regions and the effect of aging. (Adapted with permission from Fastelic J, Baer E: Deformation in tendon collagen, in *The Mechanical Properties of Biological Materials.* Cambridge, MA, Cambridge University Press, 1980.)

Materials for Artificial Ligaments

The search for a synthetic ligament is motivated by the problems of availability and harvesting morbidity that complicate the use of biologic grafts. The immediate postoperative strength and stability of synthetic grafts facilitate early rehabilitation.

Variations in polymer structure and orientation can be used to create fibers of different properties. Textile-manufacturing technologies are used to fabricate ligaments with a wide range of properties and sizes. Mimicking the load-deformation behavior of natural ligaments or tendons (Fig. 46) is only a first step in developing a useful synthetic structure for ligament repair or replacement. Yield strength and fatigue endurance must also be addressed.

Artificial ligaments have been developed from polyethylene terephthalate (for example, Dacron) and polytetrafluoroethylene (for example, Teflon). An augmentation device made of polypropylene braided into a flat structure is available. A permanent open-weave polyester design that serves as a true replacement and as a scaffold for bioingrowth is under review. Two other devices have failed in clinical trials. A bovine xenograft, cross-linked with glutaraldehyde to retard enzymatic attack, was not granted FDA approval after mixed clinical results in early trials. A carbon ligament designed to serve as a biodegradable scaffold for host tissues was withdrawn because of inconsistent clinical results and a documented release of carbon fibers with abrasion.

Ceramics

Traditional ceramic materials are those composed of inorganic, nonmetallic elements held together by ionic bonding. Vitreous and glassy materials are also now considered within the realm of ceramic materials. Most have at least some metallic oxide component and most form crystalline or polycrystalline solids.

The typical ceramic material is very stiff, brittle, and insoluble. Household pottery is the most familiar ceramic material and demonstrates well the properties of many ceramics. Orthopaedic interest is raised by their excellent biocompatibility (a function of their insolubility and chemical inertness) and their exceptional wear resistance. The brittle nature of ceramics and the difficulty of forming defect-free devices have limited their use in the past. Improved understanding of ceramic technology and processing has opened new avenues for the application of ceramics to clinical orthopaedics.

Alumina

Aluminum oxide (Al_2O_3) has excellent abrasion resistance and, when coupled with itself in congruent geometries, has the lowest coefficient of friction of any man-made bearing. For these reasons it has been used for the articulated components of total hip arthroplasties, particularly in Europe. Ceramic femoral heads can be produced with a smoother surface than can metal components; this decreased surface roughness is one factor in reducing friction and surface wear.

Alumina is brittle and has a low tensile strength, resulting in a low material toughness. Its low resistance to stress concentration makes alumina very sensitive to microstructural flaws. Improved processing technology has helped to overcome these problems, and alumina heads for modular femoral components are available from several manufacturers. They can be articulated against either UHMWPE or an alumina acetabular cup.

Zirconia

A second generation of ceramic femoral heads has been manufactured from zirconium oxide (ZrO_2). This ceramic exists in three crystalline forms, depending on the temperature. The tetragonal form, stable at elevated temperatures, is the most desirable configuration for orthopaedic applications because of its toughness. This form can be stabilized by the addition of metallic oxide to produce an alloy that is metastable at physiologic temperatures. Calcium oxide (CaO), magnesium oxide (MgO), and yttrium oxide (Y_2O_3) have all been used for this purpose, producing a class of materials referred to as partially-stabilized zirconia. Yttrium-stabilized zirconia is commercially available for surgical use. It has a much smaller grain size than surgical-grade alumina (0.5 μm versus 7 μm) and has superior strength and toughness. The wear rate of zirconia-zirconia bearings has been found to be much greater than that of alumina-alumina couples, although it is still quite low compared to other man-made bearing surfaces. The biocompatibility of stabilized zirconia, particularly long-term effects, is not yet fully documented.

Calcium Phosphate/Hydroxyapatite

The mineral component of bone is a calcium phosphate compound, so the biocompatibility of synthetic calcium-phosphates is predictably excellent. Some reports indicate a chemical bonding between hydroxyapatite [$Ca_{10}(PO_4)_6(OH)_2$] and bone; recent work has demonstrated the degradation of hydroxyapatite by osteoclasts. The use of these materials as a coating on metallic implants currently is being investigated. The results observed depend on the purity, grain size, and exact composition of the ceramic coating. The stoichiometry of the compound produced is strongly influenced by processing conditions; therefore, a chemical characterization of each batch is needed for an accurate assessment of observed results. The Ca/P ratio needs to be measured and reported; hydroxyapatite has a Ca/P ratio of 1.67. Other calcium phosphates have different ratios; one of the most common is tricalcium phosphate, where the Ca/P ratio is 1.5. Because of the wide variety of compositions that can be produced, it is often difficult to interpret conflicting experimental results.

Bioactive Glasses

A class of vitreous materials has been developed that will bond to bone. These materials partially solubilize in vivo, forming a surface hydrogel that is rich in calcium and phosphate ions. This surface gel is an inhomogeneous mixture that is very difficult to identify accurately. The two best known bioactive glasses have similar compositions. One is composed of 45 weight percent (wt%) silicon dioxide (SiO_2), 24.5 wt% each of calcium oxide (CaO) and sodium monoxide (Na_2O), and 6 wt% phosphoric anhydride (P_2O_5). The other has less sodium, more phosphorus, and additions of magnesium and potassium oxides (MgO, K_2O). Both are produced in purely vitreous forms or with microcrystalline fillers. Small differences in composition have a major effect on properties. The brittleness of these materials restricts their use to nonstructural applications such as coatings and fillers. Other glass-ceramics being developed have improved mechanical properties.

Composites

Composites are multiphase materials that gain their strength through the combining of two materials with different, often complementary, properties to produce a material that has the positive attributes of both without the defects of either. The most familiar examples are fiberglass resin and reinforced concrete. The components of a composite are usually classified as the matrix material and the fillers. The latter may be particles, fibers, or more complex structures imbedded in the matrix. The possibilities are unlimited, and composites are usually developed for a specific application. The mechanical properties of a composite often depend largely on the bonding between the matrix and the filler. Composites differ from solutions, alloys, and blends in that each component of a composite retains its chemical, structural, and material identity.

Composite materials can be strengthened by alternating the orientation of the reinforcing fibers. The anisotropic behavior of these oriented structures is obscured when several layers at different orientations are bonded together. A biologic example of this is the alternating collagen orientation in successive layers of haversian bone. Each osteon is a multilayered composite, and the entire bone is a composite of osteons in a mineralized matrix. The bond between layers is a potential weak point in composites fabricated from multiple layers.

Industrial composites usually have a wide variety of chemical moieties added either to enhance the bond between the filler and the matrix or to improve handling and processing. The biocompatibility of implant materials is seriously affected by such low molecular weight compounds. Composite materials are slowly being developed specifically for medical applications. Some of the biodegradable materials are self-reinforced composites in which the fibers and the matrix have identical composition to avoid debonding problems. The only composites commonly used in orthopaedic practice are casting materials.

Orthopaedic casts and splints have traditionally been made from plaster. This composite material is used because it is inexpensive, readily available, and easily moldable during the setting phase. Bulk plaster is brittle and relatively weak, particularly in tension; the mechanical integrity of a cast is derived from the gauze mesh used as a carrier, from the laminated structural composite made at the time the cast is applied, and from the structural properties of the cast geometry. (On a strength-to-weight basis, a tube is much stronger than a solid rod in its resistance to bending and torsional stresses.) Because the strength comes primarily from the structure rather than the material, the skill of the individual forming the cast or splint is a crucial factor. Plaster is formed by roasting crushed gypsum at 120° to 130°C to decrease the naturally occurring water content from 21 wt% to about 6 wt%. This fine powder is then bonded to a gauze mesh using either methylcellulose or polyvinyl acetate. An accelerator often is added to decrease the setting time; potassium sulfate (K_2SO_4) is one such accelerator.

When a plaster impregnated bandage is immersed in water and fully hydrated, usually after five to ten seconds, the plaster absorbs water and begins to set. The setting reaction produces crystalline calcium sulfate dihydrate:

$$(CaSO_4)_2{\cdot}H_2O + 3H_2O \rightarrow 2[CaSO_4{\cdot}2H_2O] + \text{heat.}$$

This reaction is exothermic and the heat generated accelerates the setting process. Within four to five minutes, a soft solid cast has formed but this construct has only 35% to 50% of its ultimate strength. After the heat given off by polymerization has peaked, the cast feels cold and clammy because a large volume of excess water still is trapped in the mesh. Over a period of hours or days, depending upon cast thickness and environmental conditions, this excess water evaporates and the crystalline structure achieves its full mechanical properties.

Fiberglass casts substitute a polyurethane resin for the plaster. A fabric carrier is used for structural integrity, and water is used to initiate the polymerization process. Fiberglass is more expensive than plaster and more difficult to mold. Its advantages include radiolucency, improved strength, decreased weight, improved endurance, and water resistance.

Porous Materials

Porous materials that allow the ingrowth of bone, and the biologic development of a mechanical interlock between bone and prosthesis are an alternative to cement for the fixation of prosthetic devices. Metals, polymers, and ceramics in porous forms have been investigated for this purpose. Metallic porous materials have attained the greatest acceptance.

Porous materials usually are used as a surface layer that is bonded onto a central load-bearing stem to form a composite prosthetic device. Porous metal surface coatings have been manufactured by attaching preformed beads or fibers to a prosthesis component or by flame spraying techniques in which molten metal is sprayed at high velocity at a surface and forms a rough, porous coat. Each of these techniques involves a heating operation called sintering, which is necessary to bond the porous layer to the solid portion of the prosthetic device. Points of contact between particles and between the particles and the solid substrate become metallic bonds. The size and shape of the particles and their degree of compaction determine the eventual diameter of the pores and interconnecting channels. Multiple layers or beads usually are used for Co-Cr prostheses, whereas fiber metallurgy techniques are more suitable for nonalloyed titanium. The fibers are cut to a short length, kinked, and consolidated by compaction in dies. The sintering temperature and time, and the surrounding atmosphere control the bond formed between the coating and the base component. Sintering parameters also have a profound effect on the structure and properties of the solid alloy. Grain growth and a general degradation of mechanical properties occur as a result of the solid alloy's exposure to high temperatures. With Co-Cr alloys, the final product has properties that are similar to those of cast Co-Cr alloy, the strength of which is much inferior to that obtained by forging or hot isostatic pressing. Degradation also occurs with titanium and is of serious concern because of the high notch sensitivity of titanium. Careful control of the sintering conditions is required to minimize this effect. Commercially-pure titanium fibers are often diffusion bonded onto titanium alloy components. Consideration must be given to the mechanical properties of the solid metal alloys whenever a sintering process is included in the manufacture of a prosthesis. Failure to recognize this potential problem has resulted in stem fractures that could have been avoided.

One serious concern regarding the use of porous ingrowth fixation is the development of secondary osteoporosis in the surrounding femoral cortex. This development has been documented following femoral head surface replacements, segmental long bone implants, and total joint arthroplasties in animal models. The mechanical properties of the porous layer may play a significant role, along with the stiffness of the underlying stem, in the resulting remodeling process. Studies involving softer, more flexible porous layers of various types, including meshes, fabrics, and porous plastics, have yielded mixed results.

Important considerations in the use of metallic porous material are the expanded surface areas present and the potential for crevice corrosion with significant metal ion migration into the surrounding tissues. Biocompatibility and corrosion resistance of the alloys used are important design considerations. Titanium migration has been found following long-term implantation of titanium fiber composites; concentrations of titanium ions in the urine and the lungs were found to be up to six times greater than in the controls. Similar results have been found in studies involving cobalt-chromium alloys. Although toxic effects from titanium ion migration have not been shown, the large surface areas seen with porous materials and the resultant increase in metal ion release are causes for concern. Stainless steel, because of its known propensity for crevice corrosion, is not a suitable candidate for use in porous-coated devices. Many clinical trials of total joint prostheses designed for cementless implantation, whether or not approved for that application, are underway. The results of these experiments will allow the assessment of the proper indications for the use of porous-coated implants for biologic fixation.

Biodegradable Materials

Bioabsorbable materials have been used in surgery as sutures for several decades. The manufacturing process, applications, degradation reactions, and biochemical interactions with living tissues have been described extensively in the general surgery and specialty literature. Therefore, suture materials will not be dealt with in this chapter.

Terminology is not yet standardized in this evolving field of materials science but the differences between the terms bioabsorbable, biodegradable, and bioresorbable, which are often used synonymously, should be pointed out. Biodegradable refers to any material that breaks down when placed in a biologic environment. Obviously, this is a function of both the material and the environment chosen. A material that is biodegradable in one physiologic condition might not be in another. While all three terms typically apply to polymers, a metal that corrodes in vivo is a biodegradable material. Bioresorbable specifies a material that not only is broken down in vivo but also is removed from the site, whereas bioabsorbable denotes a material whose breakdown products are incorporated into normal physiologic and biochemical processes. The distinctions are important in some applications and when discussing toxicity of materials and their degradation products. Naturally, most research has focused on bioabsorbable materials. In addition to the loss of mechanical properties with degradation, concern must also be given to the metabolic load imposed by the absorption of the breakdown products of these materials.

Attempts to use absorbable materials for fracture fixation have been, and continue to be, motivated by the disadvantages of rigid plate fixation—stress shielding and subsequent weakening of the underlying bone, the stress risers created in cortical bone by empty screw holes left after removal of the hardware, and the increased risk of infection associated with long-term implantation of a metallic object. Avoiding the risks and costs associated with hardware removal surgery is another advantage to using bioabsorbable devices.

The major difficulties in developing a reliable bioabsorbable fracture fixation device have been the relatively low strength of the available materials and the rapid rate at which the mechanical properties degrade. Progress has been made toward developing stronger materials by the use of composite technology. Attempts to retard the degradation rate are a current research focus. Only a few materials have been used extensively in experimental studies of bioabsorbable materials for the fixation of fractures, and each will be discussed briefly.

Polyglycolic/Polylactic Acids

The first absorbable suture approved for human clinical use was polyglycolic acid (PGA).

$$-\left[-CH_2-\overset{\overset{\displaystyle O}{\|}}{C}-O-\right]_n-$$

The biocompatibility of this material, at least in small amounts, has been documented thoroughly. PGA at high molecular weights is a hard, tough, crystalline polymer with a melting point of 224°C. It is insoluble in most solvents, but slowly hydrolyzes in water to glycolic acid, which is then enzymatically transformed to glyoxylate and subsequently to glycine. The glycine is used in protein synthesis or the synthesis of serine, which becomes pyruvate and is incorporated into the tricarboxylic acid cycle. The initial, and rate determining, hydrolysis occurs by the same method in vivo and in vitro.

Polylactic acid (PLA) also has a long history of clinical use as a suture material.

$$\left[-\underset{\displaystyle CH}{\overset{}{CH}}- \overset{\displaystyle O}{\overset{\|}{C}} - O - \right]_n$$

PLA undergoes hydrolytic deesterification into lactic acid, which becomes incorporated into the tricarboxylic acid cycle and is excreted as carbon dioxide by the lungs. Lactic acid contains a chiral center at the α-carbon, and the enzymatic biochemistry recognizes only the levorotatory form. Devices designed to be absorbed and excreted must be of this isomer. This material is often specified as poly-l-lactic acid or PLLA, but even when not explicitly stated, it can be assumed that polylactic acid used for implants refers to the levorotatory isomer. Much of the mechanical testing of PGA and PLA materials, and numerous copolymers of the two, have involved sutures in which material characterization is complicated by several processing variables (such as draw ratio, draw speed, and degree of orientation) as well as the standard variables important to polymer testing (molecular weight, crystallinity, strain rate, etc.).

Bulk PGA is much less stiff than metallic fracture fixation devices. This lower stiffness has the potential to increase load sharing by the bone and, thereby, decrease stress shielding and cortical osteoporosis. As the PGA material is slowly degraded and absorbed, it is replaced by bone; at no time is there an empty screw hole to act as a stress riser. The mechanical properties of PGA deteriorate over a period of four to six weeks. Bulk PLA is less stiff than PGA but has the advantage of a much longer degradation time, between six and 12 months. Numerous copolymers of PGA and PLA have been developed and tested to find a polymer system that optimizes both initial strength and strength retention.

High molecular weight is crucial not only to material properties but also is found to decrease the rate of degradation. Low temperature annealing increases crystallinity and slows biodegradation. Residual monomer and sterilization by irradiation degrade polymers and result in faster loss of mechanical characteristics, but ethylene oxide sterilization does not cause polymer degradation.

Experiments with skeletal applications of PGA and PLA devices have been ongoing for almost 20 years, first in maxillofacial reconstruction and then in orthopaedics. Fracture healing continues virtually unaffected by these materials and their degradation by-products. Good clinical results have been achieved with rapidly healing fractures.

Research has focused on ways to enhance the strength of these materials and on ways to slow the loss of properties under physiologic conditions. The material properties, particularly bending and torsional strength, of PGA have been greatly enhanced by the formation of self-reinforced composites in which oriented fibers of PGA suture are compacted and subjected to differential melting. This gives a rigid, fiber-reinforced composite without any chemical discontinuity at the fiber-matrix interface. Self-reinforced PGA rods have achieved a bending modulus up to 17 GPa with a bending strength of 400 MPa and a shear strength of 250 MPa. Extensive clinical experience with malleolus fractures and a small series of other fractures has been mostly positive. The aseptic serous drainage seen with PGA sutures has been reported in about 15% of these patients as a closed, serous bursitis, usually over portions of rod that have not been imbedded in bone. The intraosseous reaction is uniformly benign.

Polyorthoesters

Active research continues into a group of polymers with a phosphoester linkage in the backbone of the chain.

$$\left[-C_6H_4-\underset{\displaystyle CH_3}{\overset{\displaystyle CH_3}{\overset{|}{\underset{|}{C}}}}-C_6H_4-O-\underset{\displaystyle R}{\underset{|}{\overset{\displaystyle O}{\overset{\|}{P}}}}-O- \right]_n$$

The pentavalent phosphorus allows for a wide range of aliphatic and aromatic side chains (R) that can be modified to achieve the desired physical and material properties. These polymers degrade by hydrolytic cleavage of the phosphoester. The side chain affects the degradation rate by limiting access to the cleavage site; therefore, both properties and endurance can be controlled to some extent. A material with adequate strength and strength retention has yet to be developed, but the research continues.

Carbon Fiber

Carbon and carbon composites have all shown a high degree of tissue compatibility. Carbon fibers and carbon fiber-reinforced composites have been used to replace ligaments, and they have had mixed success in inducing the growth of new fibrous tissue. Abrasion during functional loading has led to debonding of the carbon fibers and subsequent synovitis and/or lymph node infiltration. The compatibility of carbon with tissues and with numerous polymers encourages further work with this class of materials.

Calcium Phosphate Ceramics

Biodegradable calcium phosphate ceramics have been used to fill osseous defects, and they serve well as a scaffold for the ingrowth of bone. Their brittle nature and structural weakness have prevented these materials from finding a use in fracture fixation devices.

Selected Bibliography

General

Asher MA (ed): *Orthopaedic Knowledge Update I: Home Study Syllabus.* Chicago, IL, American Academy of Orthopaedic Surgeons, 1984.

Black J: *Orthopaedic Biomaterials in Research and Practice.* New York, Churchill Livingstone, 1988.

Fitzgerald RH, Jr (ed): *Orthopaedic Knowledge Update II: Home Study Syllabus.* Park Ridge, IL, American Academy of Orthopaedic Surgeons, 1987.

Frymoyer JW (ed): *Orthopaedic Knowledge Update IV: Home Study Syllabus.* Rosemont, IL, American Academy of Orthopaedic Surgeons, 1993.

Park JB: *Biomaterials Science and Engineering.* New York, Plenum Press, 1984.

Poss R (ed): *Orthopaedic Knowledge Update III: Home Study Syllabus.* Park Ridge, IL, American Academy of Orthopaedic Surgeons, 1990.

von Recum AF (ed): *Handbook of Biomaterials Evaluation: Scientific, Technical and Clinical Testing of Implant Materials.* New York, Macmillan, 1986.

Materials Science

Crandall SH, Dahl NC, Lardner TJ: *An Introduction to the Mechanics of Solids,* ed 2. New York, McGraw-Hill, 1978.

Ralls KM, Courtney TH, Wulff J: *Introduction to Materials Science and Engineering.* New York, John Wiley & Sons, 1976.

Van Vlack LH: *Elements of Materials Science and Engineering,* ed 6. Reading, MA, Addison-Wesley, 1989.

Tribological Properties

Dumbleton JH (ed): *Tribology of Natural and Artificial Joints.* Amsterdam, Elsevier Scientific Publishing Co, 1981.

Lubrication and wear in living and artificial human joints. *Proc Inst Mech Eng* 1967;181:part 3J.

McKellop HA, Clarke IC: Evolution and evaluation of materials-screening machines and joint simulators in predicting in vivo wear phenomena, in Ducheyne P, Hastings GW (eds): *Functional Behavior of Orthopedic Biomaterials: Applications.* Boca Raton, FL, CRC Press, 1984, vol 2, pp 51–86.

Mow VC, Soslowsky LJ: Friction, lubrication, and wear of diarthrodial joints, in Mow VC, Hayes WC (eds): *Basic Orthopaedic Biomechanics.* New York, Raven Press, 1991, pp 245–292.

Rabinowicz E: *Friction and Wear of Materials.* New York, John Wiley & Sons, 1965.

Metals

American Society for Testing and Materials: *Annual Standards,* vol 13.01, Philadelphia, American Society for Testing and Materials, 1990.

Fontana MG, Greene ND: *Corrosion Engineering,* ed 2. New York, McGraw-Hill, 1978.

Polymers

Charnley J: *Acrylic Cement in Orthopaedic Surgery.* Baltimore, Williams and Wilkins, 1970.

Lautenschlager EP, Stupp BI, and Keller JE: Structure and properties of acrylic bone cement, in Ducheyne P, Hastings GW (eds): *Functional Behavior of Orthopedic Biomaterials: Applications.* Boca Raton, FL, CRC Press, 1984, vol 2, pp 87–120.

Saha S, Pal S: Mechanical properties of bone cement: A review. *J Biomed Mater Res* 1984;18:435–462.

Ceramics

Jarcho M: Calcium phosphate ceramics as hard tissue prosthetics. *Clin Orthop* 1981;157:259–278.

Zarb GA, Schmitt A: Implant materials, in O'Brien WJ (ed): *Dental Materials: Properties and Selection.* Chicago, Quintessence, 1989, pp 449–459.

Porous Materials

Fitzgerald RH Jr (ed): *Non-Cemented Total Hip Arthroplasty.* New York, Raven Press, 1988.

Lemons JE (ed): *Quantitative Characterization and Performance of Porous Implants for Hard Tissue Applications.* Philadelphia, American Society for Testing and Materials, 1987, Series: ASTM STP; 953.

Biodegradable Materials

Böstman OM: Absorbable implants for the fixation of fractures. *J Bone Joint Surg* 1991;73A:148–153.

Hirvensalo E: *Absorbable Synthetic Self-Reinforced Polymer Rods in the Fixation of Fractures and Osteotomies.* Helsinki, Valmmala, 1990.

Vainionpää S: *Biodegradation and Fixation Properties of Biodegradable Implants in Bone Tissue.* Helsinki, Multiprint, 1987.

Chapter 11
Conditions Affecting Orthopaedic Surgical Practice

Thomas A. Einhorn, MD
Tyler S. Lucas, MD
Robert W. Molinari, MD
Louis Flancbaum, MD
Jean C. Burge, PhD
John L. Esterhai, Jr, MD
Dempsey S. Springfield, MD
Lawrence B. Bone, MD

Chapter Outline

Introduction

The health and disease of musculoskeletal tissue are influenced by changes in the structure and function of the tissue and by alterations in other organ complexes. As such, injury and repair mechanisms in bone, cartilage, tendon, and ligament can affect vascular, cardiopulmonary, hematologic, and immunologic functions. The nutritional toll that musculoskeletal injury or elective surgery exacts on the body may also influence tissue healing. Osteomyelitis, implant infections, and the general prevention and treatment of musculoskeletal sepsis remain ever present concerns in daily clinical practice.

This chapter will address the basic scientific principles that underlie the interactions between various organ complexes and the musculoskeletal system. While it is not possible to present an exhaustive discussion of the subject in this space, the more common and relevant conditions that impact on orthopaedic surgical practice will be addressed.

Thromboembolic Disease

Venous thromboembolism remains a major cause of morbidity and mortality among adults after lower extremity orthopaedic surgery. Each year an estimated 700,000 Americans experience asymptomatic pulmonary embolism and 200,000 die from this complication. Approximately 70,000 of these deaths occur within one hour of the appearance of symptoms. The magnitude of thromboembolic risk has been well documented in the orthopaedic literature. Patients undergoing hip surgery have the highest risk of mortality; without anticoagulation therapy, as many as 75% will show deep vein thrombosis by radiographic criteria and as many as 20% will develop clinically significant pulmonary embolism with a mortality of 1% to 3%. Patients undergoing knee surgery are at significant risk as well; without anticoagulation therapy, as many as 80% will show deep vein thrombosis by radiographic criteria and pulmonary embolism will develop in approximately 8% of cases. Fatal pulmonary embolism is less common after knee surgery, occurring in less than 1% of patients (Table 1).

Survival after a thromboembolic event depends heavily on whether the diagnosis is made early and the therapy is started promptly (Fig. 1). Most patients who die from pulmonary embolism will have had an otherwise favorable prognosis for their preexisting medical condition, and in these cases, pulmonary embolism is a potentially preventable complication.

The pathophysiology by which venous thromboembolism develops depends on the interaction between biochemical and physiologic events within a specific anatomic milieu. Therefore, this complication must be discussed within the context of defined anatomic sites. Unless otherwise stipulated, this chapter will refer to venous thromboembolic events that occur in the lower extremities after total knee or hip arthroplasty or long bone or hip fracture surgery.

Table 1
Frequency of fatal pulmonary embolism and deep vein thrombosis (diagnosed by venography)

Unprotected Patients	Deep Vein Thrombosis	Fatal Pulmonary Embolism
Elective hip arthroplasty	70%	2%
Elective knee arthroplasty	80%	1%
Open meniscectomy	20%	?
Hip fracture	60%	3.5%
Spine fracture with paralysis	100%	~1%
Polytrauma patients	35%	?
Pelvic/acetabular fracture	20%	?

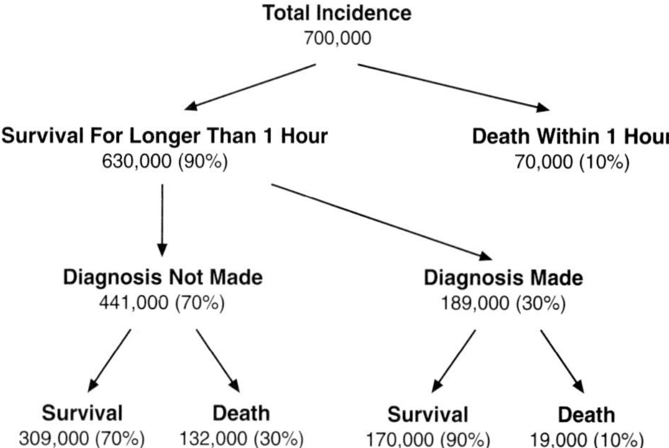

Figure 1
Survival rates in patients who have experienced asymptomatic pulmonary emboli.

Coagulation

The coagulation of blood entails the formation of fibrin through the interaction of more than a dozen proteins in a cascading series of proteolytic reactions (Fig. 2). At each step, a clotting factor undergoes limited proteolysis and itself becomes an active protease. Each clotting factor enzyme activates the next clotting factor until an insoluble fibrin clot is formed. Two initially independent pathways (the intrinsic and extrinsic pathways) for the initiation of clot formation converge to share a common clotting pathway. The extrinsic system, monitored clinically by the prothrombin time, is activated by the release of thromboplastin into the

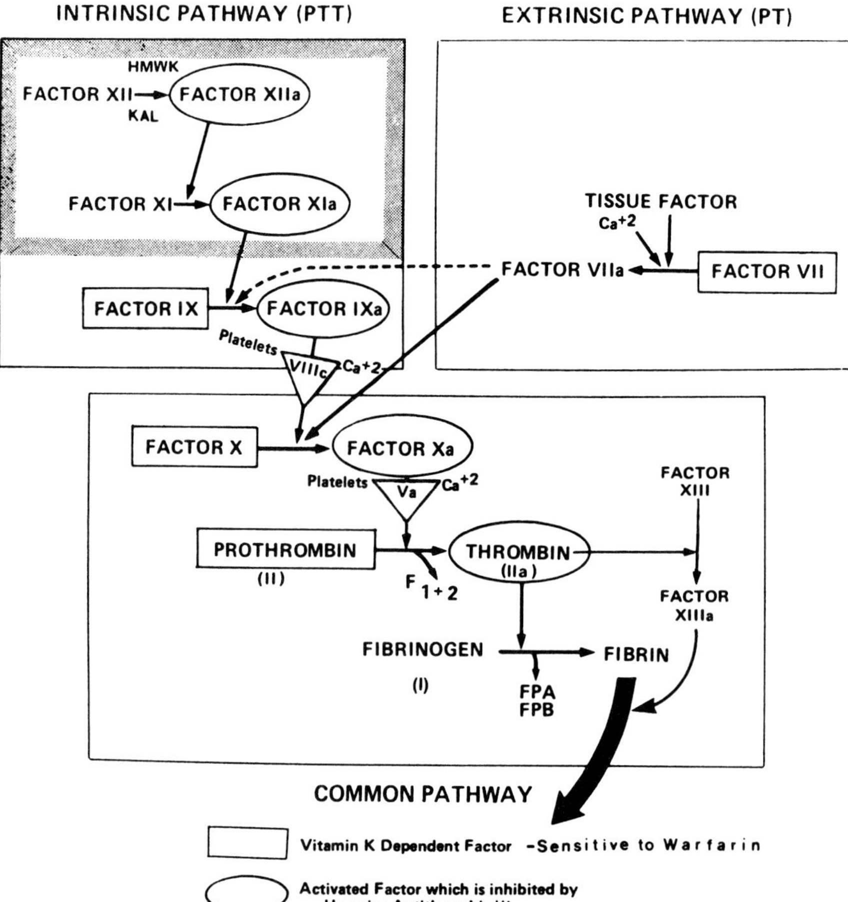

Figure 2
The coagulation pathways. Important features include the contact activation phase, vitamin K-dependent factors (affected by warfarin), and the activated serine proteases that are inhibited by heparin-antithrombin III. Prothrombin measures the function of the extrinsic and common pathways; the partial thromboplastin time measures the function of the intrinsic and common pathways. (Reprinted with permission from Stead RB: Regulation of hemostasis, in Goldhaber SZ (ed): *Pulmonary Embolism and Deep Venous Thromboembolism.* Philadelphia, WB Saunders, 1985, p 32.)

bloodstream during cell damage, as from bone and soft tissue during surgical dissection. The intrinsic pathway, monitored clinically by the partial thromboplastin time, is activated by the contact of factor XII with collagen on the exposed subendothelium of damaged vessels. This pathway may be further augmented through platelet-related mechanisms whereby platelets, which have been exposed to collagen or adenosine diphosphate, accelerate the activation of factors XI and XII. Both the intrinsic and extrinsic pathways lead to the formation of factor X. Prothrombin (factor II) is converted to thrombin by activated factor X in the presence of factor V, Ca^{2+}, and phospholipid. Thrombin then catalyzes the conversion of the soluble circulating substrate, fibrinogen (factor I), to fibrin. The clotting cascade can therefore be simplified into three "falls," or stages: (1) triggering of prothrombin-converting activity through the intrinsic or extrinsic pathways; (2) converting prothrombin to thrombin; and (3) converting fibrinogen to fibrin by the catalyzing activity of thrombin complex, during which an initially loose fibrin plug entangles to form a tight fibrin clot in the presence of factor XIII.

The fibrinolytic system prevents clot propagation and allows clot dissolution as healing takes place. In the normal state, there is a very delicate and precise balance between the coagulation and fibrinolytic systems. Without the action of the fibrinolytic system, the fibrin clot would propagate indefinitely. The key element in the fibrinolytic mechanism is the conversion of plasminogen to plasmin (Fig. 3). Plasmin dissolves the fibrin stroma and prevents the activation of certain coagulation factors. The tissue activators factor XIIA and thrombin must be present to convert plasminogen to plasmin so that the latter can act on fibrin, factor V, factor VIII, and fibrinogen.

Pathogenesis of Venous Thromboembolism

Many factors play a role in maintaining the delicate balance between the coagulation and fibrinolytic systems. Hypercoagulability, venous stasis, and endothelial damage, generally known as Virchow's triad of factors, leads to the generation of venous thrombosis.

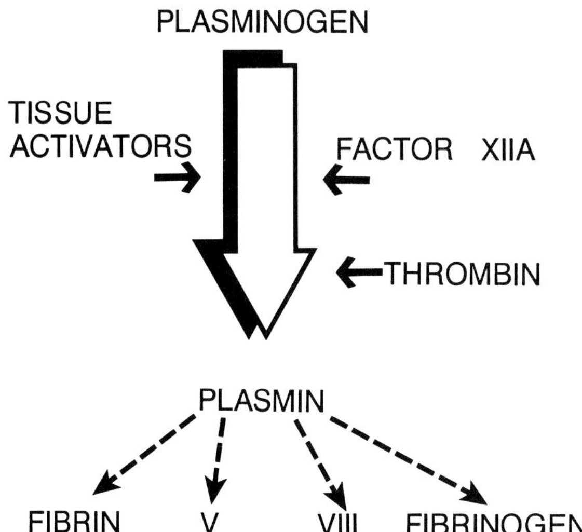

Figure 3
Schematic diagram of fibrinolytic mechanisms.

Hypercoagulability exists when coagulation dominates over fibrinolysis. Tissue trauma increases the levels of procoagulating substances, such as collagen fragments, tissue thromboplastin, and fibrinogen, in the plasma and enhances platelet activity and number. These changes tip the coagulation-fibrolytic system's balance toward coagulation and, eventually, venous thrombus formation. The patient is in a procoagulant state as soon as the surgical or traumatic event takes place, and thrombosis occurs during the surgical procedure.

Both the intrinsic and extrinsic coagulation systems have been implicated in studies concerning deep vein thrombosis and total hip replacement. A significant increase in the circulating levels of thromboplastin antigen has been noted during the reaming of the acetabulum, preparation of the femur, and impaction of the prosthesis, implicating the activation of the extrinsic system. Furthermore, an acute drop in the circulating levels of antithrombin III during and immediately after total hip replacement surgery has been reported. Antithrombin III is a naturally occurring inhibitor of thrombin, activated factor X, and possibly the other activated factors of the intrinsic system. The depletion of antithrombin III increases the amount of thrombin released during and immediately after surgery, thus creating a favorable environment for thrombus formation.

The classic view of deep vein thrombosis in the lower limb is that of a clot forming in the small veins of the calf, and then propagating proximally past the popliteal area into the larger veins of the thigh and pelvis. It has been demonstrated, however, that patients who undergo hip surgery often develop proximal thrombi de novo and that these thrombi may be more dangerous than those that occur in the calf.

Endothelial damage and venous stasis, the two remaining components of the triad, have been documented during hip surgery. Several investigators have demonstrated microscopic evidence of endothelial damage associated with total hip replacement. They postulated that endothelial tears are caused by excessive venodilation (resulting from venous smooth muscle relaxation due to bloodborne vasoactive substances), which leads to cell separation and exposure of subendothelial collagen. Filling of the long saphenous vein has been shown to increase during hip dislocation, suggesting a pressure differential across the twisted part of the vein and increasing vasodilation distally as a result of increased intraluminal pressure. Routine anesthetics, inactivity, and positioning also can have a vasodilatory effect.

Platelets also play a central role in the development of a thrombus because their adhesiveness and activity are increased after tissue trauma. Platelets accumulate behind small valve cusps, where the blood flows more slowly. An aggregated nidus develops, over which fibrin forms; as fibrin accumulates across the vessel, a clot develops (Fig. 4). Platelets also adhere and accumulate in the areas where the subendothelial portions of the veins have been damaged. In addition, fibrin formation is more easily triggered if blood contains procoagulant substances secondary to tissue trauma (Fig. 5).

Once vascular damage has occurred and the vessel endothelium has been exposed, the clotting cascade is set into motion. Although clot development may be initiated by these events, it is not known how long a clot continues to propagate and enlarge. Moreover, it is unclear how the use of antithrombotic drugs and physical modalities alter this process. It is well known, however, that physical inactivity significantly favors clot propagation, because venous perfusion tends to be reduced. Physical activity leads to increased blood flow. In an area that is perfused with fresh blood, there is a relative dilution in the concentration of activated coagulation, and an exposure of these factors to their natural biochemical inhibitors.

Surgery, trauma, obesity, malignancy, myocardial infarction, congestive heart failure, older age, and oral contraceptive use are well known risk factors for venous thrombosis. Outline 1 lists intrinsic and extrinsic risk factors. Thus, these risk factors (extensive surgery, trauma, burns, for example) cause vascular damage, which activates the coagula-

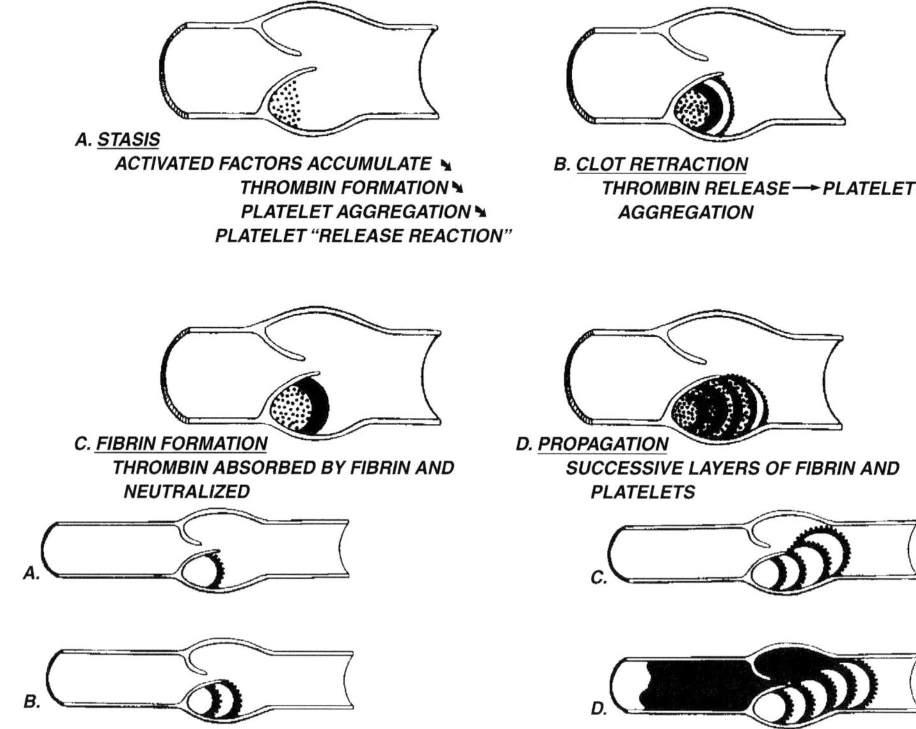

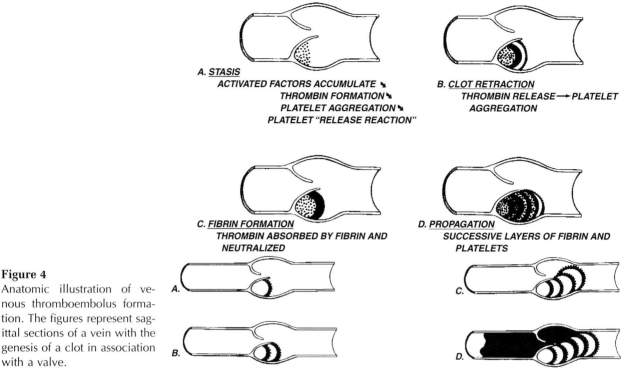

Figure 4
Anatomic illustration of venous thromboembolus formation. The figures represent sagittal sections of a vein with the genesis of a clot in association with a valve.

PATHHOGENESIS

PLATELET NIDUS

STATSIS → PLATELET ADHESIVENESS → PLATELET AGGREGATION → RELEASE ACTION

HYPERACTIVE PLATELETS → INITIATION OF INTRALUMINAL COAGULATION → PROTECTION OF ACTIVE CLOTTING ACTIONS → CATALYSIS OF INTRINSIC REACTIONS → THROMBIN → FIBRIN

FIBRIN → RELEASE ACTION → CATALYSIS OF INTRINSIC REACTIONS

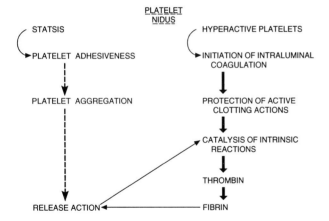

Figure 5
Flow diagram of the formation of postoperative venous thrombosis.

Outline 1
Risk factors for thromboembolism after surgery or trauma

- Intrinsic factors
  - Age
  - History of prior thromboembolism
  - Varicose veins
  - Malignant tumors
  - Oral contraceptive use
  - Inherited factors
  - Congestive heart failure
  - Smoking
  - Obesity
- Extrinsic factors
  - Increased blood viscosity
  - Extent of tissue trauma
  - Immobility
  - Lower extremity or pelvic involvement
  - Paralysis

tion pathways. In hip surgery, for example, this may occur locally as a result of damage to the wall of the femoral vein. In patients with disseminated malignant disease, studies have shown that extracts of malignant tumor cells contain cysteine proteases, which may activate factor X directly, thus accelerating the conversion of prothrombin to thrombin.

Venous thrombosis in the lower extremities can develop in the superficial leg veins, the deep veins of the calf (calf vein thrombosis), the deep veins above the knee (popliteal vein thrombosis), and the more proximal veins in the thigh (proximal vein thrombosis). Thromboses of the superficial veins generally occur in varicosities and are usually benign and self-limiting. Deep calf vein thrombosis is less serious than proximal vein thrombosis because the thrombi are smaller and less frequently associated with clinical disability or major complications.

When patients with venous thrombosis develop local symptoms, the symptoms usually occur as a result of large occlusive thrombi and approximately 80% of these are located in the proximal veins of the thigh, or extend into the popliteal region. Pulmonary embolism occurs more frequently in patients with proximal vein thrombosis compared with patients with calf vein thrombosis. Most clinically significant and fatal emboli arise from thrombi in the proximal veins of the leg.

Natural History of Thrombosis and Embolization

Once a thrombus has formed, it will evolve in one of three ways. (1) The thrombus will undergo partial or complete lysis, ultimately with complete or near complete recanalization of the thrombosed blood vessel. (2) The thrombus will become more organized, resulting in further occlusion of the vessel. (3) The thrombus will become dislodged, in whole or in part, and carried to a proximal site in the vascular system as an embolus.

Changes that lead to the eventual dissolution of a thrombus are already manifest within 48 hours of formation. In these situations, the platelet mass will become loose, fibrin will extend into the spaces between the platelet remnants, and neutrophils and monocytes will invade the thrombus mass and begin phagocytosis. After one week, up to 10% patency may be reestablished. As the process continues and endothelial cells proliferate and begin to extend over the receding thrombus mass, 50% to 70% patency may be achieved after 12 weeks.

Prophylaxis in Thromboembolic Disease

Several prophylactic regimens have been proposed to prevent and limit the development of thromboembolic disease. The best method of prophylaxis is yet to be determined; the literature provides conflicting information on the various drug regimens. The American Academy of Orthopaedic Surgeons recommends some form of prophylaxis for all patients who undergo total hip surgery.

Heparin

The use of heparin in the treatment of thromboembolic disease is directed at hypercoagulation. Heparin, which is derived from porcine and bovine lung tissue, is a heterogeneous mixture of polysaccharide chains of varying molecular weights. As a highly charged anion, heparin binds to antithrombin III and enzymatically increases by a factor of 1,000 its affinity for factor Xa and thrombin, both elements of the common coagulation pathway. Although heparin does not lyse clots directly, it decreases coagulation, which allows the fibrinolytic system to lyse clots more effectively. Less heparin is required to neutralize factor Xa than to neutralize the thrombin that is produced once the thrombotic process has begun. This is the rationale for the prophylactic antithrombotic regimens in which heparin is administered subcutaneously in very low doses. Heparin molecules larger than 5,000 to 8,000 daltons may affect platelet interactions, leading to hemorrhagic side effects. As a result, preparations of low-molecular-weight heparin have become increasingly popular.

The precise clinical control of heparin's effects is difficult. Peak plasma levels occur anywhere from two to four hours after subcutaneous injection, and the half-life is highly variable. In addition, partial thromboplastin time, which is used to monitor heparin's effect on the intrinsic system, also varies significantly because of laboratory reagents and protocol differences. Therefore, patients placed on heparin therapy must be observed closely.

Low-Dose Heparin

Fixed, low-dose heparin is used to lessen the hypercoagulable state induced by the presence of factor Xa and thrombin and to allow normal clotting to take place. This regimen can be effective when started preoperatively because the concentration of factors is low and coagulation and fibrinolysis activities are balanced. Low-dose heparin administered after surgical activation of the clotting cascade is less effective because activated factor Xa has already stimulated production of a high level of thrombin.

The use of low-dose heparin in surgery has evolved into two standard regimens beginning with 5,000 U given subcutaneously and administered preoperatively, followed by 5,000 U administered two times per day. In early clinical trials of low-dose heparin therapy measured using fibrinogen scanning, there was an average decrease in the incidence of deep vein thrombosis from 25% to 7% when compared with placebo. However, in clinical trials using venography, low-dose heparin has been shown to be ineffective in prophylaxis, probably because 5,000 U administered twice daily has a subtherapeutic effect, and the same dose administered thrice daily carries the risk of overanticoagulation.

The difference in effectiveness of heparin prophylaxis noted between patients undergoing general surgery and those undergoing orthopaedic surgery may be related to the greater endothelial damage and venous stasis experienced in limb surgery.

Adjusted-Dose Heparin

Adjusted-dose heparin therapy for total hip replacement was developed when the failure of low-dose heparin became apparent. In regimens of two or three times daily, the adjusted dose schedule is intended to maintain the partial thromboplastin time in the upper range of normal (50 seconds). For a partial thromboplastin time less than four seconds above control, the heparin dose is increased by 500 U. No change is made for partial thromboplastin times between 5 and 7.5 seconds longer than control. Heparin is decreased by 1,000 U for partial thromboplastin times that are more than eight seconds longer than control.

Several published reports suggest that adjusted-dose heparin is effective in the prophylaxis of deep vein thrombosis and that it reduces by a factor of three the incidence of this problem compared with regimens using fixed, low dosages. The advantages of this regimen are the immediate onset of action, the ability to reverse the action with protamine, and the dosage schedule, which can be written as a titratable sliding scale. The disadvantage is that the partial thromboplastin time must be monitored daily.

Both normal and increased intraoperative and postoperative bleeding have been reported with adjusted-dose heparin. The incidence of postoperative wound hematoma or remote bleeding with heparin is approximately 8%. Severe cases can be reversed with protamine sulfate infusion. Conventional heparin preparations have the potential to stimulate platelet aggregation and are associated with a small decrease in the platelet count in 30% of cases. Severe heparin-associated thrombocytopenia and arterial thrombosis are rare complications.

Heparin-Dihydroergotamine

Dihydroergotamine, when given subcutaneously in low doses, directly stimulates venous smooth muscle, causing venous constriction. In addition, dihydroergotamine prevents excessive intraoperative venodilation and postoperative venous pooling. The administration of 0.5 mg of dihydroergotamine subcutaneously produces approximately 4 mm of femoral venoconstriction (from 16 mm to 12 mm) and 2 mm of popliteal venoconstriction (from 18 mm to 16 mm). Several studies have used venography to demonstrate that the incidence of proximal vein clot formation is decreased in treated patients. This suggests that the venoconstrictive effects of dihydroergotamine lessen venous dilation and intimal wall damage. A combination of dihydroergotamine and heparin has been reported to effectively counter Virchow's triad and to reduce the risk of deep vein thrombosis by 50% when compared to fixed, low-dose heparin alone.

Contraindications to dihydroergotamine prophylaxis include hemodynamic instability, sepsis, compromised hepatic or renal function, recent arterial surgery, age younger than 40 years, peripheral vascular disease, and coronary artery disease. In Europe, proponents of dihydroergotamine therapy report that the incidence of vasospasm is only 0.003% annually, probably because they strictly adhere to contraindications in its use.

A theoretical drawback to the use of dihydroergotamine has been the risk of arterial vasospasm, causing ischemia or ergotism. Nine cases of ergotism have been reported in the literature, although none were reported after less than six doses of dihydroergotamine.

The rationale for the use of heparin-dihydroergotamine is to counteract endothelial damage, venostasis, and platelet inhibition during total hip replacement. Because the highest risk of clot formation occurs when the hip is dislocated during this procedure, heparin-dihydroergotamine is administered by subcutaneous injection two hours before surgery. Dihydroergotamine alone is currently the only agent available to reduce the extent of subendothelial collagen damage. Dihydroergotamine is not currently available for clinical use in the United States.

Low-Dose Warfarin

Warfarin interferes with the metabolism of vitamin K in the liver. Vitamin K is necessary for the synthesis of clotting factors II, VII, IX, and X. Specifically, vitamin K is required as a cofactor for the liver microsomal enzymes, which catalyze the gamma-carboxylation of certain glutamate residues in the precursor proteins for these clotting factors. Gamma-carboxyglutamyl residues must be present in the clotting factors for the normal activation of prothrombin, a process that is mediated by calcium ions and phospholipids. The clotting factors in patients who receive warfarin lack this biologic activity and thus have a reduced thrombotic potential. In order to act as a cofactor, vitamin K must be transformed to a quinone and then to hydroxyquinone. Warfarin blocks both transformations, probably by the noncompetitive inhibition of epoxide reductase, the enzyme responsible for this transformation (Fig. 2).

Factor VII has the shortest half-life and is the first clotting factor to be affected by warfarin therapy. The prothrombin time, which is used to measure the activity of the extrinsic coagulation system, is directly prolonged by the inactivity of factor VII. The time is affected in the early stages of warfarin therapy, before the common coagulation pathway is inhibited. There is a window of vulnerability during the first three to five days, where the prothrombin time may be prolonged but no true anticoagulation protection exists.

Oral warfarin is absorbed rapidly from the alimentary tract. It is bound almost wholly in plasma and is metabolized entirely in the hepatic microsomes. The action of warfarin can be reversed by a massive dose of vitamin K in the inactive, oxi-

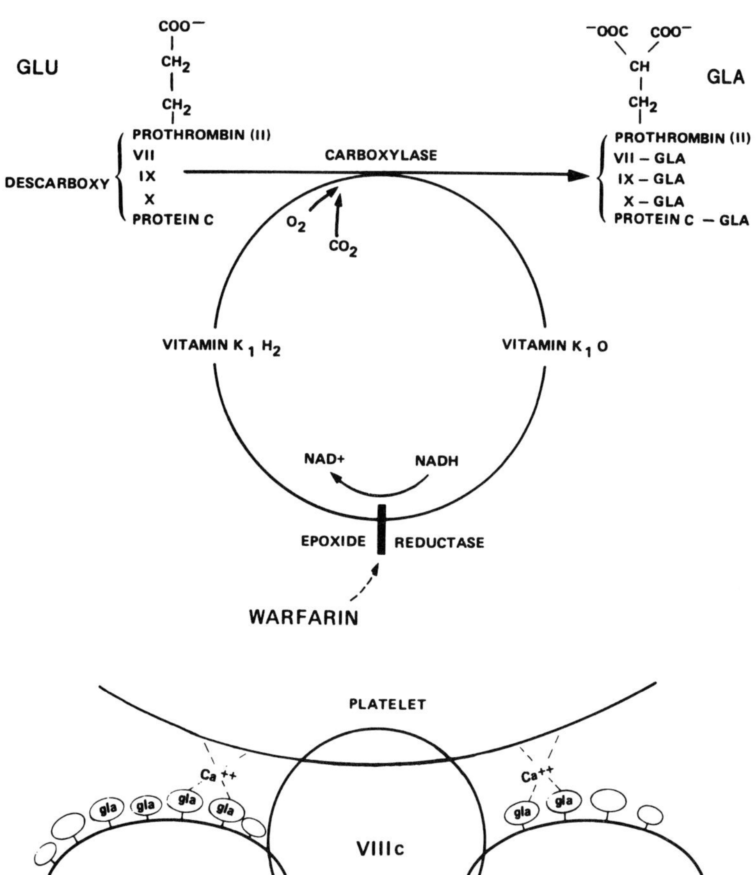

Figure 6
The mechanism of action of warfarin. Warfarin inhibits the reduction of the oxidized storage form of vitamin K_1. The reduced form (K_1H_2) functions as a co-enzyme in the carboxylation of factors II, VII, IX, and X and proteins C and S. Carboxylation of the glutamic acid residues of the vitamin K-dependent factors must occur for effective coagulation of platelet and endothelial phospholipid templates. (Reprinted with permission from Stead RB: Clinical pharmacology, in Goldhaber SZ (ed): *Pulmonary Embolism and Deep Venous Thromboembolism.* Philadelphia, WB Saunders, 1985, p 107.)

dized form, which induces the NADH-dependent vitamin K quinone reductases. These enzymes are less sensitive to warfarin than is epoxide reductase, and they mediate the reduction of vitamin K to its active form (Fig. 6). The presence of an agent that potentiates vitamin K or antagonizes warfarin activity must be suspected whenever oral anticoagulation is difficult to control (Outline 2).

Several trials have demonstrated that warfarin decreases by between two and four times the incidence of deep vein thrombosis while decreasing the incidence of fatal pulmonary embolism to less than 1%. The risk of major hemorrhagic complications has been reported to range between 4% and 14%. The risk is directly proportional to the dosage and the elevation of the prothrombin time. This risk is reduced significantly if the target prothrombin time is limited to between 1.3 and 1.5 times that of control values. Based on current data, low-dose warfarin is as safe and efficacious as any other recommended prophylaxis. It is clearly superior in terms of cost-effectiveness when used either for 12 weeks without routine venography or for the postoperative hospital stay prophylaxis.

Outline 2
Pharmacologic agents that interact with warfarin anticoagulation

Potentiating agents
- Cefamandole
- Cimetidine
- Disulfuram
- Moxalactam
- Phenylbutazone
- Phenytoin
- Trimethoprim

Antagonists
- Cholestyramine
- Griseofulvin
- Phenobarbital
- Rifampin
- Vitamin K-rich foods

Low-Molecular-Weight Dextran

Dextran consists of partially hydrolyzed polymers of glucose that are obtained from the bacterium *Leuconostoc mesenteroides.* When added to blood, dextran is used as a plasma expander. It has no in vitro effect on platelet function; however, the bleeding time, polymerization of fibrin, and platelet function are impaired in vivo.

Infusions of dextran increase the colloid osmotic pressure. This effect makes this drug somewhat dangerous for use in patients with pulmonary edema, congestive heart failure, and decreased renal function. Dextran also is contraindicated in patients who have significant anemia, severe thrombocytopenia, or reduced concentrations of fibrinogen in plasma. Side effects include occasional urticaria, wheezing, tightness in the chest, mild hypotension, and, rarely, severe anaphylaxis. Bleeding is dose-dependent and occurs in 7% to 8% of cases.

Low-molecular-weight dextran appears to be as effective as warfarin in reducing the incidence of deep vein thrombosis. It is an alternative to heparin for patients who develop complications related to heparin therapy.

Aspirin

The efficacy of aspirin prophylaxis in orthopaedic surgery remains controversial. It is inexpensive, easy to administer, and does not require monitoring. It is used mainly as an antiplatelet agent. In vitro, aspirin reduces platelet adhesiveness to glass, interferes with platelet aggregation, and inhibits prostaglandin production and prostacyclin synthesis. The latter two actions have a paradoxical effect; that is, to prevent deep vein thrombosis.

Some have championed aspirin prophylaxis as an effective alternative for prophylactic anticoagulation. Although aspirin has been reported to be as effective as warfarin and dextran in preventing clinically important thromboembolic complications following total hip arthroplasty, these findings seem to be limited to men. Unfortunately, other researchers have been unable to reproduce these results, finding no difference between aspirin and placebo. A benefit from aspirin as a prophylactic agent in women has not been reported. On the basis of available published data, there is conflicting evidence that aspirin is effective in the prophylaxis of deep vein thrombosis in orthopaedic surgery.

Intermittent Pneumatic Compression

The benefits of intermittent pneumatic compression have been attributed to the prevention of venous stasis and an increase in fibrinolytic activity in plasma. Intermittent calf compression devices increase the emptying of the lower extremity veins and clearance of the valve sinuses. In addition, intermittent venous flow is high with these devices, thereby eliminating one component of Virchow's triad.

Intermittent pneumatic compression has been shown to reduce by a factor of two the rate of deep vein thrombosis compared with controls and to be comparable to warfarin for effective prevention of deep vein thrombosis in patients who undergo total hip surgery. The documented decreased rate of DVT in all hip surgery patients ranges anywhere from 3% to 27% when compared to controls.

Intermittent pneumatic compression is not expensive, nor is it associated with bleeding complications. Because intermittent pneumatic compression is beneficial at the time of application, it is useful as an early prophylactic treatment while a pharmacologic agent is producing its effect. The use of sequential compression devices alone in the lower extremity has been shown to be less effective in preventing DVT in patients who have abnormal preoperative venograms.

Diagnosis of Thromboembolic Disease

The sensitivity, specificity, and accuracy of the commonly used methods for diagnosis of thromboembolic disease vary considerably. These characteristics assist the practitioner in choosing the diagnostic procedure or test that will provide information required for successful treatment of a specific disease or condition. Sensitivity, specificity, and accuracy are expressed as a percent value and are defined in the following equations.

$$\text{sensitivity} = \frac{\text{no. true positives}}{\text{no. true positives} + \text{false negatives}} \times 100$$

$$\text{specificity} = \frac{\text{no. true negatives}}{\text{no. true negatives} + \text{false positives}} \times 100$$

$$\text{accuracy} = \frac{\text{no. true positives} + \text{true negatives}}{\text{total number}} \times 100$$

Although not used in this chapter, the positive and negative predictive values can quantitate test performance. In practice, the ability to predict the presence or absence of disease based on test results depends on the prevalence of the disease in the population tested, as well as on the sensitivity and specificity of the test. The higher or lower the prevalence, the more likely it is that a positive or negative test is predictive of the disease. This measure is referred to as the "predictive value."

$$\text{positive predictive value} = \frac{\text{no. true positives}}{\text{no. true positives} + \text{false positives}}$$

The positive predictive value is the proportion of diseased individuals among all those who have positive test results. Similarly, the negative predictive value is the proportion of nondiseased individuals among all those who have negative test results.

$$\text{negative predictive value} = \frac{\text{no. true negatives}}{\text{no. true negatives + false negatives}}$$

The first three terms described above are used to assist in the evaluation and choice of the diagnostic procedures or tests described below.

Physical Examination

The classical findings of pain, tenderness, swelling, and discomfort with passive dorsiflexion of the ankle (Homan's sign), or of a palpable cord in the thigh or calf are not specific for deep vein thrombosis. In fact, deep vein thrombosis can occur without any clinical symptoms or signs. Clinical examination carries a sensitivity of between 30% and 50% and a specificity of 50% for total hip replacement performed without prophylaxis.

Radiocontrast Venography

The diagnostic standard for the localization and characterization of deep vein thrombosis in the calf and thigh continues to be radiocontrast venography. The venogram has an accuracy of 97%, which decreases to approximately 70% for visualization of clots in the iliac veins. Approximately 4% of patients are not candidates for venography because there is no venous access. In addition, allergic hypersensitivity to the contrast agent precludes the use of this test in 0.02% of cases.

Duplex Ultrasonography

Duplex ultrasonography assesses the patency of a blood vessel using B-mode ultrasound and Doppler shift principals. The ultrasonic component provides an image of the blood vessel wall and its contents while the Doppler component measures the blood flow at a precise location in the vessel. The data obtained from this test provide both anatomic and physiologic information with regard to blood flow.

The test is performed with the patient lying comfortably in bed. The duplex probe is applied to the femoral triangle and is oriented to provide a longitudinal image of the common femoral vein just below the inguinal ligament. The Doppler gate is adjusted to lie in the center of the venous channel and is oriented such that its angle is parallel to the direction of blood flow. To test for the presence of blood clots within the vein, the examiner uses the probe to apply direct pressure on the vein such that the vessel wall is occluded. The orientation of the probe is then rotated until it is aligned perpendicular to the long axis of the vein and the test is then repeated. This procedure is repeated along the entire length of the vein.

A normal duplex ultrasonograph will result only if the probing maneuver will produce total collapse of the vessel walls. Partial compressibility or incompressibility in either the longitudinal or transverse directions will result in an abnormal test and is indicative of the presence of a thrombus. Incompressibility in both directions coupled with absence of Doppler evidence of blood flow is strong evidence for the presence of an occlusive thrombus. The test is generally applied to the entire extremity length of the common femoral, superficial femoral, and popliteal veins. In recent clinical trials, duplex ultrasonography showed an accuracy of more than 90% for diagnosing deep vein thrombosis proximal to the trifurcation of the popliteal artery.

Fibrinogen I 125 Labeling

Fibrinogen I 125 has an accuracy of 90% in detecting thrombosis of the calf after total hip replacement. However, because fibrin is present in the proximity of the surgical wound, this scan may be falsely positive in the thigh after hip surgery or in the calf after knee surgery. Fibrinogen I 125 is not a useful examination tool in these instances.

Impedance Plethysmography

Plethysmography records the changes either in the volume of arterial filling in an extremity after systolic contraction of the heart, or in the emptying of the fluid volume from an extremity during venous return. The normal plethysmographic recording will be altered when a vein is occluded by the presence of a thrombus.

The test is administered by inflating a pneumatic tourniquet and measuring fluid volume distal to the tourniquet before and after deflation. A change in limb dimension is measured by an impedance plethysmograph transducer and recorded. This procedure is repeated until a consistent outflow tracing is obtained. The presence of a venous thrombus will produce an abnormal tracing.

This technique has been shown to be useful in detecting thigh clots after hip surgery. However, a significant number of clots may go undetected by this method. In a prospective study of patients undergoing elective hip surgery, impedance plethysmography showed a sensitivity of 30% for large thigh thrombi demonstrated by routine venography. The sensitivity of impedance plethysmography is further reduced for the smaller thrombi in the thigh and calf and by the corresponding small gradient in venous flow. This method also has failed to detect iliac thrombi.

Doppler Imaging

Doppler imaging remains an inexpensive and easy immediate bedside diagnostic tool in the diagnosis of deep vein thrombosis. It has a relatively poor sensitivity in the asymptomatic high risk patient, and results tend to vary depending on the experience of the examiner. With an experienced examiner, the sensitivity of a good Doppler examination is approximately 70%.

Pulmonary Embolism

Pulmonary embolism results from the obstruction of the pulmonary artery or one of its branches by a clot or foreign body that has been brought to the site of lodgement by blood current. After the embolus has lodged and interrupted pulmonary blood flow, the ratio of regional ventilation to perfusion increases. The lung responds with bronchoconstriction to reduce wasted ventilation. This response is mediated by a local reduction in CO_2 output. Other vasoactive agents, such as histamine, serotonin, and prostaglandins, may play a role in this process, but the net effect is to reduce the size of peripheral airways, the lung volume, and the static pulmonary compliance. The hypoxemia that is associated with this ventilation-perfusion imbalance may show some improvement after supplemental oxygen is administered; however, the effects are usually minimal. Pulmonary infarction, as a consequence of embolism, is relatively rare and is associated clinically with problems of poor systemic perfusion, such as shock and congestive heart failure. The symptoms and signs of an embolic episode depend primarily on the size of embolus involved and on the cardiopulmonary status of the patient.

Pulmonary embolism can involve any combination of a broad spectrum of nonspecific associated symptoms and signs (Tables 2 and 3). Dyspnea is the most frequent symptom followed by pleuritic chest pain. Tachypnea is the most common clinical sign followed by rales, tachycardia, and fever of greater than 37°C. These symptoms and signs are nonspecific and must be interpreted in light of the risk factors for thromboembolism that each patient shows. Figure 7 shows a flow diagram for the workup and treatment of a patient suspected of having a pulmonary embolism.

Table 2
Symptoms in patients with pulmonary embolism

Symptoms	Percent
Dyspnea	-
Chest pain	-
Cough	53
Hemoptysis	16
Altered mental status	13
Dyspnea, Chest Pain, Cough	14

Table 3
Signs in patients with pulmonary embolism

Signs	Percent
Tachypnea	90
Tachycardia	59
Recent fever	43
Rales	42
Leg edema-tenderness	23
Elevated venous pressure	18
Shock	11
Accentuated PO_2	11
Cyanosis	9
Pleural rub	8

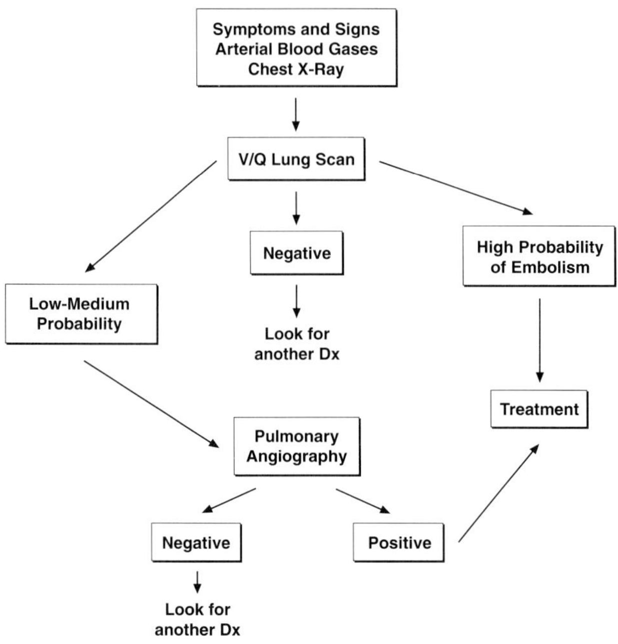

Figure 7
Treatment algorithm based on the clinical evaluation of a patient with suspected pulmonary embolism.

Diagnosis of Pulmonary Embolism

In any setting in which pulmonary embarrassment is suspected, an electrocardiogram will address the possibility of concomitant myocardial infarction. The electrocardiogram tends to show abnormalities characteristic of pulmonary embolism only in patients with extensive embolization. Changes such as ST segment depression, T wave inversions in lead III, increased P waves, right bundle branch block, or right axis deviation occur in only 25% of patients with documented pulmonary embolism.

A chest radiograph must be obtained. A radiograph that is normal in a severely dyspneic patient is strongly suggestive of pulmonary embolism. Classic radiologic abnormalities associated with massive pulmonary embolism include a relative local hyperlucency in a region of segmental arterial occlusion or an engorged hilar artery. The more common, highly nonspecific abnormalities include pleural effusion, atelectasis, or an elevated hemidiaphragm.

Arterial blood gas analysis measures pH, PCO_2, PO_2, HCO_3, the percent O_2 saturation, and temperature of blood. These data can be helpful in the management of patients with suspected pulmonary embolism, but they are not useful for the diagnosis because the findings are nonspecific in patients who have any preexisting pulmonary disease. Although an arterial PO_2 of less than 60 mm Hg is highly suggestive of respiratory distress, a normal PO_2 does not exclude the diagnosis of pulmonary embolism. Approximately 15% of patients with angiographically documented pulmonary emboli have a mean arterial PO_2 greater than 85 mm Hg.

Radionuclide ventilation-perfusion scanning (V/Q scan) is currently the most widely used diagnostic test for the detection of pulmonary embolism. The test charts the perfusion of technetium 99m-labeled human albumin isotope through the pulmonary tree. Areas of reduced perfusion as small as 2 cm in diameter can be detected. The specificity of this part of the test, however, is low, because disturbance in pulmonary flow from any cause can produce an abnormal scan. The test becomes more specific with the use of ^{99m}Tc-labeled microaerosols. When inhaled, these microaerosols disperse mainly to the peripheral airways. If the radioactive gas enters the areas of perfusion defects and then is cleared, this mismatch of ventilation and perfusion is characteristic of vascular obstruction. If, however, ventilation is also abnormal (ventilation-perfusion match), no reliable diagnostic conclusion can be reached and pulmonary angiography is required.

Pulmonary angiography is the reference standard by which the presence of pulmonary embolism can be established or excluded. The technique is invasive and requires specialized personnel. A radiopaque material is injected through a cardiac catheter that has been advanced into the pulmonary artery, affording direct visualization of the filling defect caused by pulmonary emboli. The presence of a constant intraluminal filling defect or a sharp cutoff in a vessel greater than 2.5 mm in diameter is diagnostic for pulmonary embolism.

Treatment of Pulmonary Embolism

Most patients who have had an acute episode of venous thrombosis and pulmonary embolism will be treated successfully by heparin followed by oral anticoagulant therapy with warfarin. The most widely used protocol calls for seven to ten days of continuous intravenous infusion of heparin. This therapy is monitored by the partial thromboplastin time. The frequency of clinically significant recurrence and the risk of major bleeding during this period are both less than 5%. This treatment is followed by three months of oral anticoagulant therapy with warfarin. Anticoagulation is monitored by the prothrombin time. The frequency of recurrence during this period is approximately 3%, and the risk of bleeding is between 2% and 20%. After three months, anticoagulant therapy is discontinued. With this protocol, the risk of recurrence over the following 12 months has been shown to be between 6% and 10%.

Shock

Shock is characterized by symptoms and signs that arise when the capillary blood flow is insufficient to perfuse vital organs and tissue. The four categories of shock are hypovolemic, cardiogenic, vasogenic, and neurogenic. Shock results when the normal physiologic operation of one or more of the following interrelated organs and mechanisms fails: (1) heart; (2) fluid or blood volume; (3) arteriolar resistance; and (4) capacity of the venous system (Fig. 8, *top*).

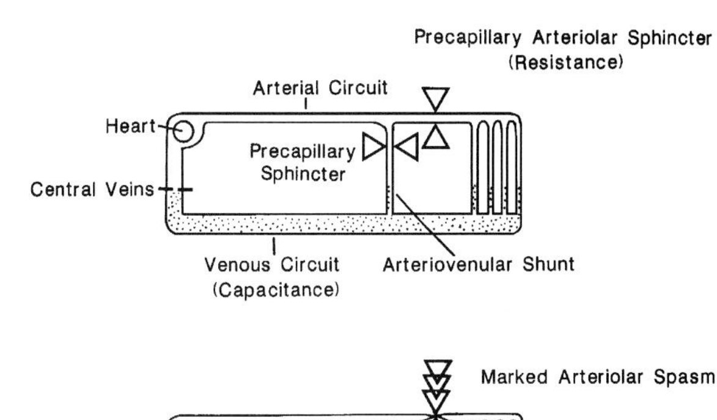

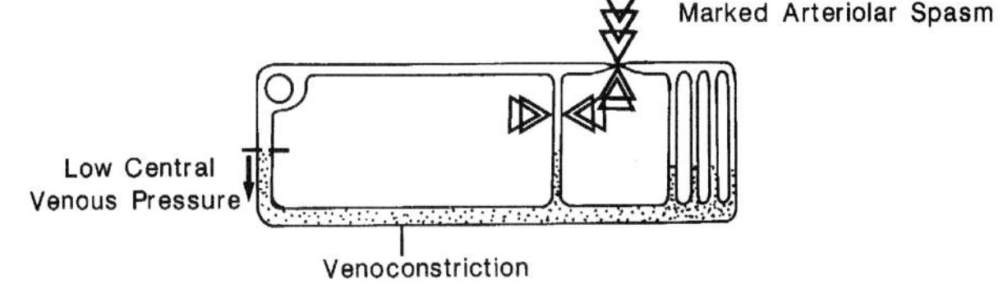

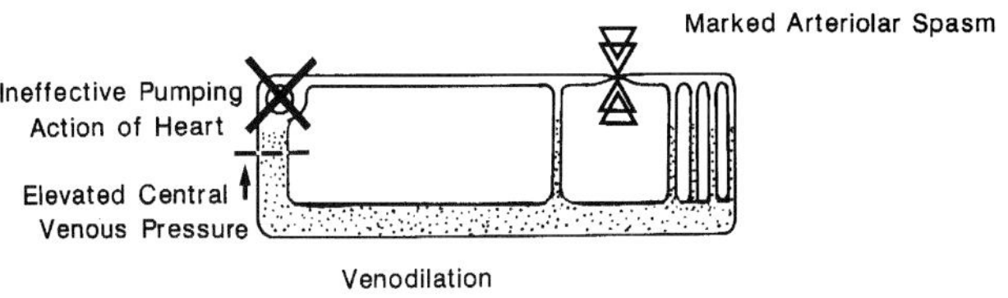

Figure 8
Schematic representation of physiologic compensatory reactions in hypovolemic shock.

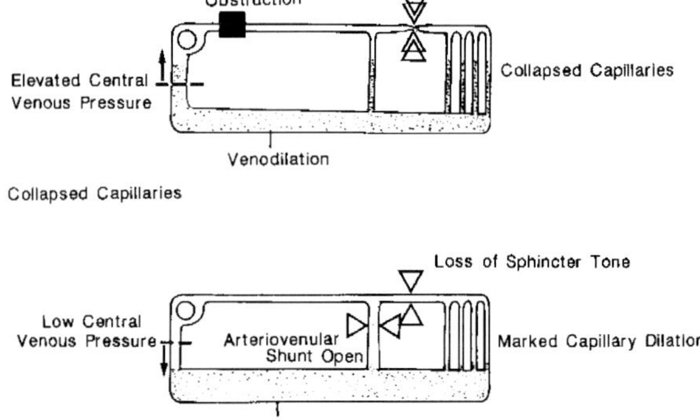

Figure 9
Schematic representation of physiologic compensatory reactions in hypovolemic shock.

In hypovolemic shock (Fig. 8, *center*), the low cardiac output results from limitation of diastolic filling and systolic emptying. When cardiac output falls, the arteriolar sphincters contract as a compensatory mechanism, increasing peripheral vascular resistance. At the same time, venous constriction forces more blood into the heart to maintain cardiac output. The degree of cardiac emptying in systole depends on the effectiveness of the systolic contraction, the arteriolar pressure against which ejection must occur, and the function of the valves and the rhythm of the heart.

In cardiogenic shock (Fig. 8, *bottom*), the ineffective pumping action of the heart leads to a loss of volume in the arterial system. Blood pressure is improved after peripheral vascular resistance is increased. Because the heart fails, a large volume of blood collects in the dilated venous system. Vasogenic shock, which develops from pulmonary emboli or pericardial tamponade, produces its result by the same mechanism; that is, dilated venous system and arteriolar constriction (Fig. 9, *top*).

Shock resulting from neurogenic causes or sepsis (Fig. 9, *bottom*) is characterized by venous and capillary dilation with pooling of blood, loss of the sphincter tone in the arterioles, and open arterial venous shunts.

Biochemical changes that occur in shock usually fall into three categories: (1) the pituitary-adrenal response to stress; (2) changes secondary to reduction in tissue perfusion; and (3) changes secondary to organ failure. The immediate effect of shock, adrenal sympathetic activity, is characterized by increased circulating epinephrine levels and can be documented by findings of eosinopenia, lymphocytopenia, and thrombocytopenia. At the same time, there is a striking negative nitrogen balance, retention of sodium and water, and increased excretion of potassium.

The algorithm shown in Figure 10 depicts neurohumoral control of volume restitution. Hypovolemia stimulates baroreceptors in the right atrium that relay impulses to the medullary nuclei and hypothalamus. The sympathetic nervous system responds with vasoconstriction and the release of cortisol and aldosterone by the adrenal gland, causing the kidney to retain fluids. Once initiated, these responses can be interrupted only by exogenous volume restoration in the form of intravenous fluids.

The changes secondary to the low-flow state result in decreased oxygen delivery to vital organs. Consequently, there is a shift from aerobic to anaerobic metabolism. An example of this shift is in the increase in lactic acid production.

The major organ involved in compensatory changes during shock is the kidney, because 25% of the cardiac output normally perfuses this organ. The kidney's response to hypovolemia is to release renin by the juxtaglomerular apparatus. Renin acts as an enzyme in the conversion of angiotensin (a hepatic

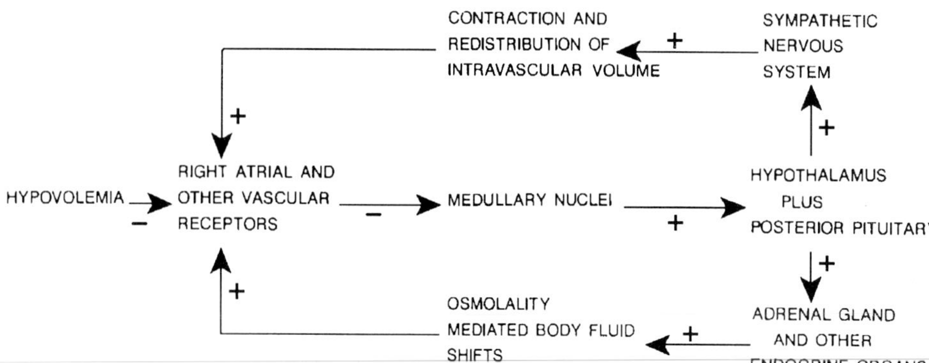

Figure 10
Schematic representation of the neurohumoral control of volume restitution in hypovolemic shock.

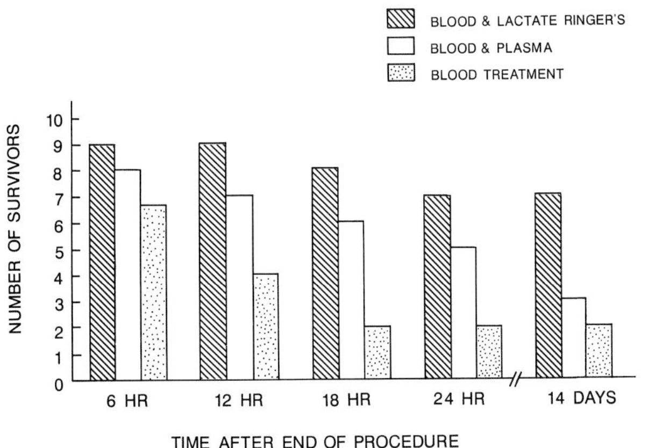

Figure 11
Survival after using crystalloid and/or colloid solution and blood replacement to restore extracellular volume.

α_2-globulin) to angiotensin I, which is converted to its active form, angiotensin II, by a converting enzyme in the lung. Angiotensin II, a potent vasoconstrictor, stimulates the adrenal cortex to secrete aldosterone, which increases the tubular reabsorption of sodium and water in an attempt to restore fluid volume. The bicarbonate concentration in plasma is the best single biochemical index of the adequacy of cardiac output relative to the body's needs. The bicarbonate level is calculated from the blood gas data on the basis of the measurement of PCO_2 and pH. In reversible hemorrhagic shock, the volume of the extracellular fluid decreases and shifts into the vascular tree and associated tissue cells. As noted in Figure 11, survival is improved by using crystalloid and/or colloid solution and blood replacement to restore fluid volume.

Adult Respiratory Distress Syndrome and Fat Embolism

The adult respiratory distress syndrome (ARDS) is characterized by hypoxemia relatively unresponsive to elevations in inspired oxygen, decreased pulmonary compliance, and radiographic changes showing areas of minimal to widespread consolidation in the lungs. The possible causes of ARDS are listed in Outline 3. In addition, ARDS may be associated with long bone fractures in the multiply injured patient who is treated while in a supine position. The supine position leads to the development of an area of high capillary hydrostatic pressure in the posterior lungs, which can contribute to progressive edema and atelectasis. Causes of hypoxemia include hypoventilation, diffusion defects, and ventilation/perfusion abnormalities (Fig. 12).

Outline 3
Possible causes of adult respiratory distress syndrome following injury

Ischemic pulmonary injury
- Pulmonary infection
- Systemic infection (sepsis)
- Aspiration
- Fat embolism
- Microembolism
- Fluid overload
- Oxygen toxicity
- Microatelectasis
- Direct pulmonary injury
- Cerebral injury

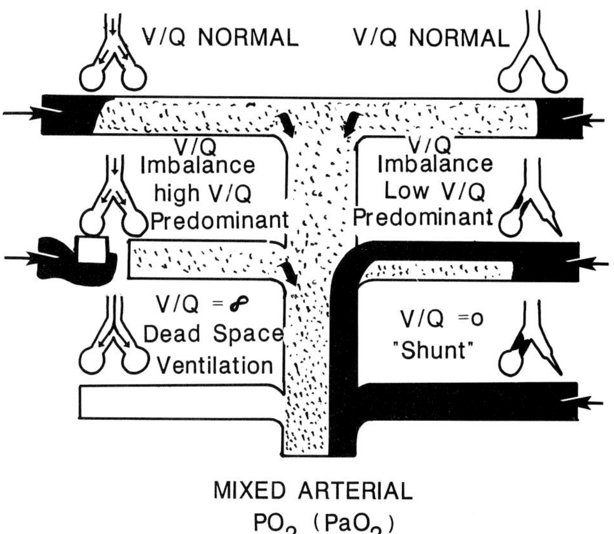

Figure 12
Schematic representation of ventilation/perfusion abnormalities.

Extracellular release of the lymphocytic enzymes and cytokines can damage the lung at the air/blood interface. In addition, peripherally activated aggregates of leukocytes and platelets may be transported as emboli to the lung, where they release their destructive factors, such as oxygen-free radicals and lysosomal enzymes, directly into the pulmonary tissue (Table 4). The embolic problems are clearly increased by delayed or inadequate resuscitation.

The pathophysiology of fat embolism is related to several factors. First, the pulmonary capillaries appear to be mechanically blocked by fat, resulting in arteriovenous (AV) shunting and alveolar hypoperfusion. This leads to hypoxia. Second, inflammation occurs as neutral fats are broken down into free

Table 4
Pathways of mediators generated or released during injury

Cascades	Activator	Active products
Coagulation	Collagen, cellular enzymes, tissue factor, platelet, endotoxin	Kallikrein, Fragment D, bradykinin, plasmin
Complement	Cellular enzymes, plasmin kallikrein, endotoxin, cell surfaces, antigen-antibody	C3a, C5a, C5, 6, 7, C3b
Cellular	Cell dependent-membrane perturbation	Cyclic endoperoxides, prostaglandins, thromboxane, prostacyclin, leukotrienes
Macrophage	Endotoxin, particulates, antigen, cytokines, C3a, activated T-cells	Plasminogen activator, Interleukin-1, TNF, thromboxane, PGE, oxygen radicals
Mast cell	Trauma, bradykinin endotoxin, anaphylatoxins, cationic proteins, antigen	Stored: histamine, heparin, ECF-A, NCF, generated: leukotrienes, PAF, LCF, prostaglandins
Neutrophil	Ingestible particles, noningestible particles, chemotactic factors, Interleukin-1	Acid hydrolases, neutral proteases, cationic proteins, elastase, cathepsin D, E, myeloperoxidase, lysozyme, oxygen free radicals, PAF, leukotrienes
Platelet	Collagen, ADP, thrombin, thromboxane A_2	ADP, serotonin, histamine, catecholamines, prostaglandins, hydrolases, platelet factors 3 and 4

fatty acids by lipases contained in the lung. Third, the platelets that are adherent and found among these fat globules break apart, releasing serotonin, which causes further vasoconstriction and bronchoconstriction, again leading to hypoxia. Because fatty acids are very toxic to lung cells, their release may disrupt the alveolar-capillary membrane and lung surfactant and lead to alveolar collapse, hemorrhage, and edema. All of these conditions can result in a ventilation/perfusion deficit and a constellation of findings consistent with ARDS (Fig. 13).

Musculoskeletal Infection

Basic Science of Bacterial Interactions

The composition of the cell wall of gram-positive and gram-negative bacteria differs significantly. The cell wall of gram-positive bacteria is

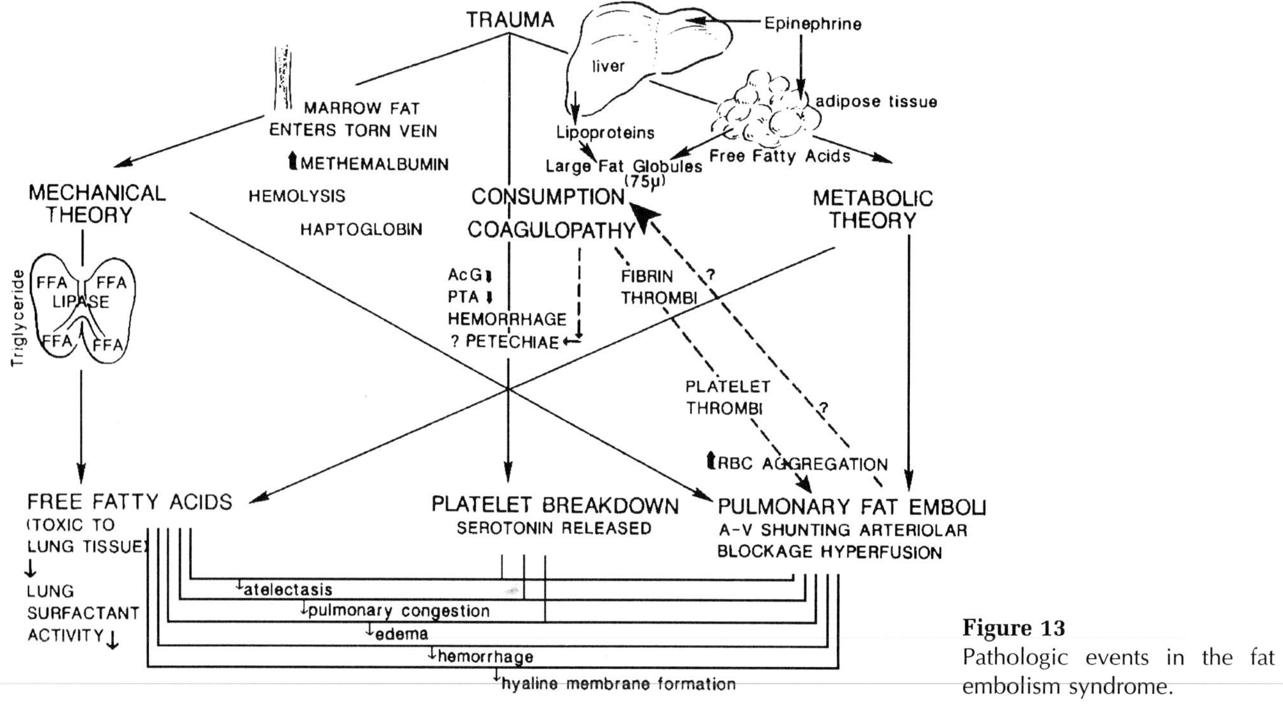

Figure 13
Pathologic events in the fat embolism syndrome.

composed of teichoic acids, while that of gram-negative organisms is composed of a lipoprotein core containing a lipopolysaccharide called endotoxin. The molecular structure of the polysaccharide confers a unique antigenic form that can be used not only to identify the organism, but also as the instigator of fever, cardiovascular shock, disseminated intravascular coagulation, tissue necrosis, increased susceptibility to stress, and death. Gram-negative organisms also secrete protein exotoxins.

Many bacteria express adhesions on their cell walls. These adhesions are specific proteins that bind to tissue surfaces and body secretions. Adhesin-receptor interactions are analogous to antibody-antigen or enzyme-substrate interactions. Some adhesins may be derived from enzymes by proteolytic cleavage, which removes the catalytic site while leaving the binding site intact. There are three useful criteria for identifying an adhesin or receptor: (1) a stereochemical adhesin-receptor interaction is saturable; (2) adhesin-receptor binding is reversible; and (3) the adhesin should exhibit the same binding specificity as the intact bacterial cell, and antibodies to the adhesion should block adhesin of the bacterium to the tissue surface. A single bacterium may possess several thousand adhesin molecules that can interact with several receptors to produce high-affinity binding. The receptors on mammalian cells contain an enormous amount of molecular information. A disaccharide can exist in more than 50 isomeric configurations.

Bacteria adhere to surfaces as a survival mechanism. Bacterial cells possess a net negative surface charge and can become associated with surfaces by nonspecific electrostatic or hydrophobic forces. Aside from being gram-positive and gram-negative, bacteria are structurally different and also have different adherence mechanisms. Gram-negative bacteria have proteinaceous structures, called pili and fimbriae, that extend from the cell wall and specifically bind to cellular proteins, matrix proteins, and glycolipids. Bacterial adherence is also species-specific. For example, *Staphylococcus epidermidis* binds more readily to hydrophobic surfaces than to hydrophilic ones.

The receptors for bacterial adhesins are found on several tissue surfaces and in a variety of components of body fluids and secretions. The in situ attachment of a bacterium then becomes a function of the relative concentration of receptor molecules on the tissue surface and the number of competing molecules in the secretions or body fluids in which the bacteria are suspended. These adhesin-receptor interactions provide the molecular biologist with an opportunity to construct receptor analogues that may bind with higher affinity than the bacteria. Such potent inhibitors of bacterial attachment could be useful in controlling bacterial adhesion.

In their adherent state, bacteria can form microcolonies that become enshrouded in biofilm, an extracellular matrix of polysaccharides, ions, nutrients, and other environmental constituents. Of the bacteria found in natural ecosystems, 90% exist in adherent biofilm. Bacteria on surfaces or within microcolonies are different physiologically from free-floating organisms. Biofilm protects the bacteria, acts as a virulence factor, and may aid in intercellular communication, transfer of genetic material, and concentration of valuable metabolic requirements. Bacterial cells possess a net negative surface charge and can become associated with surfaces by nonspecific electrostatic or hydrophobic forces. Adherent organisms are more resistant to antibiotics than are planktonic forms. This phenomenon is due not only to simple biofilm inhibition of antibiotic penetration but, more importantly, also to changes in cell phenotype that accompany cell attachment.

Bone and Joint Infection

Staphylococcus aureus remains the leading cause of osteomyelitis and nongonococcal bacterial arthritis. When musculoskeletal infections arising from contiguous foci are considered, *S epidermidis* is the predominant pathogen. The virulence of *S epidermidis* is limited to infections involving indwelling medical appliances. It causes more such infections than *S aureus,* despite the latter's greater tissue invasiveness. Although the primary reservoir for staphylococcal infections related to surgery is the patient's own skin, musculoskeletal tissues are quite susceptible to bacteremic, hematogenous infection. A secondary bacteremia is one that arises from an obvious peripheral focus, such as an abscess or contaminated intravascular catheter. A primary bacteremia has no evident origin. Unlike *S aureus,* which rarely causes primary bacteremia, the coagulase-negative staphylococci are frequently recovered from blood cultures of asymptomatic people. Approximately 51% of prosthetic joint infections are contiguous in origin while 34% are hematogenous.

The overall incidence of polymicrobial infections in orthopaedics is probably underestimated. There is good evidence that *S aureus* and group A beta-hemolytic streptococci act synergistically, making an abscess or cellulitis more severe than would be the case if the two bacterial strains were acting independently. The combination of a gram-positive organism, *S aureus,* and a gram-negative enteric organism, *Pseudomonas,* frequently occurs in wounds associated with open fractures. This combination is generally associated with a much more severe infection than would occur if the wound housed either organism alone. Similarly, aerobic and anaerobic organisms in combination can cause resistant infections. The best-studied combination is

Bacteroides and *Escherichia coli. Bacteroides* are obligate anaerobes. *E coli* are facultative and can grow under both aerobic and anaerobic conditions. The isolation of more than one organism in the same sample is indicative of polymicrobial infection.

Antibiotic-resistant bacteria are very important in medicine. There are two types of antibiotic resistance. Intrinsic resistance refers to inherent features of the cell that prevent antibiotic action on that cell, such as the absence of an enzyme or metabolic pathway that would be affected by the antibiotic in question. Acquired resistance occurs when resistant strains emerge from previously sensitive populations. Antibiotic resistance is more commonly mediated by plasmids (extrachromosomal genetic elements) and transposons than by chromosomal alteration. Transposons are mobile DNA sequences which, unlike plasmids, are not capable of self-replication. They must exist within a plasmid or chromosome. It is possible for a bacterium to obtain several different resistance genes by a series of transposon interactions. Selective pressure following exposure to an antibiotic will ensure that resistant plasmid-carrying bacteria will survive and replicate.

Infections Surrounding Implants

Biomaterials have transformed musculoskeletal surgery. The two major barriers to an even more expanded use of these devices are the lack of successful tissue integration and bacterial adhesion. Integration is the chemical bonding and compatibility of a noninflammatory host cell system in response to a biomaterial. A stable and nontraumatized integrated tissue cell surface is resistant to bacterial colonization because of its viability, intact cells, extracellular polysaccharides, and host defense mechanisms. True integration is believed to represent homeostasis, prolonging implant life and decreasing the risk of infection. Failure of implant integration is indicated by inflammation and necrosis at the interface between the biomaterial and soft tissue or bone. This inflammatory layer is more extensive in the presence of polymers, such as polymethylmethacrylate, than in the presence of metal alloys. An inflammatory interface leads to failure of soft-tissue cohabitation and results in pain and prosthetic failure. Failed integration allows bacterial colonization of the biomaterial surface. The molecular processes involved in eukaryotic integration and prokaryotic adhesion are similar and are directed not only by outer membrane molecules and receptors but also by surface geometry at the atomic level.

At the time of implantation, biomaterials are placed into a fluid environment that contains serum proteins, cellular debris, and, possibly, bacteria. Fibronectin is a ubiquitous, 440-kd serum and matrix protein that binds dissimilarly to a variety of common orthopaedic biomaterials, depending on the biomaterial's composition. It binds to the hydrocarbon polymers in greater quantities per unit area than to the metals that have been tested. Recent reports have shown that bacterial binding to fibronectin occurs at the arginine-glycine-aspartate (RGD) sequences in the fibronectin molecule.

To date there is no experimental evidence that any additional infection risk is associated with the use of porous ingrowth rather than standard prostheses. Musculoskeletal infection resulting from microbial colonization of the biomaterial and adjacent damaged tissue is extraordinarily resistant to treatment. Bone is a composite structure composed of calcium hydroxyapatite crystals embedded in a predominantly collagenous matrix. Proline-rich proteins found in the collagenous matrix act as ligands for bacterial adhesion. Traumatized cortical bone may be devoid of normal periosteum and blood supply, exposing the collagen-protein matrix and acellular calcium hydroxyapatite crystals to bacteria. The pathogenic mechanism in musculoskeletal infection can be shown experimentally. Immature rabbit metaphyseal bone exposed first to microscopic trauma and then to bacteremia invariably develops osteomyelitis. Similarly, recent studies indicate that the pathogenesis of intra-articular sepsis is based on the ability of certain strains of staphylococci to bind preferentially to cartilage matrix; for example, collagen receptors exist on the surfaces of strains of *S aureus.* The acellular articular cartilage surface offers no resistance to colonization. The mechanisms involved in bacterial adhesion to collagen epitopes in articular sepsis and to bone collagen in osteomyelitis are also relevant to allograft infections.

One of the problems with debridement surgery is the difficulty that the surgeon has in determining in the operating room whether the procedure has been completely thorough. Limited debridement of an established infection, without complete removal of involved bone, has led to a high incidence of recurrence. This can be described in terms of adhesive or cohesive failure. Adhesive failure occurs when two dissimilar materials are separated cleanly and completely (for example, when a strip of adhesive tape is removed from a surface, without leaving any tape on the surface or taking any surface material with it). Cohesive failure occurs when some part of one of the materials remains attached to the other material (for example, when a peanut butter and jelly sandwich is separated by pulling apart the two pieces of bread and some jelly remains attached to the peanut butter). Even if the infecting bacteria are successfully removed from a surface, it is unlikely that all of the macromolecular conditioning film will be removed. Thus, when the adhesive strength of the bacteria is strong, cohesive failure of the interface at the time of debridement may cause torn cellular fragments to remain on the surface.

Antibiotics in Bone and Joint Infection

Antibiotics can be used prophylactically to prevent infection in elective, clean surgical procedures; to provide initial care of a traumatic open injury; or to treat established infection. In the first two uses, the goal of parenteral antimicrobial therapy is to provide a sufficient concentration of antibiotic in the tissues to protect the clean tissue surrounding an open wound or surgical site from infection and to reduce or eliminate the contaminating bacteria in the damaged tissue. There is no blood-bone barrier. For antibiotics delivered systemically, bone interstitial fluid antibiotic concentration depends on plasma concentration, protein binding, and the ability of the antibiotic to cross the capillary membrane. In essence, the interstitial concentration of the antibiotic within viable bone equals the serum concentration of that drug once a steady state has been achieved. However, there is no indication that antibiotics effectively penetrate large bony sequestra or fibrotic scar.

The goals of prophylactic treatment of established joint infections include sterilization of the joint and decompression; removal of all inflammatory cells, enzymes, debris, or foreign bodies; elimination of destructive pannus; and return to full functional recovery. When given systemically, all antibiotics, with the exception of erythromycin, achieve intra-articular concentrations in excess of the level necessary to inhibit or kill the organisms causing the infection. Although direct instillation of the antibiotic into the joint is deleterious because it can cause an additional chemical synovitis, irrigation of an open wound with antibiotic (polymyxin/bacitracin) or dilute antiseptic (povidone iodine) may be beneficial.

The mechanism of action has been defined for seven antibiotic classes. The β-lactam antibiotics inhibit peptidoglycan synthesis by binding to the PBP (penicillin-binding proteins), which are located on the surface of the bacterial membrane. Aminoglycosides inhibit protein synthesis by binding to ribosomal RNA. Clindamycin and macrolides bind to 50S-ribosomal subunits and inhibit the dissociation of peptidyl-tRNA from ribosomes during translocation. Tetracyclines inhibit protein synthesis on 70S- and 80S-ribosomes. Glycopeptides (vancomycin and teicoplanin) interfere with the insertion of glycan subunits into the cell wall. Rifampicin inhibits RNA synthesis in bacteria. Quinolones inhibit DNAgyrase.

Three antibiotics, clindamycin, quinolones, and rifampin, can penetrate macrophages and kill already ingested bacteria. This property extends their usefulness because *S aureus* can survive within macrophages in a protected state, safe from the actions of other antimicrobials that cannot enter host cells.

The duration of antibiotic therapy for most musculoskeletal infections remains controversial and arbitrary. There are no controlled studies documenting the optimal length of treatment or the appropriate time to effect the transition from intravenous to oral therapy.

The results of recent studies suggest that the use of adjunctive nonsteroidal anti-inflammatory medication (naproxen) in conjunction with antibiotics and joint lavage decreases the glycosaminoglycan and collagen loss in septic arthritis.

Antibiotics in Prophylaxis and Treatment of Implant Infections

The treatment options for an infected orthopaedic biomaterial implant include antibiotic suppression, aggressive wound debridement accompanied by hardware removal and antibiotic therapy, and amputation. In the case of an infected total joint arthroplasty, additional options include resection arthroplasty, arthrodesis, one- or two-stage reimplantation of the prosthesis, or amputation. The presence of an implant acting as a foreign body limits the ability of the host's immune system to combat the infection. In this context, prevention is of utmost importance.

Although intravenous, perioperative antibiotic therapy is the current clinical standard during joint replacement arthroplasty, depot administration of antibiotics in a methylmethacrylate or biodegradable carrier has two advantages: high local concentration without systemic side effects and prolonged drug release. Antibiotic release does vary with the antibiotic chosen, carrier type, and manufacturing technique. Studies in an animal model comparing neomycin wound irrigation, intravenous antibiotic therapy, and gentamicin-impregnated methylmethacrylate have documented the effectiveness of the latter against *S aureus, S epidermidis,* and *E coli.* The combination of systemic and local release antibiotic therapy is effective in many implant infection situations. Routine use of prophylactic antibiotics for total joint replacement patients undergoing bacteremia-producing procedures remains controversial. Bacteremia can produce prosthetic joint infections in animal models. It is not known whether prophylaxis would be effective. A well-designed study using an animal model would provide additional data and very likely answer the question.

Radioisotope Imaging

Because plain radiography often fails to detect early subtle alterations in bone that occur as a result of infection, metastatic disease, or trauma, radionuclide studies are generally used in conjunction with, and after, a standard radiograph. Radionuclide studies are used to assess cellular activity in the musculoskeleton.

The technetium scan is the most common type of radionuclide study and it is used to evaluate osteoblastic activity caused by an injury or disease process. A gallium scan is used to evaluate soft tissues and to distinguish inflammation from other causes of bone diseases and soft-tissue masses. The indium scan is used to detect areas of infection. White blood cells radiolabeled with indium 111 provide a pictorial representation of the inflammatory response. Sulfur colloid scans are used in the assessment of inflammatory and infectious processes because sulfur colloid binds to reticuloendothelial cells. In addition to imaging the liver and spleen, it is extremely useful in studying bone marrow.

In each type of scan, the patient is injected with an isotope that is bound either to a ligand or to a white blood cell. At a given time after injection, the patient is placed within the confines of a gamma camera. Beginning at the patient's head or feet, the camera moves continuously along a track until it reaches the opposite end of the patient. As it moves, the camera records scintillation events either on film or in computer memory.

Gamma cameras contain energy discriminators that allow only those photons within a specified energy range to be recorded. Most detectors used in nuclear medicine are scintillation detectors, which are based on the property of a crystal, usually sodium iodide, that emits a photon [scintillate] after it is bombarded by ionizing radiation. These light photons are converted into an electrical signal, which is translated into the image viewed on a film. Images of either a whole body or of multiple spot views may be obtained. Whole body survey scans save time and display the entire skeleton; however, these data are inferior to those provided by spot views.

Technetium-99m (^{99m}Tc) is a readily available, inexpensive isotope that allows large quantities of activity to be administered with a low radiation dose. The isotope emits a monoenergetic infogamma ray of 140 keV, has a half-life of six hours, and emits no particulate radiation. Technetium-99m is bound to one of at least five phosphate compounds: polyphosphate, ethylenehydroxydiphosphonate, pyrophosphate, methylene diphosphonate (MDP), and hydroxymethylene diphosphonate (HMDP). The latter two compounds are stable and cleared from the blood and tissues quickly, therefore providing the best phosphate compounds for bone scanning.

The mechanism leading to the concentration of the technetium-99m-phosphate complex in bone is not fully understood, although the observation that the technetium phosphate ion is concentrated in areas where bone is being formed suggests that it is incorporated into new hydroxyapatite crystals. The technetium-99m scan represents an expression of the skeleton's response to various stimuli, such as trauma, physical stress, tumor, changes in perfusion, endocrine effects, and infection.

Although the scan appearance is rarely specific for a given disease process, certain distinctive scan patterns can suggest the type of process involved. If osteomyelitis is suspected, for example, a three-phase study helps to delineate between bone and soft-tissue inflammation and acute and chronic causes of new bone formation. The three phases are a perfusion phase, an equilibrium or "blood pool" image phase, and a delayed (standard) image phase showing bone metabolic activity. The equilibrium image is obtained immediately after completion of the perfusion study and represents the rapidly exchanging extracellular distribution of the tracer. Areas of abnormality suggest perfusion abnormalities. Regions of increased activity indicate a hyperemic process suggesting active infection or inflammation. Increased activity in the delayed scan shows increased bone formation. Thus, a normal delayed scan in conjunction with increased activity in early phases would suggest an inflammatory process limited to the soft tissue. Alternatively, increased activity in the delayed scan with normal early phases would suggest reactive bone without an inflammatory response. Examples of this type of response are seen in degenerative joint disease and chronic inactive osteomyelitis. The three-phase technetium scan also may be used as a noninvasive monitor of perfusion and the viability of vascularized or nonvascularized bone grafts.

Gallium 67 emits gamma photons and has a half-life of 78 hours. It is chemically similar to indium (both of these elements are metals in the same group on the periodic table). Because it is chemically similar to iron, gallium forms a strong bond with transferrin in the plasma. Gallium 67 is bound to citrate and, after injection into the patient, becomes 90% bound to transferrin. It is later concentrated in liver, soft-tissue abscesses, active bone and joint infections, and some tumors (particularly soft-tissue sarcomas). The mechanism for this concentration is not fully understood.

Indium 111 has a half-life of 67 hours and emits gamma photons of 172 KeV and 245 KeV. The indium compound is lipophilic and diffuses freely throughout cell membranes. Once inside the white blood cell, the indium binds to cellular proteins. Leukocyte labeling requires whole blood centrifugation and separation of the buffy coat containing white blood cells. As soon as labeling is complete, the white blood cells are reinjected and images are taken 24 hours later. This interval allows time for the cells to migrate to zones of inflammation.

Technetium-99m-labeled sulfur colloid is the most commonly used radiolabeled colloid in nuclear medicine. Its use is based on its unique ability to be cleared by the reticuloendothelial system (liver, spleen, and bone marrow). The effective half-life is almost equal to the physiologic half-life of ^{99m}Tc. A particularly relevant use of this type of scan in orthopaedics can be made in the detection of periprosthetic infection. Indium-labeled WBC activity extending along the femoral stem may be seen in patients without infection for some time after hip replacement surgery. This is apparently related to an altered distribution of reticuloendothelial cells. However, if both the sulfur colloid scan and the indium scan are used together, the diagnostic power of the study is significantly improved. Because the physiologic distributions of ^{99m}Tc-sulfur colloid and labeled leukocytes in marrow are similar, and because infection typically stimulates leukocyte accumulation, incongruence of the findings on the two scans (such as positive indium, negative sulfur colloid) shows increased sensitivity, specificity, and accuracy over indium scanning alone, when making a diagnosis of infection.

Nutrition and Metabolism

Early Principles of Nutritional Support

Clinical nutritional support was first introduced into medicine in about 1970, after the feasibility of total parenteral nutrition was demonstrated in animal studies. Widespread malnutrition in hospitalized patients, first documented in 1974, was recognized to be iatrogenic, resulting from the inadequate feeding practices prevalent at the time. This has led to dramatic efforts to understand more fully the effects of illness on nutritional status and to enhance the nutritional status of hospitalized patients.

In the 1970s, the principles of nutrition support therapy were based largely on the biochemistry of starvation, with emphasis on restoration of lean body mass, nitrogen balance, and visceral protein stores. Nutritional requirements were derived from data gathered using normal healthy male subjects, with protein dosages of approximately 1.0 g/kg/day and nonprotein calorie to nitrogen ratios of 150:1. Carbohydrate (hypertonic glucose) was the predominant energy source because safe intravenous fat formulations were not available for use in the United States until the mid 1970s. At that time, fat was given only to prevent essential fatty acid deficiency.

Over time, indications for nutritional support were expanded and these same regimens were applied to increasingly sick and diverse groups of patients (trauma, burns, and sepsis, for example). Standard nutritional regimens consisting of hypertonic (25%) dextrose with caloric loading frequently exceeding 40 to 50 kcal/kg/day and nonprotein calorie to nitrogen ratios of greater than 150:1 produced several metabolic complications, including increased CO_2 production leading to increased minute ventilation and respiratory failure, hyperglycemia with or without hyperosmolar nonketotic coma, metabolic acidosis, and hepatic steatosis. The common denominator for most of these complications appeared to be feeding of carbohydrate calories in excess of metabolic demand. A better understanding of the metabolic changes resulting from injury and stress has since led to several modifications in nutritional support to these patients. Since that time, the nutritional management of surgical patients has evolved tremendously. A number of different feeding modalities are now available that allow the nutritional management of patients to be tailored more precisely to their specific clinical condition. The basic nutritional requirements of surgical patients, the tools available to meet those needs, and their indications, contraindications, and complications will be outlined below.

Basic Nutrient Requirements

The basic nutrients required for maintenance of the human body are carbohydrate, protein, fat, vitamins, minerals, and water. Although energy in the form of ATP can be derived from carbohydrate, protein, or fat, the efficiency of ATP formation depends on the source from which it is derived. Glucose and glycogen (carbohydrates) are the most efficient sources, followed by protein and fat. Protein is important because it is the basic structural component of all significant organic machinery of the body (Table 5). Protein, fat, vitamins, minerals, and water provide substrates for the synthesis of structural proteins, enzymes, and hormones.

Protein

Amino acids, the basic building blocks of protein, are required in sufficient quantities to permit protein synthesis. An amino acid is composed of an amino group and a keto acid. The amino group, which is the same for all amino acids, cannot be synthesized by the body, but it can be removed from

Table 5
Nutrient composition of some common foods

	Amount	Protein (grams)	Carbohydrate (grams)	Fat (grams)	Calories	Major Nutrient
Skim milk	1 c	9	12	0	88 kcal	Calcium, riboflavin
Tomatoes	½ c	1	5	0	24 kcal	Potassium, vitamin C
Potatoes	½ c	2	13	0	59 kcal	Potassium, vitamin C
Carrots	½ c	1	9	0	37 kcal	Vitamin A
Orange juice	½ c	1	12	0	49 kcal	Vitamin C
Raisins	½ oz	0	11	0	40 kcal	Iron
Whole wheat bread	1 sl	2	15	0	75 kcal	Fiber, vitamin B
Oatmeal	½ c	2	15	0	75 kcal	Phosphorus, fiber, vitamin B
Rice	⅓ c	2	15	0	75 kcal	Vitamin B
Pasta	½ c	2	15	0	75 kcal	Vitamin B
Meat	3 oz	22	0	15	240 kcal	Iron, phosphorus
Chicken	3 oz	27	0	6	150 kcal	Niacin, phosphorus
Fish	3 oz	21	0	6	150 kcal	Niacin, phosphorus
Egg	1	7	0	5	82 kcal	Vitamin A, iron
Cheese	1 oz	7	0	9	113 kcal	Vitamin A, riboflavin
Soft drink	6 oz	0	19	0	75 kcal	None
Margarine	1 tsp	0	0	5	45 kcal	Vitamin A

another amino acid and transferred to an existing keto acid (transamination). In this way, the body is able to synthesize new amino acids from existing amino acids.

The keto acid provides uniqueness to an amino acid. There are 20 amino acids, each with its own unique keto acid or R group. The body can synthesize all but eight of the keto acids necessary for amino acid synthesis. The eight essential amino acids for adults are lysine, tryptophan, isoleucine, leucine, valine, phenylalanine, methionine, and threonine. In addition, the keto acids for histidine and arginine may not be synthesized in sufficient quantities during periods of rapid growth or severe stress, making them, in effect, "conditionally" essential amino acids as well.

Proteins are metabolized to peptides for absorption into the intestinal mucosa, where they are further broken down because only free amino acids can pass into the portal system and the liver. Three quarters of the circulating amino acids are extracted by the liver, where they are used for the synthesis of proteins, plasma proteins, and transport proteins, which are released by the liver. Small amounts of free amino acids are released into the general circulation, where they are taken up by muscle and other metabolically active tissues for protein synthesis. The branched chain amino acids (valine, leucine, and isoleucine), however, are not metabolized by the liver to any significant extent; rather, they are preferentially metabolized in skeletal muscle.

Amino acids are important in the synthesis of new proteins, catabolic reactions leading to the production of adenosine triphosphate (ATP) and CO_2, the conversion of the keto acid to glucose or fat, the conversion of nitrogen to urea, or the use of nitrogen for the synthesis of nonessential amino acids, purines, and pyrimidines.

All 20 amino acids must be present in sufficient quantity for protein synthesis to occur. Deficiencies in one or more of the essential amino acids will limit protein synthesis. Protein quality is based on the concentration of essential amino acids present within a particular food. Animal foods, such as meat, milk, and eggs, are considered to be proteins of high biologic value, whereas vegetable proteins, which are deficient or low in one or more of the essential amino acids, are thought to have low biologic value.

Protein requirements are based on the stage of growth, level of stress, and composition of the other major nutrients in the diet. In a normal healthy adult, 0.8 g protein/kg/day is considered adequate to maintain nitrogen balance (protein intake equals protein excretion). In severely stressed patients, protein requirements are increased to 1.0 g/kg/day or more. Protein requirements also may be expressed in terms of nitrogen content. The nitrogen content of most proteins is approximately 16%; therefore, the amount of nitrogen (in grams) multiplied by 6.25 equals the amount of protein (in grams). A nonprotein calorie to nitrogen ratio of between 100 and 150:1 in relatively normal patients is usually sufficient to obtain a positive nitrogen balance. In patients with renal impairment, more calories may be needed (250:1). Occasionally, the requirement for nitrogen is so high as to require a nonprotein calorie: nitrogen ratio of less than 100:1.

Carbohydrate

Storage of carbohydrate in the human body provides a readily available source of energy for a relatively short period of time. The human body stores carbohydrate as glycogen, a bulky hydrated molecule, in the liver and muscle. Approximately 150 g of glycogen, which provides approximately 600 calories, can be stored in the liver. This reserve is expended within the first 24 hours of starvation. Muscle glycogen does not contribute to the overall energy needs of the body because it cannot be transferred into the general circulation.

Glucose is the preferred fuel for the central nervous system, erythrocytes, leukocytes, bone marrow, and the adrenal medulla. These tissues do not adapt to ketone utilization as well as skeletal muscle, heart, and kidney. Because there is no net conversion of fat to glucose, requirements for glucose must be met entirely from carbohydrate or protein sources. Endogenous protein can be catabolized to meet the body's need for glucose; however, lean body tissue is jeopardized by this process. During normal starvation, visceral proteins tend to be catabolized; during stress, skeletal muscle is preferentially catabolized, although visceral proteins will also be decreased.

Fat

In a healthy 70 kg man, approximately 60,000 calories are stored as body fat. However, this huge caloric store is misleading for a number of reasons. Some body fat is essential for normal functioning of body organs. In addition, the energy derived from fat is in the form of ketone bodies, which only can be used by selected body tissues. Even in normal adapted starvation, the energy derived from fat does not approach 100%, as significant amounts of protein will also be catabolized for energy.

Fat in the diet provides a highly concentrated caloric source (approximately 9 kcal/g), a vehicle for fat-soluble nutrients (such as vitamins A, D, E, and K), and a source of essential fatty acids. Linoleic acid is the predominant essential fatty acid, although linolenic and arachidonic acids may not be supplied in sufficient amounts to the body during stress and/or periods of rapid growth. These fatty acids, especially arachidonic acid, are precursors of prostaglandins, which play a role in mediating the response to stress.

The respiratory quotient (RQ) is defined as the amount of CO_2 produced per oxygen consumed and provides a useful method for determining the primary fuel being used by the body. An RQ of 1 indicates carbohydrate is the primary fuel; 0.75 to 0.85 indicates mixed fuel use; and 0.7 indicates pure fat. An RQ above 1.0 indicates that lipogenesis is occurring; that is, the patient is being overfed. Theoretically, the RQ can be as high as 9, but this rarely occurs. Elevation of RQ above 1, however, does signify additional stresses on the respiratory system, because the patient must be able to eliminate the excess carbon dioxide produced by increasing minute ventilation.

Vitamins and Minerals

In 1975, the Nutrition Advisory Group of the American Medical Association established guidelines regarding formulations for parenteral administration of vitamins. Vitamin requirements for enterally fed patients are based on the current US Recommended Dietary Allowances (RDA). Although these recommendations have been designed to provide adequate nutrition to normal healthy Americans, no other organized data are available for individuals who are stressed (Table 6). The vitamins and minerals of greatest concern in stressed patients are ascorbic acid, vitamin B_6, vitamin A, folate, thiamin, iron, and zinc. Other vitamins and minerals play important roles in specific stress situations and their requirements must also be addressed.

Nutrient Metabolism

Starvation

Starvation, to some degree, is the most common state to which the body adapts. Carbohydrates, in the form of glycogen stored in the liver, constitute the body's primary fuel source during a short fast, intraprandial (between meals), or overnight. The liver normally contains about 150 g of glycogen, which is rapidly mobilized to glucose in the fasted state. Additional precursors for gluconeogenesis are derived from amino acids (predominantly alanine) that have been shunted to the liver from skeletal

Table 6
Vitamin requirements in nutritional support

Nutrient	Recommended Daily Allowance	American Medical Association Recommendations
Thiamin (mg)	1.5	3.0
Riboflavin (mg)	1.7	3.6
Niacin (mg)	19.0	40
Vitamin B_6	2.0	4.0
Pantothenol (mg)	4-7*	15
Folate (µg)	200	400
Vitamin A µg RE	1,000	1,100
Vitamin D (µg)	5	2.5
Vitamin E (mg)	10	10
Vitamin B_{12} (µg)	2.0	5.0
Vitamin C (mg)	60	100

*Safe and adequate daily intake (SADI)

muscle via the alanine cycle. Fatty acids and glycerol, which are liberated from the breakdown of stored adipose tissue, also make a small contribution to gluconeogenesis.

After seven to ten days, the body further adapts to starvation by shifting its predominant fuel source from glucose to fat, in the form of ketone bodies. A decrease in circulating insulin levels accompanied by an increase in the levels of circulating glucagon make free fatty acids more available as fuel. Ketone bodies serve as the predominant energy source for the brain and other metabolically active regions, such as kidney, heart, etc. Overall, these metabolic alterations result in a marked decrease in muscle protein breakdown, thereby providing hepatic gluconeogenic precursors, a subsequent fall in urinary nitrogen excretion, a decrease in the rate at which lean body mass is lost, and a decrease in the rate of metabolic expenditure.

Generally, these homeostatic mechanisms are readily reversed (termed "auto" or "servo" regulation) by providing a modest amount of glucose daily. This forms the basis for the current practice, often referred to as "protein sparing," of supplying 100 g of intravenous glucose daily to hospitalized patients.

Stress and Trauma

The physiologic/metabolic response to trauma and stress is markedly different from that due to starvation (Table 7). Numerous mediator-effector systems are activated (particularly those involving cytokines and eicosanoids), producing a "hypermetabolic" and catabolic state (Outline 4) and an altered hormonal milieu. Insulin levels are increased, as are those of the counterregulatory hormones (glucagon, cortisol, growth hormone, and epinephrine), resulting in increased gluconeogenesis, hyperglycemia, suppression of lipolysis, and use of protein as a primary fuel. This hypermetabolic state is characterized by an increased basal metabolic rate (proportional to the magnitude of the stress), increased caloric expenditure, and increased oxygen consumption. It is accompanied by tachycardia, increased cardiac output, and decreased systemic vascular resistance. There is a shift in fuels from carbohydrates and ketone bodies (the predominant fuels during starvation) to a "mixed fuel" combination with markedly increased protein catabolism, primarily from skeletal muscle breakdown. Branched-chain amino acids (isoleucine, leucine, and valine) are preferentially oxidized directly in skeletal muscle, while other amino acids are converted to alanine and glycine and transported to the liver for gluconeogenesis. Lactate production from pyruvate or due to anaerobic metabolism may also be increased. However, even when recycled to glucose via the Cori cycle, lactate is an inefficient source of energy (ATP). Overall, hepatic gluconeogenesis and hepatic synthesis of acute phase proteins are increased, but total body (or net) protein synthesis declines; ie, catabolism increases.

Unlike starvation, where the body is able to autoregulate its metabolic response, "hypermetabolism" resulting from trauma, stress, or sepsis is characterized by a loss of substrate-metabolite control. This inability to "turn off" the response to stress leads to progressive, relentless muscle protein breakdown, which has been termed "autocannibalism," and eventually to multisystem organ failure and death. Nutritional therapy in critically ill patients is designed to provide support for these al-

Outline 4
Physiologic changes characteristic of hypermetabolism and multisystem organ failure

Increased energy expenditure
Increased O_2 consumption
Increased CO_2 production
Increased urinary nitrogen excretion and protein catabolism
Increased cardiac output
Decreased systemic vascular resistance

Table 7
Comparison of metabolic changes in starvation and stress

	Starvation		Stress	
	Early	Late	Hypermetabolism	Multisystem
Energy expenditure	↓	↓↓	↑↑	organ failure
Mediator activation	None	None	++	++
Metabolic responsiveness	Intact	Intact	Abnormal	Abnormal
Primary fuel	CHO	KB	"Mixed" (no KB)	"Mixed" (no KB)
Hepatic gluconeogenesis	↓	↓	↑	↑ or ↓
Hepatic protein synthesis	↓	↓	↑	↑ or ↓
Whole body protein catabolism	sl. ↑	sl. ↑	↑↑	↑↑↑
Urinary nitrogen excretion	sl. ↑	sl. ↑	↑↑	↑↑↑
Malnutrition	slow	slow	rapid	rapid

tered metabolic processes while definitive treatment of the primary disease process is undertaken.

Multisystem Organ Failure

Multisystem organ failure (MSOF) is a clinical syndrome involving progressive sequential failure of several organ systems, of which lung, liver, and kidney are the most common. However, it also can be expressed by failure of the central nervous system, cardiovascular system, immune system, coagulation pathway, barrier function of the skin's submucosa, tracheobronchial lining, and urinary bladder. The onset of adult respiratory distress syndrome (ARDS), characterized by hypoxemia, increased pulmonary shunting, and decreased compliance usually heralds the onset of MSOF.

Liver failure with abnormal liver function studies is common following sepsis. Jaundice is an indicator of MSOF. It is important to rule out other causes of jaundice, such as perihepatic infection and acute acalculous cholecystitis. Acute renal failure characterized by oliguria or polyuria, mild azotemia, elevated serum creatinine, and abnormal free water clearance may also occur early.

The incidence of MSOF has been reported to be between 7% and 12% in injured or critically ill patients. It is the leading cause of death in those patients who survive longer than 48 hours. The onset of MSOF varies depending on the presentation of overt bacterial infection. Patients at highest risk for MSOF are those with more severe injuries, as indicated by the extent of hypovolemic shock. Direct organ injury, such as pulmonary contusion or liver damage or infection, increases the risk of MSOF. The metabolic response following hypovolemic shock is characterized by increased levels of catecholamines and other counterregulatory hormones, such as cortisol and glucagon.

Preexisting disease may increase the risk of MSOF because patients with recurrent illness, such as chronic pulmonary or hepatic failure, are unable to meet the metabolic demands of stress response to injury or sepsis. Critically reduced cardiac output is a predisposing factor to infection because of increased hypoxia to the injured tissue. Chronic lung disease will increase the patient's susceptibility to pneumonia because the barrier function of the airways has been damaged. In addition, metabolites, such as hydroxyl ions or peroxides, resulting from reperfusion and reoxygenation of tissues have been found to mediate tissue damage in MSOF. These tissue-damaging metabolites may be derived from polymorphonuclear leukocytes that infiltrate the wounds or inflamed tissue as part of the primary host response to injury.

The patient with chronic liver failure, renal failure, or immune system suppression is at increased risk of MSOF. Multisystem organ failure is a problem of the injured patient following hypovolemic shock and resuscitation. The injured patient is febrile, vasodilated, hypertensive, and tachycardic. This partially reflects the response by the microcirculation in the large capillary beds of the body (namely skeletal muscles and the splanchnic bed) to the inflammatory response set up by the wound. Inflammatory mediators released by phagocytic cells after circulating particulates and cellular products of damaged tissue are identified as partly responsible for this hypermetabolic state. These mediators have been identified as cytokines, such as tumor necrosis factor (TNF) and interleukin-1, and arachidonic acid metabolites, such as prostaglandin E_2 (PGE_2). The body's response to the injury may be maintained within a tolerable physiologic limit if either of two scenarios are realized: (1) the responses by the mediators and the hormonal changes that result from the injury can be controlled, such as resuscitation from shock, early fixation of long bone fractures, or excision of burn wounds; or (2) if the mediators can be modulated, for example, with aggressive protein nutrition or drainage of abscesses. Without these interventions, a progression and decompensation to septic shock and overt MSOF will result.

The Nutritional Needs of Patients With Trauma and Stress

Nutritional Assessment

In surveys of hospitalized patients, the incidence of protein-calorie malnutrition has been shown to approach 40%. Although a number of factors contribute to this high incidence among patients, major factors are inadequate surveillance of nutritional status and the failure to recognize the increased metabolic needs due to trauma and stress. Before the specific nutritional prescription for a patient can be determined, it is important to identify individuals who are at increased nutritional risk. A number of factors must be evaluated to obtain a complete assessment of the nutritional status of an individual. Table 8 defines the major components of a nutritional assessment, which include anthropometric, biochemical, dietary, and clinical parameters.

Nutrition/Metabolic Support in Trauma and Stress

Patients with significant physiologic stress should be supported with enteral or parenteral formulations designed to provide for substrate abnormalities that are known to occur (Table 9). A "mixed fuel" regimen provides about 30% to 40% of calories as fat, 40% to 50% as carbohydrate, and 20% as protein. Protein content is increased to provide between 1.3 and 2.0 g protein/kg/day (normal is 0.8-1.0 g/kg/day) with nonprotein calorie to nitrogen ratios reduced to between 75:1 and 125:1. These

Table 8
Commonly used parameters for nutritional assessment

Parameters	Measure
Anthropometric	
Height	cm
Weight	kg
Age	
Sex	
Skinfold thickness	
Arm circumference	
Ideal body weight	
Female	100 lb (first 5 ft) + 5 lb/in ± 10%
Male	106 lb (first 5 ft) + 6 lb/in ± 10%
Usual body weight	%
Biochemical	
Serum albumin	4 to 5.5 g/dl
Total iron-binding capacity	250 to 410 mg/dl
Serum transferrin	170 to 250 mg/dl
Lymphocytes	25% to 33%
White blood cells	4.5 to 11 × 10^3
Total lymphocyte count	2,500/m^3
24-hr urinary nitrogen	10 to 17 g/24 hr
24-hr urinary creatinine	1.0 to 1.5g/24 hr
Total protein	6 to 8 g/dl
Clinical	
General physical appearance of patient	
Clinical signs of protein/calorie deficiencies	
Clinical signs of vitamin/mineral deficiencies	
Significant weight loss	
Edema	
Fatigue, lassitude, weakness	
Dietary	
24-hr diet recall and nutrient assessment, past and present	
Food frequency and nutrient assessment quantitative food frequency	

formulations tend to differ substantially from those used previously, which were based on the metabolic changes occurring during starvation.

More recently, attention has focused on the use of nutrition as a therapeutic modality to try to prevent or reverse some of the deleterious changes that occur during hypermetabolism and lead to MSOF. Solutions enriched in branched-chain amino acids, because of their preferential use by skeletal muscle, have been documented to improve the rate of achieving positive nitrogen balance, but are not yet established to improve outcome. Arginine, an essential amino acid in rapidly growing tissues, has been shown to be thymogenic and improve T cell function (cell-mediated immunity) and wound healing. Similarly, glutamine is now known to play an important role in maintaining gut mucosal integrity and immunologic function and may help prevent bacterial translocation. Another area of intense investigation involves altering the fat content of nutritional formulations by increasing the ratio of omega-3 to omega-6 fatty acids in order to avoid some of the deleterious effects of the latter. Omega-6 fatty acids, predominantly linoleic acid, are metabolized to PGE_2 and thromboxane A_2 via the arachidonic acid cascade and have adverse effects on immune function and the vasculature. Preliminary data suggest that solutions enriched with omega-3 fatty acids, such as linolenic acid, lead to production of PGE_3 and thromboxane A_3, which are inactive eicosanoid derivatives and do not produce the adverse effects associated with PGE_2 and thromboxane A_2. Overall, these trends indicate that nutrition/metabolic support is increasingly being viewed as a true therapeutic modality, similar to any other drug therapy employed in the management of critically ill patients.

Enteral versus Parenteral Administration of Nutritional Support

Decisions regarding the use of enteral or parenteral feedings are based on the basic principle: If the gut works, use it! Postoperative ileus has been the classic reason for postponing the introduction of nutrients into the gut for as long as three to five days after surgery. Ileus, however, may be segmental and may not involve the entire gut, so that many patients can be fed directly into the duodenum or jejunum far earlier than previously thought. In addition, use of the gastrointestinal tract maintains the integrity and function of the gut mucosa, with its attendant immunologic benefits, such as production of secretory IgA, which may help prevent bacterial translocation, a possible etiologic mechanism for the genesis of occult sepsis and MSOF. The types of enteral formulations currently available are summarized in Table 10.

A simple decision tree can be used when determining the appropriate mode of nutritional therapy (Fig. 14). Regardless of the mode of feeding, the determination of specific nutrient requirements remains the same. Energy expenditure should be measured using indirect calorimetry or estimated using either the Harris-Benedict Equation with appropriate stress and activity factors or other appropriate energy formulas (Curreri formula for burns, for example). In general, 30 to 35 kcal/kg/day is sufficient for most stressed patients. Of these calories, up to 60% may be delivered as fat depending on the specific clinical condition.

Once energy needs are known, protein requirements must be addressed. These can be determined

Table 9
Basic nutrient requirements in normal to severe stress

	Requirements for Stress			
	Normal	Mild	Moderate	Severe
Protein (g/kg)*	0.8	0.8 to 1.2	1.3 to 1.5	1.5 to 2.0
Calories (kcal/g)+	25 to 30 (REE × 1.2)	30 to 32 (REE × 1.3)	32 to 36 (REE × 1.5)	36 to 40++ (REE × 2.0)

*The objective of nutrition support is to obtain a positive nitrogen balance. Therefore, protein intake should be adjusted in response to the measurements of nitrogen balance.
+ REE (Harris-Benedict Equation)
males 66 + [(13.7 × st in kg) + (5 × ht in cm) − (6.8 × age)]
females 665 + [(9.6 × st in kg) + (1.7 × ht in cm) − (4.7 × age)]
++ Generally reserved for major burns.

Table 10
Enteral formulations

Type	Description
Basic low-calorie formulas (1 calorie/ml)	Supplemental; can be orally consumed
Basic high-calorie formulas (1.5 to 2.0 kcal/ml)	Supplemental; can be orally consumed
High nitrogen formulas	Supplemental; most can be orally consumed
Low osmolarity formulas	Used as full support in patients unable to tolerate higher osmolar loads; most cannot be consumed orally except by tube
Elemental diets	Composed of protein hydrolysates (polypeptides) or free amino acids used for patients with impaired gastrointestinal function, most must be fed via tube
Disease-specific formulas	
Renal	Composed of essential amino acids; limit nitrogen intake
Liver	Enriched with branched-chain amino acids; low nitrogen content
Pulmonary	High fat/lower carbohydrate formula
Stress	Higher kcal levels; high nitrogen; medium-chain triglycerides; enriched branched-chain amino acids
Immune System	Contains omega-3 fatty acids; arginine; RNA; high nitrogen; high kcal

by adjusting the appropriate nonprotein calorie: nitrogen ratio or by using a protein stress factor multiplied by the weight of the patient in kilograms (1.0 to 1.2 g/kg in mild stress, 1.3 to 1.5 g/kg in moderate stress, and 1.6 to 2.0 g/kg in severe stress).

Electrolyte and trace elements are supplied to maintain normal acid-base balance and prevent deficiencies of these essential elements. The volume administered should be determined based on the patient's clinical condition. Ideally, the provision of nutrient substrate should be determined independently of volume considerations.

Patients receiving nutrition support should be monitored for efficacy of therapy and for complications (Table 11). This usually entails following serial measurements of nitrogen balance and visceral protein status, as determined by serum albumin, transferrin, total iron-binding capacity, retinol binding globulin, and other factors. Therapy is adjusted as needed.

Complications associated with nutrition support are classified as either metabolic or technical. Metabolic complications occur with both enteral and parental routes of therapy and include, for example, hyperglycemia, hypoglycemia; electrolyte and fluid imbalances; deficiencies in vitamins, trace minerals, and/or essential fatty acids; and liver function abnormalities. Technical complications vary with the mode of therapy, but occur with both routes. Those associated with parenteral nutrition are related to the need for central venous access and include both mechanical and infectious

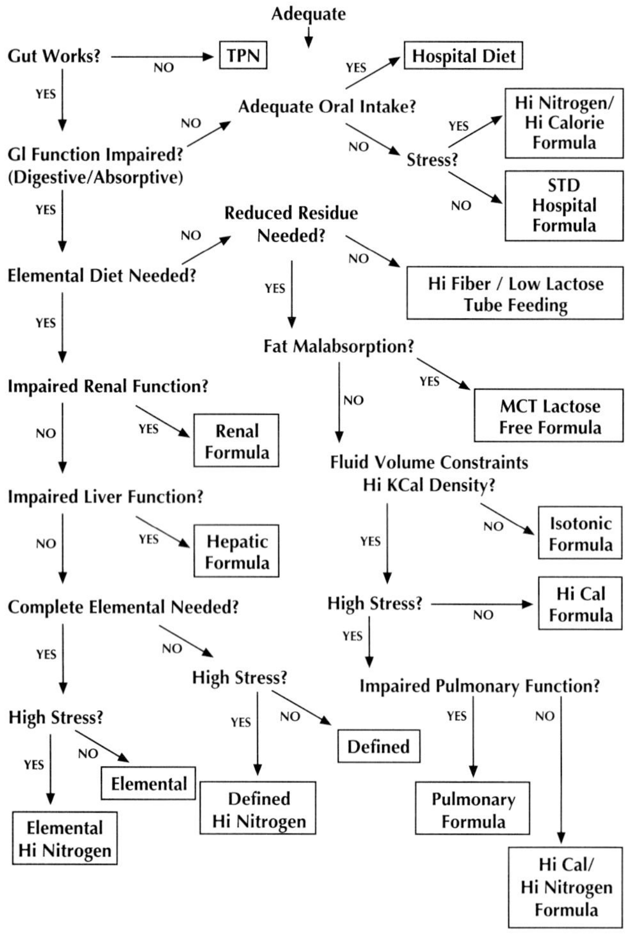

Figure 14
Decision tree for the selection of an enteral diet.

problems. Those associated with enteral feedings are related to tube placement, tube patency, and tolerance of the osmotic load of the feeding solution (Table 11).

Nutrition and Fracture Healing

It has been shown both clinically and experimentally that nutrition plays an important role in the healing of soft-tissue wounds. However, the influence of nutrition on fracture healing has received far less attention. As early as 1936, negative nitrogen balance, tissue wasting, and weight loss were shown to develop in patients with long bone fractures. The role of dietary protein and calcium in fracture healing was studied by assessing the mechanical properties of fracture calluses in rats fed diets that were deficient in or enriched by these nutrients. Supplementation of dietary protein and minerals in excess of the calculated requirements neither improved nor impaired fracture healing. Stiffness, a mechanical property acquired early in the course of normal fracture healing, was found to develop independently of alterations in dietary protein or minerals. Strength, that property of fracture callus acquired later in the course of healing, was found to depend somewhat on adequate dietary mineral content but showed a much greater dependence on adequate dietary protein.

Table 11
Complications associated with nutrition support therapy

Complication	Enteral support	Parenteral support
Metabolic	hypo-/hyperglycemia hypophosphatemia acid/base balance abnormalities hypo-/hyperkalemia hypo-/hypernatremia liver function abnormalities diarrhea nausea/vomiting	hypo-/hyperglycemia hypophosphatemia acid/base balance abnormalities hypo-/hyperkalemia hypo-/hypernatremia liver function abnormalities fatty acid deficiency bone disease
Technical	nasopharyngeal erosion esophagitis intestinal obstruction aspiration pneumonia otitis media esophageal perforation hemorrhage inadvertent insertion into trachea tube obstruction puncture of stomach or duodenum abdominal/ileus distention	subcutaneous emphysema skin bleeding local hematoma pneumothorax hydrothorax hemothorax thoracic duct injury (chylothorax) artery puncture brachial plexus injury air embolism catheter embolus failure of cannulation bacteremia/fungemia

Selected Bibliography

Thromboembolic Disease

Bergqvist D: Dextran and haemostasis: A review. *Acta Chir Scand* 1982;148:633–640.

Cranley JJ, Canos AJ, Sull WJ: The diagnosis of deep venous thrombosis: Fallibility of clinical symptoms and signs. *Arch Surg* 1976;3:34–36.

DeLee JC, Rockwood CA Jr: Current concepts review: The use of aspirin in thromboembolic disease. *J Bone Joint Surg* 1980;62A:149–152.

Eriksson BI, Eriksson E, Gyzander E, et al: Thrombosis after hip replacement: Relationship to the fibrinolytic system. *Acta Orthop Scand* 1989;60:159–163.

Evarts CM: Prevention of venous thromboembolism. *Clin Orthop* 1987;222:98–104.

Flanc C: An experimental study of the recanalization of arterial and venous thrombi. *Br J Surg* 1968;55:519–524.

Gilman AG, Goodman LS: *Goodman and Gilman's The Pharmacological Basis of Therapeutics,* ed 7. New York, Macmillan, 1985, pp 1338–1341.

Greenfield LJ: Pulmonary embolism: Diagnosis and management. *Curr Probl Surg* 1976;13:1–52.

Gruber UF, Saldeen T, Brokop T, et al: Incidences of fatal postoperative pulmonary embolism after prophylaxis with dextran 70 and low-dose heparin: An international multicentre study. *Br Med J* 1980;280:69–72.

Harris WH, Salzman EW, Athanasoulis CA, et al: Aspirin prophylaxis of venous thromboembolism after total hip replacement. *N Engl J Med* 1977;297:1246–1249.

Harris WH, Salzman EW, DeSanctis RW, et al: Prevention of venous thromboembolism following total hip replacement: Warfarin vs. Dextran 40. *JAMA* 1972;220:1319–1322.

Hull RD, Hirsh J, Carter CJ, et al: Pulmonary angiography, ventilation lung scanning and venography for clinically suspected pulmonary embolism with abnormal perfusion lung scan. *Ann Intern Med* 1983;98:891–899.

Kakkar V: The diagnosis of deep vein thrombosis using the 125-I fibrinogen test. *Arch Surg* 1972;104:152–159.

Kakkar VV, Hose CT, Flanc C, et al: Natural history of postoperative deep vein thrombosis. *Lancet* 1969;2:230–232.

Leyvraz P, Bachmann F, Vuilleumier B, et al: Adjusted subcutaneous heparin versus heparin plus dihydroergotamine in prevention of deep vein thrombosis after total hip arthroplasty. *J Arthroplasty* 1988;3:81–86.

Lotke PA, Elia EA: Thromboembolic disease after total knee surgery: A critical review, in Green WB (ed): American Academy of Orthopaedic Surgeons *Instructional Course Lectures XXXIX.* Park Ridge, IL, American Academy of Orthopaedic Surgeons, 1990, pp 409–412.

Paiement GD, Beisaw NE, Harris WH, et al: Advances in prevention of venous thromboembolic disease after elective hip surgery, in Green WB (ed): American Academy of Orthopaedic Surgeons *Instructional Course Lectures XXXIX.* Park Ridge, IL, American Academy of Orthopaedic Surgeons, 1990, pp 413–421.

Scott GB: A quantitative study of the fate of occlusive red venous thrombi. *Br J Exp Path* 1968;49:544–550.

Smith JB: The prostanoids in hemostasis and thrombosis: A review. *Am J Pathol* 1980;99:743–804.

Stamatakis JD, Kakkar VV, Lawrence D, et al: Failure of aspirin to prevent postoperative deep vein thrombosis in patients undergoing total hip replacement. *Br Med J* 1978;1:1031.

Walsh PN, Griffin JH: Contributions of human platelets to the proteolytic activation of blood coagulation factors XII and XI. *Blood* 1981;57:106–118.

Wilner GD, Nossel HL, Leroy EC: Activation of Hagemen factor by collagen. *J Clin Invest* 1968;47:2608–2615.

Shock

Behrman SW, Fabian TC, Kudsk KA, et al: Improved outcome with femur fractures: Early vs delayed fixation. *J Trauma* 1990;30:792–798.

Goldfarb RD: Evaluation of ventricular performance in shock. *Circ Shock* 1985;4:281–301.

Lane PL, McLellan BA, Johns PD: Etiology of shock in blunt trauma. *Can Med Assoc J* 1985;133:199–201.

MacLean LD: Shock: Causes and management of circulatory collapse, in Sabiston DC Jr (ed): *Davis-Christopher Textbook of Surgery,* ed 12. Philadelphia, WB Saunders, 1981, pp 58–90.

Messmer KF: Mechanisms of traumatic shock and their consequences, in Border JR, Allgöwer M, Hansen ST Jr (eds): *Blunt Multiple Trauma.* New York, Marcel Dekker, 1990, pp 39–49.

Mucha P Jr, Welch TJ: Hemorrhage in major pelvic fractures. *Surg Clin North Am* 1988;68:757–773.

Shires GT III, Fantini GA, Shires GT: Management of shock, in Mattox KL, Moore EE, Feliciano DV (eds): *Trauma.* Norwalk, CT, Appleton & Lange, 1988, pp 139–157.

Wyngaarden JB, Smith LH Jr: *Cecil Textbook of Medicine,* ed 17. Philadelphia, WB Saunders, 1985.

Adult Respiratory Distress Syndrome and Fat Embolism

Amato JJ, Rheinlander HF, Cleveland RJ: Post-traumatic adult respiratory distress syndrome. *Orthop Clin North Am* 1978;9:693–713.

Coris JA, Gimbrere JSF: The ARDs prevention scale, in Border JR, Allgöwer ST, Hansen ST Jr, et al (eds): *Blunt Multiple Trauma.* New York, Marcel Dekker, 1990, pp 701–705.

Gossling HR, Pellegrini VD Jr: Fat embolism syndrome: A review of the pathophysiology and physiological basis of treatment. *Clin Orthop* 1982;165:68–82.

Montgomery AB, Stager MA, Carrico CJ, et al: Causes of mortality in patients with the adult respiratory distress syndrome. *Am Rev Respir Dis* 1985;132:485–489.

Moore FD, et al: *Post-Traumatic Pulmonary Insufficiency.* Philadelphia, WB Saunders, 1969.

Riede U, Sandritter W, Mittermayer C: Circulatory shock: A review. *Pathology* 1981;13:299–311.

Riseborough EJ, Herndon JH: Alterations in pulmonary function, coagulation and fat metabolism in patients with fractures of the lower limbs. *Clin Orthop* 1976;115:248–267.

Shapiro BA, Cane RD, Harrison RA: Positive end-expiratory pressure therapy in adults with special reference to acute lung injury: A review of the literature and suggested clinical correlations. *Crit Care Med* 1984;12:127–141.

Shapiro BA, Harrison RA, Trout CA (eds): *Clinical Application of Respiratory Care,* ed 2. Chicago, Year Book Medical Publishers Inc, 1979, pp 87–97.

Basic Science of Bacterial Interactions

Christensen GD, Baddour LM, Simpson WA: Phenotypic variation of Staphylococcus epidermidis slime production in vitro and in vivo. *Infect Immun* 1987;55:2870–2877.

Nichols WW, Evans MJ, Slack MPE: The penetration of antibiotics into aggregates of mucoid and non-mucoid Pseudomonas aeruginosa. *J Gen Microbiol* 1988;135:1291–1303.

Voytek A, Gristina AG, Barth E, et al: Staphylococcal adhesion to collagen in intra-articular sepsis. *Biomaterials* 1988;9:107–110.

Whalen JL, Fitzgerald RH Jr, Morrissy RT: A histological study of acute hematogenous osteomyelitis following physeal injuries in rabbits. *J Bone Joint Surg* 1988;70A:1383–1392.

Infections Involving Implants

Black J: Does corrosion matter? *J Bone Joint Surg* 1988;70B:517–520.

Gristina AG: Biomaterial centered infection: Microbial adhesion versus tissue integration. *Science* 1987;237:1588–1595.

Oga M, Sugioka Y, Hobgood CD, et al: Surgical biomaterials and differential colonization by Staphylococcus epidermidis. *Biomaterials* 1988;9:285–289.

Antibiotics in Bone and Joint Infections

Baker AS, Greenham LW: Release of gentamicin from acrylic bone cement: Elution and diffusion studies. *J Bone Joint Surg* 1988;70A:1551–1557.

Hall BB, Fitzgerald RH Jr: The pharmacokinetics of penicillin in osteomyelitic canine bone. *J Bone Joint Surg* 1983;65A:526–532.

Norden CW: Lessons learned from animal models of osteomyelitis. *Rev Infect Dis* 1988;10:103–110.

Rosenstein BD, Wilson FC, Funderburk CH: The use of bacitracin irrigation to prevent infection in postoperative skeletal wounds: An experimental study. *J Bone Joint Surg* 1989;71A:427–430.

Smith RL, Schurman DJ, Kajiyama G: Effect of NSAID and antibiotic treatment in a rabbit model of staphylococcal infectious arthritis. *Trans Orthop Res Soc* 1990;15:296.

Worlock P, Slack R, Harvey L, et al: The prevention of infection in open fractures: An experimental study of the effect of antibiotic therapy. *J Bone Joint Surg* 1988;70A:1341–1347.

Antibiotics in Prophylaxis and Treatment of Implant Infections

Gristina AG, Naylor PT, Myrvik QN: Mechanisms of musculoskeletal sepsis. *Orthop Clin North Am* 1991;22:363–371.

MacMillan M, Petty W, Hendeles L: Effect of irrigation and tourniquet application on aminoglycoside antibiotic concentrations in bone. *J Orthop Res* 1988;6:311–316.

Petty W, Spanier S, Shuster JJ: Prevention of infection after total joint replacement: Experiments with a canine model. *J Bone Joint Surg* 1988;70A:536–539.

Radioisotope Imaging

Bernier DR, Christian PE, Langan JK, et al (eds): *Nuclear Medicine Technology and Techniques,* ed 2. St. Louis, MO, CV Mosby, 1989.

Palestro CJ, Kim CK, Swyer AJ, et al: Total-hip arthroplasty: Periprosthetic indium-111-labeled leukocyte activity and complementary technetium-99m-sulfur colloid imaging in suspected infection. *J Nucl Med* 1990;31:1950–1955.

Nutrition and Metabolism

Alexander JW, Peck MD: Future prospects for adjunctive therapy: Pharmacologic and nutritional approaches to immune system modulation. *Crit Care Med* 1990;18:S159–S164.

Cerra FB: Hypermetabolism, organ failure, and metabolic support. *Surgery* 1987;101:1–14.

Cuthbertson DP: Further observations of the disturbance of metabolism caused by injury, with particular reference to the dietary requirements of fracture cases. *Br J Surg* 1936;23:505–520.

Einhorn TA, Bonnarens F, Burstein AH: The contributions of dietary protein and mineral to the healing of experimental fractures: A biomechanical study. *J Bone Joint Surg* 1986;68A:1389–1395.

Flint LM: Sepsis and multiple organ failure, in Mattox KL, Moore EE, Feliciano DV (eds): *Trauma.* Norwalk, CT, Appleton & Lange, 1988, pp 879–894.

Fry DE (ed): *Multiple System Organ Failure.* St. Louis, MO, Mosby Year Book, 1992.

Gibson RS: *Principles of Nutritional Assessment.* New York, Oxford University Press, 1990.

Jensen JE, Jensen TG, Smith TK, et al: Nutrition in orthopaedic surgery. *J Bone Joint Surg* 1982;64A: 1263–1272.

Kinsella JE, Lokesh B, Broughton S, et al: Dietary polyunsaturated fatty acids and eicosanoids: Potential effects on the modulation of inflammatory and immune cells: An overview. *Nutrition* 1990;6:24–44.

Lacy JA, Yost M: A key to the literature of nutrition and immunology. *Nutr Clin Prac* 1990;5:200–206.

Long CL, Jeevanandam M, Kim BM, et al: Whole body protein synthesis and catabolism in septic man. *Am J Clin Nutr* 1977;30:1340–1344.

Recommended Dietary Allowances, ed 10. Washington, DC, National Academy of Sciences, National Academy Press, 1989.

Rombeau JL, Caldwell MD (eds): *Clinical Nutrition Volume 1: Enteral and Tube Feeding.* Philadelphia, WB Saunders, 1984.

Rombeau JL, Caldwell MD (eds): *Clinical Nutrition Volume 2: Parenteral Nutrition.* Philadelphia, WB Saunders, 1986.

Saito H, Trocki O, Alexander JW, et al: The effect of route of nutrient administration on the nutritional state, catabolic hormone secretion, and gut mucosal integrity after burn injury. *J Parenter Enteral Nutr* 1987;11:1–7.

Chapter 12
Kinesiology

Sheldon R. Simon, MD
Hannu Alaranta, MD, PhD
Kai-Nan An, PhD
Andrew Cosgarea, MD
Richard Fischer, MD
Joel Frazier, MD
Christopher Keading, MD
Michael Muha, MD
Jacquelin Perry, MD
Malcolm Pope, PhD, DMSc
Peter Quesada, PhD

Chapter Outline

Introduction

Kinesiology is the study of motion of the human body and encompasses such acts as walking or throwing a baseball. Although such motions are quite complex, they are governed by the movements of each separate component of the musculoskeletal system. The biologic and biomechanical/structural properties of these components have been described in previous chapters. This chapter describes the role and function of each of these components in the creation of human motion. It will be seen how biologic form and structure result from function and how the sum of the individual parts of this system create human functional abilities that far exceed those of any one part.

Kinematics

Kinematics is the study of the movements of rigid structures, independent of the forces that might be involved. Two types of movement, translation and rotation, occur within three orthogonal planes; that is, movement has six degrees of freedom.

Humans belong to the vertebrate portion of the phylum Chordata, and as such possess a bony endoskeleton that includes a vertebral spine and paired extremities. Each extremity is composed of articulated skeletal segments linked together by connective tissue elements and surrounded by skeletal muscle. Motion between skeletal segments occurs at joints. Most joint motion is minimally translational and primarily rotational. The deviation from absolute rotatory motion may be noted by the changes in the path of a joint's "instantaneous center of rotation." These paths have been measured for most of the joints in the body and vary only slightly from true arcs of rotation. For human motion to be effective, one comparatively rigid limb segment must not only rotate its position relative to an adjacent segment, but many adjacent limb movements must interact. Whether the hand reaches for a cup or the foot must be lifted high enough to clear an obstacle on the ground, the activity is achieved via coordinated movements of multiple limb segments.

Kinesiology, thus, is first a study of kinematics between each of many limb segments. To provide for the greatest possible function of an extremity, the proximal joint must have the widest range of motion to position the limb in space. This joint must allow for rotatory motions of large degrees in all three planes about all three axes. A means is also provided to alter the length of the limb, so that an extremity can function at all locations within its global range. Rotational motion of the elbow and knee joints allows such overall changes as adjacent limb segments move. Finally, to fine-tune the use of this mechanism with respect to the extremities, for their functional purposes, the hand and foot are required to have a vast amount of movement about all three axes, albeit relatively small. Such movement requires the presence of relatively universal joints at the terminal aspect of each extremity.

Kinetics

The study of the forces that bring about these movements is part of the mechanics discipline called kinetics. Because kinetics provides insights into the cause of the observed motion, it is essential to the proper interpretation of human movement processes. Forces and loads are not visually observable; they must be either measured with instrumentation or calculated from kinematics data. Kinetic quantities studied include such parameters as the forces produced by muscles; reaction loads between body parts as well as their interaction with external surfaces; the load transmitted through the joints; the power transferred between body segments; and the mechanical energy of body segments. Inherent to such studies are the functional demands imposed on the body.

The structure and stability of each extremity and their joints reflect different systems and functional demands. The functional demands on the upper extremity are quite different from those on either the upper and lower axial skeleton or those on the lower extremity. Depending on which joint and/or structures are addressed, different types and degrees of rotational motion are allowed and are functional. How much structural strength is needed versus how much movement is allowed in each area dictates the nature of the material, size, shape, and infrastructure of the joint system established to perform a given movement. Kinesiology depends upon anatomy in that anatomy is a study that covers the appearance, structure, and location of the various parts of the body, and kinesiology is a study of the function of the musculoskeletal elements.

Joint Stability

Human motion is governed by Newton's three laws of motion: (1) an object will change velocity only if a force is applied; (2) the change in velocity is proportional to the force; and (3) forces always exist in pairs that are equal and opposite in direction, such that if one body pushes against another, the second body will push back against the first with a force of equal magnitude. Newton's third law is especially significant because purposeful functional movements could not exist without it. Many movements of limb segments and the motion of the body as a whole could not take place without interaction with external surfaces based on Newton's third law. Applied to human internal movement, this law suggests muscles cannot impart movement to a limb segment without the segment's interaction with another bone and without a joint structure that will allow the desired rotational direction and force. If stability or directional constraints are provided through such a mechanism, translational movements, which serve to "dislocate" one rigid bony limb segment from another, are avoided.

Joint stability is created by bony configurations, ligaments, and muscles; combinations of these constructs differ between joints. Bone primarily constrains translational motions. Where rotation is needed, there is no bony blockage. Because bone is the most rigid anatomic structure, the greater the circumference of the joint enclosed by bone, the greater the amount of inherent translational stability that exists in the joint. This point is illustrated by the contrast between the spherical head of the femur (which is enclosed by a hemispheric arc of bony acetabulum) and the flatter radius of curvature of the glenoid (which encloses less of the humeral head) and the relative ease of dislocation or subluxation of the latter as compared to the former.

Ligaments can restrict or constrain rotational or translational motions. By the tension developed in it when it is stretched, a ligament resists motion along the axes in which it lies. Unlike bone, however, ligaments allow some motion to occur, and thus, cannot be considered rigid constraints. The position of the ligament is the key to the type of motions it limits. For example, at the knee, the cruciate ligaments limit the anteroposterior (AP) translation of the tibia on the femur, while at the ankle, the interosseous ligament prevents translational motion between the tibia and fibula, as compared to the deltoid or talocalcaneofibular ligaments, which prevent rotational motions as well as translational motions between these two bones and the calcaneus.

Muscle-tendon complexes are also semirigid restraints and complement the action of ligaments to stabilize joints. However, because ligaments are only passive stabilizers, muscles, which are active in controlling joint motion, have an obvious advantage. Muscle action, in fact, can protect ligaments from tearing in most instances. Muscle contraction produces compressive force across the joint tending to squeeze the joint together. This compressive force maintains stability against forces that might pivot a joint open. Where the compressive forces of a muscle are parallel to those exerted by the tensile forces occurring in the ligament, they provide load sharing. Where their direction of force is opposite, muscles can work in concert with the ligaments and serve to protect the joint when disruption of the ligament occurs. An example of this interaction is the protection the hamstrings provide when the anterior cruciate ligament is torn. Thus, not only are muscles the force actuators at joints that initiate or prevent a desired movement, but they also can limit motions caused by external body weight or antagonist muscles harmful to joint stability.

Without joint stability, true functional motion cannot exist because much displacement will occur between the two rigid members at the joint surface. The extent to which each of the three structures—bone, ligaments, and muscles—contributes to joint stability differs at each joint. These differences are illustrated throughout this chapter with the discussions of the various joints. The spine, perhaps, illustrates the most intricate balance of contributions between the three structural stabilizers.

Control of Movement

Kinesiology also concerns understanding how the musculoskeletal system provides the means to initiate a movement, control the movement's magnitude and direction, and, when the desired goal is achieved, end the movement. This implies interactions not only of adjacent limb segments, but also between multiple segments. Human motions require the use of force actuators and a control mechanism to determine the placement, timing, and magnitude of force generation. These determinations are made via a dynamic system related not only to the muscle, but also to all aspects of the neurologic system. The force causing joint rotation about an axis is not merely the contracting or stretching force produced by the muscle, but is a product of this force multiplied by the distance between the joint center of rotation and the tendon. The magnitude of the muscle force depends on the functional activity, the speed at which it occurs, and the number of other muscles contributing to the effort. For example, during locomotor activities, quadriceps activation is needed to prevent the knee joint from collapsing during initiation of weightbearing. The amount of force required differs markedly during walking, running, initiating the next step during stair climbing, or getting up from a chair. In all these activities, the quadriceps muscle does not create the movement. During kicking, quadriceps activation is needed to create the motion, the quadriceps operates in a concentric mode, and the magnitude of force required will vary depending on whether the kicking is part of a game of soccer or that required to score a field goal in a football game.

The nature of how much effort a single muscle or several muscles acting about one or more joints produces is dictated by neurocontrol. For many types of functions, the exact mechanism of neurocontrol remains a puzzle; it is the subject of intensive basic research in the field of neurophysiology. The amount of effort needed at each joint can also be viewed as a mechanical problem that has an almost infinite number of solutions. Yet, the body does not use an infinite number of solutions; it operates in a finite way, thereby suggesting that human biologic systems have developed an optimal way of performing these tasks. This area has aroused intense interest in fields of engineering and modeling, not only because of interest in biologic systems, but also because of efforts in robotics. For example, in a two-legged robot similar to humans, with hip, knee, and ankle joints, appropriate activations of springs or brakes at each of these joints would be required to maintain the robot in an upright position. If fully understood, this neurocontrol system would benefit not only the treatment of a variety of human disorders, but also the creation of mechanical robotic systems. These aspects of human movement are discussed more fully below when the mechanisms of throwing, standing, and walking are described.

Kinesiology is thus a study of how the musculoskeletal system has adapted to kinetics and kinematics on a micro- and macroscopic scale between adjacent and across multiple limb segments. It is a study and understanding of how motions are produced by forces at individual joints as well as what characterizes their integration when a specific function is desired. Like any movement involving multiple parts, it requires different types of contributions from different components and a means for controlling and integrating the various activities of the individual parts. This chapter will present current knowledge of various representative parts of the process. This is not a comprehensive representation of the entire subject of kinesiology as it is related to human movement. For that, the reader is advised to refer to the many existing texts that relate to various aspects of the system.

Structure and Function of the Shoulder Joint

The shoulder joint allows the arm to move with respect to the thorax. This motion normally occurs through a complex interaction of the individual motions of the acromioclavicular, sternoclavicular, and glenohumeral joints as well as the scapulothoracic articulation. The biomechanics of the shoulder joint really is a study of these four different articulations, which make up the shoulder complex.

The shoulder complex allows the greatest range of motion of any "joint" in the body. Traditional descriptions of humeral thoracic motion involve measuring the angle formed by the humerus and the thorax in the sagittal plane (flexion and extension) and the coronal plane (abduction). Axial rotation of the humerus is conventionally described by the measurement in degrees of internal or external rotation when the humeral axis is parallel to the thorax (Fig. 1), or perpendicular to the thorax (abducted 90°). Horizontal abduction and adduction, also known as horizontal extension and flexion, respectively, are commonly used to describe arm position when the axis of the humerus is perpendicular to the thorax.

Theoretically, 180° of elevation of the arm is possible, but very few individuals ever attain this degree of motion. Normal arm elevation in men has been reported as 167° or 168° and in women from 171° to 175°. Average extension or posterior elevation has been shown to be approximately 60° (Fig. 2). With the arm adducted by the side of the body, approximately 180° of rotation is possible with approximately 60% of that being in external rotation. With abduction of the arm to 90°, however, the total arc of rotation is reduced to 120° with relatively more internal rotation possible at that arm position. The range of motion of the shoulder decreases with normal aging. A comparison of two groups of males whose mean collective ages differed by only 12.5 years indicated that the younger group averaged 3.4° greater flexion, 3.4° greater internal rotation, 8.4° greater external rotation, and 10.2° greater extension.

Although measurements of the range of motion of the shoulder have commonly been made in specific planes such as flexion and extension, very few activities of daily living or recreation involving humeral thoracic motion are limited to these single planes. The most common plane for humeral elevation in daily living is 50° to 60° anterior to the coronal plane. This approximates the line of the

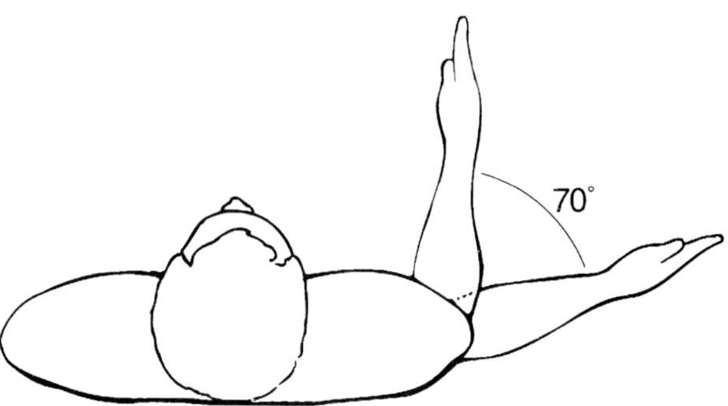

Figure 1
External rotation of the shoulder from 0° to 70° with the arm adducted.

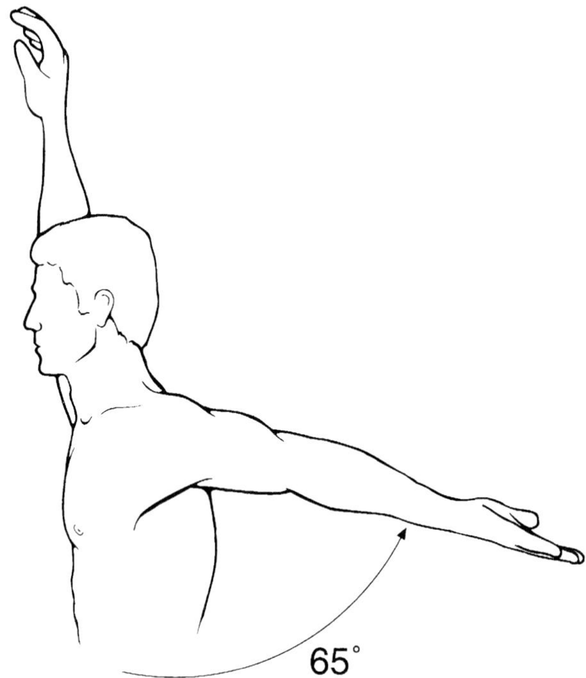

Figure 2
Extension of the shoulder to 65°.

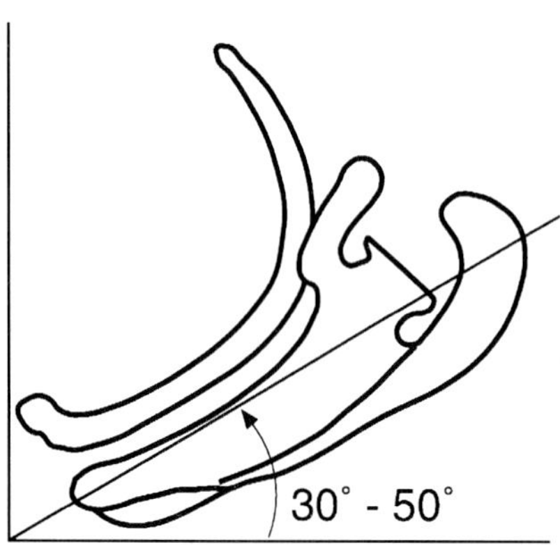

Figure 3
The plane of the scapula is approximately 30° to 50° anterior to the coronal plane of the body.

scapula or the scapular plane, which is described as being anywhere from 30° to 50° anterior to the coronal axis (Fig. 3). The act of combing one's hair requires an average of 148° of elevation in this plane, whereas the act of eating requires only an average of 52° of elevation in the same plane.

Clinical terms such as flexion, adduction, horizontal adduction, and extension are descriptive, but insufficient in their ability to portray the position of the arm with respect to the thorax, because more than one modifying word applies to virtually every arm position in space. In order to describe the position of a military salute, for example, conventional terminology would include 80° of abduction, 30° of horizontal adduction or horizontal flexion, and 40° of internal rotation of the humerus. Conversely, it could be described as forward flexion to 80°, 30° anterior to the coronal plane, with 40° of internal rotation of the humerus. Such language can be cumbersome and inconsistent. A cornerstone to the understanding of the kinematics of a joint is the ability to measure and describe its motion in an accurate and reproducible fashion. One method to achieve this accuracy in description is to designate various vertical planes available for elevation of the humerus similar to the segments of an orange or the longitudinal demarcations of a globe. The plane of pure abduction in the coronal plane is defined as the 0° plane and pure flexion in the anterior sagittal plane is +90° (Fig. 4). Maximum horizontal adduction of the shoulder occurs at +124° with maximum extension and horizontal abduction occurring at −88° (Fig. 5). Therefore, 212 different planes of humeral elevation are possible. Humeral elevation within a given plane is then quantified by measuring the angle formed between the unelevated humerus and the elevated humerus. Pure abduction to 90° is described as (0, 90) whereas pure flexion to 90° is described as (+90, 90). For example, the act of washing the contralateral axilla requires the 104° plane as well as 52° of elevation of the humerus within that plane (+104, 52).

The final determinant of shoulder position is the axial rotation of the humerus described by the angle formed between the forearm (elbow flexed to 90°) and a line perpendicular to the plane of elevation (Fig. 6). If the forearm is perpendicular to the plane of elevation, rotation is defined as 0°. External rotation from that position is designated as positive (+), and internal rotation from that position is designated as negative (−). In this system, the military salute position previously discussed can be described as (+30, 80, +40). The act of combing the hair requires 57° of external rotation and could be described in this system as (+50, 110, +57).

Biomechanics of the Glenohumeral Joint

The glenohumeral joint demonstrates a normal range of laxity in virtually every direction. Average passive glenohumeral translation of 11.5 mm, both anteriorly and posteriorly, has been demonstrated in cadaver shoulders. A study of normal unanesthetized volunteers has demonstrated that passive humeral translation on the glenoid averaged 8 mm anteriorly, 9 mm posteriorly, and 11 mm inferiorly. Up to 2 cm of glenohumeral translation has been documented in some unanesthetized volunteers

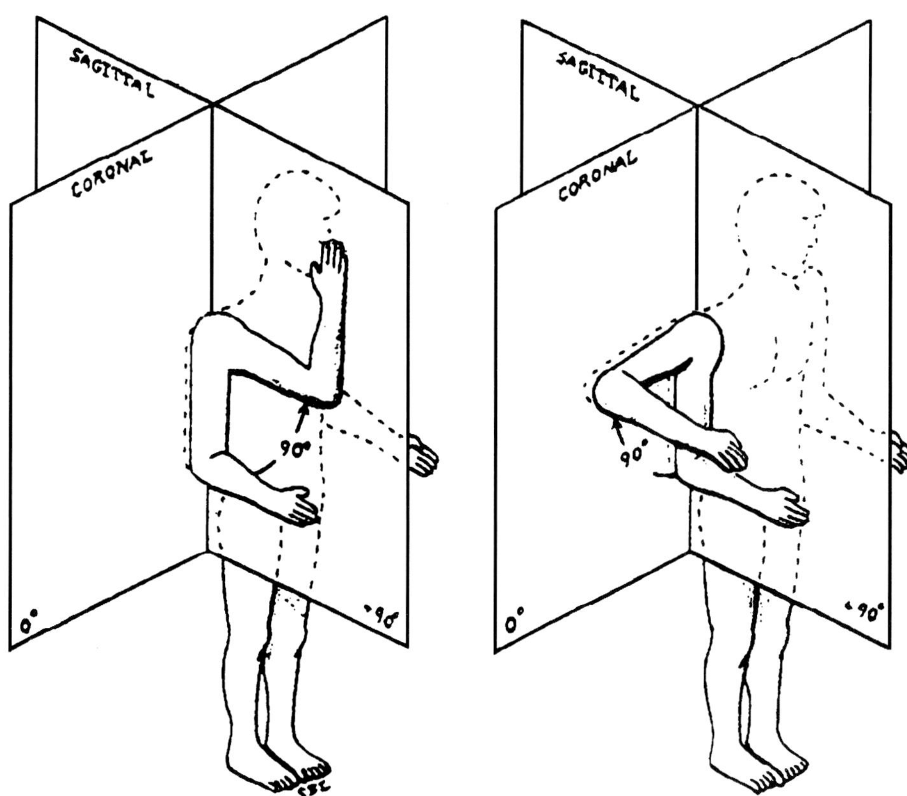

Figure 4
Left, Elevation of the arm in the sagittal plane (flexion) may be defined as occurring in the +90° plane. Flexion to an angle of 90° within that plane is then described as (+90, 90). **Right,** Elevation of the arm in the coronal plane (abduction) may be defined as occurring in the 0° plane. Abduction to an angle of 90° within that plane is described as (0, 90). (Reproduced with permission from Pearl ML, Harris SL, Lippitt SB, et al: A system for describing positions of the humerus relative to the thorax and its use in the presentation of several functionally important arm positions. *J Shoulder Elbow Surg* 1992;1:114.)

with no history of shoulder instability. These evaluations of glenohumeral laxity were performed in the absence of any significant compressive force across the glenohumeral joint. They represent possible passive translation when an externally applied passive force acts on the humerus and, therefore, do not represent normal physiologic glenohumeral kinematics. These studies do demonstrate the great potential laxity in the glenohumeral joint.

Glenohumeral translation occurs to a significantly smaller degree during arm elevation and rotation than during drawer or laxity testing. In cadaver shoulders with a rigidly fixed scapula, passive forward elevation of the humerus up to 55° in the sagittal plane has demonstrated no translation between the center of rotation of the humeral head and the center of rotation of the glenoid. Up to 35° of passive extension was also possible without any translation. Throughout this total arc of 90°, essentially pure rotation between the humerus and glenoid occurred. Translation began to occur beyond 55° of flexion or 35° of extension. However, the rigidly fixed scapula prevented normal scapular motion. Simulated active forward elevation of the cadaver shoulder using cables attached to the deltoid and rotator cuff insertions has demonstrated an initial superior translation of 1 mm, from 0° to 30° of forward elevation. However, between 30° and 180° of elevation, the center of rotation of the humeral head has been shown to translate only 0.94 mm in the AP direction and 1.29 mm in the superoinferior direction.

Radiographic analysis of normal volunteer subjects has shown that precise centering of the humeral head in the glenoid is maintained in all positions in the horizontal plane except when the arm is in maximum horizontal extension and simultaneous external rotation. At that point, 4 mm of posterior translation with respect to the center of the glenoid occurred. Radiographic analysis of active forward elevation in the plane of the scapula has shown that superior humeral head translation of 1 mm occurs for each 30° increment of forward elevation of the arm. These studies demonstrate in various ways that the center of rotation of the humeral head stays within a few millimeters of the center of rotation of the glenoid during normal glenohumeral range of motion despite the great potential for passive laxity in the glenohumeral joint. Rotational motion predominates in the glenohumeral joint despite the great potential for translation. The structure and methods for stabilizing the glenohumeral joint provide the basis for explaining how this potentially large translation is held to a minimum in this joint.

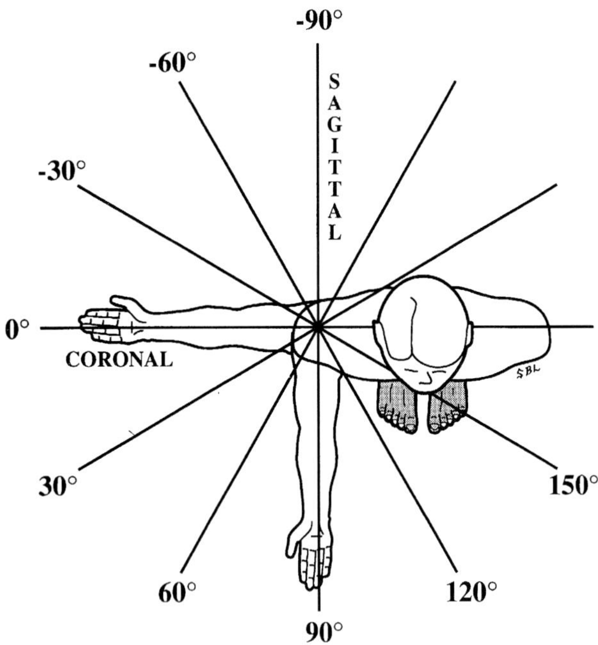

Figure 5
Planes of elevation of the arm. In normal individuals, the available planes of elevation are from -88° to +124°, therefore there are 212 different planes of humeral elevation. (Reproduced with permission from Pearl ML, Harris SL, Lippitt SB, et al: A system for describing positions of the humerus relative to the thorax and its use in the presentation of several functionally important arm positions. *J Shoulder Elbow Surg* 1992;1:115.)

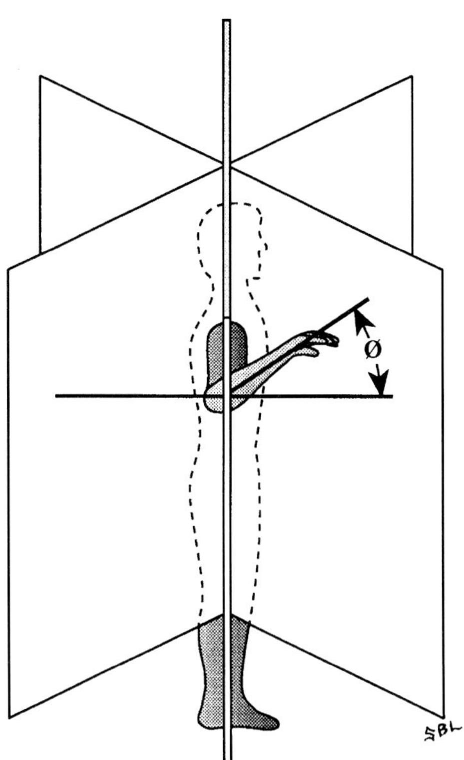

Figure 6
Rotation of the humerus is described by the angle formed by the forearm and a line perpendicular to the plane of elevation. (Reproduced with permission from Pearl ML, Harris SL, Lippitt SB, et al: A system for describing positions of the humerus relative to the thorax and its use in the presentation of several functionally important arm positions. *J Shoulder Elbow Surg* 1992;1:115.)

Anatomy of the Glenohumeral Joint

The glenoid is an oval or bean-shaped shallow socket that is retroverted approximately 7° with respect to the plane perpendicular to the plane of the scapula (Fig. 7). However, because the plane of the scapula is anterior to the coronal plane, the glenoid is anteverted 30° to 40° with respect to the coronal plane of the body (Fig. 3). The glenoid also faces superiorly approximately 5° when the scapula is in the normal resting position (Fig. 8). This superior inclination has been shown to significantly contribute to inferior stability of the glenohumeral joint, probably because of a cam effect that potentiates tightening of the superior capsule during inferiorly directed stress on the humerus. The surface area of the glenoid socket is approximately one third that of the surface area of the humeral head. The depth of the glenoid socket has been measured to be 9 mm in a superoinferior direction and 5 mm in the AP direction. Of the total depth of the glenoid socket, 50% is provided by the surrounding glenoid labrum and 50% is provided by the configuration of the bone and articular cartilage. The articular cartilage of the glenoid is thicker peripherally than centrally, and this further deepens the glenoid socket (Fig. 9). Thus, the actual joint surface of the glenoid is more concave than the concavity of the subchondral bone seen on radiographic analysis of the glenoid.

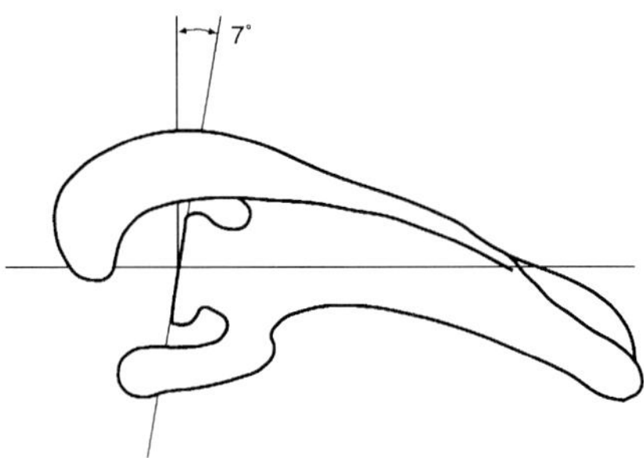

Figure 7
The glenoid is retroverted 7° with respect to the plane perpendicular to the scapular plane.

The articular surface of the proximal humerus is approximately one third of a sphere and it is

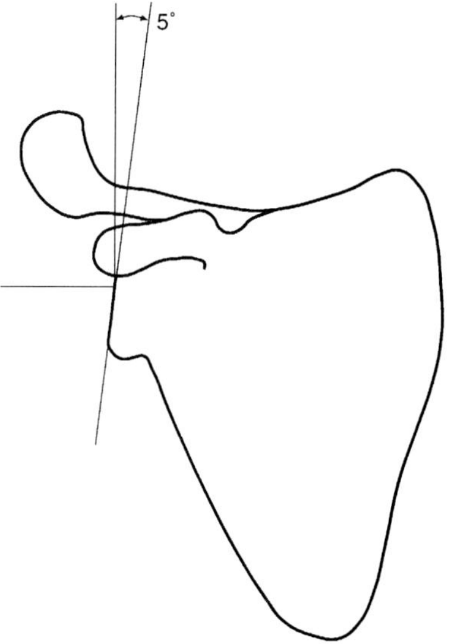

Figure 8
The glenoid faces superiorly approximately 5°.

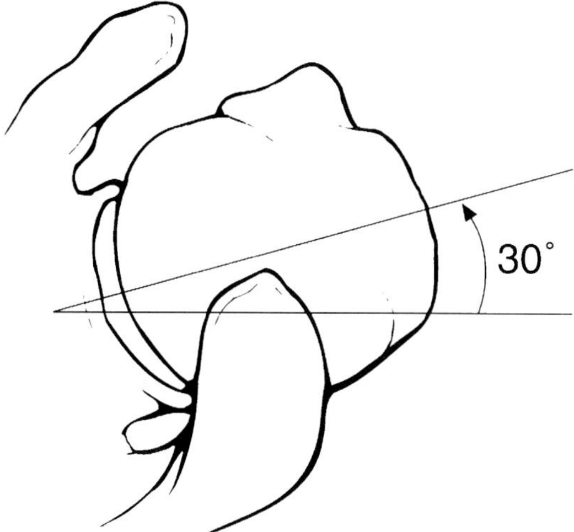

Figure 10
The humeral head is retroverted 30° to 40° with respect to the intercondylar plane of the humerus.

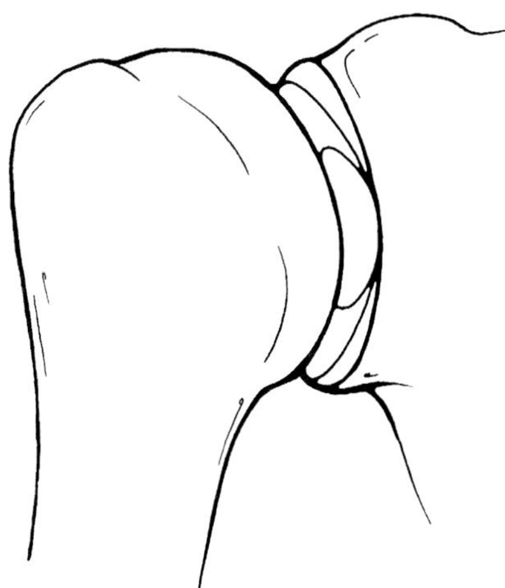

Figure 9
The glenoid labrum provides 50% of the depth of the glenoid socket. The articular cartilage is thicker peripherally than centrally, which increases the concavity of the articular surface of the glenoid.

retroverted 30° to 40° with respect to the intercondylar plane of the distal humerus (Fig. 10). Recent stereophotogrammetric studies of the curvature of fresh frozen human cadaver shoulders have demonstrated that the deviation from sphericity of the convex humeral articular surface and concave glenoid articular surface was less than 1%. Therefore, these two articular surfaces are highly congruent. Traditionally, the glenohumeral joint has been likened to a large ball articulating with a small flat platform; for example, a golf ball on a tee. The glenohumeral joint, however, is actually composed of two closely fitting spherical surfaces. The lack of stability of the humeral surface against the glenoid surface is not caused by a discrepancy in radii, but rather is a reflection of the smaller surface area of the glenoid, which cannot capture the humeral head. Because of the decreased articular surface area of the glenoid, the glenohumeral joint depends primarily on soft tissues for maintenance of a stable articulation. A combination of muscles, capsule, and ligamentous forces is necessary for normal glenohumeral motion to occur, but a variety of passive mechanisms enhance the stability of the glenohumeral articulation as well.

Glenohumeral Stability

Passive Constraints

Because of the conformity of the radii of curvature of the glenoid and the humeral articular surfaces, and because of the synovial fluid present, adhesion and cohesion act together to stabilize the glenohumeral articulation. Synovial fluid adheres to the articular cartilage via the principle of adhesion, and this thin film of fluid between the two joint surfaces allows sliding motion to occur between these surfaces. Concomitantly, because of the principle of cohesion, the two joint surfaces cannot easily be pulled apart. This works in the same way that a drinking glass can slide in a film of water on a glass tabletop, but momentarily sticks during attempts to lift the glass off the table top. In the glenohumeral joint, the compliant glenoid labrum that surrounds the rim of the glenoid further potentiates this passive stabilizing effect.

The intra-articular pressure in the glenohumeral joint is slightly negative under normal conditions. This negative intra-articular pressure probably arises as a result of high osmotic pressure in the surrounding tissues, which acts to draw water from the joint. The glenohumeral joint normally contains less than 1 cc of fluid, although it can accommodate more than 30 cc of fluid. The watertight capsule of the glenohumeral joint is pulled inwardly by this negative intra-articular pressure, thereby keeping the capsule and ligaments under continuous stretch and helping to maintain the stability of the joint. Joint effusions or venting of the capsule interferes with this mechanism. If an inferiorly directed translation force of 16 N is applied to the humerus in a cadaver shoulder, an inferior translation of 2 mm has been demonstrated. If the capsule of that cadaver shoulder is then punctured, the resultant inferior translation increases to 28 mm during application of the same 16-N force. The integrity of the capsule around the shoulder is important for the maintenance of this negative intra-articular pressure.

Considering that the arm is one twelfth of body weight, it would seem that in the normal resting position, with the arm hanging by the side, some degree of muscular activity would be necessary to maintain the glenohumeral joint in a reduced position. Electromyographic (EMG) analysis of the deltoid, supraspinatus, infraspinatus, triceps, and biceps muscles in young male volunteers has demonstrated that no activity occurs in these muscles when the arm is quietly maintained by the side. Inferior translation of the humerus is not present on normal AP radiographs of the shoulder. Spontaneous translations of the humerus on the glenoid do not occur when patients in the operating room are administered general anesthesia. Therefore, either passive stabilizing mechanisms or the ligamentous and capsule static constraints are responsible for maintaining the reduction of the glenohumeral articulation. An examination of the static capsular ligamentous constraints of the glenohumeral joint will augment understanding of how the glenohumeral joint maintains a stable reduction during resting posture.

Static Constraints

The capsule and ligaments are the most important stabilizers in preventing dislocation of the glenohumeral joint. The capsuloligamentous structures form a truncated cone of collagenous tissue with the smaller of the two circular attachments surrounding the glenoid and the larger of the two circular attachments surrounding the humeral head. The glenohumeral ligaments are thickenings or condensations of the glenohumeral capsule and are located primarily anteriorly and inferiorly in the capsule itself. The coracohumeral ligament represents a folded thickening of the glenohumeral capsule in the area of the rotator interval between the subscapularis and supraspinatus muscles. Although the capsule extends circumferentially around the glenoid, the posterosuperior quadrant of the capsule is devoid of ligamentous condensations.

Superior glenohumeral ligament The superior glenohumeral ligament (SGHL) originates just anteriorly to the long head of the biceps origin on the superior glenoid, and it inserts on the proximal aspect of the lesser tuberosity of the humerus. The SGHL is present in approximately 90% of shoulders, and is well developed in approximately 50% of shoulders. However, there is variability in its development. It is the main capsular structure resisting inferior translation of the humerus in the adducted shoulder. It is less important in stabilizing the glenohumeral joint against AP translation.

Middle glenohumeral ligament The middle glenohumeral ligament (MGHL) demonstrates the greatest variability of the glenohumeral ligaments and, in fact, is absent in up to 30% of shoulders. The MGHL originates from the glenoid or the labrum just inferior to the SGHL and inserts just medial to the lesser tuberosity of the proximal humerus (Fig. 11). It acts as a secondary restraint to inferior glenohumeral translation in the adducted and externally rotated shoulder as well as to anterior glenohumeral translation in the shoulder abducted to 90°. The MGHL limits anterior translation of the humerus on the glenoid to a more significant degree when the arm is

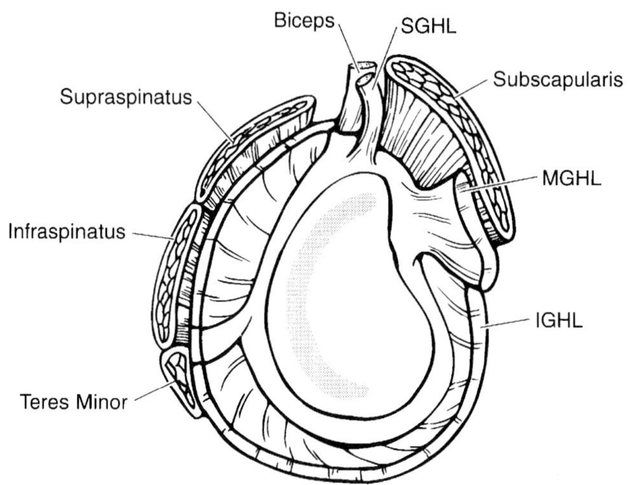

Figure 11
The relationship of the glenohumeral ligaments as they attach to the glenoid. Although the posterosuperior capsule is devoid of ligamentous condensations, this portion of the glenohumeral joint is bolstered by the presence of the rotator cuff tendons.

abducted 45° than when the arm is either at 90° or 0° of abduction.

Inferior glenohumeral ligament The inferior glenohumeral ligament (IGHL) is the most important static restraint in the glenohumeral joint. The anterior aspect of the IGHL originates on the anterior aspect of the glenoid or glenoid neck at approximately the three o'clock position. The posterior aspect of the IGHL originates from the glenoid at approximately the nine o'clock position. The IGHL is a complex structure consisting of anterior and posterior thickenings or bands with a sling-like pouch in between (Fig. 11). This pouch is referred to as the axillary pouch. The IGHL is the primary stabilizer of the abducted shoulder against AP translation. The stabilizing role of this complex ligament increases with increasing arm abduction. During external rotation of the humerus, the anterior band of the IGHL fans out and tightens, whereas the posterior band fans out and tightens during internal rotation of the arm (Fig. 12). This reciprocal tightening and loosening of the anterior and posterior bands of the IGHL, with respect to various arm positions, has been likened to the function of a hammock during asymmetric loading. The IGHL is also an important structure in providing superoinferior stability to the glenohumeral joint, especially with increasing amounts of abduction. In fact, the IGHL is the primary restraint to inferior translation of the humerus on the glenoid in a position of 90° of abduction of the arm.

Mechanical testing performed on the anterior glenohumeral capsule and IGHL has indicated that the tensile strength of the anterior capsular attachment in cadavers is approximately 70 N. When tested in tension, the IGHL complex undergoes significant plastic deformation prior to failure. The strain-to-failure of the IGHL in cadaver shoulders averages 27.9%, with a range of 15% to 61.2%.

Coracohumeral ligament The coracohumeral ligament (CHL) originates from the base of the coracoid process and attaches to the lateral aspect of the bicipital groove on the greater tuberosity of the humerus. The importance of the CHL in limiting inferior translation of the adducted humerus is unclear. Some have demonstrated that the CHL has little significance in stabilizing the adducted shoulder, although others have found that it significantly limits inferior humeral translation.

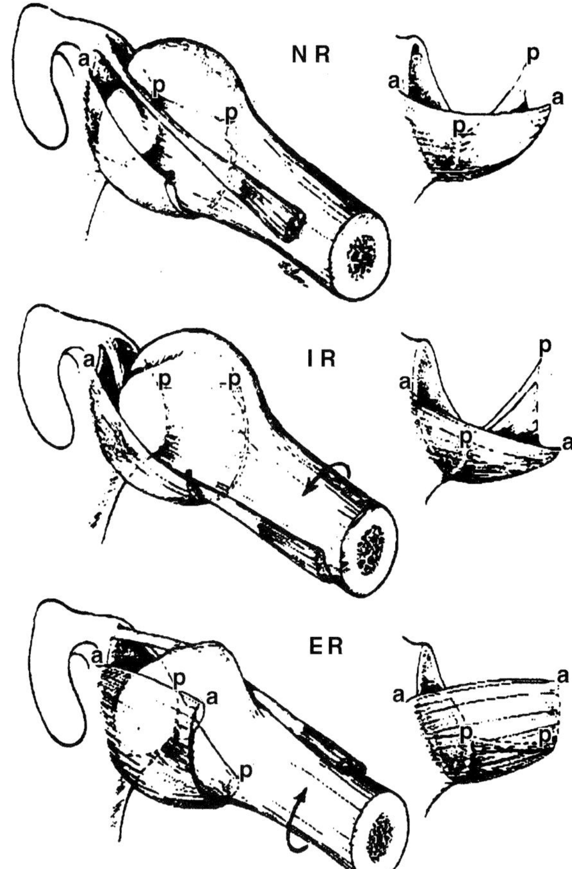

Figure 12
The anterior and posterior portions of the IGHL complex reciprocally tighten and loosen depending on the rotation of the humerus. With external rotation (ER), the anterior band (a) of the IGHL tightens and moves superiorly on the humeral head. During internal rotation (IR) of the humerus, the posterior band (p) of the IGHL tightens and moves superiorly. NR = no rotation. (Reproduced with permission from Warner JJP, Caborn DNM, Berger R, et al: Dynamic capsuloligamentous anatomy of the glenohumeral joint. *J Shoulder Elbow Surg* 1993;2:131.)

The Relationship of Static and Passive Constraints

Ligaments function in tension and are of little stabilizing effect when lax. To limit anterior translation of the humerus on the glenoid, capsuloligamentous structures would have to be under tension. If the ligamentous structures around the glenohumeral joint were responsible for eliminating translation of the humerus on the glenoid during normal motion, these structures would have to be taut. Yet, large amounts of translation are possible in the glenohumeral joint in virtually all directions. Moreover, the center of rotation of the humeral head varies only a few millimeters from the center of rotation of the glenoid during glenohumeral motion. Therefore, some mechanism exists to maintain the pure rotation of the glenohumeral joint through a great range of motion while the ligaments remain relatively lax. This pure rotation is maintained by the passive stabilizing mechanisms, such as adhesion, cohesion, and negative intra-articular pressure, as well as by the dynamic stabilizing forces that cross the glenohumeral joint when those forces are combined with the ability of the glenoid to move in space in synchrony with the humerus.

The complex bony architecture and muscular arrangement of the shoulder girdle allow the minimally constrained glenohumeral joint to maintain concentric reduction throughout the huge range of motion necessary for activities of daily living. However, pathologic translation of the humerus on the glenoid certainly occurs, especially in clinical instability of the shoulder. Most joints in the human body dislocate only when ligamentous structures are torn or periarticular fractures occur. The glenohumeral joint can dislocate without actual tearing of ligamentous tissue if capsuloligamentous structures are significantly stretched. It can be safely stated, however, that glenohumeral dislocations do not occur in the presence of efficiently functioning glenohumeral ligament structures. Selective cutting experiments have helped to clarify the role of the various capsuloligamentous structures around the glenohumeral joint.

Stabilization of the Glenohumeral Joint

The role of selective cutting experiments The primary stabilizer of the glenohumeral joint in the superoinferior direction of the adducted arm appears to be the superior capsular structures, especially the SGHL. With increasing abduction of the arm, however, the inferior capsular structures, especially the IGHL, become the most significant stabilizers against inferior translation. The primary stabilizer of the glenohumeral joint against anterior translation is the IGHL; at lower degrees of abduction, the MGHL and subscapularis also contribute. The primary stabilizer of the glenohumeral joint against posterior translation also appears to be the IGHL. If the entire posterior capsule of the glenohumeral joint is incised, posterior translation increases, but posterior dislocation does not occur. With an additional incision anteriorly, from twelve o'clock to three o'clock, through the anterosuperior capsule (SGHL, MGHL), posterior dislocation of the flexed and internally rotated humerus can occur. Posterior humeral translation increases when the anterior band of the IGHL is incised, if the arm is maintained in 30° of extension. Posterior translation increases when the anterior portion of the IGHL is detached from the glenoid (Bankart lesion).

Bankart's concept of a single essential lesion producing shoulder instability is attractive, but too simplistic. The creation of a Bankart lesion in the cadaver shoulder leads to increased glenohumeral translation of several millimeters, although anterior glenohumeral dislocation does not occur. Translation of the glenohumeral joint increases with injury to the capsule on one side of this joint, but in order for dislocation to occur, the capsule must be injured or stretched on both sides of the glenohumeral joint. This fact is important during surgical reconstruction of the ligaments around the unstable shoulder. Individuals demonstrating increased clinical laxity in the musculoskeletal system become more at risk for glenohumeral dislocation with minor trauma to their glenohumeral ligaments. In an individual with generalized joint laxity, inherent laxity of the posterior capsule combined with a small amount of injury to the IGHL anteriorly may allow a dislocation of the glenohumeral joint anteriorly. In another individual with normal ligamentous laxity a relatively greater degree of trauma to the IGHL anteriorly would be required to effect an anterior glenohumeral dislocation.

When interpreting selective cutting experiments, it is important to remember that the interaction of muscle forces, intra-articular pressure, and the degree of plastic deformation of the capsuloligamentous structures are clinically important and are difficult to replicate during experiments in cadaver shoulders. Dynamic stabilizers of the glenohumeral joint, that is, muscular forces, significantly affect glenohumeral stability as well. Selective cutting experiments in the shoulder, as opposed to some of the other joints in the human body, help to clarify ligamentous function, but must be interpreted cautiously regarding the etiology of clinical instability.

Unlike the acetabulum of the hip joint, the glenoid socket is quite mobile. This allows the relatively shallow glenoid to be placed advantageously so that it can most effectively resist the joint reaction forces generated by the muscle contractions crossing the glenohumeral joint. In this way, the glenoid can be likened to a mobile backstop. The motion required for this effect is possible because of the complex architecture of the clavicle and scapula, the coordinated activities of the musculature controlling the scapula, and the unconstrained acromioclavicular and sternoclavicular joints.

The clavicle The clavicle acts as a strut that effectively maintains the scapula and glenoid lateral to the thorax despite a variety of arm and body positions. This strut allows muscles, such as the pectoralis major and latissimus dorsi, to move the humerus powerfully without effectively changing the position of the glenoid in relation to the midline of the body. The prime movers of the humerus compress the humeral head against the glenoid and, in so doing, cause a chain reaction across the acromioclavicular joint, the scapular thoracic articulation, and, finally, the sternoclavicular joint.

The acromioclavicular joint The acromioclavicular (AC) joint is a true diarthrodial joint that allows the articulation of the medial aspect of the acromion with the lateral aspect of the clavicle. The joint surfaces are not perfectly congruent, and a fibrocartilaginous meniscus is interposed between the clavicle and the acromion. The AC capsule is thickened superiorly, forming the AC ligament. The AC ligament and AC capsule are the most important stabilizers of the AC joint in the AP direction and are important stabilizers for axial rotation of the clavicle as well. The AC capsule and ligaments are the most important stabilizers of the AC joint when this joint is subjected to relatively light loads of daily activity and recreation; however, when greater forces are applied to the AC joint, the most important stabilizing structures become the coracoclavicular ligaments composed of the trapezoid and conoid ligaments.

The scapula is essentially suspended from the clavicle by way of these two strong ligaments that span from the undersurface of the clavicle to the coracoid process of the scapula. Although the trapezoid is larger and stronger, it has been shown that during large displacements of the AC joint, the conoid resists almost four times as much force (70%) as does the trapezoid (18%). The trapezoid ligament, because of its oblique fibers, more effectively resists AC joint compression during loading of the glenohumeral joint, such as in weight lifting. This tough sling of ligamentous tissue effectively decreases the compression of the acromion against the lateral end of the clavicle.

The sternoclavicular joint The sternoclavicular joint forms the only true skeletal articulation or bridge between the upper extremity and the thorax. This diarthrodial joint is composed of reciprocally saddle-shaped, but incongruous, articular surfaces with an interposed fibrocartilaginous disc or meniscus. Ligamentous restraints surround the sternoclavicular joint anteriorly, posteriorly, superiorly, and inferiorly.

Motion of the clavicle The clavicle rotates in the AP and superoinferior directions as well as actually rotating both anteriorly and posteriorly during normal motion of the arm. Greater motion occurs at the sternoclavicular joint than at the AC joint. Approximately 35° of superior rotation, anterior rotation, and posterior rotation occurs in the sternoclavicular joint, and this unconstrained, saddle-shaped articulation allows 45° to 50° of axial rotation to occur. The clavicle has been shown to rotate 40° to 50° during active forward elevation of the arm. Although the clavicle rotates this amount with respect to the fixed sternum, it rotates only 5° to 8° with respect to the acromion at the AC joint because of the concomitant synchronous rotation of the scapula during forward elevation of the arm.

Biomechanics of the Shoulder

Muscular Activity of the Shoulder Joint Complex

Twenty different muscles act on the shoulder girdle. Some of these muscles can be further subdivided according to differing functional heads into the three heads of the deltoid, two heads of the biceps brachii, two portions of the pectoralis major, and three portions of the trapezius. The muscles affecting the shoulder girdle can be classified as glenohumeral, scapulothoracic, or thoracohumeral based on their origins and insertions (Outline 1).

The effectiveness of any muscle depends on its physiologic cross-sectional area, angle of pull, and intensity of contraction. Electromyography can demonstrate and quantify the amount of activity in a particular muscle group during dynamic conditions. The percentage of recorded EMG activity indicates the level of activity of a given muscle, but does not indicate the force generated by that muscle. For complete understanding of the force generated by a particular muscle about the shoulder, the moment arm (distance of the muscle pull from the instantaneous center of the joint rotation) and the physiologic cross-sectional area (the volume of the muscle divided by the muscle length) must be known. In the shoulder, the bones and both the

Outline 1
Muscles affecting the shoulder girdle

Glenohumeral muscles
- Deltoid
- Supraspinatus
- Infraspinatus
- Teres minor
- Subscapularis
- Teres major
- Coracobrachialis
- Biceps brachii (short head)
- Triceps brachii (long head)

Scapulothoracic muscles
- Trapezius
- Serratus anterior
- Rhomboid major
- Rhomboid minor
- Levator scapulae
- Pectoralis minor

Thoracohumeral muscles
- Pectoralis major (sternal head)
- Latissimus dorsi

Other
- Biceps brachii (long head)
- Pectoralis major (clavicular head)
- Subclavius
- Omohyoid
- Sternocleidomastoid

origins and insertions of the muscles all move simultaneously. Therefore, changes in the muscle volume, length, and moment arms occur constantly throughout the entire range of motion. The great arcs of motion in multiple planes with multiple arm rotations produce constant changes in the relationship of a given muscle to the joint's instantaneous center of rotation. The quantification of muscle forces about the shoulder is, therefore, an arduous task.

Even the most basic movement requires at least two opposing muscles. The prime mover, or agonist, initiates and produces a desired movement when contracted. A stabilizing muscle is required to oppose the prime mover so that instability or imbalance around the joint will not result. The stabilizing muscle is often referred to as the antagonist and often acts through eccentric muscle contraction. Muscles that contract together, not in opposition, to produce a particular skeletal function, are classified as synergists. The torque and the stiffness produced in the shoulder are controlled by the interaction of the agonist and the antagonist muscle groups working simultaneously. The stiffness of the joint will be high if the agonist and antagonist muscles are activated concomitantly. However, if the agonist activity or the sum of activities is greater than that of the antagonists, a net torque will be produced and the stiffness of the joint will decrease, allowing the joint to move. The degree of torque, as well as the angular velocity of the joint are then controlled by the interplay of the agonist and antagonist muscle groups. No joint in the human body demonstrates these concepts better than the shoulder. The relatively unconstrained glenohumeral joint and "floating" scapula critically depend on finely balanced muscle forces to maintain rhythm and synchrony of arm motion relative to the thorax.

Specific muscular activity about the shoulder complex has been studied anatomically and through stereophotogrammetry and dynamic EMG. The change in lever arms and orientation of musculature for the different positions of the arm with respect to the thorax have been demonstrated. The cross-sectional area of the musculature around the shoulder girdle has been studied (Table 1).

By combining knowledge of the cross-sectional area and the orientation of particular muscles, muscle forces can be approximated.

Elevation of the arm with respect to the thorax has been studied more than any other specific shoulder motion. Forward elevation of the humerus has been studied using a combination of stereophotogrammetry to analyze motion during forward elevation and EMG to record muscular activity. Although the subscapularis was not studied by EMG, the shoulder girdle muscles have been categorized into four groups of variable importance according to the relative contributions of muscular activity during elevation of the arm.

Table 1
Cross-sectional area of shoulder girdle musculature

Muscle	Area (cm^2)
Deltoid	18.17
Deltoid posterior	5.00
Supraspinatus	5.72
Subscapularis	16.30
Infraspinatus and teres minor	13.74
Pectoralis major	13.34
Latissimus dorsi	12.00
Teres major	8.77
Triceps (long head)	2.96
Biceps (long head)	2.01
Biceps (short head)	1.11
Coracobrachialis	1.60

Group 1 consisted of the essential muscles for forward elevation: deltoid (anterior and lateral head), trapezius (inferior portion), supraspinatus, and serratus anterior. Loss of any two of the muscles in group 1 results in the inability to elevate the arm appreciably. Group 2 muscles included the trapezius (middle portion), infraspinatus, and biceps brachii. The next most important group of muscles, group 3, consisted of the deltoid (posterior head), pectoralis major (clavicular head), and trapezius (superior portion). Finally, the least important muscles for forward elevation constituted group 4 and included the pectoralis major (sternal head), latissimus dorsi, and triceps.

The interrelationship between the supraspinatus and the deltoid muscles during elevation of the arm has been studied by a variety of investigators. In 1944, it was demonstrated that the supraspinatus muscle acts synergistically with the deltoid during elevation of the arm, while the infraspinatus, teres minor, and subscapularis muscles provide the humeral depressor effect necessary to prevent cephalic migration of the humeral head during forward elevation. The deltoid muscle possesses a dominant pull that is oriented vertically and amounts to 89% of the muscle's total force. This results in a vertical sheer force imparted by the deltoid. The infraspinatus, teres minor, and subscapularis have a net inferior sheer force that amounts to 71% to 82% of the total force of these muscles.

The specific contributions of the supraspinatus and the deltoid muscles, respectively, have been reported variably. The supraspinatus muscle has been thought to initiate abduction of the arm, allowing the deltoid to continue this abduction once it gained an advantageous moment arm. Dynamic EMG investigations have demonstrated that the deltoid and all four rotator cuff muscles are active throughout the full range of forward elevation in the scapular plane: flexion, as well as abduction. Investigators, using selective Xylocaine nerve blocks of either the axillary or suprascapular nerves to study torque production in the arm during flexion and abduction, demonstrated that the deltoid and the supraspinatus muscles were equally responsible for torque production. Others demonstrated that full arm abduction was possible under the influence of an axillary nerve block; however, the strength of such abduction was approximately 50% of normal. Suprascapular nerve block, by eliminating the supraspinatus and infraspinatus, still allowed full abduction of the arm, although it was significantly weaker. Under suprascapular nerve block, the remaining teres minor and subscapularis muscles provide glenohumeral compression and humeral depression.

Simultaneous axillary and suprascapular nerve blocks render active abduction of the arm impossible; this observation supports the concept of the essential muscles for elevation of the arm. Under suprascapular nerve block, isometric strength in abduction decreases approximately 50% at 30° of forward elevation in the scapular plane, and 35% at 90° of forward elevation in the scapular plane. At 120° of forward elevation, suprascapular nerve block produces a decrease in isometric abduction strength of approximately 25%.

Both the supraspinatus and deltoid are necessary for normal elevation of the arm, and although both muscles are active through the entire range of motion, the deltoid becomes progressively more effective with increasing elevation as the moment arm of the deltoid insertion progressively improves. The required lifting force of the deltoid muscle drops from 50% of maximum at 30° elevation to 43% of maximum at 90° of elevation and becomes only 18% of maximum at 150° of elevation. At 0° of abduction, the percentage of deltoid force that is directed vertically is 90%. However, as the arm is elevated to the horizontal, the percentage of vertical force of the deltoid decreases to 55% owing to the improvement of pull of the deltoid muscle (Fig. 13). The supraspinatus, however, maintains a consistent 75° angle between its line of pull and the glenoid surface. Of the muscle force of the supraspinatus, 97% is directed towards compression of the glenohumeral joint (Fig. 14). The subscapularis and infraspinatus have an angle of pull of approximately 45° directed inferiorly, and the teres minor has an angle of pull directed inferiorly approximately 55° (Fig. 14). These vectors of pull result in muscle forces that are nearly equally divided between glenohumeral joint compression and humeral head depression.

Pure arm abduction and pure arm flexion demonstrate the same basic synergy between the rotator cuff and the deltoid. In flexion, the prime movers are the anterior and middle deltoid, with 73% and 62% activity, respectively. The prime stabilizers are the infraspinatus, supraspinatus, and the latissimus dorsi. The latissimus dorsi demonstrates up to 25% activity as flexion continues above the horizontal plane. In pure abduction, a very similar relationship is demonstrated; however, the subscapularis assumes a more important stabilizing role.

External rotation The infraspinatus muscle is the primary external rotator of the humerus. It is assisted by the teres minor and the posterior deltoid. EMG studies have indicated that the infraspinatus is the most active of all shoulder muscles during external rotation in all positions of arm abduction. The activity of the infraspinatus is approximately 50% throughout external rotation; that of the subscapularis is just below 50%, indicating its importance as the primary stabilizer during external rotation.

After suprascapular nerve block, isometric external rotation strength, performed at 30° of abduction, decreased by 74%. In these same shoulders, however, the decrease in external rotation strength after suprascapular nerve block became less noticeable as the amount of abduction increased. The posterior deltoid becomes a more efficient external

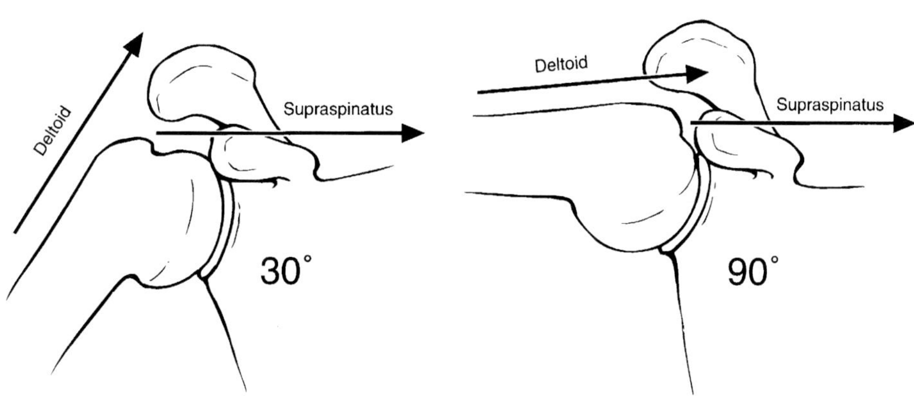

Figure 13
As the arm is abducted to 90°, the direction of pull of the deltoid approximates that of the supraspinatus. Therefore, patients with a large tear of the rotator cuff can often actively maintain the arm abducted to 90°, but may not be capable of actively abducting to 90°.

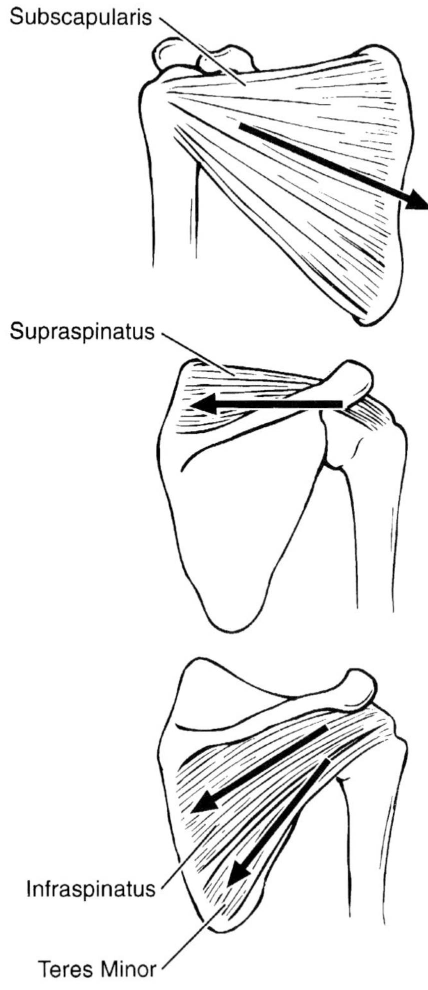

Figure 14
The angle of pull of the subscapularis **(top)** is approximately 45°. The angle of pull of the infraspinatus **(bottom)** is also approximately 45°, and the teres minor **(bottom)** is approximately 55°. These vectors result in nearly equal glenohumeral joint compression and humeral head depression. The supraspinatus (**center**) is essentially horizontal in its orientation, resulting in compression of the glenohumeral joint.

rotator of the humerus with increasing abduction of the arm, especially when combined with some degree of extension of the arm. The deltoid accounts for 60% of the strength in horizontal abduction of the arm.

Internal rotation The prime movers for internal rotation of the arm with respect to the thorax are the pectoralis major, especially the sternal head; the latissimus dorsi; and the subscapularis muscle groups. In addition, the teres major assists in this internal rotation. The subscapularis demonstrates activity in all positions during internal rotation, but its activity tends to decrease with increasing abduction. At 0° of abduction, the subscapularis activity has been shown to be 34%; whereas at 90° of abduction, it decreases to 21%. Activity in the pectoralis major during internal rotation also decreases with increasing abduction from 30% at 0° of abduction to 2% to 3% at 90° of abduction. The latissimus dorsi demonstrates a similar activity during internal rotation with a decrease from 20% at 0° of abduction to 7% at 90° of abduction. During internal rotation, EMG activity in the middle and posterior deltoid tends to increase when tested at positions of increased abduction of the arm.

Extension During extension of the arm, the prime movers are the posterior and the middle deltoid. The posterior head of the deltoid has demonstrated 70% to 74% activity on EMG during extension, with the middle head demonstrating 57% activity. The subscapularis is active throughout extension with 53% activity. The supraspinatus demonstrates increasing activity (35%) as the degree of extension increases. The subscapularis and supraspinatus are considered the prime stabilizers during extension of the arm.

Scapulothoracic motion The glenoid and, therefore, the scapula, rotate in an upward fashion as elevation of the arm occurs (Fig. 15). This rotation is important for maintenance of a constant fiber length of the deltoid muscle, thereby allowing the deltoid to remain powerful despite a variety of arm positions. Upward rotation of the scapula increases the stability of the glenohumeral joint in overhead activities and also decreases the tendency for impingement of the rotator cuff tendons beneath the coracoacromial arch. The upper trapezius, levator scapulae, and upper portion of the serratus anterior muscles contract concomitantly with the lower trapezius and lower digitations of the serratus anterior to produce a scapular rotating force couple (Fig. 16). The synergistic action of the serratus anterior and trapezius must be present for a full forward elevation of the arm to occur.

The relative contributions of scapular, thoracic, and glenohumeral motion during forward elevation have been studied extensively. The ratio of glenohumeral motion and scapulothoracic motion has been determined to be from 1.1:1 to 4.3:1. Most of the variability in this ratio occurs during the initial 30° of arm elevation. Scapulothoracic motion during this phase of elevation is highly variable and sometimes is even absent. Once the scapulothoracic motion is underway, the rhythm becomes more linear, and the relationship between glenohumeral and scapulothoracic becomes more constant. The setting

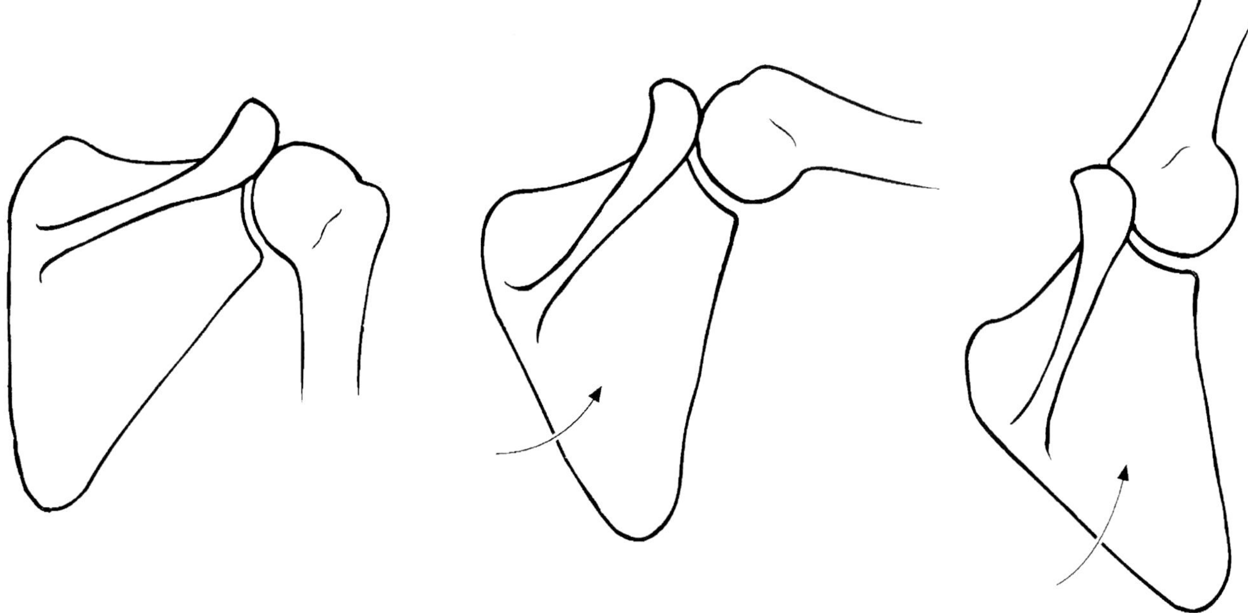

Figure 15
Forward elevation or abduction of the arm requires synchronous rotation of the scapula.

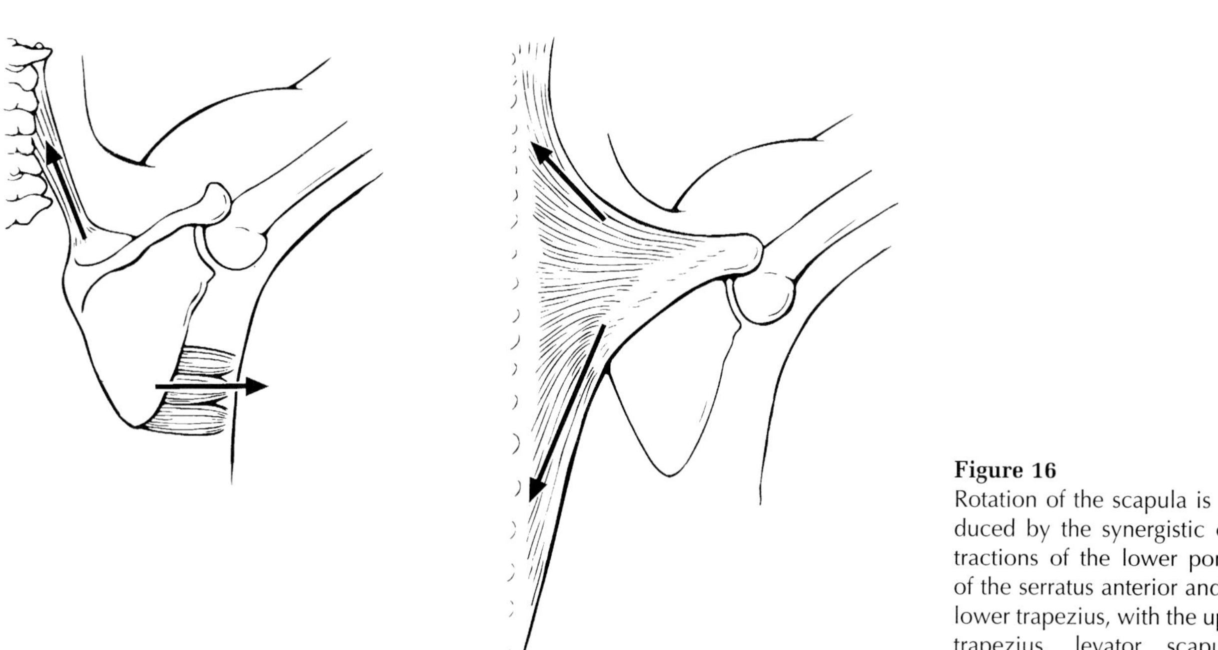

Figure 16
Rotation of the scapula is produced by the synergistic contractions of the lower portion of the serratus anterior and the lower trapezius, with the upper trapezius, levator scapulae, and upper serratus anterior.

phase of scapulothoracic motion during the first 30° of abduction is more pronounced and longer than during forward flexion. The variability observed in scapulothoracic motion during elevation of the arm can occur in one individual. This motion has been shown to be three-dimensional, complex, and task-dependent. Optimal scapular position for heavy lifting or pushing may require a different glenoid orientation to minimize glenohumeral sheer, as well as to optimize muscle length/tension relationships. Therefore, the ratio of glenohumeral scapulothoracic motion seems to be variable, but roughly 2° of glenohumeral motion occurs for each 1° of scapulothoracic motion during elevation of the arm.

Structure and Function of the Elbow Joint

Introduction

The elbow is a complex joint that acts as a component link of the lever arm system in placing the hand. As a fulcrum for the forearm lever, it provides the power to perform lifting activities. With crutch walking, the elbow is a weightbearing joint. In power and fine work activities, the elbow stabilizes the upper extremity linkage. Thus, the biomechanics of the elbow relate to the kinematics, forces across the joint, and stability.

Kinematics and Joint Stability

The elbow has two degrees of freedom: flexion-extension and axial rotation, or pronation-supination. The normal range of motion is between 0° and 140° to 160° of flexion-extension and forearm rotation with about 70° to 80° of pronation and 80° to 85° of supination. The functional arc of motion for most activities of daily living is 100° from 30° to 130° of flexion-extension with 50° of pronation and 50° of supination (Figs. 17 and 18). The rotational axis of flexion-extension occurs about a tight locus of points (instantaneous axes of rotation), measuring only 2 to 3 mm in the broadest dimension, and is located at the center of the lateral projected curvature of the trochlea and capitellum (Fig. 19). The axis of forearm rotation passes through the capitellum and head of the radius, extending to the distal

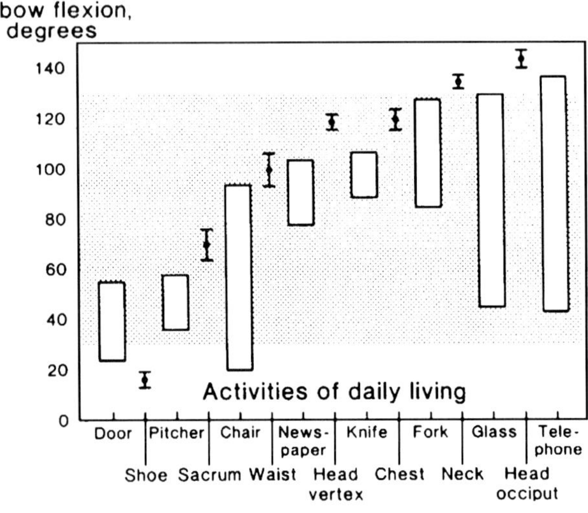

Figure 17
Functional arc of elbow motion for activities of daily living is approximately 100°, between 30° and 103°. (Adapted with permission from Morrey BF, Askew LJ, An KN, et al: A biomechanical study of functional elbow motion. *J Bone Joint Surg* 1981;63A:872.)

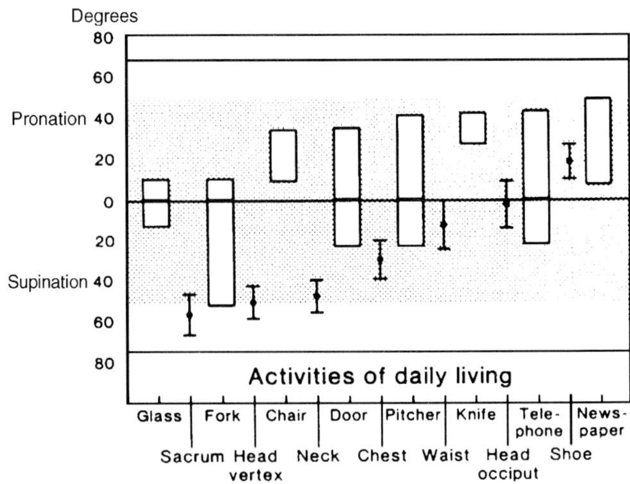

Figure 18
Functional arc of forearm rotation is approximately 50° of pronation and 50° of supination for most activities of daily living. (Adapted with permission from Morrey BF, Askew LJ, An KN, et al: A biomechanical study of functional elbow motion. *J Bone Joint Surg* 1981;63A:872.)

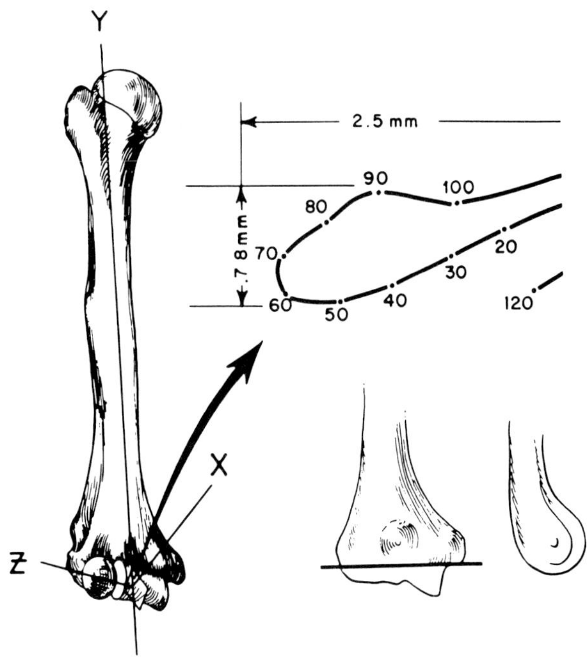

Figure 19
The very small locus of instant center of rotation for the elbow joint demonstrates that the axis may be replicated by a single line drawn from the inferior aspect of the medial epicondyle through the center of the lateral epicondyle, which is in the center of the lateral projected curvature of the trochlea and capitellum. (Modified with permission from Morrey BF, Chao EY: Passive motion of the elbow joint. *J Bone Joint Surg* 1976;58A:501.)

ulna, and defines a cone. The carrying angle, the angle formed by the long axis of the humerus and the long axis of the ulna, is measured in the frontal plane with the elbow extended, and averages 7° in men and 13° in women. This angle decreases with elbow flexion and there is a slight axial rotation of about 5°, first internal and then external rotation of the ulna with reference to the humerus (Fig. 20).

Varus/valgus rotational motions at the elbow are restricted. Motion produced in this plane constitutes joint instability. The greatest resistance to rotational forces exists at the elbow on the medial side, where the medial collateral ligament is the most important stabilizer, especially the anterior oblique fibers. The anterior oblique ligament is taut throughout the flexion-extension range, whereas the posterior oblique ligament is taut only during flexion. At 90° of flexion, the medial collateral ligament contributes 54% of the resistance to valgus stress. The remainder is supplied by the shape of the articular surface and the anterior capsule. The articular congruity provides partial stability. The radial head provides about 30% of valgus stability and is more important in 0° to 30° of flexion and pronation. In extension, the olecranon becomes locked in its fossa. Equal contributions from the medial collateral ligament, shape of joint surfaces, and anterior capsule are important to resisting valgus stress in extension.

Stability to varus stress is provided by the lateral collateral ligament, anconeus, and joint capsule. The lateral ligament contributes only 9% of restraint to varus stress at 90° of flexion. Approximately 78% is provided by joint articulation and 13% by the joint capsule. In extension, the lateral ligament contributes 14% of restraint to varus stress, with 54% provided by the joint surface shape and 32% by the capsule.

Because the elbow functions as a link to position the hand in space, no single position is considered optimal for function. To understand this it is important to recognize that the shoulder functions as a ball joint, allowing the hand to describe a portion of a surface of a sphere in space. With each

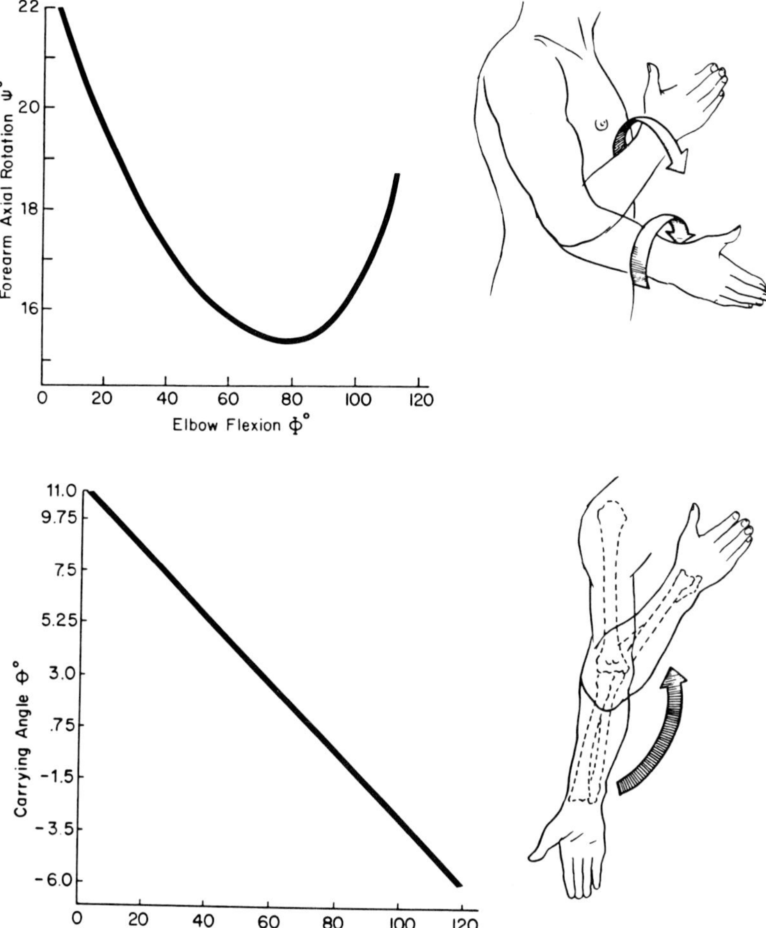

Figure 20
Top, During elbow flexion, the ulna demonstrates a slight axial rotation referable to the humerus with an amplitude of less than 10°. **Bottom,** During elbow flexion and extension, a linear change in the carrying angle is demonstrated, typically going from valgus in extension to varus in flexion. (Reproduced with permission from Morrey BF, Chao EY: Passive motion of the elbow joint. *J Bone Joint Surg* 1976;58A:501.)

successive change in the degree of rotational flexion/extension position of the elbow, a sphere of a different radius is described. The elbow thus allows the upper extremity to operate at different distances away from the body. Loss of motion at the elbow can then be described as a loss of reach length. This reach length can be described as the cosine of the angle of elbow flexion multiplied by the length of the forearm and hand. If the elbow is in full extension, then the cosine function is one and the reach length is at its maximum. With an elbow contracture smaller than 30° the cosine function remains near one, but as the angle progresses past 30° the cosine function rapidly decreases, as does the ability to reach in space. In actuality, the ability to reach not only is related to the diameter of the sphere but also affects the amount of the circumference of the sphere in which the hand can operate; that is, the volume of the sphere (Fig. 21). Thus, reach capacity is not linear, but is calculated as a function of the third power of the radius. Patients can tolerate flexion contractures of about 30° with about a 20% functional loss; when loss is more than 30° of extension, patients readily complain of functional impairment.

Elbow Kinetics

Muscle forces that act about the elbow have short lever arms; thus, they are relatively inefficient kinetically but very efficient kinematically—that is, a small muscle excursion can produce a large arc of motion at the hand. Rapid distal motion of the limb is possible by short excursions of proximal muscles lying close to the axis of joint rotation to permit actions such as throwing. Yet, large muscle forces are needed to produce large flexion or extension torques. Because the flexor moment arm is shortest at full extension, a large muscle force is necessary to initiate a flexion movement, and the joint compressive load at this position is relatively large.

For elbow flexion, the maximum isometric torque created at the elbow joint is, on average, 7 kg·m for men and 3.5 kg·m for women. Overall, men are about 50% stronger than women and the dominant extremity is 5% to 10% stronger than the nondominant side (Table 2). Muscle power is greatest during flexion at joint positions between 90° and 110°. At elbow angles of 45° to 135°, only approximately 75% of the maximum elbow flexion strength is generated. Maximum flexion strength is generated in forearm supination. The mean pronation strength is 86% of supination. Most of the torque occurs from the biceps, brachialis, and brachioradialis function.

The isometric force of the flexors is about 40% greater than the isometric force of the extensors. The maximum flexor muscle force per unit cross-sectional area is in the range of 10 to 14 kg/cm^2. About one third or one half of the maximum lifting force can be generated with the elbow in the extended or 30° flexed position. At these positions, a compressive force three times the body weight can be encountered in the elbow joint during strenuous

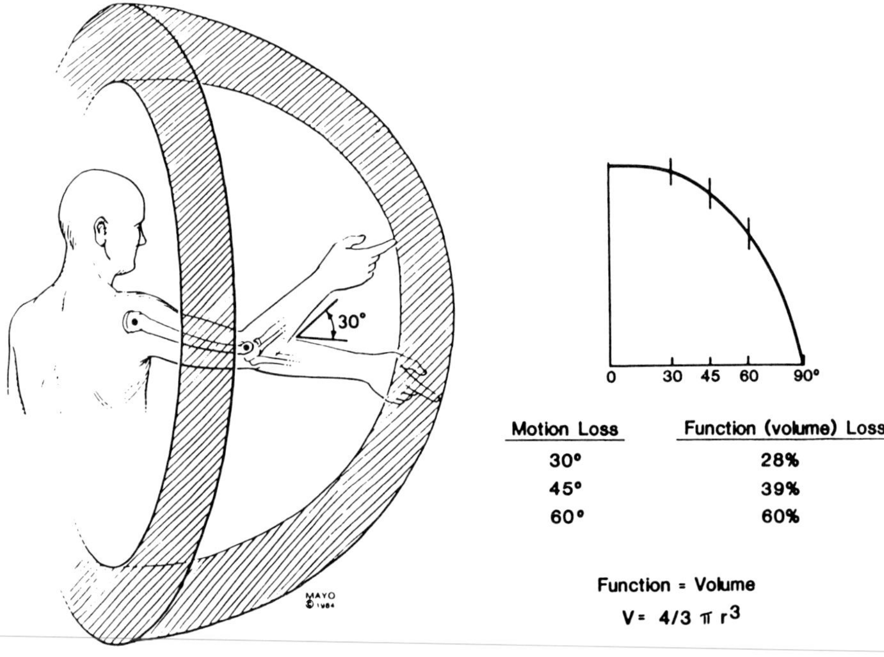

Figure 21
Restricted elbow motion limits the sphere of influence of the hand in space. Flexion contractures over 30° are associated with a rapid loss of effective reach area. (Reproduced with permission from An K-N, Morrey BF: Biomechanics, in Morrey BF, Chao EYS (eds): *Joint Replacement Arthroplasty.* New York, Churchill Livingstone, 1991, p 261.)

Table 2
Isometric Elbow Strength of 104 Normal Subjects

		Men	Women	M - W / M	Dom - Non / Dom
Flexion	Dom	725 ± 154	336 ± 80	0.54	
(Kg-cm)	Non	708 ± 156	323 ± 78	0.54	0.03
Extension	Dom	421 ± 109	210 ± 61	0.50	
(Kg-cm)	Non	406 ± 106	194 ± 50	0.52	0.04
Pronation	Dom	73 ± 18	36 ± 8	0.51	
(Kg-cm)	Non	68 ± 17	33 ± 10	0.51	0.07
Supination	Dom	91 ± 23	44 ± 12	0.52	
(Kg-cm)	Non	80 ± 21	41 ± 10	0.49	0.08
Grip	Dom	53 ± 12	30 ± 10	0.43	
(Kg)	Non	51 ± 11	27 ± 9	0.47	0.06

(Reproduced with permission from Askew LJ, An KN, Morrey BF, et al: Isometric elbow strength in normal individuals. *Clin Orthop* 1987;222:264.)

lifting. Thus, the magnitude of the force crossing the elbow joint justifies consideration of the elbow as a weightbearing joint.

The distribution of force transmission on ulna and radius with the elbow extended and axially loaded is approximately 40% across the ulnohumeral joint and 60% across the radiohumeral joint. The greatest force transmission occurs between 0° and 30° of flexion, and it consistently decreases with increased flexion. Force transmission is also greater with the forearm in pronation (Fig. 22). The varus-valgus pivot point with the elbow extended is also noted to closely approximate the line of action of the brachial muscle, which crosses near the center of the lateral portion of the trochlea.

The orientation of the resultant joint force is quite sensitive to changes of the muscle force line of the upper arm muscles. The orientation of the resultant joint force moves from the central portion of the trochlea toward the rim as the direction of muscle pull relative to the forearm changes from perpendicular to parallel. The direction of force produced by the forearm muscles with respect to the trochlear notch, on the other hand, is relatively constant, so the direction of the resultant joint forces is reasonably constant. For example, when the forearm muscles (eg, brachioradialis) carry the dominant forces, the resultant joint force on the proximal ulna is consistently toward the rim of the coronoid process throughout the elbow flexion angle.

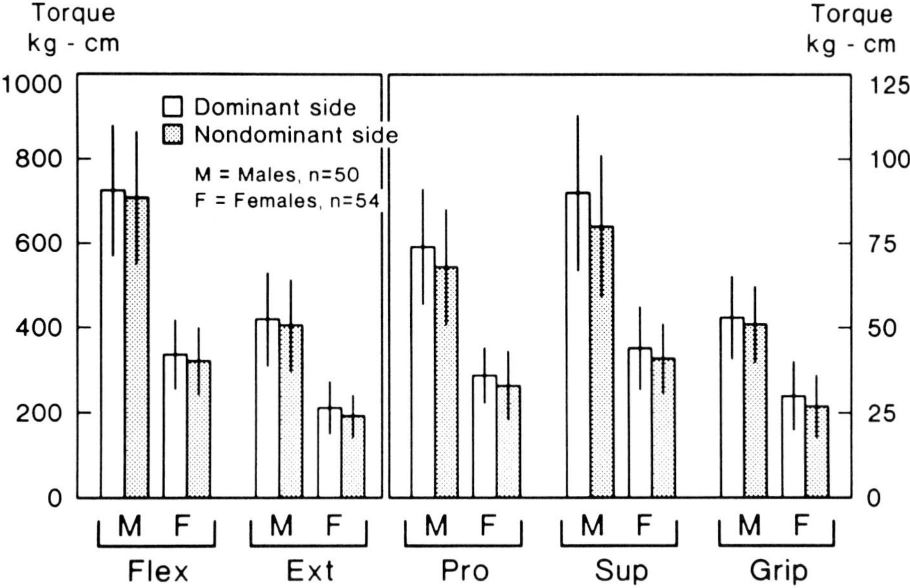

Figure 22
Isometric elbow strength in normal individuals. (Reproduced with permission from Askew LJ, An KN, Morrey BF, et al: Isometric elbow strength in normal individuals. *Clin Orthop* 1987;222:264.)

The average maximum torque strength for elbow extension is 4 kg·m for men and 2 kg·m for women. Although peak extension strength occurs between 60° and 140°, the 90° position generates the greatest isometric extension force. Elbow extension strength obtained from the prone position is significantly greater than that in the supine position.

Measurements during forearm supination and pronation demonstrate a linear relationship between strength and forearm rotation. The greatest supination strength is generated from the pronated position; the converse is also true. The average torque of supination exceeds that of pronation by about 15% to 20% for men and women throughout the majority of shoulder-elbow positions. The average pronation and supination strengths for men are 80 and 90 kg·cm, respectively, and for women, 35 and 55 kg·cm, respectively. The difference between dominant and nondominant strength averages about 10%.

Structure and Function of the Hand and Wrist

The Hand

The two primary functions of the hand as an organ are touch and prehension. Prehension has been defined as the grasping or taking hold of an object between any two surfaces of the hand, or when an object is seized within the cup of the hand. Prehension may or may not include the thumb. The fundamental requirement of prehension is a firm grip. It is performed in different fashions according to the purpose of the grip, and it is described as either power grip or precision grip.

Power grip is defined as forceful finger flexion used to maintain an object against the palm. The ulnar two digits, which are innervated by the ulnar nerve, are more related to power grip; they provide support instead of control during power grip.

Precision grip requires fine kinesthetic control and usually is associated with fine tactile sensibility at the finger tips. It is formed by the clamp of the fingers and thumb, with the object held at the tips of the digits such that the palm is not involved. In this position, maximum sensation and speedy movement are available. The thumb, index, and middle fingers, which have medial nerve innervation, are more related to precision grip. This radial side of the hand has been referred to as the "dynamic tridactyl" and is concerned with balance, such as in holding a coffee cup.

Power and precision grips can be further differentiated according to the way that each grip is performed or by describing the individual phases composing the grip. Power grip involves the formation of a finger-palm vise and, therefore, has been described as proceeding through a sequence of four stages. The first three are dynamic; that is, during these stages muscles act to change the wrist and finger positions. Stage one consists of opening the hand; this is primarily a function of the long extensors and lumbricals. Stage two, which involves positioning of the fingers for closure about the object, is followed by stage three, actual finger closure to approach and grasp the object. These two stages will be described in the finger kinetics section. The final stage involves the use of muscles to maintain the grip on the object; because there is no motion, this activity can be considered static. In this final static phase, the digits surround the object and maintain a flexed posture. In power grip, the palm is cupped and the fingers are flexed against the thenar eminence, producing an oblique grip at approximately 45° to the transverse axes of the hand. The obliquity is produced in part by the ulnar deviation and rotation of the digits at the metacarpophalangeal (MP) joints of the fingers together with flexion at the carpometacarpal (CMC) joints of the ring and little fingers. The thumb base provides the fixed buttress, with the thumb itself usually controlling the leverage of the object being gripped.

The steps of precision grip are similar to the first three steps of power grip; however, it does not include a final static gripping phase that is either similar in appearance or prolonged in time. Rather, there is a constant alteration at the fingertips between static activity to grip the object and a dynamic component to manipulate the object. Hence, precision grip is often termed precision handling.

Power grip has been divided into three subtypes: cylindrical grip, spherical grip, and hooked grip (Fig. 23). Lateral prehension is also included under power grip because it involves a static holding phase.

In cylindrical grip, the hand makes a fist around a handle such as a baseball bat. The fingers are flexed with the thumb flexed over the index and middle fingers. This involves primarily function of the flexor digitorum profundus. The flexor digitorum sublimis and interosseous muscles assist when greater force is required. The interossei are important in providing metacarpophalangeal flexion as well as abduction and rotation of the phalanges to accommodate the objects. The hypothenars are active and lock the little finger into positions. The flexor pollicis longus and thenars are active.

Spherical grip is used when gripping a baseball. It is similar to cylindrical grip except that there is greater spread at the fingers. Metacarpophalangeal joints are more abducted, resulting in more interosseous activity.

Hooked grip usually involves flexion of the proximal interphalangeal (PIP) joints of all the fingers, with an abducted thumb. This is the grip

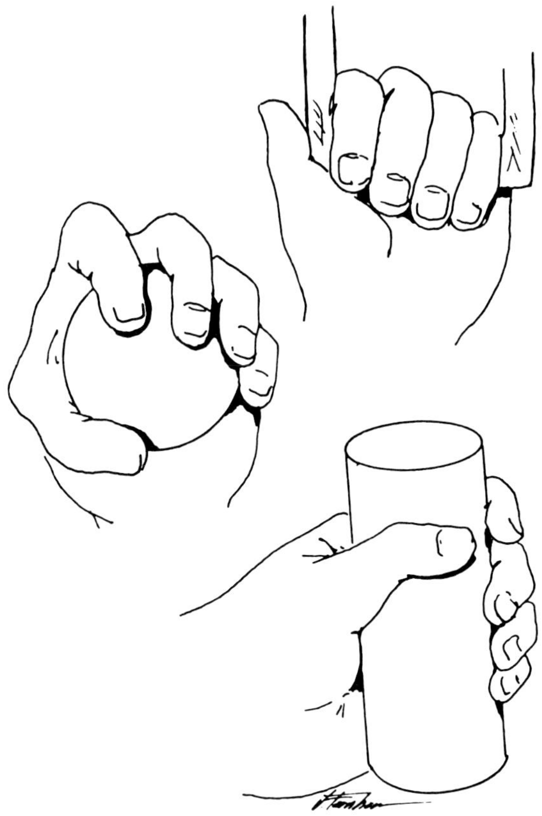

Figure 23
Power grip: hook grip **(top),** spherical grip **(center),** and cylindrical grip **(bottom).** (Reproduced with permission from Norkin C, Le Vangie P: *Joint Structure and Function: A Comprehensive Analysis.* Philadelphia, FA Davis Co, 1990, p 243.)

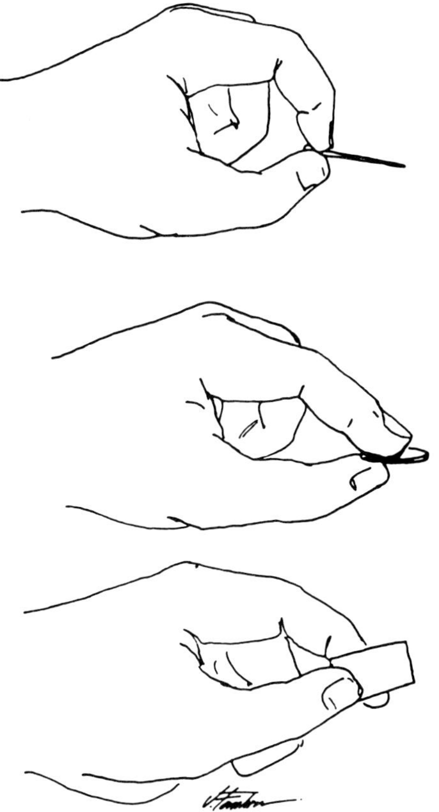

Figure 24
Precision grip or handling: tip-to-tip prehension **(top),** pad-to-pad prehension **(center),** and pad-to-side prehension **(bottom).** (Reproduced with permission from Norkin C, Le Vangie P: *Joint Structure and Function: A Comprehensive Analysis.* Philadelphia, FA Davis Co, 1990, p 248.)

normally used to carry a suitcase and is specialized in that it can be maintained for long periods of time. It is the function, primarily, of the flexor digitorum profundus and superficialis muscles of the fingers. Thumb use is excluded.

In lateral prehension, the MP and interphalangeal (IP) joints of adjacent fingers are extended. Simultaneous abduction or adduction of the adjacent MP joints brings the digits together to produce a static holding phase such as that commonly used in holding a cigarette. This form of prehension is relatively weak. It is unique in that it is the only form of prehension in which the extensors play a role in sustaining posture.

Precision grip or handling requires finer control and sensibility using the radial digits; static holding is kept to a minimum. Precision grip is divided into three subtypes: pad-to-pad, tip-to-tip, and pad-to-side prehension (Fig. 24).

Pad-to-pad prehension involves true opposition of the pulp of the thumb to that of the fingers. It is commonly referred to as two- or three-point pinch or chuck pinch through opposition of the thumb to the index or index and middle fingers, respectively, and is responsible for nearly 80% of precision handling. The pulps of the fingers supinate when the MPs are flexed or the index finger is abducted for optimum opposition and function. Pad-to-pad prehension normally involves dynamic manipulation in which the volar and dorsal interossei work reciprocally to move the objects among the fingertips. This is in contrast to power grip in which the interossei work synergistically (at the same time).

Tip-to-tip prehension is the most precise of all the prehensions. It differs from pad-to-pad prehension in that there is full interphalangeal joint flexion of the fingers and thumb. The flexor digitorum profundus, the pollicis longus, and interosseous muscles are all active.

Pad-to-side prehension, also known as key pinch, involves an adducted and extended thumb opposed to the radial side of the index. It differs from other precision handling in that the thumb is more adducted and less rotated. There is increased activity of the flexor pollicis brevis and adductor pollicis with decreased activity in the opponens pollicis. Pad-to-side prehension has more power available than in the pulp-to-pulp pinch, but it is the least precise prehension.

Power grip is applied primarily by the extrinsic musculature, with the flexors playing the major role. The interossei serve to act as MP joint flexors and rotators of the proximal phalanges. The lumbricals are not normally involved in power grip.

Precision handling also uses the extrinsic muscles to transmit force to the objects being grasped. However, the interossei act reciprocally to adduct and abduct the digits to rotate the objects at the fingertips. The lumbricals are active as are the extensors of the interphalangeal joints. Also, the thumb is motored primarily by the superficial three thenar muscles, which receive predominantly median nerve innervation as opposed to power grip, which usually involves the adductor pollicis and receives ulnar nerve innervation.

It is an important general principle to realize that, like many other places in the body during a coordinated functional movement, the flexors and extensors to the hand are in balanced opposition so that all hand movements are synergistic; that is, many muscles having opposing actions are active at the same time.

The extrinsic wrist and finger muscles, in a somewhat oversimplification, can be divided into three systems of agonist-antagonist forces. The extensor carpi ulnaris muscle acting at the same time as the abductor pollicis longus and extensor pollicis brevis muscles prevents radial deviation of the wrist and allows the action of these muscles to be directed entirely to the thumb. The action of the extensor digitorum communis, the extensor indicis proprius, and extensor digiti minimi opposed by simultaneous activity of the flexor carpi radialis and flexor pollicis longus muscles allows finger extension without causing these muscles to dissipate energy in producing wrist extension. The third group of forces involve the extensor carpi radialis brevis and longus. These are antagonized by cocontractile activity of the flexor carpi ulnaris, preventing radial deviation with the occurrence of wrist extension.

Additionally, the extensor carpi radialis brevis and longus, functioning synergistically, cocontract with the flexor digitorum profundus and superficialis muscles. Because the wrist's position optimizes the power of finger flexors through its tenodesis effect, maintaining extension of the wrist through this cocontraction enhances the excursion of the long flexor tendons required for efficient flexion of the fingers.

Optimal hand function is, therefore, the result of mobile balance of the wrist and fingers with their respective muscles. Motions occur around variable axes to facilitate precise positioning of the digits for prehension. Optimal hand function thus requires a complex interaction between the wrist, thumb, and fingers. Each of these three components will be addressed separately below for the ease of discussion. However, it must be emphasized that their functions are quite integrated and are difficult to separate clinically. Included within each section is a description of wrist and hand anatomy so essential to the comprehension of wrist and hand kinematics and kinetics. Because the scope of this section is limited, only the relevant anatomy is reviewed.

The Wrist

The wrist or carpus provides a stable support for the hand, allowing for the transmission of grip forces as well as positioning of the hand and digits for fine movements. The main function of the wrist is to fine tune grasp by controlling the length-tension relationship in the extrinsic muscles to the hand. For example, the self-selected wrist position for maximal power grip has been shown to be 35° of extension with 7° of ulnar deviation. Furthermore, full wrist flexion reduces the efficiency of the finger flexors and the grip strength to 25% of that available when the wrist is in extension. Martial arts experts have used this finding for a long time to disarm assailants. When the wrist is positioned in flexion, the combination of a passive extensor tenodesis effect, increasing resistance to flexion, and decreasing excursion of the flexors results in a weakened grip. The assailant, therefore, is unable to maintain a grip on the weapon.

Wrist Stability

Traditionally, the carpal bones are described as being arranged in two anatomic rows. The proximal carpal row consists of the scaphoid, lunate, and triquetrum, and the distal row is formed by the trapezium, trapezoid, capitate, and hamate. The pisiform lies within the flexor carpi ulnaris tendon and, through its articulation with the trapezium, functions as a sesamoid; therefore, it is not included as a functional member of the proximal carpal row. The scaphoid links the proximal and distal rows. Both rows move with respect to each other in the midcarpal joint, and the proximal row moves on the radius in the radiocarpal joint.

The carpus may also be considered in terms of three functional columns (Fig. 25). The central or flexion-extension column is formed by the distal carpal row and the lunate. This column functions as a longitudinal link between the radius and metacarpals and its integrity depends on the carpal ligaments because the muscles that produce wrist motion attach distal to the central column. The lateral

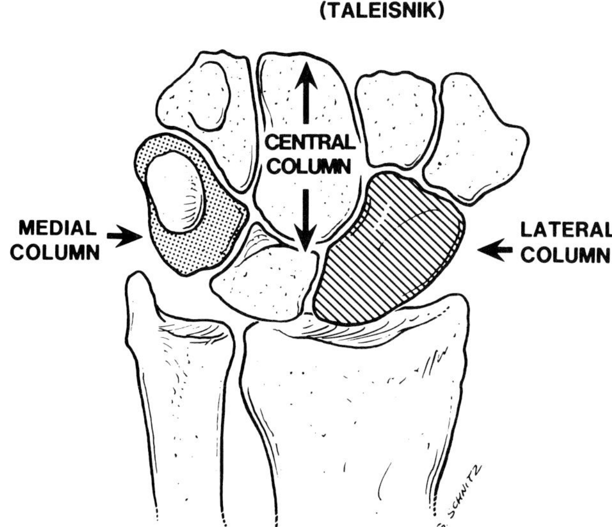

Figure 25
Three columns of the wrist with the bones in each are as follows: central, lunate and entire distal carpal row; lateral, scaphoid; and medial, triquetrum. (Reproduced with permission from *Regional Review Courses in Hand Surgery,* ed 4. Aurora, CO, American Society for Surgery of the Hand, 1991)

or mobile column is the scaphoid. The medial or rotational column is the triquetrum.

The arrangement of the carpal bones and their ligaments is crucial to wrist stability. The two carpal rows articulate to form the midcarpal joint, which consists of three different types of articular surfaces. On the radial side, the trapezium and trapezoid are concave with their articulations to the distal scaphoid and lateral capitate. The head of the capitate in the center of the midcarpal joint is convex. The ulnar-sided hamate-triquetral articulation is helicoid in nature.

The proximal carpal row has a single biconvex joint surface that articulates with a shallower, concave distal radius with two facets and a triangular fibrocartilage complex. The radiocarpal joint, therefore, appears relatively incongruent. The distal radius has an average of 14° of palmar tilt, and 22° of radial inclination. This structure probably contributes to the limitation of motion such that flexion is greater than extension and ulnar deviation greater than radial deviation. The radial articular surface of the wrist affords no real bony stability; stability is provided primarily by the soft-tissue envelope of the wrist.

Ligaments are the primary stabilizers of the wrist. They usually are classified into palmar and dorsal ligaments as well as extrinsic and intrinsic ligaments (Fig. 26). The palmar ligaments, which are more numerous and substantial than the dorsal ligaments and are considered the principle stabilizers of the wrist, function principally to resist hyperextension forces. The majority of the extrinsic ligaments, which arise from the radius and ulna and attach to the carpus, insert on the proximal carpal row. The important extrinsic ligaments are the radioscaphocapitate, radiolunotriquetral, and ulnolunate. The radioscapholunate ligament is relatively thin and offers little stability, but contains blood vessels. The palmar and dorsal radiocarpal ligaments are obliquely oriented to resist the tendency of the proximal carpal row to slide down the palmar and ulnar inclined surface of the distal radius.

The intrinsic ligaments originate and insert on the carpus. The scapholunate ligament and the lunotriquetral ligament are important links in the proximal carpal row and provide additional stability to the wrist.

The stability provided by the volar intrinsic and extrinsic ligaments may be best described by the double V configuration that they form (Fig. 27). The arcuate ligaments, consisting of the radioscaphocapitate and ulnocapitate ligaments, converge on the capitate to form the distal V. The proximal V is formed by the radiolunotriquetral, radioscaphoid, ulnolunate, and ulnotriquetral ligaments. With ulnar deviation, the proximal V changes to an L configuration. The ulnolunate ligament assumes a more transverse orientation to essentially limit lunate displacement, and the radiolunate ligament assumes a more longitudinal configuration to limit lunate extension. The distal V ligamentous configuration similarly assumes an L configuration, but in the opposite direction. The scaphocapitate ligament becomes transverse to limit ulnar translation of the capitate, and the triquetral capitate ligament assumes a longitudinal configuration to prevent capitate flexion. The opposite is felt to occur in radial deviation.

In addition to creating movement, the extrinsic muscles of the wrist offer a dynamic component to wrist stability. There are six dedicated wrist muscles: the extensor carpi radialis brevis and longus, extensor carpi ulnaris, flexor carpi radialis, flexor carpi ulnaris, and palmaris longus muscles. The extensor carpi radialis brevis and longus are usually considered in combination, and there is agreement that together they generate the largest fraction of wrist extension torque. The extensor carpi radialis brevis is the key extensor of the wrist. It inserts onto the base of the third metacarpal and is essentially a pure wrist extensor that has a minimal radial deviation moment. Although the tendon of the extensor carpi radialis brevis has a larger extension moment than that of the extensor carpi radialis longus, there is some controversy about which generates greater overall torque. This controversy exists

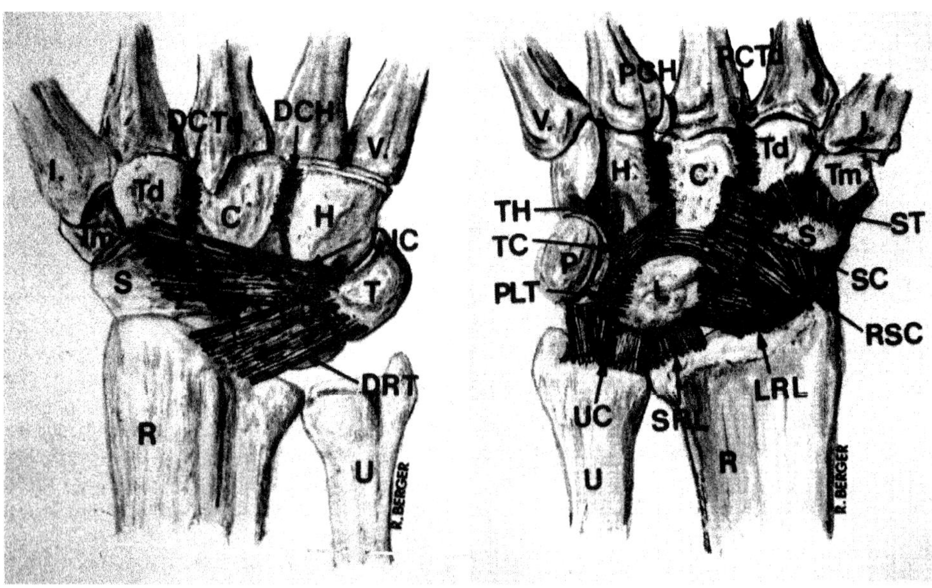

Figure 26
Left, Extrinsic ligaments of the wrist (dorsal): dorsal intercarpal ligament (DIC) and dorsal radiotriquetral ligament (DRT). **Right,** Extrinsic ligaments of the wrist (volar): scaphotrapezial (ST), radioscaphocapitate (RSC), scaphocapitate (SC), long radiolunate (LRL), short radiolunate (SRL), ulnocarpal (UC), palmar lunotriquetral (PLT), triquetral-capitate (TC), triquetral-hamate (TH), lunate (L), scaphoid (S), pisiform (P). Trapezium (Tm), trapezoid (Td), capitate (C), hamate (H), scaphoid (S), triquetrum (T). (Reproduced with permission from Cooney WP III, Linscheid RL, Dobyns JH: Fractures and dislocations of the wrist, in Rockwood CA Jr, Green DP, Bucholz RW (eds): *Rockwood and Green's Fractures in Adults,* ed 3. Philadelphia, JB Lippincott, 1991, p 564.)

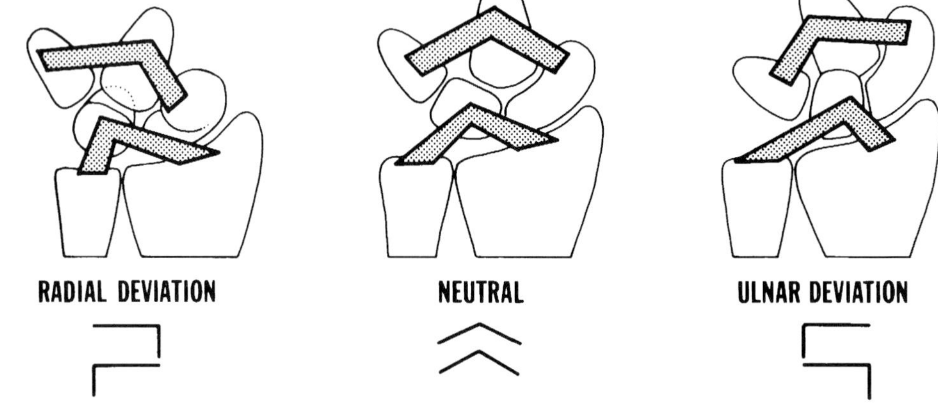

Figure 27
Diagrammatic representation of changes in orientation of palmar radiocarpal ligaments. (Illustration by Elizabeth Roselius,© 1985. Reprinted with permission from Taleisnik J: *The Wrist.* New York, Churchill Livingstone, 1985, p 26.)

because the extensor carpi radialis longus inserts onto the second metacarpal, and some of the torque it produces generates a radial deviation moment along with an extension moment. When the radial deviation force of the extensor carpi radialis longus is balanced by the extensor carpi ulnaris, some consider this combination of muscles to be the most effective manner of producing wrist extension.

The extensor carpi ulnaris tendon is unique in that its fulcrum and moment arm relative to the ulna are fixed by the fixed extensor compartment; it thus maintains a relatively constant relationship and is also an important stabilizer of the ulnar head. It is felt to be an effective wrist extensor only when the wrist is supinated, because, in pronation, the extensor carpi ulnaris tendon lies lateral to the carpus and provides an ulnar deviation moment.

The flexor carpi ulnaris is a flexor and ulnar deviator of the wrist. It inserts into the pisiform with an extension into the hook of the hamate. The intratendinous pisiform functions as a sesamoid to increase the flexion and extension moments, thus allowing the flexor carpi ulnaris to achieve the highest tension of any muscle crossing the wrist, with the least excursion. This is the muscle that powers karate chops and hammer strokes, as well as resisting the radial deviation forces produced by firing a handgun. Its ulnar deviation forces are second only to those of the extensor carpi ulnaris in a pronated wrist.

The flexor carpi radialis, through its insertion onto the base of the second metacarpal, flexes the wrist and is also active during radial deviation. It is approximately 60% as strong as the flexor carpi ulnaris.

The palmaris longus is a pure, but relatively weak, wrist flexor. It is absent in approximately 15% of the population. Its insertion into the palmar fascia often spreads over the thenars and may assist in thumb abduction. The wrist flexors, as a group, have approximately greater than twice the work capacity of the extensors (Table 3).

The long flexors and extensors of the fingers and thumb are secondary wrist muscles. To effect motion at the wrist, these muscles depend on the antagonistic forces to prevent their action on distal joints.

Wrist Kinematics

Although the wrist is usually described as having three degrees of freedom with flexion-extension rotational movement, radioulnar deviation, and pronosupination, these isolated movements do not occur around three fixed mutually perpendicular axes. The primary axis of motion is an oblique screw axis within the head of the capitate (Fig. 28).

The average amount of flexion-extension motion of the wrist is variable (Table 4) with a range of 84° to 169° and an average of 140°. The average range of flexion is 65° to 80° and of extension, 55° to 75°. Flexion usually exceeds extension by approximately 10°. The average combined radioulnar deviation is 65°, with a range of 15° to 25° of radial deviation and 30° to 45° of ulnar deviation. At rest, there is physiologic ulnar deviation of the wrist. The average arc of pronation-supination is 150° with a pronation range of 60° to 80° degrees and a supination range of 60° to 85°. For most activities of daily living, the functional range of motion for the wrist is 5° to 40° of flexion, 30° to 40° of extension, and 10° of radial deviation to 15° to 30° of ulnar deviation.

Studies have shown that there appears to be less than 12° of intercarpal motion among the distal carpal row, supporting the theory that this row can be viewed as a single functional unit. Intercarpal motion between the scaphoid and lunate has been shown to range between 24° and 34°. Similarly, motion between the lunate and triquetrum has been shown to range between 12° and 18°. This mobile proximal carpal row, with its lack of tendon or

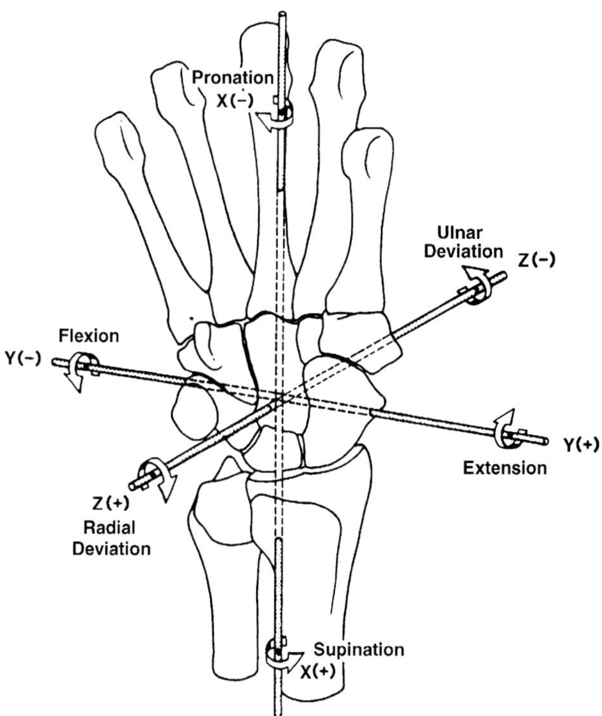

Figure 28
A coordinate system to describe the screw axis of the wrist, which passes through the head of the capitate for flexion Y(-) and extension Y(+); radial deviation Z(+) and ulnar deviation Z(-); and pronation X(-) and supination X(+). (Reproduced with permission from Cooney WP III, Linscheid RL, Dobyns JH: Fractures and dislocations of the wrist, in Rockwood CA Jr, Green DP, Bucholz RW (eds): *Rockwood and Green's Fractures in Adults,* ed 3. Philadelphia, JB Lippincott, 1991, p 564.)

Table 3
Relative muscle power

Muscle	Relative Power
Flexor digitorum pollicis	4.5
Flexor carpi ulnaris, brachoradialis, extensor digitorum communis	2.0
Palmaris, flexor pollicis longus, extensor carpi ulnaris, extensor carpi radialis longus	1.1
Extensor carpi radialis brevis, flexor carpi ulnaris, flexor carpi radialis	0.9
Palmaris longus, abductor pollicis longus	0.1

Table 4
Range of motion (axis middle finger)

Motion*	Wrist	Finger	Thumb
Extension**	55°-75°		
MP		30°-45°	0°
PIP		0°	
DIP		10°-20°	
CMC			0°
IP			0°-20°
Flexion	65°-80°		
MP		85°-100°	0°-90°
PIP		100°-115°	
DIP		80°-90°	
CMC			45°-70°
IP			85°-90°
Ulnar deviation	30°-45°		
Radial deviation	15°-25°		
Supination	60°-85°		
Pronation	60°-80°		
Abduction/adduction		20°-60°/0°	
Palmar abduction			
CMC			40°-70°
MP			0°-20°
Dorsal adduction			
CMC			0°-30°
MP			0°
Axial rotation			
CMC			17°-20°

* MP = metacarpophalangeal; PIP = proximal interphalangeal; DIP = distal interphalangeal; CMC = carpometacarpal; IP - interphalangeal.
** Thumb extension is radial abduction.

muscle attachments, is an intercalated segment, which readily responds to transmitted angular forces from the more rigid distal row and CMC joints where the wrist muscles attach at the metacarpal bases. The row's stability depends on the complex ligament structure and articular surface contours described above. With flexion-extension motion (Fig. 29), there is synchronous angulation of each carpal row in the same direction. The radiocarpal joint contributes 66% of wrist extension with 34% from the intercarpal joint. With flexion, the radiocarpal joint contributes 40%, with 60% at the intercarpal joint.

As a result of the relative strength of the wrist extensors and flexors, the wrist does not normally move on a single axis of flexion and extension in respect to the forearm; instead, it rotates about an axis creating dorsal-radial extension to the ulnar-palmar flexion axis. This motion is described as a dart-thrower's motion. Flexion and extension are closely integrated with radial and ulnar deviation in the wrist, and their separation in describing the kinematics of the wrist is somewhat of an oversimplification.

All the primary muscles of the wrist except the flexor carpi ulnaris are attached to the metacarpals. It is hypothesized that the mechanism of flexion-extension of the wrist is initiated at the distal carpal row. In proceeding from flexion to extension, the

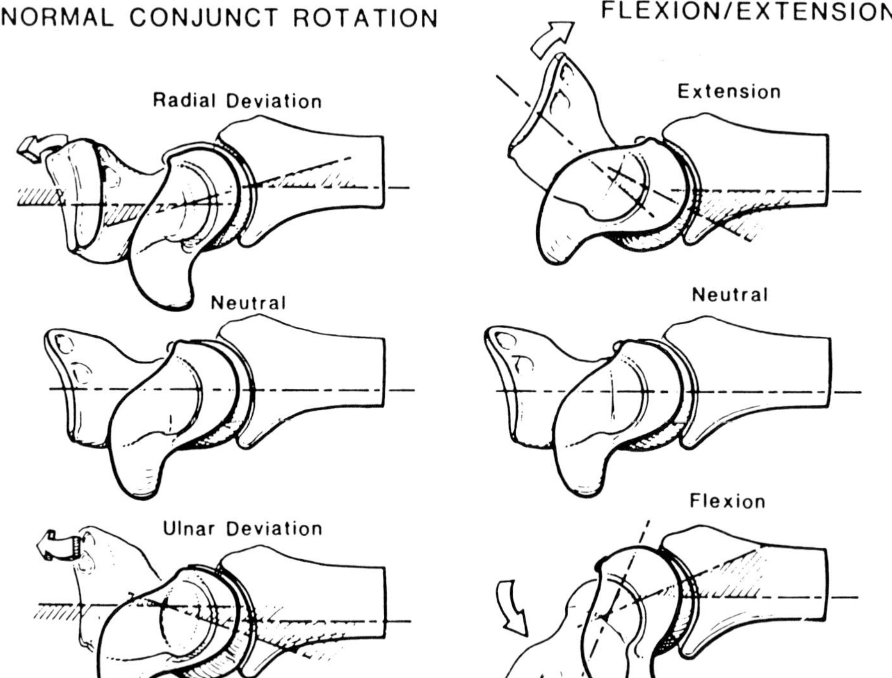

Figure 29
Conjunct rotation of the proximal carpal row occurs in flexion during radial deviation **(top left).** The axes of the radius and carpal rows are colinear in neutral **(center left),** and the proximal row extends with ulnar deviation **(bottom left).** Angulatory excursions of the proximal and distal rows are essentially equal in amplitude and direction during flexion **(bottom right)** and extension **(top right).** This may be described as synchronous angulation. (Reproduced with permission from Cooney WP III, Linscheid RL, Dobyns JH: Fractures and dislocations of the wrist, in Rockwood CA Jr, Green DP, Bucholz RW (eds): *Rockwood and Green's Fractures in Adults,* ed 3. Philadelphia, JB Lippincott, 1991, p 578.)

distal carpal row rotates on the proximal row. At neutral, the radioscaphocapitate ligament is thought to functionally link the scaphoid with the distal carpal row so that they move as a unit. With further extension, the intercarpal ligament brings the scapholunate joint into a closed packed position so that the entire distal and proximal rows now essentially move as one. Further extension then proceeds at the radiocarpal joint. The reverse occurs in proceeding from extension to flexion. The scaphoid travels through an arc of about 40° during flexion and extension. This motion exemplifies how the scaphoid is a link between the proximal and distal rows.

A similar complex interaction between the proximal and carpal distal rows occurs with radioulnar deviation. During radioulnar deviation, each carpal row demonstrates not only synchronous motion in the AP/coronal plane, but also conjoint rotation in the sagittal plane (Fig. 29). In radial deviation (Fig. 30, *left*), the obliquely oriented scaphoid flexes as the trapezium approaches the radius. During the return towards full ulnar deviation, the proximal row extends, including the scaphoid. More importantly, the hamate migrates proximally forcing the triquetrum to displace volarly and extend the lunate. This variable geometry of the proximal carpal row, which includes varying length and contour, allows for the excursion of the wrist with longitudinal stability. During radial deviation, there is primarily intercarpal motion with the distal row moving radially and negligible proximal row motion ulnarly. During ulnar deviation (Fig. 30, *right*), there is both intercarpal and radiocarpal motion, with the distal row moving ulnarly and the proximal row radially. In proceeding from ulnar deviation to radial deviation, the distal carpal row rotates in a radial direction and translates from a dorsal to a palmar direction. Simultaneously, the proximal carpal row flexes and, in a reciprocal motion, slides ulnarly on the distal radioulnar joint.

One theory holds that with radial deviation, the scaphoid initiates movement of the proximal carpal row. It flexes to avoid impingement against the radial styloid and, thus, allows greater motion. The remaining carpals of the proximal row follow in flexion by virtue of their intercarpal ligamentous attachments. The second theory holds that motion proceeds from the ulnar side of the wrist at the triquetral-hamate joint with radioulnar deviation. With radial deviation, the triquetrum is felt to slide radially, dorsally, and proximally through its articulation with the hamate. Through its intercarpal attachment, the lunate flexes followed by the scaphoid. The reverse occurs with ulnar deviation. The triquetrum slides palmarly only distal on the hamate accompanied by lunate and scaphoid extension. The proximal carpal row as a whole slides on the radial carpal joint in a direction opposite that of the hand movement.

While 90% of the pronation-supination motion occurs in the forearm, the remaining 10% (15°) is divided between the radiocarpal and intercarpal motion.

Wrist Kinetics

To further the understanding of the kinematics of the wrist, a tendon-shift mechanism has been described in which the wrist continuously rebalances its flexion and extension forces by controlling their moment arms. As previously noted, the axis of

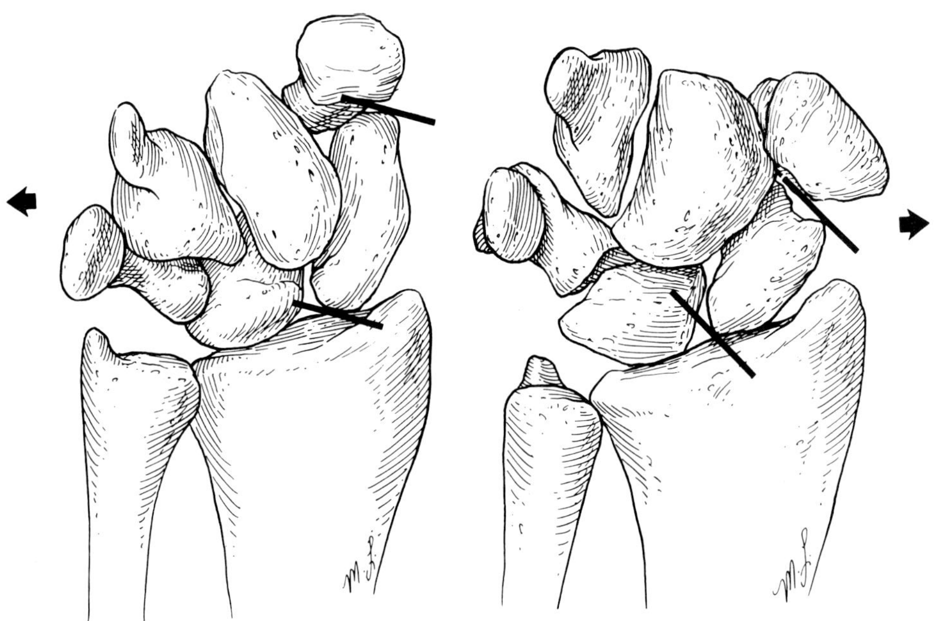

Figure 30
Right, Radial deviation. **Left,** Ulnar deviation. (Reproduced with permission from *Regional Review Courses in Hand Surgery,* ed 4. Aurora, CO, American Society for Surgery of the Hand, 1991.)

motion of the wrist is normally from extension with radial deviation to flexion with ulnar deviation. With radial deviation, the scaphoid flexes to increase the diameter on the radial side of the wrist. As the scaphoid flexes, the distal pole acts as a pulley to increase the moment arm of the flexor carpi radialis tendon. This action optimizes the force for return from extension and radial deviation to flexion. With ulnar deviation, the scaphoid extends and the wrist AP diameter decreases on the radial side. The flexed proximal carpal row and radius form a convex pulley over which the extensors pass (Fig. 31). The extensors are thus moved away from the wrist, increasing their moment arm for return to extension. The tendon-shift mechanism ensures large moment arms by maintaining a given distance between the flexors and extensors, thereby ensuring optimal wrist stability and function. To further this concept, with radial deviation-extension the flexed scaphoid distal pole forms a pulley for the finger flexors to create a moment for return to ulnar deviation (Fig. 32). The hook of the hamate similarly forms a pulley for the finger flexors when the wrist is ulnarly deviated. This tendon-shift mechanism would be disturbed by limited carpal fusions, proximal row carpectomies, or other surgeries that alter normal carpal movement.

The distal radius in the ulnar neutral wrist normally bears about 80% to 85% of the load across the distal radioulnar carpal complex and the distal ulna, 15% to 20%. Of the force transmitted across the radiocarpal joint, 46% to 50% of total radioulnar carpal complex force has been shown to be transmitted by the radioscaphoid fossa and the remaining 30% to 35% by the radiolunate fossa. The amount of force transmitted across the lunate fossa can be increased, and a slight increase can be produced in

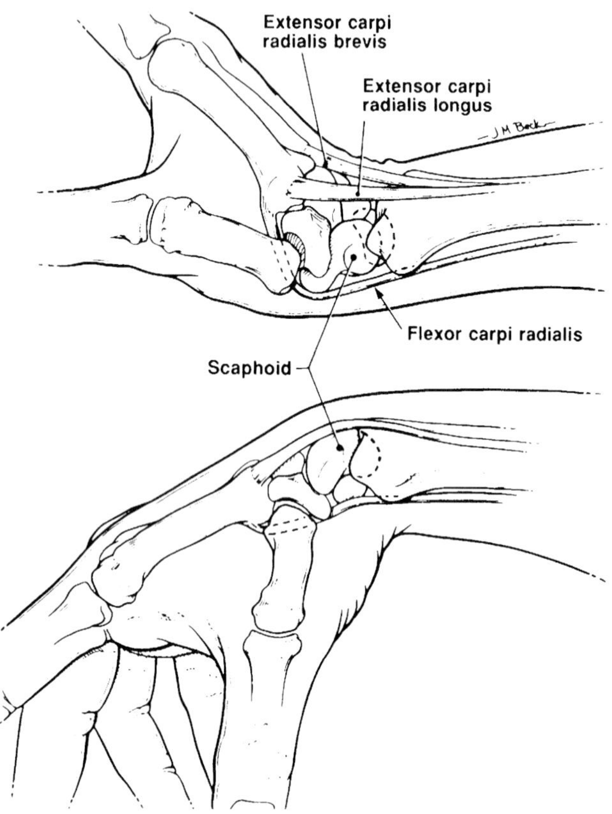

Figure 31
Top, The wrist extensors bowstring for maximal extensor moment arms while the vertical scaphoid carries the FCR tendon palmarward with the radial side of the carpus. **Bottom,** Wrist flexion creates a "convex pulley" from the combined shape of the distal radius and the repositioning of the scaphoid. This convex pulley lifts the radial wrist extensor tendons to preserve their moment arms for the return cycle into wrist extension. Simultaneously, the repositioned scaphoid moves the FCR tendon dorsally, shortening its moment arm to complement hand opening, precision digital functions, and so forth. (Reproduced with permission from Brand PW, Hollister A: *Clinical Mechanisms of the Hand,* ed 2. St. Louis, CV Mosby, 1993.)

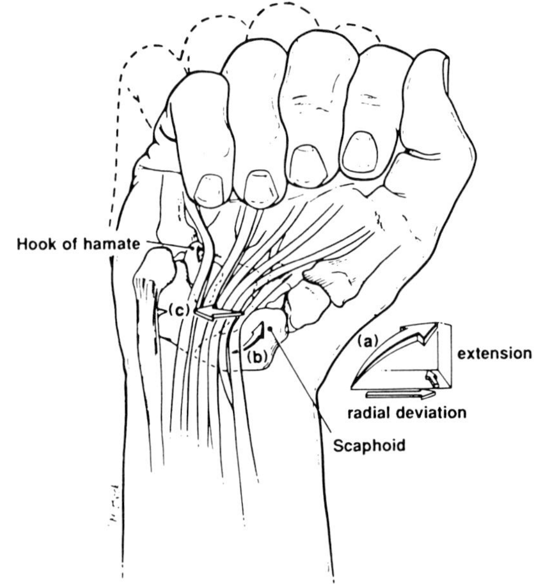

Figure 32
Radial deviation in extension (a) positions the scaphoid as a vertical "finger" of bone to define the dorsal radial wall of the carpal tunnel as a fulcrum for the digital flexor tendons. By actively sweeping into a vertical position (b), it displaces all nine digital flexor tendons toward the palmar ulnar border of the wrist (c), thereby widely separating the wrist flexion effect of the digital flexors from the radial wrist extensor tendons. Wide separation of the high tension forces transmitted by these tendons is an essential element in creating the stable wrist necessary for forceful grasp by the digits. (Reproduced with permission from Brand PW, Hollister A: *Clinical Mechanisms of the Hand,* ed 2. St. Louis, CV Mosby, 1993.)

ulnocarpal force through ulnar deviation of the wrist. The ulnocarpal force also increases with the increase in the ulnar variance associated with forearm pronation.

The triangular fibrocartilage complex (TFCC) essentially serves as a spacer between the distal ulna and carpus. An inverse linear relationship between ulnar variance and the thickness of the TFCC has been demonstrated. Forced transmission through the distal ulna changes significantly only when two thirds or more of the horizontal portion of the TFCC is excised. Therefore, partial TFCC debridement or excision is recommended in central perforations.

The total surface area of the radiocarpal joint from the carpal aspect ranges from 320 to 480 mm^2. The lunate fossa accounts for 46%, the scaphoid fossa for 43%, and the TFCC for 11% of the area. The contact area of the radiocarpal joint covers only approximately 20.6% of the total joint surface, with a range from 14% in radial deviation, pronation, and either neutral or 20° of flexion to 32% in radial deviation, supination, and 20° of extension. The separate and distinct scaphoid contact area is 1.47 times that of the lunate. The scaphoid contact area generally is greatest in ulnar deviation, when the scaphoid is vertical. The scaphoid-lunate contact area ratio usually increases as the wrist moves from radial to ulnar deviation and/or flexion to extension. The contact area is palmar when the wrist is in flexion and dorsal when the wrist is in extension at 40°, but initially from 20° of flexion to 20° of extension, the contact area shifts palmarly. The area will increase to a maximum of 40% of the available articular surface with increasing pressure. In a similar fashion, the midcarpal joint pressure contact area covers an average of 8%, up to a maximum of 15%, of the available contact area. Of this area, approximately 50% proceeds on a path from the capitate to its articulations with the scaphoid and the lunate. Carpal instabilities can significantly alter the joint contact areas and pressures. A scapholunate dissociation with an associated dorsal intercalated segmental instability deformity and palmar flexed scaphoid will result in decreased joint contact area and increased scaphoid fossa pressure. However, the lunotriquetral dissociations that have an associated palmar intercalated segmental instability are not significantly altered for the pressure distribution in the radiocarpal joint. This fact is consistent with the clinical course of this instability.

Similarly, limited intercarpal fusions for these disorders change force transmission. Scaphotrapezial-trapezoid and scaphocapitate fusions transfer loads to the scaphoid fossa. The scaphoid essentially acts as a component at the distal carpal row and is unable to flex or extend with radial and ulnar deviation. This results in increased compressive stresses at the radiocarpal joint with radial deviation that leads to assumed degenerative changes. In ulnar deviation, these limited intercarpal fusions produce a tensile stress on the scapholunate ligament, resulting in increased gapping between the scaphoid and lunate. This gapping is caused by the inability of the scaphoid to extend. Scapholunate, scapholunocapitate, and capitolunate intercarpal fusions all have less effect on load distributions at the radial carpal joint, but still are not entirely normal. Load distribution is further affected by the relative position at which the carpals are fused. On the other hand, alteration of load transmission across the radiocarpal joint may be desirable. Joint leveling by radial shortening or ulnar lengthening is a viable treatment option in the Kienböck's disease associated with a negative ulnar variant. Two and one half millimeters of ulnar lengthening have been shown to increase the ulnar load to 42%. The remaining 58% of the load transmission across the radiocarpal joint is redistributed to increase pressure across the radioscaphoid joint and decrease the pressure across the radiolunate facet.

Experimentally, the total transmitted force though the radiolunate joint can be significantly decreased by an average of 45% by a joint leveling procedure. Although this procedure results in an increased force through the TFCC, the radioscaphoid joint slightly increases and the lunocapitate force decreases to about 13% of the normally transmitted force. Reciprocally, when distal ulnar decompression is needed, ulnar shortening of 2.5 mm results in a decrease from an average of 20% to 4% of the total radioulnar force.

The Thumb

The thumb is undeniably the most important digit on the hand because of its ability to oppose the fingers as a result of its movable metacarpal.

Kinematics and Joint Stability

The thumb ray is thought to start with the trapezium and its articulation with the first metacarpal, because there is no significant motion among the carpals with thumb motion. The flexion-extension plane of motion for the thumb is described as being approximately parallel to the palm. Flexion is motion towards the hypothenar eminence, whereas palmar abduction-adduction occurs in a plane perpendicular to the flexion-extension plane. The trapeziometacarpal joint allows approximately 45° to 70° of flexion, accompanied by some pronation. Overall thumb motion also includes approximately 0° to 30° of adduction to 40° to 70° of palmar abduction. The palmar abduction is divided between the CMC joint with an average of 42° and the MP joint with a range of 0° to 20°.

Thumb opposition consists of the composite motions of abduction, which lifts the thumb away from the hand, and rotation of the thumb into pronation. Thumb pronation is rotation of the thumb so that the pulp surfaces of the thumb and fingers face one another. Opposition occurs as a unit involving the interphalangeal (IP), MP, and trapeziometacarpal joints, and sequentially proceeds through abduction, flexion, and adduction accompanied by simultaneous pronation. The motion of the thumb forms a cone. The rotation is not around the axis of the first metacarpal, but is the result of an arc around a central point in the palm. It is this swinging movement in abduction that is used to draw the thumb in front of the palm and then hold an object between the thumb and finger. Full opposition proceeds approximately through 110° from full extension to complete abduction-flexion and rotation. Opposition occurs primarily at the trapeziometacarpal joint, making it the most important joint in the hand.

The trapezium is angled volarly; placing the rest of the thumb in a position palmar to the plane of the hand. In a resting position, the first metacarpal then forms an angle of approximately 45° to 60° with the second metacarpal. Opposition of the thumb consists of abduction and internal rotation of the thumb as a unit. This rotational motion primarily occurs through movement at the trapeziometacarpal joint and is enhanced by MP joint abduction/internal rotation.

The trapeziometacarpal joint is a double-saddle configuration with a ridge on the surface of the trapezium; it is concave in one plane and convex in another. This geometry permits primarily two degrees of freedom, flexion-extension and abduction-adduction; however, with distraction an average of 17° of axial rotation occurs. The prime stabilizer of the trapeziometacarpal joint is the anterior-oblique ligament, which is taut in abduction, extension, and pronation. The first intermetacarpal, ulnar-collateral, and posterior-oblique ligaments make up the secondary stabilizers. The dorsal-radial facet provides the main resistance to dorsal subluxation and becomes eroded early in degenerative arthritis.

The MP joint of the thumb has a condylar configuration with two degrees of freedom. It has variable flexion-extension ranging from 0° to 90° and an average flexion of 55°. Although these motions at the MP joint aid in opposition, if MP joint motion is lost or the joint is fused, it is well compensated for by the adjacent joints in the thumb. Similarly, if the CMC joint is lost or fixed in an opposed position, the MP joint, having good intrinsic control, can take over as the prime mobile joint. The MP joint is statically stabilized by the collateral ligaments and volar plate. In addition, the thenar intrinsics, by inserting onto the two sesamoids and the extensor mechanism, provide dynamic restraints to hyperextension and excessive abduction and adduction.

The IP joint is a true hinge joint with one degree of freedom. It is similarly stabilized by a volar plate and two collateral ligaments. It allows an average of 85° to 90° of flexion, which is accompanied by slight pronation. The joint also allows an average of 0° to 20° of hyperextension to increase the surface area of the thumb pad available to pinch.

Kinetics

The thumb is powered by four extrinsic and four intrinsic muscles. The extrinsic muscles consist of the abductor pollicis longus, extensor pollicis brevis, extensor pollicis longus, and flexor pollicis longus. Excluding the flexor pollicis longus, the main function of these extrinsic muscles is to retrieve the position of the thumb from the opposed position in the palm. The abductor pollicis longus tendon inserts by a variable number of tendinous slips into the base of the first metacarpal. There is approximately an 80% occurrence of multiple slips. This tendon acts as a dynamic stabilizer of the CMC joint when the thumb metacarpal is adducted. With reference to the plane of thumb motion, the abductor pollicis longus primarily extends the first metacarpal, but its direction of pull also allows it to flex the wrist.

The extensor pollicis brevis inserts into the dorsal base of the proximal phalanx. Its action is to extend the proximal phalanx and secondarily abduct the thumb. The extensor pollicis brevis is always narrower than the abductor pollicis longus and is absent in 5% to 7% of people. Both the extensor pollicis brevis and abductor pollicis longus will assist in radial deviation of the wrist. The extensor carpi ulnaris normally functions synergistically with these two muscles to prevent radial deviation of the wrist and allow strong function of the thumb.

The extensor pollicis longus inserts into the base of the distal phalanx to extend the IP joint. On continued action, the extensor pollicis longus will extend the proximal phalanx, metacarpal, and wrist. The extensor pollicis longus is the most powerful of the three extrinsic muscles inserting on the dorsum of the thumb; its unique position around Lister's tubercle allows it to secondarily adduct the thumb. The extensor pollicis longus primarily positions the thumb in extension to produce a flat, open hand such as is used in clapping, slapping, or pushing. This muscle's secondary actions of adduction and supination make it the direct antagonist to opposition. It is important to note that all three dorsal extrinsics (abductor pollicis longus, extensor pollicis brevis, and extensor pollicis longus) also supinate or rotate the pulp surface of the thumb away from the finger pulp surfaces, so that the thumb pulp faces flat and parallel with the palm surface.

The flexor pollicis longus is the only extrinsic muscle on the flexor surface of the thumb. It inserts into the base of the distal phalanx, and it not only flexes the IP joint, but also flexes and adducts the first metacarpal. It is the strongest of the extrinsic muscles and provides power to thumb flexion once the thenar muscles have set the direction.

The four intrinsic muscles, collectively referred to as the thenar muscles, include the abductor pollicis brevis, opponens pollicis, flexor pollicis brevis, and the adductor pollicis. They may best be viewed as a fan of muscles originating from the carpals, metacarpals, and the transverse carpal ligament and inserting on the thumb to produce a continuum of motion from flexion-abduction to the stronger flexion-adduction. The thenar muscles are primarily responsible for producing opposition of the thumb.

There is extensive interaction between the muscles of the thumb to facilitate opposition. The abductor pollicis longus, extensor pollicis brevis, abductor pollicis brevis, and opponens pollicis work in conjunction to open the first web space. The addition of the extensor pollicis longus further opens the thumb. The extrinsics (abductor pollicis brevis, extensor pollicis brevis, and extensor pollicis longus) are responsible primarily for repositioning the thumb by extension and supination away from the palm. The intrinsics (abductor pollicis brevis and opponens pollicis) serve to position the thumb in abduction and pronation with the maximally functional force of the flexor pollicis brevis.

The activity of each of the thumb muscles varies with the force of opposition. With simple opposition in which the thumb gently contacts the finger, the activities of the opponens pollicis predominate followed by the abductor pollicis brevis, and then the flexor pollicis brevis. In forced opposition against the index and middle fingers, the activity of the flexor pollicis brevis exceeds that of the opponens pollicis. However, activity of the opponens pollicis increases to approximately equal that of the flexor pollicis brevis, as opposition proceeds ulnarly towards the little finger, because of the increased requirement for thumb metacarpal abduction and pronation. Similarly, adductor pollicis activity increases as resistance increases and as opposition progresses towards the ulnar digits. With further resisted opposition, the extrinsics (flexor pollicis longus, abductor pollicis brevis, extensor pollicis brevis, and extensor pollicis longus) assist the maximal joint control of the thenars. Thumb involvement in power grip can be distinguished from that during precision handling by high activity of the adductor pollicis. The limiting factor in grip strength may be related to the ability of the thumb to oppose loads. Thumb position is most variable during cylindrical grip. In hooked grip, thumb use is excluded.

During simple pinch, it has been shown that compressive forces averaging 3, 5.4, and 12 kg develop in the IP, MP, and CMC joints of the thumb, respectively. During power grip, however, the compressive force of the thumb's CMC joint can increase up to tenfold. Average grip strength is 50 to 53 kg and 25 to 30 kg in men and women, respectively; three point pinch strengths are 8 kg for men and 5 kg for women. Grip and pinch strengths required for activities of daily living are 4 kg and 1 kg, respectively. This may be significant in the predilection of this joint to osteoarthritis.

The abductor pollicis brevis is the most important muscle of opposition and weakest of the thenars. Through its insertion into the radial side of the proximal phalanx, lateral MP joint capsule, and extensor apparatus, the abductor pollicis brevis functions to abduct and flex the first metacarpal, slightly flex the proximal phalanx, and extend the IP joint. It acts to position the thumb for function.

The opponens pollicis inserts into the radial side of the metacarpal and is the only thenar to insert on the metacarpal. It positions the metacarpal by means of abduction, flexion, and slight pronation.

The flexor pollicis brevis consists of two parts: (1) a superficial head innervated by the median nerve and inserting via the radial sesamoid into the radial base of the proximal phalanx and extensor apparatus; and (2) a deep-ulnar head innervated by the ulnar nerve and inserting into the ulnar base of the proximal phalanx. The action of the flexor pollicis brevis is to flex the metacarpal and proximal phalanx; and through the insertion on the extensor apparatus, extend the IP joint. Secondarily, it assists in adduction and, with the thumb in a flexed position, provides slight pronation. The flexor pollicis brevis adds power to both forced opposition and abduction.

The adductor pollicis muscle usually assists in reinforcing grip. It has two heads (transverse and oblique) that converge and insert via the ulnar sesamoid into the ulnar aspect of the volar plate and proximal phalanx. It acts to adduct the metacarpal and slightly flex the MP joint. By its aponeurosis inserting into the dorsal extensor mechanism, the adductor pollicis muscle also contributes to IP joint extension.

The Fingers

Kinematics and Joint Stability

Each of the four finger rays is composed of a metacarpal, its three phalanges, and their interposed articulations.

The metacarpals themselves provide a space, in length and width, to allow objects of size to be grasped. Palmar cupping allows the hand to conform to objects to increase the surface area of contact and improve application of gripping forces. This cupping is made possible by three arches of the hand. A longitudinal arch is formed by the metacarpals and flexed fingers. This arch is supplemented by two transverse arches. One is a relatively immobile structural arch, formed by the carpals and supported by the transverse carpal ligament. The second transverse arch is distal, and is formed by the metacarpal heads, and allows the hand to have greater adaptability. The progressive motion of the ulnar digits along with the hypothenar muscles flex and adduct the fifth metacarpal and finger to assist in cradling objects. The palm cups with metacarpal flexion and, reciprocally, the palm flattens with metacarpal extension.

Proximally, the metacarpals of each digit articulate with the wrist via the CMC joints. The primary function of the these joints is to stabilize the metacarpals and, on the ulnar side, control hollowing of the palm. Those of the index through the ring fingers are considered to be plain synovial joints with one degree of freedom, flexion and extension. The fifth CMC joint is described as a shallow saddle joint with two degrees of freedom. The CMC joints are stabilized by tough transverse intermetacarpal and longitudinal CMC ligaments. The dorsal CMC ligaments are stronger than the volar ligaments. The second CMC joint is relatively immobile, but progressively more mobility is seen in the fourth and fifth metacarpals. The fourth CMC joint exhibits 8° to 10° of motion, whereas the fifth exhibits 15° to 20° of flexion with supination.

The MP joints are considered the key element in the kinematic chain of the fingers as they position the IP joints in space. Their surfaces are described as being condyloid, with predominantly two degrees of rotational freedom. Motion is primarily in the flexion-extension axis followed by abduction-adduction and accompanied by slight rotation. The metacarpal head has an eccentric articular surface that is broader on the palmar surface. This structure combined with the eccentric insertion of its collateral ligaments permits more abduction and adduction with the joint in extension than flexion. Collateral ligaments tighten with flexion, making this the most stable position. This eccentricity of the metacarpal head is the major reason the MP joints are more likely to become stiff in extension than in flexion. In addition to the collateral ligaments, the MP joints are stabilized by the volar plate, sagittal bands of the extensor apparatus, and the deep transverse metacarpal ligament. The deep transverse metacarpal ligament or intervolar plate ligament is continuous with the volar plate and holds them together. These joints show a slight increase in the range of motion into flexion proceeding from the radial side to the ulnar side with the index showing approximately 90° of flexion and the fifth MP showing approximately 110° of flexion. The MP joints have an average passive hyperextension range of 30° to 45°. Although this is relatively constant between digits, it varies greatly between individuals and is commonly used as a measure of general flexibility.

In full extension, the tips of the fingers lie on the circumference of a circle formed in the plane of the hand, the center of which is the head of the third metacarpal. In closing the hand, the fingers flex and adduct to converge towards the base of the thenar eminence. This movement is facilitated by increased motion in the ulnar digits.

A MP-IP flexion-extension curve has been described as an equiangular spiral (Fig. 33). The lengths of the osseous components of each finger ray have been noted to approximate a Fibonacci series of 2, 3, 5, 8. These numbers show a sequence of progression with a ratio of approximately 1 to 1.618, the significance of which is that each number is the sum of the two previous numbers. This means that the length of the distal and middle phalanges approximate the length of the proximal phalanx. Similarly, the metacarpal is approximately equal to the sum of the length of the proximal and middle phalanges. In addition, the mathematical center of finger motion coincides with the PIP joint axis, making this the anatomic center of finger function. These provide the structural basis for the equiangular curve. The significance of this curve is that it allows for a smooth arc of a progressively diminishing radius with finger flexion.

There are two separate functional positions that exist as the fingers flex to grasp an object. The first is the formation of the placement arc, which occurs at a position where there is full MP flexion and is responsible for 77% of total finger flexion. The position when the fingers grasp an object, known as the final encompassment, arises from motion of the PIP and distal IP (DIP) joints and makes up the remaining 23% of finger flexion. The PIP joint con-

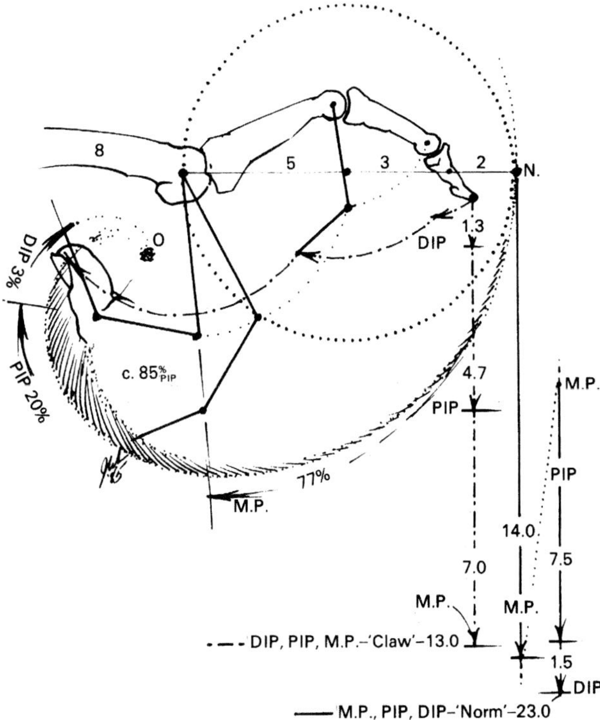

Figure 33
Metacarpophalangeal-interphalangeal extension curve. (Reproduced with permission from Littler JW, Thompson JS: Surgical and functional anatomy, in Bowers WH (ed): *Hand and Upper Limb: 1. The Interphalangeal Joints.* New York, Churchill-Livingstone, 1987, p 15.)

tributes 85% and the DIP joint 15% of this motion. Thus, it can be deduced that the PIP joint is the critical joint in final encompassment, emphasizing the importance of its motion.

The IP joints, both PIP and DIP, are true hinge joints with one degree of freedom in flexion-extension. These joints are stabilized by collateral ligaments as well as by a strong volar plate that prevents hyperextension. The collateral ligaments of the IP joints are relatively taut in all positions of flexion, such that the joint is relatively stable throughout its range of motion. Consistent with the other joints of the finger rays, the IP joints show a similar pattern of increased range of motion from radial to ulnar. PIP joint flexion averages 100° to 115° at the index finger and progressively increases to approximately 135° at the little finger. Similarly, the DIP joint of the index finger has a flexion mean of 80°, which increases to 90° at the small finger. The adjacent condyles of the heads of the proximal phalanges vary such that with flexion, the middle through small fingers deviate radially at the PIP joints while the index finger's IP joint deviates ulnarly. This deviation, along with the progressive range of motion in the ulnar digits, helps to angulate these digits when flexed towards the scaphoid tubercle, thereby assisting in the opposition to the thumb as well as providing a tighter ulnar grip.

The joint orientation angles for index finger functions are presented to reinforce the overall range that is required in different joints for various functions (Table 5).

Kinetics

The muscles of the fingers can be divided into flexors and extensors, both extrinsic and intrinsic. The flexor digitorum profundus and flexor digitorum superficialis make up the long extrinsic flexors of the fingers.

The flexor digitorum profundus inserts on the distal phalanx of each finger and is the only flexor at the DIP joint. Although the long flexors provide synchronous flexion of the proximal and distal phalanges, they contribute little to MP joint flexion. The profundus tendon also assists in adducting the finger during flexion. The tendon to the index finger is relatively independent, allowing this to be the only digit that can generate maximum profundus force even while the others are extended. The ulnar three digits have limited independent motion because of the common origin of the flexor digitorum profundus tendons as well as common origins of the third and fourth lumbricals. This conjoined nature of the profundi and lumbricals is responsible for the limited independent extension of the ring finger that is commonly annoying to piano players.

The flexor digitorum superficialis inserts on the base of the middle phalanx and flexes the PIP joints. Each superficialis can act in isolation from each other and the profundus. By preventing hyperextension, the action of the sublimis contributes to PIP joint stability. Hook or baggage grip is essentially IP flexion, is a load bearing grip, and can be sustained for long periods. Most of the sustained power comes

Table 5
Joint orientation angles for index finger functions

Function	Joint Flexion Angle (°)*		
	DIP	PIP	MP
Tip pinch	25	50	48
Key pinch	20	35	20
Pulp pinch	0	50	48
Grasp	23	48	62
Baggage/hook grip	55	72	23
Holding glass	20	48	5
Opening big jar	35	55	50

* DIP - distal interphalangeal; PIP = proximal interphalangeal; MP = metacarpophalangeal. (Reproduced with permission from An KN, Chao EY, Cooney WP, et al: Forces in the normal and abnormal hand. *J Orthop Res* 1985;3:202–211.)

from the flexor digitorum superficialis, which keep the PIP joints at about 90° with DIP control as necessary from the profundi.

Extrinsic finger extension is provided through the four tendons of the extensor digitorum communis, assisted by the extensor indicis proprius and the extensor digiti quinti (Fig. 34). The extensor digitorum communis tendon is centered by sagittal bands that insert into the deep transverse metacarpal ligament and volar plate complex. This circumferential sling extends the MP joint, because the extensor digitorum communis has no direct insertion into the proximal phalanx. It has an indirect insertion via connections to the dorsal capsule of the MP joint and via the volar sling formed by the sagittal bands to the volar plate. The extensor tendon proceeds through the extensor expansion to insert on the middle phalanx base as the central slip. The central slip's lateral fibers and intrinsic tendons form the lateral bands that insert at the base of the distal phalanx as the terminal tendon (Fig. 35).

The extensor indicis proprius inserts in a similar fashion on the index finger ulnar to the dorsally central extensor digitorum communis. The extensor digiti quinti also inserts ulnar to the midline on the fifth digit. It is considered the main extensor because the extensor digitorum communis tendon usually is absent more than 50% of the time and is replaced by a junctura tendinum from the ring finger extensor digitorum communis.

The primary function of the long extensors is to extend the MP joints. There is some controversy as to their contribution in extending the PIP joint. When the long extensors are isolated anatomically, full hyperextension of the MP joints is required before the PIP joints will start to extend. The extrinsic extensors stabilize the proximal fingers so that the intrinsics can function and can abduct with extension of the fingers as the hand opens. The extensor indicis proprius and extensor digiti quinti allow independent extension of the index and small fingers, respectively.

The intrinsic muscles of the hand are made up of the palmar and dorsal interossei, lumbricals, and hypothenars. The interossei arising from the metacarpals pass palmar to the MP joint axis flexion to insert into the proximal phalanx and extensor hood. As a group, the interossei most consistently produce MP joint flexion with simultaneous extension of the IP joints. In addition, adduction of the digits is provided by the four dorsal interossei, whereas the three palmar interossei are responsible for adducting the digits. The middle finger is the accepted axis of reference for these motions.

The dorsal interossei as a group are stronger, having twice the muscle mass of the palmar interossei. The first dorsal interosseous, being the strongest, provides the main resistance to ulnar directed forces applied by the thumb. The first

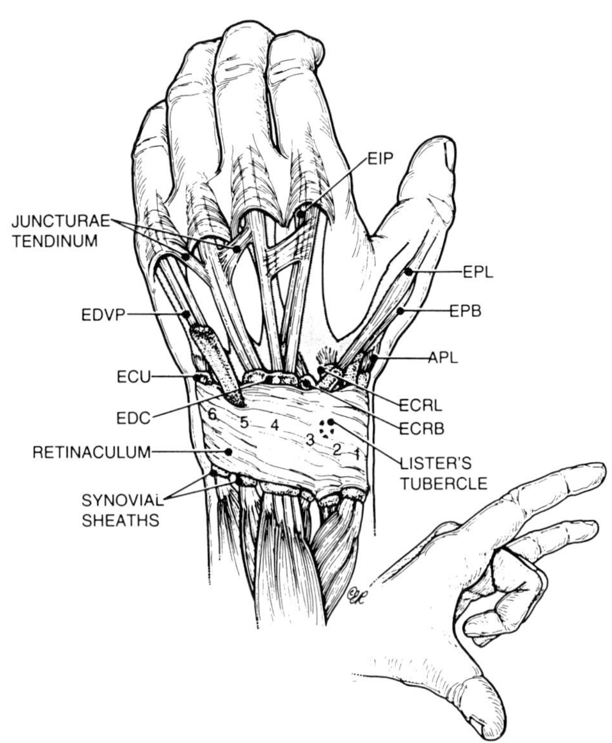

Figure 34
Left, The extensor tendons gain entrance to the hand from the forearm through a series of six canals, five fibro-osseous and one fibrous (the latter is the fifth dorsal compartment, which contains the extensor digit quinti proprius [EDQP]). The first compartment contains the abductor pollicis longus (APL) and extensor pollicis brevis (EPB); the second, the radial wrist extensors; the third, the extensor pollicis longus (EPL), which angles around Lister's tubercle; the fourth, the extensor digitorum communis (EDC) to the fingers, as well as the extensor indicis proprius (EIP); the fifth, the EDQP; and the sixth, the extensor carpi ulnaris (ECU). The communis tendons are jointed distally near the MP joints by fibrous interconnections called juncturae tendinum. These juncturae are usually found only between the communis tendons and may aid in surgical recognition of the proprius tendon of the index. The proprius tendons are always positioned to the ulnar side of the adjacent communis tendons. Beneath the retinaculum, the extensor tendons are covered with a synovial sheath. **Right,** The proprius tendons to the index and little fingers are capable of independent extension, and their function may be evaluated as depicted. With the middle and ring fingers flexed into the palm, the proprius tendons can extend the ring and little fingers. Independent extension of the index, however, is not lost following transfer of the indicis proprius. ECRB, extensor carpi radialis brevis; ECRL, extensor carpi radialis longus. (Illustration by Elizabeth Roselius, © 1993. Reproduced with permission from Doyle JR: Extensor tendons: Acute injuries, in Green DP (ed): *Operative Hand Surgery,* ed 3. New York, Churchill Livingstone, 1993, vol 2, chap 52, pp 1925–1954.)

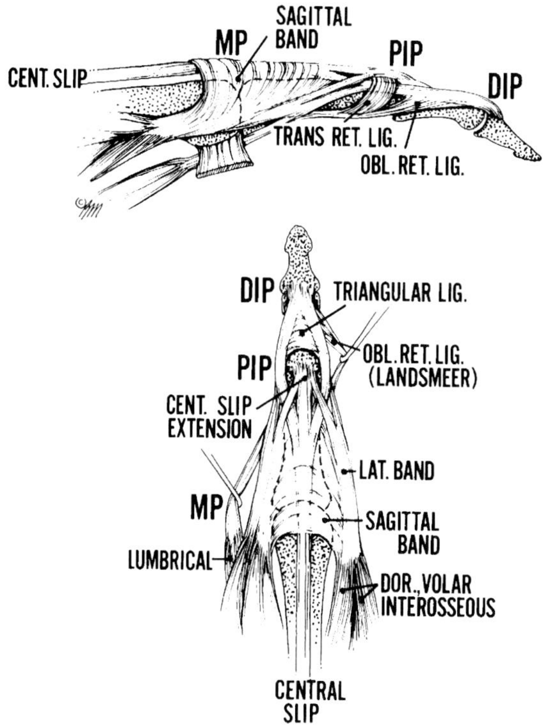

Figure 35
The extensor tendon at the MP joint level is held in place by the transverse lamina or sagittal band, which tethers and centers the extensor tendons over the joint. This sagittal band arises from the volar plate and the intermetacarpal ligaments at the neck of the metacarpals. Any injury to this extensor hood or expansion may result in subluxation or dislocation of the extensor tendon. The intrinsic tendons from the lumbrical and interosseous muscles joint the extensor mechanism at about the level of the proximal and midportion of the proximal phalanx and continue distally to the DIP joint of the finger. The extensor mechanism at the PIP joint is best described as a trifurcation of the extensor tendon into the central slip, which attaches to the dorsal base of the middle phalanx, and the two lateral bands. These lateral bands continue distal to insert at the dorsal base of the distal phalanx. The extensor mechanism is maintained in place over the PIP joint by the transverse retinacular ligaments. (Illustration by Elizabeth Roselius, © 1993. Reproduced with permission from Doyle JR: Extensor tendons: Acute injuries, in Green DP (ed): *Operative Hand Surgery,* ed 3. New York, Churchill Livingstone, 1993, vol 2, chap 52, pp 1925–1954.)

dorsal interosseous is unique among the interossei in that its insertion is entirely into the base of the proximal phalanx. In addition to abducting, it also supinates the finger to facilitate opposition to the thumb.

The four lumbricals are unique in that they all arise and insert via tendons. The lumbricals take origin from the flexor digitorum profundus tendons, pass palmarly to the MP joint axis, and insert into the radial aspect of the extensor apparatus at a point distal to that of the interossei. Their unique origin provides them with a greater contractile range. In fact, their origin actually moves more than their insertion during motion. In referring to the intrinsics as a group, it can be said that the interossei are more effective as MP flexors, while the lumbricals are more effective as IP extensors.

The hypothenar muscles are made up of the abductor digiti minimi, the flexor digiti minimi brevis, and the opponens digiti minimi. The abductor digiti minimi has a dual insertion into the ulnar base of the proximal phalanx and into the extensor apparatus of the fifth digit. It is a strong abductor and slight flexor of the proximal phalanx and secondarily extends the distal two phalanges of the fifth digit. The flexor digiti minimi brevis inserts into the ulnar base of the proximal phalanx and is a strong flexor of the MP joint. It also slightly adducts and flexes the metacarpal. The opponens digiti minimi, similar to the opponens pollicis, inserts entirely onto the fifth metacarpal to flex and adduct it. It is the most active muscle during opposition to the fifth finger. The activity of the opponens digiti minimi exceeds that of the flexor pollicis brevis with resisted opposition. The hypothenar muscles combine to flex and adduct the metacarpal, flex the proximal phalanx, and extend the middle and distal phalanges to cup the palm and enhance opposition.

It is important to mention that three primary retinacula in the hand (the extensor, flexor, and digital sheath) act as pulleys and are responsible for all direction changes of the tendons. They serve to maintain functional axes of motion and contribute to stability of the wrist and digits by preventing bow stringing, thereby ensuring functional moment arms in the hand.

Finger flexion is a combination of active muscle forces opposing the passive viscoelastic forces of the extensor apparatus. The flexor digitorum profundus is the primary flexor during synchronous flexion of the fingers. EMG studies have shown that when such flexion is produced without external resistance, the flexor digitorum profundus is the only active flexor at the IP joints. The flexor digitorum sublimis is activated when flexion against resistance is required. In a similar fashion, the interossei are responsible for MP flexion against resistance. Passive forces are primarily provided by the oblique retinacular ligament (Fig. 35). This ligament arises from the palmar aspect of the proximal phalanx and the adjacent flexor sheath, passing volar to the axis of PIP flexion and then dorsal along the sides of the middle phalanx, and dorsal to the axis of the DIP joint to insert into the distal lateral bands. The ligament's function is to coordinate motion of the middle and distal phalanges.

Finger flexion occurs first at the PIP joint by the action of the flexor digitorum profundus. This is followed by flexion at the MP and then the DIP joints. These motions are quite integrated and are difficult to separate clinically. Action of the flexor digitorum profundus produces tension in the oblique retinacula ligament, which in turn prevents DIP flexion as long as the PIP is extended. The pull of the profundus, thus, does not first cause DIP flexion; instead, its action is transferred proximally causing flexion of the PIP joint. This motion pulls the extensor apparatus distally, placing the intrinsic tendons on stretch and subsequently leading to MP joint flexion via passive viscoelastic forces. With continued flexion of the PIP joint, the oblique retinacula ligament relaxes to allow flexion at the DIP joint. Flexion of the PIP joint then proceeds along with that of the DIP joint, but does so at a faster rate. DIP joint flexion is complete only at the end, producing a locking grip.

Flexion of the fingers also is regulated by a synergistic activity of the long extensors as well as the passive forces of the lumbricals. The extensor digitorum communis acts to restrain MP and PIP flexion, effectively causing motion at these two joints to occur in a synchronous fashion. The lumbricals do not actively participate in producing flexion, but play a significant coordinating role. When finger flexion occurs unopposed by an external resistance, the passive viscoelastic forces of the lumbricals, via their insertion into the extensor apparatus, prevent full IP joint flexion prior to MP joint flexion. This allows the hand to surround an object. The importance of lumbrical function is evident in ulnar nerve palsy with intrinsic paralysis. In this situation, the finger flexes at the IP joints before flexing the MP joints, preventing the hand from grasping any object of a reasonable size.

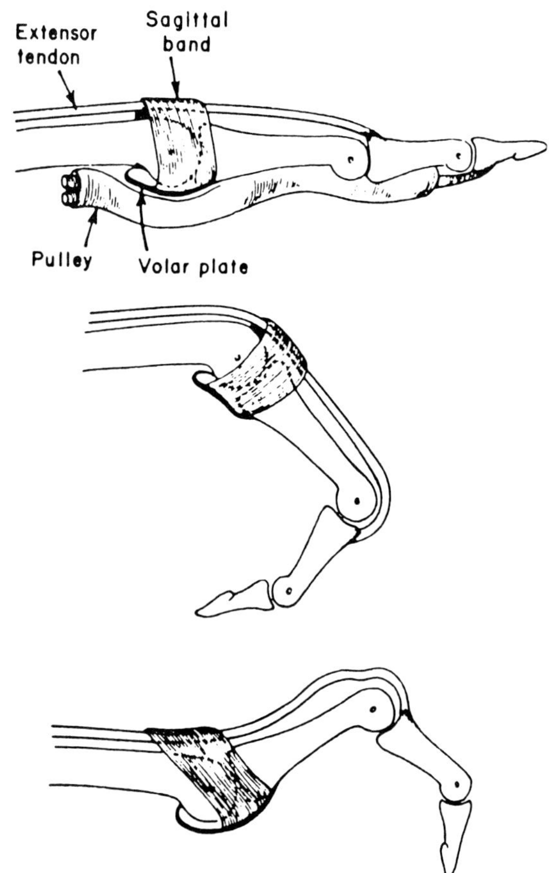

Figure 36
Diagrammatic representation of the sagittal bands. The sagittal bands are attached dorsally to the extensor tendon and volarly to the volar plate. **Top,** In extension, the bands overlie the metacarpophalangeal (MP) joint. **Center,** With flexion, the bands migrate distally. In this position the extensor tendon can extend the proximal interphalangeal (PIP) joint. **Bottom,** In hyperextension, the extensor tendon distal to the MP joint is lax and the PIP joint falls into flexion. (Reproduced with permission from Smith RJ: Balance and kinetics of the fingers under normal and pathological conditions. *Clin Orthop* 1974;104:92–111.)

Extension of the fingers is less well understood and more involved than flexion. Digital extension is similar to flexion in that it is a combination of active and passive forces. EMG studies confirm that the lumbricals and extensor digitorum communis provide the active component of extension. As with flexion, a passive component of extension is provided by the viscoelastic forces of the oblique retinacula ligament that coordinate extension of the middle and distal phalanges. In a fully flexed finger, the proximal phalanx serves as a kinetic link to extension.

With full finger flexion, the sagittal band connecting the extensor digitorum communis to the proximal phalanx is distal to the MP joint (up to 16 mm) and lax (Fig. 36). The extensor digitorum communis is thus unable to directly extend the MP joint at the beginning of extension. Extension begins at the MP joint by an indirect mechanism, which occurs through the combined forces of the central slip of the extensor digitorum communis and the flexor digitorum sublimis acting on the base of the middle phalanx. With the PIP flexed, action of these muscles transmits a force from the base of the middle phalanx through the PIP joint to the head of the proximal phalanx, which will tend to rotate this bone into extension about the MP joint. Simultaneous action of the flexor digitorum superficialis is essential to prevent extension of the PIP joint and allow the generation of the compressive force at the head of the proximal phalanx. As the MP joint extends, the extensor aponeurosis shifts proximally. The extensor digitorum communis insertion becomes tense and allows it to act directly through the sagittal band on the proximal phalanx to further extend the MP joint. At the same time, the lumbricals actively extend the IP joints. As the PIP joint extends, the oblique retinacula ligament coordinates the extension of the distal phalanx. Lumbrical muscle contraction pulls the flexor digitorum profundus tendons distally, decreasing their passive resistance to extension. The lumbricals are often considered the workhorses of finger extension, because of their dual role. As in digital flexion, the interossei are inactive during unopposed extension.

Because hand function depends intimately on the balance of its muscles, it is more appropriate to be concerned with the relative power of these muscles with respect to each other than with their individual absolute strengths (Tables 6 and 7). In general, the flexors have a work capacity three times that of the extensors. The flexor digitorum profundus muscles are on an average 50% stronger than the flexor digitorum superficialis. Tension in the flexor digitorum profundus tendons varies little from the second to the fifth digit, whereas the superficialis strength varies widely. The strength of the flexor profundus is approximately equal to that of the sublimis in the middle finger, whereas, in the small finger, the profundus is approximately three times as strong as the sublimis. It follows that the middle finger is the strongest of all the fingers to flex and resist extension. In fact, for the middle finger, the strength of the flexor digitorum profundus and superficialis together is equal to the strength of all the extensors.

When examining finger muscle forces (Tables 8 and 9) the flexor digitorum profundus and flexor digitorum superficialis consistently demonstrate high force values in comparison to other muscles in most functions. In lateral key pinch, the flexor digitorum superficialis has minimal load, but the extensor digitorum communis and two radial intrinsic muscles contribute large forces. In key pinch the radial interosseous balances the MP joint by preventing ulnar deviation. This high force-generating ability of the flexor digitorum profundus, flexor digitorum superficialis, and radial interosseous is reflected in their higher physiologic cross-sectional area. The ulnar deviation force of the radial interosseous creates a large flexion moment at the MP joint that is counteracted by the extensor digitorum communis for balance. The intrinsic muscles appear to produce more force during pinch function than grasp function to stabilize the MP joint. The muscle forces in simulated activities of daily living are similar to those of basic pinch functions.

The joint contact forces (Table 10) are comparable in both the PIP and MP joints. In lateral pinch, such forces become significantly larger in the MP joint than in the PIP joint because of muscle forces that prevent ulnar deviation of the MP joint (radial interosseous in association with the balancing force of the extensor digitorum communis). The contact forces are large for both tip and pulp pinch, and should not be overlooked. Volar-dorsal shear forces are directed dorsally, implying that under most activities of daily living the proximal phalanx tends to sublux volarly on the metacarpal head. The radial-ulnar shear forces at the MP joint are directed radially to counteract the slight tendency to shift ulnarly. The proximal phalanx also tends to shift ulnarly, loading the radial support structures.

Table 6
Muscle excursion

Muscle	Excursion (cm)
Finger flexors	7
Finger and thumb extensors	5
Wrist muscles	3
Extensor pollicis brevis, abductor pollicis longus	3
Tenodesis effect of wrist*	2.3

* Increases tendon excursion

Table 7
Ratios and aggregate muscle-tendon forces generated by the flexor digitorum profundus and superficialis in 40 normal hands

Finger	Mean (kg)	SD*
Profundus: superficialis		
Index	0.97	0.45
Middle	0.79	0.32
Ring	0.95	0.58
Little	1.50	0.73
Profundus + superficialis		
Index	13.22	3.87
Middle	13.40	4.26
Ring	11.75	5.95
Little	9.01	3.15

* Standard deviation

Table 8
Physiologic cross-sectional areas (PCSA) of muscles across index finger joint

Muscle	PCSA (cm^2)
Flexor digitorum profundus	4.10
Flexor digitorum sublimis	3.6
Extensor digitorum communis	1.39
Extensor indicis	1.12
Radial interosseous	4.16
Lumbrical	0.36
Ulnar interosseous	1.60

Table 9
Muscle forces of index finger under isometric hand function

Function	Muscle Force*					
	FDP	FDS	RI	LU	UI	EDC
Tip pinch	1.93-2.08	1.75-2.16	0.0-0.99	0.0-0.72	0.21-0.65	—
Pulp pinch	1.53-3.14	0.32-1.32	0.0-1.61	0.0-1.17	0.62-1.19	—
Lateral key pinch	1.37-5.95	—	1.01-7.04	0.0-6.10	—	7.45-15.95
Grasp	3.17-3.47	1.51-2.14	0.0-1.19	0.0-0.91	0.0-0.49	—
Baggage/hook grip	0.0-0.02	1.70-1.78	0.0-0.45	0.0-0.33	0.11-0.27	—
Holding glass	2.77-2.99	1.29-1.57	—	0.48-0.53	0.28-0.38	—
Opening big jar	3.50-5.49	—	4.2-4.53	0.0-1.15	0.0-1.00	9.48-16.23

*Forces in units of applied force; that is, magnitude or multiple times the applied force and not the exact applied force. FDP = flexor digitorum profundus; FDS = flexor digitorum sublimis; EDC = extensor digitorum communis; EIP = extensor indicis; RI=radial interosseous; LU = lumbrical; UI = ulnar interosseous.

Table 10
Joint constraint forces of index finger under isometric hand function

Function	Compressive Force* X	Dorsal Shear Force* Y	Radial Shear Force* Z
Distal interphalangeal joint			
Tip pinch	2.4-2.7	0.2-0.3	-0.1 - -0.1
Key pinch	2.9-12.5	0.7-3.2	0.7 - 0.9
Pulp pinch	3.0-4.6	0.0--0.2	-0.1 - -0.2
Grasp	2.8-3.4	0.5-0.7	-0.2 - -0.2
Baggage/hook grip	0.0-0.0	0.0-0.0	0.0 - 0.0
Holding glass	2.5-2.9	0.2-0.3	-0.2 - -0.2
Opening big jar	5.2-9.5	1.7-3.3	0.3 - 0.5
Proximal interphalangeal joint			
Tip pinch	4.4-4.9	0.9-1.1	0.0-0.1
Key pinch	4.9-19.4	1.1-4.5	0.3-1.1
Pulp pinch	4.8-5.8	1.1-1.4	0.0-0.0
Grasp	4.5-5.3	1.0-1.3	0.0 - -0.1
Baggage/hook grip	1.7-1.9	0.0-0.02	0.0-0.0
Holding glass	4.3-4.4	1.1-1.1	0.0 - -0.1
Opening big jar	7.2-14.2	2.4-4.9	0.2-0.8
Metacarpophalangeal joint			
Tip pinch	3.5-3.9	2.1-2.3	0.1-0.2
Key pinch	14.7-27.1	3.9-5.7	0.0-0.1
Pulp pinch	4.0-4.6	2.2-2.4	0.1-0.1
Grasp	3.2-3.7	2.9-3.1	0.3-0.4
Baggage/hook grip	1.0-1.3	0.6-0.7	0.0-0.0
Holding glass	4.0-4.1	0.9-0.9	02.-0.2
Opening big jar	14.8-24.3	6.5-9.9	0.2-0.3

*In units of applied force; negative sign represents force in the opposite direction.

The actual average forces in the index finger (Table 11), particularly with pinching, are considerable. Especially important are the relatively higher forces at the distal phalanx, which contribute to the etiology of osteoarthritis at the DIP joint, sparing the PIP and MP joints.

Loss of the flexor digitorum superficialis force (Table 12) has more than an additive effect on flexor digitorum profundus force required for tip pinch. With flexor digitorum superficialis loss, the flexor digitorum profundus force requirement more than doubles and the previously inactive extensor digitorum communis contributes very high forces with the increased force from the IP extensors (lumbrical and ulnar interosseous) to balance the finger.

Structure and Function of the Spine

The spine is a flexible column with a multicurved shape that is important in absorbing energy.

Table 11
Average strengths of index finger in isometric hand functions

Function	Average Strength (N)
Tip pinch	24-95
Key pinch	37-106
Pulp pinch	30-83
Grasp: distal phalanx	38-109
middle phalanx	7-38
proximal phalanx	23-73

Table 12
Muscle forces (in units of applied force) in index finger during tip pinch with and without laceration of flexor sublimis

	Normal	FDS Laceration
Flexor digitorum profundus	2.20	5.46
Flexor digitorum sublimis	1.77	—
Radial interosseous	1.26	1.43
Lumbrical	0.15	1.85
Ulnar interosseous	0.74	2.37
Extensor digitorum communis	—	7.38

It is a dynamic system composed of motion segments and having four major functions: support, mobility, housing, and control. The spine supports the mass of the body and withstands external forces. At the same time it allows for mobility and enough flexibility to absorb energy and to protect against impact. The spine architecture protects the spinal cord and nerves and the vertebral artery in the cervical area. Trunk muscles and ligaments, acting on individual vertebrae, provide postural control and spinal stability. Trauma, dysfunction, pain, or surgical intervention can affect any of these functions. Healthy spine function depends on the interplay among spinal structure, stability, and flexibility, as well as on muscular strength, endurance, and coordination.

Kinematics of the Spine

General Kinematics

The normal curves of the spine include cervical lordosis, thoracic kyphosis, and lumbar lordosis. This curvature arises naturally from the shape of the vertebrae and disks, the rib cage, and the inclination of the sacral end plate. However, variation in the inclination of the sacral end plate produces considerable individual variation in the shape of vertebrae and disks and, thus, in the curvatures of the spine.

In the spine, two types of motion, translation and rotation, are possible about each of the three orthogonal planes. These motions are usually coupled. For example, in a flexion movement, the vertebra rotates in the sagittal plane and simultaneously undergoes AP translations. In general, in vitro measurements can be made more accurately and under more controlled loading conditions than in vivo measurements, but they may not duplicate in vivo conditions (that is, muscle excitations, fluid environment, temperature, etc).

Figure 37 shows the relative motion in vivo within and between the different parts of the spine, as summarized from the literature. The main determinant for range of motion is the orientation of the facet or zygapophyseal joints and intervertebral disks. Flexion-extension predominates in the cervical region, but considerable axial rotation and lateral bending are possible. Flexion-extension movement and lateral bending mainly occur in the midcervical region, and axial rotation occurs primarily in the upper part of the cervical spine.

The thoracic region is stabilized by the rib cage and there is generally little motion. The lumbar spine permits considerable lateral bending in the middle portion, while flexion-extension is greatest in the lumbosacral motion segment. Rotation is minimal in the lumbar region because of the orientation of the facet joints. Compared with the thoracic spine, the greater mobility in the cervical and

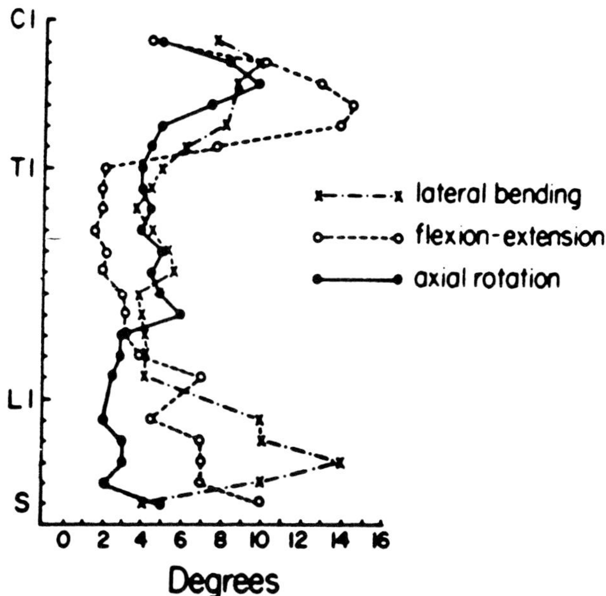

Figure 37
Range of motion within and between the different motion segments of the spine. (Reproduced with permission from Pope MH, Frymoyer JW, Lehmann TR: Structure and function of the lumbar spine, in *Occupational Low Back Pain: Assessment, Treatment, and Prevention.* St. Louis, CV Mosby, 1991.)

lumbar regions corresponds with greater stresses and more clinical complaints.

Clinical measurement of spine mobility is difficult because the hips and lumbar spine move together. Simple goniometric techniques are most commonly used, but reliability can be improved with the dual inclinometer technique and the flexicurve technique. The latter method involves reproducing a curve and taking tangents to it. Segmental axial rotation is the most difficult motion to study in vivo; however, reasonably accurate results are obtained with pins inserted into the vertebrae, or with biplane or stereo radiography.

Most researchers report less mobility of the spine among older subjects. For example, using a dual inclinometer technique, measurements of spinal mobility have been made among white- and blue-collar workers, ranging in age from 35 to 54 years. Range of motion was found to be lower among the older subjects. Women had a slightly greater range of motion in the cervical area and men showed greater mobility in the lumbar area, but not all measurements followed this pattern. A large industrial study in the United States found no evidence of a relationship between mobility and subsequent back disability; reduced spinal mobility in combination with pain or tenderness, however, is useful in predicting subsequent disability. Increased sagittal plane translation and coupled translatory and axial motion may be an early sign of disk degeneration and low back problems.

Understanding the movements of the spine, like those of other joints of the body, requires an appreciation of instantaneous axes of rotation (IARs). IARs based on in vitro studies in the cervical, thoracic, and lumbar regions are presented in Figure 38.

The Motion Segment

The motion segment is the basic anatomic unit of the spine. It comprises two adjacent vertebrae and their intervening soft tissues. This structure, sometimes called a functional spinal unit (FSU), is viscoelastic and absorbs energy. It moves with six degrees of freedom (three translations and three rotations) (Fig. 39, *top*). However, because each motion segment depends on its two bony elements with six articulate faces and multiple ligamentous components for its stability, its motions are complex. Loads and torques applied to an FSU along or about the AP, lateral, or axial axes not only produce pure simple motions but also coupled translations and rotations about several axes. This coupling behavior is present in most functional movements and varies greatly among individuals, depending on such factors as age and (where pathology exists) the level of degeneration.

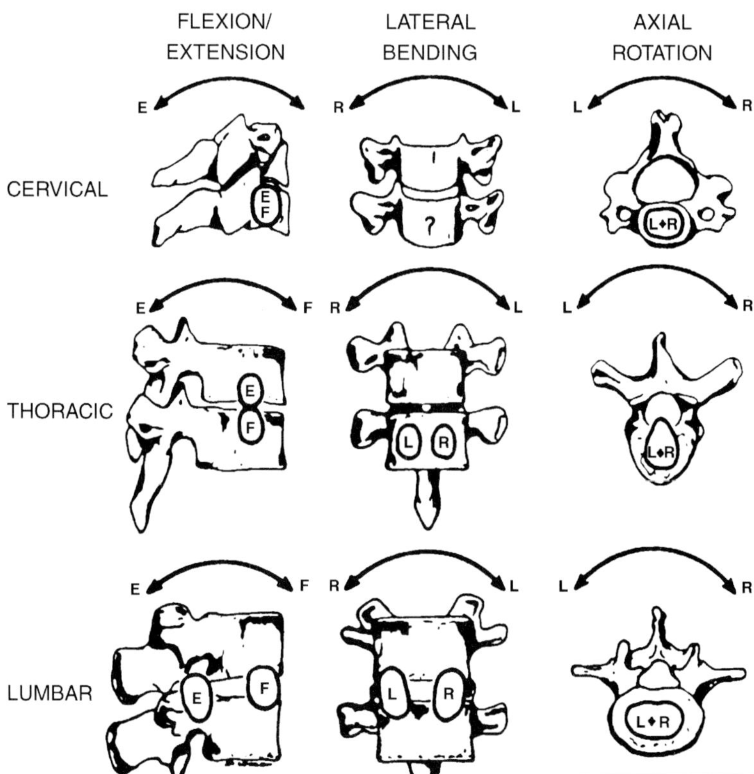

Figure 38
Approximate locations of instantaneous axes of rotation (IAR) in the three regions of the spine undergoing rotation in the three traditional planes. E = approximate location of IARs in extending from neutral position. F = IARs in flexion from neutral position. L = IARs in left lateral bending or left axial rotation. R = IARs in right lateral bending or right axial rotation. (Reproduced with permission from White AA III, Panjabi MM (eds): *Clinical Biomechanics of the Spine.* Philadelphia, JB Lippincott, 1978.)

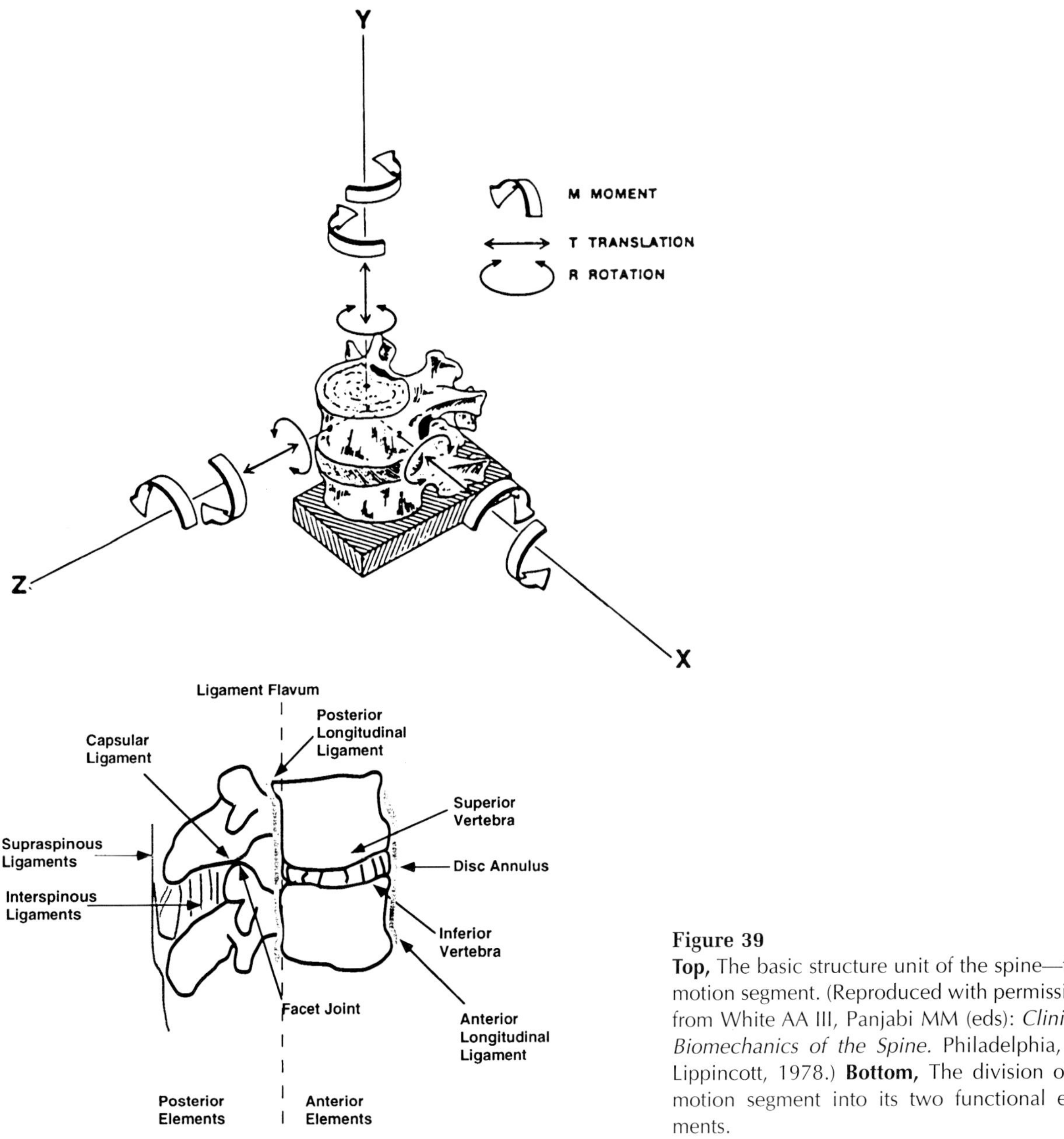

Figure 39
Top, The basic structure unit of the spine—the motion segment. (Reproduced with permission from White AA III, Panjabi MM (eds): *Clinical Biomechanics of the Spine.* Philadelphia, JB Lippincott, 1978.) **Bottom,** The division of a motion segment into its two functional elements.

It is convenient to divide the motion segment into anterior and posterior elements or columns (Fig. 39, *bottom*). The dividing line is just behind the vertebral body. The anterior elements include the vertebral body, the disk, and the anterior and posterior longitudinal ligaments. These provide the major support for the spinal column and absorb impact. In so doing they restrict vertical translational motion. The neural arch and its processes and the zygapophyseal joints lie to the posterior and, with the disk, control patterns of motion about the other axes.

Intervertebral disk The disk forms the primary articulation between the vertebral bodies and is the major constraint to motion of the FSU. The disk is composed of two morphologically separate parts. The outer part, the annulus fibrosus, is made up of about 90 collagen sheets bonded to one another. Each sheet is made of collagen fibers oriented vertically at the peripheral layer, but becoming progressively more oblique with each underlying layer (Fig. 40). The fibers in adjacent sheets run at approximately 30° angles to each other. The lamination of these layers strengthens the annulus. The inner or central part of the disk is the nucleus pulposus. In young individuals, it is nearly 90% water, with the remaining structure comprising collagen and proteoglycans, which bind water. Normally, the adult

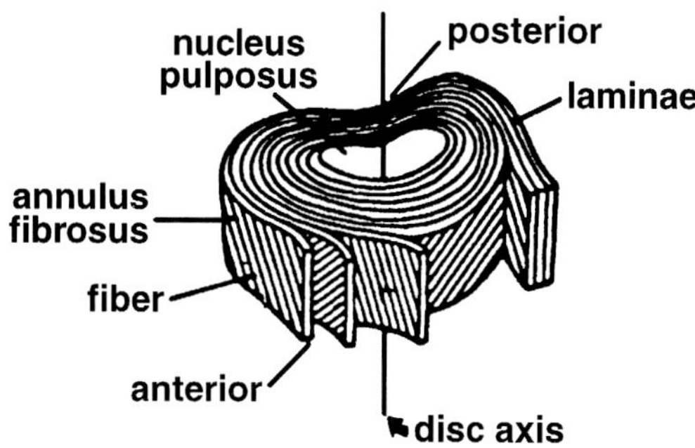

Figure 40
The intervertebral disk. (Reproduced with permission from Pope MH, Frymoyer JW, Lehmann TR: Structure and function of the lumbar spine, in *Occupational Low Back Pain: Assessment, Treatment, and Prevention.* St. Louis, CV Mosby, 1991.)

disk is avascular, but end-plate microfractures can result in vascular ingrowth, the formation of granulation tissue, and alterations in the chemistry and mechanical behavior of the disk.

In young, healthy disks, positive pressure within the nucleus pulposus increases as loads are applied to the spine. This pressure is approximately 1.5 times the mean applied pressure over the area of the end plate. The disk is actually quite flexible at low compression loads, but provides increasing resistance at high loads. Its major role in weightbearing is reflected by the fact that disk area increases as a direct function of body mass in all mammals.

Many relationships have been reported between disk height, disk bulge, pressure, and mobility. When the disk is loaded, the nucleus deforms and transfers the force to the annulus. In axial compression, the increased intradiskal pressure is counteracted by annular fiber tension and disk bulge, rather analogous to the bulging in the sides of a tire. Some disk space narrowing also occurs. To describe the internal displacements of the intervertebral disk, with only minimal disruption of normal function, the displacement of injected radiopaque beads can be determined from sagittal plane radiographs taken before and during load application. For the intact disk in compression, the intradiskal bead displacements are predominantly anterior. In flexion, the beads in the center of the disk move posteriorly, whereas the beads closer to the periphery of the disk move anteriorly. In extension, the central beads move anteriorly and the beads closer to the periphery of the disk move posteriorly. After denucleation, the bead displacements for compression and flexion suggest an inward bulging of the inner wall of the annulus, despite outward bulging of the disk surface.

Flexion, extension, and lateral bending all produce a small displacement of the nucleus. Asymmetric and cyclic loading in combined lateral bend, compression, and flexion are risk factors for disk herniation. The lumbar motion segment can resist a combination of bending moment and shear force of 156 N·m and 620 N, respectively, before complete disruption occurs. This is much less than the failure load in compression. The tension force acting on the posterior structures is 2.8 kN. The bone mineral content in the vertebrae appears to be a good predictor of ultimate strength of the lumbar motion segment. About 35% of its torque resistance is provided by the disk and the remaining resistance by the posterior elements and ligaments. Therefore, any defect in the posterior structures increases the risk of disk failure. Several reports have emphasized that little or no nucleus should be removed in surgery so as to maintain stability.

An increase in fluid content increases the stiffness of the disk. The disk is separated on both sides from the vertebral bodies by hyaline cartilage end plates. The condition of the end plates influences the nutrition of the disk. Nutrients and fluid enter the disk by diffusion through the end plates or the annulus, which is essential because the disk lacks vascular tissue. Glucose diffuses mainly through the end plates, whereas sulfate ions diffuse mainly through the annulus. The diffusion is influenced by mechanical factors. When the load on the disk increases, there is an outflow of fluid and there is a fluid influx when load decreases. Disk nutrition can also be affected by changes in end-plate permeability. Smoking and vibration decrease nutrition and dynamic exercise enhances it.

Range of motion usually is measured on the basis of a brief force application. However, if a force is applied to a collagenous viscoelastic structure for a prolonged period, further movement can be detected. This movement is small in amplitude, occurs slowly, and is known as creep. Creep is not just a laboratory phenomenon; it occurs in static postures, such as prolonged sitting or standing. Many workers must assume positions that subject the lumbar spine to prolonged load bearing or vibration in a fixed bent or stooped posture.

Time-dependent (viscoelastic) intervertebral disk changes have been demonstrated both in vitro and in vivo. It is postulated that an increase in height occurs if there is a reduction in the overall disk compressive pressure; the reduced intradiskal osmotic pressure allows water to flow into the intervertebral disk. The reverse is true if intradiskal pressure is increased. Reported diurnal changes in the overall height of individuals range from 6.3 mm to 19.3 mm, with an average of 15.7 mm. The average person is 1% shorter in the evening than in the morning; children are 2% shorter in the evening; and the elderly are 0.5% shorter in the evening.

Fifty percent of total length change occurs during the first two hours in the upright posture. Thus, for most people, the first two hours out of bed in the morning are critical for disk metabolism. Additionally, some have recommended that those who do heavy manual work have short rest periods during which they can recline. Higher loads produce greater creep, which might be associated with long-lasting, higher intradiskal pressure (Fig. 41). Healthy disks creep slowly as compared to degenerated disks, which have less ability to absorb shock; this is one reason why degeneration can increase risk of back disorders.

Physical changes, including disk herniations, have also been caused in lumbar motion segments by exposure to cyclic loading at high loads. In vivo whole-body vibration studies have established the motion characteristics and natural frequency of the lumbar region. The tissues of the motion segment may be at risk for injury at the whole-body natural frequency of 5 Hz. Many vehicles produce vibration at the body's natural frequency, possibly placing drivers at risk for low back pain or injury. The behavior is that of a classic fatigue curve: at loads above 70%, specimens sustain only a few cycles; at loads below 30%, almost all specimens sustain 5,000 load cycles without fracture. Under axial compression, fracture invariably occurs in the end plates, but the annulus is not damaged. Repetitive loading of a flexed lumbar column and cyclic torsional loads may exaggerate failure in the end plates, facets, laminae, and capsular ligaments.

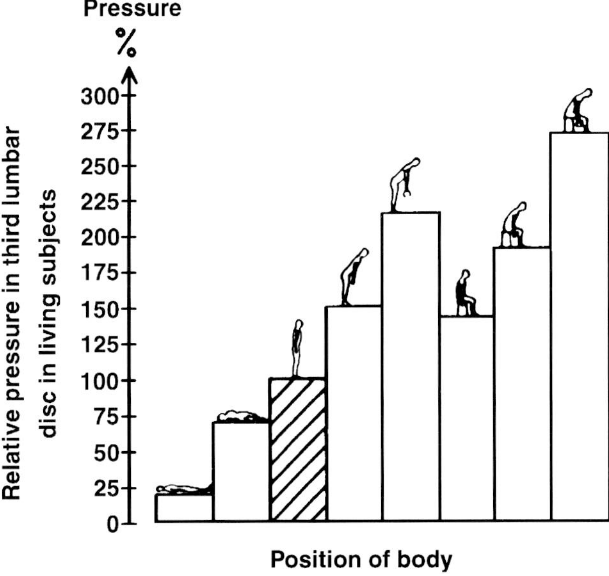

Figure 41
Relative increase and decrease in intradiskal pressure in different supine, standing, and sitting postures compared to the pressure in upright standing (100%). (Reproduced with permission from Nachemson A: Lumbar mechanics as revealed by lumbar intradiscal pressure measurements, in Jayson MIV, Dixon AS (eds): *The Lumbar Spine and Back Pain,* ed 4. Edinburgh, Churchill Livingstone, 1992, pp 157–171.)

Compression failures promote disk degeneration. A degenerated disk has increased mobility and increased bulge, and appears to behave like a thick-walled cylinder rather than a pressure vessel. In such cases, the stresses in the annulus become large compressive stresses instead of relatively small tensile stresses, and the annulus becomes distorted. Similar types of changes can occur in the denucleated disk and those that have undergone chemonucleolysis.

The Vertebral Bodies

When a pure compressive load is applied to a healthy motion segment, translational motions within an FSU will cause the two vertebral bodies to come closer together. Failure of the unit occurs first in the end plate, then in the vertebral bodies, and then in the disk. During compressive loading, pressure is higher in the center of the end plate than in the periphery. This higher concentration of pressure in the center often results in failure from the nucleus rupturing the end plate. However, as noted above, considerably higher loads are needed to disrupt the FSU by compressive loading than by any other type of loading. This is because the vertebral body is well designed for weightbearing, as reflected in its superior and inferior surfaces and internal structure.

If a vertebra had only an outer layer of cortical bone, it would not be strong enough to sustain longitudinal compression, and would tend to collapse like a cardboard box. To complete the metaphor of the box, the outer structure can be reinforced by vertical struts, similar to the vertical trabeculae between the superior and inferior surfaces. A strut can sustain high longitudinal loads, provided it does not buckle. By introducing a series of crossbeams, such as the horizontal trabeculae, the strength of a box can be further increased. When a load is applied, the crossbeams hold the struts in place, preventing them from deforming and preventing the box from collapsing.

The type of failure resulting from an injury depends on whether the spine is loaded in flexion or extension, with flexion tending to cause anterior collapse where the trabeculae are weaker. This phenomenon occurs because the basic structure just described is modified by Wolff's law (Fig. 42) in that oblique trabeculae sweep up or down to aid in load bearing. These trabeculae come together at the pedicles to resist the tensile forces. The trabeculae sweep toward the superior and inferior facets to support the compressive and shear forces in the facets, and outward to the spinous process to withstand the tensile and bending forces applied to the

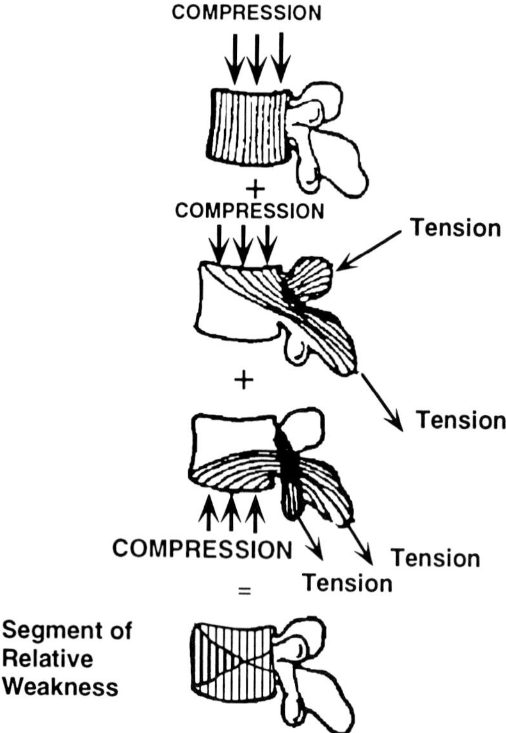

Figure 42
Trabecular directions in the vertebrae. (Reproduced with permission from Pope MH, Frymoyer JW, Lehmann TR: Structure and function of the lumbar spine, in *Occupational Low Back Pain: Assessment, Treatment, and Prevention.* St. Louis, CV Mosby, 1991.)

spinous process. Additionally, in vivo, the vertebrae are filled with blood and, thus, they behave like hydraulic shock absorbers, providing greater strength.

Compression tests reveal decreases in vertebral body load and stress with age in both men and women. However, because of their greater cross-sectional area, load failure values are higher in men than in women up to the age of 75. The load-to-failure actually increases with age, with men showing a significantly greater cross-sectional area and a significant increase in vertebral body size, as a result of continuous periosteal growth. This phenomenon is particularly significant for older people who have diminished bone strength, usually as a result of osteoporosis. Osteoporosis involves a reduction of bone volume, which is inversely related to the load to fracture. Measured bone mass thus should not be the sole index of the biomechanical competence (that is, stiffness and stress) of trabecular bone. Measurements of bone density must be considered in combination with a detailed description of the architecture.

Posterior elements and facet joints (zygopophyseal joints) The posterior elements are the components of the vertebral arch: pedicles, lamina, facet joints, and spinous and transverse processes. The spinous, transverse, accessory, and mammillary processes are levers with muscle attachments. The longer levers are the transverse and spinous processes. Every muscle acting on the lumbar vertebral column is attached somewhere on the posterior elements. The forces acting on the spinous and articular processes are ultimately transmitted to the lamina. Thus, the stability of the lumbar spine can be compromised if a lamina is weakened by disease, injury, or surgery.

The pedicles transmit all forces sustained by the posterior elements, such as tension and bending, to the vertebral bodies. If a vertebra slides forward, the inferior articular processes of that vertebra are resisted by the superior articular processes of the inferior vertebra. This resistance is transmitted to the vertebral body through the pedicles. In addition, all muscles that act on a lumbar vertebra pull downward. This action is transmitted to the vertebral body through the pedicles, which are subjected to bending. The lower parts of the pedicle are compressed, but the upper parts are under tension. The pedicles are designed to withstand these moments because they are thick-walled cylinders.

The lamina between the superior and inferior articular process on each side is the pars interarticularis, meaning "interarticular part." Because it must withstand considerable bending forces, the pars is generally thicker than the rest of the lamina. The pars is a common site of fatigue (stress) fracture, or spondylolysis, perhaps because the cortical bone is thin. Such fractures may heal by fibrous union, which weakens the motion segment and sets the stage for spondylolisthesis. Whether failure occurs primarily because of flexion or extension is widely debated. Excessive loading of the spine in extension, however, is more likely to cause loads transmitted through the facet joints to produce high strain in the pars interarticularis, eventually leading to spondylolysis.

The zygapophyseal joints, found between the articular processes, are usually called facet joints, or facets. These articulations of the superior and inferior articular processes are lined with hyaline cartilage. The facets have a major role in controlling motion. They are important in resisting torsion and shear, and they have a role in compression. Normally, the lumbar facets and disks together contribute about 80% of the torsional load resistance, with the facets contributing one half of that amount. The remaining 20% of resistance is from the passive ligamentous structures.

Load sharing between facet and disk also occurs under shear loads and axial compressive loads. This load bearing is markedly reduced by excision of a single facet. The amount of load bearing by the facet joints is related to whether the motion segment is loaded in flexion or extension. When one sits, lumbar lordosis is often unsupported and reduced, and intradiskal pressure is higher than when one stands. The increase in lumbar flexion reduces the load-bearing ability of the facets.

Ligaments The seven ligaments of the spine can be divided into three systems. The nonsegmental longitudinal system includes the anterior and posterior longitudinal ligaments and the supraspinous ligaments. The segmental longitudinal system includes the interspinous, intertransverse ligaments, and the ligamenta flava (yellow ligaments). The articular, or capsular, system comprises the capsular ligaments. At the cephalad and caudal ends of the spine, there are specialized ligaments that attach the skull and the iliac bones, respectively.

Ligaments aid in the control of motion and are vital for the structural stability of the motion segment. The ligaments are also the primary tensile load-bearing elements, acting as passive elements to prevent excessive motion. Ligaments are viscoelastic, which means that their deformation and type of failure depend on the rate at which loads are applied. Their strength also depends on the number of deformations applied. Repetitive loading cycles may cause fatigue failure.

The posterior and anterior longitudinal ligaments traverse the length of the spine, further supporting the vertebral body and disk (Fig. 39). They are interlinked at each level by the disk. These ligaments are richly supplied by pain-sensitive nerve endings. The tensile strength of the anterior longitudinal ligament is about twice that of the posterior longitudinal ligament.

The remaining ligaments support and link the posterior elements. Of great functional importance is the ligamentum flavum, which joins the lamina of adjacent vertebrae. The ligamentum flavum is highly elastic and strong compared to other ligaments, and has a large number of elastic fibers. Its elastic properties allow it to lengthen with spine flexion and shorten with extension. Considerable flexion is required before permanent failure occurs. The ligamentum flavum is normally pretensed to about 6% to 15% of its tensile strain. In patients with severe spinal degeneration the ligamentum flavum becomes thickened and less elastic. These changes produce narrowing of the spinal canal in extension, because the ligament buckles into the spinal canal.

The tip and edges of the spinous process are joined by the interspinous and supraspinous ligaments. Because they are far from the disk, and therefore act on long moment arms, these ligaments play an important role in resisting spine flexion. The ligamenta flava and lumbodorsal fascia are more important in resisting flexion. The iliolumbar ligament, at the lumbosacral junction, also resists flexion-extension and axial rotation. Intertransverse ligaments join the transverse processes of the vertebra. Capsular ligaments limit the excursion of the facet joints. Like all other joints, they are richly supplied with pain-sensitive nerve endings.

Specialization of the Functional Spinal Unit

Cervical Spine

There is an almost infinite number of possible head postures, each produced through the action of different combinations of cervical muscles. The spinous processes increase in length between C-3 and T-1 or T-2. This is consistent with morphologic adaptation to an increase in torque along the spine that is needed to resist a given load on the head. The longer the spinous process, the greater the leverage of the attached muscle.

The orientation of the articular surfaces is almost transverse at C-1 to C-2; at C-2 to C-4, it is at 45° to the longitudinal axis, and it remains approximately constant to C-7 to T-1. Below C-3 to C-4, the facet joint plates are perpendicular to the sagittal plane. At C-2 to C-3, however, the joint planes also slope downward laterally by 10° to 20°. The occipitoatlantoaxial complex is a specialized articulation that allows a relatively large range of motion between the head and torso without any intervertebral disks. Flexion-extension predominates at C-3 to C-7, axial rotation at C-1 to C-2, and lateral bend at C-3 to C-7. The flexion-extension for occipital to C-1 occurs about an axis approximately at the center of curvature of the occipital condyles. Flexion-extension for C-1 to C-2 entails motion of the anterior arch of C-1 cephalad and slightly posteriorly, because of the curved anterior surface of the odontoid. It is possible to gain additional motion by exerting external forces on the fully flexed or extended neck (Fig. 43).

Approximately 60% of the axial rotation of the entire cervical spine and occiput is found in the upper region (occiput to C-1 to C-2), and 40% is found in the lower region. Axial rotation for the occiput to C-1 region requires that one occipital condyle slide anteriorly on C-1 and that the contralateral one slide posteriorly. This is difficult because of the relatively deep fit of the condyles. In contrast, axial rotation is a major function for C-1 to C-2. The IAR is close to the spinal cord, permitting rotation without bony impingement on the spinal cord. Motion after alar ligament transection in-

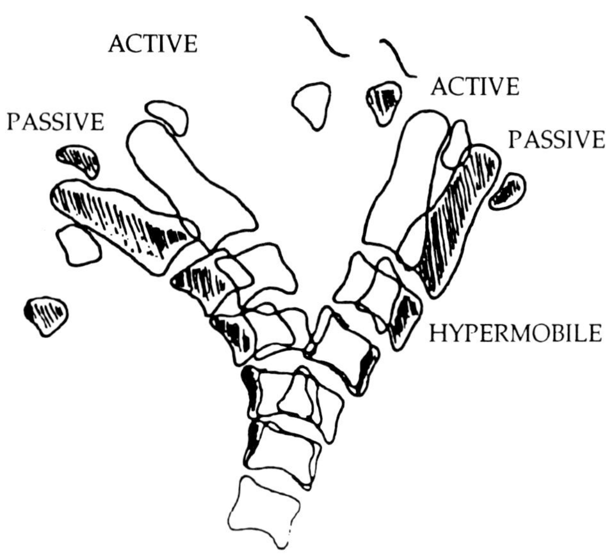

Figure 43
This diagram depicts the active and passive motions of the cervical spine. (Reproduced with permission from Dvorak J, Fraeklich D, Penning L, et al: Functional radiographic diagnosis of the cervical spine. *Spine* 1988;13:748.)

creases at both the occiput to C-1 and C-1 to C-2 joints.

Lateral bending occurs only to a small extent between occiput to C-1 because the alar ligaments force rotation about the odontoid. This, in turn, requires some stretching out of the transverse ligament.

Most of the motion in flexion-extension is in the central region. The largest range and the highest incidence of cervical spondylosis is found in C-5 to C-6. For flexion-extension, the location of the IAR for each pair of vertebrae is generally within the body of the lower vertebra, but gradually shifts from a position in the lower dorsal quadrant of C-3 to the middle of the upper end plate of C-7. The IAR is at the center of a circle passing through the articular surface of the facet joint. Full extension can cause enough foraminal closure to produce increased arm symptoms in a patient with disk herniation or osteophytic encroachment into the foramen. For lateral bending and axial rotation, there is a smaller range of motion in the more-caudal segments. The maximum sagittal plane translation occurring in the lower cervical spine under simulated flexion-extension is in the middle and lower cervical spine. The middle cervical spine region has a distinct characteristic coupling pattern, in which lateral bending and axial rotation are coupled. The coupling occurs in such a way that the spinous processes point in the direction opposite to the lateral bend, as a result of either soft-tissue tensions or the orientation of the facet joints. For lateral bending, the IAR is located in the upper vertebral body. For axial rotation, both the uncinate processes and the facet joints constrain motion. Because the facet joint plates are perpendicular to the sagittal plane, these joints must either open up slightly (for example, the right joint opens with right axial rotation) or must undergo some coupled lateral bending.

In flexion and extension of the neck, there is a sliding movement between vertebrae; in extension, the posteroinferior margin of the upper vertebral body approximates the arch of the subjacent vertebra and protrudes into the cervical canal, narrowing the sagittal diameter by 1 to 2 mm. The posterior longitudinal ligament and the ligamenta flava are lax in extension, becoming stretched and thinner in flexion. The value for the intradural sagittal diameter is 2 to 3 mm lower in extension than in flexion. This, coupled with the fact that the cord is thicker in extension than in flexion, is important clinically because the cord has less play in extension than in flexion. Fortunately, the canal is widest at the atlanto-axial level and narrows at C-5. A generally accepted average figure for the sagittal diameter of C-4 to C-7 is 17 mm, whereas that for the transverse diameter is 30 mm (measured on AP radiographs as the interpedicular distance).

Thoracic Spine

The thoracic spine is a transition between the more mobile cervical and lumbar regions. It is relatively rigid and facilitates the mechanical activities of the lungs and rib cage. The vertebral bodies and disks are larger in the lower thoracic spine. The spatial orientation of the facets in the thoracic spine changes from the upper to the lower region. In a given individual, the orientation of the facet joints may change abruptly to that of the lumbar region anywhere between T-9 and T-12.

In flexion-extension, there are 4° of motion in the upper portion of the thoracic spine and 6° in the middle segments. In the lower portion, there are 12° of motion at each segment. In lateral bending, there are 6° of motion in the upper thoracic spine, with 8° or 9° in the two lower segments. In axial rotation, there are 8° of motion in the upper half of the thoracic spine and 2° for each interspace of the three lower segments.

Abnormalities in coupling of the thoracic spine between lateral bending and axial rotation may be relevant in scoliotic deformities. In the upper and lower thoracic spine, the two motions are strongly coupled, but in the middle portion of the thoracic spine, the coupling is inconsistent. In vitro studies have shown that all six degrees of freedom demonstrate coupling patterns of varying degrees.

Lumbar Spine

The lumbar spine, in conjunction with the hips, is responsible for much of the mobility of the trunk. The flexion-extension range of motion may be attributed to the sizable intervertebral disk coupled with a lack of facet constraint. Sagittal plane translation is frequently used to determine whether or not there is instability. In symptom-free subjects, 2 to 3 mm or even larger translation of anterior sagittal plane is normal for the lumbar spine. Some reports mention that even 5-mm translational motion in the L-3 to L-4 and L-4 to L-5 segments and 4 mm in the L-5 to S-1 segment may be normal.

There are several coupling patterns in the lumbar spine such as coupling of axial rotation with +y-axis translation, coupling of three degrees of freedom translation with axial rotation (Fig. 44) and coupling of axial rotation and lateral bending with flexion-extension. Because the spinal column is symmetrical about the sagittal plane, coupled rotations in association with sagittal plane motions might not be expected. The observed coupled motions may be due to facet asymmetry, disk degeneration, or suboptimal muscle control.

One of the strongest coupling patterns is that of lateral bending with axial rotation. The pattern is such that the spinous processes point in the same direction as the lateral bending, the opposite of that in the cervical spine and the upper thoracic spine. There is also a coupling pattern of lateral bending with axial rotation at the lumbosacral joint, which is the opposite of that found in the lumbar spine and the same as that observed in the cervical and upper thoracic spine (below C-2). In vitro experiments have shown that coupling patterns are affected by the preload in the spine and by posture.

Recent analyses of in vivo flexion-extension radiographs have determined that the center of rotation lies somewhere in the posterior half of the disk near the inferior end plate (Fig. 45). However, there is considerable disagreement regarding its precise location, possibly because the center of rotation moves during flexion-extension. The path described by the moving center of rotation is called the centrode. The axes are in the right side of the disk during left lateral bending and in the left side of the disk during right lateral bending. An in vivo study of lateral bending shows much scatter in the computed instantaneous axes of rotation.

For axial rotation, the IARs are located in the region of the posterior nucleus. In the presence of disk degeneration, there is a tendency for the axes to be spread out. It might be possible to use abnormalities in the IARs to diagnose disk degeneration or other disorders.

Experiments on whole, cadaveric lumbar spines and on male volunteers have been conducted to determine whether axial rotation changes when subjects bend forward and whether rotation is affected

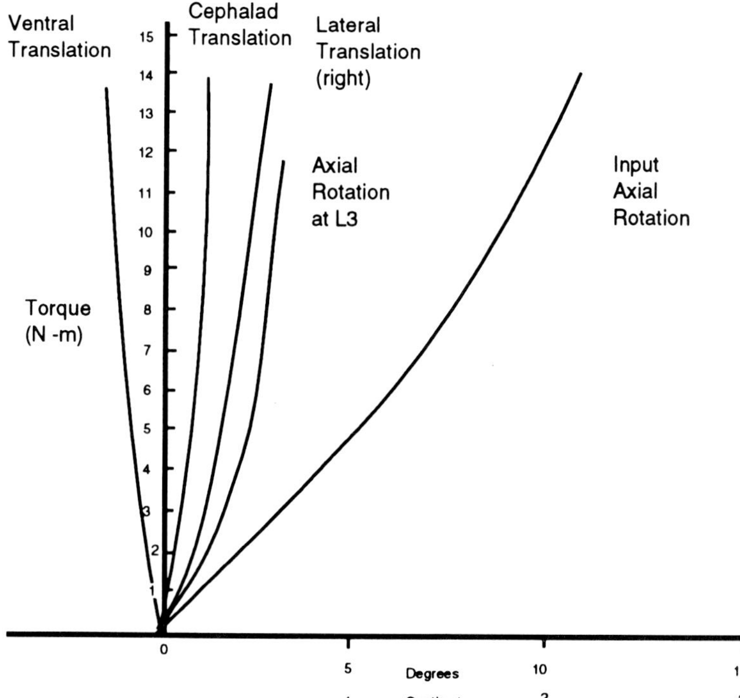

Figure 44
This illustration further demonstrates coupling of motion. Input axial rotation referred to L-3 produces axial rotation at L-3, lateral translation to the right, cephalad translation, and ventral translation. (Reproduced with permission from Pope MH, Wilder DG, Matteri RE, et al: Experimental measurements of vertebral motion under load. *Orthop Clin North Am* 1977;8:155–167.)

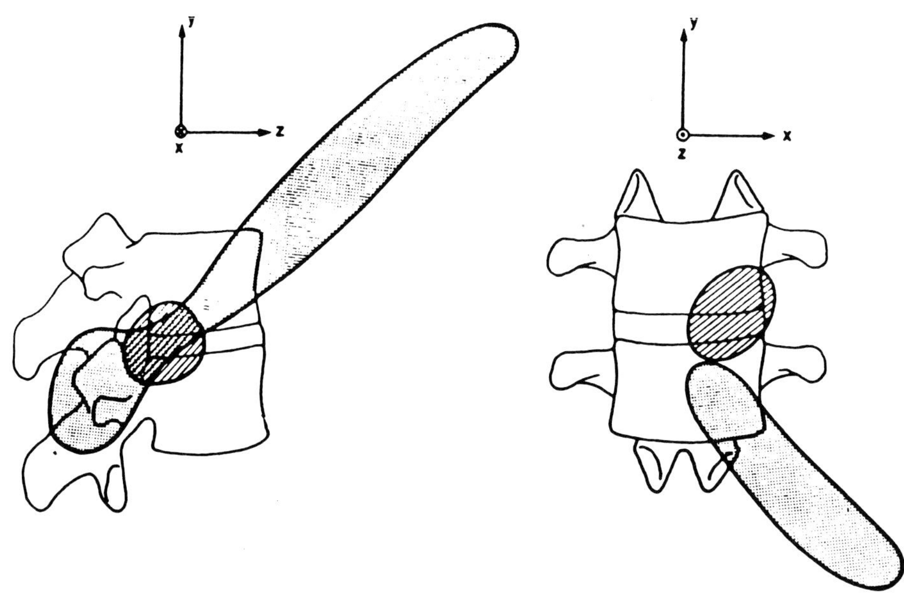

Figure 45
The changes in the location of the instantaneous axes of rotation in the lumbar spine motion segment, with and without degenerative disk disease in flexion **(left)** and right lateral bending **(right).** The axes for the normal disks are shown in the dark areas with longitudinal lines, and those for the degenerated disks are shown in the lighter gray areas. (Reproduced with permission from Rolander SD: Motion of the lumbar spine with special reference to the stabilizing effect of posterior fusion. *Acta Orthop Scand* 1966;90:1-144.)

by articular tropism. Axial rotation of implanted wires was measured while the spine was rotated in a torsion apparatus. Pins were inserted into the spinous processes of L-3, L-4, and L-5 of the volunteers, and the axial rotation of the pins was measured while the subjects rotated in a torsion apparatus. Axial rotation was found to be less when combined with forward flexion, and articular tropism did not influence the amplitude of rotation.

The Sacroiliac Region

The kinematics of the sacroiliac (SI) joint is poorly understood despite the importance of this joint. The SI joint is partly synovial and partly syndesmotic. It is completely ankylosed in as many as 76% of subjects older than 50 years of age. However, even among normal subjects, these are rather stiff joints, the overall motion and stability of which are affected by the coarse interdigitating articular surfaces.

A pelvic shift that occurs when an individual supports his weight on one leg suggests that there may be SI joint motion in the stance phase of gait. Vertical translations of 2 to 3 mm and rotations of up to 3° are reported at the pubic symphysis with standing. The symphysis motion is slightly greater in multiparous females. Patients with sacroiliac joint disorders have been studied with roentgen stereophotogrammetry. The rotations have been small, averaging 2.5°, with translations averaging 0.7 mm. Because of these very small motions, it has been suggested that external fixation of the pelvis is useful in assessing painful sacroiliac joint instability and should precede surgical intervention.

There is scatter of the IARs of the SI joint in both the sagittal and frontal plane motions. Because of the irregular contour of a portion of the joint surface, it is believed that separation must occur with enough force to overcome ligamentous resistance.

Spine Kinetics

Kinetics of the spine is best understood in terms of the spine's response to external load moments. The spine is unstable without the support of the muscles. An osteoligamentous spine without the muscles buckles under very small compressive forces. Although clinical and radiographic criteria are increasingly accurate for predicting instability, there is no consensus regarding a definition of segmental instability. Instability is defined biomechanically as a decreased stiffness of the motion segment, increased mobility, or abnormal motions. Segmental instability also has been defined in terms of a loss of stiffness such that the application of force produces pain and greater displacements than would otherwise be seen. However, there are considerable individual differences in spinal structures and motions. In order to understand low back problems, the spine must be understood as more than the sum of its parts.

Muscles allow the trunk to move and retain the position of the spinal segments. Vertebral muscles can be classified as anterior, posterior, or lateral (Table 13). The muscles of the back also can be distinguished as deep or superficial. In addition to the dorsal muscles, the anterior and lateral abdominal muscles and the gluteal muscles help to control trunk motion and support the ligamentous spine.

Cervical Muscles

The role of muscles in the neck is to control head position. The passive elements (bone, disk,

Table 13
Vertebral muscles and their motor functions

Function	Muscles
Anterior	
Muscles in front flex the spine.	Longus collis*
If the muscle runs a little obliquely and contracts independently of the corresponding muscle on the opposite side, it rotates and bends the spine laterally, as well as flexes it.	Longus capitis Rectus capitis anterior Rectus capitis lateralis+ Obliquus externus abdominis* Obliquus internus abdominis* Psoas major+ Psoas minor+ Iliacus Quadratus lumborum
Posterior	
Muscles in back extend the spine.	Superficial stratum
If the muscle runs a little obliquely and contracts independently of the corresponding muscle on the opposite side, it rotates and bends the spine laterally, as well as extends it.	Splenius capitis*+ Splenius cervicis+ Erector spinae (sacrospinalis) Iliocostalis*+ Longissimus*+ Spinalis*+ Deep stratum Semispinali Thoracis* Cervicis* Capitis* Multifidi* Rotatores* Interspinales Intertransversarii*
Lateral	
Muscles on the side bend the spine laterally.	Trapezius Sternocleidomastoid* Quadratus lumborum Scalenus* Anterior Medial Posterior

*Muscles with axial rotation function
+Muscles with lateral bending function

ligament, joints) exert important control over translations, as well as the location of the centers of rotation. However, angle rotation is controlled by the muscles, except at the end of the range of motion.

The general structure of the neck is similar to that of the rest of the axial skeleton: some gross-function muscles span several motion segments and fine-function muscles cross only one or two segments. The anterior gross-function muscles are the longus colli, longus capitis, and scalenes, which attach either to the vertebral bodies or to transverse processes. The anterior fine-function muscles are the intertransversarii, which span just one segment. The posterior gross-function muscles attached to the spinous processes are the splenius capitis and semispinalis cervices. Muscles oriented parallel to the longitudinal axis can efficiently extend or bend laterally, but other muscles are needed to produce other motions. Determination of muscle site attachments and measurements of muscle forces in vivo and in vitro have provided a basis for developing biomechanical models of the neck.

The longissimus is made up of the longissimus cervices, which inserts into transverse processes, and the longissimus capitis, which inserts into the mastoid process. The spinalis muscle, absent in the lumbar region, is also divided into two parts: spinalis cervices, which connects the transverse processes, and spinalis capitis, which inserts into the occipital. The erector spinae controls movements of both the neck and head. It lies superficial to the semispinalis, multifidus, and rotator muscles, covering them completely. The interspinales connect the adjacent spinous process, and the intertransversarii connect adjacent transverse processes. They provide intrinsic stability to individual spinal levels.

The sternomastoid muscle is the most prominent of the anterior neck muscles arising from the sternum and the clavicle and inserting into the mastoid process. This muscle is a strong rotator and lateral flexor of the head; in addition, when acting together, the sternomastoid muscles flex the neck.

Thoracolumbar Muscles

The small intersegmental muscles found at every lumbar intervertebral joint are the interspinalis and intertransversarii. The polysegmental muscles of the lumbar spine are the multifidus and the longissimus thoracis, the iliocostalis lumborum, and the spinalis thoracis (or spinalis dorsi). The lumbar multifidus is the most medial of the lumbar back muscles and consists of five segmental bands. Each segmental band stems from a spinous process and consists of several individual fascicles with various caudal insertions (Figs. 46 and 47). The spinalis thoracis is relatively small and is principally a muscle of the thoracic region. Only its lowest fibers enter the lumbar region to insert onto the L-1 to L-3 spinous processes. It has little functional role in the lumbar region.

The longissimus thoracis and iliocostalis lumborum are massive muscles and major flexors of the lumbar spine (Fig. 48). Only the thoracic fibers of the longissimus thoracis and iliocostalis lumborum contribute to the erector spinae aponeurosis. The lumbar fibers that form the lumbar erector spinae arise from individual lumbar vertebrae and insert into the iliac crest independent of the erector spinae aponeurosis.

The four abdominal muscles are the rectus abdominis, the external and internal obliques, and the

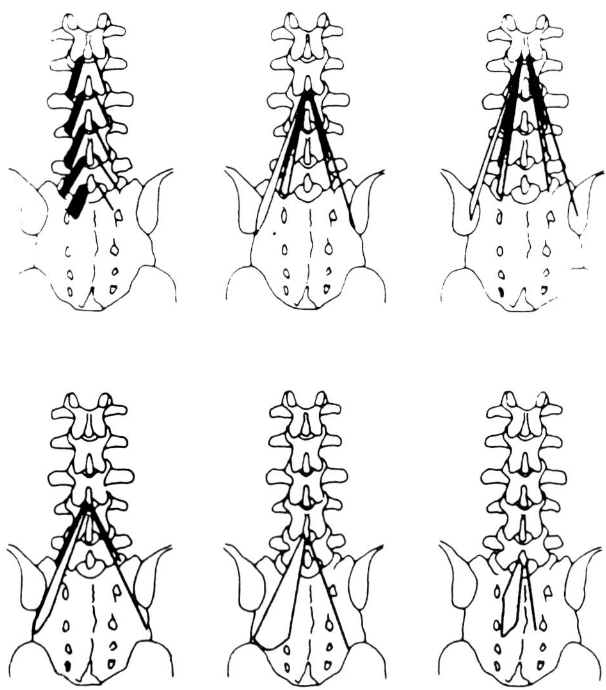

Figure 46
Schematic illustrations of the fascicles of the lumbar multifidus as seen in a posteroanterior view. A illustrates the laminar fibers at every level. B-F illustrate the longer fascicles from the caudal edge and tubercles of the spinous processes at levels L-1 to L-5. (Reproduced with permission from McIntosh JE, Bogduk N: The biomechanics of lumbar multifidus. *Clin Biomechanics.* 1986;1:205–213.)

transverse abdominal muscle. The rectus abdominis runs as a wide strong band from the xiphoid process to the pubic arch. The external oblique is the largest of the three lateral muscles and runs from the ribs to the inguinal ligament, rectus sheath, and ilium. The internal oblique is fanshaped, running caudolaterally in the superior aspect and mediolaterally in the inferior aspect. The transversus abdominis muscle is deep to the obliques and runs transversely from the rectus sheath to the six lower ribs, the thoracolumbar fascia, and the ilium.

Several other muscles that are functionally important to the spine are the quadratus lumborum, psoas, trapezius, and latissimus dorsi. The quadratus lumborum and the psoas muscle attach to the dorsal part of the vertebral bodies of T-12 to L-5 as well as to the disks, and then combine with the iliacus muscle to form the iliopsoas, which attaches to the minor trochanter. The latissimus dorsi arises from the iliac crest and lower vertebral spinous processes and ribs to insert into the humerus.

Muscle strength Strength is the ability of a muscle or a group of muscles to exert force. The type of contraction determines the force output and, therefore, calls for different measurement techniques. Strength is measured concentrically, isometrically (static strength), eccentrically, isotonically (concentric strength), isokinetically, and isoinertially. Maximum strength is the most frequently used clinical measure. Because strength varies as a function of joint angle, it can be defined as a curve displaying the force output as a function of the angle (Fig. 49). Strength curves are affected by such factors as age, gender, motivation, pain, and muscle and joint physiology and geometry.

Isometric techniques include manual muscle testing and involve the use of spring and strain gauges as well as dynamometers. Typically, the pelvis is strapped in and the subject is fitted with a harness; the subject is then asked to exert force against resistance. Isotonic strength measurement techniques, most of which are concentric, include using free weights in a controlled movement system or using a constrained system that allows unequal effort. Both the lever arm and speed of movement are important to an isotonic strength measurement. Because isotonic means the same force, a pure isotonic exercise requires changing the resistance throughout the range of motion in proportion to changes in moment arm, referred to as a variable resistance exercise. Assessment occurs throughout the range of motion, but reliability is a problem, and isotonic resistance tasks often are unfamiliar to those being tested. Isokinetic assessment requires a subject to move the trunk or limbs at a controlled speed. The systems are controlled with a dynamometer, which is either passive, allowing only concentric movement, or active, allowing both concentric and eccentric movement.

Approximately half of all compensable low back injuries are associated with manual lifting tasks. Some studies suggest a relationship between lifting strength and back injury rates. In jobs that require heavy lifting, workers with inadequate strength are probably at a higher risk of injury.

Muscle endurance Another important attribute of muscle is endurance. Endurance is defined as the point at which muscle fatigue is observable; for example, when a contraction can no longer be sustained at a certain level (isometric fatigue), or when repetitive work can no longer be maintained at a certain output (dynamic fatigue). The mechanical events are preceded by biochemical and physiologic changes within the muscle, but these changes do not necessarily immediately influence the mechanical performance of the muscle.

Mechanical tests of trunk muscle fatigue generally include maintaining a posture or performing an

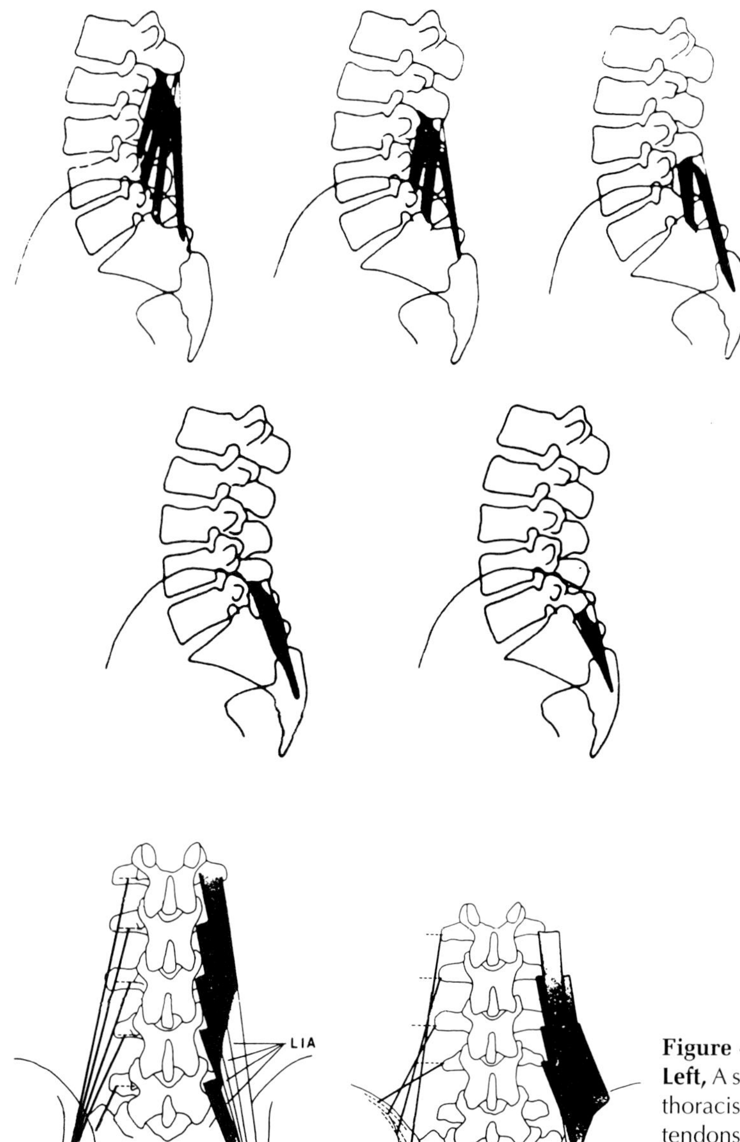

Figure 47
Schematic illustrations of the fascicles of the lumbar multifidus as seen in lateral views. A-E show the fascicles present at levels L-1 to L-5, respectively. (Reproduced with permission from McIntosh JE, Bogduk N: The biomechanics of lumbar multifidus. *Clin Biomechanics* 1986;1:205–213.)

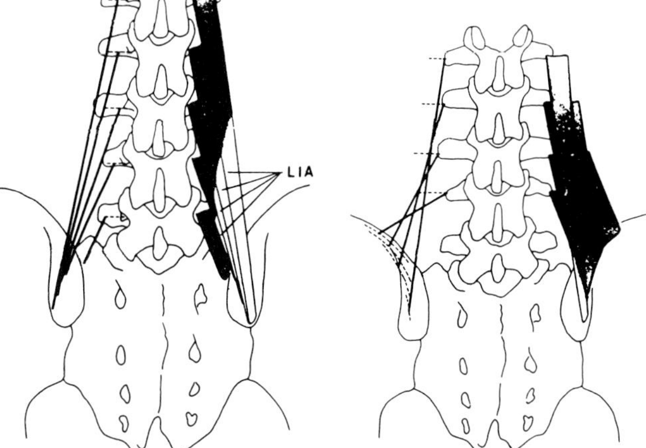

Figure 48
Left, A schematic illustration of the fascicles of the longissimus thoracis pars lumborum. Fascicles L-1 to L-4 have long caudal tendons that form the lumbar intermuscular aponeurosis (LIA). The dotted lines marked the extent of the rostral attachments. **Right,** A schematic illustration of the lumbar fascicles of iliocostalis lumborum. The dotted lines mark the extent of each attachment. (Reproduced with permission from MacIntosh JE, Bogduk N: The morphology of the lumbar erector spinal. *Spine* 1978;12:658–668.)

activity repeatedly. Endurance studies sometimes use a dynamic test in which, for example, subjects move a padded bar connected to an isokinetic dynamometer at a paced rate. In these studies, trunk flexor muscles fatigue more rapidly than trunk extensor muscles, and women have a higher endurance level than men. The trunk muscles fatigue more easily when isometric contractions are performed and the abdominal muscles fatigue more readily than the back muscles. In postural endurance tests, in which subjects maintain an unsupported trunk in a horizontal position for a defined period of time, patients with ongoing low back pain have significantly less endurance than healthy controls. Patients with injured backs also fatigue faster than do volunteers with unaffected backs when asked to maintain 60% of a maximum isometric voluntary contraction of the trunk muscles. Some studies have used an isoinertial device to study force output and movement patterns in three dimen-

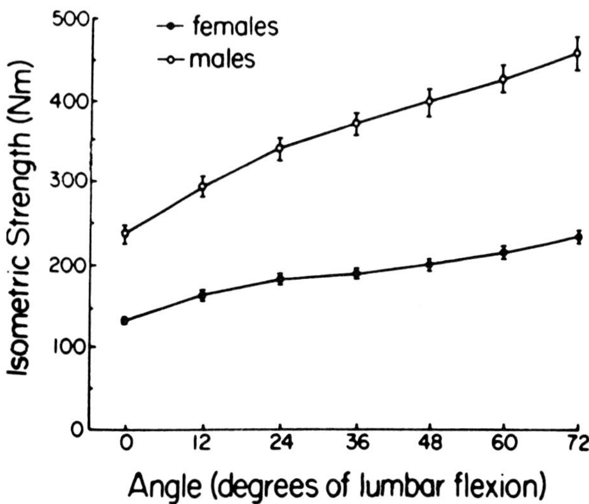

Figure 49
Isometric trunk strength as a function of joint angle. (Reproduced with permission from Graves JE, Pollock ML, Carpenter DM, et al: Quantitative assessment of full range-of-motion isometric lumbar extension strength. *Spine* 1990;15:289–294.)

sions when subjects performed a flexion-extension movement. Out-of-plane movements increased with fatigue and torque, angular excursion, and angular velocity decreased. The neuromuscular adaptation to fatigue appears to include reduced accuracy, control, and speed of contraction.

Electromyographic data analysis holds much promise as an objective method of measuring muscle fatigue. Early EMG studies relied on the amplitude of the signal as an index of muscle fatigue. However, recent developments indicate that the power density spectrum is a better index of fatigue. Lower frequencies are produced by sustained isometric contractions. Also, back pain patients can be distinguished from pain-free controls by both the initial value of the median frequency and by the rate of change in median frequency over time.

Coordination Musculoskeletal performance capacity implies not only joint stability, but also flexibility, strength, and endurance. Impairment of neuromuscular coordination may also lead to musculoskeletal disability and some suspect that poor coordination plays a role in back pain. Because no single test measures coordination, it is assessed through several independent motor ability components.

Muscular response includes both preparatory muscle activity and anticipatory postural adjustments. The body's center of gravity is shifted so as to offset the resultant forces and moments generated in an upcoming movement. Muscles have been found to be activated in anticipation of a loading event. Under sudden loading conditions, muscle activity begins earlier when adequate warning time is available. Muscle activation might be considered a pretensioning response analogous to preloading springs. Thus, slack is removed from the system, allowing for a quicker and stiffer response.

The standing human can be modeled in the sagittal plane as a three-segment linkage. The model predicts that a specific proportional relationship is necessary between the hip, knee, and ankle torques in order to maintain balance. Moreover, a fixed relationship between joint torques may be required to restore balance.

Electromyographic Activity

An understanding of the internal loading of the spine requires the estimation of the tensions in the trunk muscles in addition to considering the external forces and moments acting on the body. Both in vivo experimental and mathematical modeling studies have been performed to characterize the trunk muscle recruitment patterns during various work- or leisure-related activities. For the latter studies, time domain analysis of EMG signals consisting of quantifying the temporal and amplitude patterns of muscle activities, has been used. The underlying premise is that the tension developed in the muscle has a monotonic relationship with the EMG. Hence, with appropriate signal processing, the biologic EMG signals measured by noninvasive surface electrodes can be used to indicate muscle tension. This topic will be considered in the next section.

The majority of the EMG studies reported in the spine literature address the identification of motor control strategies for execution of trunk movement and/or biomechanical considerations, such as estimation of the compression and shear forces during physical activities. The ergonomists have used EMG studies as a tool to reduce the stresses in the spine by modifying the workplace or redesigning the task. The studies of optimal inclination angles between seat and backrest, or the beneficial role of the lumbar support are examples of how seat design has evolved. The rehabilitation experts have also used EMG of trunk muscles in addition to intra-abdominal pressure (IAP) measurements to optimize physical exercises in the treatment of low back pain. These studies have led to modification of exercises to tax the intended muscles maximally while reducing the load in the spine; for example, sit-up with flexed hip and knee joints. A brief overview follows of recent literatures on EMG studies of the trunk musculature during relaxed standing, slow trunk flexion and extension, lifting, axial rotation, and fast movements against the resistance.

Slight myoelectric activity in the paraspinal muscles have been reported during upright standing. Because postural sway is present, small activities are recorded in either paraspinal or abdominal muscles, but not simultaneously in both. The internal and external oblique muscles show very low activities during relaxed standing. The activities of muscles during unsupported sitting are very similar to those during standing. The inclination of the seat has been shown to influence trunk muscle activities. A marked reduction in activities of trunk muscles is reported as the back inclination is increased to 110°.

EMG activity in back muscle increases as a function of the trunk flexion angle, because the moment generated by the weight of the head, arm, and trunk is progressively increased at more flexed postures. At the same flexion angle, the higher the external load the greater the back muscle activity; these observations lead to one of the few universally accepted lifting recommendations: keep the load close to your body to lower the stresses in the spine. The large mass of the upper body poses postural perturbations that are anticipated and compensated by the central nervous system (CNS). During slow spinal flexion or extension movements, after a brief agonist activity initiates the movement, body weight is used to maintain the movement while antagonist muscles control the movement by their eccentric action. The pelvis and spine rhythm has been considered an important clinical sign and should be considered during routine spine mobility measurement. This coordination pattern is controlled by the trunk, pelvic, and thigh muscles. An orderly recruitment of the lower extremity muscles has been found, ensuring stability of the pelvis and lower spine during flexion or extension of the spine. At full flexion, healthy subjects will have reduced activities in the back muscles, and in some cases complete silence is observed. Patients with low back problems may not present this flexion-relaxation phenomenon. Possible explanations have been postulated to be loss of reflex inhibition, abnormal muscle reaction to lengthening, and inability to fully flex because of pain. In one study, a positive relation was found between the disability and the loss of flexion-relaxation among patients. Such relaxation has been documented during lateral bending for the trunk muscles.

Lateral bending and axial rotation movements are produced by a higher level of coactivation than sagittal plane movements. This is partly caused by the higher trunk stabilization required and the complex line of actions of trunk muscles. During lateral bending, the EMG activities of ipsilateral trunk muscles in the lumbar region increase, but the contralateral muscles have a larger increase. However, in the thoracic region, the ipsalateral muscles show the main increase in activity. The highest activities during axial rotations are found in the external oblique and erector spinae muscles.

Because of the association between manual material handling tasks and low back injuries, the interest shown in examining and quantifying trunk muscle activities during lifting has been considerable. Recent investigations using computerized dynamometers have shown that trunk muscle activities are affected by the trunk posture (including its postural asymmetry), velocity, and level of resisted force. The muscles of the back, buttocks, and hamstring are all active during the lift. The lifting mode is less important than where the load is placed and the speed of lifting. However, whether lifting should be done with the back in a position of lordosis, kyphosis, or in the straight position continues to be debated. During the fast movement of the spine, with or without external resistance, a more impulsive loading takes place with a set of agonist and antagonist recruitment patterns showing a predominantly reciprocal pattern. A very task-specific recruitment pattern is evident in these studies. The level of coactivation, in particular among the latissimus dorsi and oblique muscles, is a function of the speed, amplitude of movement, and resistance levels.

Determination of Muscle, Ligament, and Joint Forces

Figure 50 provides the computations necessary to evaluate the forces in the lumbar spine in simple sagittal plane lifting. The muscles are the primary internal source of force resulting in motion of the vertebrae. Any shift in the center of gravity of the trunk must be balanced by muscle force to maintain equilibrium. Muscle forces also are required to balance the moment caused by an arm, an external weight, or any other force applied to the trunk, head, and upper extremities. If the combined effect of all the body weight and external forces on the spine are assumed to produce a moment that must be balanced by a single spinal muscle group to maintain equilibrium, the force in that muscle group can be calculated. Such representations provide valuable information. For example, such a model illustrates that to maintain low muscle forces, and consequently low stresses, on the spine structures when standing, an upright symmetric posture is preferred and all loads should be as close to the body as possible.

However, there are a number of three-dimensional (3-D) models in the literature—most of which determine equilibrium through a cutting plane, usually at the L-3 level—in which the weights of the body segments, the moments of those weights, and any forces and moments externally

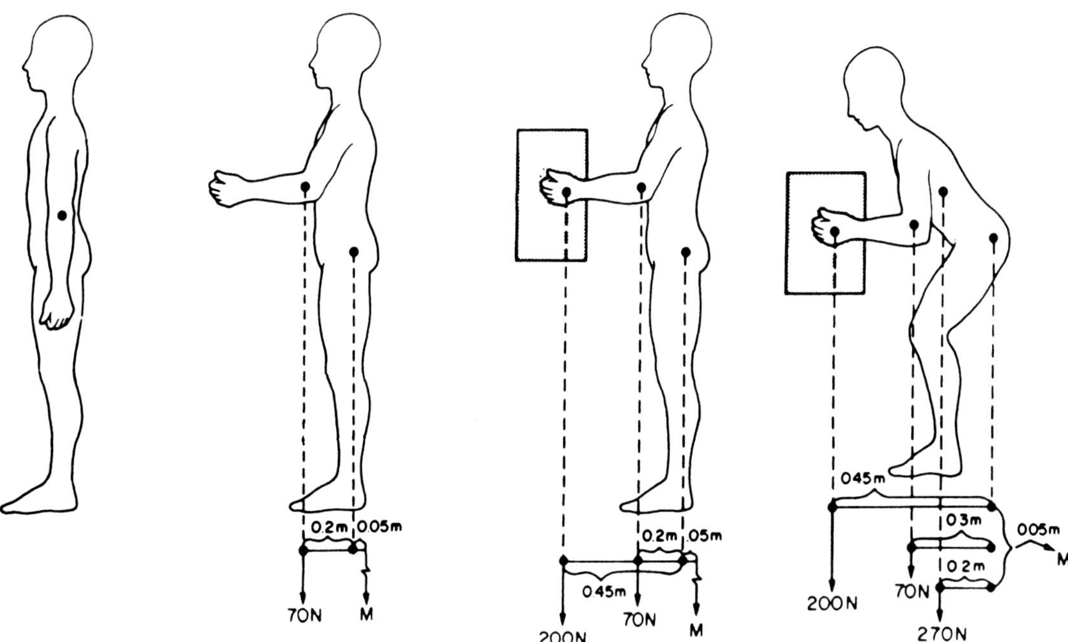

Figure 50
Left, In upright standing the body segments are well aligned with respect to the center of gravity and little muscular effort is required to maintain equilibrium. **Left center,** An elevated arm causes a load moment of about 70 N × 0.2 m (14 N·m), which must be equilibrated by the back muscles acting with an average moment arm of 0.05 m (muscle tension = 280 N). An additional object with a weight of 200 N held at 0.45 m **(right center)** causes an additional moment of 90 N·m (total muscle tension = 2,080 N). When leaning forward holding no weight **(right),** the trunk moment (270 × 0.21 = 54 N·m), arm moment (70 × 0.3 = 21 N·m), and with hand weight of 37 N·m, the hand moment (37 × 0.45 = 17 N·m) act together, causing a total load moment of 92 N·m (muscle tension = 1,840 N). An additional weight causes an additional moment of 200 × 0.45 = 90 N·m, (plus 92 N·m body load moment 182 N·m (muscle tension = 3,640 N). (Reproduced with permission from Pope MH, Andersson GBJ, Frymoyer JW, et al: Occupational biomechanics of the lumbar spine, in *Occupational Low Back Pain: Assessment, Treatment, and Prevention.* St. Louis, CV Mosby, 1991.)

applied superior to that plane are equilibrated (resisted) by moments provided by the passive tissues; that is, disks, ligaments, and several active muscle forces. These models are a more accurate representation of the problem and are used to acquire information regarding the stresses arising in each of the components sharing the load. When the load moment is applied in asymmetric postures, a much more complex situation occurs. However, in such cases, without further information, the distribution of load among the active muscles is statically indeterminate because the number of unknown muscle forces is larger than the six available equations describing the static equilibrium condition. Therefore, additional means must be provided to solve the problem.

Optimization techniques are used to select the optimal solution among the infinite number of solutions resulting from the statically indeterminate condition. An objective function (that is, the energy expenditure of muscular effort is to be minimized, the force produced by each muscle is proportional to its cross-sectional area) is chosen and a set of internal loads is calculated to minimize that function. The most common means of validating muscle activity in these models is by EMG signals. The second validation technique is to measure intradiskal pressures. The latter technique has been shown to relate directly to spine compression; however, such measurements are both invasive and difficult.

Recently, dynamic models have been considered to calculate a resultant moment at the L-4 to L-5 or L-5 to S-1 levels as a means of predicting disk compression and shear forces at the same time as considering the inertial effects caused by body acceleration.

Representation of more realistic anatomic lines of action of muscles in these models has improved the fidelity of the results. For example, L-4 to L-5 compression estimates were reduced by up to 35% with a more realistic anatomic model of the erector spinae muscle group. The shear force estimates could be altered from more than 500 N, with L-4 tending to shear anteriorly on L-5, to less than 300 N, with L-4 tending to shear posteriorly on L-5. A single "equivalent" extensor soft-tissue moment arm of 7.5 cm, rather than 5 cm would be needed to equate the compression.

More recently, the temporal and amplitude patterns of measured muscle activity have been quantified by integrating the rectified EMG signal (IEMG) to infer muscle tensions. The resulting measurements have been used in mathematical models to estimate the internal loading of the spine given the anatomic line of actions of the muscles and their cross-sectional areas. This class of models is called EMG-driven models. Some controversy exists with regard to the nature of the relationship between the IEMG and the muscle force because both linear and nonlinear relationships have been reported and actual measurements of muscle force have not been verified.

Nevertheless, these EMG-driven models have been used to quantify the loads (compression and shear forces) during dynamic activities. The main advantage of these models is their ability to account for coactivation of muscles, which is not predicted by optimization-based models. Thus, EMG-driven models will not underestimate the loads because they incorporate any coactivation that may be present. In addition, they capture inter- and intra-individual variations present in the recruitment patterns during performance of the repetitive tasks. Finally, there is no need to assume that a mathematical criterion or an objective function is being maximized (or minimized). The advantage of the optimization models is that they are suitable for simulation and design because the changes in the loading conditions can be handled by varying the input to the mathematical model. EMG-driven models, on the other hand, require an elaborate experimental setup to collect the necessary muscle activities. The future may well belong to the hybrid systems.

Intra-Abdominal Pressure

For many years IAP has been widely believed to have a beneficial role in spine biomechanics. During lifting, the amount of weight lifted is linearly related to IAP as measured in the stomach or rectum. This correlation between IAP and trunk effort forms the basis for supposing that IAP reduces loads in the trunk. IAP may help reduce compression in two ways: by directly decreasing the contribution of the muscular extensor and by creating a spinal tensile force on the diaphragm. The belief that abdominal pressure is a source of spinal support provides the rationale for flexion exercises and for the wearing of corsets and support belts during weight-lifting. Some have proposed that spinal support and alleviation of compression are achieved through action on the lumbodorsal fascia, but other researchers maintain that the theory reflects inaccurate assumptions about anatomy.

Because it is not possible to increase abdominal pressure without abdominal wall activity and a closed glottis, the associated costs of contracting the muscles cannot be neglected. The extensor forces and moments created by IAP do not offset the compression and flexor moment generated by abdominal activation. The frontal muscles must contract, producing a flexion moment in order to produce an increase in IAP. A Valsalva maneuver contracts the internal and external obliques, but the rectus abdominis contracts to a much lesser degree. There is still no direct evidence to support the hypothesis that intra-abdominal pressure reduces tension in the back muscle and compressive loads on the disk during trunk effort. Currently most of the evidence appears to be growing against the suggested role of IAP to relieve activity of the back muscles by providing an extension moment. However, the literature does point to the significance of IAP to provide stability for the trunk during peak external loading.

Structure and Function of the Hip Joint

Introduction

The hip joint is a ball-and-socket joint in which the head of the femur resides in the acetabulum of the pelvis. The surface area and the radius of curvature of the articular surface of the acetabulum closely match those of the articular surface of the femoral head. The hip joint is a highly constrained joint. Because of the inherent stability conferred by its bony architecture, this joint is well suited for performing the weightbearing supportive tasks that are required of it. The femoral ball is captured by the acetabular socket, allowing rotation to occur with virtually no translation. The constraint imparted by the bony architecture minimizes the need for ligamentous and soft-tissue constraints to maintain the stability of the hip articulation. Although this increased constraint confers stability on the hip, it does so at the expense of limiting the global range of motion of this joint at the fulcrum of the lower extremity. Fortunately, the lower extremities do not need to be placed in a variety of positions in space during activities of daily living. During most ambulatory activities, the lower extremity is positioned anteriorly in the sagittal plane with only small rotations necessary in the other two planes. Activities such as sitting, rising from a chair, and dressing require greater degrees of flexion and rotation at the hip joint.

Anatomic Structure

The acetabulum has a hemispheric shape, and is composed of portions from all three sections of the pelvis (the ilium, ischium, and pubis). It faces in

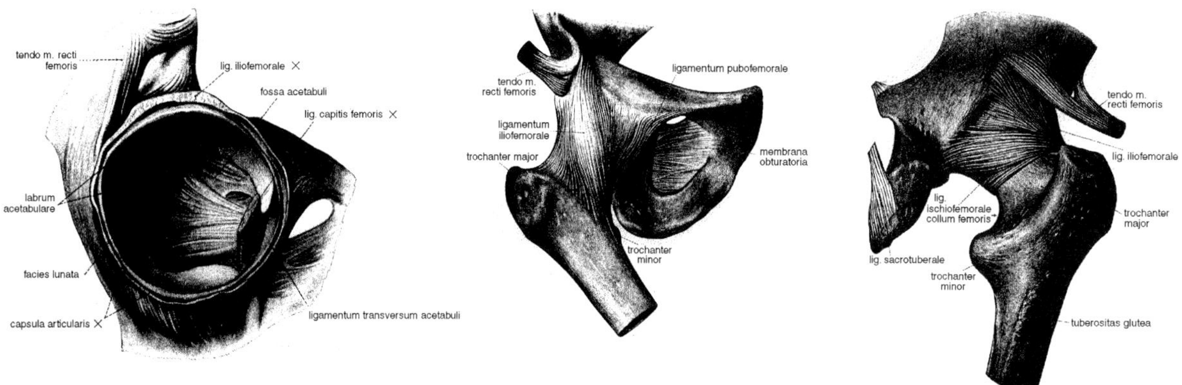

Figure 51
Anatomy of the hip. (Reproduced with permission from Figge FHJ: *Atlas of Human Anatomy: Vol. I. Atlas of Bones, Joints, and Muscles.* New York, Hafner, 1968.)

an inferior and anterolateral direction (Fig. 51, *left*). The articular cartilage is situated about the anterior, lateral, and posterolateral acetabular periphery, encompassing approximately two thirds of the surface of the hemisphere. With its underlying bone it is more prominent than the recessed medial acetabular fossa and defines a diameter that is approximately equal to that of the femoral head. It thereby encapsulates the femoral head. The acetabular labrum is a fibrocartilaginous lip around the rim of the acetabulum; it contributes to the shape and depth of the acetabulum and provides additional femoral head coverage. The matching size and spherical shape of the femoral head and acetabulum provide for a highly stable articulation. This stability and the large size of this joint are consistent with the substantial loads that must be borne by the hip. The femoral head forms approximately a 125° angle of inclination with the femoral shaft. This angle is greater in the child, often 140° at 5 years of age. The angle of femoral torsion is the angle between the transverse axes of the head and neck and that of the condylar axes at the lower end of the femur. In the adult this measures 12° to 15° whereas it measures approximately 40° at birth. Together these two angles cause the femoral neck and head to face cephalad medial and anteriorly. Thus, this direction is not in line with that of the acetabulum as both face anteriorly.

The articulation of the femoral head in the acetabulum permits three degrees of rotational freedom of the femur about the pelvis, while essentially eliminating relative translation between the femoral head and acetabulum. A smooth articulation is provided by articular cartilage. The cartilage on the femoral head is thickest at the center, while the acetabular cartilage is thickest at the superior portion of the acetabular wall. This cartilage orientation is consistent with the load-bearing and translational requirements anticipated at the hip joint. The smooth relative rotation between the acetabulum and femoral head is aided by synovial fluid lubrication as well as by the articular cartilage.

Although the bony constituents of the hip joint provide conformity and much of the joint's stability, other passive anatomic structures are required to completely restrain relative translation between femoral head and acetabulum. The capsule, reinforced by ligaments, is one of the strongest joint capsules in the entire body. External to its synovial membrane it is composed of fibers oriented in a deep circular and a superficial longitudinal layer extending from the rim of the acetabulum to the femoral neck (Fig. 51, *right*). The deep obicular band derives some of its fibers from the deep tendons of the gluteal region as well as the reflected head of the rectus. The longitudinal fibers cover the circular zone anteriorly forming a mass that varies in thickness and direction. Additional passive restraint is provided by several ligaments connecting the pelvis and femur. The ligamentum capitis (ligamentous teres) is a weak synovial attachment extending from the acetabular fossa and transverse acetabular ligament to the fovea capitis on the femoral head. The exceedingly thick band termed the iliofemoral band (or Y ligament of Bigelow) extends from the anterior superior iliac spine to the femoral intertrochanteric line. The bands extending from the upper pubic ramus to the lower intertrochanteric line are thinner and termed the pubofemoral band. The iliofemoral, pubocapsular, and ischiocapsular ligaments lie external to the articular capsule and connect the iliac, pubic, and ischial portions of the acetabular rim to the femur. Together these tissues form an exceedingly strong group of soft tissues, preventing relative acetabular/femoral head translation. These passive restraints do not prevent rotation, but they do limit it to some extent.

Musculature

Requiring movement and strength in all rotational planes about the joint, the hip is enclosed circumferentially by a large mass of 20 muscles. Their origin is from a broad spherical volume of the pelvis located anterior, medial, superior, and posterior to the hip joint. The range of excursion and power of these muscles is increased by the length of the neck, the prominence of the trochanters, and the relatively long moment arms produced by their origin and insertional positions relative to the center of the hip joint.

Anatomically these muscles may be classified by their source of innervation, the quadrant (anterior, posterior, medial, or lateral) in which they cross about the hip joint, or their primary rotational function. As in the case of the ligaments, the actions of these muscles depend significantly on the rotational position of the hip joint. This relates not only to the location of the origin of these muscles but also to their insertion.

Although muscles encapsulate the hip joint, their insertions onto the femur are at small sites about the femur and their line of action is not directly oriented parallel to the longitudinal axes of the femur when the hip joint is in a neutral position. For example, when the hip is in a neutral position, the iliopsoas, which inserts into the lesser trochanter of the femur (posteromedially), has a line of action that is directed anteromedially as it crosses the joint. Just distal to the posterior aspect of the femoral neck and slightly laterally is the gluteal ridge, where the gluteus maximus tendon inserts. This tendon insertion continues distally as the intermuscular septum. This septum with its bony ridge attachment (linea aspera) extends almost to the lateral supracondylar ridge and biceps septum. Along the linea aspera on the posterior aspect of the femur is the insertion site for the hip adductors. The iliacus and pectineus insert just medial to the linea aspera at the level of insertion of the gluteus maximus. The adductor longus, brevis, and magnus all insert below this along its ridge, extending almost halfway down the femur. Thus, these muscles not only adduct the thigh, but produce external rotation. The greater trochanter, which has a wide circumference anterolateral to posterolateral, provides the insertion area for the gluteus medius. The gluteus minimus inserts closer to the joint, but in line with the gluteus medius and combines with the ligamentous portion of the capsule. Depending on the relative position of the hip, these muscles can be internal or external rotators or assist in hip flexion, extension, or abduction. These muscles are listed in Table 14.

Kinematics

Kinematic measurements at the hip joint typically focus on describing only joint rotations, because relative translations between the articulating components are generally small and difficult to measure dynamically. These joint motions are described, commonly, in terms of flexion-extension rotation, internal-external rotation, and abduction-adduction rotation.

To quantify the 3-D motion of a body segment relative to a global reference, or the relative motion between two body segments as a joint, local coordinate systems (LCSs) for the segments must be defined. Specification of an LCS for a given segment requires that the positions of at least three points on the segments be known (Fig. 52). The first axis of an LCS can be obtained along a line connecting two known points. The second axis then can be defined along a line that is mutually perpendicular to the first axis and connecting the third point and one of the first two points. The third axis then could be defined as mutually perpendicular to the first two axes.

The most common means of expressing lower limb joint motions is through Cardan angles. Cardan angles essentially quantify the relative positions of two segments (for example, thigh and lower leg), or perhaps more specifically, the relative positions of the LCSs of two segments (Fig. 53). The vectors in Figure 52 are the unit vectors that describe the segments' LCSs. Each LCS unit vector has a magnitude of one and a direction that is mutually perpendicular to the other two LCS unit vectors for the given segment. The directions of the LCS unit vectors can be obtained as described above. The three Cardan angles represent the deviations of the LCSs for the segments about three axes (Fig. 53). These axes include one axis from each of the two segments' LCS axes. The third axis is determined as being mutually perpendicular to the first two axes. The selection of the first two axes is arbitrary; however, a common convention in motion biomechanics is to select the mediolateral axis of the more proximal segment as the flexion-extension axis, and the longitudinal axis of the more distal segment as the internal-external rotation axis. Consequently, the axis that is mutually perpendicular represents an abduction-adduction axis (Fig. 53).

Clinically, flexion rotation of the femur with respect to the trunk averages approximately 135° (knee to chest), and extension averages approximately 30°. Although this is commonly described as the range of hip flexion-extension, some of this motion relates to pelvic-vertebral motion. Estimates as to the true range of hip joint flexion-extension

Table 14
Hip muscles

Action	Muscle	Origin	Insertion
Flexor	Iliopsoas	Entire medial aspect of the ilium to the anterolateral vertebral column L-3 to L-5	Lesser trochanter
	Sartorius	Anterior iliac spine	Medial margin of tibial tuberosity
	Rectus femoris	Anterior inferior iliac spine	
Extensor	Gluteus maximus	Posterior lateral ilium to post aspect of sacrum, coccyx, and sacrotuberous ligament	Gluteal tuberosity of the posterior femur and iliotibial tract of fascia lata
	Biceps femoris long head	Ischial tuberosity	Head and lateral condyle of the tibia
	Semitendinosus	Ischial tuberosity	Tibial tuberosity
	Semimembranosus	Ischial tuberosity	Oblique popliteal ligament posterior knee capsule to medial condyle of the tibia
Adductor	Obturator externus	Lateral side of obturator membrane and medial and caudal margins of obturator foramen	Floor of trochanteric fossa
	Pectineus	Pectin of pubis	Pectineal line
	Adductor brevis	Inferior pubic ramus near symphyses	Pectineal line and proximal third of medial lip of linea aspera
	Adductor longus	Between superior and inferior pubic rami near symphyses	Middle third of medial lip of linea aspera
	Adductor magnus	Lower part of inferior pubic ramus:ramus of ischium; ischial tuberosity pubic rami near symphyses	Medial side of gluteal tuberosity along entire length of linea aspera to the medial supracondylar ridge and strong tendon to the adductor tubercle
	Gracilis	Inferior pubic ramus near symphyses	Anterior medial surface of tibia near tibial tuberosity
Abductor	Gluteus medius	Broad origin spanning external aspect of entire ilium between the anterior and posterior gluteal lines	Cephalocaudal oblique ridge on greater trochanter
	Gluteus minimus	Broad and deep origin across lateral external surface of ilium caudal to gluteus medius	Greater trochanter and hip joint capsule
	Tensor fascia latae	Iliac crest to anterior superior	Iliotibial tract
External rotator	Piriformis	Sacrum at S-2, S-3, S-4	Greater trochanter
	Quadratus femoris	Ischial tuberosity	Greater trochanter and quadrate line of femur
	Obturator internus	Posterior aspect of obturator foramen and membrane	Medial surface of greater trochanter
	Superior and inferior gemelli	Ischial spine and ischial tuberosity	Conjoint tendon with obturator internus to greater trochanter

vary; this variance is related partly to the definition of the reference axes of the pelvis with respect to its anatomic landmarks. The anatomic axes of the pelvis commonly used clinically are the line connecting the two anterior superior iliac crests and a line perpendicular to it connecting the midpoint of the pubis symphyses and the midline of the spine. The third axis is difficult to define anatomically; Nelaton's line, the line between the anterior superior iliac spine and the ischial tuberosity, is commonly used. Viewed from a lateral perspective, the proximal tip of the greater trochanter usually passes through this line. When the hip is in maximum extension, considered 0°, the long axis of the femur forms a 50° angle with Nelaton's line. The maximum possible position of hip flexion when the pelvifemoral angle is measured using these same axes is 125°. Thus, the true range of hip flexion-

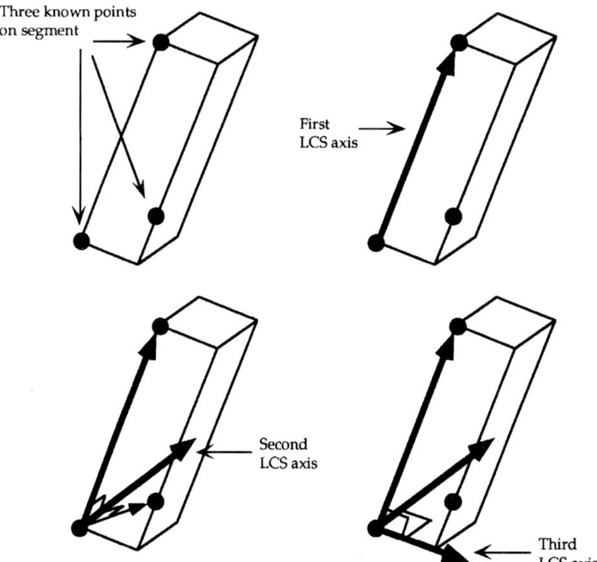

Figure 52
Local coordinate system (LCS) axes.

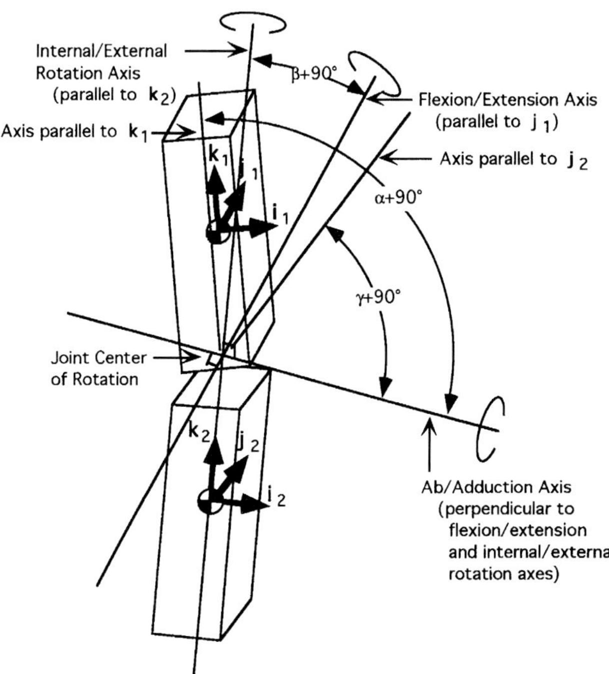

Figure 53
Cardan angles. α represents the flexion-extension angle, β represents the internal-external rotation angle, and γ represents the abduction-adduction angle.

extension is considered to be about 75° to 80°. This is truly less than the range of motion that can be achieved by rotating the femur in the acetabulum in the absence of the joint capsule and ligaments and illustrates the passive restraining action of these tissues during normal motions. In actuality, because of the orientation and strength of these tissues (architecture), the range of motion about any axis can vary with the position of the thigh.

Internal-external rotation of the femur at the hip joint occurs around a longitudinal axis passing through the head of the femur and intercondylar region at the lower end. With the the axis of the femur parallel to the trunk, the femur can rotate through a possible total arc of approximately 50°. In most circumstances, this is composed of about 35° of external rotation and 15° of internal rotation. This rotation varies depending on whether the axis of the femur is parallel or perpendicular to the trunk. When the joint is in more "flexion" the range of these movements may be increased to 40° and 60°, respectively. Finally, rotation of the femur with respect to the midline of the trunk in the coronal plane, termed abduction and adduction, also occurs. Abduction averages approximately 45° and adduction approximately 25°. With the joint in flexion, a greater range of abduction-adduction rotation is permitted.

The kinematics of the hip joint during functional activities requires a knowledge of joint positions at multiple intervals of time. As the time interval between joint position measurments decreases, the kinematic profiles of the joint become more complete. For cyclic activities, such as walking, kinematics typically are reported for a single period. Although the determination of the beginning and end of a periodic activity is generally somewhat arbitrary, standards have evolved for the delimitation of a cycle for a number of motions.

For a number of common activities, nonpathologic hip joint motion is confined primarily to a single rotation. Daily tasks involving the hip joint, such as walking, running, sitting, and bending, primarily involve motion in the sagittal plane in the form of flexion and extension. During walking and cycling, for example, hip joint rotation is mostly in flexion-extension. "Jumping jack" exercises generally involve abduction-adduction rotation. At times, however, flexion-extension, internal-external, and abduction-adduction rotations can be present in a single activity, such as soccer style kicking. Tasks that involve a single primary rotation under nonpathologic conditions can include two or all three rotations in substantial quantities under certain pathologic, or even suboptimal states. Walking for an individual with arthritis at the hip might include a raising of the contralateral hip during stance, which would be measured as a hip abduction. Increasing hip abduction during swing phase of walking could be used to compensate for reduced knee flexion in order to obtain foot clearance.

The motion at the nonpathologic hip and knee joints associated with typical daily activity (for example, walking, stair climbing) illustrates the substantial consistency between anatomic structure and essential function (Table 15). Similarly, the right-left symmetry of joint anatomy and common daily motions is not a matter of pure coincidence. Conversely, the motions of hip and knee joints with pathologic conditions (for example, arthritis, muscle spasticity or contracture, hip dislocation) often can be related directly to the specific pathology, as well as involve dramatic asymmetries. The process of relating abnormal joint motions to pathologies, however, is not always a straightforward matter, because such primary abnormal joint motions are associated, typically, with secondary compensatory motions at otherwise nonpathologic joints.

Kinetics

The kinetics at the hip joint relate to the loads associated with this joint. These loads include the forces between the articulating components of the joint, as well as the torques acting about the joints to generate or oppose rotational motion.

In addition to quantifying the relative motion between two segments at a joint, it is also beneficial to quantify, independently, the motions of body segments. Such information is particularly useful for subsequent calculations of joint reaction loads and moments. Euler angles and screw operators are techniques that have been applied frequently to motion biomechanics for representing the positions of body segments.

The Euler angles refer to a set of three specific rotations of a body in space (Fig. 54, *top* and *center*). These rotations follow after a translation of the body segment that places the LCS origin coincident with the global coordinate system (GCS) origin. As a common convention, the first rotation is by an angle ϕ about the initial local coordinate system z-axis; the second rotation is by an angle θ, about the local coordinate system x′-axis (the orientation of the LCS x-axis after the first rotation); and the third rotation is by an angle ψ, about the local coordinate system z″-axis (the orientation of the LCS z-axis after the second rotation). In biomechanics, applications of the Euler angle rotations are intended to align the segment LCS with the GCS. Consequently, the values of the Euler angles quantify the position of the segment in the GCS. To align the LCS and the GCS with the three Euler rotations, the first rotation, ϕ about the GCS z-axis, must bring the GCS x′-axis coincident with a "line of nodes" that is defined as a line mutually perpendicular to the GCS z-axis and the initial orientation of the LCS z-axis.

The screw operator involves the displacement of a body from an initial position to a final position via a rotation, ϕ, about a single axis with unit vector u and a translation δ parallel to the same axis (Fig. 54, *bottom*). This axis is referred to as the screw axis or the helical axis. Subsequently, by determining the proper direction for the screw axis, angle for the rotation, and distance for the translation, a segment can be moved in a way that aligns its LCS with the GCS. Thus, the screw operator also can be used to define the position of a segment with respect to a GCS. The screw operator is used less commonly than Cardan and Euler angles. This descriptive approach is often used at the knee joint.

Determination of joint kinetics requires considerably greater information than does the calculation of joint kinematics. In addition to body segment positions, the calculation of joint kinetics requires knowledge of body segment parameters, external

Table 15
Hip and Knee Kinematics During Various Activities

Activity Joint	Maximum Flexion	Maximum Extension	Maximum Range	Maximum Adduction	Maximum Abduction	Ab/Adduct. Range	Max. Internal Rotation	Max. External Rotation
Walking								
Hip	20°-40°	0°-20°	40°-52°	2°-10°	0°-8°	8°-14°	2°-12°	4°-10°
Knee	57°-65°	(-3)°-0°	54°-65°	2°-18°	0°-7°	5°-18°	(−5)°-10°	5°-20°
Cycling								
Knee	110°	(-45)°	65°					
Stair Ascending								
Hip	40°	(-5)°	35°					
Knee	80°	(-5)°	75°					
Stair Descending								
Hip	30°	5°	35°					
Knee	90°	(-5)°	85°					

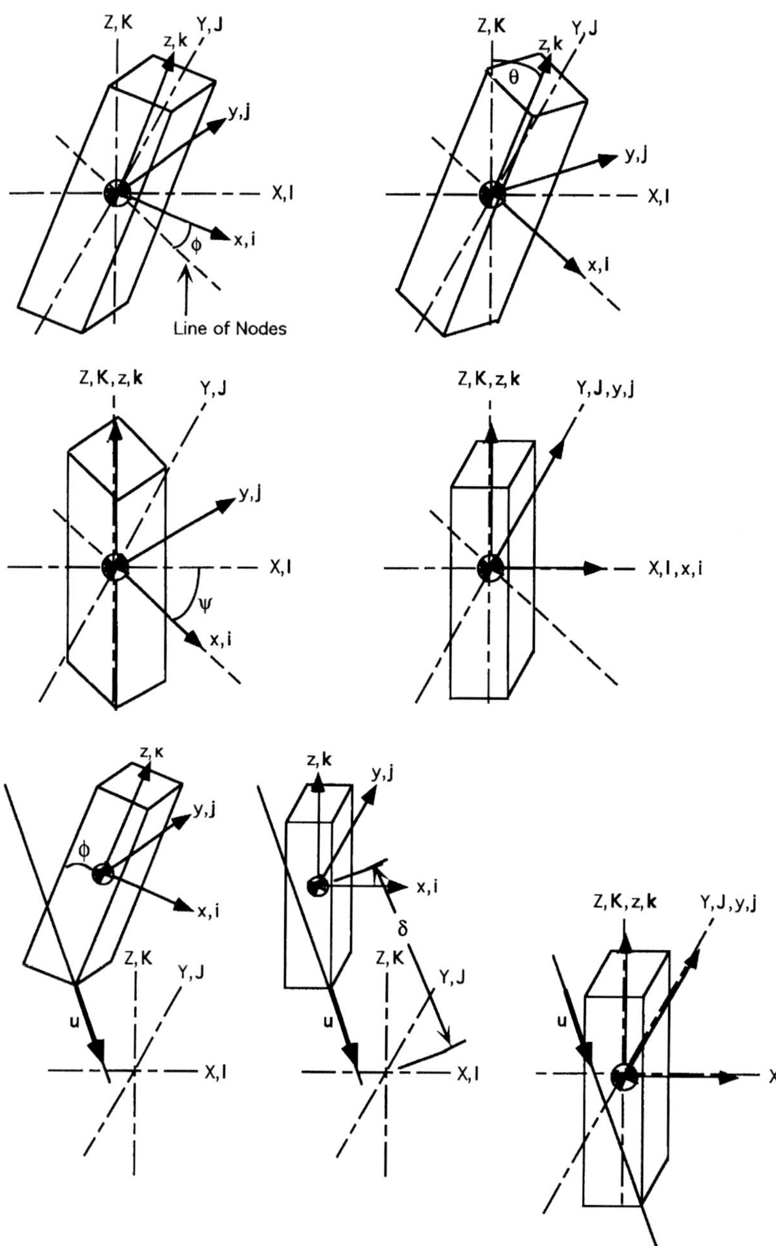

Figure 54
Top and center, Euler angles. **Bottom,** The screw operator.

loading, and segment velocities and accelerations. Body segment parameters that are typically used include mass, volume, length, diameter, and moment of inertia. External loading generally includes ground-reaction forces and gravity during weightbearing portions of activities (for example, stance phase of walking), although only gravity is involved in most nonweightbearing activities. Segment velocities and accelerations are obtained commonly by numerically differentiating positional data, however, these data can be measured directly at times.

Joint torques can be in the direction of motion, in the direction opposite to motion, or in directions for which motion is negligible. Muscles at the hip joint can contribute to joint torques in any of these generally described directions. Muscular torque contributions about the hip joint also can be active (due to contraction) or passive (due to lengthening). Torque resulting from muscular exertion can be concentric (muscle shortening during contraction), eccentric (muscle lengthening during contraction), or isometric (muscle length constant). Hip joint torques also may have contributions from passive structures (for example, ligamentous and capsular restraints); however, such contributions are generally in directions from which motion is restrained.

At the hip joint, active muscular contraction is primarily responsible for joint torque generation.

During many less strenuous activities (for example, walking), lengthening or stretching of the passive elements on a nonactivated muscle, or ligamentous stretch, is all that is required for much of the hip joint torque generated. For example, passive lengthening of the hip extensors contributes to the early deceleration of the flexing hip during mid-to-late swing. Often, it is not until very late swing, or at times not at all, that the hip extensors will actively generate torque to decelerate the hip in terminal swing. In other more demanding tasks (for example, stair climbing), active hip torque generation must be used throughout most of the activity. As with the joint kinematics, however, much of the commonly observed hip joint kinetics can be substantially altered in the presence of pathology.

Hip Joint Forces

Joint torques at the hip are calculated more reliably than joint forces. The difficulty of calculating the joint forces arises from the indeterminancy of the individual muscle forces resulting from the large number of muscles acting at the hip joint. Although a number of techniques have been devised for apportioning the loads among the various muscles, none of these techniques have been incorporated into widespread clinical use. While hip joint forces are difficult to calculate directly, it is evident that muscular contractions can contribute substantially to the generation of compressive hip joint forces, if the forces of gravity are to be neutralized by the counterforces of muscles. This has been discussed in the chapter related to biomechanics. For example, in the presence of arthritis at the hip, compensations, such as Trendelenburg lurch or hip hike, reduce the muscular exertion about the hip, and, thereby, reduce the compressive force.

Forces that act across the hip joint during dynamic activities have been investigated by several authors. Two approaches have been used. Some have made external measurements of kinetic and kinematic quantities and inferred the internal forces via the use of mathematical computation and models. Others have used internal measurement, affixing the proper instruments to a total joint prosthesis, nail plate, or femoral endoprosthesis. Although neither approach ideally depicts the exact forces present in the average person, their similarities suggest the magnitude of the forces incurred during different activities. During quiet single-leg stance, the forces transmitted across the hip joint are estimated to be between two and 2.8 times body weight. Some have predicted this force to be as high as six times body weight. During two-legged stance, the forces in each hip joint are about half that in single-leg stance. During gait, these forces can be as high as three times body weight; although, estimates as high as six times body weight again have been suggested. The difference in results relates in part to the speed at which the subject walks. In addition, internal instrumented measurements are often lower than mathematically predicted values because the former are based on early postoperative measurements of subjects who had pathologic conditions (for example, arthritis), whereas the latter use data from healthy subjects. Two peaks usually are noted in these studies; one just after foot strike at the inception of single-limb stance and the other at opposite foot strike. Forces also exist in swing phase and, generally, have been determined to be about half of the average force seen in stance phase. Getting in and out of bed, raising onto a bedpan, and transferring to a wheelchair all involve high forces of at least two times body weight. A summary of the range of motions and estimates of joint forces for the hip and the knee gleaned from the literature for different activities is presented in Tables 15 and 16.

In quiet standing and in gait, the joint-contact force varies over a limited range of the anterosuperior aspect of the femoral head, bounded by a cone. In quiet standing, the direction of this cone closely parallels that of the femoral neck. For activities that require greater hip flexion, the polar angle undergoes a greater anterior excursion consistent with altered out-of-phase increased muscular forces. The joint-contact force, however, does not seem uniform in its pressure distribution and area of contact on the acetabular or femoral cartilage. Although these surfaces represent parts of spheres of identical radius it has been demonstrated in vivo that, at low loads, the contacting area of the acetabulum is about its periphery. As the load is increased, the contacting area spreads to more central areas with a "flaring out" of the acetabular wall. This flaring, in association with the configuration of the hip joint, explains the constant changes, with changing hip position and activity level, in size and location of femoral surface contacting area.

These changes are significant to "hip containment" and actual surface pressures. Hip containment generally implies either a relative increase in acetabular coverage of the lateral femoral head or an absolute increase in contact of the femoral head with the acetabulum. The maximum potential area of the femoral head that can be in contact with the acetabulum has been estimated to be approximately 65% to 75%. This percentage changes little with changes in hip position, i.e. abduction. However, the area of the femoral surface in contact does change.

Table 16
Hip and Knee Kinetics During Various Activities

Activity Joint	Max. Joint Force (BW)	Max. Flexion Moment (N·m)	Max. Exten. Moment (N·m)	Max. Adduct. Moment (N·m)	Max. Abduct. Moment (N·m)	Max. Internal Rot. Moment (N·m)	Max. External Rot. Moment (N·m)	Max. Conc. Power (W)	Max. Ecc. Power (W)	Max. Ener. Generation (J)	Max. Ener. Absorption (J)
Walking											
Hip	3-8.5	40-80	30-130	10-100	10-105	3-20	0-13				
Knee	1.2-7.7	20-40	15-47	0-30	0-45	2-10	10-20	42	92	3.7	9.6
Cycling											
Hip		35	10					70-150		20	5
Knee	1.2	10-30	25-40	3	25			110-190		30	3
Stair Ascent											
Hip		10	125	5	60	5	15				
Knee		60	125	15	30-40	10	5				
Stair Descent											
Hip		20	115	15	85	5	20				
Knee		20-30	125-150	15	30-60	5-15	5-15				

Structure and Function of the Knee

Introduction

The knee actually consists of two joints: the femorotibial joint and the patellofemoral joint. The femorotibial joint is the largest joint in the body and is considered to be a modified hinged joint containing the articulating ends of the femur and tibia. The patellofemoral joint consists of the patella, the largest sesamoid bone. Taken together, the knee joint functions to control the distance between the pelvis and the foot. Because of its role in weightbearing and its location between the two longest bones in the body, the forces generated at the knee are larger than those at the elbow. During such activities as walking and such athletic activities as running, landing, and pivoting, the knee functions to maintain a given leg length and act as a shock absorber. In other situations, such as going up and down stairs, getting in and out of chairs, crouching, and jumping, large propulsive forces at the knee are needed to generate a lengthening of the leg or restraining forces are needed to control the amount and speed of shortening of the leg. In these situations, knee stability is a dynamic process maintained through fixed bony and ligamentous constraints and modified by the action of the muscles crossing the joint.

The bony architecture of the femur, tibia, and patella contributes to joint stability, but to a lesser extent than that of other more constrained joints, such as the hip. In contrast to shoulder stability, which is maintained primarily through the dynamic action of the surrounding muscles, static constraints play a greater role in knee stability. The cruciate and collateral ligaments are the major structures limiting motion at the knee. The posteromedial and posterolateral capsular complexes also have important roles, and, in addition to their shock absorbing function, the menisci play a role in the static restraint of the knee.

Femorotibial Joint

Architecture

Bone The femoral condyles can be thought of as having a tibial facet as well as a patella facet. Although the entire femoral condyle has a varying radius of curvature, if the tibial and patella facets are isolated (using the base of the trochlear groove), the radius of curvature of each of these facets is much more uniform, that is, closer to a circle. The condyles of the femur can be thought of as having two distinct, nearly circular cams. The central portion between these cams is flatter (has a greater radius of curvature) than either the anterior or posterior portions.

The lateral condyle is smaller than the medial one in both the AP and proximodistal directions and contributes to the valgus and AP alignment of the knee joint. This configuration, in conjunction with only a slight lateral inclination of the tibia in relation to the joint line (3° valgus and 9° posterior slope), creates an overall valgus and slightly posterior inferior alignment of between 10° and 12° in most knees. The shape of the condyles also plays a critical role in maintaining tension in the ligamentous structures about the knee in all positions of flexion and extension, and loss of architecture can lead to lack of function of the ligaments, joint instability, and alterations in muscle effort.

In cross section, the medial and lateral tibial plateaus are roughly ovoid in shape. In the coronal plane they are nearly flat; even when considered in conjunction with the menisci, they are only slightly concave.

The menisci The fibrocartilaginous medial and lateral menisci are thick peripherally and taper to thin edges centrally. Although they deepen the tibial plateaus only slightly, this deepening provides for a somewhat more congruent and constrained surface with the femoral condyles.

Cruciate ligaments Although the cruciate ligaments are intracapsular, they are covered by a synovial fold; therefore, strictly speaking, they are extra-articular.

Many authors have studied the bony attachments of the anterior (ACL) and posterior cruciate ligaments (PCL). The origin of the ACL is posterior in the femoral notch and oriented primarily in the longitudinal axis of the femur. Its insertion is wide and is oriented in the AP axis of the tibia; it occupies about one third of the width of the tibia between the anterior and middle thirds. As the ACL passes from its origin to insertion, its fibers rotate approximately 90°. This rotation leads to the development of differential tension in the ACL fibers and causes the ligament to twist as the knee flexes (Fig. 55). The ACL can be differentiated functionally into two bundles: anteromedial and posterolateral. With flexion, the anteromedial fibers develop more tension; in extension, the posterolateral bundle is tighter. Likewise, the PCL's femoral origin lies in an AP orientation in the anterior portion of the femoral notch. The PCL inserts, in a broad mediolateral span, into the posterior sulcus of the tibia between the medial and lateral joint surfaces. It can be differentiated into anterolateral and posteromedial bands. Anterolateral fibers become taut in flexion and posteromedial fibers become taut in extension.

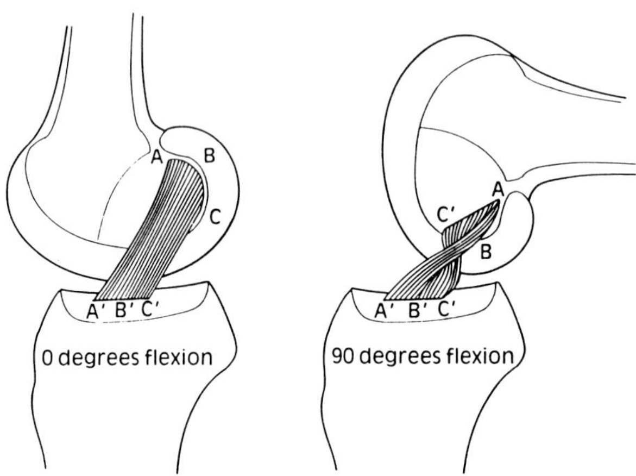

Figure 55
Schematic drawing representing changes in shape and tension of anterior cruciate ligament (ACL) components in flexion and extension. In flexion, there is lengthening of the anteromedial band (A-A′) and shortening of the posterolateral aspect of the ligament (C-C′). Also present, however, is an intermediate component (B-B′), which represents transition between the anteromedial band and posterolateral bulk, with fascicles in varying degrees of tension. (Modified with permission from Girgis FG, Marshall JL, Monajem ARS: The cruciate ligaments of the knee joint: Anatomical, functional and experimental analysis. *Clin Orthop* 1975;106:216–231.)

Capsuloligamentous restraints The capsuloligamentous structures surrounding the joint play a primary role in controlling normal joint motion. These structures include the medial (MCL) and lateral collateral ligaments (LCL), the joint capsule, and the posteromedial and posterolateral complexes.

These supporting structures surrounding the knee can be considered to be divided into three discrete layers. On the medial side, the most superficial layer (layer 1), is the deep fascia. Posteriorly this layer overlies the two heads of the gastrocnemius and serves as a support for the neurovascular structures in the popliteal fossa. Anteriorly it blends with layer 2 and the medial patellar retinaculum.

Layer 2 contains the superficial MCL. Of the two components that make up the MCL (superficial and deep), the superficial MCL is clinically more important, and it is the primary medial stabilizer of the knee. It originates on the medial epicondyle and runs approximately 10 cm to its insertion on the tibia, deep to the gracilis and semitendinosus tendons. The posterior oblique fibers of the MCL blend posteriorly into the capsule (layer 3) and, along with contributions from the semimembranosus tendon, form the oblique popliteal ligament.

Layer 3 is the knee joint capsule. It is composed of fibrous tissues of varying thickness, many of which have been identified as specific ligaments. The capsule is quite thin anteriorly. Deep to the superficial MCL, there is a distinct capsular thickening, the deep MCL. This short band of vertical fibers extends from the femur to the periphery of the medial meniscus and tibia. Along the posterior margin of the deep MCL, layer 3 merges with layer 2, forming the reinforced posteromedial capsule.

The lateral structures of the knee are also divided into three layers. The most superficial layer, the lateral retinaculum, is made up of superficial oblique and deep transverse components and provides strong lateral support for the patella. The middle layer is made up of the LCL, the fabellofibular ligament, and the arcuate ligament. The LCL originates on the lateral epicondyle and inserts on the lateral surface of the fibular head. The arcuate ligament is a complex mass of fibers running in various directions. The most consistent fibers form a triangular sheet diverging proximal from the fibular head. The strong lateral limb attaches proximally to the femur, whereas the weaker medial limb arcs over the popliteus muscle. Both blend into the posterior capsule. The deepest lateral layer is again the capsule. It is a thin, weak layer anteriorly that is reinforced posteriorly by the arcuate ligament complex.

Kinematics

The tibial femoral articulation has six degrees of freedom in three geometric axes. In each of these axes, (longitudinal, AP, and mediolateral), the tibia can either translate or rotate with respect to the femur. This results in the following six paired motions: flexion-extension, varus-valgus, and internal-external rotation; compression-distraction, AP translation, and mediolateral translation. Although this very complex joint is far from being a pure hinged joint, its rotation in the sagittal plane (flexion-extension) greatly dominates both clinical and kinematic study of the knee joint.

Sagittal range of motion In the sagittal plane, the arc of flexion-extension is greatly affected by the individual's generalized ligamentous laxity status as well as body habitus. In a normal population, knee extension varies from a few degrees short of 0 to as much as 20° of recurvatum. Knee flexion varies from 125° to 165°. A consensus normal functional range of knee motion would be from approximately 3° to 4° of hyperextension to 140° of flexion.

Like that of other joints in the body, the range of knee motion used during various activities of daily living and recreation varies with the activity. For example, during normal walking the knee is flexed approximately 10° at heel strike and has a maximum of 65° of flexion in swing. In contrast, with sprinting the knee is flexed about 35° at foot strike and requires about 130° of maximal flexion in swing. At intervening speeds, knee flexion increases both at heel strike and at maximum flexion during swing phase, and there is a smooth correlation of increasing flexion requirements for the knee with increasing speed of gait. Actually, 130° of flexion are required for most competitive athletic activities. Studies have also shown that for other routine activities of daily living, such as getting in and out of chairs and stair climbing, 115° of maximum knee flexion are required.

Total anterior and posterior translation of the tibia on the femur in an uninjured knee is also greatly affected by the general ligamentous laxity status of the individual. Measurement of translation of the tibia with respect to the femur is affected by the rotational position of the knee at the time of the measurement. The measurement depends on the degree of flexion of the knee, the amount of its internal or external rotation, and the concomitant amount of joint compression. The measurement also depends on the amount of force used to create the translational motion. The AP translation of the tibia on the femur is minimal at full extension and does not become appreciable until after the screw home mechanism (see below) has been unlocked. AP laxity in the knee is greatest between 30° and 90° of flexion, and beyond 90° it starts to diminish again. Anterior translation of the tibia is maximal at approximately 30° of flexion when the anterior restraints are most lax. This anterior translation can vary from 2 to 10 mm. Posterior translation is most apparent at 90° of flexion and can vary in magnitude from 0 to 6 mm.

The above figures represent attempts to use instrumented measuring devices to measure the passive translational AP translation. To compare translational motions between individuals, and between right and left sides in individuals, a standard position of the knee and amount of force has been used. Generally, these standards have been 20° to 30° of knee flexion, neutral internal-external and varus-valgus rotation, and approximately 90 N (about 20 lbs) of translational force. Regardless of the instrument used, it has been found that a mean anterior displacement of about 6 mm and a mean posterior displacement of approximately 3 mm are present in most subjects without ligamentous pathology. More importantly, the right and left knees in greater than 90% of subjects have a side-to-side difference of no more than 2 mm.

AP translation—instantaneous centers of rotation The concept of centers of motion has been used to describe rotational and translational motion of the articular surface of the femur relative to the tibia as the two bones move in the sagittal plane. If one rigid body rotates about another rigid body, its motion at any instant can be described by a point or axis of rotation called the instantaneous center of rotation (See the chapter on biomechanics). If the existing motion is purely rotational, this axis (point in two dimensions) remains fixed in space as motion progresses, and the contacting surfaces slide relative to each other. Rolling occurs when the instant center of rotation translates commensurate with the translation of the contacting point between the two surfaces. With pure rolling, no sliding or shear forces occur between the two surfaces; at each additional instant, the two surfaces touch via perpendicular contact. If, on the other hand, rotation of one body with respect to another occurs at the same time that rolling occurs, the center of rotation must also change at each instant proportional to the degree of translation occurring, and, at the contacting surfaces, both rolling and gliding occur and shear and compressive forces are present.

Relative motion between the femur and the tibia is both rotational and translational. If the distance between the contact point on the tibial plateau at full extension and at full flexion is measured, the distance between these two points is much less than the distance along the surface of the femoral condyle between the contact points of full extension and full flexion. The femoral condyles thus perform a combination of rolling and gliding as they articulate with the tibial plateaus. By mapping the pathway of the instant center or flexion axis of the knee in the sagittal plane, it is possible to see that, as the knee moves from full extension to full flexion, the instant center moves posteriorly relative to both the femur and the tibia. The fact that it is important to keep the surface contact point beneath the instant center to reduce sliding leads to the conclusion that the surface contact point must also move posteriorly as the knee moves from flexion to extension; this is, indeed, what happens. Different investigators have measured the amount of posterior movement of the surface contact point during flexion on both the medial and lateral tibial plateaus. This posterior movement of the contact point has been estimated to be between 5 and 12 mm in each compartment, with less translation in the lateral compartment than in the medial one. This difference is a reflection of the fact that the lateral condyle is smaller than the medial one and, additionally, results in simultaneous internal-external rotation of the femur about the tibia during flexion-extension.

As the knee rotates, the menisci move posteriorly with flexion and anteriorly with knee extension. Anterior meniscal translation with extension is caused by the larger surface area of the anterior femoral condyles pushing the anterior portion forward. The extent of translation is limited by the size of the condyle as well as by increased tension in the capsule posteriorly. Posterior translation of the medial meniscus is aided by its attachments to the MCL and semimembranosus, and posterior translation of the lateral meniscus by the popliteus and meniscofemoral ligaments. Each of these tissues translate posteriorly in flexion, with relatively greater displacement than the tibia itself. Translation of the meniscus allows a maximum contact area and distributes compressive loads evenly across the joint during most positions of femoral rotation.

A common convention used to describe the relative motion between the femur and tibia is one of the tibia remaining stationary and the femoral surface rolling and sliding on the surface of the tibia. The distance traversed on the tibia reflects the degree of rolling that occurs, and the difference between this distance and that on the femur to some degree reflects the amount of gliding. A slip ratio has been defined as the ratio of the distance between two successive contact points on the femoral articular surfaces to the distance between the corresponding two contact points on the tibial surface for a given arc of motion. The greater the slip ratio, the more gliding that occurs for any given amount of roll. In order for the articulation to have true roll and no slip, the slip ratio would be 1. In the human knee, at no point during flexion or extension in the sagittal plane is the slip ratio 1. As the knee moves from full extension to flexion, the surface contact point moves posteriorly on the tibia, but the femoral condyles slide anteriorly diminishing the posterior progression of the rolling effect. The exact ratio of rolling to gliding differs between individuals and does not remain constant throughout all degrees of flexion. It is estimated to be one to two in early flexion and to increase to one to four by the end of flexion.

The direction of movement of the femoral surface contact with the tibia is perpendicular to a line connecting the instant center of rotation with the point of surface contact (Fig. 56). In order to maintain a smooth sliding action of the femoral surface on the tibial plateau, this direction of movement must be parallel to the tibial plateau. In the normal knee, as the femur rolls and glides on the tibial surface, the multiple directional lines generated always remain parallel to the tibial surface. If, for any

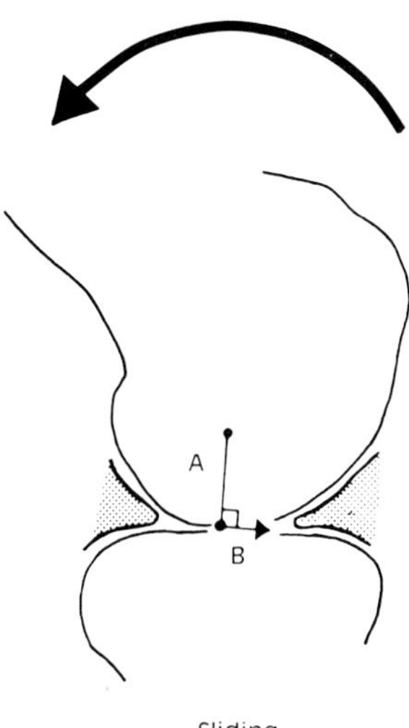

Figure 56
In the normal knee, a line drawn from the instant center of the tibiofemoral joint to a tibiofemoral contact point (line A) forms a right angle with a line tangential to the tibial surface (line B). The arrow indicates the direction of displacement of the contact points. Line B is tangential to the tibial surface, indicating that the femur slides on tibial condyles during a measured interval of motion. (Reproduced with permission from Frankel VH, Nordin M: *Basic Biomechanics of the Skeletal System*. Philadelphia, Lea & Febiger, 1980.)

reason, the relationship between the instant center and surface contact point is altered, femoral movement will be directed either into the plateau, crushing the surfaces together, or away from the plateau, producing a lift off (Fig. 57). It has been found that displacement of either the instant center or the normal contact point can occur with either internal derangement, ligamentous disruption, joint surface loss, or abnormal external constraints, such as a knee brace or nonphysiologic ligament reconstruction, and that this displacement results in disruption of the normal roll-glide mechanism with impairment of knee flexion and extension. The result is analogous to an improperly hung door in which the two hinges are not parallel to each other and, depending on the severity of the malalignment, the door will not open smoothly. A knee in which the path of the instant center has been altered will experience either marked increased joint compressive forces, blocking of motion, or stretching of its surrounding soft tissue constraints, with consequent loss of stability.

Frontal plane Rotation of the tibia on the femur in the frontal plane, also known as varus and valgus angulation, again varies greatly in a normal knee depending on the degree of flexion of the knee as well as the general ligamentous status of the patient. In the normal knee during passive testing, minimal varus-valgus movement of the tibia exists at terminal extension. Maximal varus and valgus rotation of the tibia occur at approximately 30°. As a general rule, varus motion is greater than valgus rotation because the LCL is lax in flexion, while parts of the MCL remain tight. At 30° of flexion, medial joint distraction with a valgus stress ranges from one to 10 mm, with an average of 4 mm; lateral joint opening to a varus stress has been found to be 2 to 14 mm, with an average of 6 mm. During the dynamic activity of walking at a freely selected speed, maximum valgus rotation occurs at heel strike and maximum varus movement occurs during swing phase with an average total varus-valgus rotation during gait of 11°. No significant mediolateral translation of the tibia on the femoral condyles occurs in the normal knee, passively or actively.

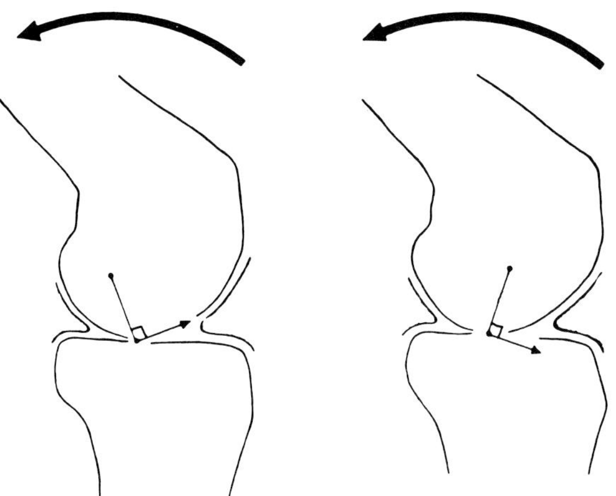

Figure 57
Surface motion in two tibiofemoral joints with displaced instant centers. In both joints, the line that is at a right angle drawn between the instant center and the tibiofemoral contact point describes the direction of displacement of the contact points. **Left,** The arrow in the joint indicates that the tibiofemoral joint will be distracted with further flexion. **Right,** The arrow in the joint indicates that the tibiofemoral joint will become compressed with further flexion. (Reproduced with permission from Frankel VH, Nordin M: *Basic Biomechanics of the Skeletal System.* Philadelphia, Lea & Febiger, 1980.)

Transverse plane Internal-external rotation of the tibia on the femur is minimal at full extension. The amount of internal tibial rotation on the femur increases progressively from negligible at 0° to a maximum at between 90° and 120° of flexion. No significant rotation becomes apparent until after the first 10° to 20° of flexion. The range of maximum external rotation can vary from 0° to 45°, whereas maximum internal rotation ranges from 0° to 25°. During normal gait, the tibia undergoes internal rotation during the swing phase and external rotation during the stance phase. When skeletal pins were used to measure total tibial rotation in normal gait total rotation was found to be between 4° and 13° with an average of 8°.

Obligatory external rotation of the tibia on the femur occurs during the terminal degrees of knee extension and is caused, in part, by the differential in radius between the medial femoral condyle and the smaller lateral femoral condyle. This phenomenon has been referred to as the "screw home mechanism." Because the medial femoral condyle is larger than the lateral femoral condyle, the distance from the extreme flexion contact point to the extreme extension contact point of the medial femoral condyle has been found to be approximately 17 mm greater than that of the lateral femoral condyle. As the tibia travels from flexion into extension, the medial tibial plateau must cover a greater distance and thus the tibia externally rotates. This screw home mechanism in terminal extension results in a tightening of both cruciate ligaments and locks the knee such that any movement of the tibia on the femur is minimized and the tibia is in the position of maximal stability with respect to the femur.

Kinetics

Theoretically, the tibia has six degrees of freedom in relation to the femur. In practice, the dynamic and static constraints limit motion to sagittal rotation (flexion-extension) and minimize sagittal translation (AP translation), coronal rotation (varus-valgus), and rotation in the transverse plane (internal-external rotation). The range of motion normally allowed at the knee is limited by the forces developed by bony and joint surface congruity to prevent axial compressive displacement and, primarily, by the tensile strength of the ligaments augmented by muscle contraction to limit all other types of motion.

Ambulatory use of the lower extremity results in ground-reaction forces being transmitted through the tibia. The direction and magnitude of the moment created by these forces depends on the magnitude of the force and the distance of the force line from the instant center of rotation. In order to limit adverse motions of the knee, this externally-generated moment is to some extent counteracted by the moments generated by muscle contraction (Fig. 58). Muscle forces so generated in combination with the ground-reaction force create the joint-reaction force. If this joint-reaction force is perpendicular to the joint surfaces, only an increased joint compressive load results. If the joint-reaction force is not perpendicular to the joint surfaces, translation of the tibia on the femur will occur unless restrained by other passive soft-tissue structures. It is a combination of ligament-generated and joint-reaction load-sharing forces that resists these applied loads and limits the motions about the knee.

For example, the most stable position for the knee is full extension. Extension brings the flatter central (distal) femoral articular surface into contact with the tibial plateaus. This contact makes the joint surfaces more congruent, allowing body weight to be distributed over a greater surface area of the joint and menisci and providing greater resistance to shear. The bony shapes of the femoral condyles and tibial plateau create forces to resist translational motion, mainly when the joint reactive forces are compressive. The menisci, in association with their soft-tissue attachments to the tibia, are felt to also help limit femoral translation by acting as a buttress. This stabilizing buttress effect is even greater with increasing axial loads. An anteriorly directed force on the tibia produces greater displacement of the lateral tibial plateau than of the medial tibial plateau. This difference may be a reflection of the firmer fixation of the medial meniscus via the coronary and posterior oblique ligaments versus the greater mobility of the lateral meniscus and the less congruent surface of the lateral tibial plateau. In an ACL-deficient knee the posterior horns act as a buttress to prevent further anterior translation (Fig. 59). Stability in extension is augmented by increased tension in the collateral and cruciate ligaments as well as the posterior capsule. The knee is

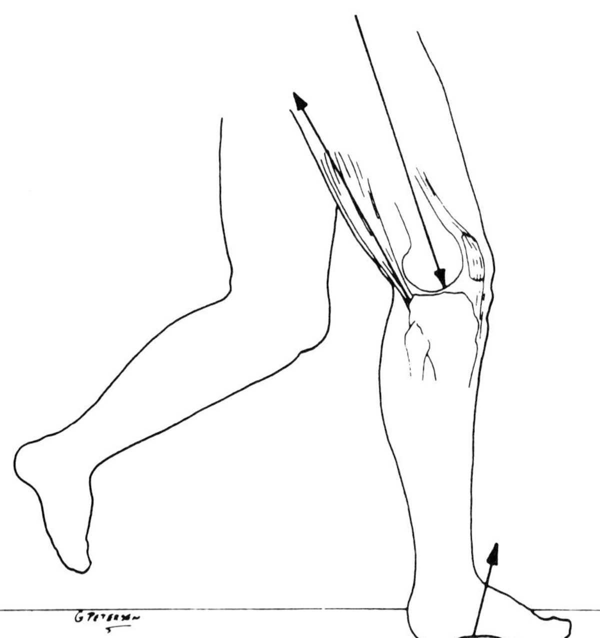

Figure 58
When the foot is in midstance, the foot-floor reaction lies anterior to the bone joint. This force tends to extend the knee and is resisted by muscle forces that tend to flex the knee. These forces in combination require a joint reaction force on the tibial plateau, which is located in the anterior region of the plateau. (Reproduced with permission from Daniel DM, Akeson WH, O'Connor JJ (eds): *Knee Ligaments: Structure, Function, Injury, and Repair.* New York, Raven Press, 1990, p 44.)

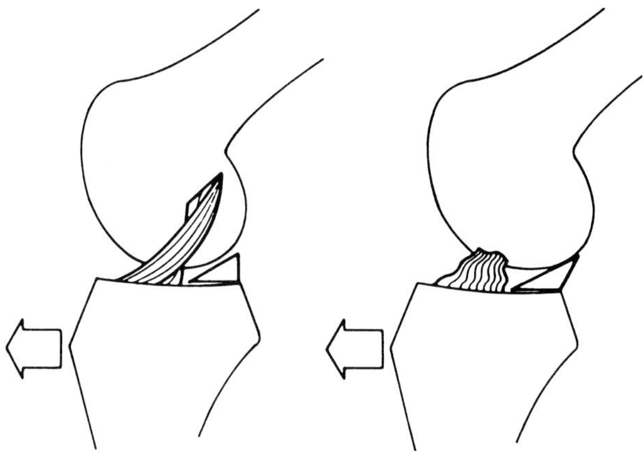

Figure 59
Left, With an intact anterior cruciate ligament (ACL), forward translation of the tibia stops before contact with the medial meniscus. **Right,** However, with disruption of the ACL, the posterior horn contacts the femoral condyle and acts as a wedge that resists further anterior tibial translation. (Reproduced with permission from Levy IM, Torzilli PA, Warren RF: The effect of medial meniscectomy on anterior-posterior motion of the knee. *J Bone Joint Surg* 1982;64A:883–888.)

further stabilized during standing by gravity, and with the center of gravity lying anterior to the knee joint, the entire posterior capsule offers resistance to hyperextension.

Specific restraints Conceptually, the same interplay between the various soft tissues about the knee exists regardless of the nature of rotational forces present and the position of the knee. However, over the past decade, a concept of primary and secondary ligamentous restraints has been developed to explain how the soft tissues about the knee provide shared forces to restrict motion and maintain joint stability. By sectioning knee ligaments and measuring the resultant motion, then varying the order of sectioning, the relative importance of specific ligaments in preventing abnormal motion can be identified. The ligament with the greatest role in preventing motion is designated as the primary restraint, those with a less important role are considered secondary restraints.

AP translation, four-bar cruciate linkage, and the roll-glide mechanism The ACL is the primary restraint to anterior translation. The deep MCL (middle medial capsule) is a major secondary restraint. The primary restraint to posterior translation is the PCL. The LCL, posterolateral capsule, and superficial MCL are minor secondary restraints. Contraction of the tensor fascia lata has questionable significance.

The rotation of the tibia about the femur in the sagittal plane can be described by a four-bar mechanical linkage system. In this model, the two ligamentous links are the ACL and PCL. The two bony links are the lines connecting the ACL and PCL attachments on the femur as well as their attachments on the tibia (Fig. 60). The femoral link roughly describes the roof of the intercondylar notch. Computer simulation studies of this four-bar linkage system have shown how the femur can roll and slide on the tibia and still allow full flexion and extension while not creating undue compressive force across the articular surfaces. Each of the cruciate ligaments as a whole is isometric during the arc of motion, although no single fiber of the cruciate ligament may be truly isometric. Thus, none of the four bars in the linkage change in length during flexion and extension of the knee, but the geometric angle between the bars does change. It can be shown that in full extension, the ACL is nearly parallel with the roof of the intercondylar notch or femoral link, whereas in full flexion, the PCL link is nearly parallel with the femoral link. During 140° of flexion, the ACL moves through an angle of approximately 100° with respect to its femoral link and approximately 40° with respect to the tibial link. During 140° of knee flexion, the PCL moves through

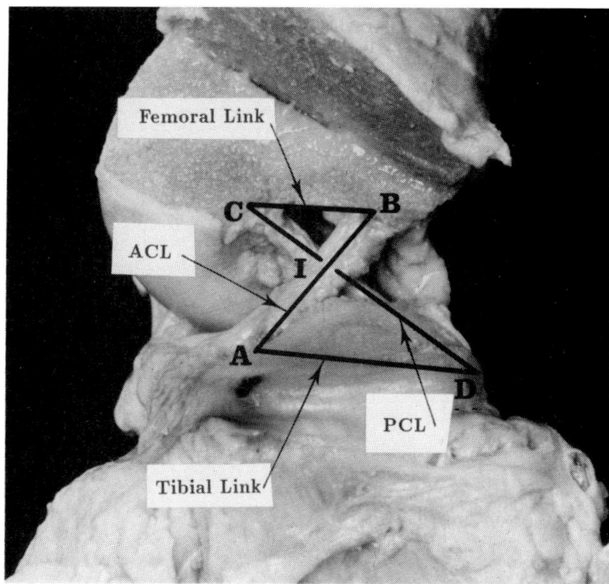

Figure 60
A human knee with the lateral femoral condyle removed, exposing the cruciate ligaments. Superimposed is a diagram of a four-bar linkage comprising the anterior cruciate ligament (ACL) AB, the posterior cruciate ligament (PCL) CD, the femoral link CB joining the ligament attachment points on the femur, and the tibial link AD joining their attachment points on the tibia. (Reproduced with permission from O'Connor J, Shercliffe T, FitzPatrick D, et al: Geometry of the knee, in Daniel DM, Akeson WH, O'Connor JJ (eds): *Knee Ligaments: Structure, Function, Injury, and Repair.* New York, Raven Press, 1990, pp 163–169.)

an arc of approximately 100° with respect to the femoral link and 40° with respect to the tibial link.

The center of rotation (or instant center) in the four-bar linkage model is where the two cruciate ligament links cross. Because both cruciates pass through the instantaneous axis of rotation and not anterior or posterior to it, they are unable to generate a flexion or extension moment in the knee during normal range of motion (Fig. 61, left). Although the cruciates are unable to produce a rotational force in the sagittal plane, they do play a major role in restraining translation in this plane. Because neither the ACL nor the PCL is parallel to the tibial surface, they resist AP translation in two ways. The component of the resultant tension force in these ligaments provides a force that directly resists translation. In addition, the component of the ACL resultant force vector perpendicular to the tibia produces a compressive force that increases joint congruency (Fig. 61, *right*). It is the ligamentous four-bar linkage mechanism of the knee that differentiates the kinetics and kinematics of the knee as being largely influenced by ligamentous restraints in contrast to the hip joint in which bony geometry plays the major role.

With any given four-bar linkage system, a multitude of articular surfaces for a femur and tibia

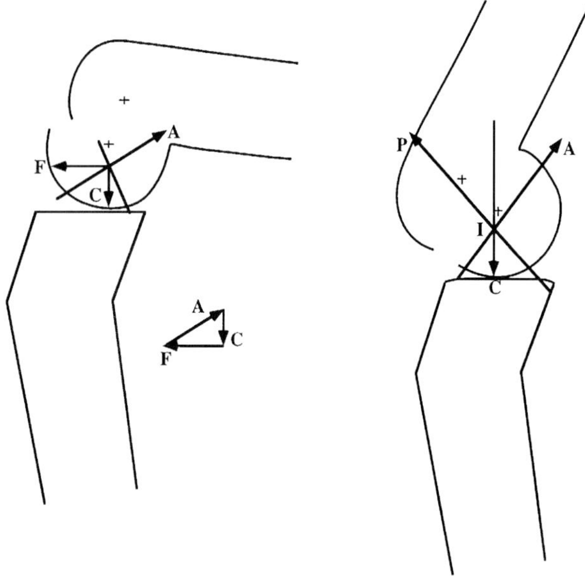

Figure 61
The cruciate ligament forces A and P and the tibiofemoral contact force C intersect at the flexion axis I. They have no moment about that axis. (Reproduced with permission from Daniel DM, Akeson WH, O'Connor (eds): *Knee Ligaments: Structure, Function, Injury and Repair.* New York, NY, Raven Press, 1990, p 202.)

could be designed that would be compatible with a functional roll-glide mechanism. Once an arbitrary articular surface replacement or new four-bar linkage system has been designed for one side of the joint, the geometry of the four-bar linkage system will describe the appropriate corresponding movement of the articulating surfaces. Each of these different articular contours for a given four-bar linkage may describe a different roll-glide ratio during the arc of motion.

Varus-valgus The LCL is the primary restraint to varus angulation. Because it is located posterior to the axis of flexion-extension rotation, it is tightest in extension and relaxes with flexion beyond 30°. In extension, the fibers of the iliotibial band are probably the most important lateral stabilizers. The posterolateral capsule is the major secondary restraint. The superficial and deep MCL are the primary restraints to valgus angulation. Increasing tension in the MCL is a manifestation of the geometry of the femoral condyles and origin of the collateral ligaments. The tension in the MCL increases beyond a certain flexion angle as the distance between the origin and insertion increases. With knee flexion, the femur and proximal end of the superficial MCL translate posteriorly relative to the proximal tibia. As flexion progresses, the anterior fibers of the superficial MCL develop increased tension, whereas the obliquely oriented posterior fibers show decreased strain. With loss of either of these two ligaments, secondary restraints to varus-valgus stresses come from the cruciate ligaments.

Internal-external rotation The superficial and deep MCL are the primary restraints to internal rotation of the tibia on the femur. The ACL is a secondary restraint. The LCL and posterolateral capsule are the primary restraints to external rotation. The PCL is a major secondary restraint.

Dynamic restraints As the knee moves through a given arc of motion, forces acting across the knee constantly change. In addition, the magnitude of forces acting on the knee for a given knee motion varies greatly with the specific activity involved. For example, forces acting on the knee during supine knee extension are different from the forces generated during a squat or a running jump. Such requirements mandate constant changes in muscle activity for the 14 muscles that cross the knee joint.

In each case, the dynamic action of the muscles occurs in conjunction with the static ligamentous restraints. An obvious example of this muscle-ligament interaction is the effect of the knee flexor-extensor muscle groups on anterior and posterior tibial translation. Anterior knee translation is strongly influenced by the quadriceps muscles. When the quadriceps contract to extend the knee, they create a line of force along their tendinous insertion into the tibia. There is one angle for each muscle in each knee at which the tendon's force is perpendicular to the tibial plateau and no translational force is created. This angle has been termed the critical angle. For the quadriceps, this is approximately 70° to 80° of flexion. When this angle is less acute, the tendon's force will have an anterior component directed at creating anterior tibial translation. This force will be counteracted by the component of the tensile forces developed in the ACL parallel to the tibial plateau as well as by a joint contact force. Similarly, when the knee is flexed, the hamstrings exert a large posteriorly-directed translational force with contraction counteracted by the PCL; the gastrocnemius can also be effective in creating posterior femoral translation, which is counteracted by the ACL. The force is greatest with marked knee flexion.

When knee extension is created by activity of the quadriceps, anterior translation of the tibia occurs during the terminal 45° of active extension. This translation shifts the starting point of the surface contact point and instant center posteriorly, resulting in an initial increased quadriceps lever arm. Correspondingly, as the hamstrings pull the tibia posteriorly, moving the initial surface contact point and instant center anteriorly, the lever arm and mechanical advantage of the hamstrings are increased at the inception of knee flexion. This ability of the human knee to shift its instant center anteriorly and posteriorly to increase or decrease the moment arm of the extensors or flexors decreases the magnitude of muscle force required to overcome the externally applied load, and results in a reduction in joint compressive and shear loads when it is most needed. It would seem that this phenomenon is important both in energy and muscle efficiency as well as in protecting the joint from excessive loads.

If a functional externally applied load to the lower extremity produces a flexion moment at the knee, this rotational force will be counterbalanced by a quadriceps contraction. This phenomenon occurs, for example, during the initiation of stance phase in walking or running, where the ground-reaction force is located posterior to the knee joint. If the knee is flexed less than its critical angle, the patella tendon force will also produce an anteriorly directed vector on the tibia, resulting in adverse shear stress at the joint. Cocontraction of the knee flexor and extensor muscles is the primary mode of dynamic knee stabilization to external flexion-extension, as well as to the concomitant varus-valgus and internal-external rotational forces. This cocontraction maintains stability of the joint during times of marked changes in stresses. However, as stated earlier, the passive ligamentous contribution to stability in these directions is clinically more important. At footstrike and early stance phase, the knee progresses from about 10° to about 15° to 20° of flexion, with the body's weight tending to be directed posterior to the knee joint. Both the hamstrings and quadriceps muscle groups are active at this time. Such activity has the overall effect of increasing the joint's reactive force and, hence, the importance of static components, such as the bony congruence and the buttress effect of the menisci, in providing joint stability. It is important to realize that this complex interplay of joint reaction and muscle and tendon forces occurs in all three planes simultaneously and that this interplay is different at each position of the tibia on the femur.

The ability of muscle contraction to stabilize the knee is readily apparent to anyone who has tried to evaluate an acute knee-ligament injury. Involuntary muscle contraction or spasm may minimize abnormal anterior translation when stress is applied to an ACL-deficient knee, limiting the usefulness of the Lachman test. Likewise, inability of the subject to relax his or her muscles during knee arthrometer testing is the major cause of spurious ligament laxity measurements.

Patellofemoral Joint

The patellofemoral joint is important to knee stability primarily through its role in the extensor mechanism. The patella increases the mechanical advantage of the extensor muscles by transmitting the force across the knee at a greater distance (moment) from the axis of rotation. Stability of the patella in the trochlear groove is a function of bony, ligamentous, and muscular components.

The patella is a sesamoid bone in the quadriceps tendon, which increases the functional lever arm of the quadriceps as well as changing the direction of the pull of the quadriceps mechanism. The patella articulates with the trochlear groove of the femoral condyle as it slides a distance of approximately 7 cm from full extension to full flexion. Geometric congruence between the patella and femoral trochlea varies during the flexion arc. In addition, there is considerable anatomic variation at the patellofemoral joint. Significant patellofemoral contact does not occur until approximately 20° of flexion, and "capture" of the patella between the trochlear ridges may require even more flexion.The contact area in the trochlear groove moves from proximal to distal as the knee flexes. On the patella, the contact point moves distal to proximal with knee flexion. At greater than 90° of flexion, the quadriceps tendons start to contact the trochlear articular surface. Individuals with abnormalities of the bony architecture, such as patella alta, a flat trochlear groove, or hypoplastic lateral condyles, are predisposed to instability.

The role of the patella in increasing the quadriceps muscle lever arm varies depending on the degree of knee flexion. In full flexion, when the patella is entirely in the intercondylar notch, it increases the lever arm of the quadriceps by only 10%. As the knee starts to come into extension, the patella's contribution to the extensor lever arm increases until approximately 45° of flexion, at which the patella lengthens the lever arm by approximately 30%. From 45° of flexion to full extension, the patella's contribution to the lever arm slowly decreases. Study results have indicated that greater quadriceps muscle force was required for the last 15° of knee extension.

The patellofemoral joint reaction force is determined not only by the magnitude of the quadriceps contraction, but also by the amount of knee flexion at the time of the contracture. When the leg is positioned horizontally to eliminate the effect of gravity, as the knee is extended from 90° of flexion to 0° and the quadriceps is used to pull against a constant resistance applied to the distal tibia, quadriceps muscle force increases and the joint reaction force decreases. Normal walking has been estimated to create joint compressive forces of approximately one half body weight. Walking upstairs increases joint compression loads to between 2.5 to 3.3 times body weight, and doing deep-knee bends produces loads up to seven to eight times body weight across this joint. The articular cartilage of the patella is one of the thickest in the body in order to accommodate these great compressive loads.

Structure and Function of the Foot and Ankle

Introduction

The ankle and foot have long been thought of as an unsophisticated appendage that joins the leg to the ground. While the foot may have fewer functions than the hand, in many respects its intricate construction and complex dynamic organization, which provide shock absorption, stability, and propulsion for the body during upright posture and ambulation, are more elaborate than those of the hand.

Ground-reaction forces are a response to the muscular actions and the weight of the body transmitted through the feet. As the foot hits the ground during bipedal locomotion, forces transmitted to the foot begin at the heel, rapidly shift to the entire foot, dwell there during mid-support, and then rapidly move to the forefoot and end at the medial aspect of the forefoot as the leg ends stance and prepares for swing. The direction of the ground-reaction force varies as stance phase progresses. Up and down oscillations of the vertical-reaction force occur during stance as the body decelerates and then accelerates. Changes in the horizontal shear reaction forces correlate with progressional and lateral accelerations of the eccentrically placed body and provide additional force to initiate and bring to an end periods of locomotion and to change the speed or direction of walking. At the initiation of stance, the supporting foot is ahead of the body's center of mass, requiring a backward shear as well as vertical force to brake the movement of the foot and absorb shock. As the body passes medially over the supporting foot, lateral shear forces persist; fore-aft shear forces drop to zero, then are directed forward as the body's center of mass moves ahead of the foot. As the horizontal distance between the supporting foot and the body's center of mass increases, an increase in walking speed, which normally increases both the step length and width (distance between the right and left feet), results in an increase in the peaks of all components of the ground-reaction forces. Changes in functional activities (running, jumping, and stair climbing) or terrain will also alter the magnitude, direction, and primary location of these forces on the foot.

Thus, for proper function, the foot and ankle must withstand high loads at different times and locations during various body speeds, changes of direction, and conditions of terrain. It successfully performs this task by forming a kinematic chain with the lower leg. This chain transmits forces and motions in the sagittal direction via translations and rotations, the axes of which are not in the body's orthogonal axes. Furthermore no true hinge joints exist in the foot; rather, through the constrained and unconstrained interaction of 26 bones, 21 functional joints, 30 muscles, and over 100 ligaments, the foot and ankle illustrate how form is dictated by function.

The Ankle Joint

General Description

The ankle joint consists of the saddle-shaped lower end of the tibia and fibula, and its inferior transverse ligament encloses the superior aspect of the body of the talus (the trochlea) (Fig. 62). The tibial surface forming the superior dome of the ankle is concave sagittally, is slightly convex from side to side, and is oriented about 93° from the long axis of the tibia (is higher on the lateral than the medial

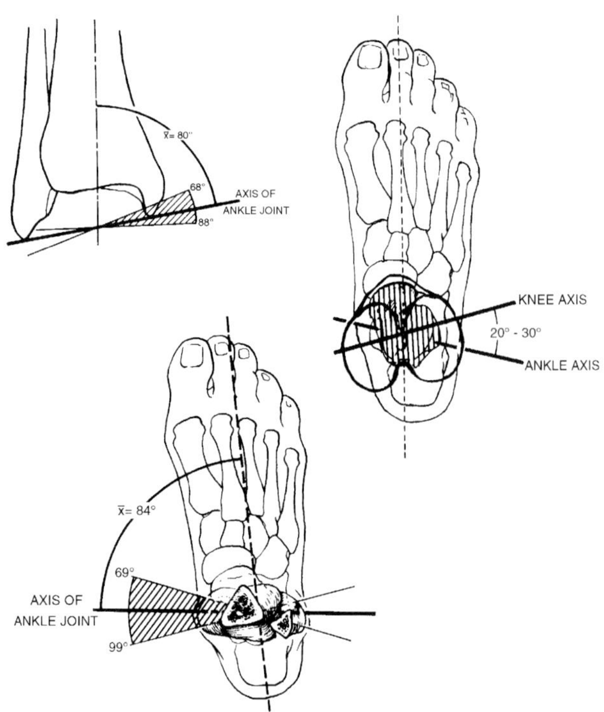

Figure 62
Top left, Variations in the frontal axis of the ankle joint. **Top right,** Relationship of the knee and ankle axes. **Bottom,** Relationship of the ankle axis to the long axis of the foot. (Reproduced with permission from Mann RA: Biomechanics of the foot, in *American Academy of Orthopaedic Surgeons: Atlas of Orthotics,* ed 2. St. Louis, MO, CV Mosby, 1985.)

side). The shape of the cavity formed by the tibiofibular mortise appears to match closely that of the upper articulating surfaces of the talus. The superior part of the body of the talus (trochlea) is wedge-shaped; it is about one-fourth wider in front than behind, with an average difference of 2.4 ± 1.3 mm and a maximal difference of 6 mm. From front to back, the articular surface spans an arc of about 105°. This surface contour has been likened to a section or rostrum of a cone, having a smaller diameter medially than laterally.

The primary motion of the ankle joint is dorsiflexion-plantarflexion (Table 17). Its axis of rotation is obliquely oriented with respect to all three anatomic planes. Passing through the inferior tips of the malleoli, the axis extends from anterior, superior, and medial to inferior, posterior, and lateral. It is at angles of 93° with respect to the long axes of the tibia and about 11.5° to the joint surface. However, rather than a true single IAR, the ankle has been noted to have multiple instant centers, all of which fall very close to a single point within the body of the talus. Through a complete arc of ankle rotation, the center may shift anywhere from 4 to 7 mm. Because the axis of rotation is obliquely oriented to the sagittal, coronal, and transverse planes, translation of the talus in the mortise can occur in all three directions.

The talus has been observed in vitro to rotate easily in the ankle mortise implying relative movement between the malleoli. Because the trochlea is wider anteriorly than posteriorly, some believe that lateral play of the talus within its mortise occurs only when the ankle is in plantarflexion. Others believe that instability exists in dorsiflexion, while still others believe that with intact ligaments translation occurs only in the sagittal direction. These differences can be explained by behavior of the ligaments and by the roles played by the subtalar joint, the kinematic chain of the hindfoot, and the muscles that traverse this area in transmitting forces across this area during plantarflexion and dorsiflexion.

The talus is unique because this bone, which lies between the foot and the leg, contains no muscular attachments and has seven articulations that connect it to four other bones. The stability of the talus and its articulations, therefore, relies heavily on the ligamentous attachments and musculotendinous complexes that traverse the talus and attach distally. Passive stability of the ankle joint, thus, results from a variety of factors. First is the bony stability provided by contact of the trochlea with the tibial plafond. Second are the medial and lateral cartilaginous slightly concave surfaces that articulate with the two malleoli. Third are the ligamentous connections between the tibia, fibula, talus, and calcaneus.

Ligaments of the Ankle Joint

The ankle joint has a fibrous capsule that encircles the joint completely and is thickened laterally. The posterior and anterior tibiofibular ligament (Fig. 63) attaches the fibula to the tibia to strengthen the tibiofibular syndesmosis. The origin of the posterior tibiofibular ligament is broad, covering most of the horizontal distal surface of the tibia. As the

Table 17
Type and position of the axis of rotation for the ankle

Investigators	Position with respect to the anatomic planes		
	Frontal	**Sagittal**	**Transverse**
Elftman (1945)		67.6° ± 7.4°	
Isman and Inman (1969)		84° ± 7°	10° ± 4°
	8 mm anterior, 3 mm inferior to the distal tip of the lateral malleolus to 1 mm posterior, 5 mm inferior to the distal tip of the medial malleolus		
Inman and Mann (1979)		78° ± 12°	
Allard and associates (1987)	95.4° ± 6.6°	77.7° ± 12.3°	17.9° ± 4.5°
Parlasca and associates (1979)	96% within 12 mm of a point 20 mm below the articular surface of the tibia along the long axis		
Hicks (1953)	Dorsiflexion: 5 mm inferior to tip of lateral malleolus to 15 mm anterior to tip of medial malleolus		
	Plantarflexion: 5 mm superior to tip of lateral malleolus to 15 mm anterior, 10 mm inferior to tip of medial malleolus		

(Adapted with permission from Allard P, Stokes IA, Salathe EP, et al: Modeling of the foot and ankle, in Jahss MH (ed): *Disorders of the Foot and Ankle: Medical and Surgical Management,* ed 2. Philadelphia, WB Saunders, 1991, pp 432–468.)

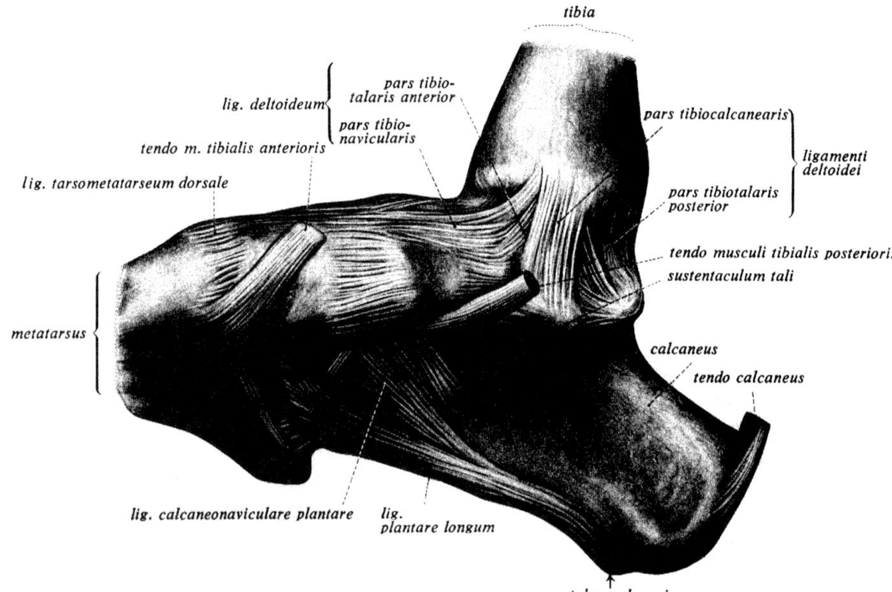

Figure 63
Ligaments of the ankle and foot. (Reproduced with permission from Figge FHJ: *Atlas of Human Anatomy: Vol. I. Atlas of Bones, Joints, and Muscles.* New York, Hafner, 1968.)

ligament fibers sweep laterally and distally to insert on the fibula they fit over the trochlea. The deltoid (medial collateral) ligament is a strong triangular ligament made up of superficial and deep components that arise from the anterior, distal, and posterior borders of the medial malleolus (Fig. 64). The superficial portion consists of three parts; the tibionavicular, tibiocalcaneal (inserting onto the sustentaculum tali of the calcaneus), and posterior tibiotalar ligaments. The deep portion consists only of the anterior tibiotalar ligament.

From the lateral malleolus, three ligaments fan out to provide stability. The relatively weak anterior talofibular ligament passes from the anterior surface of the fibula malleolus to the talus. The calcaneofibular ligament, which is attached proximally to the lateral malleolus and distally to the tubercle of the lateral surface of the calcaneus, is long and strong, resembling a collateral ligament of other hinged joints. The posterior talofibular ligament runs horizontally from the posterior process of the talus to the posterior process of the fibula malleolus.

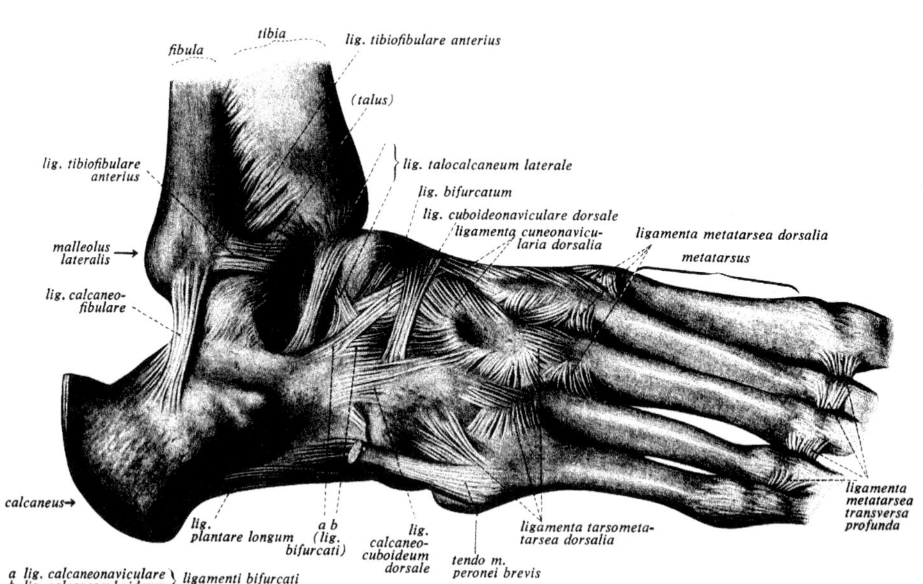

Figure 64
Ligaments of the foot. (Reproduced with permission from Figge FHJ: *Atlas of Human Anatomy: Vol. I. Atlas of Bones, Joints, and Muscles.* New York, Hafner, 1968.)

Thus, of seven ligaments arising from the two malleoli, only four connect to the talus, and none of these four are the strongest ligaments surrounding the ankle joint. The other three ligaments connect more distally to the calcaneus, and are the strongest. This structure has led to the concept that the subtalar joint must be considered a constrained joint and its inversion-eversion movements are integrally involved in the stability of the ankle. This concept will be discussed further after the stability of the foot is described.

Stabilizing Mechanisms of The Foot

Arches of the Foot

The longitudinal vault structure of the foot is considered to be built up by medial and lateral longitudinal arch systems (Fig. 65). The lateral arch system, the lower and shorter one, is composed of the calcaneus, the cuboid, and two lateral rays. This system is the more stable, weightbearing portion of the arch; it carries the longer and higher medial arch system, which consists of the calcaneus, talus, navicular, cuneiforms, and three medial rays. Both arches are prolonged into the five shorter kinematic chains of the toes. A transverse arch configured by the shape of the midtarsal bones (cuneiforms and cuboid) and the bases of the metatarsals is also described. A second transverse arch is suggested to exist at the metatarsal heads when no weight is being borne; it does not exist during weightbearing.

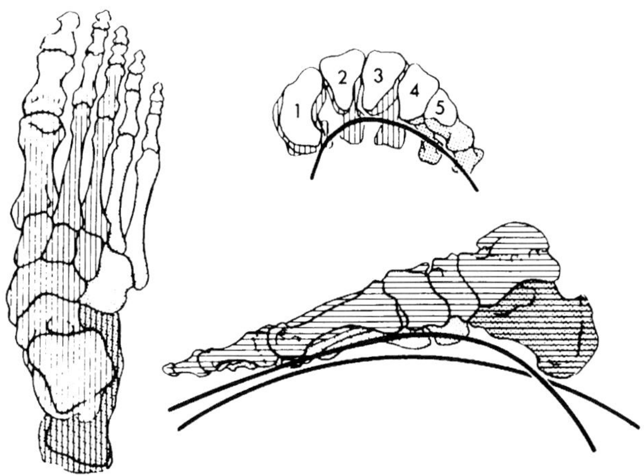

Figure 65
The arches of the foot. **Left,** The medial longitudinal arch (lines) is the active portion of the arch. The lateral longitudinal arch (stippled) is the static portion of the arch. The calcaneus is common to both arches. **Top right,** Curvature of the transverse arch. **Bottom right,** Curves of the medial and lateral longitudinal arches. (Reproduced with permission from Mann R, Inman VT: Structure and function, in DuVries HL (ed): *Surgery of the Foot,* ed 2. St. Louis, MO, CV Mosby, 1965.)

The longitudinal arch is not intrinsically stable owing to the shape of the bones and their intervening joints; it is, in fact, stabilized by heavy ligamentous structures surrounding the joints. This arch is reduced somewhat during weightbearing. However, for short periods, the tension developed in the large mass of ligamentous structure on the plantar surface of the foot can protect it from completely collapsing. EMG studies performed during quiet standing reveal minimal to no activity of intrinsic muscles.

Plantar Aponeurosis

The longitudinal arch is passively stabilized further by the plantar aponeurosis. The plantar aponeurosis arises from the tubercle of the calcaneus, passes distally, and inserts into the base of the proximal phalanges of all the toes. Classically, its mechanism of action has been described as a windlass type. This aponeurosis is most functional on the medial side of the foot; excision of the proximal phalanx or the metatarsal heads causes loss of its function. The breaking load of the aponeurosis varies between 1.7 and 3.4 times body weight, depending on which toe insertion is broken.

If stance is simulated by applying a downward force to the tibia and an upward force in the Achilles tendon, it has been suggested that the applied load is carried partially by a bending moment in the tarsometatarsal arch and partially by tension in the plantar aponeurosis. The plantar aponeurosis may account for about one-quarter of the applied load. If the plantar aponeurosis is divided, at least three times body weight can be supported by the bony ligamentous arch without damage to the metatarsal bones or attachments.

Dynamic Support

The intrinsic muscles of the foot, like the plantar aponeurosis, help stabilize the longitudinal arch. The flexor digitorum brevis helps to stabilize both the medial and lateral arches; the abductor hallucis and abductor digiti minimi help stabilize the medial arch and the lateral arch, respectively. Thus, when the toes are forced into dorsiflexion, this enhances the function of the plantar aponeurosis and the intrinsic muscles.

The flexor hallucis longus and flexor digitorum longus (extrinsic muscles) do not directly stabilize the arch. These muscles help to produce inversion of the heel and to maintain the ankle in plantarflexion. However, contributions from the posterior and anterior tibialis and the peroneus longus may serve a more direct function in maintaining the arch. Tendons from these muscles run parallel to the ligaments and insert in an area of the first cuneiform and base of the first metatarsal. By enveloping its medial, plantar, and lateral aspects, they strongly assist in constraining movement of the proximal half of the foot. The peroneus longus, and the slip of the posterior tibialis inserting onto the cuboid, in association with the oblique and transverse heads of the adductor hallucis brevis, maintain the transverse arch and stabilize the link between the medial and longitudinal arches. Added support of the arch can be obtained by small rotations of the individual joints via external rotation of the tibia, inversion of the calcaneus, and adduction of the forefoot.

Kinematics and Kinetics of the Foot

The axis of rotation of the subtalar joint is obliquely oriented (Fig 66). The joint forms angles of about 41° to the horizontal in the sagittal plane and 23° to the midline axis of the foot in the transverse plane. Forces transmitted across this joint, thus, tend to create inversion with slight plantarflexion and adduction or eversion with slight dorsiflexion and abduction with respect to orthogonal axes about the tibia. However, translational motions occur with rotational motions about this joint. As high as a 10-mm lateral shift in the axis has been noted between maximum eversion and inversion, resulting in variations of up to 13° with respect to the position of the rotational axis. Although this shift suggests a variable axis rather than a fixed one, there is still controversy about whether its movement is about a hinge or a screw-like mechanism.

The transverse tarsal joints lying distal to the subtalar joint are two joints that form a continuous line across the foot. Medially and superiorly, the talonavicular joint can be characterized as a ball-and-socket joint that has considerable rotational mobility (Fig. 67). Inversion-eversion induces the greatest rotation in this joint. Laterally and inferiorly, the calcaneocuboid joint can be classified as a saddle joint that allows mostly translation.

Proximally, the plantar calcaneonavicular (spring) ligament is the most important ligament supporting the medial arch (Fig. 68). The short and long plantar ligaments, the strongest ligaments of the foot, connect the calcaneus, cuboid, and lateral metatarsals. Predominantly vertically oriented fibers that belong not only to the talocalcaneal ligaments, but also to the tarsal crural ligaments keep the

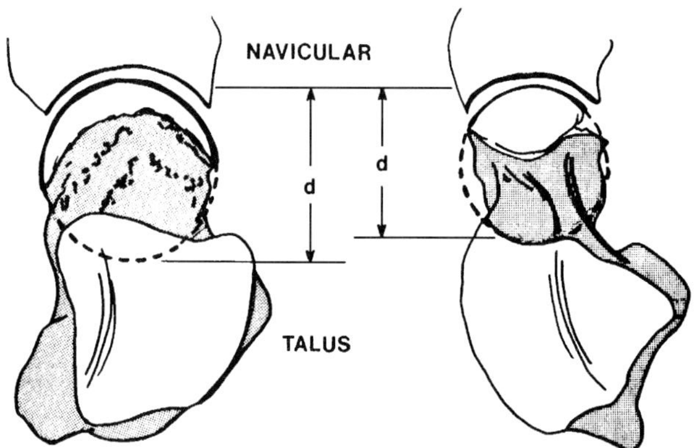

Figure 67
Superior view **(left)** and lateral view **(right)** of the relationship of the head of the talus to the navicular bone showing differing diameters of the head of the talus.

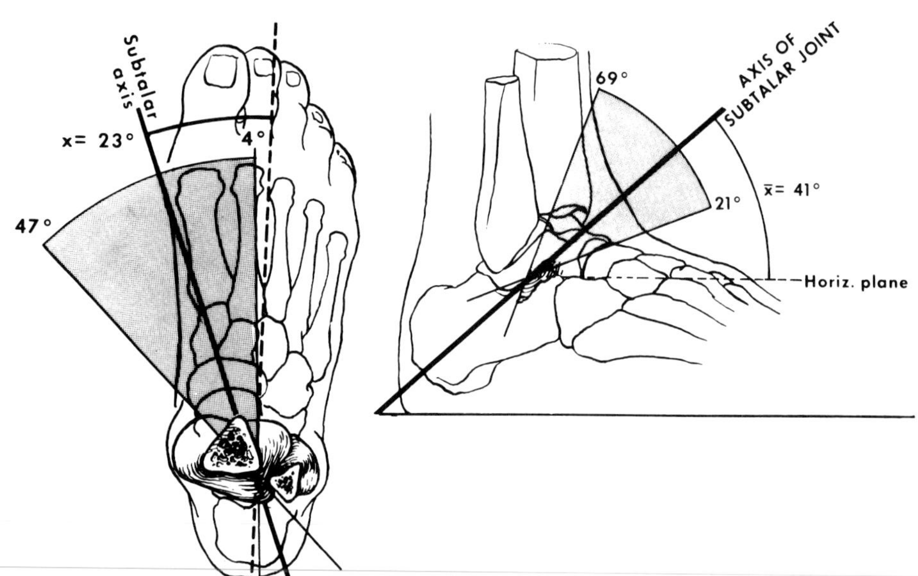

Figure 66
Variations in the axes of the subtalar joint. **Left,** Transverse plane. **Right,** Horizontal plane. (Reproduced with permission from Mann RA: Biomechanics of the foot, in *American Academy of Orthopaedic Surgeons: Atlas of Orthotics,* ed 2. St. Louis, MO, CV Mosby, 1985.)

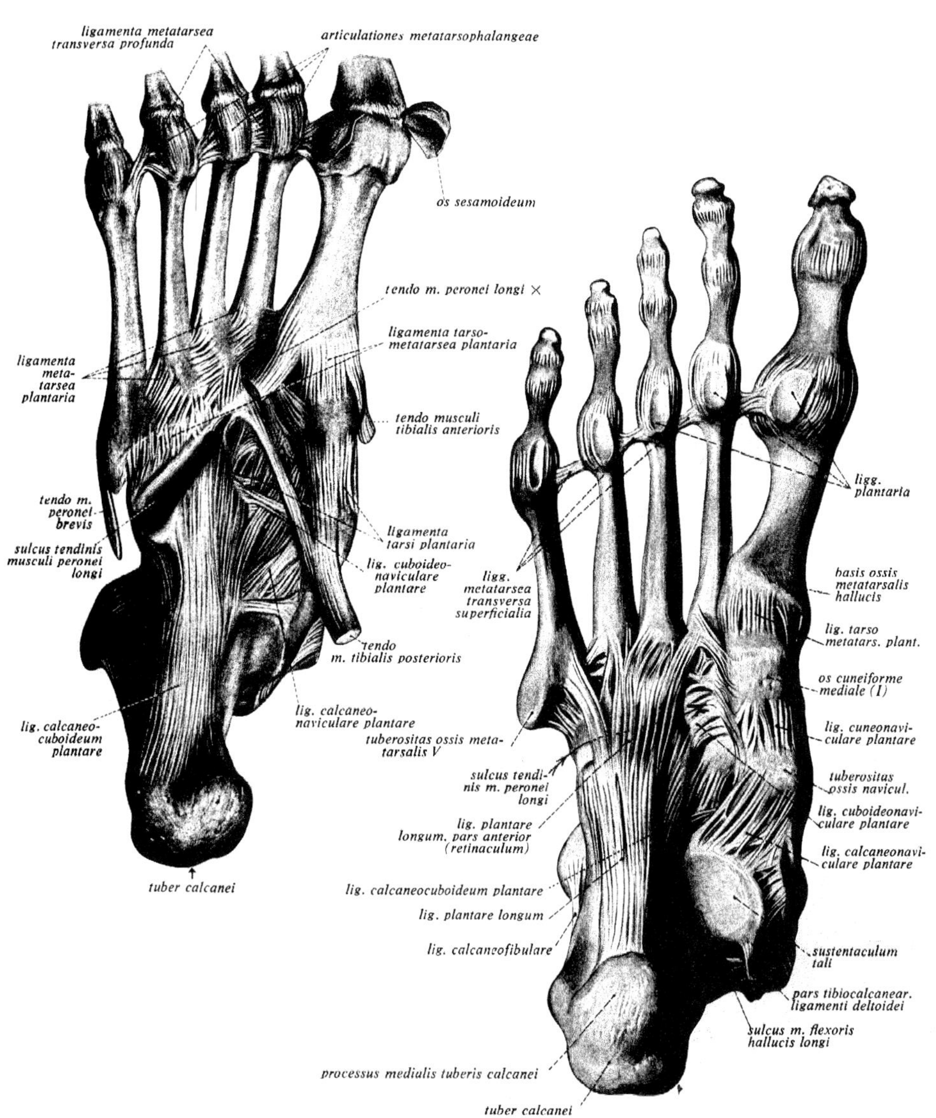

Figure 68
Left, Ligaments of the foot and ankle. **Right,** Ligaments of the plantar surface of the foot. (Reproduced with permission from Figge FHJ: *Atlas of Human Anatomy: Vol. I. Atlas of Bones, Joints, and Muscles.* New York, Hafner, 1968.)

medial and lateral arches together where the medial arch is mounted on the lateral arch. Oblique and some transverse fibers, especially in the region of the navicular, cuboid, and cuneiform bones and at the bases of the metatarsals, keep the parallel rows of the arch systems together.

In the proximal part of the foot composed of the tarsal bones, the static longitudinal arch system is integrated kinematically into what can be called a closed kinematic chain with interdependent movements at the different joints. The mechanical coupling of the talus, calcaneus, cuboid, and navicular as a result of their arrangement in a closed kinematic chain is known as the tarsal mechanism. The ligaments surrounding these joints, especially horizontal fibers of the talofibular ligament, are crucial structural elements in this mechanism.

During activities of daily living, motions at these joints are induced primarily by varus-valgus ground-reaction force and forces tending to rotate the lower leg in internal-external rotation. The transverse rotation of the leg alone or in combination with sideward swaying motions is converted by the tarsal mechanism into inversion-eversion motions of the foot.

These rotational as well as dorsiflexion-plantarflexion motions are transmitted from the leg to the rest of the foot through a number of different but closely cooperating osteoligamentous mechanisms in addition to the tarsal mechanism. These mechanisms include: (1) the midtarsal mechanism; (2) the tarsometatarsal mechanism; and (3) the metatarsophalangeal mechanism.

Tarsal Mechanism

The subtalar and talo-navicular-calcaneo-cuboid joints are most involved with the mechanics of inversion and eversion. The navicular and cuboid bones move as a single unit, whereas the calcaneus articulates with both the talus and the cuboid navicular piece by means of separate hinges. Although this mechanism is structurally complex, it is routinely conceptualized mechanically as a simple hinge of the subtalar joint. In actuality, the axis of rotation of motions of these tarsal joints are best described as a fan-shaped or cone-shaped bundle of discrete axes representing the successive positions of a moving axis in reference to the subtalar joint. All of the axes have an oblique direction with respect to the foot.

In vivo the foot inverts in response to external rotation of the leg. Starting from a neutral position, this response has been found to be far more extensive than the limited eversion response to internal rotation. In addition, a delayed response of relative external rotation of the talus during external rotation of the leg occurs, resulting from a "lock" of the tarsal mechanism that prohibits further eversion.

Because no muscles can move the talus directly, forces transmitted through the contact surfaces and the ligaments of the talocrural joint must impose the input motion on the talus. The horizontally running fibers of the anterior talofibular ligament play a crucial role in bringing the talus into an external rotation, which is converted into inversion by the tarsal mechanism. Thus, in stance, via this mechanism the tibialis posterior is an effective invertor together with the flexor digitorum longus, whereas the peronei and the extensor digitorum longus have the opposite effect. Under these conditions, the tibialis anterior seems to be a less effective invertor. The abductor hallucis muscle is an example of an intrinsic foot muscle acting directly on the tarsal mechanism. Through its attachments toward distal elements and proximally to the calcaneus, it has a notable inversion effect.

These features support the clinical experience that patients with permanent ligament defect after injury may regain stable joint function through specific and careful muscle training. It has also been noted during the initial phase of external rotation of the tibia that the talus does not follow the tibia immediately, and this has been described as the tibial talar delay. This delay may be ascribed to a variable laxity in the horizontal talocrural ligament fibers and it is supposed that these fibers have to build up an initial tension before they can transmit the pulling forces from the leg to the talus. After this initial delay, talar rotation increases generally. In most cases, after having reached a plateau, talar rotation decreases again during the last phase of tibial rotation.

The anterior talofibular ligament thus plays an important role in talocrural transmission; this ligament permits different people to have different degrees of rotational motion. Joints with rather lax talocrural ligaments seem to be characterized by a delay that is greatest from 0° to 10° of external rotation of the tibia and increases with the increase of plantarflexion. Joints with rather stiff talocrural ligaments feature a delay that occurs mainly at the end of external rotation and especially in 25° to 30° of plantarflexion. Tibial talar delay can increase markedly after severing the anterior talofibular ligament with its adjacent capsular structures.

Ankle joint stability can now be viewed in light of this tarsal mechanism. One commonly accepted theory is that, because of the talar mechanism, ligaments play the following role during plantarflexion. The stability of the ankle is achieved mainly by the tibionavicular fibers of the deltoid and the lateral ligaments. The lateral ligaments maintain the intrinsic stability of the talus and its mortise by developing a fairly uniform ligamentous force about it. As plantarflexion occurs, all the lateral ligaments remain taut, and because of this passive talar mechanism, movement of inversion and adduction occurs. This movement is assisted dynamically in the early phases of gait by the intrinsic plantarflexors on the medial side of the ankle, which are active throughout stance as are all the extrinsic ankle and foot plantarflexors (Fig. 69).

Because of this talar mechanism, in the absence of muscular contracture the talus still cannot move freely in its mortise during passive plantarflexion. The anterior talofibular ligament and the similarly oriented fibers of the deltoid ligament are brought into tension during plantarflexion and contribute equally to ankle stability. In dorsiflexion, medial and lateral stretch of the middle and posterior ligamentous fibers plays the predominant role. The differences in ankle stability may thus be related to interpersonal variation in the strength of the ligaments and the orientation of the axes of rotational and translational motions of the ankle joint and tarsal mechanism.

Moreover, the tendons of the dorsiflexors, restrained in part by the inferior extensor retinaculum, have a horizontal force component preventing forward displacement of the talus. In plantarflexion, the posterior shift of the talus is limited by the lower tibial margin and the posterior talar-tibial and talofibular ligaments, as well as by possible external rotation of the fibula.

The Midtarsal Mechanism

The bones of the midtarsal area consist of the cuneiforms and the cuboid. Chopart's joint, the articular connection of these bones to the tarsal mechanism, shares a common synovial cavity that is continuous with the second and third cuneiform-metatarsal joints. The bones across these joints are connected by strong dorsal, plantar, and interosseous ligaments, making them relatively immovable with respect to each other. Forces and motions created proximal or distal to this unit thus

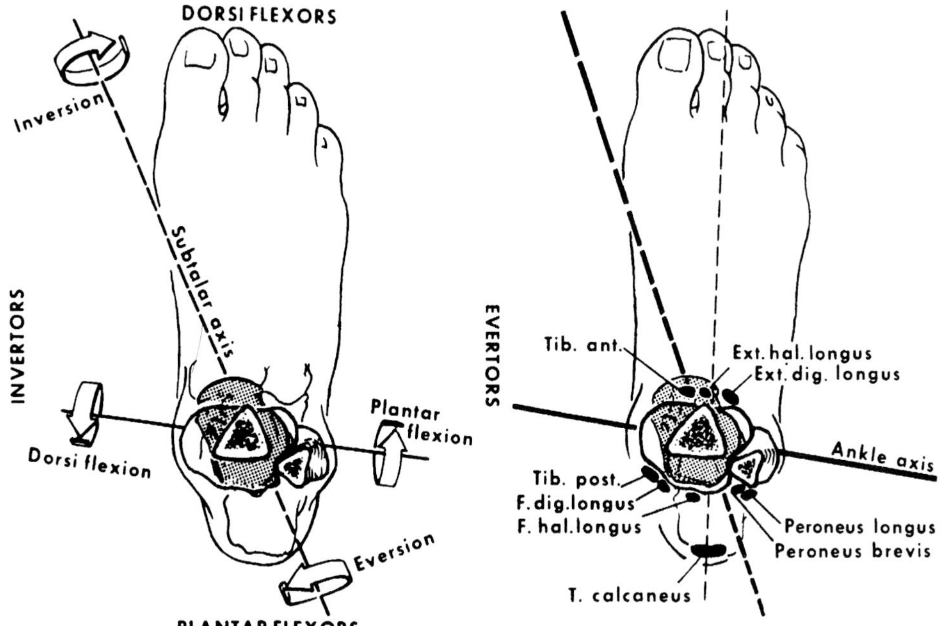

Figure 69
Left, Rotation occurs about the subtalar and ankle joint axes. **Right,** The relationship of the various muscles about the subtalar and ankle joint axes. (Reproduced with permission from Mann RA: Biomechanics of the foot, in *American Academy of Orthopaedic Surgeons: Atlas of Orthotics,* ed 2. St. Louis, MO, CV Mosby, 1985.)

may be considered to be transferred across it, unchanged by these constrained joints.

The Tarsometatarsal Mechanism

A single line of bones proximally, the longitudinal arch systems split up distally to form the most dynamic portion of the arch. In this part of the foot, the individual longitudinal tarsometatarsal chains can be moved in dorsal or plantar directions, more or less independently. Thus, the concept of the foot as a mobile weightbearing vault structure seems to be related predominantly to motion initiated at the tarsometatarsal joints and reflected in the distal part of the foot comprising the metatarsophalangeal joints.

A striking functional anatomic feature of the tarsometatarsal region is the relatively immobile connection of the second metatarsal to its surrounding tarsal bones; the other metatarsal bones are far more mobile. Because the base of the second metatarsal is "locked" in a socket formed by the cuneiform bones, the distal half of the foot can be twisted around the longitudinal axis formed by the second metatarsal (Fig. 70). This possible twisting mobility, which is seated mainly in the tarsometatarsal joints with a possible contribution from the talonavicular joint and calcaneocuboid joint, is known as the supination or pronation twist of the forefoot. This twisting change of shape of the metatarsal part of the foot is produced by small gliding motions with different ranges of each of the lateral three metatarsals and gliding and rotations of the first metatarsal in dorsal and plantar directions.

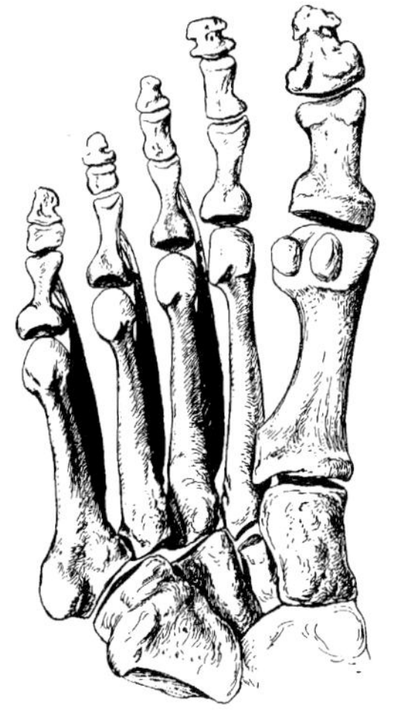

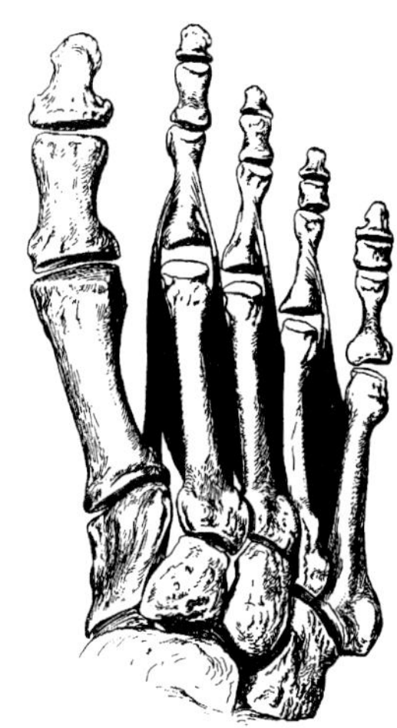

Figure 70
The interosseous muscles of the foot. **Left,** plantar. **Right,** dorsal. (Reproduced with permission from Figge FHJ: *Atlas of Human Anatomy: Vol. I. Atlas of Bones, Joints, and Muscles.* New York, Hafner, 1968.)

The asymmetry of the torsional tarsometatarsal mobility at both sides of the second metatarsal can be recognized in the structural relationships between the metatarsal heads. In this sense, there seems to be a principal difference between the connections between the first and second and between the second, third, fourth, and fifth metatarsals. Proximal interosseous ligaments and distal transversely running ligaments (the transverse metatarsal ligament) are found only between the heads of the second to the fifth metatarsals; they are absent between the first and second metatarsals. This is similar to the hand. Only the insertion of the transverse part of the adductor hallucis muscle provides an obvious anchorage of the first metatarsal to the other metatarsals distally. Moreover, the belly of the transverse adductor originates from the deep transverse metatarsal ligaments, and these origins are restricted to the spaces between metatarsals two, three, four, and five. These features allow greater mobility of the first metatarsal ray than of the lateral three and relative immobility of the second.

The Metatarsophalangeal Mechanism

The actively stabilized phalangeal arches of the toes are of paramount importance for proper function of both the support of the arch and the mechanism of pronation-supination of the forefoot. The five metatarsophalangeal joints together with their phalangeal chains form five separate nonconstrained mechanisms.

The stabilization of the multiarticulated chain occurring in each metatarsophalangeal joint and toe against external forces appears to be similar to that described for the hand. The flexor digitorum brevis and interossei, which are major force-generating structures at the end of stance, are essential to maintain the stability of this arch. The powerful abductor, adductor, and flexor hallucis brevis are present not only for stabilization of the first metatarsal joint, but also, by virtue of their far proximal origin, have a stabilizing effect on the metatarsal cuneiform connections and even more proximal joints. The proximal origin of the interossei, unlike those in the hand, is beyond the metatarsals from the tarsal ligamentous meshwork so that the pole of the interossei is transferred across the transmetatarsal joints. This structure suggests that the interossei are stabilizers of the forefoot rendering the tarsometatarsal joints rigid when weight is carried on the ball of the foot. An intrinsic minus foot, therefore, not only affects the metatarsal joints, but also deprives more proximal joints of a plantar stabilizing force.

Finally, the plantar aponeurosis bowstrings all three mechanisms and is connected to their bony parts as well as to the sole of the foot in an anatomically complex way. By its windlass action, it raises the longitudinal arches of the foot when the toes are dorsiflexed as well as stiffening the fibrous skeleton of the ball of the foot during push-off (Fig. 71). This effect is most evident in the medial arch and it also can be seen by dorsiflexion of the great toe. Because inversion of the tarsal mechanism leads mostly to a rise of the medial longitudinal arch, the use of this windlass mechanism is accompanied by a slight inversion of the tarsus and external rotation of the leg.

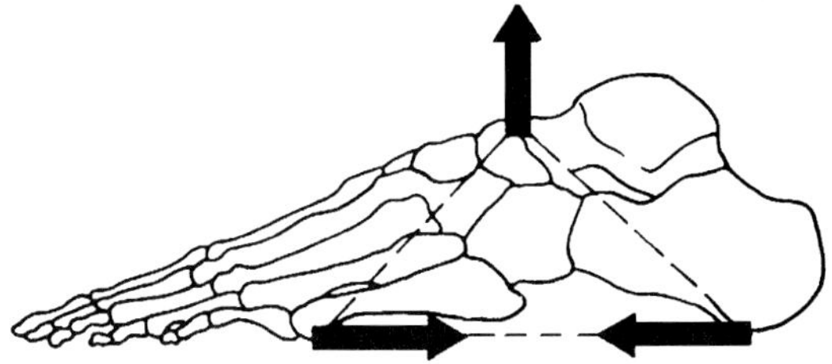

Figure 71
The intrinsic muscles of the foot, which stabilize the longitudinal arch of the foot and aid in the elevation of the arch along with the plantar aponeurosis. (Reproduced with permission from Saunders JBCM, Inman VT, Eberhart HD: The major determinants in normal and pathological gait. *J Bone Joint Surg* 1953;34A:552.)

Coordinated Functions

Control of Human Movement

Human movement and central nervous system (CNS) involvement in the control of skilled movements both have been active areas of research in recent years. Based on experimental results obtained using cats and apes, it is now accepted that commands for skilled voluntary movements are initiated from the higher centers of the CNS, descend the spinal pathways, and are decoded and executed at the muscle level. Proprioceptive feedback to the higher centers of the brain and the spinal cord is not considered essential to the performance of skilled movements. The propagation and synaptic delays involved in this process preclude the possibility of active closed-loop regulation in the course of normal movements. Such feedback is, however, useful in improving the learning proficiency of the movement or in situations in which unfamiliar movement conditions are encountered.

Spring-like behavior of the muscle plays an important role in the maintenance of posture and in the formation of movement trajectories. The muscle-joint system is dynamically similar to a mass-spring system with controllable equilibrium length. The spring-like properties of the muscle cause the joint trajectories to exhibit stable equilibrium behavior in the absence of any kind of sensory feedback; however, this spring-like behavior also exists in the presence of proprioceptive feedback.

Human movements involve active control of trajectory as well as the final position achieved by continuously varying the firing rate commands issued to the motoneurons of antagonist muscle pairs. The intrinsic muscle feedback that evolves from the spring-like behavior of the muscle provides primary movement stability during trajectory formation. Stretch reflex can be used to compensate for the asymmetries in muscle behavior away from the operating point. The spinal level controller regulates the skilled movements through the feedback servomechanism known as motor servo. The motor servo consists of the muscle spindle, the sensory pathways, and the skeletal muscle. The muscle spindle senses instantaneous changes in the spinal controller, which modulates the motoneuron firing rates. The muscle spindle receptors involved in the motor servo exhibit a nonlinear dynamic behavior characterized by low fractional power of velocity during the stretch phase.

CNS control of skilled movements involves choosing one among a number of muscle synergies available to perform the same task. A number of hypotheses have been advanced regarding the selection criteria used by the CNS. These hypotheses include energy optimal controls, quadratic cost optimization, impedance control, dynamic optimization, or, simply, the minimization of the number of muscles involved. There is little evidence that the CNS always controls any of the muscle variables in a fixed manner. Instead, there is much evidence for the flexible control of any and all variables so as to achieve the required adjustments.

Throwing

The shoulder complex is subjected to significant physical demands during the act of overhand throwing, an activity that is integral to many sports and recreational activities. Similar demands occur during stroke activities and racquet sports. Recent investigations involving dynamic EMG have significantly increased the level of understanding of the muscular activity of the shoulder complex as it relates to sports activities.

To throw a baseball, an athlete must generate kinetic energy and apply this energy to the ball; direct this force in order to steer the ball towards a target; and, after release of the ball, dissipate the retained energy. This is all accomplished through a complex series of coordinated muscle contractions involving both the lower and upper extremities as well as the trunk. The baseball-throwing motion has been divided into separate phases (Fig. 72). The first phase is the windup, which is characterized by the preparation activities performed by the athlete up until the time the ball is removed from the baseball glove. The second phase is the cocking phase, which is further divided into early cocking and late cocking. During early cocking, the arm is elevated and externally rotated. Late cocking occurs after the "lead" or "kick" leg becomes planted on the ground. After this foot hits the ground, late cocking continues until the maximum amount of external rotation of the arm is attained. This signals the end of the cocking phase and begins the acceleration phase. The acceleration phase of throwing is characterized by the rapid internal rotation and adduction of the arm, which results in the release of the ball. After the ball is released, the final phase of throwing is the follow-through. During the follow-through phase, the remainder of the energy in the system is dissipated.

During the windup, dynamic EMG of the shoulder muscles does not demonstrate a consistent pattern of activity. However, during cocking, all three heads of the deltoid demonstrate peak activity while holding the arm at 90°. The biceps brachii maintains appropriate elbow flexion during the cocking phase. During late cocking, amateur pitchers tend to demonstrate significantly greater activity in the supraspinatus muscle as compared to professional pitchers. The supraspinatus, infraspinatus, and teres minor all fire during cocking but begin to relax during late cocking. As the arm reaches the limit of external rotation late in cocking, the pectoralis major, latissimus dorsi, and subscapularis muscles decelerate the arm through eccentric muscle contraction.

The acceleration phase of the throw is characterized by relatively little activity in the rotator cuff and deltoid musculature. The pectoralis major, latissimus dorsi, and serratus anterior muscles contract strongly during the acceleration phase as the arm is adducted and internally rotated. Professional base-

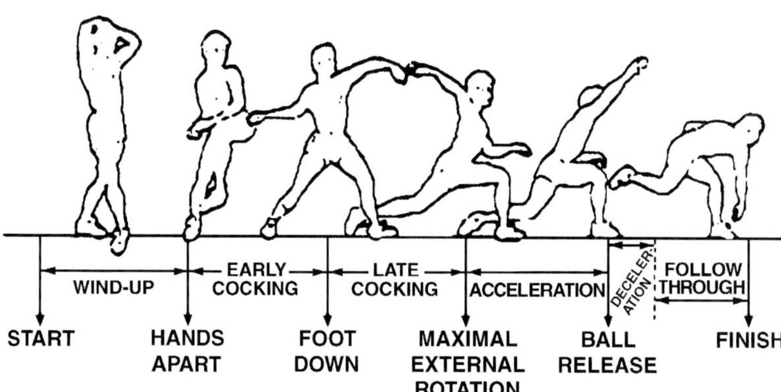

Figure 72
Six phases of pitching. (Reproduced with permission from Di Giovine NM, Jobe FW, Pink M, et al: An electromyographic analysis of the upper extremity in pitching. *J Shoulder Elbow Surg* 1992;1:16.)

ball pitchers have demonstrated significantly greater subscapularis activity during the acceleration phase when compared to amateur pitchers. Furthermore, amateur pitchers have demonstrated a tendency to use the biceps brachii more commonly during the acceleration phase

Throughout the throwing motion, the trapezius and, especially, the serratus anterior control the scapula. This is important for the maintenance of a stable platform (glenoid) for the humeral head, as well as for the maintenance of the optimal orientation of this platform with respect to the ever-changing joint reaction forces. Fatigue of the scapular rotators jeopardizes the synchrony of the shoulder complex during throwing and may precipitate injuries to the shoulder musculature.

Once the ball has been released, deceleration of the arm is required, and this is accomplished through eccentric contraction of the infraspinatus and teres minor muscles, as well as the supraspinatus, subscapularis, and posterior deltoid muscles. Protraction of the scapula is countered by eccentric contractions of the trapezius during follow-through. The entire throwing sequence usually takes less than one second from the start of the activity to ball release. The acceleration phase accounts for approximately 2% of the entire throwing motion. The arm internally rotates 7,000° to 8,000° per second during the acceleration phase. The ball has been calculated to accelerate from 0 mph at the onset of the acceleration phase to greater than 90 mph in approximately 80 ms. During this acceleration phase, the kinetic energy in the arm is 27,000 in-lb, which is approximately four times the kinetic energy in the kicking leg. This difference results from the angular velocity of the throwing arm being twice that of the kicking leg (the kinetic energy varies proportionately with the square of the angular velocity). All of this energy does not instantly dissipate with release of the ball. The arm, still moving forward after release of the ball, must be rapidly decelerated in order that capsular ligamentous injury to the glenohumeral joint not occur. The dynamic constraints, especially the rotator cuff muscles, are the critical decelerators to prevent excessive distraction forces at the glenohumeral joint during the follow-through of each pitching motion.

Posture

Posture is the position of the total body or an individual segment relative to gravity. Posture can be thought of in static (anatomic) or dynamic (physiologic) terms. As a static term, it describes the position of the body in space or the position of the parts of the body relative to one another. Dynamically, posture denotes the precise control and neuromuscular activity that function to maintain the body's center of mass over its base of support. Even in the static-appearing condition of dual-limb stance, postural control mechanisms work constantly to maintain stability. For instance, low voltage EMG activity can be recorded intermittently in calf muscles throughout simple stance. A continuous sway mechanism is at work, with postural muscle activity in the calf counteracting and maintaining the sway. This sway and the concomitant muscle contractures are theorized to be one way in which the body in stance guards against orthostatic circulatory insufficiency.

Balance is a term that describes the control by the CNS and muscles of the inertial state of the body or any of its segments. The complex mechanism of postural control is not fully understood. Present models and thoughts concerning posture are based on experimental studies, neuromuscular theory, principles of biomechanics, and understanding of the nervous system.

Force-platform studies use the center of pressure, defined as the center of distribution of total force applied to the platform, to determine indirectly the vertical projection of the location of the body's center of mass or center of gravity. In normal dual-limb stance the center of mass is in the vicinity of the sacral promontory. Technically, movement of the center of pressure depends on movement of the center of mass and the distribution of muscle forces responsible for that movement. Platform study has shown that in maintained, motionless dual-limb stance, the body's center of pressure (measured at 0.2-s intervals) fluctuates continuously around its mean center of pressure and traverses large total excursions (measured over 30 seconds of maintained stance) while remaining extremely close to the mean center of pressure.

Fluctuations of the body's center of pressure may be indicative of the sway mechanism, with total excursion indicative of total sway. With each individual sway, the center of pressure stays remarkably close to the mean center of pressure. The data show that in normal adults, the body does not deviate from its mean center of pressure, and seems to stay very close to that point automatically. Platform studies also have been used to measure differences between groups of adults. For instance, centers of pressure measured incrementally deviate farther from the mean center of pressure in the elderly patient than in younger adults. Stroke victims' centers of pressure may be very poorly tuned, with very large excursions and an inability to stay close to the mean center of pressure. The center of pressure also shifts away from the weaker extremity in a hemiplegic.

Force-platform studies also allow researchers to describe an area of stability or cone of stability. The area is defined as all points from which the body can return to a point of origin without taking a step or changing the base of support. Another way of explaining this area is as the area over which weight can be safely shifted and maintained. This area is enclosed within the margin defined by the position of the center of pressure during weight shifting. Normal adults apparently are aware of the limits they can or cannot exceed to safely perform this task. Again, the elderly and stroke patients show a poorer aptitude for this task, with a resultant smaller measured area of stability.

Force-platform measurements have shown how a person can precisely maintain the center of gravity over his or her base of support during sustained weightbearing and weightshifting. Investigation, using EMG measurements, of the maintenance of posture via movement, has led to the addition of synergies to postural control theory.

In experiments in which the base of support of a person in stance is moved rapidly and unexpectedly, the nervous system and body have a problem to solve. There appears to be an inordinate number of ways for the body to solve this problem, that is, potential muscle contractions or limb motions to maintain balance. The nervous system is thought to simplify this potentially complex postural problem by choosing among a set of prestructured, well-timed combinations of muscle contracture, or postural synergies. The chosen synergy is the one that optimally solves the problem.

Synergies originally were theorized to simplify situations in which the body has little time (sometimes on the order of milliseconds) to react. These synergies now are thought to be important in all aspects of postural maintenance, and seem to be developed early in life. EMG studies of infants show a cephalocaudal development of synergies, with muscle timing and patterns for reliable head control developing first, followed by trunk control and then stance control. Not until an organized synergistic pattern is developed can these developmental landmarks be attained. Maturing of synergies appears to occur as the child's nervous system matures, as the body's size and muscle strength develop, and through experience. By 7 years of age, the synergistic patterns (as measured by EMG) and postural ability of the child are much like those of the normal adult.

Synergies occur around certain postural joints. The predominant synergies or joint strategies of stance occur around the ankle and hip joints. On a stable base of support in dual-limb stance, the ankle strategy predominates, with perturbations that cause the center of gravity to move forward counteracted by organized distal-to-proximal firing of the gastrocnemius-soleus and hamstrings (with turning off of the tibialis anterior). The posterior muscle firing counters the forward movement of the body and uses rotation about the ankle joint to maintain a stable center of gravity. A similar distal-to-proximal synergistic response is seen with posterior perturbation, with the tibialis anterior and rectus femoris firing sequentially to oppose the movement. The hip strategy occurs with a less stable base of support, such as a person standing on a balance beam, with trunk and hip muscles acting in a synergic proximal-to-distal sequence to maintain the center of gravity over the base of support by bending the trunk about the hip joint.

The chosen synergies appear not only to be neurologically and muscularly the optimal solution to the problem, but also work to minimize and, therefore, optimize biomechanical considerations (and perhaps energy requirements) during the adjustment. With more extreme perturbations, the hip and ankle strategies may be inadequate. The body tries to maintain its balance by lowering the center of gravity by knee bending (vertical strategy), or by changing the base of support by taking a step (step strategy).

These posture studies describe a feedback control: the body senses the perturbation and reacts via feedback using the appropriate synergy. This postural synergy feedback mechanism has been termed a postural reaction. The postural accompaniment that occurs just prior to or simultaneously with a voluntary movement might be called a "feedforward" mechanism. Feedforward involves anticipating the effect of a voluntary movement and coordinating precisely the postural adjustment (accompaniment) required to minimize the displacement of the center of gravity. Via EMG measurement, feedforward (postural accompaniment), like feedback (postural reaction), has been shown to use postural synergies.

The voluntary movement of standing up on one's toes can be used as an example of feedforward. Without the appropriate postural accompaniment, the subject will push himself or herself upward and backward, off balance. To prevent this, just prior to firing the gastrocnemius-soleus for the desired focal movement, the postural accompaniment turns off the soleus very briefly and fires a short burst of the tibialis anterior. The tibialis anterior moves the center of gravity slightly anteriorly in anticipation of the focal movement that will tend to move the center of gravity posteriorly. Postural accompaniments also occur with focal arm movements. A postural accompaniment of some sort occurs with any focal movement that alters the center of gravity, thereby keeping the center of gravity as unchanged as possible. Interestingly, the body has been shown experimentally to turn off a postural accompaniment if it senses that stability is provided from another source, such as if the subject is grasping a handrail.

Another mechanism of postural control occurs sequentially well before a postural accompaniment and is called a postural preparation. Examples of this are an athlete widening his or her stance or stiffening his or her postural joints prior to an anticipated collision, or an elderly or unsteady individual grabbing a handrail before arising from a chair. Postural mechanisms are thought to combine safety with efficiency. Whereas postural reactions by necessity are efficient, they may not be safe; the reaction may not be of sufficient magnitude. Postural preparations are safe, but not necessarily efficient. Postural accompaniments are both safe and efficient.

Postural maintenance through synergies is intimately integrated with all focal movements of the body. In gait, as steps are taken, the center of mass is constantly maintained safely and efficiently over the center of pressure. Postural synergies are active in undisturbed gait in the form of postural accompaniments. Evidence shows that older individuals have an altered ability to control balance and subsequent posture. For the elderly, acceleration of the head in the AP plane is significantly greater, while that noted for the hip is significantly less than in younger individuals. Acceleration of the head is only 23% of that of the hip in the AP plane in young adults, whereas it appears to be about 42% in the elderly. Furthermore, from stride to stride, variance of these numbers as well as for lower joint moments and power, is greater for the elderly than for young adults. It is quite possble that the decrease in velocity, step length, push off, and the increase in double support, seen in the elderly, is a compensation to maintain balance and control during gait. EMG studies of gait show more consistent motor patterns in the elderly than in the young adult population, and kinematic observations show more consistency from stride to stride in a given individual and between individuals, with mild motion deviations, mostly at the time of double support at the hip knee, and ankle, of about 5° to 10° compared to younger adults.

Sensory input is an important contributor to postural maintenance. Visual, vestibular, and somatosensory inputs are all involved. In stance, somatosensory input depends predominantly on the body sensing its base of support. This input can influence the choice of postural strategy; for example, the sensing of a narrow base of support causes the body to choose the hip strategy over the ankle strategy. Experiments have shown that normal, healthy adults can maintain posture with vestibular input alone (while receiving altered or inhibited visual and somatosensory inputs). Elderly adults and children have problems when depending solely on vestibular input. Children also appear to choose visual cues over somatosensory cues, perhaps because the fine-tuning of sensing ankle and foot position takes longer to develop. Normal adults depend more on somatosensory input than visual input. Investigation of the effects of sensory contributions on posture control is continuing.

Experience clearly appears to be involved in postural control. The improvement of postural maintenance from childhood to adult levels, in addition to being dependent on maturity of the nervous system and the development of synergies, may best be explained by experience. Even in the normal adult, new or unusual tasks or movements may require new or unusual postural accompaniments via new synergies or novel combinations of synergies. Improvement in these new postural mechanisms develops with experience or practice. Experience may also explain why the elderly choose to maintain a smaller area of stability in platform testing. Previous experience (a fall) may prevent them from taking risks. Of course, this decreased performance in the elderly may also result from a number of factors, including a deteriorating sensory input (poor vision, neuropathy), diminishing CNS control, and decreased muscle strength. Nevertheless, experience cannot be denied as an important factor, and it is an important tool used by physical therapists to help stroke victims improve their levels of postural development.

Other factors that seem to contribute to posture are muscle strength and joint range of motion. The tibialis anterior has been found to be weaker in the elderly, and this weakness may contribute to more frequent falling. Children's development of posture may depend on the development of sufficient strength for body size in addition to the aforementioned factors. Patients with neuromuscular disease (dystrophies) show deterioration of postural ability. Hemiplegics' decreased strength affects the location of the center of pressure, away from the weak extremity. Joint range of motion (ROM) also plays a role. Postural synergies that might work for normal adults via an appropriate ankle strategy will not work for someone with a decreased joint ROM (stroke victims, cerebral palsy). The ability of such patients to develop new synergies or strategies is key to their ability to maintain some level of posture.

The CNS plays a major role in postural control, as a place where sensory input is processed, experience is stored, and neuromuscular postural synergies are developed and dictated. In addition, highly abnormal postural control is found in certain CNS deficiencies. Patients who have Parkinson's disease, which affects the basal ganglia, or cerebellar disorders show decreased ability to perform simple postural tasks. Patients who have cerebellar disease have shown absent postural responses to simple focal movements, while those who have Parkinson's disease show delayed or prolonged postural synergies. The heavy network of inputs and outputs from both the cerebellum and basal ganglia to and from the cerebral cortex (the center of motor and sensory input for the body) explains why deficiencies in these areas cause postural problems. It is thought that the cerebellum and basal ganglia are involved with timing, appropriateness, and gain of postural responses. Further study is needed to better understand their respective contributions.

A recently published central control model summarizes currently accepted knowledge of postural control: (1) The human body can precisely and automatically maintain its center of mass over its base of support under a variety of conditions. (2) Postural control centers on the CNS, which transmits motor output and receives sensory input. Additionally, certain CNS diseases provide the most challenging questions and problems of postural maintenance. (3) Postural synergies are ways in which the CNS (with the postural muscles) derives optimal solutions for potentially complicated postural problems and combinations. (4) Sensory input plays an important role via visual, vestibular, and somatosensory inputs both in the choice of postural strategies and in providing the feedback and, therefore, the experience from which a person modifies and fine-tunes the postural strategies. (5) Joint ROM and muscle strength contribute only as much as the body is aware of any deficiencies in these areas and can thereby make postural adjustments.

The present understanding of postural control has arisen through experience, neuromuscular theory, biomechanical principles, and knowledge of the CNS. Further experimental studies continue to enhance this understanding. The orthopaedic literature has provided little input to postural control studies. Most present knowledge comes from the neurologic, biomechanical, and physical therapy literature. Nevertheless, the orthopaedist must be aware of posture as it relates to gait and to patients with neurologic and muscular diseases. The orthopaedist also should be aware of other subsets of patients (elderly, children) who may suffer falls or trauma because of deficiencies in postural maintenance and control.

Walking

Human gait consists of a series of multiple limb segment rotational movements that produce stable forward propulsion in an energy-conserving manner (Fig. 73). Forces produced by muscles interacting with the body's gravitational and inertial properties result in joint angular changes. The effective summation of these movements is the stride length produced and, in association with the number of steps taken per minute (cadence), the overall velocity. These latter features constitute a measure of overall performance. Timing of muscle activity, joint angular changes, and time-distance parameters (step length, phase times, cadence, velocity, and so forth) are reproducible from cycle to cycle and person to person.

The natural cadence reported in the literature varies from 101 to 122 steps per minute. Women walk faster than men, having a cadence of 122 versus 116 steps per minute. The cadence of infants and children is greater than that of adults. Children aged 1 may have a cadence as high as 180 steps per minute while 7-year-olds have been reported to have a mean cadence of about 145 steps per minute. Studies of individuals between 60 and 85 years of age

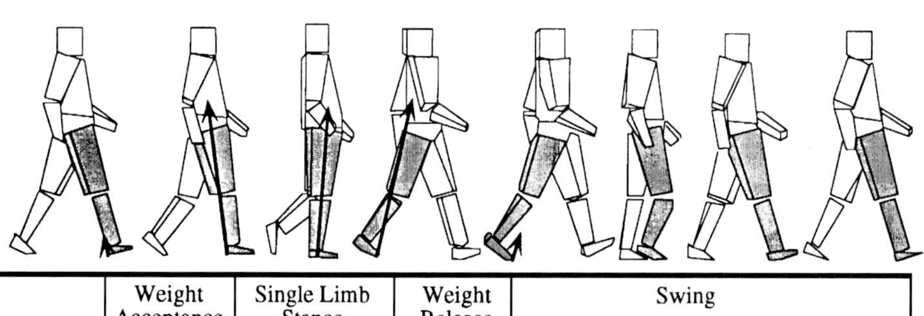

Figure 73
Limb movement in normal stride.

seem to indicate that, in the absence of pathologic conditions, cadence does not decrease, but stride length does decrease.

Kinematic measurements of joint angles of the lower extremities also differ little between men and women and between individuals 20 and 65 years of age. From cycle to cycle for a given subject, joint angular changes vary by only approximately 2° or less at any given instant in the gait cycle. Differences between subjects may be as high as 10%. These changes, which occur at the transitions of heel strikes and toe walks, are associated with differences in free walking cadence and in step length. While there is evidence that step lengths and velocities decrease for people older than 65 years of age (up to 85), this decrease does not appear to be related to marked changes in angular positions of the lower extremities. In the sagittal plane, angular changes show that mature gait is established by the age of 3. However, angular changes in the nonsagittal plane apparently take longer to achieve, and the normal degrees of rotation of adults seem to occur by the age of 7. Similarly, the walk-to-walk variability of muscle patterns seen during gait in a given subject is low although differences can be noted between the two sides. Patterns are apparently very similar from person to person and, at present, from 2- and 3-year-old children up to very old age.

Muscular activity and resulting limb positions and joint angular changes vary throughout the cycle (Fig. 74). The need for support and propulsion varies with the phase of the gait cycle. A normal CNS provides the control for gait to occur. Joint, ligament, bone, or muscle disease or injury produces a pattern that is different than normal, but is still controlled reproducibly by a normal CNS. Gait dysfunction from such disorders seems to be governed by a set of rules of compensation. The result, at times, may sacrifice energy efficiency, may increase joint forces and muscle effort, and may not fully compensate; but it does allow walking to be maintained. Diseases that affect the nervous system may not allow normal compensatory reactions and, in association with spasticity or weakness, may produce a walking pattern that is not readily understood by standard clinical methods.

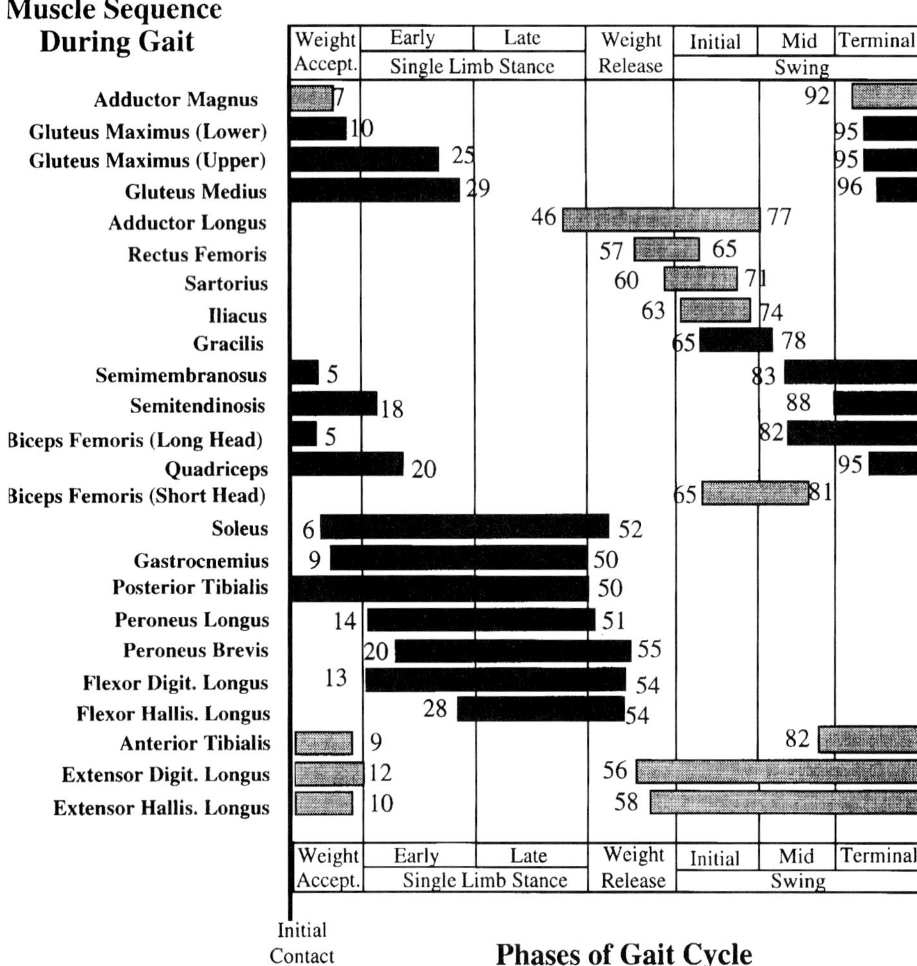

Figure 74
Muscular sequence of lower limb muscles during gait. Numbers signify percent of time in gait at which the muscle activity begins and ends.

To best understand the relationship between particular gait deviations and performance criteria, it is important to briefly review a few basic principles of gait. Whenever a person assumes an upright posture, inherent passive stability no longer exists. Unlike birds or creatures whose center of gravity lies below the pivoted hip joint, the human center of gravity is above it. A forward or backward force tends to rotate this center of gravity further away, thus making the individual susceptible to falling. Two mechanisms can prevent this. Muscles intended to reverse this trend can be activated, that is, postural reactions, or muscles intended to extend a limb outward in the direction of movement to brace or provide a stable structure under the falling object can be activated. In normal walking, a combination of the two mechanisms exists to provide stability. The leg in stance uses postural reactions. The leg in swing provides stability by reaching out a given distance at a given time. As a consequence of the latter, propulsive forces are imparted to the body to maintain forward movement. Then, this acceleration force must be decelerated when the leg hits the ground.

Thus, walking requires a greater muscular effort than quiet standing to remain stable. This dynamic stability remains only when acceleration and deceleration forces are relatively balanced. The swing of one leg may be simultaneously balanced by the stance of the opposite leg, and acceleration of one leg similarly may be simultaneously offset by deceleration of the other. Alternatively, some balancing may be done by the same leg at a later time. In normal gait, both mechanisms operate and are confined primarily to the structures of the pelvis and below.

As cadence and velocity increase, both stance and swing times decrease. As percentages of the gait cycle, stance decreases approximately 3.5 times as rapidly as swing. In absolute time, swing time decreases little as the speed of walking changes. Cadence and stride length depend on one another; both vary as the square root of the velocity. Up to approximately 120 steps per minute, speed increases are achieved equally by increasing stride and cadence. Above 120 steps per minute, step-length levels off leaving only cadence to increase to a maximum. Additionally, in contrast to kinematic data, sagittal plane moments about the hip, knee, and ankle joints are quite variable from step to step. In particular, this variability comes between the hip and the knee, and it is present both intra and inter subject. If the sum of these moments is examined as a reflection of the balance about the body's center of gravity, this sum remains relatively the same from step to step. Stability is controlled overall by changes in load sharing between different joints (predominantly the hip and knee).

These mechanisms are the reason for defining the phases of the gait cycle as weight acceptance, single limb stance, weight release (preswing), and swing, and are controlled by the neurologic system. The phases are relatively similar from person to person in the motions of limb segments and the active time of various muscles. The walking speed of various normal individuals is thus similar, efficient, and adaptable. For normal individuals, normal motions and normal muscular activity provide optimum results for all criteria of performance.

In neuromuscular disease, a peripheral defect alters a single or several bodily areas, thereby jeopardizing dynamic stability. Normal compensatory mechanisms that seek to correct the defect affect certain performance criteria more than others. For example, speed may be maintained close to normal at the expense of excess energy. Central defects, by attacking the control mechanisms as well as causing local abnormalities, jeopardize dynamic stability even more, thus creating an even wider discrepancy in what might be considered the normal values for various performance criteria. Because treatment does not restore normalcy, but substitutes for it, the orthopaedist must be sure that as many performance criteria as possible are improved. To best determine this, the physician must understand and analyze each gait pathology, closely examining both the primary defects and compensatory mechanisms and determining how they are related to each criterion of performance.

The process called walking is a repeated cycle of limb motions, controlled by selective muscle action, that carries the body forward while maintaining optimal upright stability. Included are actions directed toward absorption of the shock of floor impact and conservation of energy. Except for knee flexion in swing, most joint function depends on small, but critical, 15° to 20° arcs. A 10° deviation can be obstructive.

The clearance of the foot from the ground that occurs with each of the approximately two million steps an individual takes each year illustrates this well. The toe is the last body segment to leave the ground at the beginning of swing and, because of the angle of the leg and foot during swing, the toe rises to no more than 2.5 cm above the ground. It then drops to 0.87 cm of clearance at midswing. This minimal toe clearace occurs at the most dangerous phase of the toe trajectory, when the horizontal velocity of the foot is at a maximum, and the body is beginning its acceleration ahead of the opposite foot in stance. As the knee extends and the foot dorsiflexes, the toe rises to a maximum of 13 cm just prior to heel strike and then lowers to the floor. Altering the subject's speed essentially does not change the overall pattern nor the maximum-minimum of the displacement of the foot from the ground. At heel contact, it has been estimated that, although the forward velocity of the body center of mass is 1.6 m/s, the velocity at the heel is 4 m/s horizontally and 0.05 m/s vertically. Thus, the heel does not strike the ground but slides and must be braked in milliseconds to zero velocity. For the elderly, heel contact velocity in the horizontal direction seems to be significantly higher (30%) despite the fact that these individuals are walking with a shorter step length and slower overall velocity.

During walking, the multiple segments of the body move at different speeds. The upper and lower extremities change their speeds and displacements to the greatest degree. Another concept of control is noted by looking at the displacement of the head, the trunk, and the pelvis. As an individual walks, vertical displacement of the head increases from 3.6 cm at slow speeds to 6.2 cm at fast speeds. Yet, during this period of change in speed, the head's lateral displacement actually decreases from 4.2 cm at slow cadences to 2.7 cm at fast cadence. The thorax and pelvis do not move in unison. When the acceleration of the head is compared to that of the pelvis, the pelvic vertical accelerations are just marginally greater than those of the head despite the greater distance from the fulcrum at which the head is located. At free speed walking, the horizontal accelerations of the head are about one half those of the pelvis, whereas in the medial lateral plane, the head's acceleration and deceleration are only about three quarters those of the pelvis. Thus, it is clear that the trunk plays an active role in reducing the translational and rotational displacements and accelerations of the head relative to the pelvis. The neurocontrol to achieve all these tasks requires extremely fine tuning.

This narrow margin between normal and abnormal function makes the diagnosis of gait deviations difficult. To overcome these limitations, objective instrumented systems for evaluating gait disorders have been developed. Their value in identifying functional problems and determining the effectiveness of treatment is becoming more and more evident. Because walking is such a complex interaction of joint motions and muscle actions, a summary of the critical events is provided as background for the survey of the recent literature.

Normal Gait

During each stride (cycle) the limb moves through eight unique synergistic motion patterns (phases of gait) to accomplish three basic tasks: weight acceptance, single limb support, and limb advancement (Fig. 73). As these tasks are accomplished, the ankle and knee use four positions, and the hip two. A posture that is appropriate in one gait phase would signify dysfunction at another point in the cycle because the functional need has changed. As a result, timing often is as significant as posture. The relative significance of one joint's motion compared to the other varies among the gait phases. This factor makes observational gait analysis difficult.

Each joint has its own normal pattern of motion, moments, and joint powers as well as muscle control (Figs. 75 and 76). During stance, the stimulus is forward fall of body weight. As a result, muscle action is eccentric (that is, restraining a lengthening force). In swing, joint function is directed to clearing the floor, advancing the limb, and preparing for the next stance period. Muscle action is concentric.

Ankle The mode of foot/ankle mobility and muscular control is the most significant determinant of both limb stability and body progression.

Initial floor contact with the heel establishes the heel rocker that will be used to preserve the progression and initiate shock absorption during the limb's loading response. After heel contact, the ankle undergoes rapid plantarflexion. Vigorous deceleration of the tibialis anterior, assisted by the extensor hallucis longus, provides a controlled heel rocker. Two purposes are served: Part of the impact shock is absorbed directly and the tibia is advanced to preserve progression and accelerate knee flexion for further shock absorption.

Controlled dorsiflexion to 10° (midstance) and subsequent heel rise (terminal stance) throughout the single limb support period are the main sources of body progression. Active deceleration of the tibial advance is a critical component of knee stability. Reversal of ankle motion toward dorsiflexion immediately follows floor contact by the forefoot. The stimulus is forward momentum of the body weight. Deceleration of this motion by soleus and gastrocnemius activity provides a controlled ankle rocker. The muscles yield as they hold to allow the tibia, and thus the body, to move forward. The restraining force, however, is sufficient to make the rate of tibial advance slower than that of the femur. This allows the knee to extend. Body weight moves across the length of the foot, reaching the metatarsal head area as the ankle attains 10° dorsiflexion. Increased (strong) gastrocnemius and soleus action stabilizes the ankle and allows the heel to rise.

The forefoot becomes the final progressional rocker. During this action, the ankle moves into slight plantar flexion (5°) just before the forwardly

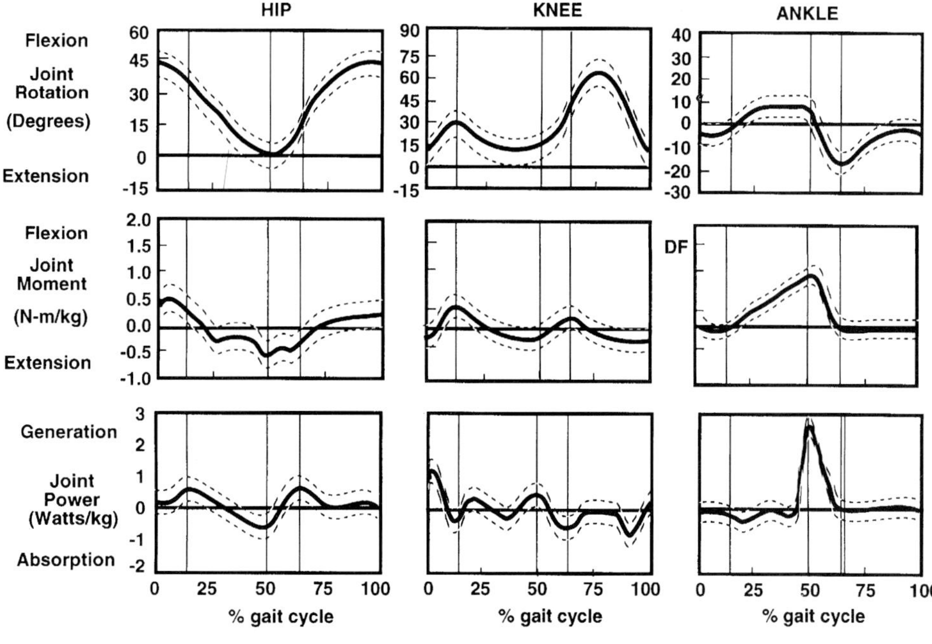

Figure 75
Joint angles, moment, and power of the hip, knee, and ankle in flexion and extension at each joint.

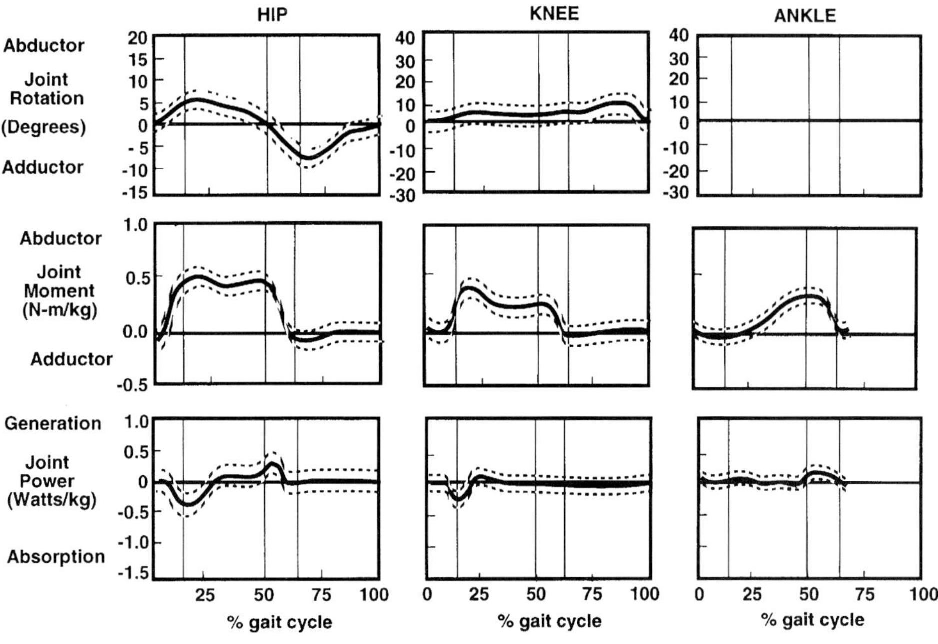

Figure 76
Joint angles, moment, and power of the hip, knee, and ankle in abduction and adduction at each joint.

aligned body weight drops onto the other foot. The limb then unloads; the muscles of the gastrocnemius-soleus group promptly relax. Hence, the functions of these muscles are to decelerate tibial advance for knee stability and to stabilize the ankle for a forefoot rocker. Push-off is not their role. The large arc of plantarflexion that occurs in pressing is functionally insignificant because the limb is virtually unloaded; it contributes to clearance but not to balance. Strength demands on the gastrocnemius-soleus musculature increase as the stride is lengthened.

Dorsiflexion to neutral in swing is the final event. It is responsible for toe clearance in midswing.

Three types of pathologic circumstance prevent effective ankle motion: (1) plantarflexion contracture; (2) weakness of plantarflexion muscles; and (3) weakness of dorsiflexion muscles.

Plantarflexion contracture is functionally significant when the ankle cannot attain a 5° dorsiflexed posture by the end of midstance. This angle is necessary for body weight to advance onto the forefoot. Dorsiflexion to 0° is not enough; this keeps body weight in the area of the ankle joint. A 15° plantarflexion contracture is not uncommon. Insensitivity to this posture stems from the fact that it is a natural event; it is the resting posture of the ankle and is a normal occurrence during the loading response. Contractures form as an incidental element of immobilization. Spontaneous positioning of the ankle will be in 15° of plantarflexion if specific efforts are not taken to avoid it. Inability to achieve dorsiflexion blocks the body's efforts to move forward over the supporting foot. Stride length and gait velocity are decreased. The knee may be strained into hyperextension. Forefoot pressure is prolonged and the intensity is increased, leading to pain and skin damage. Substitution of early heel-off (occurring in middle rather than terminal stance) improves progression but continues to strain the forefoot and knee.

Gastrocnemius-soleus insufficiency introduces tibial instability with a corresponding increase in quadriceps demand. If the body lacks the ability to restrain a dorsiflexion torque, body weight is kept close to the heel throughout the single limb support period. Stride length is shortened; endurance is reduced; and heel rise is delayed until the limb is unloaded. This is a very disabling situation that is difficult to recognize. The signs are persistent heel contact with excessive dorsiflexion at the end of single stance, persistent knee flexion in midstance, and lack of knee flexion during weight acceptance. All of these signs are subtle, and instrumented gait analysis may be needed to make the diagnosis. Because several motion patterns are possible, dynamic EMG also is indicated.

Clinical definition of gastrocnemius-soleus weakness is obscure. Manual testing is convenient but does not reproduce the force used in a single heel rise. Hence, this examination is woefully inadequate. Grade 5 strength supine is no better than grade 2 standing. The lesser perimalleolar plantarflexors (the peroneus group, tibialis posterior, and toe flexors) can meet the challenge of manual testing but not the standing demand. Repetitive, single limb heel rise (full range at least 18 times is normal) and instrumented force testing are the only valid measures.

Tibialis anterior weakness causes the familiar foot drop. This is the most frequently treated, but least significant gait error involving the ankle. Functional significance is low because there are so many ways to adjust for it (slightly increased hip flexion and contralateral vaulting, circumduction). Orthotic assistance at the onset of disability is indicated. Only the more severely disabled patients who lack an alternate means of lifting the foot continue to use the orthosis, however.

Knee Three essential actions occur at the knee: flexion to decrease the impact of floor contact, extension for weightbearing stability, and flexion for toe clearance in swing.

Weight acceptance is accomplished by knee flexion of about 15°. This flexion provides valuable shock absorption, but it also introduces postural instability. Two mechanisms are involved. Body weight is behind the foot at the time of initial contact, and the heel rocker rolls the tibia forward. Both events place the body vector line behind the knee. Quadriceps activity preserves limb stability. When the flexion is limited to 15°, the functional demand is well tolerated. Peak stance-phase knee flexion occurs just at the onset of single limb support. Throughout midstance, the knee progressively extends over the stable tibia. As the body-weight line reaches and then moves ahead of the knee axis in late midstance, the quadriceps relax and knee extension stability depends entirely on tibial control at the ankle.

Knee flexion for swing begins in the terminal double-support period (pressing). Approximately 40° is attained passively as body weight rolls beyond the metatarsal heads, and distal stability is lost. Only if the rate of knee flexion is excessive is there any restraining muscle action. Knee flexion is increased in initial swing (60°) for toe clearance. Momentum from hip flexion and slight local knee flexion action (short head of the biceps femoris) are the sources.

The final knee action is progressive knee extension to neutral in preparation for the next weightbearing period. This begins passively in midswing and is completed by quadriceps activity in terminal swing.

Assessment of knee position is complicated by the fact that two bony landmarks are eccentric to the joint axes they are supposed to indicate. The greater trochanter prominence is 3 cm behind the center of the femoral head, and the apex of the lateral malleolus is 1 cm behind the ankle axis. Use of these anatomic landmarks without corrections for their eccentric alignment can indicate 15° knee flexion when that joint is seen to be fully extended on the radiograph.

There are three significant gait errors. Each relates to the key function listed above. (1) Inadequate knee flexion during the loading response generally is not listed, but it deprives the patient of valuable shock absorption. The primary cause is quadriceps weakness. Patients substitute by using premature ankle plantarflexion to prevent the normal heel rocker. A second substitution is increased hip extensor muscle action. Slight forward lean of the trunk provides proximal stability so the hip extensors can draw the femur back. (2) Persistent knee flexion during single-limb support increases the duration of quadriceps demand. If knee position exceeds 15°, it also increases the supporting force needed. Both situations lead to premature fatigue. A flexion contracture or persistent hamstring muscle action are well-recognized causes. Weak gastrocnemius-soleus musculature must be added to this list. Walking on a flexed knee increases energy costs because the extensor muscle must remain active. (3) Insufficient knee flexion in initial swing causes a toe drag unless the patient substitutes. Possible substitutions include lateral trunk lean, circumduction, and vaulting by the other foot. All of these alternate mechanisms increase the energy cost of walking.

Hip Sagittal plane motion is simple. Starting from 45° of flexion, the hip progressively extends during stance. In swing there is rapid reversal into flexion for limb advancement. Demands on the extensor musculature are brief, lasting only during the weight-acceptance period. The dominant control is by the single joint muscles (gluteus maximus and adductor magnus). Relaxation of the hamstrings avoids excessive knee flexion. At the end of stance, the hip is drawn toward hyperextension, with iliacus activity being the restraining force. Limb advancement in early swing is accomplished by a mixture of low flexor muscle activities.

Hip control in the coronal plane is more demanding. Gluteus medius activity starts with the onset of stance and persists through most of the single-limb support period. The upper gluteus maximus also functions as an abductor. In addition, the hip is subjected to rotational forces as the trunk moves from behind to ahead of the supporting limb.

The significant functional errors are insufficient hip extension range and inadequacy of hip extensor, abductor, or flexion musculature. Flexion contractures commonly are accommodated by increased lumbar lordosis. In time, lumbosacral pain may be an additional complication. Patients who lack this range must lean forward. This introduces the need for a cane or crutch. Backward lean of the trunk (or lordosis) also is the postural substitution for hip extensor weakness. The two causes may be differentiated by timing: an extensor weakness requires accommodation at initial contact whereas demands for a flexion contracture may wait until mid or terminal stance. Hip abductor weakness leads to coronal plane instability. The immediate reaction is a drop of the contralateral side of the pelvis. Upright balance is maintained by a lateral trunk lean toward the supporting limb. Insufficiency of hip flexor strength leads to a loss of limb advancement unless the person can substitute by a contralateral lean or increased pelvic motion.

Movement Instrumentation Systems

With the dramatic improvement in types and refinements of musculoskeletal treatments, the clinician has a wide variety of options from which to select the optimal program. To best assess the proper treatment and its results, movement may now be evaluated using objective, quantifiable methods based on commercially available electronic and computer hardware and software. Recent technologic advances make clinical use of the movement laboratory feasible. Because these newer systems are becoming available and more widely used, a summary of their characteristics and principles is provided.

The function of a movement analysis laboratory is to quantify and assess an individual patient's functional performance. At present, five types of instrumentation systems are applicable to clinical use: motion analysis, dynamic EMG, force plates, foot-switch stride analysis, and measurement of energy costs. Automated motion systems are replacing photography because they are more rapid and more comprehensive. Dynamic EMG provides a direct means of identifying appropriate muscle action. This is an invaluable aid in determining the appropriate surgical plan for improving the gait of persons disabled by cerebral palsy, head trauma, and stroke. Use of this technique to identify compensatory muscle action in other types of impairment also is increasing. Definition of stride characteristics by use of foot switches or other methods classifies the patient's ability to walk, and is an excellent means of measuring the functional effectiveness of treatment. Energy-cost determination identifies the physiologic strain of gait disorder. Computer equipment is required to process the data and to allow visual checks of the functioning of the system. Moments around joints and deforming forces may be calculated from the measured variables. To avoid the inconvenience of direct oxygen measurement, calculations of mechanical work and energy are being explored. However, the excessive muscular effort that may be used to minimize a limp cannot be determined by summation of segment displacement. Consequently, the ratio between the two sets of data is low even though the correlations are good.

Like any other laboratory test, movement analysis testing yields information; the tests themselves do not provide an interpretation of the data. This is left to the clinician.

Automated Motion Analysis

To provide an accurate measurement of human movement, motion analysis systems must (1) visualize and accurately record all movements desired; (2) identify and quantify where in space each area of interest exists at every instant in the movement cycle; and (3) calculate parameters of interest to clinicians, for example, joint angles, velocity, stance times. In current systems all three steps are performed using video-type cameras, specialized electronic hardware, and computers.

Movement Visualization and Recording

As every limb segment changes its position during each instant of the movement cycle, all these systems instantaneously capture all the segment positions simultaneously and perform this task multiple times during the movement (Fig. 73). For walking, such snapshots or frames of data are obtained at least 50 to 60 times per second; for faster movements, such as sports, current systems obtain these frames at least 200 times per second. Anatomic skin areas of interest are highlighted by use of markers, shapes that can be light-contrasted from the background. The marker itself can be the light source or reflective tape can be used to highlight and intensify infrared or regular light. A second camera, which simultaneously views and records the same markers, allows the 3-D position in space (X,Y,Z) of each of the markers (after further processing) to be known. If the field of view of the camera to the marker is obscured, for example, if a crutch, cane or walker is in the way, a third camera directed at viewing the same markers often is used. Alternatively, if the view is only obscured for several snapshots or frames, computer software can later fill in the missing spots. If both sides of the body must be visualized simultaneously, careful choice of marker location is necessary to minimize the number of cameras needed.

Motion analysis systems vary as to how these visualized frames are recorded; some use VCR tape and later process and digitally record automatically or by hand off-line. In some systems, each camera is directly linked to an electronic hardware processor and the computer automatically identifies the two-dimensional (2-D) x-y position of each marker as it is imaged on-line and computer stored. This method requires seeing and numerically recording the position of up to 25 markers from two to six cameras every fiftieth of a second. It is necessary to properly identify each marker in each frame. In all systems, this is done by identifying, via a computer software program, each marker's anatomic relationship in the first few frames of the movement. A computer program then sorts out each marker's trajectory for the cycle by automatically tracking the marker as it changes its position from frame to frame or snapshot to snapshot. From each camera's 2-D marker file, all motion analysis systems using computer software programs combine the same marker site from at least two camera's files to produce a 3-D file of each marker in space.

Limb Segment and Joint Position Calculations

Recorded marker positions do not represent specific joints or limb segments. They represent only a single place on or near the skin that is related to a known anatomic location, for example, distal tip of the lateral malleolus of the ankle, tibial tubercle. This positional information must then be translated into limb segment or joint positional information (Fig. 73). Where markers are placed on the skin in a given movement study is determined by how this calculation is made. Appropriate software programs have been developed to perform these calculations. A variety of different methods exist for this process. These methods vary in their degree of mathematic and biomechanical sophistication.

Calculation of Movement Parameters

A multitude of movement parameters can be calculated from these 3-D limb segment and joint positions. Certain parameters routinely are clinically useful, for example, hip flexion/extension. Other parameters may be useful in specific movement disorders, for example, toe clearance from the floor during swing. The accuracy in measurement of such parameters depends to some degree on (1) the accuracy of the camera system used, (2) the movement addressed, (3) the trueness of the 3-D motion file established, and (4) the mathematic approach used to calculate the desired parameter.

Sagittal knee movement during gait represents large angular changes (60°), marker placement on the skin does not differ significantly from patient to patient relative to the degree of the angular error that can be produced, and the mathematics used to calculate the resulting angles use a well-defined joint axis. Knee flexion-extension in almost all motion systems thus yields very similar results. However, ankle dorsiflexion-plantarflexion can be quite variable. To calculate this parameter in the simplest manner, three markers are used: lateral side of knee, lateral malleolus, and the dorsum or lateral side of the patient's metacarpal phalangeal joint of the foot. The angle is then calculated for each data frame of the movement cycle using simple trigonometric relationships between these points. Foot abnormalities or dynamic changes in a flexible foot during gait can cause hindfoot varus-valgus, forefoot pronation-supination, and midtarsal flexion-extension. Because the ankle angle is calculated from markers spanning these joints, the calculation program includes any combination of these motions in the sagittal ankle angle calculation and does not represent true ankle dorsiflexion-plantarflexion. To overcome such limitations, differing marker configurations and more sophisticated mathematic approaches to this angle's calculations have been developed.

The attempt for greater accuracy can lead to more markers (or cameras) being used and more difficulty in tracking individual markers during the sorting process. For different reasons, similar potential measurement inaccuracies exist in determining all the joint angles at the hip and varus-valgus and internal-external rotation of the knee. Depending on the nature of the movement, the motion system used, and the specific joint angle to be evaluated, how accurately the measurement recorded reflects and needs to reflect the real motion occurring varies with the study and the information desired

Foot-Switch Stride Analyses

In contrast to joint angular determinations, many time-distance parameters of gait (cadence, stride length, single limb stance time) are less subject to processing variation when they are calculated from motion systems or from foot-switch stride analyses. From motion systems, such calculations are defined by selected single markers about the foot, for example, heel and frame number recording of well-defined gait events such as heel strike in frame number five, toe off in frame number 10. The frame in which a gait event occurs is determined by user intervention. Selecting whether a foot strike or toe off occurs in one frame or in the next one, a fiftieth of a second later is sometimes difficult. Distances traversed and time intervals are then calculated from the 3-D position of the marker at each of the gait events. It has been found that in addition to calculating the absolute time and distance of the gait cycle phases, normalizing each time interval to a percent of the gait cycle yields useful clinical data.

Dynamic EMG Measurement

Dynamic EMG recording represents the neurologic system's control of when a particular muscle is to be activated as well as the ability of the muscle to be activated. Investigations have established the fact that, during any functional movement, a particular muscle is activated only for a given period of time. For example, during an individual gait cycle, no muscle is activated for more than 30% to 40% of the entire cycle. Dynamic EMG does not represent the absolute force of the muscle, and the magnitude of EMG activity alone is not useful in comparing a muscle's force from one testing session to another or between subjects. However, the timing of EMG activity can be used to compare a subject's performance to normal values and to determine whether the performance is prolonged or continuously active from condition to condition and from subject to subject. Comparison in the same session of the magnitude of EMG activity during movement to that during a maximal voluntary contracture of the muscle has been found to provide useful clinical information.

The EMG signal recorded is a summation of multiple motor units and muscle fibers being activated. During the time of its activation, the magnitude and the frequency of the signal change. Sampling occurs from a given region of the muscle. The number of muscle fibers and motor units recorded varies with the method of sampling. One method obtains the signal using hair-thin electric (bipolar) wires (wire electrode) inserted into the muscle. It has been found that for most pathologic disorders, if the site of the EMG has been properly selected, the small number of motor units tested by this method accurately represents the entire muscle. The alternative to wire-electrode sampling is the use of surface electrodes. These electrodes represent a larger area of muscle motor units and muscle fibers.

The EMG signal recorded from either method represents the summation of the depolarization and repolarization of multiple muscle fibers. Because this occurs in individual muscle fibers at slightly different rates, the summation in the waveform represents negative and positive values. Wire electrodes represent the most accurate methods of recording EMG activity for such circumstances. This recording process is, however, time consuming and in certain cases, because of its invasive nature, may be a somewhat painful process. Surface-electrode recording minimizes the problem, but must be interpreted with caution. The signal picked up from surface electrodes represents transmission of the true signal through fat, fascia, and skin. Some signal is thereby reflected and/or refracted, yielding alterations in the signal's magnitude and frequency. Moreover, muscles in adjacent areas, whether laterally or deeply positioned, for example, the various components of the quadriceps (vastus intermedius, vastus lateralis, vastus medialis) represent part of the signal recorded from the muscle directly under the surface electrode, in this case the rectus femoris. In most cases, adjacent muscles are similar in activation and the signal recorded poses little problem in interpretation if surface electrode EMG is defined as measuring muscle groups, that is, quadriceps rather than rectus femoris, and is used to help understand whether regional muscle activity contributes to flexing or extending a given joint.

In addition to the electrode recorder, all dynamic EMG systems contain electrical components to ground the signal, minimize interference noise, transmit the signal, and record the signal. Both wire and surface electrodes pick up low-magnitude muscle electrical signals. The signal also contains electrical artifact noise produced by skin, muscle, wire, or electrode movement. Such noise can be equal to or larger in magnitude than that of the EMG signal. With all systems, careful placement of the electrode is essential, and an amplifier is provided as close to the origin of the signal as possible in order to minimize this noise. The signal can then be transmitted to a recording device via a cable wire system (dragged along as the patient walks) or via the airwaves (telemetry). The transmitted signals are immediately recorded and stored on tape or digitally converted and computer stored. Additional electronic hardware is necessary to synchronize the EMG signals recorded with the movement events or with motion analysis systems or with force platform systems, on-line or off-line.

The EMG data often are presented as a smoothed wave of hills and valleys; or they can be illustrated as a single horizontal bar that merely illustrates the on-off activity of the muscle. Mathematic processing techniques are necessary to alter the signal for such purposes.

As the use of dynamic EMG for the evaluation of movement dysfunction has gained in popularity, its usefulness in understanding normal movement has also increased. Investigation has determined that three strides of EMG data per subject provide information as reliable as that obtained from 12 strides. EMG examination of eight muscles about the ankle during manual muscle testing and three walking velocities (free, fast, slow) has shown that the intensity of muscle action during walking is related to the manual muscle test grades. Walking at the normal free velocity required fair (grade 3) muscle action. During slow gait, the muscle functioned at a poor (grade 2) level. Fast walking necessitated muscle action midway between fair and normal, which was interpreted as good (grade 4). Analysis of surface EMGs of seven major muscles in adults indicates two general types of pattern change in lower extremity muscle activity as a function of walking speed. The fundamental phasing of muscle activity never changes, but relative amplitudes within the phases are modulated as speed increases; and different phases of activity exist for different walking speeds. The timing of most phases (expressed as percentage of the stride) decreased as speed increased. This suggests that the time base should be further normalized by stance and swing phases.

Foot-Floor Force and Pressure Recordings

The changes in direction, magnitude, and area of contact of the foot-to-ground reaction forces during the stance phase of walking are among the most relevant parameters in the assessment of human gait. Body weight and inertial forces are effective in moving the body forward and providing stability only if they are resisted by the ground. Measurement of the foot-to-ground reaction forces via platforms provides an understanding of these respective forces. These platforms, embedded in the ground, provide accurate measurements of the vertical and horizontal forces of the foot against the ground in hundredths or thousandths of seconds. The force platform must be small enough to allow only the forces on a single foot to be measured. If the platform is too small, the foot could miss the force plate. Most platforms are about two feet by two feet. To obtain information from both feet, either two or more force platforms must be used or the subject must walk across the force platform several times. Measurement devices within the force platform use piezoelectric or strain-gauge electronic technology and highly-insulated wire conduction systems to transmit the force measurements (after they are amplified) to a recording device. The recording devices are similar to those of EMG or motion analysis systems.

Such signals are graphically represented as absolute time during the stance phase or are normalized to the gait cycle if that cycle is synchronized to motion analysis systems.

If the external moments about the hip, knee, or ankle joints are clinically desired, further software routines are needed to calculate the resultant vector force from the vertical and fore-aft, medial-lateral forces, as well as the force's distance (moment arm) from the joint at each instant in the cycle. This calculation requires the synchronization of force platform data and motion data and further calculation of the perpendicular distance from the force vector to the joint axis. Individual software programs have been developed for this purpose; moment calculation routines therefore vary from laboratory to laboratory.

Force platforms do not provide information about the areas of contact or pressure distribution of the foot with the ground. Assessment via Harris mat provides an inexpensive qualitative snapshot of all the areas of contact of the foot with the ground during the entire stance phase. Miniature shoe devices and in-ground pedobarographs are now available to provide quantitative means of identifying the foot's vertical forces and the area of their distribution at each instant in the stance phase. These are extremely sophisticated devices; they require multiple miniature force-measuring systems and, in one case, highly-sophisticated miniaturized amplifier and transmitting devices. The shoe-borne devices offer the advantages of not requiring the individual to walk in a confined space and of obtaining data from multiple steps and cycles. Shoe insert systems either are mats that have multiple miniature devices that come in different sizes or they use several separate small force recorders that are placed at specific locations under the foot. Based on a quantitative picture of the pressure-distribution under the human foot, a sectorial evaluation of the pressure-distribution, including an analysis of weight, area, maximum pressure, and average pressure in the different sectors, can be reported. Standardized static and dynamic pictures of the pressure-distribution of the foot can be obtained using such devices.

The normal foot-floor force pattern of a large number of normal children, young adults, and elderly people is characterized by a marked population variability, but there is a considerable step-to-step consistency and symmetry of the forces from both feet of a given subject. The force pattern in pathologic gait secondary to disorders of the foot also has shown marked repeatability.

Selected Bibliography

Shoulder

Bankart ASB: The pathology and treatment of recurrent dislocation of the shoulder joint. *Br J Surg* 1938;26:23–29.

Basmajian JV, Bazant FJ: Factors preventing downward dislocation of the adducted shoulder joint in an electromyographic and morphological study. *J Bone Joint Surg* 1959;41A:1182–1186.

Boone DC, Azen SP: Normal range of motion of joints in male subjects. *J Bone Joint Surg* 1979;61A:756–759.

Bowen MK, Warren RF: Ligamentous control of shoulder stability based on selective cutting and static translation experiments. *Clin Sports Med* 1991;10:757–782.

Bradley JP, Tibone JE: Electromyographic analysis of muscle action about the shoulder. *Clin Sports Med* 1991;10:789–805.

Colachis SC Jr, Strohm BR: Effects of suprascapular and axillary nerve blocks on muscle force in upper extremity. *Arch Phys Med Rehabil* 1971;52:22–29.

Cooper DE, O'Brien SJ, Arnoczky SP, et al: The structure and function of the coracohumeral ligament: An anatomic and microscopic study. *J Shoulder Elbow Surg* 1993;2:70–77.

Dempster WT: Mechanisms of shoulder movement. *Arch Phys Med Rehabil* 1965;46:49–70.

DiGiovine NM, Jobe FW, Pink M, et al: An electromyographic analysis of the upper extremity in pitching. *J Shoulder Elbow Surg* 1992;1:15–25.

Flatow EL: The biomechanics of the acromioclavicular, sternoclavicular, and scapulothoracic joints, in Heckman JD (ed): *Instructional Course Lectures Volume 42.* Rosemont, IL, American Academy of Orthopaedic Surgeons, 1993, pp 237–245.

Freedman L, Munro RR: Abduction of the arm in the scapular plane: Scapular and glenohumeral movements: A roentgenographic study. *J Bone Joint Surg* 1966;48A:1503–1510.

Fukuda K, Craig EV, An KN, et al: Biomechanical study of the ligamentous system of the acromioclavicular joint. *J Bone Joint Surg* 1986;68A:434–440.

Gerber C, Ganz R: Clinical assessment of instability of the shoulder: With special reference to anterior and posterior drawer tests. *J Bone Joint Surg* 1984;66B: 551–556.

Gowan ID, Jobe FW, Tibone JE, et al: A comparative electromyographic analysis of the shoulder during pitching: Professional versus amateur pitchers. *Am J Sports Med* 1987;15:586–590.

Harryman DT II, Sidles JA, Clark JM, et al: Translation of the humeral head on the glenoid with passive glenohumeral motion. *J Bone Joint Surg* 1990;72A: 1334–1343.

Harryman DT II, Sidles JA, Harris SL, et al: The role of the rotator interval capsule in passive motion and stability of the shoulder. *J Bone Joint Surg* 1992;74A:53–66.

Howell SM, Galinat BJ: The glenoid-labral socket: A constrained articular surface. *Clin Orthop* 1989;243:122–125.

Howell SM, Kraft TA: The role of the supraspinatus and infraspinatus muscles in glenohumeral kinematics of anterior shoulder instability. *Clin Orthop* 1991;263:128–134.

Howell SM, Galinat BJ, Renzi AJ, et al: Normal and abnormal mechanics of the glenohumeral joint in the horizontal plane. *J Bone Joint Surg* 1988;70A:227–232.

Inman VT, Saunders JB, Abbott LC: Observations on the function of the shoulder joint. *J Bone Joint Surg* 1944;26:1–30.

Itoi E, Motzkin NE, Morrey BF, et al: Scapular inclination and inferior stability of the shoulder. *J Shoulder Elbow Surg* 1992;1:131–137.

Jobe FW, Tibone JE, Perry J, et al: An EMG analysis of the shoulder in throwing and pitching: A preliminary report. *Am J Sports Med* 1983;11:3–5.

Kronberg M, Nemeth G, Brostrom LA: Muscle activity and coordination in the normal shoulder: An electromyographic study. *Clin Orthop* 1990;257:76–85.

Kuhlman JR, Iannotti JP, Kelly MJ, et al: Isokinetic and isometric measurement of strength of external rotation and abduction of the shoulder. *J Bone Joint Surg* 1992;74A:1320–1333.

Kumar VP, Balasubramanium P: The role of atmospheric pressure in stabilizing the shoulder: An experimental study. *J Bone Joint Surg* 1985;67B:719–721.

Matsen FA III: Biomechanics of the shoulder, in Frankel VH, Nordin M (eds): *Basic Biomechanics of the Skeletal System.* Philadelphia, Lea and Febiger, 1980, pp 221–242.

Matsen FA III, Fu FH, Hawkins RJ: *The Shoulder: A Balance of Mobility and Stability.* Rosemont, IL, American Academy of Orthopaedic Surgeons, 1993.

Matsen FA, Thomas SC, Rockwood CA Jr: Anterior glenohumeral instability, in Rockwood CA Jr, Matsen FA III (eds): *The Shoulder,* ed 1. Philadelphia, WB Saunders, 1990, vol 1, pp 526–622.

Morrey BF, An KN: Biomechanics of the shoulder, in Rockwood CA Jr, Matsen FA III (eds): *The Shoulder.* Philadelphia, WB Saunders, 1990, pp 208–245.

Ovesen J, Nielsen S: Anterior and posterior shoulder instability: A cadaver study. *Acta Orthop Scand* 1986;57:324–327.

O'Brien SJ, Neves MC, Arnoczky SF, et al: The anatomy and histology of the inferior glenohumeral ligament complex of the shoulder. *Am J Sports Med* 1990;18:449–456.

Pearl ML, Harris SL, Lippitt SB, et al: A system for describing positions of the humerus relative to the thorax and its use in the presentation of several functionally important arm positions. *J Shoulder Elbow Surg* 1992;1:113–118.

Perry J: Muscle control of the shoulder, in Rowe CR (ed): *The Shoulder.* New York, Churchill Livingstone, 1988, pp 17–34.

Perry J: Anatomy and biomechanics of the shoulder in throwing, swimming, gymnastics and tennis. *Clin Sports Med* 1983;2:247–270.

Poppen NK, Walker PS: Normal and abnormal motion of the shoulder. *J Bone Joint Surg* 1976;58A:195–201.

Poppen NK, Walker PS: Forces at the glenohumeral joint in abduction. *Clin Orthop* 1978;135:167–170.

Reeves B: Experiments on the tensile strength of the anterior capsule structures of the shoulder in man. *J Bone Joint Surg* 1968;50B:858–865.

Rockwood CA Jr, Green DP (eds): *Fractures in Adults,* ed 2. Philadelphia, JB Lippincott, 1984.

Schwartz R, O'Brien SJ, Warren RF, et al: Capsular restraints to anterior/posterior motion of the shoulders. *Orthop Trans* 1988;12:727.

Shevlin MG, Lehmann JF, Lucci JA: Electromyographic study of the function of some muscles crossing the glenohumeral joint. *Arch Phys Med Rehabil* 1969;50:264–270.

Soslowsky LJ, Flatow EL, Bigliani LU, et al: Articular geometry of the glenohumeral joint. *Clin Orthop* 1992;285:181–190.

Staples OS, Watkins AL: Full active abduction in traumatic paralysis of the deltoid. *J Bone Joint Surg* 1943;25:85–89.

Turkel SJ, Panio MW, Marshall JL, et al: Stabilizing mechanisms preventing anterior dislocation of the glenohumeral joint. *J Bone Joint Surg* 1981;63A: 1208–1217.

Warner JJP, Caborn DNM, Berger R, et al: Dynamic capsuloligamentous anatomy of the glenohumeral joint. *J Shoulder Elbow Surg* 1993;2:115–133.

Warner JJP, Deng XH, Warren RF, et al: Superoinferior translation in the intact and vented glenohumeral joint. *J Shoulder Elbow Surg* 1993;2:99–105.

Warren RF, Kornblatt IB, Marchand R: Static factors affecting posterior shoulder stability. *Orthop Trans* 1984;8:89.

Elbow

An K-N, Morrey BF: Biomechanics of the elbow, in Mow VC, Ratcliffe A, Woo SL-Y (eds): *Biomechanics of Diarthrodial Joints.* New York, NY, Springer-Verlag, 1990, vol 2, chap 34, pp 441–464.

An K-N, Morrey BF: Biomechanics, in Morrey BF, Chao EYS (eds): *Joint Replacement Arthroplasty.* New York, NY, Churchill Livingstone, 1991, chap 20, pp 257–273.

Miller MD: Basic Sciences: Part I. Biomechanics, in Miller MD (ed): *Review of Orthopaedics.* Philadelphia, PA, WB Saunders, 1992, chap 2, pp 37–48.

Morrey BF, Askew LJ, Chao EY, et al: A biomechanical study of normal functional elbow motion. *J Bone Joint Surg* 1981;63A:872–877.

Morrey BF, An K-N, Chao EYS: Functional evaluation of the elbow, in Morrey BF (ed): *The Elbow and Its Disorders.* Philadelphia, PA, WB Saunders, 1985, chap 5, pp 73–91.

Ries MD, Hurst LC, Dee R: Biomechanics of the elbow, in Dee R, Mango E, Hurst LC (eds): *Principles of Orthopaedics Practice.* New York, McGraw-Hill, 1989, chap 33, vol 1, sec B, pp 515–519.

Wrist and Hand

Anatomy and Pathophysiology of the Intrinsic Muscles and Digital Extensor Mechanism. The American Society for Hand Surgery Syllabus, 1991, chap 1.

An KN: The effect of force transmission on the carpus after procedures used to treat Kienböck's disease. *Hand Clin* 1993;9:445–454.

An KN, Chao EY, Cooney WP, et al: Forces in the normal and abnormal hand. *J Orthop Res* 1985;3:202–211.

An KN, Berger RA, Cooney WP III (eds): *Biomechanics of the Wrist Joint.* New York, NY Springer-Verlag, 1991.

Backhouse KM, Hutchings RT: *Color Atlas of Surface Anatomy: Clinical and Applied.* Baltimore, Williams & Wilkins, 1986.

Bowers WH (ed): *The Interphalangeal Joints: The Hand and Upper Limb.* Edinburgh, Churchill-Livingstone, 1987.

Brand PW, Hollister A (eds): *Clinical Mechanics of the Hand,* ed 2. St. Louis, MO, Mosby Year-Book, 1992.

Burkhalter WE: Median nerve palsy: Intrinsic replacement in median nerve paralysis, in Green DP (ed): *Operative Hand Surgery,* ed 3. New York, Churchill Livingstone, 1992, vol 2, chap 39, pp 1419–1466.

Cooney WP III, Chao EYS: Biomechanical analysis of static forces in the thumb during hand function. *J Bone Joint Surg* 1977;59A:27–36.

Cooney WP III, Linscheid RL, Dobyns JH: Fractures and dislocations of the wrist, in Rockwood CA Jr, Green DP, Bucholz RW (eds): *Rockwood and Green's Fractures in Adults,* ed 3. Philadelphia, PA, JB Lippincott, 1991, chap 8, pp 563–678.

Cooney WP, Garcia-Elias M, Dobyns JH, et al: Anatomy and mechanics of carpal instability. *Surg Rounds Orthop* 1989;3:15–24.

Doyle JR: Extensor tendons: Acute injuries, in Green DP (ed): *Operative Hand Surgery,* ed 3. New York, Churchill Livingstone, 1993, vol 2, chap 52, pp 1925–1954.

Froimson AI: Tenosynovitis and tennis elbow: DeQuervain's disease, in Green DP (ed): *Operative Hand Surgery,* ed 3. New York, Churchill Livingstone, 1993, vol 2, chap 54, pp 1989–2006.

Hall MC (ed): *Carpo-Metacarpal, Inter-metacarpal, and Inter-phalangeal Joints: The Locomotor System Functional Anatomy.* Springfield, IL, Charles C. Thomas, 1965, chap 13, pp 272–301.

Hoppenfeld S: Physical examination of the wrist and hand, in Hoppenfeld S, Hutton R (eds): *Physical Examination of the Spine and Extremities.* New York, Appleton-Century-Crofts, 1976, chap 3, pp 59–104.

Imaeda T, An KN, Cooney WP III, et al: Anatomy of trapeziometacarpal ligaments. *J Hand Surg* 1993;18A:226–231.

Kauer JM: Functional anatomy of the wrist. *Clin Orthop* 1980;149:9–20.

Lampe EW: Surgical anatomy of the hand with special references to infection and trauma. *Clin Symp* 1969;21:66–109.

Lichtman DM (ed): *The Wrist and Its Disorders.* Philadelphia, WB Saunders, 1988.

Littler JW: On the adaptability of man's hand with reference to the equiangular curve. *Hand* 1973;5:187–191.

Long C II, Conrad PW, Hall EA, et al: Intrinsic-extrinsic muscle control of the hand in power grip and precision handling: An electromyographic study. *J Bone Joint Surg* 1970;52A:853–867.

Miller MD: Basic sciences: Part 1, in *Biomechanics, Review of Orthopaedics.* Philadelphia, WB Saunders, 1992, chap 2, pp 37–48.

Norkin CC, Levangie PK (eds): *Joint Structure and Function: A Comprehensive Analysis.* Philadelphia, FA Davis, 1983.

O'Driscoll SW, Horii E, Ness R, et al: The relationship between wrist position, grasp size, and grip strength. *J Hand Surg* 1992;17A:169–177.

Palmer AK, Werner FW: Biomechanics of the distal radioulnar joint. *Clin Orthop* 1984;187:26–35.

Palmer AK, Werner FW, Glisson RR, et al: Partial excision of the triangular fibrocartilage complex. *J Hand Surg* 1988;13A:391–394.

Palmer AK, Werner FW, Murhy D, et al: Functional wrist motion: A biomechanical study. *J Hand Surg* 1985;10A:39–46.

Posner MA: Ligament injuries in the wrist and hand. *Hand Clin* 1992;8:603–828.

Ries MD, Hurst L: Biomechanics of the hand and wrist, in Dee R, Mango E, Hurst LC (eds): *Principles of Orthopaedic Practice.* New York, McGraw-Hill, 1989, vol 1, chap 33, sec c, pp 519–529.

Ruby LK, Cooney WP III, An KN, et al: Related motion of selected carpal bones: A kinematic analysis of the normal wrist. *J Hand Surg* 1988;13A:1–10.

Ryu JY, Cooney WP III, Askew LJ, et al: Functional ranges of motion of the wrist joint. *J Hand Surg* 1991;16A:409–419.

Sarrafian SK, Melamed JL, Goshgarian GM: Study of wrist motion in flexion and extension. *Clin Orthop* 1977;126:153–159.

Spinner M (ed): *Kaplan's Functional and Surgical Anatomy of the Hand,* ed 3. Philadelphia, JB Lippincott, 1984.

Steindler A (ed): *Kinesiology of the Human Body: Under Normal and Pathological Conditions.* Springfield, IL, Charles C. Thomas, 1955.

Stern P: Fractures of the metacarpals and phalanges,in Green DP (ed): *Operative Hand Surgery,* ed 3. New York, Churchill Livingstone, 1993, vol 2, p 695.

Taleisnik J (ed): *The Wrist.* New York, Churchill Livingstone, 1985.

Tubiana R (ed): *The Hand.* Philadelphia, WB Saunders, 1981, vol 1.

Viegas SF, Tencer AF, Cantrell J, et al: Load transfer characteristics of the wrist: Part I. The normal joint. *J Hand Surg* 1987;12A:971–978.

Youm Y, Flatt AE: Kinematics of the wrist. *Clin Orthop* 1980;149:21–32.

Youm Y, McMurtry RY, Flatt AE, et al: Kinematics of the wrist: I. An experimental study of radial-ulnar deviation and flexion-extension. *J Bone Joint Surg* 1978;60A: 423–431.

Spine

Adams MA, Hutton WC: The relevance of torsion to the mechanical derangement of the lumbar spine. *Spine* 1981;6:241–248.

Ahmed AM, Duncan NA, Burke DL: The effect of facet geometry on the axial torque-rotation response of lumbar motion segments. *Spine* 1990;15:391–401.

Anderson CK, Chaffin DB, Herrin GD, et al: A biomechanical model of the lumbosacral joint during lifting activities. *J Biomech* 1985;18:571–584.

Andersson GBJ: Evaluation of muscle function, in Frymoyer JW, Ducker TB, Hadler NM, et al (eds): *The Adult Spine: Principles and Practice.* New York, Raven Press, 1991, vol 1, pp 241–274.

Andersson GBJ, Chaffin DB, Pope MH: Occupational biomechanics of the lumbar spine, in Pope MH, Andersson GBJ, Frymoyer JW, et al (eds): *Occupational Low Back Pain: Assessment, Treatment and Prevention.* St. Louis, MO, Mosby Year Book, 1991, pp 20–43.

Andersson GBJ, Ortengren R, Nachemson A, et al: Lumbar disc pressure and myoelectric back muscle activity during sitting: I. Studies on an experimental chair. *Scand J Rehabil Med* 1974;6:104–114.

Andersson GB, Ortengren R, Herberts P: Quantitative electromyographic studies of back muscle activity related to posture and loading. *Orthop Clin North Am* 1977;8:85–96.

Andersson GB, Ortengren R, Schultz A: Analysis and measurement of the loads on the lumbar spine during work at a table. *J Biomech* 1980;13:513–520.

Berkson MH, Nachemson A, Schultz AB: Mechanical properties of human lumbar spine motion segments: Part II. Responses in compression and shear; influence of gross morphology. *J Biomech Eng* 1979;101:53–57.

Bland JH, Boushey DR (eds): *Disorders of the Cervical Spine: Diagnosis and Medical Management.* Philadelphia, PA, WB Saunders, 1987.

Bouisset S, Zattara M: Biomechanical study of the programming of anticipatory postural adjustments associated with voluntary movement. *J Biomech* 1987;20:735–742.

Broberg KB, von Essen HO: Modeling of intervertebral discs. *Spine* 1980;5:155–167.

Crisco JJ III, Panjabi MM: The intersegmental and multisegmental muscles of the lumbar spine: A biomechanical model comparing lateral stabilizing potential. *Spine* 1991;16:793–799.

De Luca CJ: Myoelectrical manifestations of localized muscular fatigue in humans. *Crit Rev Biomed Eng* 1984;11:251–279.

Eklund JA, Corlett EN: Shrinkage as a measure of the effect of load on the spine. *Spine* 1984;9:189–194.

el Bohy AA, Yang KH, King AI: Experimental verification of facet load transmission by direct measurement of facet lamina contact pressure. *J Biomech* 1989;22: 931–941.

Freivalds A, Chaffin DB, Garg A, et al: A dynamic biomechanical evaluation of lifting maximum acceptable loads. *J Biomech* 1984;17:251–262.

Frymoyer JW, Frymoyer WW, Wilder DG, et al: The mechanical and kinematic analysis of the lumbar spine in normal living human subjects in vivo. *J Biomech* 1979;12:165–172.

Goel VK, Nishiyama K, Weinstein JN, et al: Mechanical properties of lumbar spinal motion segments as affected by partial disc removal. *Spine* 1986;11:1008–1012.

Goode JD, Theodore BM: Voluntary and diurnal variation in height and associated surface contour changes in spinal curves. *Eng Med* 1983;12:99–101.

Graves JE, Pollock ML, Carpenter DM, et al: Quantitative assessment of full range-of-motion isometric lumbar extension strength. *Spine* 1990;15:289–294.

Gregersen GG, Lucas DB: An in vivo study of the axial rotation of the human thoracolumbar spine. *J Bone Joint Surg* 1967;49A:247–262.

Gunzburg R, Hutton W, Fraser R: Axial rotation of the lumbar spine and the effect of flexion: An in-vitro and in-vivo biomechanical study. *Spine* 1991;16:22–28.

Hansson TH, Keller TS, Spengler DM: Mechanical behavior of the human lumbar spine: II. Fatigue strength during dynamic compressive loading. *J Orthop Res* 1987;5:479–487.

Hirsch C, Nachemson A: New observations on the mechanical behavior of lumbar discs. *Acta Orthop Scand* 1954;23:254–283.

Horst M, Brinckmann P: 1980 Volvo award in biomechanics: Measurement of the distribution of axial stress on the end-plate of the vertebral body. *Spine* 1981;6:217–232.

Hukins DW, Kirby MC, Skoryn TA, et al: Comparison of structure, mechanical properties, and functions of lumbar spinal ligaments. *Spine* 1990;15:787–795.

Jensen KS, Mosekilde L, Mosekilde L: A model of vertebral trabecular bone architecture and its mechanical properties. *Bone* 1990;11:417–423.

Kahanovitz N, Nordin M, Verderame R, et al: Normal trunk muscle strength and endurance in women and the effect of exercises and electrical stimulation: Part 2. Comparative analysis of electrical stimulation and exercises to increase trunk muscle strength and endurance. *Spine* 1987;12:112–118.

Kazarian LE: Creep characteristics of the human spinal column. *Orthop Clin North Am* 1975;6:3–18.

Keller TS, Hansson TH, Abram AC, et al: Regional variations in the compressive properties of lumbar vertebral trabeculae: Effects of disc degeneration. *Spine* 1989;14:1012–1019.

Keller TS, Holm SH, Hansson TH, et al: 1990 Volvo Award in experimental studies: The dependence of intervertebral disc mechanical properties on physiologic conditions. *Spine* 1990;15:751–761.

Konttinen YT, Gronblad M, Antti-Poika I, et al: Neuroimmunohistochemical analysis of peridiscal nociceptive neural elements. *Spine* 1990;15:383–386.

Krag MH: Biomechanics of the cervical spine, in Frymoyer JW, Ducker TB, Hadler NM, et al (eds): *The Adult Spine: Principles and Practice.* New York, Raven Press, 1991, vol 2, pp 929–965.

Krämer J: Pressure dependent fluid shifts in the intervertebral disc. *Orthop Clin North Am* 1977;8:211–216.

Kulak RF, Belytschko TB, Schultz AB, et al: Nonlinear behavior of the human intervertebral disc under axial load. *J Biomech* 1976;9:377–386.

Lavender SA, Mirka GA, Schoenmarklin RW, et al: The effects of preview and task symmetry on trunk muscle response to sudden loading. *Hum Factors* 1989;31:101–115.

Lin HS, Liu YK, Adams KH: Mechanical response of the lumbar intervertebral joint under physiological (complex) loading. *J Bone Joint Surg* 1978;60A:41–55.

Liu YK, Goel VK, Dejong A, et al: Torsional fatigue of the lumbar intervertebral joints. *Spine* 1985;10:894–900.

Lorenz M, Patwardhan A, Vanderby R Jr: Load-bearing characteristics of lumbar facets in normal and surgically altered spinal segments. *Spine* 1983;8:122–130.

Macintosh JE, Bogduk N: 1987 Volvo award in basic science: The morphology of the lumbar erector spinae. *Spine* 1987;12:658–668.

Macintosh JE, Bogduk N: The biomechanics of the lumbar multifidus. *Clin Biomech* 1986;1:205–213.

Maroudas A, Stockwell RA, Nachemson A, et al: Factors involved in the nutrition of the human lumbar intervertebral disc: Cellularity and diffusion of glucose in vitro. *J Anat* 1975;120:113–130.

Mayer TG, Kondraske G, Mooney V, et al: Lumbar myoelectric spectral analysis for endurance assessment: A comparison of normals with deconditioned patients. *Spine* 1989;14:986–991.

Mayer TG, Tencer AF, Kristoferson S, et al: Use of noninvasive techniques for quantification of spinal range-of-motion in normal subjects and chronic low-back dysfunction patients. *Spine* 1984;9:588–595.

Moroney SP, Schultz AB, Miller JA, et al: Load-displacement properties of lower cervical spine motion segments. *J Biomech* 1988;21:769–779.

Mosekilde L, Mosekilde L: Sex differences in age-related changes in vertebral body size, density and biomechanical competence in normal individuals. *Bone* 1990;11:67–73.

Nachemson A: Lumbar intradiscal pressure, in Jayson M (ed): *The Lumbar Spine and Back Pain.* New York, Grune & Stratton, 1976, pp 257–269.

National Institute for Occupational Safety and Health: *Work Practices Guide for Manual Lifting.* Cincinnati, OH, US Department of Health and Human Services, 1981, Tech Report 81-122.

Nies N, Sinnott PL: Variations in balance and body sway in middle-aged adult: Subjects with healthy backs compared with subjects with low-back dysfunction. *Spine* 1991;16:325–330.

Ogston NG, King GJ, Gertzbein SD, et al: Centrode patterns in the lumbar spine: Baseline studies in normal subjects. *Spine* 1986;11:591–595.

Panjabi M, Aburni K, Duranceau J, et al: Spinal stablity and intersegmental muscle forces: A biomechanical model. *Spine* 1989;14:194–200.

Panjabi MM, Andersson GB, Jorneus L, et al: In vivo measurements of spinal column vibrations. *J Bone Joint Surg* 1986;68A:695–702.

Panjabi MM, Brand RA Jr, White AA III: Mechanical properties of the human thoracic spine as shown by three-dimensional load-displacement curves. *J Bone Joint Surg* 1976;58A:642–652.

Panjabi M, Dvorak J, Dranceau J, et al: Three-dimensional movements of the upper cervical spine. *Spine* 1988;13:726–730.

Panjabi MM, Krag MH, Chung TQ: Effects of disc injury on mechanical behavior of the human spine. *Spine* 1984;9:707–713.

Panjabi MM, White AA III, Johnson RM: Cervical spine mechanics as a function of transection of components. *J Biomech* 1975;8:327–336.

Parnianpour M, Nordin M, Kahanovitz N, et al: 1988 Volvo award in biomechanics: The triaxial coupling of torque generation of trunk muscles during isometric exertions and the effect of fatiguing isoinertial movements on the motor output and movement patterns. *Spine* 1988;13:982–992.

Parnianpour M, Li F, Nordin M, et al: A database of isoinertal trunk strength tests against three resistance levels in sagittal, frontal, and transverse planes in normal male subjects. *Spine* 1989;14:409–411.

Pearcy MJ, Bogduk N: Instantaneous axes of rotation of the lumbar intervertebral joints. *Spine* 1988;13: 1033–1041.

Penning L: Functional anatomy of joints and discs, in The Cervical Spine Research Society Editorial Committee (eds): *The Cervical Spine,* ed 2. Philadelphia, PA, JB Lippincott, 1989, pp 33–56.

Pope MH, Andersson GB, Broman H, et al: Electromyographic studies of the lumbar trunk musculature during the development of axial torques. *J Orthop Res* 1986;4:288–297.

Pope MH, Frymoyer JW, Lehmann TR: Structure and function of the lumbar spine, in Pope MH, Andersson GBJ, Frymoyer JW, et al (eds): *Occupational Low Back Pain: Assessment, Treatment and Prevention.* St. Louis, MO, Mosby Year Book, 1991, pp 3–19.

Pope MH, Svensson M, Andersson GB, et al: The role of prerotation of the trunk in axial twisting efforts. *Spine* 1987;12:1041–1045.

Pope MH, Wilder DG, Matteri RE, et al: Experimental measurements of vertebral motion under load. *Orthop Clin North Am* 1977;8:155–167.

Posner I, White AA III, Edwards WT, et al: A biomechanical analysis of the clinical stability of the lumbar and lumbosacral spine. *Spine* 1982;7:374–389.

Reid JG, Costigan PA: Trunk muscle balance and muscle force. *Spine* 1987;12:783–786.

Ritchie JH, Fahrni WH: Age changes in lumbar intervertebral discs. *Can J Surg* 1970;13:65–71.

Roy SH, De Luca CJ, Casavant DA: Lumbar muscle fatigue and chronic lower back pain. *Spine* 1989;14:992–1001.

Schultz A, Andersson GB, Ortengren R, et al: Analysis and quantitative myoelectric measurements of loads on the lumbar spine when holding weights in standing postures. *Spine* 1982;7:390–397.

Schultz A, Cromwell R, Warwick D, et al: Lumbar trunk muscle use in standing isometric heavy exertions. *J Orthop Res* 1987;5:320–329.

Schultz AB, Warwick DN, Berkson MH, et al: Mechanical properties of human lumbar spine motion segments: Part I. Responses in flexion, extension, lateral bending and torsion. *J Biomech Eng* 1979;101:46–52.

Seidel H, Beyer H, Brauer D: Electromyographic evaluation of back muscle fatigue with repeated sustained contractions of different strengths. *Eur J Appl Physiol* 1987;56:592–602.

Seroussi RE, Pope MH: The relationship between trunk muscle electromyography and lifting moments in the sagittal and frontal planes. *J Biomech* 1987;20:135–146.

Smidt GL, Blanpied PR, White RW: Exploration of mechanical and electromyographic responses of trunk muscles to high-intensity resistive exercise. *Spine* 1989;14:815–830.

Smith JL, Smith LA, McLaughlin TM: A biomechanical analysis of industrial manual materials handlers. *Ergonomics* 1982;25:299–308.

Snook SH: Low back pain in industry, in White AA III, Gordon SL (eds): *American Academy of Orthopaedic Surgeons Symposium on Idiopathic Low Back Pain.* St. Louis, MO, CV Mosby, 1982, pp 23–38.

Soukka A, Alaranta H, Tallroth K, et al: Leg-length inequality in people of working age: The association between mild inequality and low-back pain is questionable. *Spine* 1991;16:429–431.

Thurston AJ, Harris JD: Normal kinematics of the lumbar spine and pelvis. *Spine* 1983;8:199–205.

Urban JP, Holm S, Maroudas A, et al: Nutrition of the intervertebral disc: An in vivo study of solute transport. *Clin Orthop* 1977;129:101–114.

White AA III, Panjabi MM: The basic kinematics of the human spine: A review of past and current knowledge. *Spine* 1978;3:12–20.

White AA III, Panjabi MM (eds): Kinematics of the spine, in *Clinical Biomechanics of the Spine,* ed 2. Philadelphia, PA, JB Lippincott, 1991.

Wilder DG, Pope MH, Frymoyer JW: The biomechanics of lumbar disc herniation and the effect of overload and instability. *J Spinal Disord* 1988;1:16–32.

Yang JF, Winter DA, Wells RP: Postural dynamics in the standing human. *Biol Cybern* 1990;62:309–320.

Zetterberg C, Andersson GB, Schultz AB: The activity of individual trunk muscles during heavy physical loading. *Spine* 1987;12:1035–1040.

Hip

Crowninshield RD, Johnston RC, Andrews JG, et al: A biomechanical investigation of the human hip. *J Biomech* 1978;11:75–85.

Das De S, Bose K, Balasubramaniam P, et al: Surface morphology of Asian cadaveric hips. *J Bone Joint Surg* 1985;67B:225–228.

Davy DT, Kotzar GM, Brown RH, et al: Telemetric force measurements across the hip after total arthroplasty. *J Bone Joint Surg* 1988;70A:45–50.

Figge FHJ: *Atlas of Human Anatomy,* ed 8. New York, Hafner Publishing, 1968, vol 1.

Hardt DE: Determining muscle forces in the leg during normal human walking: An application and evaluation of optimization methods. *J Biomech Eng* 1978;100:72–78.

Hodge WA, Carlson KL, Fijan RS, et al: Contact pressures from an instrumented hip endoprosthesis. *J Bone Joint Surg* 1989;71A:1378–1386.

Patriarco AG, Mann RW, Simon SR, et al: An evaluation of the approaches of optimization models in the prediction of muscle forces during human gait. *J Biomech* 1981;14:513–525.

Paul JP, McGrouther DA: Force actions transmitted by joints in the human body. *Proc R Soc Lond [Biol]* 1976;192:163–172.

Pedotti A, Krishnan VV, Stark L: Optimization of muscle-force sequencing in human locomotion. *Math Biosci* 1978;38:57–76.

Rydell NW: Forces acting on the femoral head-prosthesis: A study on strain gauge supplied prostheses in living persons. *Acta Orthop Scand Suppl* 1966;88:1–132.

Knee

Arms S, Boyle J, Johnson R, et al: Strain measurement in the medial collateral ligament of the human knee: An autopsy study. *J Biomech* 1983;16:491–496.

Bartel DL, Marshall JL, Schieck RA, et al: Surgical repositioning of the medial collateral ligament: An anatomical and mechanical analysis. *J Bone Joint Surg* 1977;59A:107–116.

Brantigan OC, Voshell AF: The tibial collateral ligament: Its function, its bursae, and its relation to the medial meniscus. *J Bone Joint Surg* 1943;25A:121–131.

Butler DL, Noyes FR, Grood ES: Ligamentous restraints to anterior-posterior drawer in the human knee: A biomechanical study. *J Bone Joint Surg* 1980;62A: 259–270.

Daniel DM, Akeson WH, O'Connor JJ (eds): *Knee Ligaments: Structure, Function, Injury and Repair.* New York, Raven Press, 1990.

Daniel DM, Malcom LL, Losse G: Instrumented measurement of anterior laxity of the knee. *J Bone Joint Surg* 1985;67A:720–726.

Feagin JA Jr: *The Crucial Ligaments: Diagnosis and Treatment of Ligamentous Injuries About the Knee.* New York, Churchill Livingstone, 1988.

Frankel VH, Nordin M: *Basic Biomechanics of the Skeletal System.* Philadelphia, PA, Lea & Febiger, 1980.

Fukubayashi T, Torzilli PA, Sherman MF, et al: An in vitro biomechanical evaluation of anterior-posterior motion of the knee: Tibial displacement, rotation, and torque. *J Bone Joint Surg* 1982;64A:258.

Girgis FG, Marshall JL, Al Monajem ARS: The cruciate ligaments of the knee joint: Anatomical, functional and experimental analysis. *Clin Orthop* 1975;106:216–231.

Hollinshead WH: *Anatomy for Surgeons: The Back and Limbs.* New York, Hoeber-Harper, 1954, vol 3.

Hughston JC, Bowden JA, Andrews JR, et al: Acute tears of the posterior cruciate ligament: Results of operative treatment. *J Bone Joint Surg* 1980;62A:438–450.

Insall JN, Scott WN, Kelly M, et al (eds): *Surgery of the Knee,* ed 2. New York, Churchill Livingstone, 1993.

Kaplan EB: The iliotibial tract: Clinical and morphological significance. *J Bone Joint Surg* 1958;40A:817–832.

Nicholas JA, Hershman EB: *The Lower Extremity and Spine in Sports Medicine.* St. Louis, MO, CV Mosby, 1986.

Odensten M, Gillquist J: Functional anatomy of the anterior cruciate ligament and rationale for reconstruction. *J Bone Joint Surg* 1985;67A:257–262.

Warren LF, Marshall JL: The supporting structures and layers on the medial side of the knee: An anatomical analysis. *J Bone Joint Surg* 1979;61A:56–62.

Foot and Ankle

Allard P, Thiry PS, Duhaime M: Estimation of the ligaments' role in maintaining foot stability using a kinematic model. *Med Biol Eng Comput* 1985;23: 237–242.

Allard P, Eng P, Stokes IAF, et al: Modelling of the foot and ankle, in Jahss ME (ed): *Disorders of the Foot & Ankle: Medical and Surgical Management,* ed 2. Philadelphia, WB Saunders, 1991.

Andrews JG: On the specification of joint configurations and motions. *J Biomech* 1984;17:155–158.

Attarian DE, McCrackin HJ, Devito DP, et al: Biomechanical characteristics of human ankle ligaments. *Foot Ankle* 1985;6:54–58.

Barnett CH, Napier JR: The axis of rotation at the ankle joint in man: Its influence upon the form of the talus and the mobility of the fibula. *J Anat* 1952;86:1–9.

Bonink RJ: The constraint mechanism of the human tarsus: A roentgenological experimental study. *Acta Orthop Scand Suppl* 1985;569(Suppl 215]:1–135.

Bojsen-Møller F: Calcaneocuboid joint and stability of the longitudinal arch of the foot at high and low gear push off. *J Anat* 1979;129:165–176.

Cass JR, Morrey BF, Chao EYS: Three-dimensional kinematics of ankle instability following serial sectioning of lateral collateral ligaments. *Foot Ankle* 1984;5:142–149.

Castaing J, Delplace J, Le Roy JD: *La Cheville.* Paris, Edition Vigot, 1960.

Cavanagh PR, Rodgers MM: Pressure distribution underneath the human foot, in Perren SM, Schneider E (eds): *Biomechanics: Current Interdisciplinary Research.* Doredrecht, Martinus Nijhoff Publishers, 1985.

Close JR, Inman VT, Poor PM, et al: The function of the subtalar joint. *Clin Orthop* 1967;50:159–179.

Close JR, Todd FN: The phasic activity of the muscles of the lower extremity and the effect of tendon transfer. *J Bone Joint Surg* 1959;41A:189–208.

Duckworth T, Betts RP, Franks CI, et al: The measurement of pressures under the foot. *Foot Ankle* 1982;3:130–141.

Dul J, Townsend MA, Shiavi R, et al: Muscular synergism: I. On criteria for load sharing between synergistic muscles. *J Biomech* 1984;17:663–673.

Dul J, Johnson GE, Shiavi R, et al: Muscular synergism: II. A minimum fatigue criterion for load sharing between synergistic muscles. *J Biomech* 1984;17: 675–684.

Grundy M, Tosh BP, McLeish RD, et al: An investigation of the centres of pressure under the foot while walking. *J Bone Joint Surg* 1975;57B:98–103.

Hicks JH: The mechanics of the foot: I. The joints. *J Anat* 1953;87:345–357.

Hicks JH: The mechanics of the foot: II. The plantar aponeurosis and the arch. *J Anat* 1954;88:25–30.

Hicks JH: The mechanics of the foot: IV. The action of muscles on the foot in standing. *Acta Anat* 1956;27:180–192.

Hicks JH: The foot as a support. *Acta Anat* 1955;25:34–45.

Huson A: Functional anatomy of the foot, in Jahss MH (ed): *Disorders of the Foot & Ankle: Medical and Surgical Management,* ed 2. Philadelphia, PA, WB Saunders, 1991.

Huson A, Van Langelaan EJ, Spoor CW: The talocrural and tarsal mechanism and tibiotalar delay. *Acta Morphol Neerl-Scand* 1986;24:296.

Mann R, Inman VT: Phasic activity of intrinsic muscles of the foot. *J Bone Joint Surg* 1964;46A:469–481.

Mann RA, Baxter DE, Lutter LD: Running symposium. *Foot Ankle* 1981;1:190–224.

Mann R: Overview of foot and ankle biomechanics, in Jahss MH (ed): *Disorders of the Foot & Ankle: Medical and Surgical Management,* ed 2. Philadelphia, PA, WB Saunders, 1991.

Rasmussen O: Stability of the ankle joint: Analysis of the function and traumatology of the ankle ligaments. *Acta Orthop Scand* 1985;(Suppl 211):1–75.

Stiehl JB (ed): *Inman's Joints of the Ankle,* ed 2. Baltimore, MD, Williams & Wilkins, 1991.

Stott JR, Hutton WC, Stokes IA: Forces under the foot. *J Bone Joint Surg* 1973;55B:335–344.

Wright DG, Desai SM, Henderson WH: Action of the subtalar and ankle-joint complex during the stance phase of walking. *J Bone Joint Surg* 1964;46A:361–382.

Coordinated Functions

Frank JS, Earl M: Coordination of posture and movement. *Phys Ther* 1990;70:855–863.

Friedli WG, Cohen L, Hallett M, et al: Postural adjustments associated with rapid voluntary arm movements: I. Electromyographic data. *J Neurol Neurosurg Psychiatry* 1984;47:611–622.

Friedli WG, Hallett M, Simon SR: Postural adjustments associated with rapid voluntary arm movements. II. Biomechanical analysis. *J Neurol Neurosurg Psychiatry* 1988;51:232–241.

Horak FB: Clinical measurement of postural control in adults. *Phys Ther* 1987;67:1881–1885.

Mann RA, Hagy J: Biomechanics of walking, running and sprinting. *Am J Sports Med* 1980;8:345–350.

Mansour JM, Lesh MD, Nowak MD, et al: A three-dimensional multi-segmental analysis of the energetics of normal and pathological human gait. *J Biomech* 1982;15:51–59.

Martin JP: A short essay on posture and movement. *J Neurol Neurosurg Psychiatry* 1977;40:25–29.

Morrison JB: Bioengineering analysis of force actions transmitted by the knee joint. *Biomed Eng* 1968;3:464–470.

Murray MP: Gait as a total pattern of movement. *Am J Phys Med* 1967;46:290–333.

Murray MP, Seireg AA, Sepic SB: Normal postural stability and steadiness: Quantitative assessment. *J Bone Joint Surg* 1975;57A:510–516.

Nashner LM: Balance adjustments of humans perturbed while walking. *J Neurophysiol* 1980;44:650–664.

Nashner LM, McCollum G: The organization of human postural movement: A focal basis and experimental synthesis. *Behav Brain Sci* 1985;8:135–172.

Nashner LM: Adaptations of human movement to altered environments. *Trends Neurosci* 1982;3:358–361.

Pedotti A, Krishnan BV, Stark L: Optimization of muscle-force sequencing in human locomotion. *Math Biosci* 1978;38:57–76.

Perry J: *Gait Analysis: Normal and Pathological Function.* Thorofare, NJ, SLACK, Inc, 1992.

Pierrynowski MR, Morrison JB: Estimating the muscle forces generated in the human lower extremity when walking: A physiological solution. *Math Biosci* 1985;75:43–68.

Saunders JB, Inman VT, Eberhart HD: The major determinants in normal and pathological gait. *J Bone Joint Surg* 1953;35A:543–558.

Seireg A, Arvikar RJ: The prediction of muscular load sharing and joint forces in the lower extremities during walking. *J Biomech* 1975;8:89–102.

Sutherland DH, Olshen R, Cooper L, et al: The development of mature gait. *J Bone Joint Surg* 1980;62A:336–353.

Thorstensson A, Nilsson J, Carlson H, et al: Trunk movements in human locomotion. *Acta Physiol Scand* 1984;121:9–22.

Winter DA: *The Biomechanics and Motor Control of Human Gait: Normal, Elderly and Pathological.* Waterloo, Ontario, Canada, University of Waterloo Press, 1991.

Woollacott MH, Shumway-Cook A: Changes in posture control across the life span: A systems approach. *Phys Ther* 1990;70:799–807.

Chapter 13
Experimental Design and Statistical Analysis

Richard L. Lieber, PhD

Chapter Outline

Introduction

Improved understanding of the musculoskeletal system results from the search for general truths and the desire to understand the general laws that regulate the system. Building such an understanding requires that experiments be conducted to observe how the system operates under different conditions. The way such observations are made depends on the type of phenomenon observed. In certain circumstances, a phenomenon can be considered deterministic; that is, every time it is observed the outcome is exactly the same. For example, a ball with a known size and weight dropped from a certain height will always hit the ground with the same force, no matter how many times it is observed. In this situation, only one observation is needed to know what the results will always be. However, certain phenomena may occur only sometimes; each time one of these phenomena occurs or is tested, different results can be obtained. Because these results occur with a certain probability, such phenomena are considered probabilistic. To determine whether there is some consistency in the effects produced, or whether relationships or associations occur, such phenomena must be observed many times, and the data obtained must be analyzed.

Analysis of such results must distinguish between causality and chance occurrence. These distinctions are made using statistical analysis. Inherent in this analysis is the fact that conclusions are reached by repeatedly observing a subset of members of an entire population. For example, members of the entire population of a given fish species must be examined many times to be sure that a color or design pattern is, indeed, inherent in that species. Observing one member of that species once would not necessarily provide such a conclusion. Because it is often either impractical, costly, or inefficient to examine the entire population, a representative group is selected, and the phenomenon is tested only the number of times with each representative member that suffices to ensure its validity. Statistics provides the objective methodology to assure adequate performance of this task. The reliability of statistics and the conclusions drawn from it are based on the science of probability.

This chapter defines and describes many terms and techniques used in statistics. Its purpose is to provide the reader with the basis for understanding, appreciating, and evaluating conclusions that may be drawn from clinical or basic science studies. In addition, it will provide the reader with the means to recognize both the validity and limitations of the conclusions that are drawn. All topics of statistics are not covered in this chapter; it covers only those that are current or that more particularly demonstrate principles that apply to the extraction of valid conclusions for musculoskeletal system phenomena.

Hypothesis Testing

If we are to examine a phenomenon and try to extract information from observations of it, where the chance of its occurring each time it is observed is not 100%, we must first describe it in a quantitative form. We often have a preconceived notion of how a group of individuals will respond to a treatment. We thus formulate a hypothesis. A hypothesis, simply stated, is a supposition that appears to describe a phenomenon and acts as a basis of reasoning and experimentation. Hypotheses may be extremely basic—for example, growth factor binding to extracellular matrix proteins activates cellular protein synthesis—or very applied—for example, use of the patellar tendon for surgical reconstruction of the anterior cruciate ligament results in loss of quadriceps strength.

A hypothesis is an untested statement based on previous information, a hunch, or an intuition. It can be stated for any group of observations. However, to ensure that the observations noted are appropriate, the measurements made are accurate, the experiment is performed efficiently, and the conclusions drawn are accurate, the hypothesis must be stated in a quantitative form and in a specific manner. Clearly stating the hypothesis focuses attention on the central issues and assures that a given phenomenon can properly be evaluated and reexamined.

A hypothesis to be tested using statistical methodology is presented in terms of the null hypothesis. The null hypothesis states that experimental treatment has no effect; that is, is null. As an example, we could propose the following null hypothesis: There is no difference in ultimate tensile strength between a patellar tendon that is a surgically repaired substitute for the anterior cruciate ligament and a normal anterior cruciate ligament. To test this hypothesis, ultimate tensile strength from a control group that has no ligament injury is compared to ultimate strength from an experimental group that was surgically repaired using the patellar tendon.

In one of the most common embodiments, an experiment based on a null hypothesis is designed with a control group that receives no treatment, and one or more experimental groups that receive treatment (Fig. 1).

Four conclusions can be drawn from the use of the null hypothesis (Table 1). The null hypothesis

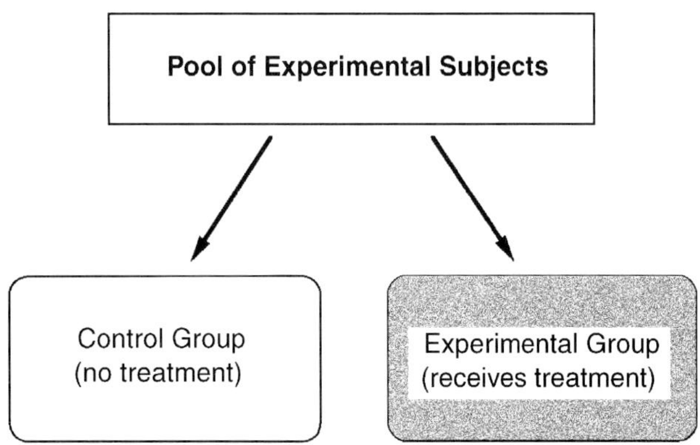

Figure 1
Schematic illustration of the simplest experimental design in which experimental subjects are divided into a control and an experimental group.

Table 1
Statistical errors related to the null hypothesis

	Null Hypothesis	
	Accepted	**Rejected**
True	Correct decision	Type I error
False	Type II error	Correct decision

can be either true or false. In addition, each of these can be accepted or rejected (that is, believed or not believed). Of the four potential decisions, two are correct and two are incorrect (Table 1). Suppose, in our ligament strength example, that the null hypothesis is true; that is, there really is no difference in ligament strength between experimental and control groups. But suppose also that, based on our analysis or limited sample, we choose to believe that there is a difference (that is, we reject a true null hypothesis). In statistics, rejection of a true null hypothesis is an incorrect conclusion known as type I error. In this experiment, committing type I error would imply that there is a significant effect of surgical repair when, in fact, there is not. This error can be viewed in more clinical terms as a false positive (Table 2).

An alternate possibility is that the null hypothesis is false; that is, surgical repair has a significant effect on ligament strength. If, for similar reasons, we chose to believe that there was no effect on ligament strength, we would be falsely accepting the null hypothesis. Accepting a false null hypothesis is known as a type II error. In this experiment, committing a type II error would imply that surgery had no effect when, in fact, it actually had an effect. This can be viewed in clinical terms as a false negative (Table 2).

Table 2
Interpretation and control of statistical error

Condition	Greek Symbol	Clinical Meaning	Controlled Using
Type I error	α	False positive	Significance level
Type II error	β	False negative	Statistical power

In the above experiment, what would it mean clinically to commit a type I or type II error, and if one did commit such errors, how serious would they be? First, if we committed a type I error, we would state there is a difference in strength with surgical repair using the patellar tendon when, in fact, there is none. We would be stating something is different when it really is not. We then would probably try to find another tendon that showed no difference in strength, and we would modify our rehabilitation program when we used the patellar tendon in the procedure. We would continue to test different tendons until we found one that showed no difference in strength. However, if we kept committing the same type of error, we might never find the right tendon. Then we would be forced to accept a procedure as a compromise—a less than desirable condition. In spite of the time and expense involved in such experimentation, we still would be left with the incorrect conclusion.

If we made a type II error, we would be stating that there is no difference in strength when the patellar tendon is used, when in fact there is a difference. We would be missing something that is really there. This is a more serious error in this example, for it can lead not only to our abandoning the attempt to find a better substitute, but also to our performing a procedure that could subsequently produce complications. Only after we knew of these complications and our patients have suffered the consequences, would we seek a substitute.

The seriousness of each type of error depends on the situation; in the best situation, we must try not to commit either type of error. If we cannot eliminate errors, we must at least try to reduce the chance of committing either type of error. The probability or chance of committing a type I error, that is, the probability of finding an effect when there really isn't one, is known as the significance level of a statistical test, termed alpha or α. The probability or chance of committing a type II error, that is, the probability of failing to find an effect when there really is one, is known as beta or β. In statistical testing, the term "significance level" is used to describe a type I error, and "statistical power" (defined as 1-β) to describe a type II error. The calculation of α, β, or power is based on the science of probability and need not be detailed here because it can readily be found in statistical tables and/or automatically calculated by a computer program. Its importance to readers of this text lies in the awareness that both types of errors can exist and in the understanding of how they are avoided. Now, let us consider many terms and definitions that are common in statistical analysis.

Statistical Definitions and Descriptions of Observations

Our ability to extract the truth from a set of observations rests on our ability to accurately describe the phenomenon and use the appropriate tools to analyze it. To do this, we must first describe the phenomenon in statistical terms, which are presented here.

Statistical Terms

Sample Versus Population

In statistics, a population is the entire collection of elements about which information is desired. A sample is a collection of observations representing the population or a collection of individual observations from the population selected by a specified procedure. Statistics are used to generalize from a sample to a population. In practice, a correct interpretation of these terms is related to a proper value for sample size; that is, the value for n.

It is important to define the "collection of elements" from which data are obtained. An example of a population could be the anterior compartment muscles of male humans in San Diego County. Additional qualifications such as age and health status might also be important. Having defined the population, it would only be appropriate to generalize from the analysis of our sample to other populations having similar traits. This fact has been recognized by the National Institutes of Health in their recent report on the paucity of scientific data that are applicable to women.

The sample concept refers both to the actual data obtained and to the procedure itself. An example of a sample is the maximum dorsiflexion torque from 40 male college-aged volunteers. Here the concept of sample includes the amount of data or number of observations or data points to be examined, termed n. This number must be explicitly determined to guard against erroneous generalizations or inflated significance levels.

Variable

A variable is the actual property measured by the individual observations. Using our example, a variable would be torque, measured in N·m.

Variate

A variate is a single reading, score, or observation of a given variable. Thus, a sample is composed of a number of variates obtained for a selected number of variables. An example of a variate would be the value 142.2 N·m from subject DJC.

Level

Level is the number of different values a grouping variable can have. For example, in an experiment where men's versus women's strength is compared, the grouping variable, sex, has two levels: male or female.

Precision

Precision is the closeness of repeated measurements of the same quantity.

Accuracy

Accuracy is the closeness of a measured variate to its true value. This definition implies that a standard is available against which a measure can be compared. A knowledge of accuracy determines the numbers of significant figures for the presentation of experimental results. Using an example, we might determine that a 2.000000-kg standard mass is shown on a balance scale as 2.011233 kg. This is probably an acceptable level of accuracy (within 1%), but it would be absurd to report mass to six decimal places. Although there is no problem in retaining all figures for intermediate calculations, the final data presentation must reflect the appropriate accuracy, in this case 2.01 or about 0.56%.

Accuracy and precision are often confused. Precision simply refers to the repeatability of a particular measurement. Thus, in our example above, the balance scale may read 2.011233 kg for one reading, 2.011210 for the next, and 2.011225 for the next. Our device is thus precise to 0.00002 kg in spite of the fact that it is only accurate to about 0.01 kg. In this age of computers and digital displays it is important to vigilantly recall that high precision does not imply high accuracy.

It is important to ensure that accurate results are obtained to enable comparison of experimental data across laboratories. For example, a balance scale used to weigh samples in one laboratory might be precise but consistently read values that are greater than another balance scale down the hall. In such a case, the two laboratories will differ with respect to their interpretation of a particular phenomenon. In addition, if an experimenter uses both balances interchangeably, experimental variability will be needlessly increased.

Conversely, we should not be quick to discard measurements that are not very precise (for example, intraoperative measurements of nerve width) believing that they do not contain useful information. For example, intraoperative measurements with a standard ruler calibrated in millimeters can be read to a fraction of a millimeter. One of the beauties of multiple measurements of the same quantity is that random errors tend to cancel out. Thus, three measurements of nerve width might be 2.5 mm, 3.0 mm, and 3.0 mm. The average value of 2.83 mm is probably closer to the true value than any of the individual measurements. It is, therefore, possible to resolve smaller differences than are actually present on a measuring device by repeated measures with this "less precise" device!

Mean

The sample mean, designated $\overline{X}$, is the average of all variates for a sample and is an unbiased estimator of the population μ. The population mean is the most probable value within the population and the one that the investigator wishes to estimate based on the mean of its representative sample. The sample mean estimates the population mean if the population is normally distributed. The values within a normally distributed sample fit into the classic bell-shaped curve (Fig. 2). The shape of the normal distribution is very specific; the curve cannot be too tail heavy if it is to be considered normally distributed. Many natural measurements, such as length, height, and mass, are usually normally distributed, whereas many others, especially ratios and percentages, are almost never normally distributed. One of the first concerns in statistical analysis of experimental data is whether or not the sample variates are normally distributed.

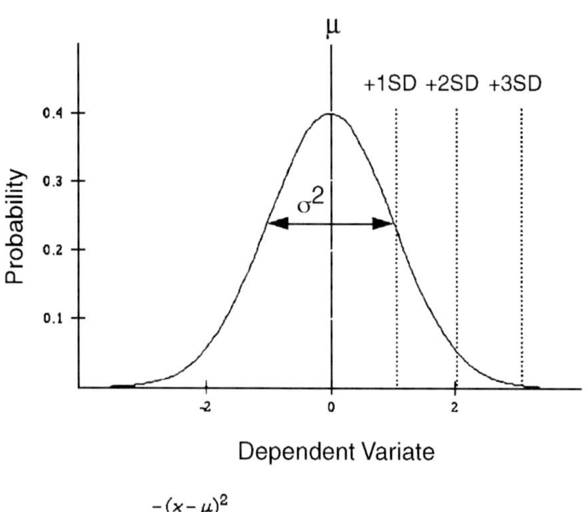

Figure 2
Graphic representation of the normal distribution. Note that the mean μ represents the most probable value and the variance σ^2 represents the population variability.

The units of the mean are the same as the units of the variable. Sample mean is calculated as:

$$\overline{X} = \frac{\sum_{i=1}^{i=n} X_i}{n} \qquad \textbf{(Eq. 1)}$$

where

$\sum_{i=1}^{i=n}$ = the arithmetic summation of all n values of X_i
X_i = the value of an individual variate (read as the "ith" variate)
n = the sample size.

An example of a sample mean would be 136.2 N·m of knee extension torque, calculated as the mean of 12 individual variates.

Median

The median is the value below which half of the values lie and above which the remaining half of the values lie. It is the middle or the fiftieth percentile of a normal distribution.

Variance

The sample variance s^2 is a measure of the spread of data about the sample mean and is an estimator of the population variance σ^2. As shown in Figure 2, each population not only has its most probable value, the mean μ, it also has a certain variability or variance σ^2 about that value. It is more difficult to extract the "truth" from a population with large variance because the likelihood of obtaining a variate near the mean is less when sample variability is high.

As an example, to determine whether a particular exercise caused an increase in quadriceps strength after surgery, two groups of individuals were used—one group receiving traditional therapy and one group receiving therapy using the new exercise. Average group strengths would be compared, and the results of the comparison would indicate whether the exercise was efficacious. Suppose that the results in one population were highly variable (Fig. 3). The high variability might make it difficult to determine whether the two samples are truly different because the exercised group has many values that overlap with the traditional therapy group. It is fairly easy to detect a difference between the two means μ_1 and μ_2 in Figure 3, *top;* however,

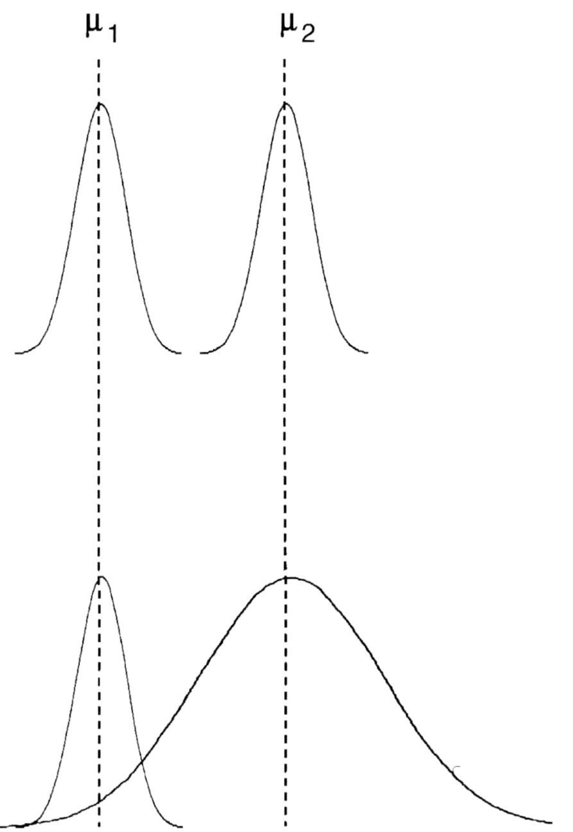

Figure 3
Graphic illustration of the difficulty in detecting a difference between the means of two populations when one population has a high variability (**bottom**) compared to when it has a lower variability (**top**).

with increased population variability (Fig. 3, *bottom*), this difference is less easy to demonstrate.

The proper units used to express variance are variable units squared. The calculation of variance uses a "sum of squared terms" as a type of expression.

$$\sigma^2 = \frac{\sum_{i=1}^{n} (\bar{X} - X_i)^2}{n - 1} \quad \text{(Eq. 2)}$$

The variance term contains a squared difference between the sample mean and the individual variate. This squared difference represents the "distance" from the mean to the value of a particular variate; it is squared to eliminate the sign of the difference (positive or negative) so that variability of either sign is summed over the entire sample. The entire summed, squared difference is divided by (n − 1) to yield a sort of "average" difference. The term n − 1 is used instead of the more intuitively appealing n because, as sample size gets small, statisticians have determined that this mathematical expression tends to slightly overestimate population variance. An example of a population variance might be 44 $(N\cdot m)^2$ which describes the variance of the mean of 12 individual knee extension torque variates.

Standard Deviation

Standard deviation (SD) is the square root of the sample variance. SD is more often used to describe population variability than sample variance because the units of SD are the same as the original variate units. An example of a SD is 6.6 N·m. This statement contains information as to the estimated population mean and has some information with respect to population variability.

The calculation of SD is simply:

$$SD = \sqrt{s^2} \quad \text{(Eq. 3)}$$

where

s^2 = the calculated sample variance.

SD has a very useful property for normally distributed data in that 66% of the variates are within one SD of the mean, 95% of the variates are within two SDs of the mean, and 99% of the variates are within three SDs of the mean (Fig. 2). Because this value refers to the variability of the original sample, it can be used to make powerful predictions regarding the variability of the original population if the sample properly represents the entire population.

An example of this type of approach is a study by investigators who were interested in understanding the normal anatomic path of the superficial branch of the radial nerve (SBRN). It was important to know where the SBRN became subcutaneous from the interval between the brachioradialis and the extensor carpi radialis longus, because external fixator pins are frequently inserted in this area and thus surgical approaches must avoid the SBRN. The researchers measured, in cadaveric specimens, the distance between the subcutaneous SBRN and an external bony landmark such as the radial styloid process, which can be palpated. They found that this distance was mean ± SD = 9.0 ± 1.4 cm, which enabled them to conclude that, in 95% of the individuals from the general population, the subcutaneous SBRN region extended from 6.2 cm (mean − 2 SD) to 11.8 cm (mean + 2 SD) proximal to the radial styloid process. Knowledge of this 95% confidence interval has significant surgical implications.

Standard Error of the Mean (SEM)

The SEM is the variability associated with estimation of the population mean. This value is used to describe the level of confidence we have that the mean, which is determined from a sample of a given population, represents the mean of the entire population. It is calculated as:

$$SEM = \frac{SD}{\sqrt{n}} \quad \textbf{(Eq. 4)}$$

where

SD = standard deviation
n = sample size.

SD is a relatively constant estimate of population variability, whereas SEM changes with sample size and does not estimate the population variability at all. Because it actually represents the accuracy of a mean estimate, it is preferable to use SEM when comparisons are made between means. SD, which is related to population variability, is preferable when it is necessary to express the variability of the original population. For example, SD might be preferred when describing the baseline characteristics of a group of experimental subjects because it would provide the reader with an idea of the level of variability in the population from which the sample was obtained. However, when comparing a treatment group to a control group, SEM may be preferable because the accuracy of the individual mean values is of interest.

Coefficient of Variation (CV)

The CV is a generic indicator of population variance. CV is calculated as:

$$CV = \frac{SD}{\bar{X}} \cdot 100\% \quad \textbf{(Eq. 5)}$$

so that the CV is expressed without the original units of measurement. Because CV is independent of units and absolute variate magnitude, it provides a general feel for a population's variability. There is no acceptable level of variability for a particular population. Thus, in a clinical experiment involving complex treatment of individuals who have variable characteristics, a CV of 50% to 100% might be expected and accepted, whereas in a laboratory experiment involving a more homogeneous species and a clearly defined procedure, a CV of 10% to 25% would be more likely. It is much easier to determine whether significant effects of a particular treatment exist when the CV of the sample is low.

Choice of Significance and Power Values

Terms such as SD, SEM, and CV and the calculation of such parameters illustrate that an experiment does not always work the way we expect. It is the variation that these terms represent that causes us to question or believe the results we obtain, and these terms give us an indication of how much we can believe the conclusions drawn. However, there is no true or ideal answer to the question of how much variability or error we can accept before we will no longer believe or disbelieve the results. The investigator and reader must decide what to accept, and their decisions will vary depending on the nature of the study. Statistics provides a means of quantifying what we wish to accept. This is expressed in the p value and α and β levels.

The p value is simply the probability (denoted α) of committing type I error in a given experiment (Table 2). When a report states that the results were significant ($p < 0.05$), the investigator is saying that type I error has been committed less than 5% of the time. Often we conclude that if a type 1 error is committed only 5% of the time we can believe the results; that is, we expect the conclusions drawn to be found not just in the representative sample but in the entire population as well. The problem with this automatic use of $p < 0.05$ as the level for statistical significance is that many times, especially in clinical situations, it may not be reasonable, nor even safe, to commit type I error 5% of the time, whereas in other cases it might be acceptable to commit a type I error a greater percentage of the time. The significance level α should actually be determined based on its meaning in the context of the experiment performed.

The p level chosen by the investigator as demonstrating significance for the results obtained from a particular experiment is called the critical p level; this level may be different from the one that actually is obtained when the study is run. While most investigators are familiar with setting limits for type I error by choosing a critical p value, they are not as familiar with limiting type II error. However, controlling type II error can be as important as, or more important than, controlling type I error, as described in the next example.

Many of us have observed presentations where a small sample size was used (for example, $n = 3$), statistical analysis was performed, and a p value greater than 0.05 was obtained. The speaker concluded that the treatment had no effect. Immediately, a protestor, believing the sample size to be too small, claimed that the speaker committed type II error.

In another presentation, we may observe a surgeon who performed an experiment using a small sample size in which he or she attempted to compare a new surgical technique to the standard technique. Based on a high p value, the surgeon concluded that there was no significant difference between the new and standard methods and that the new method should be used because it is easier and cheaper. Is this an appropriate conclusion?

Although this conclusion might be correct, we would also want to be sure that if a p value greater than 0.05 were obtained, we are not committing type II error by incorrectly accepting a false null hypothesis. In the example stated above, we may wish to design the experiment with a power of 95%. In that case, we would be 95% sure that if the surgical repair had an effect on ligament strength (the null hypothesis were false), we would not falsely conclude that it did not.

Several methods, which use graphs, tables, and equations, have been developed to allow the experimenter to set the significance level (α, the critical p value) and the statistical power for an experiment, and then to determine the sample size required to achieve that design. Using these methods, the experimenter chooses α and β, estimates the sample variance, and anticipates the magnitude of the treatment effect (Fig. 4).

A survey of the scientific literature, especially that related to biology and medicine, reveals that an overwhelming majority of investigators set the critical α value to 0.05. It should be obvious that there is nothing magical about an α value of 0.05. This value simply indicates that the investigator is willing to accept committing type I error 5% of the time and still believe that the results obtained are true. However, there may be situations where the investigator is not willing to commit type I error 5% of the time or even 1% of the time. In such cases, the critical α value should be adjusted accordingly; that is, made lower. An example of this concept is an experiment in which the investigator attempts to demonstrate a significant decrease in knee laxity using a new surgical procedure compared to an established procedure. If the critical α value is 0.05, the investigator is willing to conclude 5% of the time that the new surgical procedure is more effective, even if it actually is not. If the new procedure represents an increased risk to the patient or a significant increase in expense or rehabilitation time, the surgeon may be willing to commit type I error only 1% of the time or a fraction of a percent of the time. In such a case, a critical α value of 0.05 may be too high.

At times, type II error may be more important to an investigator than type I error. For example, suppose that a safe experimental drug were administered to prevent thrombophlebitis after knee surgery. In this case, type I error would indicate that the drug had an effect when in fact it did not. The detriment to the patient is that he or she would take a drug that had no effect and would be at risk for developing the problem that the drug was intended to avoid. However, suppose type II error were committed in the same study. Type II error would indicate that the drug had no effect when in fact it had an effect. In this case, an effective drug would be withheld from the patient, which could represent a large problem. It may be that in this example, the power of the test should be 99.9%, while the critical α value should only be 0.1. The interpretation of the meaning of the α value is therefore paramount in selecting its value and in guarding against cookbook application of statistical methods.

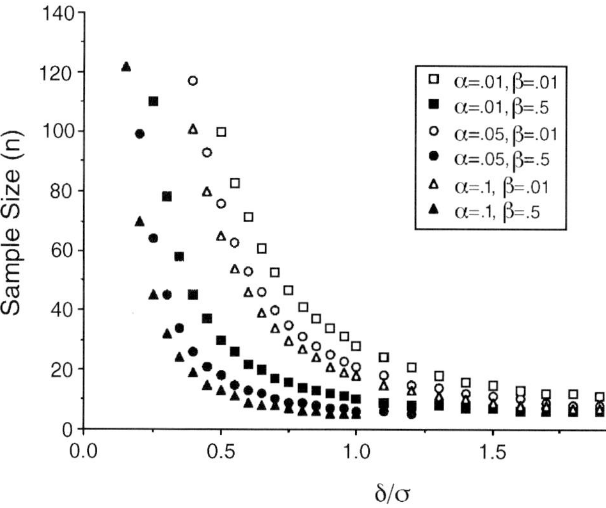

Figure 4
Relationship between sample size n, type I error rate α, type II error rate β, and the ratio of δ/σ for a t test between two groups of data. Note that as α, β, and δ/σ decrease, sample size increases.

Calculation of Sample Size

To properly test a hypothesis and ensure that the conclusions drawn accurately represent the phenomenon, we infer that our sample adequately represents the behavior of the population. Clearly the greater the n is for this sample, the greater the likelihood that our conclusions will, in general, be correct. However, the greater the sample size, the greater the amount of testing and cost will be required to perform the investigation. Therefore, a balance must be struck between adequate representation and available resources.

A number of experimental methods have been developed to calculate sample size for various experimental designs. Each method is specific for the experimental model used. Several of these are presented in the "Selected Bibliography." For purposes of illustration, we will consider the equation used for sample size calculation in the full factorial analysis of variance (ANOVA) model. This equation relates sample size to significance level and statistical power. In its most common form, the equation is represented as:

$$n = 2 \cdot \left\{\frac{\sigma}{\delta}\right\}^2 \cdot \{t_{\alpha,\upsilon} + t_{2\beta,\upsilon}\}^2 \qquad \textbf{(Eq. 6)}$$

where

n = required sample size
σ = population standard deviation
δ = difference desired to detect
α = desired significance level (type I error rate)
υ = degrees of freedom, which is related to sample size
β = desired type II error rate
$t_{\alpha,\upsilon}$ = t statistic corresponding to significance level α and degrees of freedom υ
$t_{2\beta,\upsilon}$ = t statistic corresponding to significance level 2β and degrees of freedom υ.

Both of these t values can be found in tables such as Table 3.

The meanings of σ, α, and β have already been discussed. The parameter δ represents the magnitude of the intended treatment effect. For example, in our previous discussion of quadriceps strength, the hypothesis might be that use of a particular tendon would be acceptable only if it increased strength over that of an unrepaired ligament by 30 N·m. Anything less than this would be considered as no difference. This experiment is a much different experiment than if the hypothesis were that a particular tendon would increase strength by 300 N·m. The point made here is that the value of δ is an implied part of the experimental design determined by clinical or scientific knowledge rather than statistical knowledge.

A number of observations follow from inspection of Equation 6 and Figure 4. First, as population variability σ increases, required sample size increases. Population variability can increase as a result of extrinsic variability (poor technique, instrument measuring variability) as well as intrinsic variability (variability of the population itself). Thus, the investigator's techniques should be as clean as possible.

Table 3
Critical values of student's *t*-distribution

Degrees of Freedom (υ)	Significance Level (α)								
	0.9	0.5	0.4	0.2	0.1	0.05	0.02	0.01	0.001
1	0.158	1.000	1.376	3.078	6.314	12.706	31.821	63.657	636.62
2	0.142	0.816	1.061	1.886	2.920	4.303	6.965	9.925	31.598
3	0.137	0.765	0.978	1.638	2.353	3.182	4.541	5.841	12.924
4	0.134	0.741	0.941	1.533	2.132	2.776	3.747	4.604	8.610
5	0.132	0.727	0.920	1.476	2.015	2.571	3.365	4.032	6.869
6	0.131	0.718	0.906	1.440	1.943	2.447	3.143	3.707	5.959
7	0.130	0.711	0.896	1.415	1.895	2.365	2.998	3.499	5.408
8	0.130	0.706	0.889	1.397	1.86	2.306	2.896	3.355	5.041
9	0.129	0.703	0.883	1.383	1.833	2.262	2.821	3.250	4.781
10	0.129	0.700	0.879	1.372	1.812	2.228	2.764	3.169	4.587
11	0.129	0.697	0.876	1.363	1.796	2.201	2.718	3.106	4.437
12	0.128	0.695	0.873	1.356	1.782	2.179	2.681	3.055	4.318
13	0.128	0.694	0.87	1.350	1.771	2.160	2.650	3.012	4.221
14	0.128	0.692	0.868	1.345	1.761	2.145	2.624	2.977	4.41
15	0.128	0.691	0.866	1.341	1.753	2.131	2.602	2.947	4.073
16	0.128	0.69	0.865	1.337	1.746	2.12	2.583	2.921	4.015
17	0.128	0.689	0.863	1.333	1.74	2.11	2.567	2.898	3.965
18	0.127	0.688	0.862	1.330	1.734	2.101	2.552	2.878	3.922
19	0.127	0.688	0.861	1.328	1.729	2.093	2.539	2.861	3.883
20	0.127	0.687	0.860	1.325	1.725	2.086	2.528	2.845	3.850
21	0.127	0.686	0.859	1.323	1.721	2.080	2.518	2.831	3.819
22	0.127	0.686	0.858	1.321	1.717	2.074	2.508	2.819	3.792
23	0.127	0.685	0.858	1.319	1.714	2.069	2.500	2.807	3.767
24	0.127	0.685	0.857	1.318	1.711	2.064	2.492	2.797	3.745
25	0.127	0.684	0.856	1.316	1.708	2.060	2.485	2.787	3.725
26	0.127	0.684	0.856	1.315	1.706	2.056	2.479	2.779	3.707
27	0.127	0.684	0.855	1.314	1.703	2.052	2.473	2.771	3.690
28	0.127	0.683	0.855	1.313	1.701	2.048	2.467	2.763	3.674
29	0.127	0.683	0.854	1.311	1.699	2.045	2.462	2.756	3.659
30	0.127	0.683	0.854	1.310	1.697	2.042	2.457	2.750	3.646
40	0.126	0.681	0.851	1.303	1.684	2.021	2.423	2.704	3.551
60	0.126	0.679	0.848	1.296	1.671	2.000	2.390	2.660	3.460
120	0.126	0.677	0.845	1.290	1.658	1.980	2.358	2.617	3.373
∞	0.126	0.674	0.842	1.282	1.645	1.960	2.326	2.576	3.291

Second, to resolve very small differences δ relative to the population SD σ, it will be necessary to use a large sample size. Notice how the graph curves up to higher sample sizes as the ratio of δ/σ decreases (Fig. 4). Stated another way, big differences are easy to detect and do not require large population samples. Note in Equation 6 above that one does not need to know the actual values for σ and δ, only their ratio δ/σ. This means that it is possible to predict the sample size needed for many combinations of α, β, and δ/σ (Table 4 and Fig. 4). Note that sample size must increase as the desired rates of type 1 and type II error decrease (α and β, respectively) and/or with the attempt to resolve smaller and smaller differences (ratio of δ/σ increases).

Third, high statistical power (or low β) or low significance levels (low α), which provide greater assurance against committing type II or type I errors, require a concomitant increase in sample size (Fig. 4). The understanding of the relationship between the ratio δ/σ and sample size permits almost immediate evaluation of proposed experiments. For example, if an experiment is proposed for increasing tendon suture strength by 25 N in a system where the normal tendon strength variability is 20 N, this represents a design in which δ = 25 N, σ = 20 N, and the ratio δ/σ is 1.25. Clearly, it would require a relatively small sample size to test this hypothesis (Table 4). Conversely, suppose it was hypothesized that using a new method would increase suture strength by 2 N. Now, the ratio δ/σ of 0.1 would require a sample size of several hundred, perhaps precluding the study entirely. Thus, before beginning an experiment, it is possible, and should be

Table 4
Number of observations for *t*-test of means between two groups

	α = 0.01; β =					α = 0.05; β =					α = 0.1; β =				
$\frac{\delta}{\sigma}$	**0.01**	**0.05**	**0.1**	**0.2**	**0.5**	**0.01**	**0.05**	**0.1**	**0.2**	**0.5**	**0.01**	**0.05**	**0.1**	**0.2**	**0.5**
0.05															
0.1															
0.15															122
0.2										99					70
0.25					110				128	64			139	101	45
0.3				134	78			119	90	45		122	97	71	32
0.35			125	99	58		109	88	67	34		90	72	52	24
0.4		115	97	77	45	117	84	68	51	26	101	70	55	40	19
0.45		92	77	62	37	93	67	54	41	21	80	55	44	33	15
0.5	100	75	63	51	30	76	54	44	34	18	65	45	36	27	13
0.55	83	63	53	42	26	63	45	37	28	15	54	38	30	22	11
0.6	71	53	45	36	22	53	38	32	24	13	46	32	26	19	9
0.65	61	46	39	31	20	46	33	27	21	12	39	28	22	17	8
0.7	53	40	34	28	17	40	29	24	19	10	34	24	19	15	8
0.75	47	36	30	25	16	35	26	21	16	9	30	21	17	13	7
0.8	41	32	27	22	14	31	22	19	15	9	27	19	15	12	6
0.85	37	29	24	20	13	28	21	17	13	8	24	17	14	11	6
0.9	34	26	22	18	12	25	19	16	12	7	21	15	13	10	5
0.95	31	24	20	17	11	23	17	14	11	7	19	14	11	9	5
1.0	28	22	19	16	10	21	16	13	10	6	18	13	11	8	5
1.1	24	19	16	14	9	18	13	11	9	6	15	11	9	7	
1.2	21	16	14	12	8	15	12	10	8	5	13	10	8	6	
1.3	18	15	13	11	8	14	10	9	7		11	8	7	6	
1.4	16	13	12	10	7	12	9	8	7		10	8	7	5	
1.5	15	12	11	9	7	11	8	7	6		9	7	6		
1.6	13	11	10	8	6	10	8	7	6		8	6	6		
1.7	12	10	9	8	6	9	7	6	5		8	6	5		
1.8	12	10	9	8	6	8	7	6			7	6			
1.9	11	9	8	7	6	8	6	6			7	5			
2.0	10	8	8	7	5	7	6	5			6				
2.1	10	8	7	7		7	6				6				
2.2	9	8	7	6		7	6				6				
2.3	9	7	7	6		6	5				5				
2.4	8	7	7	6		6									
2.5	8	7	6	6		6									
3.0	7	6	6	5		5									
3.5	6	5	5												
4.0	6														

required, to know the amount of time, energy, and money that will be required to achieve the desired experimental design. This decision can be based only on very approximate pilot data in which estimates can be made for the parameters discussed.

Correct sample size determinations, which represent a balance between guarantees against committing errors and the costs in time, money, and ability to perform the experiment, are not statistical in nature; rather they are clinical or scientific decisions to be made based on the clinician's understanding of the comfort level with being wrong either as a false positive or false negative. However, reviewers of an investigator's work may have a different comfort level than the investigator. This means it is prudent to be conservative in most cases.

The procedure used to calculate sample size using Equation 6 is an iterative one. It is initiated based on some information about the experiment. A first guess is made at sample size, and the expected sample size is calculated. A new, better guess at sample size is obtained, the process is repeated, and a new expected sample size is calculated. These steps continue until the repeated calculations of sample size converge on a particular value of n.

An example of such a process is taken from a study of the treatment of flexible flatfoot in children. Before performing the study, the investigators wished to determine the number of subjects required to determine whether three different treatment methods were effective. The experimental design included one control group and three experimental groups (Fig. 5). The investigators measured radiographic angles of the foot before and after treatment. Based on their previous experience with radiographic angle measurements on other children, they knew that the SD of radiographic angle within the general pediatric population was approximately 5°. In their clinical judgment, they considered an improvement in the radiographic angle of 5° to be a significant effect of treatment. The null hypothesis in this experiment was that treatment had no effect on the radiographic angle. Type I error would conclude that the treatment had an effect when, in fact, it did not. Type II error would conclude that treatment had no effect when, in fact, it did. The investigators decided to accept a type I error frequency of 5% (a critical *p* value or significance level α of 0.05), and wished to make the power of the statistical test 90% (P = 0.9, β = 0.1).

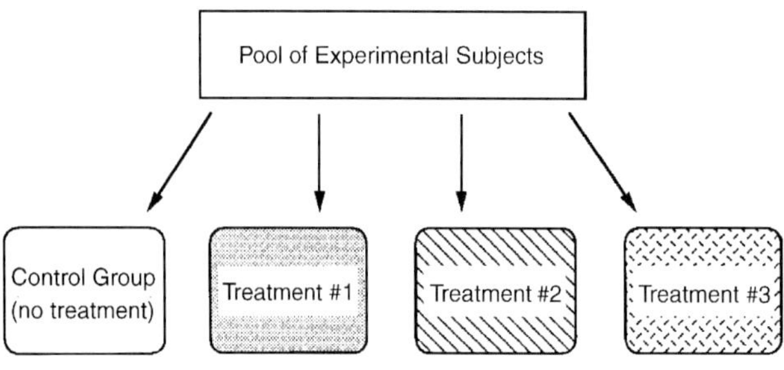

Figure 5
Schematic diagram of the ANOVA experimental design used to test three different treatments against no treatment (control) to correct flexible flatfoot in children.

To calculate the required sample size given this problem, we first make a rough guess at sample size, say n =10. We then calculate the degrees of freedom, using the following equation:

$$\upsilon = a(n - 1) \qquad \text{(Eq. 7)}$$

where

υ = the degrees of freedom
a = the number of groups
n = the number of independent samples per group.

Because we have four groups, the degrees of freedom are 4(10 − 1) = 36. We obtain from a statistical table (Table 3) the *t* value corresponding to a significance level of 0.05, 36 degrees of freedom, and a significance level of 0.2, 36 degrees of freedom. The corresponding *t* values are 2.031 and 1.308. We enter these values into Equation 6 and solve for n, obtaining n = 22.8 (Fig. 6). Based on this calculation, we now refine our guess of sample size to n = 25 and repeat the calculations. Now the degrees of freedom are 4(25 − 1) = 96. The appropriate *t* values are 1.990 and 1.292. We recalculate the sample size and n = 27.3. We then repeat the calculations with n = 30 and find that the calculated n = 27.05. Thus, as we refined our guess, the number of samples converged on a particular number. We would probably decide to perform the experiment with at least 30 independent samples per group. This may require actually entering about 35 individuals per group to allow for attrition.

To summarize, in designing this experiment, we specified the type I error rate, or the acceptable probability that we will commit a false positive. We also established the type II error rate by specifying the power. We then computed sample size, given the experimental variability and our desired difference. Having specified both type I and type II errors, interpretation of the data is straightforward. If our *p* value exceeds 0.05, we conclude that the treatment has no effect. We can be sure that if it is greater than 0.05, it is so, not because we have too few samples, but because the null hypothesis is indeed false. In fact, this latter result was the study outcome. The authors concluded that the four different methods for treating flexible flatfoot (including *no treatment*) were equally effective.

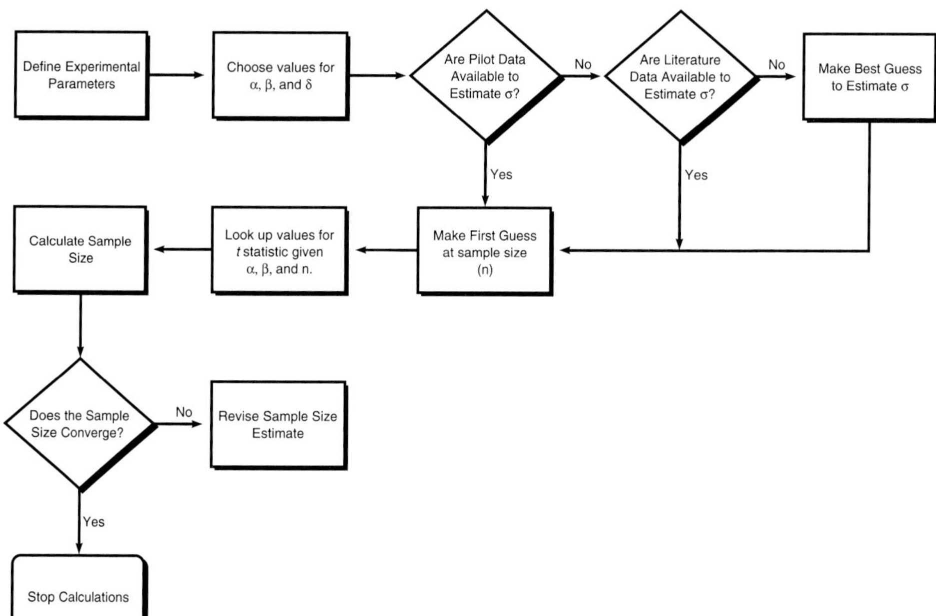

Figure 6
Logical progression for sample size calculation. Terms contained within symbols are defined in the text.

Student's *t*-Test

One of the simplest experimental designs involves the comparison of two groups—one that is treated experimentally and one that serves as an untreated control (Fig. 1). A characteristic of the experimental group is measured and is compared to the same characteristic of the control group to determine whether the particular treatment has had a significant effect. Consider a case in which the experimental sample represents the quadriceps extension strength from 15 individuals who have received conservative treatment for femoral fracture. At the end of four weeks of cast immobilization, quadriceps strengths of the treated individuals are measured and compared to quadriceps strengths of the normal legs of 15 untreated individuals. (It is hoped that these individuals would be matched for physical and socioeconomic factors.)

Suppose that the average strength of the immobilized leg was 210 ± 15 N·m (mean ± SEM) and the average strength of the control leg was 240 ± 13 N·m. Are these leg strengths significantly different? When there are one or two experimental groups, the traditional statistical analysis involves the use of Student's *t*-test. Note that analysis of variance (ANOVA) yields exactly the same results and is also generally applicable to more than two groups and to more complex designs. It is, thus, preferable to learn ANOVA. However, for the sake of completeness, we present an example of the use of the *t*-test.

The null hypothesis for the *t*-test is that $H_o: \mu_1 = \mu_2$, where μ_1 and μ_2 represent the means of the 1st and 2nd groups, respectively. If the sample sizes are equal, the statistic used to compare the two means is the *t*-statistic, which is calculated as:

$$t = \frac{\overline{X}_1 - \overline{X}_2}{\frac{s}{\sqrt{n}}} = \frac{\overline{X}_1 - \overline{X}_2}{\text{SEM}} \qquad \textbf{(Eq. 8)}$$

where

$\overline{X}_1$ and $\overline{X}_2$ = the sample means for groups 1 and 2, respectively
SEM = the average standard error of the mean for the two groups.

If the sample sizes are not equal, the equation is only slightly modifed and can be found in most statistical texts. Thus, the *t*-statistic calculates "how many" standard errors two means are apart from one another. Depending on the sample size, critical values of the *t*-distribution have been compiled (Table 3) and can be used to determine whether means are significantly different from one another. In the current example, $t = \frac{240 - 210}{14} = 2.14$.

The degrees of freedom for this experimental design is a(n − 1) = 2(14) = 28, and the critical *t*-value for a significance level of 0.05 is 2.048. Thus, the calculated *t*-value of 2.14 is (barely) statistically significant at the 0.05 level. The two-sample *t*-test is easily modified to treat the one sample case where a particular sample mean is compared to a hypothetical mean value. In this case, the *t*-statistic is calculated as:

$$t = \frac{\overline{X} - \mu}{\text{SEM}} \qquad \textbf{(Eq. 9)}$$

where

$\overline{X}$ = the sample mean
μ = the hypothetical mean to which the sample mean is compared.

For the cases in which more than two groups are to be considered, ANOVA is required to properly extract the appropriate information.

Analysis of Variance

The purpose of ANOVA is to determine whether a significant difference exists between two or more sample means. This statistical test is often used in the experimental setting to determine whether an experimental treatment has a significant effect. In practice, this analysis tests the null hypothesis that the means of "a" groups are equal. In other words, the null hypothesis for ANOVA is that

$$H_o: \mu_1 = \mu_2 = \mu_3 = \ldots = \mu_a$$

where μ_a represents the mean of the ath group and H_o is the abbreviation for the null hypothesis.

When ANOVA involves only two groups, the analysis is mathematically equivalent to the Student's *t*-test.

ANOVA Assumptions

ANOVA assumes that the various sample groups are normally distributed and that the variance between groups is equivalent. These assumptions are important because deviations from them can invalidate ANOVA results. As mentioned above, not all bell-shaped curves are normally distributed. A population that is normally distributed can be described in terms of its mean μ and its variance σ^2 (Fig. 2). The population mean of each group can be estimated by the arithmetic average and each sample variance describes each group's variability.

The ANOVA Table

An example is used to explain ANOVA and the ANOVA table. Suppose we are interested in determining whether there is a difference in average muscle fiber area between three quadriceps muscles. In this experiment we would obtain three groups of data from, for example, the vastus medialis (VM), the vastus lateralis (VL), and the rectus femoris (RF) muscles. This experimental design is similar in concept to the one presented in Figure 5 for the flexible flatfoot problem in which the three different groups were the different treatments. These raw data are presented in Table 5 and plotted in Figure 7 as the mean ± SEM. In this example, we have three groups and six samples per group. The null hypothesis in this experiment is stated as:

$$H_o: \mu_{VL} = \mu_{VM} = \mu_{RF}$$

Table 5
Fast muscle fiber area from three quadriceps muscles (μm^2)

Animal ID	Muscle		
	Vastus Lateralis	Vastus Medialis	Rectus Femoris
461	2,265	2,505	1,961
463	2,506	2,305	2,794
464	1,918	1,396	2,077
467	2,491	2,065	2,233
469	1,717	1,975	2,682
472	1,809	1,905	2,122
Mean fiber area	2,118	2,025	2,311
Standard deviation	348	380	343
Standard error	142	155	140

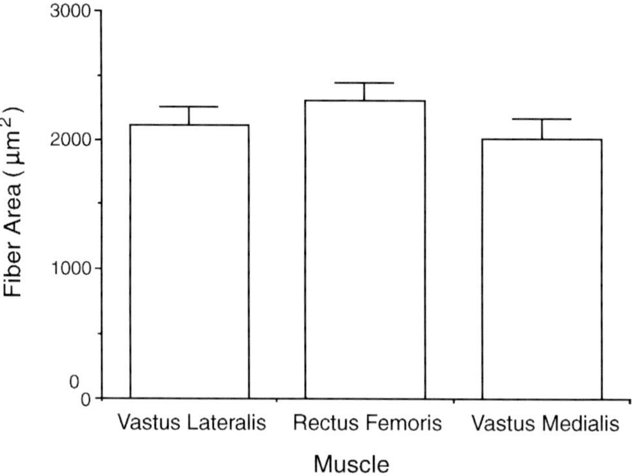

Figure 7
Bar graph of muscle fiber areas from three different quadriceps muscles. Each bar represents the group mean ± standard error of the mean (SEM). One-way ANOVA reveals no significant difference between groups ($p > 0.3$, Table 6).

where μ_{VL} is the mean of the sample obtained from the vastus lateralis muscle; μ_{VM} is the mean of the sample obtained from the vastus medialis muscle; and μ_{RF} is the mean of the sample obtained from the rectus femoris muscle.

Calculation of the ANOVA Statistics

To determine whether there is a difference in average muscle fiber area between the three muscles using ANOVA, we first calculate the variance *within* each group relative to its average by:

$$\sigma_i^2 = \frac{\sum_{i=1}^{n} (Y_i - \overline{Y})^2}{(n-1)} \qquad \textbf{(Eq. 10)}$$

which is simply a modified form of the variance equation presented above. The variance of the ith group in Equation 10 is calculated as the difference between an individual observation Y_i and the mean of that sample $\bar{Y}$. Those differences, which are calculated for each variate, are squared and summed, and the sum of squares (SS) is divided by the sample size in order to calculate variance within that group. (Actually, for mathematical reasons, the SS is divided by n − 1 to obtain the within-group variance.) This procedure in which an individual value is subtracted from another and squared is extremely common in statistical equations.

To estimate the overall variance of the entire data set including all three groups, the variances of all the individual groups are averaged. This variance is termed the mean squared error (MSE):

$$\mathrm{MSE} = \frac{\sum_{j=1}^{a}\left(\frac{\sum_{i=1}^{n}(Y_{ij}-\bar{Y}_j)^2}{(n-1)}\right)}{a} \quad \textbf{(Eq. 11)}$$

where

a = the number of groups
n = the number of variates per group
Y_{ij} = the ith variate in the jth group
$\bar{Y}_j$ = the mean of the jth group.

This value can be expressed more simply as:

$$\mathrm{MSE} = \frac{1}{a(n-1)}\sum_{j=1}^{a}\sum_{i=1}^{n}(Y_{ij}-\bar{Y}_j)^2 \quad \textbf{(Eq. 12)}$$

In this equation, the value obtained from Equation 10 for each of the "a" groups has been added and divided by the total number of groups (three in this example).

In addition to the overall or average within group variance, the variance between the three groups can be calculated as shown below:

$$\mathrm{MST} = \frac{1}{(a-1)}\sum_{j=1}^{a}(\bar{Y}_j-\bar{\bar{Y}})^2 \quad \textbf{(Eq. 13)}$$

where

$\bar{Y}_j$ = the mean of the jth group
$\bar{\bar{Y}}$ = the average of all of the means (grand mean).

Equation 13 again has a SS term, but this term is used to calculate the variability *between* groups because each group mean is compared to the grand mean. These squared differences are added, and the sum is divided by the number of groups minus one. This value is known as the mean square for treatment (MST) because this term is related to the magnitude of the treatment effect. Readers should note that the term treatment used here is a statistical term and does not specifically denote a medical treatment.

Equations 12 and 13 are used to estimate the variability within groups and between groups, respectively. Statisticians have determined that both of these terms are unbiased estimators of the population variance; that is, variability of the population from which these data were obtained.

Significance Level in ANOVA

If data obtained from a sample population represent that population, any observation should be similar to any other. The MSE and MST would be similar, and their ratio would be unity. This is a key point. This ratio of the variability between groups to the variability within groups is defined as a statistic known as the *F* distribution. It is this *F* value that is tested for significance. From the *F* value, a *p* value is obtained using a computer program or statistical tables. (Elucidation of the theory behind the calculation of the *p* level from the *F* value is beyond the scope of this chapter). In a typical ANOVA table (Table 6), all of the values that have been discussed are reported.

When the *F* value is not one, the ratio of the two mean squares (MSE and MST) reveals information relevant to our understanding of the existing variation in the study (Table 7). First, consider the within-group variance. It can be seen from Equation 12 that the within-group variance is calculated using the variability of an individual variate within a group relative to its group mean. In other words, this variance represents experimental variability, the variability in obtaining values from a given population. It is hoped that most of this variability results from the nature of the actual variability itself and not from other factors that could have been controlled, such as time of day, humidity, temperature, and so forth. That is why the SS term derived from Equation 12 is referred to as the SSE, which is the error associated with making repeated measurements from a particular population. This variability should be as small as possible. Each experimental group has its own SSE, and these are averaged to yield the MSE. ANOVA assumes that the variability of each of the groups is approximately equivalent. If it is not, other statistical tests that do not rely on equality of variance between groups are used. The

Table 6
One-way ANOVA table for control muscle example

Source of Variation	Sum of Squares	Degrees of Freedom	Mean Squares	*F* Ratio	*p*
Between	256,228	2	128,114	1.001	0.391
Within	1,920,493	15	128,032		

Table 7
Symbolic one-way ANOVA table

Source of Variation	Sum of Squares*	Degrees of Freedom	Mean Squares*	*F* Ratio
Between	SST	$\upsilon_1 = a - 1$	MST = SST/υ_1	$F_{\upsilon1,\upsilon2}$ = MST/MSE
Within	SSE	$\upsilon_2 = a(n - 1)$	MSE = SSE/υ_2	

* SST = sum of squares for treatment; SSE = sum of squares error; MST = mean square treatment; MSE = mean square error

MSE term does not depend on the absolute value of the mean for a particular group. For example, group 1 could have a mean value of approximately 1, group 2 could have a mean value of approximately 100, and group 3 could have a mean value of approximately 1,000. If the error variability of each group is the same, their individual SSE terms will be similar. The MSE term, thus, is not sensitive to the absolute mean value of the individual groups.

However, this is clearly not the case for the MST term. The MST represents the average between-group variability of the individual sample means around the grand mean. Thus, the MST term is very sensitive to differences between absolute mean values. In the previous hypothetical example, where the grand mean of the sample is the average of 1, 100, and 1,000, which is 367, the MST term would be large.

At this point, the reader should realize that as the differences between group means becomes large, given the same experimental variability in each group, the MST becomes large; whereas, the MSE remains relatively unchanged. This is the manner in which ANOVA detects differences between group means by testing variances and, therefore, why it is termed analysis of variance. When the *F* value is close to unity, there is generally not a significant difference between group means. However, as the group means become significantly different, the *F* value increases dramatically because of the increased MST term. There is, thus, a high level of probability or statistical significance that the groups are different (low *p* value).

ANOVA, as described here, in which the variates are grouped by a single classification (from which type of muscle the sample was obtained, VL, VM, or RF) is known as *single classification* or one-way ANOVA. It is important to clarify that one-way ANOVA refers only to the way in which the data are classified, not to the number of parameters or groups to be analyzed. Thus, the current example is of a one-way ANOVA on fiber area between muscles, but it is also possible to perform a one-way ANOVA on such things as capillary density, fiber type percentage, area fraction of connective tissue, and so forth, simply using one-way ANOVA again and again for the analysis of each parameter.

With this strategy, any problem can be approached using essentially the same procedure modified for the experiment at hand.

Two-Way ANOVA

As an extension of our previous example, consider the case in which each variate is classified based on two factors. This experiment, shown schematically in Figure 8, is undertaken to determine whether there is a significant difference in fiber area among the three different muscles in immobilized and nonimmobilized legs (Fig. 9). Whereas, in the previous example each variate was classified based only on the muscle from which it came (single classification), each variate is now classified by its muscle and whether or not the muscle was immobilized (two classifications). This is an example of a two-way ANOVA design (Table 8). Data are collected from each of three different types of muscle when each of these muscles is in a state of immobilization or mobilization; that is, six different combinations of the two factors need to be observed. In tabular form, data for six "cells" need to be obtained. Calculations involved in two-way ANOVA are analogous to those for one-way ANOVA. We have an MSE term, which is calculated for each group (now six) in the two-way ANOVA and, instead of a single MST term,

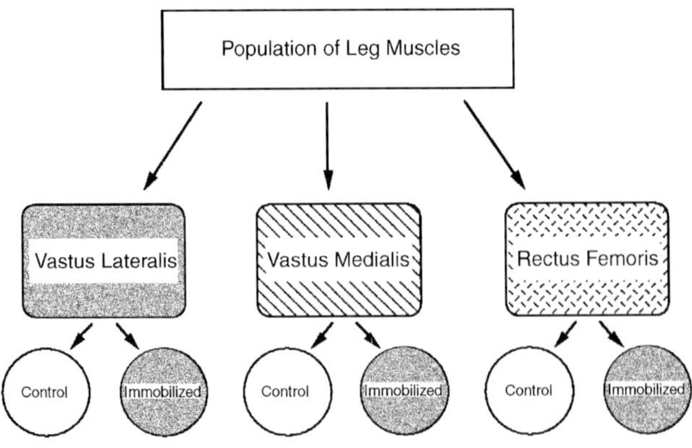

Figure 8
Schematic representation of the two-way ANOVA experimental design. Note that each variate is classified by two factors: The muscle from which it was obtained and the leg (immobilized or control) it came from.

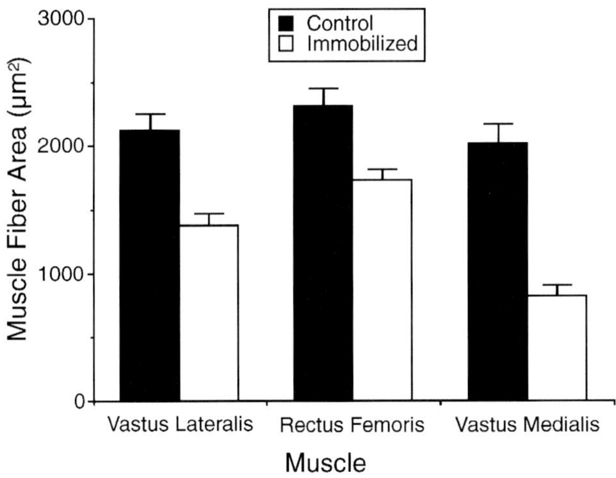

Figure 9
Graphic representation of Mean ± SEM of fiber area (µm^2) from three different muscles (VL, VM, RF) and two types of leg (control and immobilized). This 2 x 3 two-way ANOVA design is shown schematically in Figure 8. Data are from Table 8.

we have two MST terms. One MST term refers to the variance between legs (immobilized versus nonimmobilized), and the other refers to the variance between muscles (VM versus VL versus RF).

The data that led to this analysis, expanded from our previous experiment, appear in Table 8. Note that instead of three cells or groups of data, we now have six. These six cells result from two factors (muscle and state of mobilization) and three levels for each factor (three different muscles). In experimental design, this commonly is described as a 3 × 2 level ANOVA design. (If six muscles and three states of mobilization for each muscle were to be examined, this would be considered a 6 × 3 level two-way ANOVA design).

For this analysis, we establish two null hypotheses (one for each classification):

H_1: $\mu_{VL} = \mu_{VM} = \mu_{RF}$, and
H_2: $\mu_{immobilized} = \mu_{controls}$

In this example, it is possible that immobilization may have a different effect on fiber area, depending upon which muscle is examined. To understand this effect, in addition to the two main null hypotheses above, there is a *very important* interaction term that also will be calculated. This will be described below.

In the two-way ANOVA, only one error term (MSE) is determined, but six groups will be used to calculate it. However, there are now two separate treatment effects: type and muscle. The equations describing these two treatment effects are completely analogous to the MST for a one-way ANOVA. The equations are:

$$MST_{Type} = \frac{1}{(b-1)} \sum_{k=1}^{b} (\bar{Y}_k - \bar{\bar{Y}})^2 \quad \textbf{(Eq. 14)}$$

where

$\bar{Y}_k$ = the mean of the kth type
b = the number of types
$\bar{\bar{Y}}$ = the grand mean.

Similarly, the equation for the other MST is shown below:

$$MST_{Muscle} = \frac{1}{(c-1)} \sum_{l=1}^{c} (\bar{Y}_l - \bar{\bar{Y}})^2 \quad \textbf{(Eq. 15)}$$

where

$\bar{Y}_l$ = the mean of the lth muscle
c = the number of muscles
$\bar{\bar{Y}}$ = the grand mean.

The two-way ANOVA table looks very much like the one-way table, except that it has a few more rows (Table 9).

Because two MST terms exist, two *F* values are needed to test for the significance of a Type effect and a Muscle effect. These values are calculated as follows:

$$F_{Type} = \frac{MST_{Type}}{MSE} \quad \textbf{(Eq. 16)}$$

Table 8
Fast muscle fiber area from control and immobilized muscles (µm^2)

Animal ID	Vastus Lateralis		Vastus Medialis		Rectus Femoris	
	Control	Immobilized	Control	Immobilized	Control	Immobilized
474	2,265	1,755	2,505	1,000	1,961	1,780
476	2,506	1,302	2,305	450	2,794	1,599
479	1,918	998	1,396	943	2,077	2,100
481	2,491	1,442	2,065	800	2,233	1,632
483	1,717	1,364	1,975	851	2,682	1,450
488	1,809	1,421	1,905	921	2,122	1,821

(Column group header: Muscles)

$$F_{Muscle} = \frac{MST_{Muscle}}{MSE} \quad \textbf{(Eq. 17)}$$

so that, symbolically, the two-way ANOVA table (excluding the interaction row) looks like that shown in Table 10.

The Meaning of Statistical Interaction

In the current example, the data presented in Table 9 indicate there is a significant effect of immobilization, a significant effect of muscle, and a significant "interaction" term. This indicates that the effect of immobilization on fiber area depends on which muscle is examined, or, stated in statistical terms, the immobilization effect *interacts* with the muscle effect.

The interaction term demonstrates that each grouping factor or classification, whether it be the state of immobilization or which muscle is tested, is not independent of the other. From Figure 9 it can be seen that the VM shows a dramatic decrease in fiber area upon immobilization, whereas the RF shows less decrease. Stated another way, this study has demonstrated a muscle-dependent effect of immobilization.

The mean squared term for interaction represents the departure of the subgroup means from the values expected on the basis of additive combinations of data from the two grouping factors. This term is calculated from Equation 18 or 19.

The value $MST_{All\ Groups}$ represents the average MST for all six groups regardless of whether they are muscle groups or type groups. In this way, the interaction term increases as level-specific changes within a factor occur. The interaction mean squared term can be represented as:

$$MST_{M \times T} = \{MST_{All\ Groups}\} - \{MST_{Muscle} + MST_{Type}\} \quad \textbf{(Eq. 18)}$$

or,

$$MST_{M \times T} = \left\{\frac{1}{(a-1)(b-1)} \sum_{j=1}^{ab} (\bar{Y}_j - \bar{\bar{Y}})^2\right\} - \left\{\frac{1}{(a-1)} \sum_{k=1}^{a} (\bar{Y}_k - \bar{\bar{Y}})^2 + \frac{1}{(b-1)} \sum_{m=1}^{b} (\bar{Y}_m - \bar{\bar{Y}})^2\right\} \quad \textbf{(Eq. 19)}$$

The complete symbolic two-way ANOVA table is shown in Table 11.

Multiple Comparisons of Subgroups

While it is important to determine the significance of main effects and interaction terms, sometimes comparisons between specific cells within the analysis are of interest. For example, in the previous two-way ANOVA example, it is possible to say that there is a significant effect of immobilization and a significant interaction term. However, the investigator may wish to determine whether there is a significant difference between the control and immobilized leg for each muscle, that is, to determine whether there is a significant immobilization effect on a muscle-by-muscle basis. It is important to understand that although such paired comparisons are made using the Student's *t*-test, the number of comparisons and the specific comparisons to be made must be determined in the initial planning stages of the experiment. In the current example, the investigators wished to determine whether a significant immobilization effect was present for each

Table 9
Two-way ANOVA table for immobilization example

Source of Variation	Sum of Squares	Degrees of Freedom	Mean Squares	*F* Ratio	*p*
Type	6,331,094.7	1	6,331,094.7	71.2	0.0001
Muscle	2,126,327.2	2	1,063,163.6	11.9	0.0002
Type*Muscle	616,367.1	2	308,183.5	3.466	0.0442
Within	2,667,405.8	30	88,913.5		

Table 10
Symbolic two-way ANOVA table

Source of Variation	Sum of Squares	Degrees of Freedom	Mean Squares	*F*-Ratio
Between types	SST_{Types}	υ_T	$MST_T = SST_{Types}/\upsilon_T$	$F_{\upsilon_T,\upsilon_E} = MST_T/MSE$
Between muscles	$SST_{Muscles}$	υ_M	$MST_M = SST_{Muscles}/\upsilon_M$	$F_{\upsilon_T,\upsilon_E} = MST_M/MSE$
Within	SSE	υ_E	$MSE = SSE/\upsilon_E$	

Table 11
Symbolic two-way ANOVA table with interaction

Source of Variation	Sum of Squares	Degrees of Freedom	Mean Squares	*F* Ratio
Between types	SST_{Types}	$\upsilon_T = b - 1$	$MST_T = SST_{Types}/\upsilon_T$	$F_{\upsilon_T,\upsilon_E} = MST_T/MSE$
Between muscles	$SST_{Muscles}$	$\upsilon_M = c - 1$	$MST_M = SST_{Muscles}/\upsilon_M$	$F_{\upsilon_M,\upsilon_E} = MST_M/MSE$
Type*muscles interaction	SST_{MxT}	$\upsilon_{MxT} = (b - 1)(c - 1)$	$MST_{MxT} = \dfrac{SST_{MxT}}{MxT}$	$F_{\upsilon_{MxT},\upsilon_E} = MST_{MxT}/MSE$
Within	SSE	υ_E	$MSE = SSE/\upsilon_E$	

muscle, and, therefore, were interested in paired comparisons between each muscle; that is, control versus immobilized leg. In addition, the investigators were interested in determining whether fiber areas between the immobilized legs were significantly different, but not in whether the control legs differed significantly. It is not possible to extract the same information from two one-way ANOVAs as from one two-way ANOVA, nor is it valid. In other words, it is not appropriate to analyze the experimental data that were presented earlier as two one-way ANOVAs. Results obtained from the one-way ANOVAs would lead to the erroneous conclusion that there was no significant difference between muscles and no significant effect of immobilization. The results would be misleading because the differences between muscles would have been averaged out across the immobiliized and control legs. The interaction effect, which was a crucial aspect of this analysis, would have been impossible to extract from two parallel one-way ANOVAs.

The analysis thus involved six paired comparisons: control versus immobilized for each of the three muscles, and VM versus VL, VM versus RF, and VL versus RF for the three immobilized muscles. In such a situation, it is also not appropriate to simply perform six separate Student's *t*-tests because as the number of *t*-tests increases, so does the probability of obtaining a significant difference only because of chance. In other words, a correction must be made for performing this number of comparisons. One of the simplest methods for making this correction is to perform the Bonferroni approximation for multiple paired comparisons. To achieve an overall experimental significance level of 0.05, the critical *p* value for any individual test must be adjusted based on the number of comparisons as follows:

$$\text{New critical } p \text{ value} = \frac{\text{Experimental } p \text{ value}}{\text{Number of comparisons}} \qquad \textbf{(Eq. 20)}$$

In the current example, in which there are six paired comparisons, the experimental *p* value of 0.05 is divided by six to achieve a new critical *p* value of 0.0083. Then each individual *p* value obtained by Student's *t*-test is compared to 0.0083 to determine whether there is a significant difference between groups at the desired 0.05 level.

To satisfy the mathematical assumption of random sampling, the specific comparisons to be made in multiple paired comparisons must be chosen based on the experimental design, not on viewing of the data. For example, it would have been inappropriate, after looking at the data (Fig. 9), to test whether there was a significant difference between the VM control leg and the VL immobilized leg using a Student's *t*-test, although it appears from the figure that such a difference exists. However, if after performing the experiment and viewing the data, the investigators determined that this comparison was of interest, the paired comparison could be made using the Bonferroni approximation. However, it would be necessary to adjust the critical *p* value of 0.05 by the total number of possible paired comparisons in that entire data set. With six groups of data, the total number of possible paired comparisons is 15, which would make the critical *p* value 0.0033. In other words, it would be difficult to demonstrate a significant difference between these groups, but this is the price to be paid for making unplanned or a posteriori comparisons.

Potential Errors Using ANOVA

As stated above, ANOVA assumes that the groups are independent, that they are normally distributed, and that their variances are similar. Any departure from these assumptions will affect the validity of the results. Specific statistical tests are available to test these assumptions in a given experiment. The concept of group independence is subtle and, in many situations, may be difficult to appreciate. The requirement of independence can be stated as "the knowledge of a value from one group should not allow us to predict a value from another group." One common example of when groupings are related occurs when values obtained are separated only by time. These should not be considered independent. Suppose that we measure a person's weight before and after a diet program. Generally, extremely heavy people will still be heavy following a diet program, even after losing weight. The groups before and after, separated only by time, are not independent but, instead, have a high degree of covariance. This analysis requires a separate type of ANOVA design, known as a repeated measures design, in which the different groups are expected to have some degree of covariance and the covariance is adjusted for in the analysis itself.

Another common mistake made using ANOVA is to use the significant ANOVA p values to make statements about individual groups. In the example above, there was a significant difference between control and immobilized legs, no significant difference between muscles, and a significant interaction term. Based on the null hypothesis, it is obvious that if any single leg were different from its control leg, there would be a significant difference between control and immobilized legs. To simply state, therefore, that immobilization causes muscle atrophy for all legs would be incorrect. The ANOVA must be followed with multiple paired comparisons in order to make specific statements about each leg or muscle.

Another more subtle problem associated with ANOVA arises when the within-group variance (MSE) is artificially decreased. As can be appreciated from the F ratio, any factor that tends to decrease the MSE artificially will inflate the F value and produce significant results. This occurs most commonly when an n for a particular group is artificially high. Generally, this problem occurs when an investigator uses an n value that doesn't actually represent the number of independent samples obtained from a population, but rather represents the number of measurements that were made, which are not necessarily independent (for example, multiple weighing of a single sample). Repeated or replicate measurements from exactly the same sample only estimate the reproducibility of the measurement technique. Thus, repeated measurements of tumor mass obtained from the same subject simply serve to establish the mass of that tumor more accurately. No matter how many times that mass is measured, the mass of that particular tumor counts as n = 1 in the final tally because the population that we intend to generalize to is the mass of all tumors obtained from subjects. The total number of subjects in the sample must equal the sample size.

In summary, ANOVA is used to detect differences between group means. The mathematical procedure used relies on the fact that it is possible to obtain several estimates of the population variance. ANOVA tests only the null hypothesis that the group means are equal, and it generally is followed up by a multiple comparison that corrects for the number of paired comparisons made. The strength of ANOVA is in using it to design experiments in which the main and secondary effects will have great scientific meaning. These interaction terms can provide great insights into biologic and clinical phenomena but would be extremely difficult to obtain using a simple one-at-a-time experimental approach. Designs that incorporate multiple factors, as well as the investigation of interaction terms, should be encouraged.

The discussion of ANOVA has shown that ANOVA determines whether an effect is significant by creating an F ratio—a ratio of two variances. The steps generally used to test the significance of an effect are: (1) define the variances of interest; (2) define the comparisons to be made; (3) calculate the appropriate F statistics; and (4) test the F values for significance levels.

The next sections will refine our understanding of ANOVA by describing several common variations on the theme presented above.

Fractional Factorial Designs

The discussion of ANOVA demonstrated the power of examining main effects and interactions to determine the relative contribution of each to the observed effect. However, when there is an interest in knowing the effect of many factors, our traditional, full-factorial ANOVA may become extremely cumbersome.

For example, suppose an investigator were interested in determining the optimal screw design for bone fixation, and ten supposedly different factors of each screw needed to be considered, such as screw pitch, screw diameter, and so on. Performing this experiment using a full factor factorial model, that is, a 10-way ANOVA, would involve a lot of effort (Table 12). In fact, if only two different levels (values per factor) are used, multiple experiments would

Table 12
Number of experiments required for n=1 of a full factorial design

Number of Factors (k)	Levels per Factor	Number of Experiments (2^k)
2	2	4
3	2	8
4	2	16
5	2	32
6	2	64
7	2	128
8	2	256
9	2	512
10	2	1024

have to be performed, testing each value against every other value of every other factor. This would mean 1,024 experiments would have to be performed to obtain a single data point. Many investigations involve not two levels, but at least three or four levels per factor. For four levels, this could increase the number of experiments per data point to 4,096. Moreover, for a ten-factor design with two levels, to insure that an accurate mean value is obtained if five replications of each experiment are required 5 × 1,024 or 5,120 experiments would have to be performed. There must be a better way. Fractional factorial designs are that way.

Fractional factorial designs are based on the "sparsity of effects" principle, which states that any time there are more than about four factors, the system is probably driven by the main effects and a few of the low order interactions.

In ANOVA, replication generates the MSE term, which represents experimental error. In a full factorial experiment of k factors or groups and two levels per factor with n replicates per group, there are $(n)2^k$ experiments required. How many are actually needed? In the 10-way ANOVA example, 5,120 experiments is overkill. In general, statisticians have shown that only about 30 to 35 experiments are really needed for a good estimate of MSE.

The downside of our decision to perform fewer experiments is our inability to calculate higher-order interaction terms. The sparsity of effects principle suggests that because such high-order interaction terms are likely to be unimportant, it is not necessary to go to all of the trouble to perform a full factorial 2^k experiment. Thus, when it is desirable to perform a smaller number of experiments, a different statistical methodology is needed to evaluate the results. This methodology is called fractional factorial analysis.

The key to the fractional factorial experiment is to perform enough experiments to generate a reliable MSE term and to eliminate unnecessary replication, which only serves to generate high-order interaction terms. While it is beyond the scope of this chapter to describe this methodology, awareness of it and an understanding of when it is useful are important to all readers of this text.

Nested ANOVA Designs

Statistical methods of fractional factorial design can be used when a full factorial ANOVA would require such a large number of experiments that it would be impractical or too costly or time consuming to perform. In other cases, a full factorial ANOVA is not sufficient to describe the complexity of the phenomena or to fully extract all of the information from it regardless of how many experiments are performed. The nested ANOVA, sometimes referred to as a hierarchical ANOVA, is the statistical method to address this issue. In essence, it allows one or more factors to be subordinate to another factor.

In the full factorial model, the treatment effects (factors) may be either fixed (that is, defined by the investigator, as in the case of three specific surgical procedures) or random (that is, treatments chosen as interesting but not fully under the investigator's control, as in the case of three geographic locations in which blood pressure values are studied). An example of a full factorial ANOVA with two factors would be an experiment in which the investigators were interested in the effects of drug A and drug B on the blood pressure of males and females. The two factors are drug and sex. Each factor has two levels (drug A and B for the factor drug and male and female for the factor sex). This is thus commonly referred to as a 2 × 2 factorial design and is represented in Table 13.

Another example of a full factorial ANOVA would be the measurement of respiratory rate of both sexes of three species of rats at three temperatures. Each factor is a fixed effect with two levels of the factor sex and three levels each of species and temperature as shown in Table 14. This design is a 2 × 3 × 3 full factorial three-way ANOVA. The model is referred to as full factorial, because each level of each factor exists in combination with each level of every other factor. Statisticians would say that the model is "fully crossed." Also, low temperature in one cell has exactly the same meaning as low temperature in any other cell. Finally, measurements in one cell of the ANOVA are independent of measurements in another

Table 13
2 × 2 Factorial design

	Factor 1 (Sex)	
	Male	Female
Factor 2 (Drug)	Drug A Drug B	Drug A Drug B

Table 14
2 x 3 x 3 three-way ANOVA

Species	Temperature					
	Male			Female		
1	Low	Medium	High	Low	Medium	High
2	Low	Medium	High	Low	Medium	High
3	Low	Medium	High	Low	Medium	High

Table 15
Nested ANOVA example

Block	Tibialis Anterior		Gastrocnemius		Plantaris	
Block 1	Measurement 1	Measurement 2	Measurement 1	Measurement 2	Measurement 1	Measurement 2
Block 2	Measurement 1	Measurement 2	Measurement 1	Measurement 2	Measurement 1	Measurement 2
Block 3	Measurement 1	Measurement 2	Measurement 1	Measurement 2	Measurement 1	Measurement 2
Block 4	Measurement 1	Measurement 2	Measurement 1	Measurement 2	Measurement 1	Measurement 2

cell. For example, if the investigator knows something about species 2 at low temperature, he or she does not necessarily know anything about species 3 at low temperature. These points may seem subtle now, but will be contrasted with the following example of nested ANOVA design.

Consider the experiment in which the investigator is interested in determining the effect of immobilization on muscle fiber area in three different muscles. The muscles themselves differ with respect to fiber orientation and fiber type distribution (that is, percentage of fast and slow muscle fibers). Muscle fiber area is measured twice from each of four different blocks of tissue from each muscle. In this experiment (Table 15), the dependent variable is fiber area, and the factors are muscle (three levels) and block (four levels).

In this case, measurement 2 from block 2 of the tibialis anterior will not have anywhere near the same meaning as measurement 2 from block 2 of the plantaris. Block 2 of the tibialis anterior does not have exactly the same meaning as block 2 of the plantaris because the anatomy of the two muscles is different. It, therefore, would not be appropriate to analyze these data as a full factorial two-way ANOVA (effect of immobilization or mobilization) because the meaning of a particular cell, in this instance, measurement 2 from block 2, needs to be expressed in terms of the hierarchical factors from which is it obtained. If the proper statistical technique is to be used to analyze these data, the physician must realize the relative importance or weight to be given to each factor and provide this information to the statistician. Statisticians cannot be expected to understand the subtleties of different medical factors. To illustrate the nested ANOVA and the importance of choosing the correct statistical methodology, data from this experiment will be statistically analyzed in three different ways.

In our first (incorrect) analysis of these fiber area data, each of the pairs of measurements is treated as a separate "treatment" and the data analyzed as a one-way full factorial ANOVA between 12 groups (Table 16). Each of the two measurements, from each of the four blocks from each of the three muscles, is

Table 16
Sample ANOVA table obtained by incorrectly analyzing the nested problem as a one-way ANOVA with 12 independent groups

Source	df	Sum of Squares	Mean Square	*F* Value	*p* Value
Cell number	11	2,386.353	216.941	166.664	0.0001*
Residual	12	15.620	1.302		

Dependent: Fiber area
* Note the highly significant difference between "cells."

considered from a separate group (2 × 2 × 2). When this analysis is performed, a highly significant difference between cells is found. The *F* ratio, which is MST/MSE, is calculated as 216.9/1.3. This suggests there is no statistical difference between immobilization and mobilization using these four sections in these three muscles as representative of the animals' muscles. However, the MSE of 1.3 is only a result of repeated measurement of areas from a given section, but the large MST is a result of several factors such as intermuscular differences and interblock differences. Underestimating the MSE term will lead to artificial inflation of the *F* values, resulting in a very low and untrue significance level. This is another way in which a type I error can be made—by choosing an incorrect analysis method for the experimental design. The current problem is that all of the effects (muscles, blocks, and repeat measurements) have been lumped together, which makes one very large effect that cannot be sorted out. For proper experimental analysis, the MST needs to be broken down into its components.

Now the analysis is rearranged (again incorrectly) by simply pooling all of the blocks and repeated measurements for a given muscle and comparing each of these pooled data from the three different muscles using a one-way ANOVA (Table 17). There is still a significant difference between muscles, but it is less than with the previous example. The within group variability measured is now increased. The MSE now is 82.6 whereas it was only 1.3 in the first example. The MSE term now

Table 17
Sample ANOVA table obtained by incorrectly analyzing the nested problem as a one-way ANOVA with three independent groups

Source	df	Sum of Squares	Mean Square	F - Value	p - Value
Muscle	2	665.676	332.838	4.026	0.0331*
Residual	21	1736.298	82.681		

Dependent: Fiber area
* Note the significant effect of muscle, even when combining blocks.

includes all within group variability, which means that the MSE term has some between-block and between-section information within it. This leads to further breakdown of the model into its components.

The next (incorrect) approach to the phenomena could be to analyze the data as a two-way factorial ANOVA using blocks and muscles as the main factors (Table 18). The problem with this analysis is twofold. First, the F value for muscles can be calculated as the between-muscle variability divided by the MSE (332.8/1.3). This calculation is incorrect because the MSE term represents the error or variability associated with repeated measurements of different sections within a block. To know if there is a muscle effect, the between-muscle effect must be expressed relative to the next level of organization, which is the different blocks.

Finally, the data are analyzed correctly using a two-way nested ANOVA, and then the results are interpreted (Table 19). Note that the data, when analyzed correctly, actually show that there is no significant effect of muscle, but a highly significant block effect. In other words, it is not which muscle that is important, but the block from which the sample is taken. Between-block variability is actually the important factor in this experiment, not the particular muscle. This result may indicate, for example, that there is much more heterogeneity observed along a muscle in the proximal-distal direction than between different muscles. The experiment could thus be refined to ensure that the major source of variability in the data (between blocks) was accounted for in any experimental protocol. In this nested ANOVA, the F value for muscle is 1.74, which is the MST for muscle divided by the block(muscle) effect (read as blocks within muscles), or 332.8/191.2.

Use of the nested ANOVA has resulted in determination of the major sources of error in our experiment. The relative portion of each source of error can be quantified directly from the SS terms (MST and MSE) in Table 19. The total data variability is represented by the sum of all the SS terms, which, for our experiment, is:

Total variability	=	between muscle variability	+	between block variability	+	residual error

or

2,400	=	666	+	1,721	+	16

The relative contribution of each source to the total variability is thus: muscles, 27% (666/2,400); blocks, 72% (1,721/2,400); and repeated measurements, 1% (16/2,400). Thus, it makes no sense to spend the extra time and effort to make the repeated measurements when they are a minuscule part of the total variability. Conversely, the investigator may want to take several different blocks to try to understand the very large between-block variation.

This type of approach can be applied to any experimental system in which sample "aliquots" are nested. This is an excellent initial screening method for determining the major sources of experimental error in a system that is subdivided such as in this example. It is prudent not to waste time and energy "oversampling" at the levels with very low experimental variability. Thus, by analyzing the nested ANOVA, not only is a proper understanding of where the variability lies acknowledged, but the number of experiments is reduced if all the factors are considered.

Table 18
Sample ANOVA table obtained by incorrectly analyzing the nested problem as a two-way ANOVA with two grouping factors

Source	df	Sum of Squares	Mean Square	F - Value	p - Value*
Muscle	2	665.676	332.838	2.56E2	0.0001
Block	3	260.203	86.734	66.633	0.0001
Muscle*Block	6	1,460.474	243.412	1.87E2	0.0001
Residual	12	15.620	1.302		

Dependent: Fiber area
* Note the highly significant effects of muscle and block, and the significant muscle by block interaction.

Table 19
ANOVA table obtained by correctly analyzing the repeated measures problem

Source	df	Sum of Squares	Mean Square	F - Value	p - Value	Error Term
Muscle	2	665.676	332.838	1.741	0.2295*	Block(Muscle)
Block(Muscle)	9	1,720.677	191.186	146.878	0.0001	Residual
Residual	12	15.620	1.302			

Dependent: Fiber area
* Differences between muscles were not significant. Note that the description of the error term has been included for didactic reasons.

The incorrect analyses performed here illustrate an extremely important point in data analysis, which has been made even more important with the advent of microcomputer programs that make statistical analysis easy. Mathematically, the computer doesn't care about the numbers and will generate p values for just about any design that is input. In our examples, it was incorrect simply to provide block and muscle as individual factors that were assumed to be crossed. It is necessary to indicate to the computer program that blocks are nested within muscles and repeated measures nested within blocks.

The initial incorrect conclusion, that there were significant muscle effects, was obtained when the data were analyzed using the incorrect one-way ANOVA model in which each cell was considered a treatment. The incorrect conclusion was a result of testing the hypothesis that all group means were equal. This incorrect significant difference between muscles was determined because several of the cells were from different blocks, and difference between blocks really was the major source of variability.

Repeated Measures ANOVA

The nested ANOVA model presented above is used when measurements are thought to be related because large heterogeneities or variabilities are thought to be present within a factor. On the other hand, measurements are sometimes related just because they come from the same subject. For example, suppose we measured body mass of subjects before a diet program, and at five and ten weeks after the diet program, which involved three different diet foods. There are two factors: type of diet food (three levels) and time (three levels). It would not be appropriate to treat the three levels of time as independent and perform a 3 × 3 factorial, two-way ANOVA because the weights of the same subjects were measured before and during the diet treatment. To make this a full factorial design we would use three random samples of individuals obtained at different time periods. We would measure one group's mass before the diet, one group's mass at five weeks after the diet, and one group's mass at ten weeks. This design satisfies the requirement for the full factorial design because the groups are independent—knowledge about the five-week group on diet #1 would not carry over to the ten-week group on diet #1 because the subjects would be different. However, this design would be undesirable because it adds unnecessary variability to the data in that each person weighed at each interval has no relationship to the person weighed at a different time interval. The repeated measures ANOVA design is a way to minimize extraneous variability while providing an internal control for the experimental treatment. As with the nested ANOVA, the data to be obtained must be properly defined and the proper statistical methodology used to obtain meaningful results.

A typical repeated measures ANOVA data set might be set up as in Table 20 and the resulting ANOVA table might look like the one shown in Table 21. There is no significant effect of diet ($p > 0.1$), but there is a significant effect of the timing of the measurement ($p < 0.001$). Thus, all subjects probably improved, independent of the particular diet. Also note a significant timing × diet interaction term that represents a differential time-dependent effect of diet on weight loss. This term indicates that the time course of weight loss is different between the different diets.

Table 22 shows what the results might have looked like if this problem had been analyzed incorrectly as a two-way ANOVA. This situation leads to

Table 20
Repeated measures ANOVA example

Food Type	Timing of Measurement		
Diet 1	0 weeks	5 weeks	10 weeks
Diet 2	0 weeks	5 weeks	10 weeks
Diet 3	0 weeks	5 weeks	10 weeks

Table 21
ANOVA table obtained from repeated measures problem illustrated in Table 20

Source	df	Sum of Squares	Mean Square	*F* - Value	*p* - Value
Diet	2	26.751	13.376	2.154	0.1370
Subject(Group)	25	155.225	6.209		
Time	2	19.121	9.560	8.874	0.0005
Time * Diet	4	18.171	4.543	4.216	0.0051
Time * Subject(Group)	50	53.869	1.077		

Dependent: Weight loss

Table 22
ANOVA table obtained by incorrectly analyzing the repeated measures problem as a two-way ANOVA with two grouping factors.

Source	df	Sum of Squares	Mean Square	*F* - Value	*p* - Value
Food type	2	26.751	13.376	4.798	0.0109
Measurement time	2	19.121	9.560	3.429	0.0376
Food type* Measurement time	4	18.171	4.543	1.629	0.1757
Residual	75	209.095	2.788		

Dependent: Weight loss

the conclusion that food type has a significant effect because the *F*-value for food type is created using the MSE instead of the more appropriate $MSE_{Time \times Diet}$, which includes variability between the subjects themselves. In this case, this type of incorrect analysis results in a type I error.

The lesson of these presentations of ANOVA models is that the ANOVA technique is a powerful one that can extract important information from a particular experiment. However, it is equally true that a computer does not care which type of model the investigator chooses and cannot distinguish between correct and incorrect decisions based on the experimental data alone. The appropriate choice of an ANOVA model requires an understanding of how the data are organized (Fig. 10). The investigator must choose the correct model based on his or her expertise, and the person reading the report of the research must evaluate the conclusions based on the analysis of the data. This exposure to various models should provide at least an appreciation for the nature of the problem, and should encourage the investigator to approach a biostatistician for technical advice. There are numerous ANOVA models available for use, and the reader is referred to several of the excellent experimental design texts listed in the "Selected Bibliography" for further information.

Regression Analysis

Introduction

Another statistical test that is used in many experimental designs is regression analysis. The regression method is applied to a data set consisting of a group of independent variables that are measured exactly and a group of dependent variables. The analysis, known as the "least-squares" procedure, determines the equation that best fits the data and determines the relationship between the independent and dependent variables. This procedure can be performed selecting an exponential, logarithmic, polynomial, or any other equation to describe the relationship mathematically. In the interest of simplicity, we will illustrate regression analysis using linear regression; that is, best fit of the data to a straight line. The concepts learned using linear regression are applicable to other regression equations.

The most common reason for using linear regression is to test whether a relationship (not necessarily one of cause and effect) exists between two variables. This procedure may be as simple as determining the relationship between force and voltage output in the calibration of a force transducer or as complex as determining the relationship between drug dosage and a particular physiologic response in

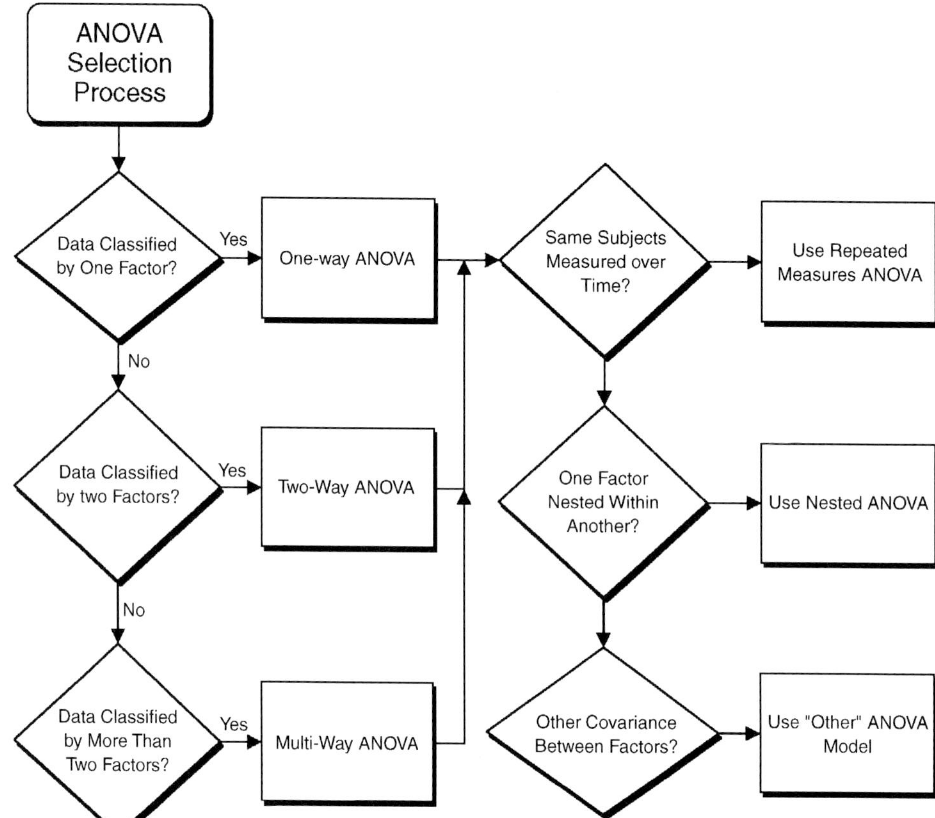

Figure 10
Flowchart for choosing appropriate ANOVA procedure.

creating a dose-response curve. Once established, a functional relationship can be statistically analyzed.

In linear equation analysis, any data set can be fit to a line. Solving for the best fit line is easily done on any type of data no matter how they appear, because the procedure simply consists of mathematical operations applied to a given data set. The pertinent questions to ask after performing linear regression are whether the data provide a good fit to the line, and whether the relationship between the two variables is significant.

The first question, dealing with goodness of fit, is answered by inspection of the correlation coefficient *r*; the second question, dealing with significance, is answered using the *p* value. All of the concepts that will be used to discuss the *r* and *p* values follow directly from the previous discussion of ANOVA. Keep in mind that both the *p* and *r* values should be reported by a linear regression program. Beware of obtaining one value without the other using pocket calculators and the like.

Statistical Significance

The method for calculating the *p* value for a regression model is a simple modification of the methods learned in the one-way ANOVA: defining SS terms and calculating variance ratios. In the case of linear regression, the SS terms are the familiar variances within and between groups, here called the unexplained SS and the new explained SS. The schematic diagram in Figure 11 illustrates the source of these terms.

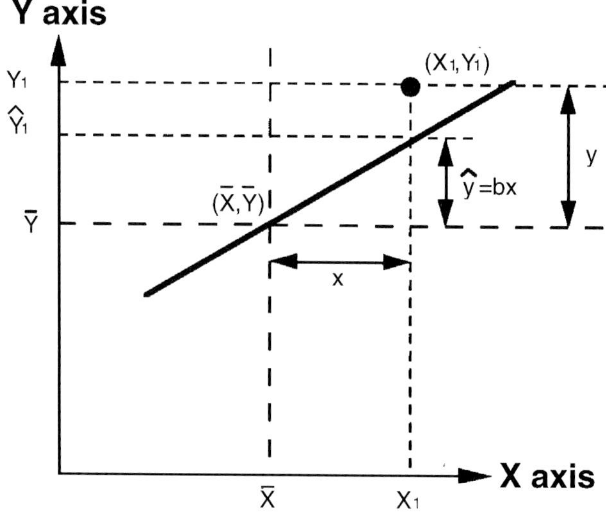

Figure 11
Graphic representation of the source of the sums of squares (SS) terms used in linear regression. $\bar{X},\bar{Y}$ represents the mean of all of the data, X_1,Y_1 represents a typical data point, and y represents the predicted values for y given x.

Following calculation of these terms, significance testing occurs in a manner similar to a one-way ANOVA in which the F value is the ratio of the two mean squares mentioned above. The data can be organized to look like an ANOVA table containing two mean squares, an F value, and a p value. The difference here relates only to what we call the terms. The MSE term used in ANOVA, here called the unexplained error, is simply the SS of the distances between the predicted data and actual observed points, or

$$\text{Unexplained variation} = \sum_{i=1}^{n} (y_i - \hat{y}_i)^2 \quad \textbf{(Eq. 21)}$$

where

y_i = predicted value of y, given a particular value of X_i.

As the predicted line approaches the data points, this term becomes small. The reason that these points deviate from the line is not known and, thus, this is termed unexplained variability.

The second mean squared term, which in ANOVA analysis was called mean square treatment MST, is here called the explained source of variability. It is the difference between the predicted values $\hat{y}_i$ and the group mean:

$$\text{Explained variation} = \sum_{i=1}^{n} (\bar{y} - \hat{y}_i)^2 \quad \textbf{(Eq. 22)}$$

The F value is calculated as the ratio of the explained/unexplained mean squared terms. Thus, the total variation is partitioned into explained and unexplained terms rather than MSE and MST as in ANOVA. The statistical significance level is then obtained using a table or computer program, and these values are expressed as a p value.

Goodness of fit

In addition to tests of significance, linear regression calculates a goodness of fit statistic called the coefficient of determination r^2. The coefficient of determination is the fraction of the total variation that our model, which in this case is a linear model, explains. In other words,

$$r^2 = \frac{\sum_{i=1}^{n} (\bar{y} - \hat{y}_i)^2}{\sum_{i=1}^{n} (y_i - \bar{y})^2} = \frac{\text{Explained variation}}{\text{Total variation}} \quad \textbf{(Eq. 23)}$$

The total variation about the mean can be represented as:

$$\text{Total variation} = \sum_{i=1}^{n} (y_i - \bar{y})^2 \quad \textbf{(Eq. 24)}$$

which can be partitioned as:

$$\sum_{i=1}^{n} (y_i - \bar{y})^2 = \sum_{i=1}^{n} (\bar{y} - \hat{y}_i)^2 + \sum_{i=1}^{n} (y_i - \hat{y}_i)^2 \quad \textbf{(Eq. 25)}$$

or

Total variation = explained variation + unexplained variation

Thus, the closer r^2 is to 1, the better is the fit of the data to the model; the relationship is represented as a line or a mathematical equation. If the fit is good, a quantitative relationship exists, which enables powerful statements to be made regarding the percentage of total experimental variability explained by a particular model. This percentage concept is equally valid for multiple regression (in which multiple independent parameters are used) as it is for simple regression.

Often the goodness of fit is expressed as a correlation coefficient rather than as the coefficient of determination. The correlation coefficient r is simply defined as:

$$r = \sqrt{r^2} \quad \textbf{(Eq. 26)}$$

where

$r > 0$ if the slope of the line is positive
$r < 0$ if the slope of the line is negative.

A correlation coefficient of -1 is a perfect fit to a negatively sloped line and a correlation coefficient of +1 is a perfect fit to a positively sloped line.

Linear Regression Example

As an example of the application of linear regression to experimental data, consider the data presented in Table 23, which were obtained from several different dogs.

Table 23
Dog mass versus dorsiflexion torque (n = 15)

Dog Mass (kg)	Left Leg Torque (N·m)	Right Leg Torque (N·m)
9.2	2.38	2.51
14.1	3.50	3.61
13.9	2.25	2.41
14.0	2.71	2.81
21.1	2.50	2.70
23.1	3.11	3.45
23.1	2.75	2.95
23.0	2.50	2.84
24.0	3.51	3.71
28.0	4.55	5.15
28.1	3.22	3.55
30.0	4.53	4.74
31.1	3.66	3.84
32.1	3.78	3.98
33.1	4.00	4.11

In this particular experiment, the investigators wanted to know whether there was a significant relationship between dog mass and dorsiflexion torque so that they would be able to predict torque simply based on dog mass. For each dog, maximum dorsiflexion torque was measured (in N·m) from each leg along with dog mass (in kg). These data were entered into a computer, and the graph shown in Figure 12 was obtained. Note that there is a fair amount of scatter to the data. The best fit equation and other relevant statistics from regression analysis were:

$$Y\ (\text{N·m}) = 0.072\ (\text{N·m/kg}) \cdot \text{mass (kg)} + 1.605\ (\text{N·m}) \quad \textbf{(Eq. 27)}$$
$(p < 0.005,\ r^2 = 0.486)$

and the corresponding ANOVA table is shown in Table 24.

The table obtained from the regression analysis is completely analogous to the table we saw in the one-way ANOVA example. The coefficient of determination of these data, as calculated from Equation 25, is 3.882/7.991 = 0.49. Thus, although the regression relationship is highly significant ($p < 0.005$), the linear relationship only explains 49% of the experimental variability. As a result, its use as a predictor of leg torque would be questionable.

Table 24
ANOVA table of torque (N·m) versus dog mass (kg)

	df	Sum of Squares	Mean Square	F - Value	p - Value
Explained	1	4.030	4.030	13.496	0.0028**
Unexplained	13	3.882	0.299*		
Total	14	7.911			

* Note low unexplained error relative to explained error, yielding a high F value.
** Note the significant effect of dog mass on torque ($p < 0.01$).

Potential Problems With Regression Analyses

Although regression provides a powerful tool for data analysis, it is possible to be fooled by the statistics or to overstate the implications of the analysis. Such errors come from an incomplete understanding of the meaning of the p value and correlation coefficients. These potential problems are discussed briefly below, and graphs illustrating the problems are shown (Fig. 13).

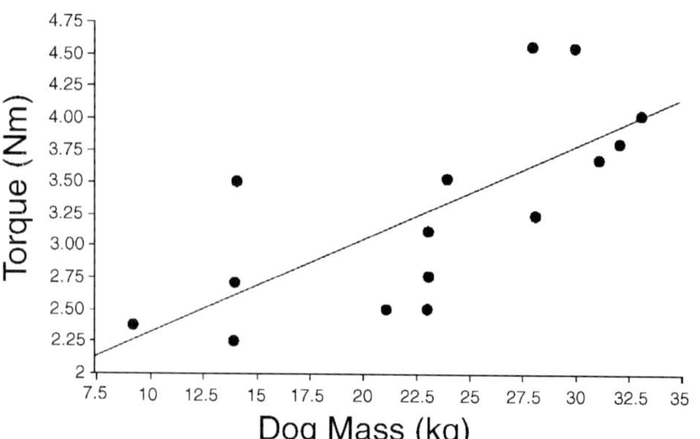

Figure 12
Scatter graph of the data in Table 23 along with linear regression best-fit line.

Extrapolating Beyond the Independent Value for the Data Set

Clearly, the predictive value of curve-fitted data applies only to the range of independent values for which the original relationship was derived (Fig. 13, *top left*). Many complex functions, exponential and logarithmic, for example, are highly linear over restricted ranges. Extrapolation beyond the range for which data are available assumes incorrectly that the relationship between the two variables is invariant for all possible values of the independent variable.

Interpolating Into a Region That Contains No Data

Similar to the argument presented above, sometimes data are obtained that cluster into two regions (Fig. 13, *top right*). An excellent mathematical fit can be obtained to two clusters of data gathered at different values for the independent variable, in spite of the fact that no information is available for the intermediate values. Again, it is incorrect to assume a relationship for which no data are available; it is better to make two groups of data and use ANOVA.

Missing a Secondary Trend Superimposed Onto a Linear Trend in Linear Regression

Very good linear fits are possible for data that are not changing in a strictly linear fashion. In Figure 13, *bottom left,* the linear fit is excellent although the overall behavior of the phenomenon has been missed. This mistake can be avoided by inspecting the residuals of the data that are obtained following analysis. Residuals are the individual errors for all of the data points. That is, the residual for a given data point is the unexplained error for that data point. If the linear fit is equally good across the entire data set, the residuals should appear as a sort of random cloud of data points. However, if an underlying trend has been missed, there will be a good deal of form to the residual plot.

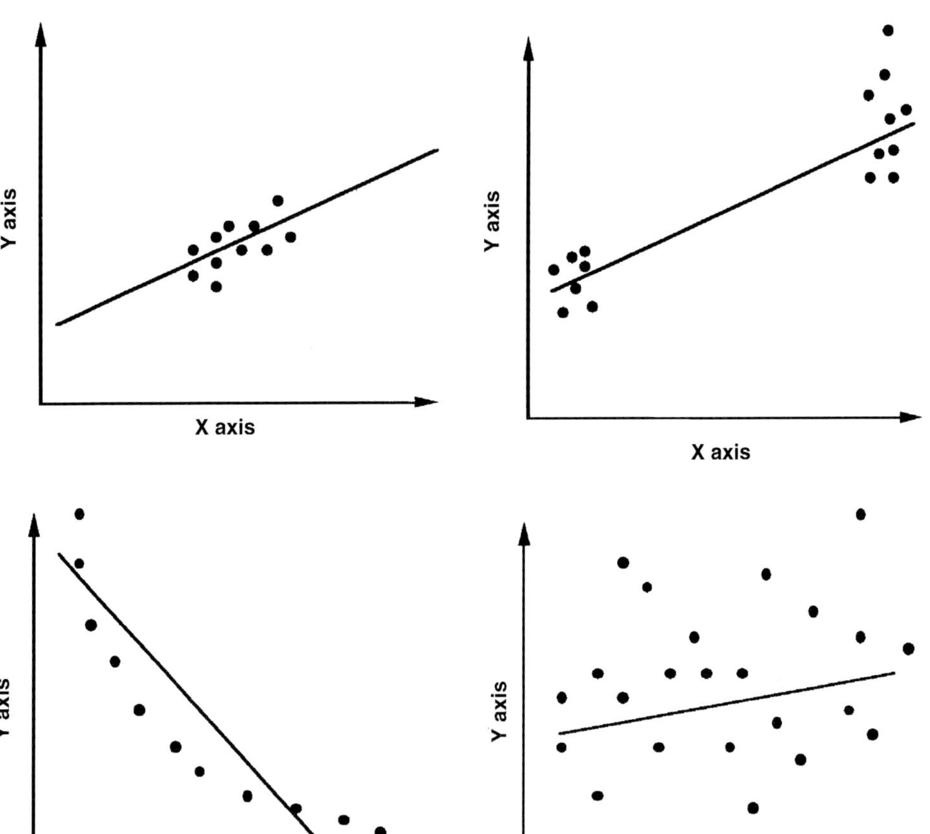

Figure 13
Schematic examples of errors that can be made using linear regression. **Top left,** Extrapolating beyond the range for which independent data values are available. **Top right,** Interpolating between two clusters of data to a region where no independent data are available. **Bottom left,** Missing a secondary trend superimposed on the linear trend. **Bottom right,** Using a regression equation when the *p* value is not significant.

Neglecting *p* Values and Implementing an Insignificant Equation

Any data set can be fit to a straight or curved line. Thus, if the *p* value is high, suggesting no significant relationship between the independent and dependent variables, there is no sense in using the regression equation for any purpose (Fig. 13, *bottom right*). The analysis should stop at this point. Often, a regression equation is used in the absence of knowledge of the *p* value, and inappropriate calculations are made using an irrelevant equation.

Neglecting r^2 and Overemphasizing a Significant *p* Value

The other extreme of misinterpretation is to rely only on the significant *p* value in deciding to implement a regression equation (Fig. 13, *top right*). As was seen in the dog leg example above, a highly significant linear relationship can still have an extremely small correlation coefficient and, thus, have no useful prognostic value.

ANOVA Versus Regression

The previous example has demonstrated a great deal of analytical and conceptual similarity between ANOVA and regression. In many cases it is difficult to decide which type of analysis is more appropriate. When the data are gathered across a continual range, regression makes more sense than ANOVA because it would be difficult to define distinct independent variables, factors, or treatment groups for the ANOVA. However, if the data are gathered either at discrete intervals (for example, age) or in fairly well-defined subgroups (for example, old and young), the ANOVA model is more applicable. This type of question is more easily answered in the context of a specific experiment. It is this type of question that can be addressed by local statisticians, provided they are made aware of the inherent characteristics of the variables (factor, treatment groups).

Analysis of Covariance (ANCOVA)

Introduction to Covariates

In contrast to ANOVA, ANCOVA is used when the value of the dependent variable is affected by additional information related to the independent variable. In this case, the dependent variable is corrected for fluctuations in the independent variable, known as the covariate, before the analysis is performed. ANCOVA is thus similar to ANOVA in that it is used to test for equality among group means. In terms of calculations, ANCOVA actually represents the combination of ANOVA and linear regression.

ANCOVA often is used when it is not possible or practical to keep all things constant between groups. For example, in comparing muscle strength between two different groups of patients, patients of different weights might necessarily have been used. Because strength (dependent variable) is highly dependent on patient weight (independent variable), there will be scatter in the data solely as a result of variability in patient weight and unrelated to the actual diet treatments. This scatter will increase the MSE term, making it difficult to obtain statistically significant results. Therefore, ANCOVA is used to correct muscle strength for patient weight and then perform the statistical comparison. Although, at first, ANCOVA appears to be a panacea for decreasing sample variability, we must remember that ANCOVA is useful only when a detailed measure of the covariate property is available. This requires not only predicting the need for a covariate but also choosing the correct covariate, in this case patient weight. Such decisions typically should be made during pilot experiments.

As an example of the use of the ANCOVA model, suppose we were interested in comparing the pullout strength of prostheses inserted into cadaveric specimens using two different bone cements—one with high-viscosity (HVC) and one with low-viscosity (LVC). Human cadaveric specimens are highly variable in their mechanical properties; therefore, we might predict that a covariate will be useful with regard to bone cement. Suppose the biomechanical experiments were performed and the data were obtained as shown in Figure 14.

Because there are two groups of data that are classified based on one factor (cement type), it is possible to compare pullout strength using a one-way ANOVA design (mathematically equivalent to an unpaired *t*-test). When this analysis is performed (Table 25), no significant difference is found between groups ($p > 0.6$).

Note that almost all of the variability is unexplained (98% to be exact, calculated as residual error divided by total variability, 2,902/2,974). However, much of the residual error term variability is simply variability between specimens, which can be accounted for by using ANCOVA.

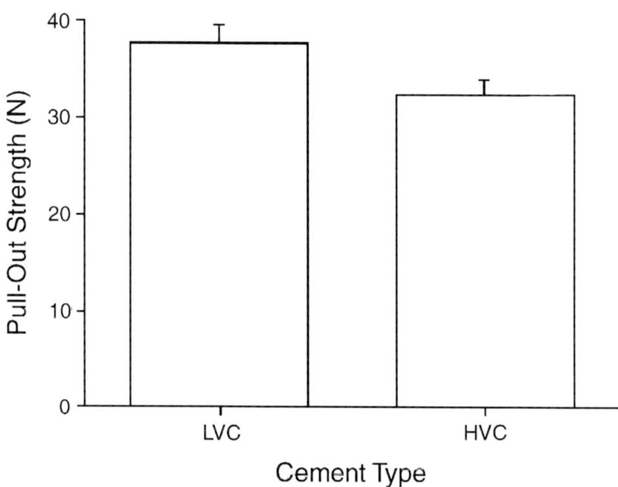

Figure 14
Bar graph of pullout strength ± SEM of prostheses that were embedded in cadaveric femurs using high-viscosity cement (HVC) and low-viscosity cement (LVC).

It is possible that the lack of significant difference between the LVC and HVC cements is being masked by variability resulting from some other factor, which must be measurable. This is particularly suited to ANCOVA. To perform the ANCOVA, an independent variable (the covariate) must be measured, which estimates something relevant about the specimen. In the present case, we might suspect that some of the variability between specimens may simply be a result of the quality of the tubercular bone. Thus, the bone density of the various specimens is measured independently, and the analysis is rerun using bone density as the covariate.

ANCOVA Calculation Method

The first step in ANCOVA is to perform a linear regression on the pullout strength of each cement versus bone density to determine the precise relationship, if any, between the dependent and independent variables. All pullout strengths then are ad-

Table 25
ANOVA table from cement example analyzed without a covariate

Source	df	Sum of Squares	Mean Square	*F* - Value	*p* - Value
Cement type	1	72.361	72.361	0.199	0.6670*
Residual	8	2,902.384	362.798		

Dependent: Pullout + 20
* There is no significant effect of cement type.

justed for bone quality based on the regression relationship. This is mathematically analogous to creating bones of similar bone density before the actual statistical test in order to decrease within-group variability. Finally, the two adjusted group means are tested for equality in a manner similar to ANOVA.

There is a very strong relationship between bone density and pullout strength for both types of cement (Fig. 15). Thus, bone density is a useful covariate in this experiment. In ANCOVA, it is important that the slopes of the two regression lines are not significantly different. In effect, then, the ANCOVA tests for differences between y-intercepts. The mean values for the HVC and LVC groups (arrows) are relatively close, but are smeared out because of variation in bone density (Fig. 15). Finally, and most importantly, the ANCOVA table (Table 26) shows a significant effect of cement type now that the variability due to bone density is accounted for as a covariate.

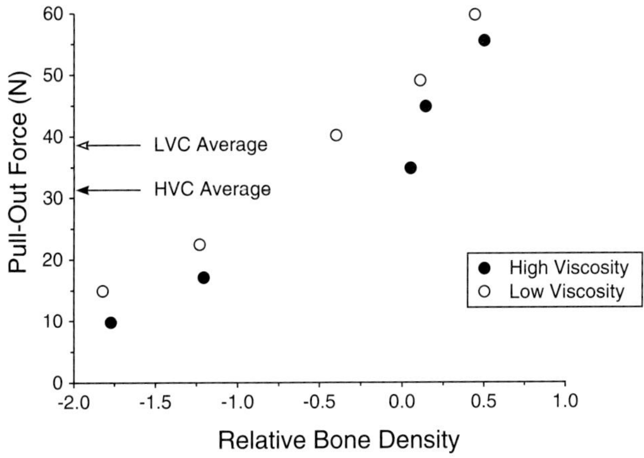

Figure 15
Scatter graph of pullout strength of prostheses that were embedded in cadaveric femurs using high-viscosity cement (HVC) and low-viscosity cement (LVC) as a function of bone quality (the covariate). Note the average values for HVC and LVC are rather close compared to the scatter in the data caused by altered bone quality.

A comparison between Tables 25 and 26 reveals the basis for the initial inability to detect differences between cements. The MSE variability (residual) in Table 25 is 2,902; whereas, in Table 26, it is only 86. Where did it go? Note that the SS due to bone density is 2,815. Thus, of the initial 2,902 residual error, 2,815/2,902 or 97% simply was caused by variations in bone density. This can be seen in Figure 14 in which the change in pullout strength is large with respect to bone density, but relatively small due to cement type. Thus, while the effect of cement type is significant, it is of smaller magnitude than the bone density effect. If it were not for the existence of the ANCOVA method, the information would have been lost completely (Fig. 16).

Generalization of the ANCOVA Model

The simple ANCOVA example described here can be extended to multiple covariates and multiple grouping factors. In fact, the basis for the general linear model (GLM) approach to ANOVA or regression, which now we see are essentially the same thing, simply requires that the experimenter choose, for a given dependent variable, any design that includes grouping variable(s), dependent variable, and independent variable(s), if any.

Judicious choice of experimental design can often demonstrate a significant effect that would otherwise be masked by unrelated variability, as seen in the above example, and can also demonstrate no significant effect of a grouping factor that is confounded by another, uncontrolled variable. Again, the importance of a clinical study of the data used in statistical analyses cannot be overemphasized.

Frequency Analysis

Sometimes there is interest in evaluating an effect that cannot be, or is not, measured using traditional, continuous variables. A continuous variable is one that can be measured to vary over a continuous range. For example, length, height, and weight are all continuous variables because they take on a continuous range of values. However,

Table 26
ANOVA table from cement example analyzed using bone density as a covariate.

Source	df	Sum of Squares	Mean Square	*F* - Value	*p* - Value
Cement type	1	109.595	109.595	7.671	0.0324*
Bone density	1	2,815.795	2,815.795	197.101	0.0001
Cement type	1	0.791	0.791	0.055	0.8018
Residual	6	85.716**	14.286		

* Note the significant effect of cement now that bone density is included as covariate.
** Note the low residual (unexplained) error (compared to Table 25) after including the bone density covariate.

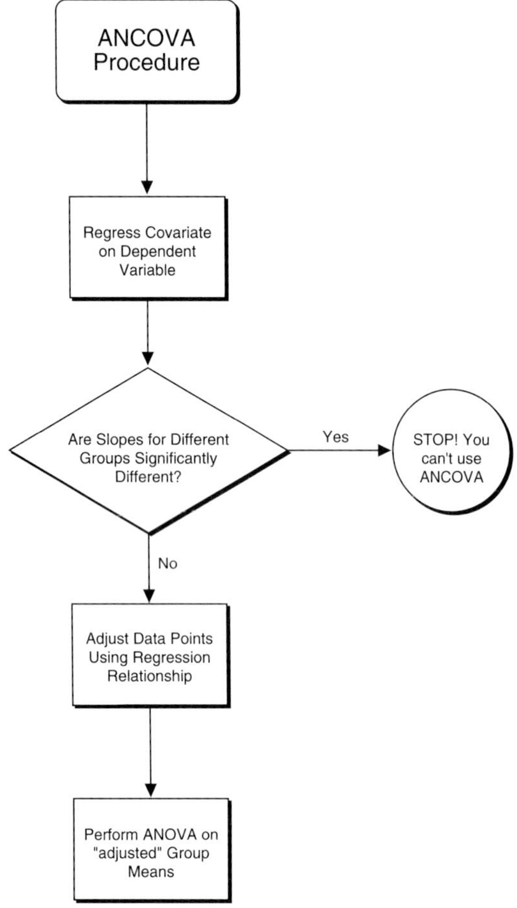

Figure 16
The flow of events included in the ANCOVA procedure. Note that if group slopes are significantly different, the procedure cannot be applied.

sometimes we are unable to measure continuous variables in an experiment and instead "measure" a discrete categorical variable that can only take on certain values (for example, surgical outcome of good, fair, or excellent; presence or absence of a disease state). In these examples, it would be inappropriate to apply ANOVA simply by assigning numbers to different portions of the scale. The assigned numbers would be completely arbitrary because the numbers in and of themselves have a distinct mathematical meaning or value different from what we arbitrarily assign to them, and this must be considered when it comes to using them for calculations. Use of such numbers in regression or ANOVA models is inappropriate. For example, an investigator might judge tissue healing on a rating scale and judge the tissues from 0 (the worst) to 5 (the best). It would be just as easy to make the scale from 0 to 100, but this would have different meaning using the various parametric statistics described above. Thus, for the case in which categorical or qualitative data are to be analyzed, traditional parametric statistics, such as ANOVA and regression analysis, are not appropriate.

Frequency tables are used to express qualitative and categorical data, and frequency analysis is used to test specific hypotheses regarding the data contained in these tables. Frequency tables can be one-way, two-way, or multiway, analogous to classification schemes in ANOVA.

The Chi-Square (χ^2) Test for Proportions

Sometimes we wish to compare a set of observed frequencies to an expected proportion. The classic examples come from genetics in which, for example, frequencies of two colors of flowers are compared with the expected proportions, 0.75 and 0.25, which represent dominant and recessive traits, respectively. A clinical example might be envisioned in which we wish to test patient choice regarding three different knee braces. The braces might differ with respect to size, shape, or color, but we are interested merely in knowing if one choice dominates over the other two. Suppose we asked 270 patients to state their choice regarding knee braces and obtained the data shown in Table 27. Note that 108 patients chose brace 2 over the other two. Does this indicate that patients choose brace 2 significantly more often? To answer this question, we use the method of χ^2 analysis. As with other statistics we have seen, the χ^2 statistic is used to measure how far a particular distribution deviates from a theoretical distribution. It is calulated according to the equation:

$$\chi^2 = \sum_{i=1}^{a} \frac{(f_i - \hat{f}_j)^2}{\hat{f}_i} \qquad \textbf{(Eq. 28)}$$

where

f_i = the observed frequency of the ith group
$\hat{f}_i$ = the expected frequency of the ith group
a = the number of groups.

Because we think each brace has an equal likelihood of being chosen, the expected frequency of observa-

Table 27
Observed and expected counts for knee brace preference

Frequency	Brace No.		
	1	2	3
Observed	69	108	93
Expected	90	90	90

tion for each of the braces, given 270 patients, is 270/3 = 90. The χ^2 statistic is calculated as:

$$\chi^2 = \frac{(69-90)^2}{90} + \frac{(108-90)^2}{90} + \frac{(93-90)^2}{90} \quad \textbf{(Eq. 29)}$$
$$= 4.9 + 3.6 + 0.1$$
$$= 8.6$$

Statisticians have compiled tables of calculated critical values for the χ^2 distribution for various sample sizes and numbers of experimental groups. We look up in such a table that, for an experiment with a = 3 groups (that is, two degrees of freedom), the critical χ^2 value corresponding to $p < 0.05$ is 5.991. Because our value of 8.6 is much greater than 5.991, we reject the null hypothesis that our observed frequency equals our expected frequency (in fact, 8.6 exceeds the critical χ^2 value corresponding to $p < 0.025$). Note that in Equation 28, it makes sense that, the larger the value for χ^2, the more probable it is that a significant difference exists between observed and expected frequencies. This is because the numerator of the statistic is calculated directly from the difference between observed and expected frequencies.

Single Classification Frequency Analysis

The general problem of numeric analysis of frequencies also can be illustrated using a basic science study in which a nerve was cut, repaired, and then allowed to grow back into a specific muscle and innervate individual muscle fibers. Prior to the transection, it was demonstrated that a normal muscle contained 50% fast and 50% slow fibers as judged using a histochemical reaction on tissue slices. Six months following nerve repair, a total of 450 muscle fibers were examined on tissue sections; 290 turned out to be fast fibers and 160 were slow fibers.

The investigator wanted to know if the muscle fibers that were reinnervated were reinnervated randomly, or if there was some type of preferential innervation of either fast or slow muscle fibers. In effect, the investigator would state the null hypothesis that the proportion of fiber type after reinnervation would be the same as the proportion before surgical transection.

If muscle fibers, which initially were present in a 1:1 ratio, were randomly innervated, a 1:1 ratio of fiber types would also be expected after reinnervation. The actual ratio, however, was 290:160 = 1.81:1. Is this significantly different from what could happen if random reinnervation occurred? To answer this question, we apply simple ideas from probability theory to the specific numbers obtained from this experiment. First, we summarize both the data expected if reinnervation were random and the observed data. The expected proportions for the fiber types were: fast = 0.50 and slow = 0.50. However, the observed proportions were fast = 290/450 = 0.64 and slow = 160/450 = 0.36. Using the terminology of frequency analysis, the expected frequency of fast fibers was E(fast) = 0.50 x 450 = 225 and the expected frequency of slow fibers was E(slow) = 0.50 x 450 = 225. The data are summarized in Table 28.

Calculation of the Likelihood Ratio

To use probability theory for determining the likelihood of the observed finding, we compare it to the expected finding. If the two results are very different, we may conclude that the observed frequency was not expected. If the two are similar, we may conclude that the observed result is expected and our hypothesis is true. Thus, probability theory is used here to test a null hypothesis. In this case the investigator is testing the null hypothesis that E(fast) = E(slow) = 0.5, making use of the expected proportion. An investigator, who had previous knowledge regarding probabilities in another muscle where the normal muscle might contain 75% fast and 25% slow fibers, would choose another value.

To test this hypothesis, the investigator first calculates the probability of observing a 290:160 frequency given a probability of occurrence of 0.5. According to probability theory, the probability of observing x occurrences out of n trials given an expected success rate of p is given by the expression:

$$E(x;n,p) = C(n,x)p^x(1-p)^{n-x} \quad \textbf{(Eq. 30)}$$

where

$C(n,x)$ = the number of possible combinations from a sample of n taken x at a time
p^x = the probability of achieving x successes
$(1-p)^{n-x}$ = the probability of achieving n - x failures.

This is a reasonable expression because, in order for the observed outcome to have occurred, we must first know the probability of 290 successes (that is, fast fibers innervated) and the probability of 160 failures (that is, slow fibers innervated) both occurring. This is represented by the expression $(1-p)^{n-x}\,p^x$ because the probability of multiple events occurring is

Table 28
Expected and observed fiber type values

Fiber Type	Observed Frequency	Observed Proportion	Expected Frequency	Expected Proportion
Fast	290	0.64	225	0.5
Slow	160	0.36	225	0.5

simply the product of their individual probabilities. Finally, this successful event can occur in $C(n,x)$ different ways. Therefore, the event probability is multiplied by the total number of different ways by which it can occur to arrive at Equation 30. In this example, the probability of obtaining the actual results when $p = 0.64$ is 0.1229, whereas the probability of obtaining the actual results when $p = 0.50$ is 0.01838.

Therefore, there is a greater probability that the observed frequencies would result if the odds of innervating a fast fiber were 0.64 than if the odds of innervating a fast fiber were 0.5. It follows that the greater the ratio between the observed and expected probabilities, the more likely it is that the observed data did not come from the hypothetical (expected) population. This is analogous to our ANOVA statistic F, in which the MST was compared to the MSE. The greater the ratio, the greater the probability of significant differences.

In frequency analysis, a statistical test based on such a ratio is called the likelihood ratio test. In this example, the likelihood ratio is L = 0.1229/0.01838 or 6.683, and it can be shown that this result is not quite significant ($p > 0.1$).

This example represents a single classification or one-way frequency analysis problem. Frequency analysis classifications can be based on one or multiple factors. In fact, a significant set of tools is available to analyze two-way frequency analysis problems.

Two-Way Frequency Analysis

As a second example of a frequency analysis problem, suppose an investigator were interested in determining the best method for repair of a meniscus following a bucket-handle tear. Ideally, a continuous variable that characterizes the state of the meniscus (for example, meniscal compression or shear strength) should be measured. However, many times, the evaluation of the success of a procedure is more often based on intuitive or subjective interpretation of repair quality, such as a subjective rating of meniscal healing based on histologic evaluation of excised menisci from experimental animals. In the former case, ANOVA would suit the problem well, whereas in the latter case, frequency analysis must be used.

As an example, we can analyze the data from an experiment in which two types of surgical repairs were performed on a canine right medial meniscus. In one group of experimental animals, a core of tissue was removed to promote vascular ingrowth from the meniscal periphery; in the other group, a section of synovial flap was sutured to the defect to promote vascular ingrowth. The measure of the success of the procedures was based on whether or not the animals were weightbearing after a certain time interval, whereupon it was assumed that the menisci of the weightbearing animals had been successfully repaired. If the repair method had no influence in whether or not the animal was bearing weight, the conclusion would be that the repair methods were not significantly different; that is, the repair method and weightbearing results were independent. However, if the surgical repair method influenced whether or not the animal was weightbearing, this result might indicate that one procedure was more effective than another. The data from this type of experiment could be scored and arranged as data shown in Table 29. Based on the numbers provided and analytical methods such as those mentioned above for one-way frequency analysis problems, the p value obtained was 0.24, which leads us to the conclusion that the surgical repair methods are equivalent in efficacy, at least as far as the experimental animals evaluated are concerned. The experimental conclusion is only as powerful as the variables measured. The methods may have significantly different abilities to cause tissue healing, but the weightbearing status of the experimental animals may not depend on whether the tissue is healed. The investigator must beware of choosing the correct variable to measure.

Ordered Two-Way Frequency Analysis

Another type of frequency analysis is useful when the observations are ordered. For example, an investigator might use two surgical treatments on a ligament and then assess tissue healing on a scale from 1 (least healed) to 3 (most healed), or poor, better, best. The scale itself is irrelevant as long as it is ordered. The data from such an experiment might be organized as shown in Table 30.

The usefulness of frequency analysis in this type of problem, in which one category is ordered and the other is dichotomous, is that it is possible not only to test for differences in the treatment methods (independence), but also to check to see if there are trends across proportions (analogous to determining whether a slope is significant in linear regression).

Table 29
2 x 2 frequency analysis example

	Weightbearing	
Method	**Yes**	**No**
Flap	21	29
Core	11	39

Table 30
Histologic appearance

	Poor	Better	Best
Sutured	11	22	30
Not sutured	14	26	23

The level of complexity of frequency analysis problems is limited only by the investigator's creativity. The key, as a designer of experiments knows, is that this tool exists and should be used when appropriate. Frequency analysis should not be used when another parametric statistical method, such as ANOVA, would be more useful. Furthermore, the investigator should try to measure the variable that is most closely related to the experimental question.

Nonparametric Statistics

Why Use Nonparametric Statistics?

For many parametric statistical tests (for example, ANOVA), certain numeric assumptions about the sample distribution must be satisfied. However, in spite of the power of mathematical transformations and all of our sophisticated experimental designs, it is not always possible to meet these requirements. Before performing statistical analyses, the assumptions of the particular test must be tested. For example, in ANOVA, the assumptions are that the groups have equal variance and that the group data are normally distributed.

Nonparametric statistical tests must be used when the requirements of parametric statistical tests cannot be satisfied. Nonparametric methods are also called distribution-free methods, because they are not dependent on any distribution, such as the normal distribution. The word nonparametric is used because the null hypothesis is not concerned with specific parameters, such as the mean in ANOVA, but only with the distribution of the variates. This point is critical, because conclusions based on nonparametric statistics cannot address differences between means. Therefore, the investigator must be careful not to use a phrase such as "the old patients were significantly heavier than the young ones ($p < 0.05$) as demonstrated by the Mann-Whitney nonparametric statistical test," because heavier implies a greater average mass and refers to a mean (a parameter that cannot be used in this test).

Advantages and Limitations of Nonparametric Statistics

Nonparametric tests pose a trade-off in terms of utility. On the one hand, there are absolutely no limitations to the characteristics of the data set to be analyzed; in fact, the data need not even be numeric. On the other hand, significant effects cannot be related back to any parametric property of the data set, such as the mean or variance.

Data that appear to be distributed as a bell-shaped curve may not be normally distributed. The two parameters usually checked in testing the normal distribution assumption are skew and kurtosis. Skew simply refers to the direction in which the data distribution leans. A normal distribution does not lean, but nonnormal distributions may lean to the right or to the left. Both of these variations are shown in Figure 17, in which it should be empha-

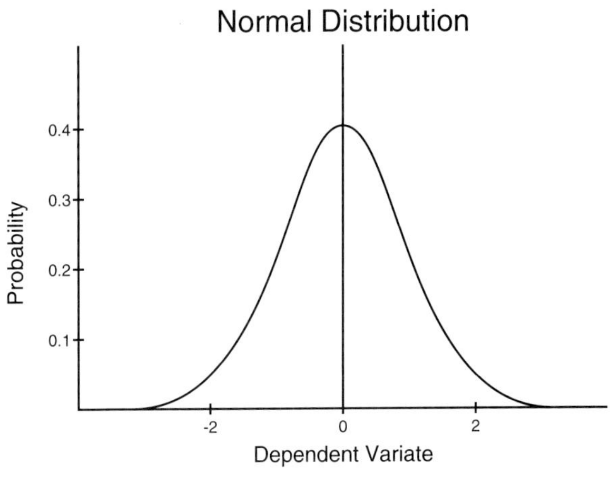

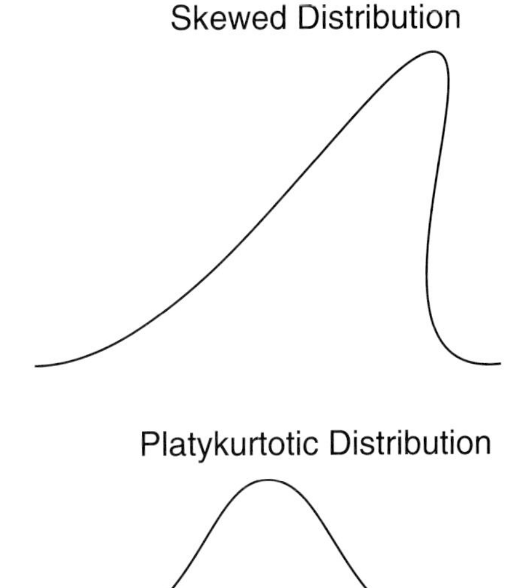

Figure 17
Alterations in the normal distribution that can be measured. **Top,** The normal distribution. **Middle,** A nonnormal distribution skewed to the right. **Bottom,** A nonnormal distribution that demonstrates platykurtosis—too much weight in the tail region of the distribution.

sized that all distributions are bell-shaped but not all are normally distributed. Because normal distribution is an assumption for all parametric statistical tests, one of the first decisions to be made in analyzing data is whether or not the data set is normally distributed. If it is not, and cannot be made to be normally distributed, then nonparametric statistics are the only option (Fig. 18). Kurtosis refers to the distribution of variates in the sample. A normal distribution has a certain weight in the tail and hump regions. Thus, a sample with too much data near the tails is said to be platykurtotic, whereas one with too much data near the hump is said to be leptokurtotic.

Common Nonparametric Tests and Their Parametric Counterparts

The five most common nonparametric statistical tests and their corresponding parametric counterparts are shown in Table 31. Fortunately, there are really no new concepts to learn when choosing a nonparametric analytic tool. The classification schemes discussed in the ANOVA section above apply also to conditions in which nonparametric statistics are used. Thus, a perusal of Table 31 reveals that numerous nonparametric tests are available for one-way, two-way, and multiway classification experiments. The decision regarding the specific test is largely a matter of preference. The degree to which each type of test tends to be conservative is also a factor.

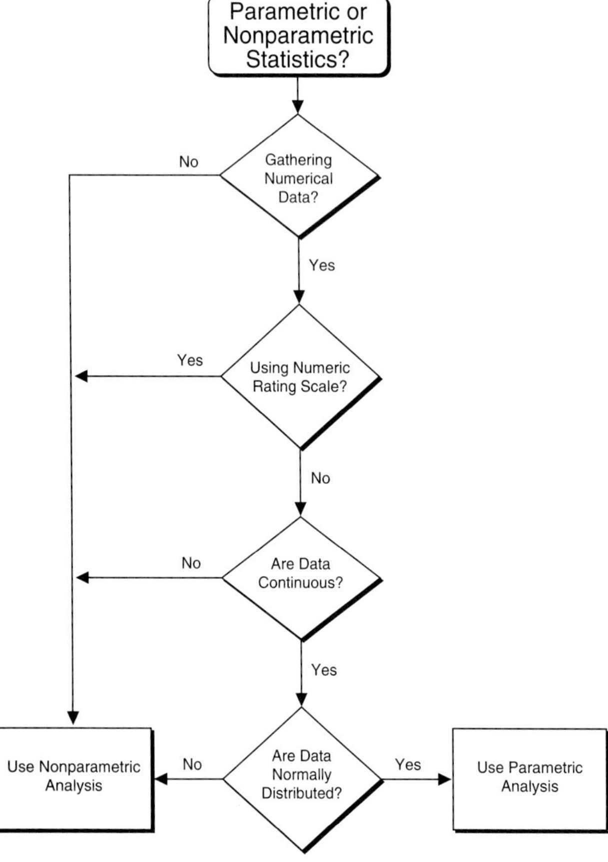

Figure 18
Logical algorithm used to decide between parametric and nonparametric statistical analysis methods.

Table 31
Corresponding parametric and nonparametric tests

Nonparametric Test	Parametric Counterpart
Mann-Whitney U-test	Student's *t*-test
Wilcoxon two-sample	Student's *t*-test
Wilcoxon's Signed-Ranks	Paired *t*-test
Kruskal-Wallis test	One-way ANOVA
Friedman test	Two-way ANOVA

Wilcoxon Two-Sample Nonparametric Statistical Test

The Wilcoxon two-sample test is a good illustration of the basis for nonparametric testing. Many other nonparametric tests involve similar calculation methods, and the reader is referred to the "Selected Bibliography" for further examples.

Suppose an investigator wanted to compare femur lengths from individuals of the same age who live in either San Diego or Boston, and, in spite of heroic efforts, found that they were not normally distributed. The investigator chose to compare them anyway using the Wilcoxon two-sample test. The data are given in Table 32 and graphed as a histogram in Figure 19. Note that the raw data are given along with their "rank" relative to the total data set.

Table 32
Sample data for Wilcoxon two-sample test

Boston Sample		San Diego Sample	
Femur Length (mm)	Rank	Femur Length (mm)	Rank
104	2	100	1
109	7	105	3
112	9	107	4.5
114	10	107	4.5
116	11.5	108	6
118	13.5	111	8
118	13.5	116	11.5
119	15	120	16
121	17.5	121	17.5
123	19.5	123	19.5
125	21		
126	22.5		
126	22.5		
128	25		
128	25		
128	25		

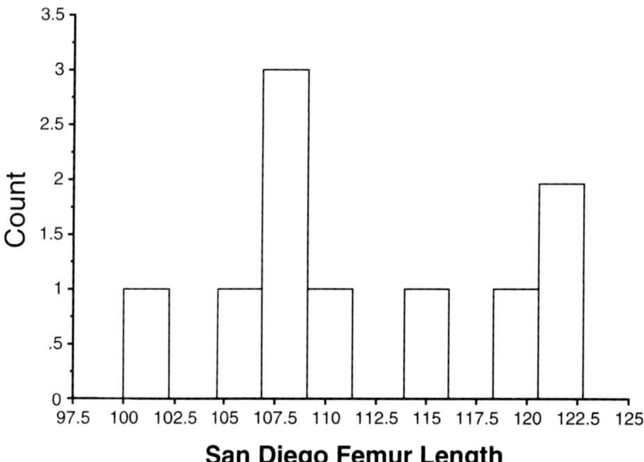

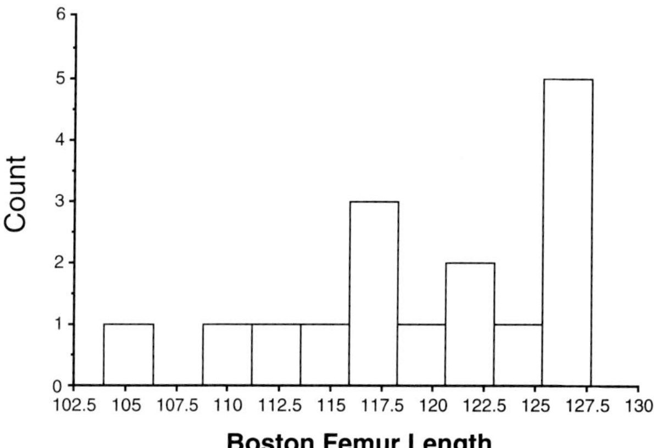

Figure 19
Histogram of data from Table 32 used in the Wilcoxon two-sample nonparametric statistical test. Nonparametric analysis reveals a significant difference between the distributions ($p < 0.03$).

A good way to understand these tests is to examine the calculation procedure, which is relatively simple. First, we rank the variates from smallest to largest, independent of group. In the case of a tie, we split the difference. Then we calculate a statistic directly from the ranks, not the variates. In this case, it's the Wilcoxon *C* statistic. The equation for this statistic is:

$$C = n_1 n_2 + \frac{n_2(n_2 + 1)}{2} - \sum_{i=1}^{n_2} R_i \qquad \textbf{(Eq. 31)}$$

where

n_1 = the size of the larger sample
n_2 = the size of the smaller sample
R_i = the individual rank.

This statistic is compared with $n_1 n_2 - C$, and the greater of the two quantities defined as the test statistic U.

In this example we find a significant difference between femur lengths from San Diego versus Boston ($p = 0.0223$ using the Wilcoxon *C* statistic). However, looking at Figure 18 would not indicate exactly what is different about the distributions. These methods do not require each variate to be a precise measurement, as long as the observations can be ranked. The actual variate measured need not be related to a particular parameter because the calculations are made based on the observation's rank. Thus, typical observations might be: arrival time of patients for surgery, time of day casts are applied, or which flavor ice cream is ordered.

Multivariate Statistical Analysis

Univariate Versus Multivariate Tests

All analyses described up to this point have operated on a single dependent variable, and thus are referred to as univariate analysis methods. For example, the ANOVA example was used to measure the effects of immobilization on muscle fiber area, and the ANCOVA example to measure the effects of cement viscosity on prosthesis pullout strength. In both cases, the analysis was performed on a single variable, fiber area or pullout strength. What if the investigator had measured and was interested in the behavior of several dependent variables? How would the analysis proceed? Obviously, using univariate analysis would require performing numerous one-way ANOVAs on each variable and interpreting the results accordingly. Two problems could occur with the use of multiple univariate analyses. Because different dependent variables may contain different types of information, it is possible that multiple univariate analyses of experimental data would yield significant differences for different reasons. Many dependent variables behave in the same manner simply because they are indicators of the same underlying phenomenon. For example, in measurement of muscle compartment pressure, an investigator might also measure limb girth, mass, and temperature. Because all of these parameters would be expected to increase with a compartment syndrome, the investigator really would like to narrow the focus onto the one parameter that best characterized the phenomenon without the "dilution" of discussing the numerous other parameters. It would be nice to be able to evaluate all dependent variables simultaneously. To perform this type of simultaneous evaluation of multiple variables requires multivariate analysis.

Stepwise Linear Regression

There are several types of multivariate analyses, just as there are many types of univariate analyses. A stepwise linear regression problem will illustrate the general method.

In the stepwise linear regression method, simple linear regression analytic methods, such as

Table 33
Sample data for multiple regression problem

Unit Number	Maximum Tension (N·m)	Innervation Ratio	Fiber Area (μm^2)	Muscle Mass (g)	Unit Cross-sectional Area (cm^2)	Specific Tension (N/cm^2)
1	23.0	60	2,149	6.40	0.001289	17.838
2	46.0	88	3,007	5.80	0.002646	17.384
3	51.0	132	2,296	7.40	0.003031	16.828
4	84.0	161	2,234	5.40	0.003597	23.354
5	94.0	188	2,451	8.00	0.004608	20.400
6	124.0	243	2,607	6.70	0.006335	19.574
7	124.0	166	3,239	6.00	0.005377	23.062
8	157.0	193	2,953	4.30	0.005699	27.547
9	270.0	281	3,694	6.10	0.010380	26.011
10	279.0	379	3,287	6.50	0.012458	22.396
11	284.0	311	3,483	6.90	0.010832	26.218

those described above, are performed on a dependent variable, but multiple independent variables are included in the linear model in a stepwise fashion. At each step, only new information adds to the fit of the model and, thus, the investigator is assured that, by including multiple independent variables in the model, each has unique information. In addition, because the coefficient of determination is calculated after each step, it is possible to quantify the relative percentage to which each independent variable that is added affects the dependent variable.

As an example of stepwise regression applied to a musculoskeletal problem, consider the situation in which the investigators want to know the factor or factors that contribute to muscle motor unit tension. It is known that some motor units develop high tensions (the dependent variable), and other units develop lower tensions. What are the anatomic factors that affect motor unit tension? It is possible to measure total motor unit muscle fiber area, number of muscle fibers per unit (innervation ratio), and muscle mass (all independent variables), as well as motor unit maximum tension (dependent variable). The raw data are presented in Table 33. The data are entered into a stepwise regression program.

By watching the stepwise process, it is possible to illustrate numerous concepts that were presented in the ANOVA and regression sections. New statistical methods are often simple extensions of familiar methods.

The first step in the analysis is to perform simple linear regression of each independent variable on the dependent variable. In statistical terminology, we regress each independent variable on the dependent variable to determine the one that accounts for the greatest explained variation. In our model, the dependent variable is maximum tension, and the independent variables are innervation ratio (IR), fiber cross-sectional area (CSA), muscle mass, and specific tension (motor unit force/motor unit area). The initial regression table (Table 34) shows that the highest F ratio belongs to the variable IR (F = 61.860). Recall that in regression, F represents the explained variation (Equation 22) divided by the unexplained variation (Equation 21) and, thus, IR explains the most variability in tetanic tension of all variables. Also note that muscle mass is not a good predictor of tetanic tension with its very low F value.

Now, the typical simple linear regression analysis is performed and the appropriate ANOVA table generated (Table 35). Note that the relationship is highly significant ($p < 0.0001$) and the coefficient of determination $r^2 = 0.873$ (Table 36). Thus, IR accounts for 87.3% of the total experimental variability. This concludes step one of the procedure and, for many investigators, would conclude the entire experiment. However, more interesting information can be extracted by proceeding to the next steps.

In step two, an analysis of covariance (ANCOVA) is performed using each remaining independent variable with IR as the covariate. The variable with the highest F value, CSA, is entered into the

Table 34
Step One: Initial calculation of F statistics for all dependent variables in the stepwise regression model

	Partial Correlation	*F*-to-Enter*
Innervation ratio	0.934	61.860
Fiber cross-sectional area	0.829	19.749
Muscle mass	0.039	0.014
Calculated specific tension	0.737	10.685

* The higher the F-value, the better the correlation between the independent variable shown and motor unit tetanic tension.

Table 35
ANOVA table generated following the first step of the multiple regression analysis

	df	Sum of Squares	Mean Square	*F* - Value	*p* - Value
Regression	1	81,584.867	81,584.867	61.860	<0.0001*
Residual	9	11,869.679	1,318.853		
Total	10	93,454.545			

* Even after entry of only a single variable into the equation, there is a highly significant effect of IR on maximum tetanic tension.

Table 36
Regression summary, step one

Count	11
Number missing	0
r	0.934
r^2	0.873
Adjusted r^2	0.859
RMS residual	36.316

Table 37
Step two: Second set of *F* calculations

	Partial Correlation	*F*-to-Enter*
CSA**	0.799	14.145
Muscle mass	-0.414	1.652
Calculated spec ten	0.667	6.403

* *F* statistics calculated following step two of the multiple regression analysis.
** The next independent variable to enter the regression model is CSA.

model (Table 37), an ANCOVA is performed, and the regression results are presented as before (Table 38).

Now the coefficient of determination has increased from 0.873 to 0.954 (Table 39), which means that the addition of CSA into the model has accounted for an additional 8.1% of the experimental variability. Because more than one independent variable contributes to the correlation coefficient, it is now termed a serial or multiple correlation coefficient. This added variability is, however, much less important than IR, which initially accounted for 87.3% of the variability.

The stepping process continues until one of two things happens: all variables are entered into the multiple regression equation or the remaining variables have *F* values that are lower than an arbitrary *F* value that is referred to as *F*-to-enter (representing the minimum *F* value required to enter the multiple regression model). In the current case, the next step included the specific tension variable and then the sole remaining variable (muscle mass) had an *F* value of 0.514, far lower than the *F*-to-enter value of 4.000, which we preselected. There is really no right or wrong F-to-enter value. This parameter can be varied and in many cases makes no difference as to the experimental outcome. Table 40 summarizes the stepping process for the stepwise regression model just described. In this case, it is clear that, unless the F-to-enter was decreased to 0.5, the same outcome would be obtained. It usually is possible, using most statistical programs, to force each variable into the equation to calculate just how much of the dependent variable can be accounted for by each independent variable.

The stepwise regression model and simple variations of it are extremely useful in clinical settings in which we desire to know the relative influence of a number of risk factors. Each risk factor is entered as an independent variable and the relative influence determined by the percentage of data variability accounted for by it. The key in multivariate analysis is to go ahead and measure numerous factors. If they are unimportant, they will not enter the equation. If they are important, valuable insights can be gained into the etiology and course of many disease or injury processes.

Importance of Statistical Analysis

It is important to understand experimental design and statistical analysis in order to extract the "truth" from an experiment. The benefits of proper planning and analysis cannot be overstated. Many potentially superb ideas have not been realized because of poor experimental design. Similarly, the significance of numerous excellent experiments has not been extracted because of shoddy or qualitative analysis. Unfortunately, while many scientists and clinicians are trained in their specialty, very few are explicitly tutored in experimental design and statistical analysis. We are thus at risk of mixing well-conceived ideas with shoddy analysis and incorrect interpretation. Clearly, this compromises our pursuit of scientific truth and our ability to prescribe appropriate clinical treatment.

Table 38
ANOVA table of stepwise regression analysis after step two

	df	Sum of Squares	Mean Square	*F* - Value	*p* - Value
Regression	2	89,166.580	44,583.290	83.178	<0.0001
Residual	8	4,287.966*	535.996		
Total	10	93,454.545			

*The residual error (4,287.966) has decreased from that shown in Table 35 (11,869.679) due to addition of CSA into the regression model.

Table 39
Regression summary, step two

Count	11
Number missing	0
r	0.977
r^2	0.954
Adjusted r^2	0.943
RMS residual	23.152

*The serial correlation coefficient has increased from 0.873 in step one (Table 36) to 0.943 in step two.

The purpose of this chapter has been to describe, by example, the basis for appropriate prospective experimental design and analysis. The two general classes of experimentation are prospective (experiments designed prior to their execution) and retrospective (experiments designed after the data have been gathered). Retrospective experiments are usually applied to clinical studies in which data from patients who have already been treated is analyzed. Retrospective experiments have two major advantages: they are relatively inexpensive and rapid to perform. These advantages exist because the time and money devoted to the experiment itself have already been spent. The investment consists of the time required to extract and analyze the data. The pitfall of retrospective clinical studies is that, because originally no experiment was envisioned, there is little control regarding the protocol used to record the data and important desired information may not be available. Because these are major drawbacks, numerous clinical journals will not publish retrospective studies and many clinicians view such studies with skepticism. For this reason, the majority of this chapter has been devoted to the description of methods used to design and analyze data from prospective studies, with the caveat that the methods discussed also allow comparisons to be made within data after they have been acquired as part of a prospective study.

Table 40
Stepwise regression summary

Step Number	Variable Entered	Coefficient of Determination	Percent of Data Variability Explained
1	Innervation ratio	0.873	87.3
2	Fiber CSA	0.954	8.1
3	Specific tension	0.972	1.8
4	None		

Proper experimental execution consists of three steps: (1) planning and designing the experiment, (2) executing the experiment, and (3) analyzing and interpreting the data obtained from the experiment. The latter depends on the proper statistical techniques based on the proper size and clinical description of sample population and nature of dependent and independent variables. If these suggestions are followed, costs are decreased, direction is maintained, and the project retains continuity. Most importantly, the data ultimately have more impact because results are concisely and accurately presented.

The following steps will help the investigator choose among the various models presented and help the reader to evaluate the research and the results presented.

1. Describe the dependent variable.
2. Define the factors.
3. Define the levels of each factor.
4. State whether the factors are fixed or random.
5. Describe the appropriate statistical method along with a rationale for your choice.

Applying these steps to the various models will be helpful to both the prospective investigator and evaluator.

Sample Experimental Designs

Example 1

Growth rate of fibroblasts in the anterior cruciate ligament (ACL) are measured using one of three growth factors. A pool of fibroblast cells from the ACL are split into three different dishes and the growth factor is added.

This is a 1 × 3 one-way ANOVA with repeated measures. The repeated measure is present because the same culture of fibroblasts was split into three dishes and, thus, the cultures have a good deal in common.

Example 2

The weight-gain of patients after total joint replacement is measured using one of four dietary regimens. Forty patients are randomly placed into one of four experimental groups. One group of ten patients receives no dietary supplement.

This is a 1 × 4 full-factorial one-way ANOVA with repeated measures. Each of the groups is independent of the other and receives only one treatment.

Example 3

A biomechanics laboratory is involved in the measurement of the stress-strain properties. The principal investigator suspects that the four technicians working for her do not obtain consistent results; therefore, she asks each technician to independently measure the strain in the same ten videotaped biomechanical experiments.

This is a 1 × 4 one-way ANOVA. Because each technician is measuring the same videotape, this experiment will determine whether there are systematic differences in the way each technician performs the measurement.

Example 4

The blood hormone levels of postmenopausal women are measured. Half of the women are taking hormone supplements and half are taking a placebo. They are blinded to the treatment. Hormone levels are measured immediately before the study, and one and six months after the study begins.

This is a 2 × 3 two-way ANOVA with repeated measures. In this case, the repeated measure is present because the same individuals are measured at different time periods.

Example 5

Bean plants are grown in four different locations within a greenhouse. Within each plot, four different fertilizers are used to induce growth. After one month, the plant heights are measured.

This is a 1 × 4 one-way nested ANOVA. This is a nested design because the soil will be slightly different in each portion of the greenhouse. Thus, the different fertilizers used in each region of the greenhouse will have a soil-dependent effect.

Example 6

Maximum bone strength is measured in an experimental animal using either a bone plate that flexes or a completely rigid plate.

This is a 1 × 2 one-way ANOVA or simply a *t*-test. Only two groups are present, and they are independent so this represents a *t*-test design.

Example 7

A force transducer is calibrated by hanging various masses on the transducer and measuring output voltage.

This is a simple linear regression example because the independent variable (mass) is related to the dependent variable (voltage) using a linear equation. The equation itself will yield the calibration factor.

Example 8

Serum levels of creatinine kinase are measured in myocardial infarction patients who receive a new drug treatment or placebo medication. Before a patient enters into the study, a complete blood panel including chemistry is obtained along with smoking history, weight, and serum cholesterol levels.

This is a one-way ANOVA model. We are interested in the differences between the drug group and placebo groups, but we will first correct these values for other suspected covariates that were measured. In this way, we will be sure that the differences measured are not simply a result of misrepresentation of certain patient characteristics in one group or the other.

Example 9

The volume of above-knee stumps are measured following amputation. The goal is to resolve postoperative swelling as soon as possible in order to permit fitting of a prosthesis as soon as possible. Three different methods of stump volume reduction are used: plaster cast wrap, ace bandage wrap, and manual massage. Stump volume is measured once per week for six months.

This is a regression model in which time is the independent variable and stump volume the dependent variable. The slope of the regression equation will yield the rate at which stump volume decreases. The method that yields the greatest rate—assuming that the three methods provide equally good fits—is the preferable method.

Example 10

ACL reconstruction is performed in professional football players using either a patellar tendon autograft or a ligament augmentation device. The trainer measures whether or not the player returns to the starting lineup after surgery.

This is a frequency analysis problem with the measurement being a yes or no answer as to whether the player returns to the starting lineup.

Example 11

ACL reconstruction is performed in professional football players using either a patellar tendon autograft or a ligament augmentation device. The trainer records how many weeks postoperatively the player returns to full practice.

This is a one-way ANOVA model because we have measured a continuous variable—time. This design is preferable to that performed in example 10 because it provides greater sensitivity to changes that can occur between players. Ideally, many variables, such as knee extension strength, time in the 40-yard dash, and length of workout, would also be measured to determine which surgical procedure provided the best results.

Selected Bibliography

General Statistical Texts

Altman DG: *Practical Statistics for Medical Research.* London, Chapman & Hall, 1991.

Bliss CI: *Statistics in Biology: Statistical Methods for Research in the Natural Sciences.* New York, McGraw-Hill, 1967.

Bliss CI: *Statistics in Biology.* New York, McGraw-Hill, 1970.

Bowerman BL, O'Connell RT: *Linear Statistical Models: An Applied Approach,* ed 2. Boston, MA, PWS-Kent Publishing, 1990.

Cochran WG, Cox GM: *Experimental Designs,* ed 2. New York, Wiley & Sons, 1957.

Dawson-Saunders B, Trapp RG: *Basic and Clinical Biostatistics.* Norwalk, CT, Appleton & Lange, 1990.

Dixon WJ, Massey FJ Jr: *Introduction to Statistical Analysis,* ed 3. New York, McGraw-Hill, 1969.

Draper NR, Smith H: *Applied Regression Analysis,* ed 2. New York, Wiley & Sons, 1981.

Dunn OJ, Clark VA: *Applied Statistics: Analysis of Variance and Regression.* New York, Wiley & Sons, 1974.

Fleiss JL: *The Design and Analysis of Clinical Experiments.* New York, Wiley & Sons, 1986.

Fleiss JL: *Statistical Methods for Rates and Proportions,* ed 2. New York, Wiley & Sons, 1981.

Montgomery DC: *Design and Analysis of Experiments.* New York, Wiley & Sons, 1966.

Mosteller F, Tukey JW: *Data Analysis and Regression: A Second Course in Statistics.* Redding, MA, Addison-Wesley, 1977.

Schefler WC: *Statistics for Health Professionals.* Redding, MA, Addison-Wesley, 1984.

Shuster JJ: *CRC Handbook of Sample Size Guidelines for Clinical Trials.* Boca Raton, FL, CRC Press, 1990.

Snedecor GW, Cochran WG: *Statistical Methods,* ed 6. Ames, IA, Iowa State University Press, 1967.

Sokal RR, Rohlf FJ: *Biometry: The Principles and Practice of Statistics in Biological Research,* ed 2. San Francisco, WH Freeman & Co, 1981.

Tatsuoka MM: *Multivariate Analysis: Techniques for Educational and Psychological Research.* New York, Wiley & Sons, 1971.

Zar JH: *Biostatistical Analysis,* ed 2. Englewood Cliffs, NJ, Prentice-Hall, 1974.

Some Details of Statistical Methodology

Bishop YMM, Fienberg SE, Holland PW: *Discrete Multivariate Analysis: Theory and Practice.* Cambridge, MA, MIT Press, 1975.

Cramer EM: Significance tests and tests of models in multiple regression. *Am Statistics* 1972;26:26–30.

Fisher RA: *Statistical Methods for Research Workers,* ed 12. Edinburgh, Oliver & Boyd, 1954.

Fleiss JL: Confidence intervals vs significance tests: Quantitative interpretation. *Am J Public Health* 1986;76:587–588.

Freiman JA, Chalmers TC, Smith H Jr, et al: The importance of beta, the type II error and sample size in the design and interpretation of the randomized control trial: Survey of 71 "negative" trials. *N Engl J Med* 1978;299:690–694.

French S: How significant is statistical significance? A critique of the use of statistics in research. *Physiotherapy (Lond)* 1988;74:266–268.

Godfrey K: Simple linear regression in medical research. *N Engl J Med* 1985;313:1629–1636.

Grubbs FE: Procedures for detecting outlying observations in samples. *Technometrics* 1969;11:1–21.

Gurland J, Tripathi RC: A simple approximation for unbiased estimation of the standard deviation. *Am Statistics* 1971;25:30–32.

Ku HH, Kullback S: Loglinear models in contingency table analysis. *Am Statistics* 1974;28:115–122.

Nelissen RG, Brand R, Rozing PM: Survivorship analysis in total condylar knee arthroplasty: A statistical review. *J Bone Joint Surg* 1992;74A:383–389.

Poole C: Beyond the confidence interval. *Am J Public Health* 1987;77:195–199.

Ratain JS, Hochberg MC: Clinical trials: A guide to understanding methodology and interpreting results. *Arthritis Rheum* 1990;33:131–139.

Ricker WE: Linear regression in fishery research. *J Fish Res Bd Can* 1973;30:409–434.

Rudicel S, Esdaile J: The randomized clinical trial in orthopaedics: Obligation or option? *J Bone Joint Surg* 1985;67A:1284–1293.

Seal HL: *Multivariate Statistical Analysis for Biologists.* New York, Wiley & Sons, 1964.

Sokal RR, Braumann CA: Significance tests for coefficients of variation and variability profiles. *Syst Zoology* 1980;29:50–66.

Spector P: Post-hocs vs. contrasts: A look at the strengths and weaknesses of both types of means comparisons. *Abacus News* Fall 1990.

Student (Gossett WS): On the error of counting with a haemacytometer. *Biometrika* 1907;5:351–360.

Thompson WD: Statistical criteria in the interpretation of epidemiologic data. *Am J Public Health* 1987;77:191–194.

Thompson WD: On the comparison of effects. *Am J Public Health* 1987;77:491–492.

Tsutakawa RK, Hewett JE: Comparison of two regression lines over a finite interval. *Biometrics* 1978;34:391–398.

Welsch RE: Stepwise multiple comparison procedures. *J Am Statistics Assoc* 1977;72:566–575.

Examples of Statistics Applied to Biology and Medicine

Bodine SC, Roy RR, Eldred E, et al: Maximal force as a function of anatomical features of motor units in the cat tibialis anterior. *J Neurophysiol* 1987;57:1730–1745.

Frank C, McDonald D, Lieber R, et al: Biochemical heterogeneity within the maturing rabbit medial collateral ligament. *Clin Orthop* 1988;236:279–285.

Lieber RL: Statistical significance and statistical power in hypothesis testing. *J Orthop Res* 1990;8:304–309.

Lieber RL, Blevins FT: Skeletal muscle architecture of the rabbit hindlimb: Functional implications of muscle design. *J Morphol* 1989;199:93–101.

Lieber RL, Brown CG: Quantitative method for comparison of skeletal muscle architectural properties. *J Biomech* 1992;25:557–560.

Lieber RL, Friden JO, Hargens AR, et al: Differential response of the dog quadriceps muscle to external skeletal fixation of the knee. *Muscle Nerve* 1988;11:193–201.

Lieber RL, Jacobson MD, Fazeli BM, et al: Architecture of selected muscles of the arm and forearm: Anatomy and implications for tendon transfer. *J Hand Surg* 1992;17A:787–798.

Golbranson FL, Wirta RW, Kuncir EJ, et al: Volume changes occurring in postoperative below-knee limbs. *J Rehabil Res Dev* 1988;25:11–18.

Wenger DR, Mauldin D, Speck G, et al: Corrective shoes and inserts as treatment for flexible flatfoot in infants and children. *J Bone Joint Surg* 1989;71A:800–810.

Glossary

accommodating resistance exercise A type of exercise that isolates a joint and constrains the muscle action so that the joint is moved at a constant angular velocity. The limits of this angular velocity can be set by a servocontrolled dynamometer (also called an isokinetic dynamometer).

accuracy The closeness of a measured reading, score, or observation to the true value.

action potential The propagating electrical potential that develops when a muscle or nerve cell is activated; the summation of nearly synchronous action potentials is referred to as a compound muscle, nerve, or sensory nerve action potential, according to the fibers activated.

active tension The amount of tension generated in muscle as a result of muscle activation (*See* passive tension).

adhesin Microbial surface antigen, usually in the form of pili or fimbriae, that binds to specific receptors on epithelial cell membranes, providing for cell attachment.

adsorption Adherence of atoms, ions, or molecules to the surface of another substance.

aerobic glycolysis The metabolism of glucose in the presence of oxygen with the final oxidation of its products through the mitochondrial Krebs cycle and electron transport.

afferent Toward the central nervous system.

aggrecan A large aggregated proteoglycan consisting of a protein core and many glycosaminoglycan chains, and possessing the ability to form aggregates with hyaluronate and link protein.

alloantigen Immunoglobulin specific for a major histocompatibility complex (HLA complexes in humans).

allograft (*also called* homograft) A tissue or an organ transplanted between individuals of the same species, but genetically nonidentical (*See* isograft).

α (significance level) The probability of Type 1 error in an experiment involving hypothesis testing.

Amonton's law Three empirical observations regarding the nature of dry friction (1699).

amplification An increase in the amount of DNA or RNA replicated; implies a stimulated process of replication meant to produce extra DNA or RNA.

anabolic steroid Natural and synthetic sex hormones that promote protein synthesis and enhance the growth of tissue, especially muscle.

anaerobic glycolysis The metabolism of glucose in the absence of oxygen with the final oxidation to lactic acid through cytosolic glycolysis.

analysis of covariance (ANCOVA) The analytic technique that compares mean values between groups after adjusting for an independent covariate.

analysis of variance (ANOVA) The analytic method for determining whether means obtained from various samples are equivalent.

anelastic material A material without a well-defined relationship between stress and strain.

aneuploid A cell or group of cells with an abnormal concentration of DNA compared with that of a normal cell, whether more or less than haploid, diploid, or tetraploid.

angiogenin A factor that stimulates vessel formation.

anisotropic material A material in which the properties differ depending on direction; for example, material with oriented fibers embedded in a matrix.

annealing Heat treatment that renders metals softer and more ductile by relieving residual stresses.

anodal block Local block of nerve conduction caused by hyperpolarization of the nerve cell membrane by an electric stimulus.

anode The positive electrode and more reactive metal in a corrosion cell or battery, it is oxidized, gives up electrons, and is degraded; the positive pole of the stimulating electrode in a nerve conduction study.

anterograde From the neuronal cell body toward the axonal target.

antibody (*also called* immunoglobulin) Immune protein made by B cells in response to the presence of antigens.

antidromic Propagation of an impulse in the direction opposite to physiologic conduction; conduction along motor nerve fibers away from the muscle and along sensory fibers away from the spinal cord.

antigen Substances capable of evoking a reaction in nonself.

antioncogene (*also called* recessive oncogene; tumor suppressor gene) Gene whose presence normally prevents neoplasia and whose absence or malfunction leads to the production of a neoplasm.

apophyseal growth plate Growth plate under tensile force that produces growth of nonlong bones.

apparent density The density (mass/total volume) of a porous material even though the mass occupies only a small portion of the total volume.

area moment of inertia (*also called* second moment of area) Resistance to bending that is solely a function of geometry, independent of material properties, and is inversely proportional to the stress caused by bending.

atactic Orientation of a polymer in which side groups are distributed on both sides of a macromolecular chain.

ATP (*Adenosine 5′-triphosphate*) A nucleotide whose high-energy phosphate bonds are used in metabolism to supply energy to many physiologic mechanisms.

attrition The wearing away of a material by friction.

autocrine A growth factor or biologically active molecule produced by a cell, it acts locally to stimulate the same cell type in a tissue.

autograft A tissue or an organ transplanted into a new position within or on the same individual.

average (X) A value, calculated from a sample, that estimates the population mean.

axon The central core of axoplasm that constitutes the conducting element of a nerve fiber; it is bounded by a surface membrane called the axolemma.

axon hillock Region of the cell body from which the axon originates, often the site of impulse initiation.

axoplasmic transport Intracellular movement of materials, both distally and centrally, within the axoplasm.

basal lamina Thin layer of extracellular matrix material, primarily collagen, laminin, and fibronectin, that surrounds muscle cells and Schwann cells; also underlies all epithelial sheets.

bending Deformation caused by transverse loading of a structure or by bending moments.

bending moment A force that tends to produce a moment to bend an object.

β (significance level) The probability of type 2 error in a hypothesis testing experiment.

beta-oxidation A metabolic pathway for the breakdown of long-chain fatty acids.

biglycan A small proteoglycan that consists of a short protein core and two dermatan sulfate side chains.

bioabsorbable material A material whose breakdown products are incorporated into normal physiologic and biochemical processes.

biocompatible material A material that can function in a biologic environment without known and/or significant detrimental effects on either the material or the living system.

biodegradable material A material that breaks down when placed in a biologic environment.

bioelectric potential An electric potential, generated by cellular elements and cellular metabolism, that depends on cellular viability.

biomaterial A natural biologic material or a synthetic material used to replace, treat, or augment tissue and/or organ function.

bioresorbable material A material that is broken down in vivo and removed from the implantation site.

biotribology Study of friction, lubrication, and wear of contacting biologic structures, particularly diarthrodial joints.

biphasic material A material composed of a solid phase and a fluid phase; for example, articular cartilage and meniscus.

bone histomorphometry Histologic quantitation of volumes, surfaces, and cell numbers involved in bone formation and resorption.

bone mass Quantity of bone in the entire skeleton.

bone modeling unit (BMU) A group of osteoblasts, osteocytes, and osteoclasts that are linked and participate in remodeling (activation, resorption, and formation) of a discrete area of bone.

bone morphogenic protein (BMP) A family of glycoproteins in the TGF-β superfamily that are found in demineralized bone matrix and participate in bone formation, stimulating the production of the cartilage that undergoes enchondral ossification to form bone; BMP-3 is called osteogenin.

boundary lubrication Separation of the sliding contacts of two bodies by a layer of adsorbed molecules on each surface.

brittle Sustaining little or no permanent deformation prior to failure.

bulk modulus Proportionality constant between change of volume per unit volume and the applied pressure, analogous to Young's modulus.

calcitonin A protein produced by parafollicular cells of the thyroid that decreases serum calcium by inhibiting osteoclast activity and accelerates growth plate calcification.

cambium The inner cellular layer of the periosteum that interfaces with bone.

capacitance (C) The property that permits storage of electrical energy as a result of electric displacement when opposite surfaces of conducting plates separated by an insulator carry opposite electrical charges; it is determined by the area of the two plates and the distance between them and is measured in farads (F); increasing or decreasing the distance between plates will increase the capacitance.

carbohydrate A compound of carbon, hydrogen, and oxygen: $(CH_2O)_n$; the most important dietary carbohydrates are starches, sugars, and celluloses.

carbohydrate loading An exercise and diet regimen that elevates muscle glycogen by regulating exercise level and emphasizing dietary carbohydrate.

carcinogen Agent associated with an increase in cancer production.

casting Fabrication of parts by pouring molten material (such as metal) into molds.

cathode The negative electrode and less reactive metal in a corrosion cell, it is reduced and does not corrode; the negative pole of the stimulating electrode in nerve conduction studies.

centroid The point at which an object's geometry may be considered to be concentrated; for an object with uniform density, the centroid is located at the center of mass.

ceramic Inorganic, ionically bonded materials often having a metallic oxide component.

channel Pathway through a membrane allowing passage of ions or molecules.

chemotaxis The movement of a cell up or down a gradient of a chemical signal.

χ^2-statistic The statistic used in frequency analysis to compare expected proportions.

chondrocalcinosis The presence of calcium salts in cartilaginous structures of joints.

chondron The region within articular cartilage that contains the chondrocyte and its pericellular and territorial matrices.

chromosome A nuclear structure containing a linear strand of DNA; humans have 46 chromosomes (23 pairs).

coefficient of determination (r^2) The "goodness of fit" statistic that represents the total fraction of the data explained by a linear relationship.

coefficient of friction The resistance of relative motion of two objects in contact measured by dividing the frictional force by the compressive load (*See* Amonton's law).

cold flow Plastic deformation during creep.

collagen A large family of genetically distinct proteins, each of which has a triple helix fibrillar component, and which form a major proportion of the organic matrix of bone, cartilage, tendon, and ligament.

collagenase Metalloproteinase that cleaves collagen enzymatically.

component of a force The magnitude of force in a specific direction; in three dimensions, a force has three components.

compliance The inverse stiffness (m/N); the motion caused by a load divided by that load.

compression A force tending to squeeze or crush an object.

concentration cell An electrochemical cell arising from unequal electrolyte concentrations between compartments.

concentric activation (*also called* concentric action) The shortening of a muscle during activation (*See* eccentric activation).

conductance (g) The readiness with which an electric current is conducted; the reciprocal of resistance: $g = 1/R$.

conduction velocity Speed of propagation of an action potential along a nerve or muscle fiber.

contact guidance Notion that axon outgrowth is directed by mechanical features of the local environment.

contact healing (*also called* primary bone healing) A term previously used to indicate healing of a fracture without callus formation when bone fragments are touching.

coordinate system The right-handed orthogonal (Cartesian) coordinate system is used throughout.

copolymer Macromolecules composed of more than one type of monomer.

correlation coefficient (*r*) The "goodness of fit" statistic that represents the degree to which the experimental data fit a line; the square root of the coefficient of determination; positive for positive slopes and negative for negative slopes.

corrosion Electrochemical destruction of a metal.

couple The moment formed by two parallel forces of equal magnitude and opposite direction; a pure moment with a resultant force of zero.

coupling Motion in which rotation or translation of a rigid body about one axis is associated with rotation or translation of that same rigid body about another axis.

covalent bond Atomic bonding produced by the sharing of a pair of electrons between two adjacent atoms.

crack A flaw or hole inside or on the surface of an object.

cramp An involuntary (painful) condition of muscle characterized by a powerful activation of the muscle.

creep A viscoelastic property of materials whereby the deformation continues to increase, without the loss of material, when subjected to a constant force.

cross-linking The chemical or mechanical connection of adjacent polymer chains.

current (I) The amount of charge moved per unit time; in biologic systems it is carried by ions and flows in the direction of the positive ions; measured in amperes (A).

cytofluorometry A method of measuring the DNA content of a cell by labeling the DNA with a fluorochrome and measuring the amount of light reflected under a microscope.

cytokine Generic term for nonantibody proteins that mediate cell function by binding to specific cell-surface receptors; a group of growth factors; this term replaces both lymphokine and monokine (*See* interleukin).

dalton (d) Measurement of molecular mass in which 1 dalton = 0.9997 mass unit or one sixteenth of the mass of oxygen 16.

Darcy's law Linear relationship between fluid flux and pressure gradient.

decorin A small proteoglycan that contains a short protein core and one dermatan sulfate side chain; it coats the surfaces of collagen fibers.

degree of freedom The number of independent quantities needed to describe the position of an object; for example, six degrees of freedom describe the position of any segment of the body in three dimensions (three angles and three coordinates of a point on the body), and when there are constraints, the degrees of freedom will be reduced accordingly; in one degree of freedom a rigid body either translates back and forth in either direction along a straight line or rotates clockwise and counterclockwise in either direction.

depolarization Reduction in the magnitude of the resting membrane potential toward zero.

descriptive statistics Numeric expressions that serve to describe a sample; for example, mean (X).

desmosome A small, discrete, circular, dense body that forms the site of attachment between certain epithelial cells.

differential melting Surface melting resulting from the brief application of heat from an external source.

diffusion bonding Adhesion of two materials in contact by the movement of surface atoms between them.

dilatation An increase or decrease in volume per unit volume.

diploid Twice haploid; the amount of DNA in a normal resting human cell (the Go/G phase of the cell cycle).

DNA (*deoxyribonucleic acid*) A nucleic acid that constitutes the genetic material of all cellular organisms and the DNA viruses; considered to be the autoreproducing component of chromosomes and of many viruses.

dominant oncogene A proto-oncogene that when mutated (altered) transforms the cell to the malignant phenotype by a variety of mechanisms; for example, acting as a growth factor.

Donnan ion distribution Concentration of counter-ions in the interstitium resulting from charges fixed on the porous-permeable solid matrix.

Donnan osmotic pressure Component of swelling pressure resulting from excess ionic particles due to Donnan ion distribution within the interstitium.

drag coefficient Proportionality factor between drag force and flow speed.

dual-energy x-ray absorptiometry (DEXA) Radiographic technique that measures bone density and cross-sectional geometry.

dual photon absorptiometry (DPA) The use of two photon beams to measure bone density.

ductile Capacity to sustain large amounts of permanent deformation without failing.

dynamic shear modulus Response of a viscoelastic material resulting from sinusoidal excitation.

dynamics Study of relationships between forces, moments, and motions of objects.

eccentric activation (*also called* eccentric action) Muscle activation with simultaneous muscle lengthening.

efferent Away from the central nervous system.

eicosanoids Biologically active substances derived from arachidonic acid, including the prostaglandins and leukotrienes.

elastic deformation Deformation that disappears when the stress is removed.

elastic limit Strain beyond which permanent deformation occurs.

elastic modulus Measure of material stiffness defined by dividing stress (measured in pascals) by strain; for linear materials, it is the slope of the stress-strain curve.

elastohydrodynamic lubrication Condition that occurs when the deformation of bearing surfaces becomes important in hydrodynamic lubrication.

electrodiagnosis Recording and analysis of responses from nerves and muscle to electric stimulation and identification of patterns of insertion, spontaneous, involuntary, and voluntary action potentials.

electromyography Recording and study of insertion, spontaneous, and voluntary electric activity of muscle.

endochondral ossification (*also called* enchondral ossification) Bone development through the formation of a cartilage matrix.

endomysium Connective tissue surrounding the muscle cell.

endoneurial tube Convenient term describing the endoneurial sheath and the column of tissue it encloses.

endoneurium Connective tissue that forms the supporting framework for the nerve fibers and capillaries inside a fascicle.

endotenon A loose connective tissue that surrounds individual fascicles of a tendon.

endurance limit Repetitive stress that can be endured indefinitely by a material; for stresses below the endurance limit, fatigue life is theoretically infinite.

engineering stress Applied force divided by unstressed (original) area.

enhancer Portion of DNA that assists in initiating transcription (constructing mRNA from DNA), but is not necessary for the process.

enzyme A protein molecule that catalyzes chemical reactions of other substances without itself being destroyed or altered during the reaction; the six main groups are oxidoreductases, transferases, hydrolases, lyases, isomerases, and ligases.

epigenesis Production of a neoplasm due to the expression of genes normally present in the genome, but not normally activated or expressed.

epimysium Connective tissue surrounding the entire muscle.

epineurium Connective tissue that envelops the nerve and extends internally to separate and enclose individual fascicles so that they are embedded in it.

epiphysis The end of a long bone formed by the secondary center of ossification and covered by articular cartilage.

equilibrium Point at which the sum of all forces and moments acting on an object equals zero; for example, $\Sigma F = 0$ and $\Sigma M = 0$.

equilibrium potential Membrane potential at which there is no net passive movement of a permanent ion species into or out of a cell.

equipollent force system System in which the action of a force about a point p is equivalent to the force acting at that point plus a couple that is equal to the moment of the force about the point p.

ergotism Poisoning from excessive or misdirected use of ergot as a medicine or from eating ergotized grain containing the fungus *Claviceps purpura;* characterized by necrosis of the extremities caused by contractions of the peripheral vascular bed.

exon Portion of mRNA that codes for protein.

***F*-statistic** The statistic created by the ratio of two variances, it can be used in ANOVA to compare whether a number of means are equivalent.

facultative Ability to live under more than one set of environmental conditions.

fascicle Bundle of nerve fibers and their related endoneurial tissue.

fasciculation Random spontaneous twitching of a group of muscle fibers or a motor unit.

fast-glycolytic (FG) fiber A fast-twitch muscle fiber characterized by low aerobic and high anaerobic capacities.

fast-oxidative glycolytic (FOG) fiber A fast-twitch muscle fiber characterized by high aerobic activity and moderate anaerobic activity.

fast-twitch (FT) muscle fiber A muscle fiber characterized by fast contraction time in response to electrical stimulation of the nerve and muscle.

fatigue Structural failure caused by repetitive stresses below the ultimate strength.

fibrillation A small, local, involuntary muscle contraction resulting from spontaneous activation of single muscle fibers.

fibroblast growth factor (FGF) Peptide hormone derived from the pituitary and from cartilage; it is a potent stimulator of proliferation.

flow-dependent viscoelasticity Creep and stress-relaxation phenomena resulting from interstitial fluid flow through a porous-permeable material, for example, articular cartilage.

flow-independent viscoelasticity (*also called* intrinsic viscoelasticity) Creep and stress-relaxation phenomena resulting from molecular rearrangement within the solid matrix of a porous-permeable material.

fluorocytometry A technique used to measure cells, nuclei, or other cellular components that are prelabeled with a fluorochrome and passed single-file through an exciting wavelength of light; the emitted fluorescence is measured and the results plotted, usually on a histogram (*See* cytofluorometry).

force A type of vector that describes a push or pull; for example, a push with a magnitude of 10-pounds, acting from left to right.

forging Fabrication by plastic deformation.

fracture Failure resulting from the unbounded growth of a crack.

fracture toughness A material property that is measured by the energy required to cause crack propagation in the material.

free-body diagram Partial model of an object that is used to isolate it from the environment to explore all the forces that act on it.

frequency analysis The analytic technique that determines the probability that certain numbers of frequencies of observations are independent.

friction Resistance to relative sliding motion between two surfaces in contact.

F wave Long-latency motor response resulting from antidromic activation of α motoneurons in the spinal cord.

gap healing Healing by bone formation across a reduced fracture where a gap exists.

gene A segment of a DNA molecule that contains all the information required for synthesis of a product (polypeptide chain or RNA molecule), including both coding and noncoding sequences.

gene enhancer Regions of a gene that regulate transcription.

gene promoter Regulatory portion of DNA that is found adjacent to the protein coding region of a gene and that controls the expression of the gene.

genome The complete complement of genetic information of an organism.

germ line defect An inherited DNA mutation that is present in the DNA of all cells in the organism; the resulting alteration is usually subtle and not recognized at birth.

glass An amorphous, undercooled liquid of extremely high viscosity that has all the appearances of a solid.

glass transition temperature (T_g) The temperature at which the behavior of an amorphous material changes from brittle to viscous.

glia Neuroglia; supporting structure of nerve tissue composed of astrocytes and oligodendrocytes in the central nervous system, Schwann cells in the peripheral nervous system, and satellite cells in ganglia.

glycosaminoglycan (GAG) Repeating units of sulfated disaccharides, including keratan sulfate, dermatan sulfate, and chondroitin 4-sulfate and chondroitin 6-sulfate, that bind to a protein core to form proteoglycans.

graded potential Local change in the membrane potential of a neuron.

groove of Ranvier Cells that surround the cartilaginous component of the growth plate at the junction between the reserve and proliferative zones and function in the circumferential enlargement of the growth plate.

ground electrode Electrode placed between the stimulating and recording electrodes in nerve conduction studies.

growth cone Specialized end of a growing axon (or dendrite) that generates the motive force for elongation.

growth factor Polypeptides that are released by certain cells and bind to specific cell wall receptor sites to influence cells to divide or remain quiescent.

growth plate (*also called* physis; epiphyseal plate) A cartilaginous structure composed of proliferating chondrocytes that produce a large extracellular matrix, which serves as a template for bone formation (*See* endochondral ossification).

haploid The amount of DNA in a normal human egg or sperm, or half that found in a normal cell.

hardness A surface property of a material that imparts resistance to penetration or scratching.

haversian bone Mature bone formed by whole or fractured osteons usually arranged longitudinally.

haversian canal Freely anastomosing channels within cortical bone containing blood vessels, lymph vessels, and nerves.

helical axis *See* screw axis.

Hertz (Hz) Unit of frequency equivalent to one cycle per second.

heterogeneous Nonuniform.

heterograft *See* xenograft.

histocompatibility complex *See* human leukocyte antigen.

homograft *See* allograft.

Hooke's law A linear relationship, F = kx, defining the response of an elastic material between load (F) and deformation (x), where k is a constant that defines the stiffness of the material.

hot isostatic pressing Consolidation under high temperature and pressure of metal powder into a fine-grained material.

H reflex Electrically-evoked spinal monosynaptic reflex involving the Ia afferent fibers from the muscle spindles and motor axons.

human leukocyte antigen (HLA) The human major histocompatibility complex, which lies on chromosome 6 and is divided into four main regions, A, B, C, and D, each encoding for different types of cell surface molecules.

hyaline cartilage Normal cartilage.

hybridoma Activated B-lymphocyte (plasma cell) combined with myeloma cell to produce an immortal population of cells capable of producing a single specific antibody.

hydrodynamic lubrication Separation of sliding contacts between two bodies by a layer of lubricant in the form of a liquid or gas.

hydrogen bond Secondary bonds in which a hydrogen atom is attracted to electrons of neighboring atoms.

hydroxyapatite (*also called* apatite) Naturally occurring mineral [$Ca_{10}(PO_4)_6(OH)_2$] found as the major inorganic constituent of bone matrix.

hyperplasia An abnormal increase in the number of cells in a tissue or organ.

hypertrophic zone That portion of the growth plate in which the chondrocytes enlarge and matrix calcification occurs.

hypertrophy An abnormal increase in the size of a cell or organ.

hypophosphatasia A genetic deficiency in alkaline phosphatase resulting in deficient cartilage mineralization and a clinical picture similar to rickets.

hysteresis Conversion of strain energy to heat during cyclic loading; that is, mechanical energy is lost during each cycle.

immunity In materials, resistance to corrosion.

indirect calorimetry A method of estimating metabolic rate and energy sources by measuring the amount of oxygen used by the body.

instant center of rotation (ICR) The point about which an object appears to be rotating; this concept is valid only for two-dimensional motion.

insulin-like growth factors (IGF) Peptides that behave similarly to insulin and stimulate cell proliferation.

integrin Transmembrane proteins that function in the attachment of cells to the extracellular matrix and in the transduction of mechanical stimuli in cellular metabolism; one of a family of cell surface molecules that play a role in the attachment of metastatic neoplastic cells to endothelial cells.

interleukin Polypeptide mediator in the class designated as cytokines; a type of growth factor.

intramembranous ossification Bone formation directly within a fibrous mesenchymal connective tissue.

interneuron Neuron that intervenes between sensory and effector neurons.

intron Portion of mRNA that does not code for proteins.

ionic bond Atomic bonding through coulombic attraction of oppositely charged ions.

isograft A tissue or an organ transplanted between genetically identical individuals.

isokinetic A term used to describe the conditions of muscle activation; when applied to isolated muscles, it implies a constant velocity of shortening or lengthening, and when applied to the action of muscles moving joints, it implies a constant angular velocity of joint rotation.

isometric A term used to describe the conditions of muscle activation; when applied to isolated muscle, it implies that the muscle length is held constant, and when applied to the action of muscles moving joints, it implies that the angular position is set at a given position and not allowed to rotate.

isotactic Orientation of a polymer in which all side groups are on one side of the carbon chain.

isotonic A term used to describe the conditions of muscle activation; when applied to isolated muscles, it implies that the load on the muscle is constant, and when applied to the action of muscles moving joints, it implies that the load-resisting angular rotation of the joint is constant.

isotropy Having the same material properties independent of direction.

jitter Variability with consecutive discharges of the interpotential interval between two muscle fiber action potentials belonging to the same motor unit.

kinematics Description of motion, regardless of how the motion came about.

kinesiology Study of motion in the human body.

kinetics Study of the forces that bring about motion.

Krebs cycle (*also called* tricarboxylic acid cycle; citric acid cycle) A sequence of chemical reactions in the metabolic pathways in which the end products of glycolysis are degraded to carbon dioxide and hydrogen atoms.

kurtosis The degree to which the variability of a distribution matches the variability of a normal distribution.

lamellar bone Organized bone so named because of its laminar appearance.

latency Interval between the onset of a stimulus and the onset of a response.

leptokurtotic Kurtosis of a distribution in which a greater number of observations are obtained near the tails of the distribution than near the mean.

lineal strain (ϵ) Change of length ($\triangle l$) divided by original length (l_0), such that $\epsilon = \triangle l/l_0$; in three dimensions, there are three lineal strains.

linear regression The analytic technique whereby a line is fit through a data set yielding a correlation coefficient and a *p* value.

link protein Small globular protein that forms intermolecular bonds between the core proteins of aggrecan molecules and hyaluronate to form a proteoglycan aggregate.

linkage analysis The use of marker genes associated with a restriction fragment length polymorphism to locate an abnormal gene in the same chromosome; the inheritance pattern of the clinical features of the disorder must be known.

loss modulus Amount of energy lost per unit volume in a viscoelastic material as a result of sinusoidal excitation over one cycle.

lubrication Reduction of frictional resistance by an interposed material (lubricant).

lyophilization (*also called* freeze drying) The process of drying a sample by freezing the solution and evaporating the ice under a vacuum.

major histocompatibility complex (MHC) A cluster of genes important in immune recognition and signaling between cells of the immune system; originally identified as a locus encoding molecules present on cell surfaces, such that animals that differed at this locus would rapidly reject each other's tissue grafts.

material property Any physical characteristic of an object's substance, for example, heat conduction, diffusivity, thermal expansion, and melting point, that is independent of the object's structure and geometry.

matrix vesicle Small trilaminar membrane sacs rich in alkaline phosphatase and derived from the plasma membrane of bone cells and chondrocytes; they sequester calcium and have a role in matrix mineralization.

maximal oxygen consumption The maximal rate at which oxygen can be consumed by an exercising individual, indicative of the the power or capacity of the aerobic system of that individual.

mean (μ) The most common observation within a population.

mechanical property A subset of material properties that relates stresses to strains; for linear elastic materials, the proportionality constants are Young's modulus, shear modulus, Poisson's ratio, etc.

membranous bone formation Bone formation without a cartilaginous template (*See* intramembranous ossification).

mesotenon (*also called* mesotendineum) The synovial layer that passes from the tendon to the wall of the tendon sheath.

messenger RNA (mRNA) An RNA fraction of intermediate molecular weight, it transmits information from DNA to the protein-forming system of the cell.

metallic bond Interatomic bond in metals characterized by delocalized electrons shared by many atoms.

metalloproteinase Class of degradative enzymes, collagenase, stromelysin (proteoglycanase), and gelatinase, that depend on zinc and calcium for enzyme activity and are important for normal matrix turnover as well as for the pathologic degradation of the cartilage matrix in both articular and growth plate tissue.

mineralization The addition of mineral deposits on already deposited mineral nuclei.

mitogen An agent that stimulates DNA production and cell division.

modulus Proportional constant between stresses and strains; for example, Young's modulus, shear modulus, bulk modulus.

molecular weight Mass, in grams, of 6.02×10^{23} (Avogadro's number) molecules; for polymers, the average molecular size; M_n is the number-average molecular weight and M_w is the weight-average molecular weight.

moment (*also called* torque) The tendency of a force, measured in N·m or ft-lb, to cause rotations about an axis; a vector having a magnitude defined by the product of the magnitude of the force and the perpendicular distance between the axis and the line of application of the force.

moment of inertia Resistance of a geometric shape to deformation; solely a function of geometry, independent of material properties (*See* area moment of inertia).

monomer The smallest repeating unit in a polymer.

motion segment The basic anatomic unit of the spine; it comprises two vertebrae and their intercalated soft tissue; functional spinal unit.

motoneuron Nerve cell that innervates skeletal muscle.

motor end plate The synapse between a motoneuron and a muscle fiber.

motor point The anatomic site at which the motor nerve enters the muscle; the point over a muscle at which a contraction may be elicited by a minimal-intensity, short-duration electric stimulus.

motor unit An alpha motoneuron and the muscle fibers innervated by it.

motor unit territory Muscle area over which muscle fibers belonging to an individual motor unit are distributed.

mucopolysaccharidoses A group of genetically inherited diseases that are characterized by a deficiency of enzymes responsible for the synthesis of proteoglycans, resulting in the accumulation of undegraded glycosaminoglycans in the lysosome.

multivariate analysis An analytic technique that operates on a number of variables simultaneously; for example, stepwise linear regression.

muscle activation The process by which muscle shortens or resists lengthening by mechanisms involving contractile protein interactions and metabolic energy.

muscle contraction The attempt of muscle to shorten and generate tension in response to activation, although the muscle may actually remain the same length or lengthen if the opposing load is large enough.

muscle fatigue Inability of muscle to maintain a given force or exercise intensity due to factors in the muscle itself or in the peripheral or central nervous systems.

muscle twitch A brief period of contraction followed by relaxation in the response of a motor unit to a stimulus (nerve impulse).

mutagen An agent that causes an alteration (mutation) in the DNA, leading to neoplasia.

mutagenesis The production of a neoplasm caused by an alteration in the DNA's structure.

M wave Short latency orthodromic response resulting from antidromic activation of alpha motoneurons in the spinal cord; compound action potential evoked from a muscle by a single electric stimulus to its motor nerve.

myositis ossificans Development of heterotopic bone in muscle.

nerve fiber The connecting unit of a nerve composed of a central core, the axon, enveloped in a complex covering comprised of a single layer of Schwann cells, a basement membrane, and a sheath of endoneurial tissue.

neuropathy Nerve lesions not caused by physical injury; may be a consequence of toxic and metabolic disturbances and primary vascular disease.

neuropraxia Failure of nerve conduction, usually reversible, caused by metabolic or microstructural abnormalities without disruption of the axon.

neurotmesis Partial or complete severance of a nerve, with disruption of the axons, their myelin sheaths, and the supporting connective tissue; results in degeneration of the axons distal to the injury site.

neutral axis The line of intersection between the plane of loading on a beam and the neutral plane.

neutral plane The plane within a bent beam on which the stress is zero; this plane divides the compressive and tensile regions within the beam.

newton A unit of force named after Sir Isaac Newton in which 1 N = 0.225 lb.

newtonian fluid A fluid in which the shear stress (τ) is linearly proportional to the rate of shear (γ), and the viscosity (η) may depend on temperature: $\tau = \eta\gamma$.

node of Ranvier Localized area devoid of myelin that occurs at intervals along a myelinated axon.

normal distribution The probability distribution described by the function:

$$y = \frac{e^{\frac{-(x-\mu)^2}{2\sigma^2}}}{\sigma\sqrt{2\pi}}$$

which represents the probability of obtaining an observation a certain distance away from the mean within a standard sample.

normal stress A force acting perpendicular to the area of interest divided by that area.

Northern hybridization (*also called* Northern blot) Detection of a particular RNA sequence (target sequence) using a fragment of radioactively labeled, single-stranded DNA (a probe), which binds to the complementary target sequence, creating a DNA-RNA hybrid (*See* Southern hybridization).

nucleation The first deposition of mineral crystal in cartilage or bone matrix.

nucleotide A compound composed of a base (purine or pyrimidine), a sugar (ribose or deoxyribose), and a phosphate group.

Ohm's law Relates current (I) to voltage (V) and resistance (R); V = IR.

oncogene Either of two types of abnormal genes (proto-oncogenes and antioncogenes) associated with the production of a neoplasm.

orthodromic Propagation of an impulse in the direction of physiologic conduction; conduction along motor nerve fibers towards the muscle and along sensory nerve fibers towards the spinal cord.

osteoblast An active bone-forming cell that produces type I collagen, responds to parathyroid hormone, and releases osteocalcin when stimulated by 1,25-dihydroxyvitamin D_3.

osteocalcin A small bone-specific, noncollagenous protein that is produced by the osteoblast and may play a role in osteoclast recruitment.

osteoclast A multinucleated bone cell that resorbs bone matrix when activated.

osteocyte A mature bone cell surrounded by bone matrix and active in bone mineral homeostasis.

osteogenesis imperfecta A genetic defect in type I collagen metabolism that results in bone fragility.

osteoid Unmineralized bone matrix.

osteomalacia Condition characterized by insufficiently mineralized bone matrix, although the mass of bone can be normal, decreased, or increased (*See* rickets).

osteon A haversian canal with its concentrically arranged lamellae.

osteopenia Generic term that describes neither a specific disease state nor a diagnosis, but a radiographic appearance of decreased bone density.

osteoporosis A decrease in bone mass per unit volume of normally mineralized bone.

outcomes research A type of clinical research in which specific outcomes (such as range of motion, patient satisfaction, or subjective pain) are used as measures of the success of a particular clinical treatment.

paracrine Local action of molecules (such as growth factors) that are produced by one cell on another cell type within the same tissue.

paramagnetic agent An atom or molecule with unpaired electrons that, when placed in a magnetic field, generates its own small magnetic field that adds and/or subtracts from the main magnetic field.

paratenon The material that separates the tendon from the sheath.

parathyroid hormone (PTH) A protein produced by the parathyroid gland, it is important in calcium metabolism and bone homeostasis.

pascal A measure of pressure or stress in the formula Pa = N/m^2; MPa = 10^6Pa = N/mm^2 = 145 psi, GPa = 10^9Pa.

passive tension The tension generated in stretched muscle due to the inherent properties of the tissue and not to muscle activation.

pennation angle The angle of muscle fibers with respect to the direction of the resultant force of the muscle-tendon unit.

perichondral ring of LaCroix The fibrous structure that surrounds the cartilaginous portion of the growth plate, is contiguous with the periosteum of the metaphysis, and lends mechanical support to the growth plate.

perimysium Connective tissue surrounding a fascicle.

perineural Around the nerve trunk.

perineurium Thin sheath of specialized perineurial or lamellar cells, arranged in concentric layers, that encircle a bundle of nerve fibers.

permeability coefficient The proportionality constant (κ) between volume flux per unit area and pressure gradient, it determines the ease of fluid flow through a porous material; it is inversely related to diffusive drag coefficient (K) by: $\kappa = \phi^2/K$, where ϕ is porosity.

p-glycoprotein A molecule embedded in the cell membrane encoded by the MOR-1 gene, it actively pumps certain classes of molecules, drugs, or toxins from the cell's cytoplasm.

phenotype Physical characteristics expressed by an individual.

phosphocreatine (PC) A chemical compound stored in muscle; when hydrolyzed, it aids in manufacturing ATP.

physeal growth plate Growth plate that produces long bone growth under compressive force (*See* growth plate).

physicochemical forces Forces derived from the charged nature of constituents within a material; for example, charged proteoglycan gives rise to Donnan osmotic pressure and charge-to-charge repulsion.

physiologic cross-sectional area (PCSA) The sum of the cross-sectional areas of all the muscle fibers in the muscle; it is calculated by dividing the muscle's volume by the length of individual muscle fibers.

piezoelectric potential An electric potential generated by the deformation of a solid material that contains fixed charges but is neutral because of the presence of counterions or electrons.

plasmid An extrachromosomal element that replicates and is transferred independently of the host (bacterial) chromosome and usually is not essential to the host's basic functioning; independent piece of DNA (usually nonhuman) that can replicate.

plastic deformation Permanent change in shape of an object even after the load has been removed.

platelet-derived growth factor (PDGF) Glycoprotein growth factor that stimulates cell proliferation and chemotaxis in cartilage, bone, and many other cell types after being produced by mesenchymal cells or released by platelets during clotting.

platykurtotic A distribution property in which a greater number of observations are obtained near the mean than near the tails of the distribution.

point mutation An alteration in the genomic DNA at a single nucleotide; depending on the base change (A to T or G to C), it may or may not alter the genetic code and resulting protein product.

Poisson's ratio A material property defining the lateral expansion (or contraction) of a deformable object transverse (at 90°) to the direction of loading; when an object is stretched, it also will contract in the transverse direction, and vice versa.

polar moment of inertia Resistance to twisting; it is solely a function of geometry, independent of material properties; the stress caused by torsion is proportional to the applied torque and inversely proportional to the polar moment of inertia.

polygeneic inheritance Effects of multiple genes and alleles interacting with environmental factors to influence form, function, and incidence of any trait.

polymer Molecule composed of many repeating units (mers).

polymerase chain reaction (PCR) A method for the repetitive synthesis of specific DNA sequences in vitro.

polymorphism The variability of molecular sequencing among different individuals, frequently used in reference to DNA.

population In statistics, the entire collection of elements about which information is desired.

porosity Ratio of void (or fluid) volume to apparent (total) volume of a porous material (*See* solidity).

power grip The forceful finger flexion used to maintain an object against the palm of the hand.

precision The closeness of repeated measurements of the same quantity; the repeatability of a particular measurement.

precision grip Grip associated with fine tactile sensibility at the fingertips; requires fine kinesthetic control; does not involve the palm.

prehension The grasping or taking hold of an object between any two surfaces of the hand.

primary bone healing *See* contact healing.

primary ossification center Site of initial bone formation in the cartilaginous template of a bone.

primary spongiosa Woven bone formed on calcified cartilage during endochondral ossification.

probe A small portion of radioactively labeled DNA that is complementary to the DNA sequence being sought and therefore able to attach to it.

proliferative zone A region of the growth plate primarily responsible for longitudinal growth through chondrocyte proliferation.

promoter Portion of the DNA that initiates transcription (constructing RNA from DNA), and is necessary for transcription.

proportional limit The end of the linear range of the stress-strain curve.

prospective study An experimental study in which the data are acquired after the experimental design is proposed.

protein Any of a group of complex organic compounds that contain carbon, hydrogen, oxygen, nitrogen, and usually sulfur, and that essentially consist of combinations of amino acids in peptide linkage.

proteoglycan Major constituent of the organic matrix of all connective tissues; it consists of a protein core and glycosaminoglycan side chains and plays a major role in the structural and biologic properties of the tissue.

proteoglycan aggregate A macromolecule composed of aggrecans, hyaluronate, and link proteins.

proto-oncogene A normal gene that when initiated becomes an oncogene; a dominant oncogene.

***p* value** The probability obtained from a statistical analysis that type 1 error will occur.

quantitative computed tomography (QCT) Quantitative measurement of bone density at various sites using CT images.

Rad (radiation absorbed dose) Unit of absorbed dose of ionizing radiation equal to an energy of 100 ergs per gram of irradiated material; 100 rads = 1 joule/kg = 1 Gy.

Rb gene (retinoblastoma gene) The oncogene (recessive) associated with retinoblastoma and an oncogene associated with some cases of osteosarcoma.

recessive oncogene An antioncogene.

reciprocal inhibition Simultaneous inhibition of antagonists and excitation of homonymous and synergistic motoneurons.

recombinant DNA A DNA fragment that is removed from its original source and ligated with DNA from another source.

recruitment An increase in muscular force by adding (recruiting) the activities of more motoneurons and motor units of the central nervous system in response to a prolonged stimulus.

recrystallization The formation of new annealed grains in metals from strain-hardened grains.

recrystallization temperature Temperature above which recrystallization is spontaneous, and which depends on the specific material and the strain state.

reference electrode electrode placed distal to the active recording electrode on the tendon during motor nerve conduction studies and over the nerve during sensory studies.

rem Dosage of ionizing radiation that will cause the same biologic effect as one roentgen of X-ray or gamma radiation dosage; for clinical diagnostic radiographic procedures, 1 rem = 1 rad.

repeated measures Measurements that are taken from a population from the same sampling element; for example, measuring blood pressure in the same individuals over time.

reserve zone Portion of the growth plate consisting of sparse regularly shaped chondrocytes in an abundant matrix; its functions are storage and matrix production.

resilience The capacity of a strained material to recover its size and shape after the deforming load is removed.

resistance (R) The hindrance to movement of electrical charges measured in ohms (Ω); its strength depends on the material through which the particles are moving. Current flowing through a resistance will produce a voltage: V = IR.

resting membrane potential Voltage across the membrane of an excitable cell at rest.

restriction enzyme Endonuclease that cleaves DNA at specific sites, producing restriction fragments.

restriction fragment length polymorphism (RFLP) Variation in the lengths of DNA restriction fragments resulting when the DNA from which the fragments are derived is altered.

retrograde From the axon terminal toward the cell body.

retrospective study An experiment in which the data are already acquired by the time the specific experiment is designed.

rickets Condition characterized by insufficient mineralization of growth plate in the immature skeleton (*See* osteomalacia).

RNA (*ribonucleic acid*) The nucleic acid composed of ribonucleotide monomers, each containing ribose, a phosphate group, and a nitrogenous base; found in all cells (in the nucleus and cytoplasm) in particulate and nonparticulate form, and also in many viruses.

roentgen (R) Unit of radiation exposure equal to 2.58×10^{-4} coulombs/kg of air; applies only to X and gamma radiation below 3 meV.

rotation Revolving motion of an object about a point or an axis.

sample A collection of individual observations selected in accordance with a specified procedure.

sample size (n) The number of independent observations that make up a sample; sample size is related to statistical power in hypothesis testing.

sarcolemma Muscle-cell membrane and its associated basement membrane.

screw axis (*also called* helical axis) Any motion can be resolved into a rotation and a translation. In three dimensions, an object's motion may be described as a combination of rotation about an axis and translation parallel to the same axis. This unique axis is called the screw axis.

scurvy A nutritional disorder caused by a deficiency of vitamin C.

secondary ossification center Located usually at the ends of bones, a site of bone formation in the cartilaginous template of a bone, which occurs after primary ossification.

secondary spongiosa Trabecular lamillary bone formed after the resorption of the primary spongiosa.

selectivity Ability of an axon to chose appropriately among potential synaptic partners.

semicrystalline A polymer conformation consisting of ordered regions in a matrix of randomly oriented chains; the degree of crystallinity has a strong effect on the mechanical properties.

shear modulus (G or μ) The proportionality constant between shear stress and shear strain.

shear strain Change of angle between two lines inscribed in a material, which were originally at 90°; in three dimensions, there are three shear strains.

shear stress A force acting parallel to the area of interest divided by that area.

shear thinning Decrease in viscosity with increasing shear rate.

SI units (*also called* System International units) Units of physical quantities; commonly force, Newton (N) = 0.225 lb; length, meter (m) = 39.37 in; time, second (s); and stress, pascal (Pa) = N/m^2 = 1.45×10^{-4} psi.

significance level (α) The probability of type 1 error in an experiment involving hypothesis testing.

single photon absorptiometry (SPA) Measurement of bone density using a single photon beam.

sintering A method by which high pressure produces the temperatures used to bond particulate matter into a solid.

sinusoidal excitation A periodic (sine function) deformation or stress imposed on a material.

size principle The principle governing an increase in muscle activation by central nervous system recruitment of motor nerves and motor units in order of size from smallest to largest.

skew The property of a distribution that "leans" either to the right or to the left; skewed distributions are, by definition, not normally distributed.

slow-oxidative (SO) fiber A slow-twitch muscle fiber characterized by fatigue resistance and high aerobic capacity.

slow-twitch (ST) muscle fiber A muscle fiber characterized by high aerobic capacity and low anaerobic capacity.

s-n curve Plot of fatigue stress (s) versus number (n) of cycles to failure.

solidity Ratio of solid volume to apparent (total) volume of a porous material (*See* porosity).

somatic defect An abnormality that is present only in the cells of the abnormal tissue of the organism with the neoplasia, not in the normal cells.

Southern hybridization (*also called* Southern blot) Detection of a specific DNA sequence (target sequence) using a fragment of radioactively labeled single-stranded DNA (a probe), which binds to the complementary target sequence, creating a DNA-DNA hybrid (*See* Northern hybridization).

splicing Removing introns from mRNA before translation can occur.

spring A linear elastic structure in which the force-deformation relationship is defined by $F = kx$, where k is the stiffness.

squeeze-film lubrication Type of lubrication in which two bearing surfaces are loaded perpendicular to each other, causing the lubricant to be squeezed from the gap.

standard deviation (s) The square root of the sample variance; a measure of population variability that is expressed in terms of the original measurement units.

standard error of the mean (SEM) The error associated with estimating the mean value of a sample.

statics Study of structures in mechanical equilibrium.

statistical power (1-β) The probability that, if a negative result is obtained, it truly represents a negative result and not simply inadequate sample size.

stiffness Resistance of a structure to a deformation.

stimulus artifact In nerve conduction studies, deflection from the baseline resulting from direct conduction of the stimulus.

storage modulus Amount of energy stored per unit volume in a viscoelastic material as a result of sinusoidal excitation over one cycle.

strain Measure of deformation having six components (three lineal strain and three shear strain).

strain energy The amount of energy stored in a loaded material associated with the deformation of the material from its undeformed state.

strain energy density Work required to produce a given strain in a unit volume of a material under load, expressed in Joules/meter^3 = Newtons/meter^2.

strain rate Speed at which a material is deformed.

streaming potentials Electrical potentials produced by the flow of an electrolyte fluid through a porous charged matrix; the material itself is neutral because of the presence of counterions and electrons.

strength Maximum resistance to strain before mechanical failure begins.

stress A physical quantity defined as force per unit area (F/A) and consisting of six components: three normal stresses and three shear stresses (*See* tensor).

stress concentration Increased level of stress around a flaw caused by the presence of that flaw, such as a crack, hole, or discontinuity (*See* stress riser).

stress relaxation Decrease in stress at constant strain by internal molecular rearrangement.

stress riser A flaw (crack, hole, or discontinuity) in a material that increases local stress (*See* stress concentration).

stress shielding A decrease in physiologic stress in a biologic material caused when a stiffer structure (such as a rod, plate, implant) acts in parallel with the stress riser.

stress-strain plot The experimental data relating stress (F/A) to strain ($\Delta l/l$).

stromelysin Metalloproteinase that degrades proteoglycans and activates procollagenase.

structure Any object of finite size and consisting of geometrically shaped materials; for example, a bridge, airplane, femur, tibia, or humerus.

subchondral bone The bone of the epiphysis underlying and supporting articular cartilage.

swelling An increase (or decrease) of size, weight, or water content of an object as a result of changing environmental conditions; for example, changes in ion concentration.

swelling pressure of cartilage Sum of Donnan osmotic pressure and charge-to-charge repulsive forces in cartilage.

synapse A specialized apposition between a neuron and its target cell for transmission of information by release and reception of a chemical transmitter agent.

syndiotactic Orientation of a polymer in which the side groups are on alternate sides of the macromolecular chain.

tan δ A property of viscoelastic materials that measures the ratio of loss modulus to the storage modulus; δ = phase angle.

temporal dispersion Relative desynchronization resulting from different rates of conduction of two or more synchronously evoked components of a compound action potential from the stimulation point to the record electrode.

tensile strength The maximum stress reached before a specimen in an uniaxial tensile test begins to fail.

tension A force tending to elongate an object; a pull.

tensor A mathematical quantity representing stresses and strains; in three dimensions it has six independent components.

tetanus The contractile condition of muscle in which a higher frequency of stimulation produces no increase in the muscle force.

tetraploid Four times haploid, or twice the amount of DNA in a normal resting human cell; the amount of DNA in a normal human cell in G2 phase of the cell cycle.

threshold Term generally used to refer to the voltage level at which an action potential is initiated in a single axon or a group of axons; operationally defined as the intensity that produces a response in about 50% of equivalent trials.

tidemark Demarcation between the deep uncalcified and calcified zones of articular cartilage; it appears as one or more wavy lines on histologically stained tissues.

tissue inhibitor of metalloproteinase (TIMP) A naturally occurring inhibitor of proteolytic enzymes found in cartilaginous tissue.

torque Synonym to moment of a force (*See* moment and couple).

torsion Deformation caused by twisting (torquing) of a shaft.

toughness Qualitative term for the ability of a material to absorb energy before failure; usually associated with large deformations; for example, rubber or plastic.

transcription The process by which genetic information contained in DNA produces a complementary sequence of bases in an RNA chain; constructing mRNA from nuclear DNA.

transformation Inserting into a bacterium a plasmid (independent self-replicating DNA) with added recombinant DNA.

transforming growth factors Peptides that transform fibroblastic cells in monolayer culture and stimulate colony formation in soft agar; two major classifications are α and β, which includes bone morphogenic proteins.

transgene A gene that is not normally found in an organism, but was artificially placed into the single-celled embryo and therefore is present in all cells of that organism.

transgenic animal An animal that develops from a fertilized egg into which a foreign gene (transgene) has been inserted.

translation (biologic) Building proteins; mRNA, which is constructed based on the order of nitrogenous bases in nuclear DNA, builds protein by joining amino acids.

translation (mechanical) Linear motion of an object without rotation.

transposon An element of bacterial DNA that can migrate from a plasmid to a chromosome or bacteriophage, allowing a specific gene sequence to be incorporated.

transverse isotropy Isotropy in a plane, with material properties distinctly different along the axis perpendicular to this plane; for example, laminated structures such as mica or cortical bone.

trophic Ability of one tissue or cell to support another; usually applied to long-term interactions between pre- and postsynaptic cells.

tropic An influence of one cell or tissue on the direction of movement or outgrowth of another.

tropism Orientation of growth in response to an external stimulus.

tropocollagen A word previously used to describe a single collagen molecule that results from the winding of three alpha chains.

***t*-statistic** The statistic used to compare two means obtained from two different samples.

tumor suppressor gene An antioncogene.

twitch A brief contractile response of a skeletal muscle elicited by a single volley of impulses in the neurons supplying it.

type I fiber A slow-oxidative (SO) muscle fiber.

type II fiber A fast-oxidative glycolytic (FOG) or fast-glycolytic (FG) muscle fiber.

ultimate strain Maximum strain sustained by the specimen prior to failure of the material.

ultimate stress Maximum stress (resistance divided by the original area) sustained by a specimen prior to failure of the material.

unit cell The smallest repetitive volume that possesses the symmetry of a crystal lattice.

univariate analysis Any statistical analytic technique that operates on a single variable at a time; for example, one-way analysis of variance.

van der Waals forces Weak secondary forces that attract neutral atoms and molecules.

variable The actual property measured by means of individual observations.

variance (s^2) The variance measure of the spread of data about the sample mean.

variate A single reading, score, or observation of a given variable.

vector Quantity such as force, having both direction and magnitude and represented graphically as an arrow, which indicates the line of application and direction of the force, and the length of which represents the magnitude of the force.

viscoelastic In biology, a property of a tissue that exhibits both viscous and elastic behavior (creep and stress relaxation); the material's stress-strain behavior depends on strain rate.

viscosity (η) Resistance (τ) offered by a fluid to shearing (γ), given by Newton's law for viscous fluids: $\tau = \eta\gamma$.

viscous A property of the fluid that offers resistance to flow; for example, frictional drag.

vitreous Glassy or amorphous.

vitrification Solidification by cooling to produce an amorphous, glassy material.

voltage The potential for separated charges to do work; the amount of work done by an electric charge when moving from one point to another measured in volts (V).

wear Unintended removal of surface material during normal functional use.

wear debris Particles produced by wear.

Wolff's law A law that states that the remodeling of bone or soft tissue is influenced and modulated by mechanical stresses.

work hardening Increased hardness (and strength) from plastic deformation at ambient temperature.

woven bone Immature bone without laminar or osteonal organization.

xenograft (*also called* heterograft) Material transplantation between individuals of different species.

yield strength (*also called* yield stress) Stress necessary to cause plastic flow.

Young's modulus (E) The intrinsic stiffness of a linear material in tension or compression expressed as the ratio of stress to strain: E = stress/strain.

Index